Companion CD Contents*

NCLEX® Examination Review Questions

- Drug Action: Pharmaceutic, Pharmacokinetic, and Pharmacodynamic Phases
- Nursing Process and Client Teaching
- Principles of Drug Administration
- Medications and Calculations
- The Drug Approval Process
- Transcultural and Genetic Considerations
- Drug Interaction and Over-the-Counter Drugs
- Drugs of Abuse
- Herbal Therapy with Nursing Implications
- Pediatric Pharmacology
- Geriatric Pharmacology
- Medication Administration in Community Settings
- The Role of the Nurse in Drug Research
- Vitamin and Mineral Replacement
- Fluid and Electrolyte Replacement
- Nutritional Support
- Adrenergics and Adrenergic Blockers
- Cholinergics and Anticholinergics
- Central Nervous System Stimulants
- Central Nervous System Depressants
- Anticonvulsants
- Drugs for Neurologic Disorders: Parkinsonism and Alzheimer's Disease
- Drugs for Neuromuscular Disorders: Myasthenia Gravis, Multiple Sclerosis, and Muscle Spasms
- Nonopioid and Opioid Analgesics
- Antiinflammatory Drugs
- Antipsychotics and Anxiolytics
- Antidepressants and Mood Stabilizers
- Penicillins and Cephalosporins
- Macrolides, Tetracyclines, Aminoglycosides, and Fluoroquinolones
- Sulfonamides
- Antituberculars, Antifungals, Peptides, and Metronidazole
- Antivirals, Antimalarials, and Anthelmintics
- Drugs for Urinary Tract Disorders
- HIV- and AIDS-Related Drugs
- Vaccines
- Anticancer Drugs
- Targeted Therapies
- Biologic Response Modifiers
- Drugs for Upper Respiratory Disorders
- Drugs for Lower Respiratory Disorders
- Cardiac Glycosides, Antianginals, and Antidysrhythmics
- Diuretics
- Antihypertensives
- Anticoagulants, Antiplatelets, and Thrombolytics
- Antilipids and Peripheral Vasodilators
- Drugs for Gastrointestinal Tract Disorders
- Antiulcer Drugs
- Drugs for Eye and Ear Disorders
- Drugs for Dermatologic Disorders
- Endocrine Drugs: Pituitary, Thyroid, Parathyroid, and Adrenal Disorders
- Antidiabetics
- Female Reproductive Cycle I: Pregnancy and Preterm Labor Drugs
- Female Reproductive Cycle II: Labor, Delivery, and Preterm Neonatal Drugs
- Postpartum and Newborn Drugs
- Drugs for Women's Health and Reproductive Disorders
- Drugs for Men's Health and Reproductive Disorders
- Drugs for Infertility and Sexually Transmitted Diseases
- Adult and Pediatric Emergency Drugs

Pharmacology Animations

- Nursing, Medical, and Pharmacology Domains
- Client Noncompliance
- Agonists/Antagonists
- Receptor Interaction
- Passive Diffusion
- Impact of Surface Area
- Overview of Pharmacokinetics: Oral Administration
- Distribution: Fat- vs. Water-Soluble Drugs
- Cytochrome P-450 Drug Metabolism
- Half-Life of Intravenously Administered Ampicillin
- Drug Movement Through the Body
- Normal Electrophysiology
- Renin-Angiotensin in Control of Blood Pressure
- Time to Steady State
- Time to Steady State: Starting and Stopping Drug
- Adenosine Infusion, Cardiac Effects
- Atropine Therapy for Sinus Bradycardia
- Diltiazem Injection, Cardiac Effects
- Epinephrine and CPR
- Amiodarone Treatment for Ventricular Tachycardia
- Amiodarone, Antiarrhythmic Drug; Treatment of Ventricular Fibrillation
- Heparin for Acute Coronary Syndrome
- Heparin for Atrial Fibrillation
- Thrombolytic Drugs; Clot Dissolving Drugs
- Acute Myocardial Infarction

IV Therapy Checklists

- Administration of Bolus Medication Through Continuous IV
- Adding Medication to a Secondary Intravenous Set (Volume Control Set)
- Intermittent Intravenous Medication Administration via a Piggyback or Secondary Set
- Changing Container of an Existing Intravenous Solution

Medication Errors Checklists

- Interpreting Medication Orders
- Transcribing Medication Orders
- Reviewing Medication Orders
- Preparing Medications
- Administering Medications
- Assessing Client Response
- Appropriate Documentation of Medication Administration
- Procedural Safeguards
- Reporting Medication Errors

Drug Calculation Problems

- Oral Medication Administration: Solid
- Oral Medication Administration: Liquid
- Injectable Medication (IM) Administration
- Intravenous Medication Administration
- Intermittent IV Administration
- IV Infusion Pump Administration
- Direct IV Injection Administration
- Pediatric Medication Administration
- Pediatric Intramuscular Administration
- Pediatric Intravenous Administration
- Pediatric IV Infusion Pump Rate

Electronic Calculators

- Absolute Neutrophil Count (ANC)
- Body Mass Index (BMI)
- Body Surface Area (BSA)—Adults
- Body Surface Area (BSA)—Pediatric
- Fluid Deficit
- Sodium Deficit
- IV Infusion Rate
- Calculated Serum Osmolality
- Predicted Peak Flow (PPF) Females
- Predicted Peak Flow (PPF) Males
- Glomerular Filtration Rate (MDRD)

Top 200 Drugs with Pronunciations

References from the Textbook

*Companion CD content prepared by Marilyn Herbert-Ashton, MS, RN, BC. Selected animations provided by Ed Tessier, PharmD, MPH, BCPS.

:• *To access your Student Resources, visit:*

http://evolve.elsevier.com/KeeHayes/pharmacology/

Evolve® Student Resources for Kee/Hayes/McCuistion: *Pharmacology: A Nursing Process Approach,* **sixth edition,** offer the following features:

■ **Case Studies**
20 case studies with answer guidelines test your ability to think critically.

■ **Content Updates**
Check back often for information updates on new drugs and changing pharmacology information.

■ **Frequently Asked Questions**
Find answers to frequently asked questions and submit questions of your own.

■ **Student Review Activities**
Utilize flash cards for terminology review and memory match puzzles, crossword puzzles, and figure labeling activities for review of key terms and concepts.

■ **WebLinks**
Link to hundreds of websites carefully chosen to supplement the content of the textbook. WebLinks are regularly updated, with new ones added as they develop.

■ **Additional Reference Material**
Find information on FDA approved, recalled, and high-risk drugs; online sources for smoking cessation; caffeine content in beverages; selected sugar-free and alcohol-free products; and more!

6TH EDITION

Pharmacology

A Nursing Process Approach

Joyce LeFever Kee, MS, RN
Associate Professor Emerita
School of Nursing
College of Health Sciences
University of Delaware
Newark, Delaware

Evelyn R. Hayes, PhD, MPH, FNP-BC
Professor
School of Nursing
College of Health Sciences
University of Delaware
Newark, Delaware

Linda E. McCuistion, PhD, RN, ANP, CNS
Professor
Division of Nursing
Our Lady of Holy Cross College
New Orleans, Louisiana

SAUNDERS

ELSEVIER

11830 Westline Industrial Drive
St. Louis, Missouri 63146

PHARMACOLOGY: A NURSING PROCESS APPROACH   ISBN: 978-1-4160-4663-9
Copyright © 2009 by Saunders, an imprint of Elsevier Inc.

Notice

Knowledge and best practice in this field are constantly changing. As new research and experience broaden our knowledge, changes in practice, treatment and drug therapy may become necessary or appropriate. Readers are advised to check the most current information provided (i) on procedures featured or (ii) by the manufacturer of each product to be administered, to verify the recommended dose or formula, the method and duration of administration, and contraindications. It is the responsibility of the practitioner, relying on their own experience and knowledge of the patient, to make diagnoses, to determine dosages and the best treatment for each individual patient, and to take all appropriate safety precautions. To the fullest extent of the law, neither the Publisher nor the Authors assumes any liability for any injury and/or damage to persons or property arising out of or related to any use of the material contained in this book.

The Publisher

Previous editions copyrighted 1993, 1997, 2000, 2003, and 2006.

Library of Congress Cataloging-in-Publication Data
Kee, Joyce LeFever.
   Pharmacology : a nursing process approach / Joyce LeFever Kee, Evelyn
R. Hayes, Linda E. McCuistion. -- 6th ed.
      p. ; cm.
   Includes bibliographical references and index.
   ISBN 978-1-4160-4663-9 (pbk. : alk. paper)
1.   Pharmacology. 2.   Nursing.   I. Hayes, Evelyn R.   II. McCuistion,
      Linda E.   III. Title.
   [DNLM: 1.   Pharmcology--Nurses' Instruction. 2.   Drug Therapy--
Nurses' Instruction.   QV 4 K26p 2009]
   RM301.K44 2009
   615'.1--dc22
                                                        2008035237

Senior Acquisitions Editor: Kristin Geen
Developmental Editor: Jamie Horn
Editorial Assistant: Jennifer Stoces
Publishing Services Manager: Jeff Patterson
Senior Project Manager: Clay S. Broeker
Design Direction: Teresa McBryan

Printed in Canada

Last digit is the print number: 9   8   7   6   5   4   3   2

Meet the Authors

Joyce LeFever Kee

Joyce LeFever Kee received her Bachelor of Science and Master of Science degree in Nursing from the University of Maryland and earned 36 postgraduate credits from the University of Delaware. She was a distinguished faculty educator at the University of Maryland for 4 years and at the University of Delaware for 27 years. The subjects she taught included pharmacology, pathophysiology, fluid and electrolyte imbalances, and medical-surgical nursing in the classroom and clinical areas. She had taught in the undergraduate and graduate programs at the University of Delaware. She retired as Associate Professor Emerita from the University of Delaware.

Joyce is a member of the Sigma Theta Tau Nursing Honor Society and Phi Kappa Phi Honor Society. She received the Excellence in Teaching Award from and was inducted into the Mentor's Circle at the University of Delaware.

Joyce gave numerous lectures and presentations throughout the United States from 1970 to 1990. She has written various articles, particularly on fluid and electrolytes, laboratory and diagnostic tests, and research projects, in the *American Journal of Nursing, Nursing Clinics of North America, Nursing Journal,* and *Critical Care Quarterly.* She has participated in several research studies on "Identification of Hypertensive Young Adults."

Joyce has authored and coauthored several text and reference books, including *Fluids and Electrolytes with Clinical Applications* (2004), seventh edition; *Handbook of Fluid, Electrolyte, and Acid-Base Imbalances* (2004), second edition; *Pharmacology: A Nursing Process Approach* (2006), fifth edition, with ancillaries including Companion CD for students, Instructor's Resource CD-ROM, and Study Guide; *Clinical Calculations in General and Specialty Areas* (2008) sixth edition, with Instructor's Manual, Testbank, and CD; *Laboratory and Diagnostic Tests with Nursing Implications* (2005), seventh edition; and *Handbook of Laboratory and Diagnostic Tests with Nursing Implications* (2008), sixth edition.

Joyce and her husband enjoy traveling, including trips to Australia, New Zealand, China, Japan, Great Britain, Russia, Greece, Italy, France, Turkey, Egypt, Spain, South America, Scandinavian countries, Mexico, the Caribbean islands, and others. They enjoy snorkeling, swimming, and playing golf.

Evelyn R. Hayes

Evelyn (Lyn) R. Hayes received her Bachelor of Science in Nursing from Cornell University—New York Hospital School of Nursing; an MPH in Public Health Nursing from the University of North Carolina, School of Public Health in Chapel Hill, North Carolina; and a PhD in Higher Education from Boston College. In addition, she completed a Post Master's Certificate as Family Nurse Practitioner at the University of Massachusetts at Amherst and is a certified family nurse practitioner. She has valuable practice experience in acute care institutions and in the community. Currently she is Professor in the School of Nursing, College of Health Sciences, at the University of Delaware. In this role, she has had teaching responsibilities at both the undergraduate and graduate levels and experience with distance learning. She also serves as Director, UD Nursing Center, and Co-Coordinator of Nurse Practitioner Program. Lyn has consulted with faculty in Taiwan and Panama.

A strong advocate of health promotion, Lyn served as Project Director and co-investigator of a U.S. Public Health Service grant Promoting Health Lifestyles in Delaware.

As author, coauthor, and collaborative team member, she has published in multiple journals. General areas of interest include smoking cessation in teens and young adults, comprehensive geriatric assessments, and preparing students for perceived threats in the community with recent publications in *MCN: The American Journal of Maternal/Child Nursing, Public Health Nursing, Journal of Nursing Education,* and *Nurse Educator;* the use of research based protocols in nursing practice in *Clinical Nurse Specialist;* and issues related to prenatal care in *Journal of Perinatal Education* and *Applied Nursing Research.*

Throughout her career, Lyn has held member and leadership positions at various levels within the University of Delaware as well as professional and community organizations. She has ably provided long-term service and leadership to Sigma Theta Tau International, American Nurses Association, National League for Nursing Accrediting Commission (NLNAC), and the Delaware Nurses Association.

Now a retired colonel in the United States Army Reserve, Lyn's last two assignments were as Principal Reservist to Deputy Commander for Nursing, Walter Reed Army Medical Center, Washington, DC, and Moncrief Army Community Hospital, Fort Jackson, South Carolina. She also is a frequent traveler, both for pleasure and business. When at her home base, she enjoys being creative with crafts and spending time with friends.

Linda E. McCuistion

Dr. Linda E. McCuistion received a Diploma of Nursing from the Lutheran Hospital School of Nursing in Fort Wayne, Indiana; Bachelor of Science in Nursing from William Carey College in Hattiesburg, Mississippi; Masters in Nursing from Louisiana State University Medical Center; and a PhD in Curriculum and Instruction from the University of New Orleans. She is licensed as an Advanced Practice Nurse and has 35 years of nursing experience, including acute care and home health nursing. Currently, Linda is a Professor in the Division of Nursing at Our Lady of Holy Cross College in New Orleans, Louisiana. She received an Endowed Professorship Award in 2000 and 2003.

Linda has served as a past president, vice president, and faculty advisor of the Sigma Theta Tau International Honor Society in Nursing, Xi Psi chapter-at-large. She is a past associate editor of the *NODNA Times*, which is the New Orleans District Nurses' Association newsletter. She is a member of Phi Delta Kappa and The American Society of Hypertension.

To ease the transition of new nursing graduates into the workforce, Linda has held the role as coordinator for the Graduate Plus Internship Program, a preceptorship program for new nursing graduates in the state of Louisiana. She has served as a legal nurse consultant and as a member of a medical review panel. Linda is a past Advisory Board Member, Consultant, and Reviewer of a software preparation company for the state licensure examination. She has served as an Advisory Board member for a School for Surgical Technicians. Linda has also served as a consultant to improve the quality of nursing care and to assist acute care facilities in preparation for accreditation.

Linda was chosen as a "Great One Hundred Nurse" by the New Orleans District Nurses' Association in 1993. She is also listed in the 2005/2006 Edition of the Empire Who's Who Executive and Professional Registry.

Linda has given numerous lectures and presentations regionally and nationally on a variety of nursing topics, particularly hypertension, orthopedic assessment, arthritis, multiple organ dysfunction syndrome, Alzheimer's disease, and intravenous workshops. She has published articles in nursing journals and authored many chapters in several nursing textbooks including *Pharmacotherapeutics: Clinical Decision-Making in Nursing* (1999), *Saunders Manual of Medical-Surgical Nursing: A Guide for Clinical Decision-Making* (2002), and the *Saunders Nursing Survival Guide: Pathophysiology* (2007). She is author and coauthor of many chapters and co-editor of the *Saunders Nursing Survival Guide: Pharmacology* (2007).

Linda enjoys cruises to the Caribbean and traveling to Europe, Aruba, and across the United States. When at home, she enjoys visiting family and friends, playing golf, and writing.

Contributors

Margaret Barton-Burke, PhD, RN
Assistant Professor
University of Massachusetts Amherst
Amherst, Massachusetts
Chapter 38

Joseph Boullata, PharmD, BCNSP
Associate Professor—Pharmacology and Therapeutics
University of Pennsylvania, School of Nursing
Philadelphia, Pennsylvania
Table 9–3: "Selected Herb-Drug Interactions"

Michelle M. Byrne, MS, PhD, CNOR
Associate Professor of Nursing
North Georgia College and State University
Dahlonega, Georgia
Chapter 6

Robin Webb Corbett, PhD, RN, C
Associate Professor
East Carolina University
School of Nursing
Greenville, North Carolina
Chapters 52, 53, and 54

Sandy Elliott, CNM, MSN
President
Woman to Woman Health Care
Milford, Delaware
Chapters 55 and 57

Judith W. Herrman, PhD, RN
Assistant Director/Assistant Professor
School of Nursing, University of Delaware
Newark, Delaware
Chapter 10

Kathleen J. Jones, RN-C, MS, ANP
Adult Nurse Practitioner
Walter Reed Army Medical Center
Washington, DC
Chapter 56

Robert J. Kizior, BS, RPh
Educational Coordinator
Alexian Brothers Medical Center
Elk Grove Village, Illinois
Chapter 34

Paula R. Klemm, PhD, RN, OCN
Professor and Coordinator of Graduate Program
University of Delaware, School of Nursing
Newark, Delaware
Chapter 36

Linda Laskowski-Jones, RN, MS, APRN-BC, CCRN, CEN
Vice President: Emergency, Trauma, and Aeromedical Services
Christiana Care Health System
Wilmington, Delaware
Chapter 58

Patricia O'Brien, MA, MSN
Clinical Research Coordinator/Nursing Instructor
Lovelace Scientific Resources/University of New Mexico
Albuquerque, New Mexico
Chapter 8

Laura K. Williford Owens, PharmD
Chief of Pharmacy Services
Carolina Family Health Centers, Inc.
Wilson, North Carolina
Chapters 52, 53, and 54

Lisa Ann Plowfield, PhD, RN
Professor and Dean
College of Nursing
Florida State University
Tallahassee, Florida
Chapter 34

Lynette M. Wachholz, MN, APRN, IBCLC
Clinical Faculty
University of Washington
Department of Family and Child Nursing
Seattle, Washington
Pediatric Nurse Practitioner and Lactation Consultant
The Everett Clinic
Everett, Washington
Chapter 35

Gail Wilkes, MS, RNC, AOCN
Oncology Nurse Educator
Boston Medical Center
Boston, Massachusetts
Chapter 38

Additional Teaching and Learning Resources

Judith W. Herrman, PhD, RN
Associate Professor and Assistant Director
University of Delaware, School of Nursing
Newark, Delaware
Test Bank and Audience Response Questions for i-Clicker and Other Systems

Marilyn Herbert-Ashton, MS, RN, BC
Grants Development and Special Projects
Coordinator, Grants Development, Special Projects, and
  Community Relations
Associate Professor
Virginia Western Community College
Roanoke, Virginia
Adjunct Faculty
Department of Nursing
Finger Lakes Community College
Canandaigua, New York
  NCLEX® Examination Review Questions, Medication Errors
  Checklists, and IV Therapy Checklists for the Companion CD

Caroline Peltz, MSN, MSHSA, RN
  with Brian J Peltz, MS, RPh
Professor of Nursing
Wayne County Community College District
Detroit, Michigan
  Evolve Case Studies and FAQs

Reviewers

Rachel Blankstein Breman, MSN, MPH, RN
School of Nursing Faculty
Brockton Hospital
Brockton, Massachusetts

Michelle M. Byrne, RN, PhD, CNOR
Associate Professor of Nursing
North Georgia College and State University
Dahlonega, Georgia

Brigitte L. Casteel, RN, MSN
Program Director, Associate Professor
Mountain Empire Community College
Big Stone Gap, Virginia

Darlene Clark, RN, MS
Senior Lecturer in Nursing
School of Nursing
Penn State University
University Park, Pennsylvania

Linda Coakley, EdD, APN
Assistant Professor of Nursing
Western Kentucky University
Bowling Green, Kentucky

Barb Diederick, MS, RN
Chair, Department of Nursing
North Dakota State College of Science
Wahpeton, North Dakota

Robert D. Ekas, PhD
Associate Director, Medical Sciences
Gilead Sciences, Inc.
New Orleans, Louisiana

Teresa S. Fox, ADN, RN, BSN
Practical Nursing Instructor
Virginia Western Community College
Roanoke, Virginia

Alice Gardner, PhD
Assistant Professor of Pharmacology/Toxicology
Department of Pharmaceutical Sciences
Massachusetts College of Pharmacy and Health Sciences
Worcester, Massachusetts

Kathleen M. Geib, DNSc, RN
Associate Professor of Nursing
Malone College
Canton, Ohio

Cene' L. Gibson, RN, MSN, ARNP
Family Nurse Practitioner
Family Healthcare and Minor Emergency Clinic
Oklahoma City, Oklahoma

Margaret M. Gingrich, RN, MSN
Professor of Nursing
Harrisburg Area Community College
Harrisburg, Pennsylvania

Mary E. Greipp, RN, EdD, FAAN
Professor of Nursing
Rutgers the State University of New Jersey
Camden, New Jersey

Rhonda Helm, RN, MSN, PhD(c)
Assistant Professor of Nursing
Western Kentucky University
Bowling Green, Kentucky

Marilyn Herbert-Ashton, MS, RN, BC
Associate Professor
Virginia Western Community College
Roanoke, Virginia

Marita Hoffart, PhD
Professor of Nursing
Minot State University
Minot, North Dakota

Susie Huyer, RN, MSN, CHPN
Administrator
Heartland Hospice
Fairfax, Virginia
Online Nursing Faculty
University of Phoenix
Phoenix, Arizona

Suzanne Jed, MSN, APRN-BC
Nurse Practitioner
Los Angeles, California

BJ Taylor Kosak, MSN, RN, CS
Assistant Professor of Nursing
Northern Kentucky University
Highland Heights, Kentucky

Wendy Likes, DNSc, ARNP-BC
Assistant Professor
Acute and Chronic Care
University of Tennessee Health Science Center
Memphis, Tennessee

Lora McGuire, RN, MS
Professor of Nursing
Joliet Junior College
Joliet, Illinois

Charles E. McPherson, III, PharmD
Clinical Assistant Professor
University of Illinois at Chicago College of Pharmacy
Chicago, Illinois

Brenda Michel, EdD, MS, RN, CDE
Professor of Nursing
Lincoln Land Community College
Springfield, Illinois

Diane Muckenhirn, RN, MSN, CNP
Nurse Practitioner
Hutchinson Medical Center
Hutchinson, Minnesota

Julie D. Painter, RN, MSN, OCN
Clinical Nurse Specialist/Adult Nurse Practitioner
Clinical Practice Education and Research
Community Health Network
Indianapolis, Indiana

Brenda Condusta Pavill, RN, PhD
Nursing Faculty
College Misericordia
Dallas, Pennsylvania

Peggy Przybycien, RN, MS
Professor of Nursing
Onondaga Community College
Syracuse, New York

Carolyn Ryan, RPh, PharmD
Tri-Regional Pharmacist, Strategic National Stockpile
Office of Public Health
Shreveport, Louisiana

Kimberly J. Sharp, RN, OHND, BA, BSN, MSc, PhD
Professor of Nursing
Cedarville University
Cedarville, Ohio

Carla Petsick Smith, MS, RN
Assistant Professor of Nursing
East Texas Baptist University
Marshall, Texas

Patricia A. Tabloski, PhD, APRN, BC
Associate Dean of Graduate Studies
William F. Connell School of Nursing at Boston College
Chestnut Hill, Massachusetts

Martha A. Tafoya, MSN, RN
Professional Specialist in Nursing
Angelo State University
San Angelo, Texas

Scott Thigpen, RN, MSN, CCRN, CEN
Assistant Professor of Nursing
South Georgia College
Douglas, Georgia

Sheryl Thomas, MSN, RN
Nursing Instructor
Wayne County Community College
Detroit, Michigan

Darlene Thomay, RN, BA, DNC
Staff Nurse
Medical Specialties Clinic
Metrohealth Medical Center
Cleveland, Ohio

Barbara Timby, MA, BSN, RN, BC
Nursing Professor
Glen Oaks Community College
Centreville, Michigan

Preface

The sixth edition of *Pharmacology: A Nursing Process Approach* is written for students in a variety of nursing programs who can benefit from its presentation of the principles of pharmacology in a straightforward, student-friendly manner. It focuses on the need-to-know content and it helps students learn to administer drugs safely and eliminate medication errors through extensive practice of dosage calculations and careful application of the nursing process.

Organization

Pharmacology: A Nursing Process Approach is organized into **19 units** and **58 chapters.** Unit One is an overview of the principles of pharmacology from the unique perspective of nursing. The unit begins with chapters on drug action, the nursing process and client teaching, and principles of drug administration. Unit Two—a comprehensive review of drug dosage calculation for adults and children—is a unique strength of this book. This extensive unit—tabbed for quick reference—consists of six sections:

- Section 4A: Systems of Measurement with Conversion
- Section 4B: Methods for Calculation
- Section 4C: Calculations of Oral Dosages
- Section 4D: Calculations of Injectable Dosages
- Section 4E: Calculations of Intravenous Fluids
- Section 4F: Pediatric Drug Calculations

Unit Two presents six methods of dosage calculation, **color-coded to identify each method:**

- Method 1: Basic Formula
- Method 2: Ratio and Proportion
- Method 3: Fractional Equation
- Method 4: Dimensional Analysis
- Method 5: Body Weight
- Method 6: Body Surface Area

Integral to Unit Two are its **clinical practice problems,** featuring **over 100 problems with 85 actual drug labels in full color,** which provide extensive practice in real-world dosage calculations. With this wide array of practice problems in a variety of health care settings, the chapter eliminates the need to purchase a separate dosage calculation book. In addition, color photographs illustrate the equipment used to deliver medications. The accompanying **Study Guide** and **Companion CD** included with the text provide additional practice problems with answers, a review of need-to-know mathematics, printable checklists, and more.

Unit Three covers contemporary issues in pharmacology, including the changing drug approval process (Chapter 5), drug interactions and over-the-counter drugs (Chapter 7), a chapter dedicated to discussion of drugs of abuse (Chapter 8), and more. The book promotes a global approach toward client care with a separate transcultural considerations chapter (Chapter 6), thoroughly updated for the sixth edition. An expanded chapter on herbal therapy (Chapter 9) discusses client self-treatment with herbal products and its nursing implications. Lifespan issues are addressed in chapters on pediatric and geriatric pharmacology (Chapters 10 and 11).

Unit Four addresses nutrition and fluids and electrolytes, with separate chapters covering vitamin and mineral replacement (Chapter 14), fluid and electrolyte replacement (Chapter 15), and nutritional support (Chapter 16).

Units Five through Nineteen are the core of *Pharmacology: A Nursing Process Approach* and cover the drug families that students will need to understand in order to practice effectively. Each drug family chapter includes a chapter outline, learning objectives, a list of key terms, at least one Prototype Drug Chart, a drug table, and an extensive Nursing Process section. For the sixth edition, a **new unit on pain and inflammation management** makes drug therapy for pain easier to find. Also, the **antibacterial and antiinfective agents are now discussed in two separate units** to differentiate and clarify this important and complex content.

The **Prototype Drug Charts**—over 100 throughout the sixth edition—are a unique tool that students can use to view the many facets of a prototype drug through the lens of the nursing process. Each prototype drug is one of the common drugs in its drug class. Each of these charts includes Drug Class, Trade Names, Contraindications, Dosage, Drug-Lab-Food Interactions, Pharmacokinetics, Pharmacodynamics, Therapeutic Effects/Uses, Side Effects, and Adverse Reactions. With these charts, students can see how the steps of the Nursing Process correlate with these key aspects of drug information and therapy.

The **drug tables** provide a quick reference to routes, dosages, uses, and key considerations for the most commonly prescribed medications for a given class. They list drug names (generic, brand, and Canadian), dosages, uses and considerations, pregnancy categories, and specific information on half-life and protein-binding.

The **Nursing Process sections** provide a convenient summary of how to assess a client, develop nursing diagnoses, determine and follow through with the plan of care, and evaluate the outcomes of your efforts. The Nursing Process sections also include highlighted **culturally sensitive content (denoted with a ❖ symbol), nursing inter-**

ventions, suggestions for **client teaching**, and relevant herbal information (✐).

New to this Edition

The sixth edition of *Pharmacology: A Nursing Process Approach* features several significant new components.

- **NCLEX Study Questions** have been added to the end of each chapter to help prepare students for the NCLEX examination, with its increasing emphasis on pharmacology; answers are listed upside-down at the bottom of the page for quick feedback.
- A **new chapter on targeted therapies to treat cancer** discusses newer, cutting-edge cancer treatments such as multikinase inhibitors, angiogenesis inhibitors, monoclonal antibodies, and more.
- **Preventing Medication Errors boxes** have been updated and expanded to include information on packaging, doses, and other types of potential medication errors.
- **Several new photos and illustrations** give the book a fresh and exciting new look.
- The **explanation of dimensional analysis** has been clarified to make this challenging content even more understandable to students.
- **Chapter objectives have been revised** to reflect more of an emphasis on the analysis level.
- **Key terms now include page numbers** and have been bolded and defined in the text to enhance this "built-in glossary" feature for students.
- As mentioned previously, **new units for pain and inflammation management, antibacterial agents, and antiinfective agents** clearly delineate and explain these important concepts more clearly.
- Additional **Canadian drug names that correspond with the generic drug names** used in the United States have been added to the Evolve website.

Additional Features

Throughout this edition, we have retained and enhanced a variety of popular features that teach students the fundamental principles of pharmacology and the role of the nurse in drug therapy:

- **Coverage of Pathophysiology.** Relevant pathophysiology is included in Units Five through Nineteen. Understanding the pathophysiology of disease processes is foundational to understanding the rationale for drug therapy.
- **Nursing Process.** In addition to the nursing considerations in the Prototype Drug Charts, each chapter includes special Nursing Process sections that clearly delineate coverage of all five steps of the nursing process, with the following headings: Assessment, Nursing Diagnoses, Planning, Nursing Interventions, and Evaluation.
- **Client Teaching.** Under Nursing Interventions, we include client and family teaching information. This

content includes helpful **teaching tips** that relate to general information, self-administration, diet, side effects, and cultural considerations.

- **Cultural Considerations.** In addition to an entire chapter discussing general cultural considerations in drug therapy, this text includes specific Cultural Considerations in the Nursing Interventions sections of the Nursing Process.
- **Critical Thinking Case Studies.** Each chapter concludes with a clinical scenario, followed by a series of critical thinking questions. These exercises challenge students to carefully consider the scenario and apply their knowledge and analytical skills to respond to the situations. Answers are provided only in the Instructor's Manual to encourage thorough consideration before seeking expert feedback.
- **Appendixes.** Also listed in the appendixes are Therapeutic Drug Monitoring, which contains over 100 drugs, their therapeutic range, peak time, and toxic level; and a list of the 200 most commonly prescribed drugs with pronunciations.
- **Electronic Resources boxes** direct students to the Evolve website and Companion CD for more in-depth researching and application of the material discussed within each chapter.
- **Herbal Alerts.** These boxes appear throughout the text, providing students with a quick reference to information on popular herbs and their side effects, drug interactions, and more.
- **Anatomy and Physiology.** Unit openers for all drug therapy chapters include illustrated overviews of normal anatomy and physiology. These introductions give students the foundation for understanding how drugs work in various body systems.
- **Bioterrorism information.** An appendix on bioterrorism agents covers potential weapons of bioterrorism, clinical manifestations, and drug treatment considerations.

Additional Teaching and Learning Resources

The sixth edition of *Pharmacology: A Nursing Process Approach* is the core of a complete teaching and learning package for nursing pharmacology. Additional components of this package include resources for students, resources for both students and faculty members, and resources just for faculty members.

For Students

A comprehensive *Study Guide* provides more than 1800 study questions and answers, including clinically-based situational practice problems, more than 160 drug calculation problems and questions (many with actual drug labels), and critical thinking exercises to help students master text-book content. A new format for each chapter begins with **Study Questions** (multiple-choice, matching, word searches, crossword puzzles, completion exercises, and so on) and is followed by a section for **NCLEX Review Questions** (now including alternate format questions!). **Critical Thinking Exercises** are provided for all drug chapters. Answers—with detailed math solutions and rationales where appropriate—are provided at the end of the *Study Guide*.

A **Companion CD** is packaged with each sixth edition text, a valuable *free* learning tool including:

- 450 NCLEX examination review questions, *now organized by chapter and including NCLEX alternate-item formats*
- 30 Pharmacology animations
- IV therapy and medication error checklists
- Drug calculation problems
- Electronic calculators
- Top 200 drugs with pronunciations
- References from the textbook

For Both Students and Faculty

A completely updated Evolve website *(http://evolve.elsevier. com/KeeHayes/pharmacology/)* provides additional resources for students and faculty, including student review activities, weblinks, content updates, answers to frequently asked questions, case studies, suggestions for using the book in various programs, teaching tips, and additional reference content. The site is updated periodically to keep both faculty members and students informed of the latest information in nursing pharmacology.

Pharmacology Online

This unique collection of ready-to-use modules and a library of online assets may be used to create or customize an online, "blended," or web-enhanced pharmacology course that corresponds to *Pharmacology: A Nursing Process Approach*. Assets include:

- **15 Self-study modules**, including 11 modules covering the basic principles of pharmacology, a concise *Drug Calculation Review* module, and three new *Drug Content Review* modules. The self-study modules include an integrated *Online Drug Handbook* and *Audio Glossary*, with pronunciations for more than 1400 drug names and terms; they also include a rich variety of interactive activities and animations, as well as a quiz to ensure content mastery
- Unit Resources, including:
  - **26 Interactive case studies** using true-to-life clinical scenarios to promote "learning by doing," with feedback for both correct and incorrect choices
  - **220 Interactive learning activities,** offering a challenging, game-like review of drug essentials
  - **20 care planning activities** that challenge you to create complete care plans
  - Online drug handbook
  - Over **800 NCLEX examination–style practice questions** (1 quiz for each chapter) that help stu-

dents prepare for the NCLEX exam with its increased emphasis on pharmacology
- **Approximately 2,000 Flashcards** that offer a handy, easy-to-use way to memorize information about major drugs, drug classes, and pharmacologic principles
- **Library of Supplemental Resources** includes unique *Roadside Assistance* video clips, all of the animations from the self-study modules, a complete audio glossary, and more; the *Roadside Assistance* video clips use humor, analogy, and memorable visuals to help clarify core pharmacology concepts in a way students and faculty will never forget!

Evolve Select

This innovative resource is available to faculty who adopt a number of Elsevier texts, including *Pharmacology: A Nursing Process Approach*. Evolve Select is an integrated electronic study center consisting of a collection of textbooks made available electronically in CD format. It is carefully designed to "extend" the textbook for an easier and more efficient teaching and learning experience. It includes study aids such as highlighting, e-note taking, and cut and paste capabilities. Even more importantly, it allows students and instructors to do a comprehensive search within the specific text or across a number of titles. Please check with your Elsevier sales representative for more information.

Evolve Reach

A complete online testing and remediation solution, Evolve Reach helps students prepare for certification examinations with reliable, valid questions and exams. Diagnostic reports pinpoint any weaknesses, and personalized remediation comes from Elsevier's trusted Mosby and Saunders textbooks.

Evolve Apply

Online case studies challenge students to apply key concepts and develop skills in critical thinking. By answering questions and viewing rationales for a range of realistic scenarios, students learn to manage complex patient conditions and make sound clinical judgments.

Just for Faculty Members

An *Instructor's Electronic Resource* is available on CD and on the faculty Evolve website. This resource includes the following:

- **Instructor's manual**: Thoroughly revised to include new chapter focus summaries, key terms, learning objectives, chapter outlines with teaching strategies, answers to the critical thinking case studies in the text, and cross-references to relevant items on the companion CD and student Evolve site
- **Test bank**: Over 1000 ExamView test questions, including over 50 NCLEX alternate-item format questions as well as rationales and page references for each question

- **PowerPoint presentations:** Approximately 800 customizable slides with images and discussion questions incorporated
- **Image collection:** Approximately 150 full-color images from the book
- **Audience response questions:** Approximately 150 questions for use with i-Clicker and other systems

It is our hope that *Pharmacology: A Nursing Process Approach* and its comprehensive ancillary package will serve as a dynamic resource for teaching nursing students the basic principles of pharmacology and their vital role in drug therapy.

Joyce LeFever Kee

Evelyn R. Hayes

Linda E. McCuistion

Acknowledgments

We wish to extend our sincere appreciation to the many professionals who assisted in the preparation of the sixth edition of *Pharmacology: A Nursing Process Approach* by reviewing chapters and offering suggestions.

We wish to especially thank the authors of the new chapters and the original authors and those who updated the established chapters: Margaret Barton-Burke, PhD, RN; Joseph Boullata, PharmD, BCNSP; Michelle M. Byrne, MS, PhD, CNOR; Robin Webb Corbett, PhD, RN, C; Sandy Elliott, CNM, MSN; Linda Goodwin, RNC, MEd; Judith W. Herrman, PhD, RN; Kathleen J. Jones, RN-C, MS, ANP; Robert J. Kizior, BS, RPh; Paula R. Klemm, PhD, RN, OCN; Anne E. Lara, RN, MS, AOCN, APRN,BC; Linda Laskowski-Jones, RN, MS, APRN, BC, CEN; Ronald J. Lefever, RPh; Patricia S. Lincoln, BSN, RN; Patricia O'Brien, MA, MSN; Laura K. Williford Owens, PharmD; Lisa Ann Plowfield, PhD, RN; Larry D. Purnell, PhD, RN, FAAN; Nancy C. Sharts-Hopko, RN, PhD, FAAN; Jane Purnell Taylor, RN, MS; Lynette M. Wachholz, MN, APRN, IBCLC; and Gail Wilkes, MS, RNC, AOCN.

Of course, we are deeply indebted to the many clients and students we have had throughout our many years of professional nursing practice. From them we have learned many fine points about the role of therapeutic pharmacology in nursing practice.

Our deepest appreciation goes to pharmaceutical companies for permission to use their drug labels. Pharmaceutical companies that extended their courtesy to this book include:

Abbott Laboratories
American Home Products
  Lederale Laboratories
American Regent
  Luitold Pharmaceuticals
Astra Zeneca Pharmaceuticals
Bayer Corporation Inc.
Bristol-Myers Squibb Co.
  Apothecon Laboratories
  Mead Johnson Pharmaceuticals
  E. R. Squibb and Sons, Inc.
DuPont/Merck Pharmaceuticals
Eli Lilly and Company
Elkins-Sinn, Inc.
  A subsidiary of A. H. Robins
Glaxo-SmithKline
Marion Merrell Dow, Inc.

McNeilab, Inc.
  McNeil Consumer Products Co.
  Ortho-McNeil Pharmaceutical
Merck and Co., Inc.
Mylan Pharmaceuticals
Pfizer Inc.
SmithKline Beecham Pharmaceutical
Warner-Lambert Consumer Health Products
  Parke-Davis
Wyeth-Ayerst Laboratories

We extend our sincere thanks to the companies and publishers who gave us permission to use photographs, illustrations, and other materials in the text. These include:

American Association of Critical-Care Nursing
Appleton & Lange
Baxter Healthcare Corp.
Becton-Dickinson Division
Ciba-Geigy Pharmaceuticals
Elsevier, Inc.
  Mosby, Inc.
  W. B. Saunders
F. A. Davis
IMED Corporation
Medical Letter, Inc.
MiniMED, Inc.
Prentice Hall Health
Pyxis System
Wyeth-Ayerst Laboratories

Our sincere and deepest thanks to the staff at Elsevier, especially Kristin Geen, Senior Acquisitions Editor; Jamie Horn, Developmental Editor; Clay Broeker, Senior Project Manager; and Jeff Patterson, Publishing Services Manager, for their suggestions and assistance. Also, thanks to Don Passidomo, librarian at the Department of Veterans Affairs, Wilmington, Delaware, for his help with library research.

Appreciation and love go out to my husband Edward D. Kee (JLK), to my parents Margaret K. and Justin F. Hayes (ERH), and to Robert Ekas, Jr. (LEM) for their support.

Joyce LeFever Kee

Evelyn R. Hayes

Linda E. McCuistion

Contents

ONE

A Nurse's Perspective of Pharmacology

Assessing a client's response to drug therapy is an ongoing nursing responsibility. To adequately assess, plan, intervene, and evaluate drug effects, the nurse needs to have knowledge of the pharmaceutic, pharmacokinetic, and pharmacodynamic phases of drug action, all of which are described in Chapter 1, Drug Action: Pharmaceutic, Pharmacokinetic, and Pharmacodynamic Phases. A drug chart organizes specific drug data needed for preparation and application of the nursing process, as discussed in Chapter 2, Nursing Process and Client Teaching. Client teaching, also discussed in Chapter 2, is essential to promoting client and family adherence to the drug regimen and therapy.

Along with understanding the three phases of drug action, the nursing process, and client teaching, two other important functions in nursing practice include application of drug administration principles and calculation of drug doses. Chapter 3, Principles of Drug Administration, contains basic learning material for the administration of medications. It describes the "ten rights" in drug administration, drug orders, drug distribution, drug charts, drug administration guidelines, and drug administration routes (with illustrated parenteral sites).

Chapter 3 and Unit Two may be used for drug administration and calculation in place of a nursing fundamentals text or a drug calculation text.

1

Drug Action: Pharmaceutic, Pharmacokinetic, and Pharmacodynamic Phases

ELECTRONIC RESOURCES

evolve

Evolve website (http://evolve.elsevier.com/KeeHayes/pharmacology/):
- *Case Studies*
- *Content Updates*
- *Frequently Asked Questions*
- *Student Review Activities*
- *WebLinks*
- *Additional Reference Material*

Companion CD-ROM:
- *NCLEX Examination Review Questions*
- *Pharmacology Animations*
- *IV Therapy Checklists*
- *Medication Error Checklists*
- *Drug Calculation Problems*
- *Electronic Calculators*
- *Top 200 Drugs with Pronunciations*
- *References from the Textbook*

Outline

Objectives

- Differentiate the three phases of drug action.
- Identify the two processes that occur before tablets are absorbed into the body.
- Describe the four processes of pharmacokinetics.
- Explain the meaning of pharmacodynamics, dose response, maximal efficacy, the receptor, and nonreceptors in drug action.
- Define the terms protein-bound drugs, half-life, therapeutic index, therapeutic drug range, side effects, adverse reaction, and drug toxicity.
- Check drugs for half-life, percentage of protein-binding effect, therapeutic range, and side effects in a drug reference book.
- Describe the nursing implications of pharmacokinetics and pharmacodynamics.

Terms

A drug taken by mouth goes through three phases—pharmaceutic (dissolution), pharmacokinetic, and pharmacodynamic—as drug actions occur. In the pharmaceutic phase, the drug becomes a solution so that it can cross the biologic membrane. When the drug is administered parenterally by subcutaneous (subQ), intramuscular (IM), or intravenous (IV) routes, there is no pharmaceutic phase. The second phase, the pharmacokinetic phase, is composed of four processes: absorption, distribution, metabolism (or biotransformation), and excretion (or elimination). In the pharmacodynamic phase, a biologic or physiologic response results.

Pharmaceutic Phase

Approximately 80% of drugs are taken by mouth. The **pharmaceutic phase** (dissolution) is the first phase of drug action. In the gastrointestinal (GI) tract, drugs need to be in solution so they can be absorbed. A drug in solid form (tablet or capsule) must disintegrate into small particles to dissolve into a liquid, a process known as dissolution. Drugs in liquid form are already in solution. Figure 1–1 displays the pharmaceutic phase of a tablet.

Tablets are not 100% drug. Fillers and inert substances, generally called **excipients**, are used in drug preparation to allow the drug to take on a particular size and shape and to enhance drug dissolution. Some additives in drugs, such as the ions potassium (K) and sodium (Na) in penicillin potassium and penicillin sodium, increase the absorbability of the drug. Penicillin is poorly absorbed by the GI tract because of gastric acid. However, by making the drug a potassium or sodium salt, penicillin can then be absorbed. An infant's gastric secretions have a higher pH (alkaline) than those of adults; therefore infants can absorb more penicillin.

Disintegration is the breakdown of a tablet into smaller particles. **Dissolution** is the dissolving of the smaller particles in the GI fluid before absorption. **Rate limiting** is the time it takes the drug to disintegrate and dissolve to become available for the body to absorb it. Drugs in liquid form are more rapidly available for GI absorption than are solids. Generally, drugs are both disintegrated and absorbed faster in acidic fluids with a pH of 1 or 2 rather than in alkaline fluids. Both the very young and the elderly have less gastric acidity; therefore drug absorption is generally slower for those drugs absorbed primarily in the stomach.

Enteric-coated drugs resist disintegration in the gastric acid of the stomach, so disintegration does not occur until the drug reaches the alkaline environment of the small intestine. Enteric-coated tablets can remain in the stomach for a long time; therefore their effect may be delayed in onset. Enteric-coated tablets or capsules and sustained-release (beaded) capsules should not be crushed. Crushing would alter the place and time of absorption of the drug.

Food in the GI tract may interfere with the dissolution and absorption of certain drugs. However, food can also enhance absorption of other drugs; thus some drugs should be taken with food. Some drugs irritate the gastric mucosa, so fluids or food may be necessary to dilute drug concentration and to act as protectants.

FIGURE 1–1 The two pharmaceutic phases are disintegration and dissolution.

TABLET   DISINTEGRATION   DISSOLUTION

Pharmacokinetic Phase

Pharmacokinetics is the process of drug movement to achieve drug action. The four processes are absorption, distribution, metabolism (or biotransformation), and excretion (or elimination). The nurse applies knowledge of pharmacokinetics when assessing the client for possible adverse drug effects. The nurse communicates assessment findings to members of the health care team in a timely manner to promote safe and effective drug therapy for the client.

Absorption

Absorption is the movement of drug particles from the GI tract to body fluids by passive absorption, active absorption, or pinocytosis. Most oral drugs are absorbed into the surface area of the small intestine through the action of the extensive mucosal villi. Absorption is reduced if the villi are decreased in number because of disease, drug effect, or the removal of small intestine. Protein-based drugs such as insulin and growth hormones are destroyed in the small intestine by digestive enzymes. **Passive absorption** occurs mostly by diffusion (movement from higher concentration to lower concentration). With the process of diffusion, the drug does not require energy to move across the membrane. **Active absorption** requires a carrier such as an enzyme or protein to move the drug against a concentration gradient. Energy is required for active absorption. **Pinocytosis** is a process by which cells carry a drug across their membrane by engulfing the drug particles (Figure 1–2).

The GI membrane is composed mostly of lipid (fat) and protein, so drugs that are lipid soluble pass rapidly through the GI membrane. Water-soluble drugs need a carrier, either enzyme or protein, to pass through the membrane. Large particles pass through the cell membrane if they are nonionized (no positive or negative charge). Weak acid drugs such as aspirin are less ionized in the stomach, and they pass through the stomach lining easily and rapidly. Certain drugs such as calcium carbonate and many of the antifungals need an acidic environment to achieve greater drug absorption; thus food can stimulate the production of gastric acid. Hydrochloric acid destroys some drugs such as penicillin G; therefore a large oral dosage of penicillin is needed to offset the partial dose loss. Drugs administered by many routes do not pass through the GI tract or liver. These include parenteral drugs, eyedrops, eardrops, nasal sprays, respiratory inhalants, transdermal drugs, and sublingual drugs.

Remember: Drugs that are lipid soluble and nonionized are absorbed faster than water-soluble and ionized drugs.

Blood flow, pain, stress, hunger, fasting, food, and pH affect drug absorption. Poor circulation as a result of shock, vasoconstrictor drugs, or disease hampers absorption. Pain, stress, and foods that are solid, hot, and fatty can slow gastric emptying time, so the drug remains in the stomach longer. Exercise can decrease blood flow by causing more blood to flow to the peripheral muscle, thereby decreasing blood circulation to the GI tract.

Drugs given IM are absorbed faster in muscles that have more blood vessels (e.g., the deltoids) than in those that have fewer blood vessels (e.g., the gluteals). Subcutaneous tissue has fewer blood vessels, so absorption is slower in such tissue.

Some drugs do not go directly into the systemic circulation following oral absorption but pass from the intestinal lumen to the liver via the portal vein. In the liver, some drugs may be metabolized to an inactive form which may then be excreted, thus reducing the amount of active drug. Some drugs do not undergo metabolism at all in the liver, and others may be metabolized to drug metabolite, which may be equally or more active than the original drug. The process in which the drug passes to the liver first is called the **first-pass effect**, or hepatic first pass. Examples of drugs with first-pass metabolism are warfarin (Coumadin) and morphine. Lidocaine and some nitroglycerins are not given orally because they have extensive first-pass metabolism and therefore most of the dose would be destroyed.

Bioavailability is a subcategory of absorption. It is the percentage of the administered drug dose that reaches the systemic circulation. For the oral route of drug administration, bioavailability occurs after absorption and hepatic drug metabolism. The percentage of bioavailability for the oral route is always less than 100%, but for the intravenous route it is usually 100%. Oral drugs that have a high first-pass hepatic metabolism may have a bioavailability of only 20% to 40% on entering systemic circulation. To obtain the desired drug effect, the oral dose could be three to five times larger than the drug dose for IV use.

Factors that alter bioavailability include (1) the drug form (e.g., tablet, capsule, sustained-release, liquid, transdermal patch, rectal suppository, inhalation), (2) route of administration (e.g., oral, rectal, topical, parenteral), (3) GI mucosa and motility, (4) food and other drugs, and (5) changes in liver metabolism caused by liver dysfunction or inadequate hepatic blood flow. A decrease in liver function or a decrease in hepatic blood flow can increase the bioavailability of a drug, but only if the drug is metabolized by the liver. Less drug is destroyed by hepatic metabolism in the presence of liver disorder.

With some oral drugs, rapid absorption increases the bioavailability of the drug and can cause an increase in drug concentration. Drug toxicity may result. Slow absorp-

FIGURE 1–2 The three major processes for drug absorption through the gastrointestinal membrane are passive absorption, active absorption, and pinocytosis.

tion can limit the bioavailability of the drug, thus causing a decrease in drug serum concentration.

Distribution

Distribution is the process by which the drug becomes available to body fluids and body tissues. Drug distribution is influenced by blood flow, the drug's affinity to the tissue, and the **protein-binding effect** (Figure 1–3). In addition, volume of drug distribution (Vd) is dependent on drug dose and its concentration in the body. Drugs with a larger volume of drug distribution have a longer half-life and stay in the body longer. See the section on metabolism, or biotransformation, later in this chapter.

As drugs are distributed in the plasma, many are bound to varying degrees (percentages) with protein (primarily albumin). Drugs that are greater than 89% bound to protein are known as highly protein-bound drugs; drugs that are 61% to 89% bound to protein are moderately highly protein-bound; drugs that are 30% to 60% bound to protein are moderately protein-bound; and drugs that are less than 30% bound to protein are low protein-bound drugs. Table 1–1 lists selected highly protein-bound drugs and moderately highly protein-bound drugs. The portion of the drug that is bound is inactive because it is not available to receptors, and the portion that remains unbound is free, active drug. Only **free drugs** (drugs not bound to protein) are active and can cause a pharmacologic response. As the free drug in the circulation decreases, more bound drug is released from the protein to maintain the balance of free drug.

When two highly protein-bound drugs are given concurrently, they compete for protein-binding sites, thus causing more free drug to be released into the circulation. In this situation, drug accumulation and possible drug toxicity can result. Also, a low protein level decreases the number of protein-binding sites and can cause an increase in the amount of free drug in the plasma. Drug overdose may then result. Drug dose is prescribed according to the percentage in which the drug binds to protein. Examples of causes of low protein levels are malnutrition and advanced aging.

With some health conditions that result in a low serum protein level, excess free or unbound drug goes to nonspecific tissue binding sites until needed and excess free drug in the circulation does not occur.

Table 1–1

Protein-Binding and Half-Life of Drugs

Drug	Protein-Bound (%)	Half-Life (t½) (h)
Highly Protein-Bound Drugs (>89%)		
amitriptyline	97	40
chlorpromazine	95	30
diazepam	98	30-80
dicloxacillin	95	0.5-1
digitoxin	90	8
furosemide	95	1.5
ibuprofen	98	2-4
lorazepam	92	15
piroxicam	99	30-86
propranolol	92	4
rifampin	89	2
sulfisoxazole	85-95	4.5-7.5
valproic acid	92	15
Moderately Highly Protein-Bound Drugs (61%-89%)		
erythromycin	70	3
nafcillin	86	2-20
phenytoin	88	10-40
quinidine	70	6
trimethoprim	70	11
Moderately Protein-Bound Drugs (30%-60%)		
aspirin	49	0.25-2
lidocaine	50	2
meperidine	56	3
pindolol	40	3-4
theophylline	60	9
ticarcillin	45-65	1-1.5
Low Protein-Bound Drugs (<30%)		
amikacin	4-11	2-3
amoxicillin	20	1-1.5
atenolol	6-16	6-7
cephalexin	10-15	0.5-1.2
digoxin	25	36
neostigmine bromide	15-25	1-1.5
terbutaline sulfate	25	3-11
timolol maleate	<10	3-4
tobramycin sulfate	10	2-3

h, Hour; >, greater than; <, less than.

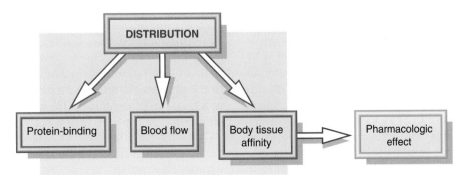

FIGURE 1–3 Drug distribution.

Some drugs bind with a specific protein component such as albumin or globulin. Most anticonvulsants bind primarily to albumin. Some basic drugs such as anti-dysrhythmics (e.g., lidocaine, quinidine) bind mostly to globulins.

Clients with liver or kidney disease or those who are malnourished may have an abnormally low serum albumin level. This results in fewer protein-binding sites, which in turn leads to excess free drug and eventually to drug toxicity. The elderly are more likely to have hypoalbuminemia.

To avoid possible drug toxicity, checking the protein-binding percentage of all drugs administered to a client is important. The nurse should also check the client's plasma protein and albumin levels, because a decrease in plasma protein (albumin) decreases protein-binding sites, permitting more free drug in the circulation. Depending on the drug the result could be life threatening.

Abscesses, exudates, body glands, and tumors hinder drug distribution. Antibiotics do not distribute well at abscess and exudate sites. In addition, some drugs accumulate in particular tissues such as fat, bone, liver, muscle, and eye tissues.

Metabolism, or Biotransformation

Drugs can be metabolized in both the GI tract and liver; however, the liver is the primary site of **metabolism**. Most drugs are inactivated by liver enzymes and are then converted or transformed by hepatic enzymes to inactive metabolites or water-soluble substances for excretion. A large percentage of drugs are lipid soluble; thus the liver metabolizes the lipid-soluble drug substance to a water-soluble substance for renal excretion. However, some drugs are transformed into active metabolites, causing an increased pharmacologic response. Liver diseases such as cirrhosis and hepatitis alter drug metabolism by inhibiting the drug-metabolizing enzymes in the liver. When the drug metabolism rate is decreased, excess drug accumulation can occur and lead to toxicity.

The **half-life (t½)** of a drug is the time it takes for one half of the drug concentration to be eliminated. Metabolism and elimination affect the half-life of a drug. For example, with liver or kidney dysfunction, the half-life of the drug is prolonged and less drug is metabolized and eliminated. When a drug is taken continually, drug accumulation may occur. Table 1–1 gives the half-life of selected drugs.

A drug goes through several half-lives before more than 90% of the drug is eliminated. If the client takes 650 mg of aspirin and the half-life is 3 hours, it takes 3 hours for the first half-life to eliminate 325 mg, 6 hours for the second half-life to eliminate an additional 162 mg, and so on until the sixth half-life (or 18 hours), when 10 mg of aspirin is left in the body (Table 1–2). A short half-life is considered to be 4 to 8 hours, and a long one is 24 hours or longer. If the drug has a long half-life (such as digoxin at 36 hours), it takes several days for the body to completely eliminate the drug.

Table 1–2

Half-Life of 650 mg of Aspirin

Number t½	Time of Elimination (h)	Dosage Remaining (mg)	Percentage Left
1	3	325	50
2	6	162	25
3	9	81	12.5
4	12	40	6.25
5	15	20	3.1
6	18	10	1.55

h, Hour; *t½*, half-life.

By knowing the half life, the time it takes for a drug to reach a steady state of serum concentration can be computed. Administration of the drug for three to five half-lives saturates the biologic system to the extent that the intake of drug equals the amount metabolized and excreted. An example is digoxin, which has a half-life of 36 hours with normal renal function. It would take approximately 5 days to 1 week (three to five half-lives) to reach a steady-state for digoxin concentration. Steady-state serum concentration is predictive of therapeutic drug effect. The half-life of drugs is also discussed under Pharmacodynamic Phase.

Excretion, or Elimination

The main route of drug **elimination** is through the kidneys (urine). Other routes include hepatic metabolism, bile, feces, lungs, saliva, sweat, and breast milk. The kidneys filter free unbound drugs, water-soluble drugs, and drugs that are unchanged. Protein-bound drugs cannot be filtered through the kidneys. Once the drug is released from the protein, it is a free drug and is eventually excreted in the urine. The lungs eliminate volatile drug substances and products metabolized to carbon dioxide (CO_2) and water (H_2O).

The urine pH influences drug excretion. Urine pH varies from 4.5 to 8. Acid urine promotes elimination of weak base drugs, and alkaline urine promotes elimination of weak acid drugs. Aspirin, a weak acid, is excreted rapidly in alkaline urine. If a person takes an overdose of aspirin, sodium bicarbonate may be given to change the urine pH to alkaline to help potentiate excretion of the drug. Large quantities of cranberry juice can decrease urine pH, causing an acid urine and inhibiting the elimination of aspirin.

With a kidney disease that results in decreased glomerular filtration rate (GFR) or decreased renal tubular secretion, drug excretion is slowed or impaired. Drug accumulation with possible severe adverse drug reactions can result. A decrease in blood flow to the kidneys can also alter drug excretion.

The most accurate test to determine renal function is **creatinine clearance (CLcr)**. Creatinine is a metabolic byproduct of muscle that is excreted by the kidneys. Creatinine clearance varies with age and gender. Lower values are expected in elderly and female clients because of their decreased muscle mass. A decrease in renal GFR results in an increase in serum creatinine level and a decrease in urine creatinine clearance.

With renal dysfunction either in the elderly or as a result of kidney disorders, drug dosage usually needs to be decreased. In these cases, the creatinine clearance needs to be determined to establish appropriate drug dosage. When the creatinine clearance is decreased, drug dosage likewise may need to be decreased. Continuous drug dosing according to a prescribed dosing regimen without evaluating creatinine clearance could result in drug toxicity.

The creatinine clearance test consists of a 12- or 24-hour urine collection and a blood sample. Normal creatinine clearance is 85 to 135 ml/min. This rate decreases with age because aging decreases muscle mass and results in a decrease in functioning nephrons. Elderly clients may have a creatinine clearance of 60 ml/min. For this reason, drug dosage in the elderly may need to be decreased. Refer to Chapter 11 for further explanation of drug dosing in the elderly.

Pharmacodynamic Phase

Pharmacodynamics is the study of drug concentration and its effects on the body. Drug response can cause a primary or secondary physiologic effect or both. The primary effect is desirable, and the secondary effect may be desirable or undesirable. An example of a drug with a primary and secondary effect is diphenhydramine (Benadryl), an antihistamine. The primary effect of diphenhydramine is to treat the symptoms of allergy, and the secondary effect is a central nervous system depression that causes drowsiness. The secondary effect is undesirable when the client drives an automobile, but at bedtime it could be desirable because it causes mild sedation.

Dose Response and Maximal Efficacy

Dose response is the relationship between the minimal versus the maximal amount of drug dose needed to produce the desired drug response. Some clients respond to a lower drug dose, whereas others need a high drug dose to elicit the desired response. The drug dose is usually graded to achieve the desired drug response.

All drugs have a maximum drug effect (maximal efficacy). For example, morphine and propoxyphene hydrochloride (Darvon) are prescribed to relieve pain. The maximum efficacy of morphine is greater than propoxyphene hydrochloride, regardless of how much propoxyphene hydrochloride is given. Propoxyphene hydrochloride has a lower maximum efficacy than morphine. The pain relief with the use of propoxyphene hydrochloride is not as great as it is with morphine.

Onset, Peak, and Duration of Action

One important aspect of pharmacodynamics is knowing the drug's onset, peak, and duration of action. **Onset of action** is the time it takes to reach the minimum effective

FIGURE 1–4 The time-response curve evaluates three parameters of drug action: (1) onset, (2) peak, and (3) duration. MEC, Minimum effective concentration; MTC, minimum toxic concentration.

concentration (MEC) after a drug is administered. **Peak action** occurs when the drug reaches its highest blood or plasma concentration. **Duration of action** is the length of time the drug has a pharmacologic effect. Figure 1–4 illustrates the areas in which onset, peak, and duration of action occur.

Some drugs produce effects in minutes, but others may take hours or days. A **time-response curve** evaluates three parameters of drug action: the onset of drug action, peak action, and duration of action. Figure 1–4 indicates these parameters by using T (time) with subscripts (e.g., T_0, T_1, T_2, T_3).

It is necessary to understand the time response in relationship to drug administration. If the drug plasma or serum level decreases below threshold or MEC, adequate drug dosing is not achieved; too high a drug level above the minimum toxic concentration (MTC), can result in toxicity.

Receptor Theory

Most receptors, protein in structure, are found on cell membranes. Drug-binding sites are primarily on proteins, glycoproteins, proteolipids, and at enzymes. There are four **receptor families**: (1) kinase-linked receptor, (2) ligand-gated ion channels, (3) G protein-coupled receptor systems, and (4) nuclear receptors. The term **ligand-binding domain** is the site on the receptor in which drugs bind.

- *Kinase-linked receptors.* The ligand-binding domain for drug binding is on the cell surface. The drug activates the enzyme (inside the cell), and a response is initiated.
- *Ligand-gated ion channels.* The drug spans the cell membrane and, with this type of receptor, the channel opens, allowing for the flow of ions into and out of the cells. The ions are primarily sodium and calcium.
- *G protein-coupled receptor systems.* There are three components to this receptor response: (1) the receptor, (2) G protein that binds with guanosine triphosphate

(GTP), and (3) the effector that is either an enzyme or an ion channel. The system works as follows:

$$\text{drug} \xrightarrow{\text{activates}} \text{receptor} \xrightarrow{\text{activates}} \text{G protein} \xrightarrow{\text{activates}} \text{effect.}$$

- *Nuclear receptors.* Cell nucleus and not on the surface of the cell membrane. Activation of receptors through the transcription factors is prolonged. With the first three receptor groups, activation of the receptors is rapid.

Drugs act through receptors by binding to the receptor to produce (initiate) a response or to block (prevent) a response. The activity of many drugs is determined by the ability of the drug to bind to a specific receptor. The better the drug fits at the receptor site, the more biologically active the drug is. It is similar to the fit of the right key in a lock. Figure 1–5 illustrates a drug binding to a receptor.

Agonists and Antagonists

Drugs that produce a response are called **agonists**, and drugs that block a response are called **antagonists**. Isoproterenol (Isuprel) stimulates the beta 1 receptor, and so it is

WEAK AGONIST   STRONG AGONIST

FIGURE 1–5 Two drug agonists attach to the receptor site. The drug agonist that has an exact fit is a strong agonist and is more biologically active than the weak agonist.

an agonist. Cimetidine (Tagamet), an antagonist, blocks the histamine (H_2) receptor, thus preventing excessive gastric acid secretion. The effects of an antagonist can be determined by the inhibitory (I) action of the drug concentration on the receptor site. IC_{50} indicates that the drug is effective in inhibiting receptor response in 50% of persons.

Nonspecific and Nonselective Drug Effects

Almost all drugs, agonists and antagonists, lack specific and selective effects. A receptor produces a variety of physiologic responses, depending on where in the body that receptor is located. Cholinergic receptors are located in the bladder, heart, blood vessels, lungs, and eyes. A drug that stimulates or blocks the cholinergic receptors affects all anatomic sites of location. Drugs that affect various sites are **nonspecific drugs** and have properties of nonspecificity. Bethanechol (Urecholine) may be prescribed for postoperative urinary retention to increase bladder contraction. This drug stimulates the cholinergic receptor located in the bladder, and urination occurs by strengthening bladder contraction. Because bethanechol affects the cholinergic receptor, other cholinergic sites are also affected. The heart rate decreases, blood pressure decreases, gastric acid secretion increases, the bronchioles constrict, and the pupils of the eye constrict (Figure 1–6). These other effects may be either desirable or harmful. Drugs that evoke a variety of responses throughout the body have a nonspecific response.

Drugs may act at different receptors. Drugs that affect various receptors are **nonselective drugs** or have properties of nonselectivity. Chlorpromazine (Thorazine) acts on the norepinephrine, dopamine, acetylcholine, and histamine receptors, and a variety of responses result from action at these receptor sites. Epinephrine acts on the alpha$_1$, beta$_1$, and beta$_2$ receptors (Figure 1–7).

Drugs that produce a response but do not act on a receptor may act by stimulating or inhibiting enzyme activity or hormone production.

DRUG	CHOLINERGIC RECEPTOR SITE		RESPONSES
Bethanechol	Eye		Constrict pupils
	Heart		Decrease heart rate
	Blood vessels		Decrease blood pressure
	Stomach		Increase gastric secretion
	Bronchus		Constrict bronchioles
	Bladder		Increase bladder contraction

FIGURE 1–6 Cholinergic receptors are located in the bladder, heart, blood vessels, stomach, bronchi, and eyes.

DRUG	RECEPTOR	SITES	RESPONSES

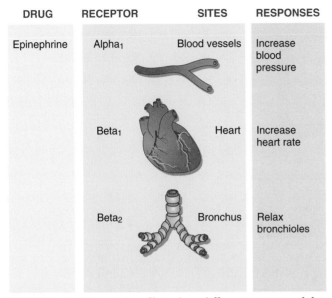

FIGURE 1–7   Epinephrine affects three different receptors: alpha₁, beta₁, and beta₂.

Categories of Drug Action

The four categories of drug action include (1) stimulation or depression, (2) replacement, (3) inhibition or killing of organisms, and (4) irritation. In drug action that stimulates, the rate of cell activity or the secretion from a gland increases. In drug action that depresses, cell activity and function of a specific organ are reduced. Replacement drugs such as insulin replace essential body compounds. Drugs that inhibit or kill organisms interfere with bacterial cell growth (e.g., penicillin exerts its bactericidal effects by blocking the synthesis of the bacterial cell wall). Drugs also can act by the mechanism of irritation (e.g., laxatives irritate the inner wall of the colon, thus increasing peristalsis and defecation).

Drug action might last hours, days, weeks, or months. The length of action depends on the half-life of the drug; therefore the half-life is a reasonable guide for the determination of drug dosage intervals. Drugs with a short half-life such as penicillin G (2 hours) are given several times a day. Drugs with a long half-life such as digoxin (36 hours) are given once a day. If a drug with a long half-life is given two or more times a day, drug accumulation in the body and drug toxicity are likely to result. If there is liver or renal impairment, the half-life of the drug increases. In these cases, high doses of the drug or too-frequent dosing can result in drug toxicity.

Therapeutic Index and Therapeutic Range (Therapeutic Window)

The safety of drugs is a major concern. The **therapeutic index (TI)** estimates the margin of safety of a drug through the use of a ratio that measures the effective (therapeutic or concentration) dose (ED) in 50% of persons or animals (ED_{50}) and the lethal dose (LD) in 50% of animals (LD_{50}) (Figure 1–8). The closer the ratio is to 1, the greater danger of toxicity.

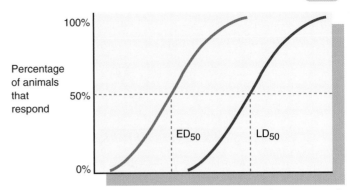

FIGURE 1–8   The therapeutic index measures the margin of safety of a drug. It is a ratio that measures the effective therapeutic dose and the lethal dose.

$$TI = \frac{LD_{50}}{ED_{50}}$$

In some cases the ED may be 25% (ED_{25}) or 75% (ED_{75}).

Drugs with a **low therapeutic index** have a narrow margin of safety (Figure 1–9, A). Drug dosage might need adjustment, and plasma (serum) drug levels need to be monitored because of the small safety range between ED and LD. Drugs with a **high therapeutic index** have a wide margin of safety and less danger of producing toxic effects (Figure 1–9, B). Plasma (serum) drug levels do not need to be monitored routinely for drugs with a high TI.

The **therapeutic range (therapeutic window)** of a drug concentration in plasma should be between the minimum effective concentration in the plasma for obtaining desired drug action and the minimum toxic concentration, the toxic effect. When the therapeutic range is given, it includes both protein-bound and unbound portions of the drug. Drug reference books give many plasma (serum) therapeutic ranges of drugs. If the therapeutic range is narrow, such as for digoxin (0.5 to 2 ng/ml), the plasma drug level should be monitored periodically to avoid drug toxicity. Monitoring the therapeutic range is not necessary if the drug is not considered highly toxic. Table 1–3 lists the therapeutic ranges and toxic levels for anticonvulsants.

Peak and Trough Drug Levels

Peak drug level is the highest plasma concentration of drug at a specific time. Peak drug levels indicate the rate of absorption. If the drug is given orally, the peak time might be 1 to 3 hours after drug administration. If the drug is given IV, the peak time might occur in 10 minutes. A blood sample should be drawn at the proposed peak time, according to the route of administration.

The **trough drug level** is the lowest plasma concentration of a drug, and it measures the rate at which the drug is eliminated. Trough levels are drawn immediately before the next dose of drug is given, regardless of route of administration. Peak levels indicate the rate of absorption of the drug, and trough levels indicate the rate of elimination of the drug. Peak and trough levels are requested for drugs that

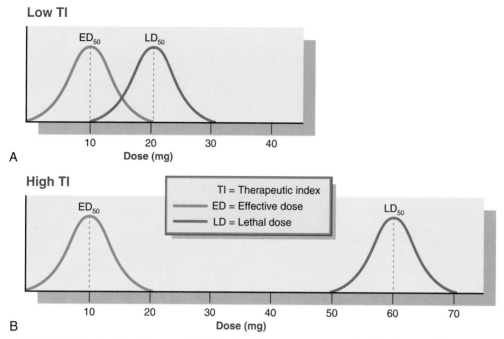

FIGURE 1-9 A, A low therapeutic index drug has a narrow margin of safety, and the drug effect should be closely monitored. B, A high therapeutic index drug has a wide margin of safety and carries less risk of drug toxicity.

Table 1-3

Anticonvulsants: Therapeutic Ranges and Toxic Levels

Drug	Therapeutic Range (mcg/ml)	Toxic Level (mcg/ml)
carbamazepine	6-12	> 12-15
ethosuximide	40-80	> 80-100
phenytoin	10-20	> 30
primidone	5-10	> 12-15
valproic acid	50-100	> 100

>, Greater than.

have a narrow therapeutic index and are considered toxic, such as the aminoglycoside antibiotics (Table 1-4). If either the peak or trough level is too high, toxicity can occur. If the peak is too low, no therapeutic effect is achieved.

Loading Dose

When immediate drug response is desired, a large initial dose, known as the **loading dose**, of drug is given to achieve a rapid minimum effective concentration in the plasma.

After a large initial dose, a prescribed dosage per day is ordered. Digoxin, a digitalis preparation, requires a loading dose when first prescribed. Digitalization is the process by which the minimum effective concentration level for digoxin is achieved in the plasma within a short time.

Side Effects, Adverse Reactions, and Toxic Effects

Side effects are physiologic effects not related to desired drug effects. All drugs have side effects, desirable or undesirable. Even with a correct drug dosage, side effects occur and are predicted. Side effects result mostly from drugs that lack specificity, such as bethanechol (Urecholine). In some health problems, side effects may be desirable (e.g., the use of diphenhydramine HCl [Benadryl] at bedtime when its side effect of drowsiness is beneficial). At times, however, side effects are called *adverse reactions*. The terms *side effects* and *adverse reactions* might be used interchangeably. Some side effects are expected as part of drug therapy. The occurrence of these expected but undesirable side effects is not a reason to discontinue therapy. The nurse's role includes teaching clients to report any side effects. Many can be managed with dosage adjustments, changing to a different drug in the same

Table 1-4

Aminoglycoside Antibiotics: Peak and Trough Levels

Drug	Peak (mcg/ml)	Trough (mcg/ml)	Toxic Peak Level (mcg/ml)	Toxic Trough Levels (mcg/ml)
amikacin	15-30	5-10	> 35	> 10
gentamicin	5-10	<2	> 12	> 2
tobramycin	5-10	<2	> 12	> 2

>, Greater than; <, less than.

class of drugs, or implementing other interventions. It is important to know that the occurrence of side effects is one of the primary reasons clients stop taking the prescribed medication. **Adverse reactions** are more severe than side effects. They are a range of untoward effects (unintended and occurring at normal doses) of drugs that cause mild to severe side effects, including anaphylaxis (cardiovascular collapse). Adverse reactions are always undesirable. Adverse effects must always be reported and documented because they represent variances from planned therapy.

Toxic effects, or **toxicity**, of a drug can be identified by monitoring the plasma (serum) therapeutic range of the drug. However, for drugs that have a wide therapeutic index, the therapeutic ranges are seldom given. For those drugs with a narrow TI, such as aminoglycoside antibiotics and anticonvulsants, the therapeutic ranges are closely monitored. When the drug level exceeds the therapeutic range, toxic effects are likely to occur from overdosing or drug accumulation.

Pharmacogenetics

Pharmacogenetics is the effect of a drug action that varies from a predicted drug response because of genetic factors or hereditary influence. Because people have different genetic makeup, they do not always respond identically to a drug dosage or planned drug therapy. Genetic factors can alter the metabolism of the drug in converting its chemical form to an inert metabolite; thus the drug action can be enhanced or diminished. Some persons are less or more sensitive to drugs and their drug actions because of genetic factors. For example, African Americans do not respond as well as Caucasians to some classes of antihypertensive medications such as ACE inhibitors.

Tolerance/Tachyphylaxis

Tolerance refers to a decreased responsiveness over the course of therapy. In contrast, **Tachyphylaxis** refers to a rapid decrease in response to the drug. In essence, tachyphylaxis is an "acute tolerance". Drug categories that can cause tachyphylaxis include narcotics, barbiturates, laxatives, and psychotropic agents. For example, drug tolerance to narcotics can result in decreased pain relief for the client. If the nurse does not recognize the development of drug tolerance, the client's request for more pain medication might be interpreted as drug-seeking behavior associated with addiction. Prevention of tachyphylaxis should always be part of the therapeutic regimen.

Placebo Effect

A **placebo effect** is a psychologic benefit from a compound that may not have the chemical structure of a drug effect. The placebo is effective in approximately one third of persons who take a placebo compound. Many clinical drug studies involve a group of subjects who receive a placebo. The nurse can increase the therapeutic effect of the drug (e.g., narcotics for pain management) but violate the truth-telling ethical principle if a nontherapeutic drug is presented as a therapeutic agent. Hence it is required that participants in drug trials be told from the start that they might receive a placebo.

Summary

The phases of drug action are pharmaceutic, pharmacokinetic, and pharmacodynamic. Figure 1–10 illustrates these three phases for drugs given orally, but drugs given by injection are involved only in the pharmacokinetic and pharmacodynamic phases. Nurses should be aware that tablets must disintegrate and go into solution (the pharmaceutic phase) to be absorbed.

To avoid toxic effects, the nurse needs to know the half-life, protein-binding percentage, normal side effects, and therapeutic ranges of the drug. This information can be obtained from drug reference books.

Nursing Process

ASSESSMENT

■ Recognize that drugs in liquid form are absorbed faster than those in solid form.

■ Assess for signs and symptoms of drug toxicity when giving two drugs that are highly protein-bound. The drugs compete for protein-binding sites, and displacement of drugs occurs. More free drug is in circulation because there are not enough protein-binding sites. Too much of a free drug can result in drug toxicity.

■ Identify side effects of drugs that are nonspecific (same receptor at different tissue and organ sites). For example, when atropine is the drug to be administered, assess for tachycardia, dry mouth and throat, constipation, urinary retention, and blurred vision. If nonspecific

FIGURE 1–10 The three phases of drug action.

drugs are given in large doses or at frequent intervals, many side effects are likely to occur.

■ Check peak levels and trough levels of drugs such as aminoglycosides that have a narrow therapeutic range. If the trough level is high, toxic effects can result.

■ Check the drug literature for the protein-binding percentage of the drug. Drugs with a high protein-binding effect have a large portion of drug bound to protein. This causes the drug to become inactive until it is released from the protein. The portion not bound to protein is a free and active drug.

NURSING INTERVENTIONS

■ Advise client not to eat fatty food before ingesting an enteric-coated tablet, because fatty foods decrease absorption rate.

■ Report to the health care provider if drugs with a long half-life (i.e., greater than 24 hours) are given more than once a day. Some drugs with a long half-life, the anticoagulant warfarin (Coumadin) for instance, can be more dangerous than others and should be monitored frequently.

■ Monitor the therapeutic range of drugs that are more toxic or have a narrow therapeutic range (e.g., digoxin).

Cultural Considerations ❖

• Be aware that individuals from some cultures metabolize drugs differently than the general population.

• Assess for adverse effects that may result from this variation in metabolism.

EVALUATION

■ Evaluate the determinants that affect drug therapy according to Figure 1–11.

Critical Thinking Case Study

As the nurse, you are preparing a teaching session for JM and his wife LM on his medication regimen. JM's long standing medications include Lanoxin, furosemide, and acetylsalicylic acid. Ibuprofen is the new drug to be added to the regimen. What basic principles need to be incorporated into your teaching plan for JM and his wife?

FIGURE 1–11   Determinants that affect drug therapy.

NCLEX Study Questions

1. The 4 sequential processes of the pharmacokinetic phase are:
   a. Distribution, metabolism, excretion, absorption
   b. Biotransformation, excretion, absorption, metabolism
   c. Absorption, distribution, metabolism, excretion
   d. Metabolism, distribution, absorption, excretion

2. A tablet undergoes which of the following two processes before it is absorbed?
   a. Metabolism, dissolution
   b. Disintegration, distribution
   c. Biotransformation. distribution
   d. Disintegration, dissolution

3. A drug that is 75% protein-bound is classified as:
   a. Highly protein-bound
   b. Moderately highly protein-bound
   c. Moderately protein-bound
   d. Low protein-bound

4. As the nurse, you notice that one of your client's drugs has a low therapeutic index. The most important nursing implication of this is:
   a. A wide margin of safety
   b. A narrow margin of safety
   c. Measured 1 hour after administration
   d. Measured 10 minutes after administration

5. The most accurate test to determine renal function is:
   a. Creatinine clearance   c. Glomerular filtration rate
   b. Blood urea nitrogen   d. Renal clearance

Answers: 1. c; 2. d; 3. b; 4. b; 5. a.

2

Nursing Process and Client Teaching

ELECTRONIC RESOURCES

Evolve website (http://evolve.elsevier.com/KeeHayes/pharmacology/):
- *Case Studies*
- *Content Updates*
- *Frequently Asked Questions*
- *Student Review Activities*
- *WebLinks*
- *Additional Reference Material*

Companion CD-ROM:
- *NCLEX Examination Review Questions*
- *Pharmacology Animations*
- *IV Therapy Checklists*
- *Medication Error Checklists*
- *Drug Calculation Problems*
- *Electronic Calculators*
- *Top 200 Drugs with Pronunciations*
- *References from the Textbook*

Outline......

Objectives......

- Differentiate the steps of the nursing process and their purpose in relation to drug therapy.
- Develop client-centered goals.
- Discuss at least eight principles for health teaching related to drug therapy plans.
- Describe at least six culturally sensitive health teaching tips.
- Analyze the nurse's role related to drug therapy plans.

Terms......

assessment, p. 14
culturally sensitive, p. 18
evaluation, p. 21

goal setting, p. 17
holistic nursing approach,
   p. 13

implementation, p. 17
nursing diagnosis, p. 15
planning, p. 17

Nurses have a significant role in the management of drug therapy. Influences on this role include technology, increased longevity of the citizenry, and survival of persons with multiple and varied biopsychosocial needs. Variables in drug therapy are numerous and, at times, unknown. A **holistic nursing approach** to care is crucial to the success of drug therapy initiation, maintenance, and evaluation.

This chapter explores the use of the nursing process as it relates to drug therapy. Careful detail to each phase of the

process fosters the client's success with the prescribed medication regimen. Considerations for the use of over-the-counter (OTC) drugs and herbal remedies are explored in Chapters 7 and 9.

Nursing Process

The four phases of the nursing process are assessment (including nursing diagnosis), planning, implementation, and evaluation. The nursing process is not linear. Each phase is discussed as it relates to health teaching in drug therapy.

Assessment

Assessment, the first phase of the nursing process, is particularly important because the data provided by the assessment form the basis on which care is planned, implemented, and evaluated. Data collection involves both subjective and objective information.

Subjective Data

The components listed below are reflective of subjective data related to the medication regimen:

Current health history, including any problems with swallowing

Client symptoms as verbalized by client

Current medications

Dosage, frequency, route, prescribing health care provider, if any

Client knowledge about drug and its side effects and for what diagnosis and symptoms client is taking the drug

Client expectation and perception of drug effectiveness

Client knowledge about what effects or drug reactions to report to health care provider

Client compliance with regimen and reasons for deviations. Are deviations based on valid data/rationale and clinically sound?

Drug allergies or reactions both past and present; also food and dye intolerance and reactions

OTC drugs

Herbal remedies

Street drugs. If used, what is their frequency of use?

Alcohol consumption

Smoking

Past health history

Past illnesses, major injuries, and drug therapy, including reactions

Medications saved from previous use; how stored; expiration date

Street drugs

Client's environment

Client's language and communication needs

History of compliance with drug therapy as prescribed (i.e., were prescriptions filled and finished?)

Does client read and follow instructions from the health care provider and the pharmacy?

Client knowledge of specific drug storage requirements, if any

Availability, willingness, and ability to administer or assist in the administration of medications. This information is essential for third-party payment for continued home visits or for admission to an extended care facility.

Household members, neighbors, friends, and their roles; ages of household members

Learning style preferences

First language, if other than English

Readiness to learn

Activities of daily living (ADLs) capabilities

Dietary patterns, cultural and economic influences, safety

Financial resources (drugs can be expensive)

Mental status

REMEMBER: Clients, even those who do not intend to withhold information, do not always tell all about their medications. Therefore, in addition to asking about prescription drugs, ask specifically about vitamins, herbal supplements, all contraceptives, aspirin or acetaminophen, and antihistamines or decongestants. Also identify caffeine and nicotine use. Ask to see the contents of the medicine chest at home (or other storage area for medications), and ask whether a pharmacist is used as a consultant.

Objective Data

The components listed below are reflective of objective data related to the medication regimen:

Gross and fine motor control, hand joint range of motion, and decreased muscle strength can interfere with client's ability to open medication containers. Visual impairment can limit a client's ability to read labels and correctly measure dosages.

Laboratory tests
Diagnostic studies   } Baseline data are essential for
Physical/health   future comparisons.
  assessment

Data collection should focus on symptoms and those organs most likely to be affected by drug therapy. For example, if a drug is nephrotoxic, the client's creatinine clearance should be assessed. Assess major body systems for any signs of reaction or interaction of drugs or ineffectiveness of therapy.

Based on assessment data, the nurse must identify high-risk clients (those likely to have adverse reactions). The client's health history, physical assessment, and laboratory test results are sources of these data. The client's attitudes and values about taking medication are very important in planning intervention to support the client's decision to adopt healthy behaviors related to taking medications. Emphasis is on assessing the client's social support system, for it is this special support system that promotes the taking of medication as prescribed or notifying the health care provider if a problem arises.

Enhancing client compliance with the drug therapy regimen is an essential component of health teaching. The client and family response to the following three questions provides the nurse with critical information unique to each client's teaching situation:

1. What things help you take your medicine as prescribed?
2. What things prevent you from taking your medicine as prescribed?
3. What would you do if you forgot to take a dose of medication?

Frequently cited factors for noncompliance include forgetfulness, knowledge deficit, side effects, low self-esteem, depression, lack of trust in the health care system, family problems, language barriers, high cost of medications, anxiety, value systems (religious and other), and lack of motivation. The nurse's role is critical to drug therapy. The nurse is most often the one person who follows the client most closely and the one who is frequently first to assess the client's response to drugs. The nurse applies knowledge of pharmacology to anticipate drug responses in the individual client.

Nursing Diagnosis

A **nursing diagnosis** is made based on the analysis of the assessment data. More than one applicable nursing diagnosis may be generated, and a nursing diagnosis may be actual or potential. The registered nurse formulates nursing diagnoses and uses them, with the assistance of others, to guide the development of a care plan. A list of nursing diagnoses accepted by the North American Nursing Diagnosis Association (NANDA) is presented in Box 2–1.

Box 2–1

NANDA-Approved Nursing Diagnoses: 2007-2008

Activity intolerance
Activity intolerance, risk for
Airway clearance, ineffective
Allergy response, latex
Allergy response, risk for latex
Anxiety
Anxiety, death
Aspiration, risk for
Attachment, risk for impaired parent/child
Autonomic dysreflexia
Autonomic dysreflexia, risk for
Behavior, risk-prone health
Body image, disturbed
Body temperature, risk for imbalanced
Bowel incontinence
Breastfeeding, effective
Breastfeeding, ineffective
Breastfeeding, interrupted
Breathing pattern, ineffective
Cardiac output, decreased
Caregiver role strain
Caregiver role strain, risk for
Comfort, readiness for enhanced
Communication, impaired verbal
Communication, readiness for enhanced
Conflict, decisional
Conflict, parental role
Confusion, acute
Confusion, chronic
Confusion, risk for acute
Constipation
Constipation, perceived
Constipation, risk for
Contamination
Contamination, risk for
Coping, compromised family
Coping, defensive
Coping, disabled family
Coping, ineffective
Coping, ineffective community
Coping, readiness for enhanced
Coping, readiness for enhanced community
Coping, readiness for enhanced family
Death syndrome, risk for sudden infant
Decision making, readiness for enhanced

Denial, ineffective
Dentition, impaired
Development, risk for delayed
Diarrhea
Dignity, risk for compromised human
Distress, moral
Disuse syndrome, risk for
Diversional activity, deficient
Energy field, disturbed
Environmental interpretation syndrome, impaired
Failure to thrive, adult
Falls, risk for
Family processes: alcoholism, dysfunctional
Family processes, interrupted
Family processes, readiness for enhanced
Fatigue
Fear
Fluid balance, readiness for enhanced
Fluid volume, deficient
Fluid volume, excess
Fluid volume, risk for deficient
Fluid volume, risk for imbalanced
Gas exchange, impaired
Glucose, risk for unstable blood
Grieving
Grieving, complicated
Grieving, risk for complicated
Growth and development, delayed
Growth, risk for disproportionate
Health maintenance, ineffective
Health-seeking behaviors
Home maintenance, impaired
Hope, readiness for enhanced
Hopelessness
Hyperthermia
Hypothermia
Identity, disturbed personal
Immunization status, readiness for enhanced
Incontinence, functional urinary
Incontinence, overflow urinary
Incontinence, reflex urinary
Incontinence, stress urinary
Incontinence, total urinary
Incontinence, urge urinary
Incontinence, risk for urge urinary

From NANDA International: *NANDA nursing diagnoses: definitions and classification 2007-2008,* Philadelphia, 2007, NANDA.

Continued

Box 2-1—cont'd

NANDA-Approved Nursing Diagnoses: 2007-2008

Infant behavior, disorganized
Infant behavior, risk for disorganized
Infant behavior, readiness for enhanced organized
Infant feeding pattern, ineffective
Infection, risk for
Injury, risk for
Injury, risk for perioperative positioning
Insomnia
Intracranial adaptive capacity, decreased
Knowledge, deficient
Knowledge, readiness for enhanced
Lifestyle, sedentary
Liver function, risk for impaired
Loneliness, risk for
Memory, impaired
Mobility, impaired bed
Mobility, impaired physical
Mobility, impaired wheelchair
Nausea
Neglect, unilateral
Noncompliance
Nutrition, imbalanced: less than body requirements
Nutrition, imbalanced: more than body requirements
Nutrition, readiness for enhanced
Nutrition, risk for imbalanced: more than body requirements
Oral mucous membrane, impaired
Pain, acute
Pain, chronic
Parenting, readiness for enhanced
Parenting, impaired
Parenting, risk for impaired
Peripheral neurovascular dysfunction, risk for
Poisoning, risk for
Post-trauma syndrome
Post-trauma syndrome, risk for
Power, readiness for enhanced
Powerlessness
Powerlessness, risk for
Protection, ineffective
Rape-trauma syndrome
Rape-trauma syndrome: compound reaction
Rape-trauma syndrome: silent reaction
Religiosity, impaired
Religiosity, readiness for enhanced
Religiosity, risk for impaired
Relocation stress syndrome
Relocation stress syndrome, risk for
Role performance, ineffective
Self-care, readiness for enhanced

Self-care deficit, bathing/hygiene
Self-care deficit, dressing/grooming
Self-care deficit, feeding
Self-care deficit, toileting
Self-concept, readiness for enhanced
Self-esteem, chronic low
Self-esteem, situational low
Self-esteem, risk for situational low
Self-mutilation
Self-mutilation, risk for
Sensory perception, disturbed
Sexual dysfunction
Sexuality pattern, ineffective
Skin integrity, impaired
Skin integrity, risk for impaired
Sleep deprivation
Sleep, readiness for enhanced
Social interaction, impaired
Social isolation
Sorrow, chronic
Spiritual distress
Spiritual distress, risk for
Spiritual well-being, readiness for enhanced
Stress overload
Suffocation, risk for
Suicide, risk for
Surgical recovery, delayed
Swallowing, impaired
Therapeutic regimen management, effective
Therapeutic regimen management, ineffective
Therapeutic regimen management, ineffective community
Therapeutic regimen management, ineffective family
Therapeutic regimen management, readiness for enhanced
Thermoregulation, ineffective
Thought processes, disturbed
Tissue integrity, impaired
Tissue perfusion, ineffective
Transfer ability, impaired
Trauma, risk for
Urinary elimination, impaired
Urinary elimination, readiness for enhanced
Urinary retention
Ventilation, impaired spontaneous
Ventilatory weaning response, dysfunctional
Violence, risk for other-directed
Violence, risk for self-directed
Walking, impaired
Wandering

Common nursing diagnoses related to drug therapy include the following:

• Cultural/language barrier or speech articulation problem leading to deficient knowledge about drug action, administration, and side effects
• Pain (acute or chronic) related to hesitancy in taking prescribed pain medications because of fear of addiction

• Ineffective health maintenance related to not having recommended preventive care
• Ineffective protection related to effects of anticoagulant medication on clotting mechanism
• Ineffective therapeutic regimen management
• Noncompliance related to forgetfulness
• Risk for injury related to side effects of drug (e.g., dizziness and drowsiness)

Wellness Nursing Diagnoses Grouped According to Functional Health Patterns

1. Health Perception–Health Management Pattern
   Health-Seeking Behaviors
   Effective Therapeutic Regimen Management
2. Nutritional–Metabolic Pattern
   Effective Breastfeeding
   Readiness for Enhanced Nutritional Metabolic Pattern
   Readiness Enhanced Skin Integrity
3. Elimination Pattern
   Readiness for Enhanced Bowel Elimination Pattern
   Readiness for Enhanced Urinary Elimination Pattern
4. Activity–Exercise Pattern
   Readiness for Enhanced Cardiac Output
   Readiness for Enhanced Diversional Activity Pattern
   Readiness for Enhanced Activity–Exercise Pattern
   Readiness for Enhanced Home Maintenance Management
   Readiness for Enhanced Self-Care Activities
   Readiness for Enhanced Tissue Perfusion
   Readiness for Enhanced Breathing Pattern
   Readiness for Enhanced Organized Infant Behavior
5. Sexuality–Reproductive Pattern
   Readiness for Enhanced Sexuality Patterns
6. **Sleep–Rest Pattern**
   Readiness for Enhanced Sleep
7. Sensory–Perceptual Pattern
   Readiness for Enhanced Comfort Level
8. Cognitive Pattern
   Readiness for Enhanced Cognition
9. Role–Relationship Pattern
   Readiness for Enhanced Relationships
   Readiness for Enhanced Parenting
   Readiness for Enhanced Role Performance
   Readiness for Enhanced Communication
   Readiness for Enhanced Social Interaction
   Readiness for Enhanced Caregiver Role
   Readiness for Enhanced Grieving
10. Self-Perception–Self-Concept Pattern
    Readiness for Enhanced Self-Perception
    Readiness for Enhanced Self-Concept
11. Coping–Stress Tolerance Pattern
    Readiness for Enhanced Individual Coping
    Readiness for Enhanced Family Coping
    Readiness for Enhanced Community Coping
12. Value–Belief Pattern
    Readiness for Enhanced Spiritual Well-Being

Modified from Weber JR: *Nurses' handbook of health assessment*, ed 5, Philadelphia, 2005, Lippincott Williams & Wilkins. All diagnoses are used with permission from North American Nursing Diagnosis Association.

- Ineffective therapeutic regimen management related to lack of finances or health care coverage to purchase medications
- Therapeutic regimen management, readiness for enhanced

The last nursing diagnosis listed above represents a wellness/health promotion diagnosis. Use of the nursing diagnosis is beneficial to the client because it facilitates the development of an individualized care plan. The abnormal data collected during the assessment serve as the defining characteristics (for actual problem) or risk factors (for high risk for problem) to support the appropriate nursing diagnosis for each client. **NOTE:** To strengthen comprehensiveness of nursing diagnoses, consider using well/health promotion diagnoses. Wellness nursing diagnoses are presented in Box 2–2.

Planning

The **planning** phase of the nursing process is characterized by **goal setting** or expected outcomes. Planning also includes development of nursing interventions that will be used to assist the client in meeting the outcome. Implementation occurs once the nursing interventions are actually put into action. Effective goal setting has the following qualities:

- Client-centered; clearly states the expected change
- Acceptable to both client and nurse (dependent on client's decision-making ability)
- Realistic and measurable
- Shared with other health care providers
- Realistic deadlines
- Identifies components for evaluation

Examples of a goal are (1) EC (the client) will independently administer prescribed dose of insulin by the end of the fourth session of instruction; (2) DZ (the client) will prepare a medication recording sheet that correctly reflects prescribed medication schedule within 3 days.

Implementation

The **implementation** phase includes the nursing actions/interventions necessary to accomplish the established goals or expected outcomes. Client education and teaching are key nursing responsibilities during this phase. In most practice settings, administration of drugs and assessment of drug effectiveness are also important nursing responsibilities. Refer to Chapter 3 for more information.

Client Teaching

Client education is an ongoing process. Teaching is more effective in an environment free of distractions, and the information should be tailored to the client's interests and level of understanding. Assessment data suggest the complexity, number, and length of teaching sessions that may be required. Be sensitive to the client's motivation to learn, attention span, and level of frustration. Readiness to learn is paramount. Readiness should be assessed first, before information is presented to the client. Use a positive approach; for example, "This narcotic is usually effective for the relief of the type of pain you have." Be an active listener and observer. The inclusion of a family member or friend in the teaching plan is an excellent idea. Assessment data guide the nurse to the appropriate persons to be included. This other person may (1) act as a psychologic support, (2) actually administer all or part of the drug therapy, (3) observe the effectiveness and side effects of drug therapy, and (4) implement other changes such as food shopping or instituting new methods of food preparation. Provide simple written materials appropriate for individual client needs. The client and family need to have the appropriate information (e.g., telephone number, email) to reach the health care provider for questions and concerns. Health care providers need to be available to provide timely responses.

Client teaching is a complex activity. As such, it might be helpful for the nurse to use an outline format. Suggested headings related to pharmacotherapeutics include the following:

- *General.* Instruct the client to take the drug as prescribed. Compliance is of utmost importance because discontinuing the drug before the course is completed may result in relapse or future ineffectiveness of the drug. Do not adjust dose, frequency, or time of day taken unless directed by the health care provider. Advise women contemplating pregnancy to check first with their health care provider before taking prescription or OTC medications and herbal products. Advise clients to consult with their health care provider about laboratory tests such as liver enzymes, blood urea nitrogen (BUN), creatinine, and electrolytes, which should be monitored when taking drugs such as antifungal agents.

- *Self-administration.* Instruct the client on the administration of the drug according to the prescribed route: eyedrops or nose drops, subcutaneous insulin injections, suppositories, swish-and-swallow suspensions, and metered-dose inhalers with and without spacers. Include demonstration and return demonstration in the instructions when appropriate, and give written instructions for the sighted client and audio instructions for the visually impaired. Instruct more than one person when possible, because this aids in reinforcement and retention of information. It also provides a "backup" if the client is unable to self-administer the drug.

- *Diet.* Instruct clients about what foods to include in their diet and what foods to avoid. For example, advise clients to eat foods rich in potassium (e.g., bananas) when taking most diuretics, unless they are on a potassium chloride (KCl) supplement, or to avoid large amounts of green, leafy vegetables if taking warfarin (Coumadin) preparations.

- *Side effects.* Instruct the client to report immediately to the designated health care provider—usually a nurse, physician, or pharmacist—if he or she experiences unusual symptoms. Also give the client instructions that help minimize any side effects (e.g., avoiding direct sunlight when there is risk of photosensitivity or sunburn). Inform the client of any expected changes in the color of urine or stool. Advise the client who has dizziness caused by orthostatic hypotension to rise slowly from a sitting to a standing position.

- *Cultural considerations.* Be **culturally sensitive**—an awareness of the implications of culture for this family and/or client. Be alert to client and family cultural expectations. For example, time may not be viewed as important;

therefore this may affect the client's adherence to taking medications at specific time intervals during the day to ensure therapeutic blood levels of the medication.

The nurse applies knowledge of cultural considerations to individualize a teaching plan. For example, respect for health care providers is a value among many Asian cultures, and the client will adopt communication behaviors that demonstrate that respect. This behavior includes not making eye contact, not asking questions, and not disagreeing with the nurse or physician. The client may nod in agreement when the nurse asks whether he or she understands what the nurse is teaching even if he or she does not understand. In this situation, it is better for the nurse to have the client do a return demonstration or repeat what he or she has learned.

NOTE: Refer to Chapter 6 for more information. Cultural content is found throughout the text and in the Nursing Process boxes sections within each chapter. Also see Box 2–3, Culturally Sensitive Health Teaching Tips.

A teaching plan with interventions that involve stimulation of several senses and active participation by the client enhances learning. Inclusion of return demonstrations by the client and others, when applicable, gives the nurse important feedback about the client's learning and gives the client confidence in carrying out the regimen or selected aspects of the regimen. Additional teaching tips include the following:

- Establish a trusting relationship.
- Incorporate interventions that involve stimulation of several senses.
- Actively involve the client.
- Provide written instructions in addition to other teaching aids.
- Use colorful charts and graphs.
- Consider using a variety of media, including compact discs and videos.
- Encourage questions from the client and family; provide time for this. Do not rush.
- Use materials and language appropriate to the client's level of understanding; access a computerized drug information system with client medication information sheets in different languages and appropriate reading levels.
- Space instruction over several sessions if appropriate.
- Review community resources related to the client's nursing diagnosis.
- Support multiagency collaboration in the mobilization of resources.
- Identify clients at risk for nonadherence with regimen. Alert health care provider and pharmacist so they can develop a plan to minimize the number of drugs and times administered.
- Evaluate client's understanding of medication regimen on a regular basis.
- Empower client to take responsibility for managing medications.

A client teaching session is shown in Figure 2–1. The use of teaching drug cards is helpful. These cards provide

Box 2-3

Culturally Sensitive Health Teaching Tips

- Flexibility in timing appointments may be necessary for those who have a circular sense of time, such as American Indian/Alaskan Natives and some Hispanic/Latino populations, rather than the dominant culture's linear sense of time.
- Make reminder calls for appointments, and encourage the client about the importance of timeliness.
- When language and cultural barriers exist, using videos and literature in the client's preferred language with pictures of that group may enhance compliance with health interventions.
- Decrease language barriers by decoding the jargon of the health care environment for those with language difficulties and for those who are not in the health care field.
- Failing to allow adequate time for information processing may result in an inaccurate response or no response. Allow time for people to respond to questions, especially for those who have language barriers. Speak clearly and slowly, giving time for translation. Obtain an interpreter if necessary.
- Although more traditional and older individuals in some cultures do not maintain eye contact, the acculturated and more educated usually do maintain eye contact. Do not assume that lack of eye contact means the client is not listening or does not care. It might indicate respect.
- Do not misunderstand loud voice volume as necessarily reflecting anger among some African Americans and Arabs, who may be merely expressing their thoughts in a dynamic manner.
- When translation is needed, discuss the ethnicity of the interpreter as well as the language desired. Provide an interpreter with the same ethnic background and gender if possible, especially with sensitive topics. Do not rely on family members, who may not fully disclose because of honor or shame.
- Speak slowly and clearly with exaggerated mouthing or use a loud voice volume, which changes the tone of words. Even though the client may appear to understand the fundamentals of the English language, provide an interpreter if in doubt.
- Do not give directions such as take one "blue" pill at a specified time. Instead, provide the name and dosage of the medication.

- Ask open-ended questions and have clients demonstrate, rather than verbalize, their understanding of treatments. Because politeness and saving face may prevail, do not assume that a positive response means a definite yes.
- Use simple and clear instructions. Ask family members to assist with translation only if an interpreter is not available. Do not use compound sentences.
- Do not take offense from a casual touch on the arm or shoulder or if clients stand closer than you are accustomed to. Do not assume that prolonged eye contact is a sign of anger.
- Health care workers should ask indirectly whether the Asian client understands instructions and should have the client or family member do a return demonstration of a procedure or repeat an instruction rather than question his or her comprehension. Speak clearly and slowly. Allow time to respond to questions, giving time for translating the dialect into English. Asking if the person understands may elicit a positive response because of cultural reluctance to say no.
- Many ethnocultural groups from countries outside the United States, and some people from within the United States as well, may be accustomed to not taking all their medications as ordered or to using medicines prescribed for other people. Emphasize that medications need to be taken as prescribed, medications are ordered specifically for each ailment, unused drugs should be discarded, and use of medications by individuals other than the intended may have serious consequences.
- When offering a prescription, instructions, or pamphlets to Asians and Pacific Islanders, use both hands to show respect.
- To establish trust among Hispanics/Latinos or Appalachians, it is necessary to demonstrate an interest in the client's family and other personal matters, to drop hints instead of giving orders, and to solicit the client's opinions and advice.
- Some individuals may respond better to verbal instructions and education with reinforcement from videos rather than printed communications.

Adapted from Purnell L, Paulanka B: A guide to culturally competent health care, Philadelphia, 2004, FA Davis.

information about a specific drug or drug group. They may be developed by the health care provider or obtained from drug manufacturers. Audiocassettes and videotapes are available from many drug companies. Group classes are useful for clients with certain diagnoses or who require certain drugs. A variety of formats can be developed. Be creative! Helpful components for the teaching drug cards include the following:

- Name of drug
- Reason for taking drug
- Dosage
- Specific times to take the drug
- What specific things should or should not be done while taking the medication; for example, tablets may or may not be crushed or may be taken with or without food

FIGURE 2-1 Client teaching session.

- Possible side effects of medication
- Possible adverse effects of medication; when to notify health care provider

General helpful and healthful points to remember and Top 10 Tips to making patient education successful are presented in Box 2–4 and Box 2–5 respectively.

Many people take multiple medications simultaneously several times each day, which presents a challenge to the client, his or her family, and the nurse. This complex activity of taking medications can be segmented into several simple tasks including the following:

- Preparation of 1 day's or 1 week's supply of medication. The day's medication can be put in one container. Sort-

ing of a day's supply allows the client and nurse to see at a glance what medications have and have not been taken. Keep in mind that a missing pill may have been dropped and not actually taken. A variation in accomplishing this task is to take a day's medication and sort or package the pills according to the time each is to be taken. Multicompartment dispensers (available at local drug or variety stores) or an egg carton may help some clients sort their drugs.

- A recording sheet may be helpful. The client or a family member marks when each medication is taken. The sheet is designed to meet the client's individual needs; for example, the time can be noted by the client or could be entered before hand, with the client marking when each dose is taken. A generic format follows:

Medication	Dosage (mg daily)	Day of Week						
		S	M	T	W	T	F	S
captopril (Capoten)	12.5							
digoxin	0.25							
furosemide (Lasix)	40							

- Figure 2–2 shows a nurse reviewing a medication record with her client. Alternatives to recording sheets are also available. Mechanical alarm reminder devices may be helpful to some clients.
- A combination of daily supply and recording may be helpful. Consider color coding. Visual acuity, manual dexterity, and mental processes have a major effect on which system works best for each client.

Throughout the teaching plan, the nurse promotes client independence. The nurse should not lose sight of the goals or outcomes and become immersed in the intervention process (e.g., teaching a client with short-term memory loss). Box 2–6 presents suggestions for a checklist for health teaching in drug therapy.

Box 2–4

Helpful and Healthful Points to Remember

- Take medication as prescribed by your health care provider. If you have questions, call.
- Keep medication in the original labeled container, and store as instructed.
- Keep all medicines out of reach of children. Remind grandparents and visitors to monitor their purses and luggage when visiting.
- Before using any over-the-counter (OTC) drugs, check with your health care provider. This includes use of aspirin, laxatives, and so on. Pharmacists are good resources to ask before buying or using a product.
- Bring all medications with you when you visit the health care provider.
- Know why you are taking each medication and under what circumstances to notify the health care provider.
- Alcohol may alter the action and absorption of the medication. Use of alcoholic beverages is discouraged around the time you take your medications and is absolutely contraindicated with certain medications.
- Smoking tobacco also alters the absorption of some medications (e.g., theophylline-type drugs, tranquilizers, antidepressants, and pain medications). Consult your health care provider or pharmacist for specific information.

Box 2–5

Top 10 Tips for Successful Teaching Sessions

1. Be focused
2. Assess the client
3. Listen to the client
4. Keep it simple
5. Know the client's motivation
6. Consider time constraints
7. Pick the appropriate strategy
8. Know your resources
9. Document your teaching
10. Trust yourself

From Weber JR: Nurse's handbook of health assessment, ed 5, Philadelphia, 2005, Lippincott Williams & Wilkins.

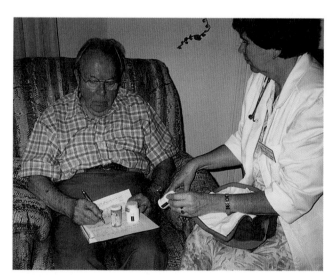

FIGURE 2–2 A client records his medications on a schedule sheet.

Evaluation

The effectiveness of health teaching about drug therapy and attainment of goals are addressed in the **evaluation** phase of the nursing process. The time at which the evaluation of a goal occurs is dependent on the time frame specified in the statement of a goal. Evaluation should be ongoing and related to progress as well as to attainment of the final goal.

If goals are not met, the nurse (in collaboration with the client when possible) needs to determine the reasons for this and revise the plan accordingly. This includes additional assessment data and the setting of new goals. If the goals are met, the plan of care has been completed.

To complete the care for any current client, follow these recommendations:

- Review with the client and family the need for follow-up care, if required.
- Encourage choices in ADLs.
- Refer the client to community resources as necessary.

Figure 2–3 shows a nurse meeting with a client and his spouse to review his therapeutic regimen.

Box 2–6

Checklist for Health Teaching in Drug Therapy

- Comprehensive drug and health history
- Reason for medication therapy
- Expected results
- Side effects and adverse reactions
- When to notify health care provider or pharmacist
- Drug-drug, drug-food, drug-laboratory, drug-environment interactions
- Required changes in activities of daily living (ADLs)
- Demonstration of learning; may take several forms, such as listening, discussing, or return demonstration of psychomotor skills (insulin administration)
- Medication schedule, associated with ADLs and drug level of action as appropriate
- Recording system
- Discussion and monitoring of access to financial resources, medication, and associated equipment
- Development and support of backup system
- Community resources

FIGURE 2–3 A nurse reviews the therapeutic regimen with a client and his spouse.

KEY WEBSITES

National Library of Medicine: _www.nlm.nih.gov_
Centers for Disease Control and Prevention: _www.cdc.gov_
Client Handouts in Spanish: _www.advancefornurses.com_ (click on "Spanish Patient Handouts" in the left bar under "Resources and Events")

Critical Thinking Case Study

MZ, a 66-year-old male, lives in a two-story home in the rural area of Vermont. He complains of shortness of breath, wheezing, and cough, primarily at night. MZ takes multiple asthma medications and one of them (albuterol) is administered via the nebulizer. He is 5 feet 11 inches tall and weighs 118 pounds. He admits to loss of appetite and reports, "I eat enough to keep going." What are the most relevant nursing diagnoses for this client?

NCLEX Study Questions

1. As the nurse, you know that you will find data for the basis of the care plan in which phase of the nursing process?
   a. assessment
   b. planning
   c. implementing
   d. evaluating

2. You record client teaching in which phase of the nursing process?
   a. assessment
   b. planning
   c. implementing
   d. evaluating

3. The most essential component of your teaching plan is:
   a. provide written instructions
   b. establish trust relationship
   c. use colorful charts
   d. review community resources

4. Common areas for health teaching include all the following except:
   a. importance of adherence to prescribed regimen
   b. how to administer the medication(s)
   c. what side/adverse effects to report to health care provider
   d. instructing client what foods must be eaten

5. The effectiveness of health teaching about the therapeutic regimen is documented in which phase of the nursing process?
   a. assessment
   b. planning
   c. implementing
   d. evaluating

Answers: 1, a; 2, c; 3, b; 4, d; 5, d.

3

Principles of Drug Administration

ELECTRONIC RESOURCES

Evolve website (http://evolve.elsevier.com/KeeHayes/pharmacology/):
- Case Studies
- Content Updates
- Frequently Asked Questions
- Student Review Activities
- WebLinks
- Additional Reference Material

Companion CD-ROM:
- NCLEX Examination Review Questions
- Pharmacology Animations
- IV Therapy Checklists
- Medication Error Checklists
- Drug Calculation Problems
- Electronic Calculators
- Top 200 Drugs with Pronunciations
- References from the Textbook

Outline

Objectives

- Describe the "five-plus-five rights" of drug administration.
- Discuss safety guidelines for drug administration.
- Describe factors that modify drug response.
- Differentiate routes of administration.
- Compare and contrast the various sites for parenteral therapy.
- Explain the equipment and technique used in parenteral therapy.
- Explain the method for charting medications.
- Describe the nursing interventions related to administration of medications by various routes.

Terms . . . .

. . . .

Administration of medications is a basic activity in nursing practice. As a result of the transition from hospitals and institutions to community-based services, an increasing number of nurses are practicing in a variety of settings. Nurses therefore must be knowledgeable about the specific drugs and their administration, client response, drug interactions, client allergies, and related resources. Safety and prevention of medication errors are highlighted.

Nurses are accountable for the safe administration of medications. Nurses must know all the components of a drug order and question those orders that are not complete, unclear, give a dosage outside the recommended range, or are contraindicated by client allergy or laboratory test results. Nurses are legally liable if they give a prescribed drug and the dosage is incorrect or the drug is contraindicated for the client's health status. In some health care settings, medical students write drug orders; these orders must be countersigned by an attending or staff physician or other prescribing health care provider before they are considered official. Once the drug has been administered, the nurse becomes liable for the predicted effects of that drug. Drug references (e.g., United States Pharmacopeia [USP], National Formulary [NF], Physicians' Desk Reference [PDR], and American Hospital Formulary drug reference handbook), human resources (e.g., pharmacists), and technology resources (Micromedix, Pyxis, Palm Pilot Epocrates) must be consulted when the nurse is unsure about the expected therapeutic effect, contraindications, dosage, potential side effects, or adverse reactions and interactions of a medication.

NOTE: Medication errors are the most frequent malpractice claims against hospitals and nurses, costing about $5000 per error. Greater than $3 million is awarded (on average) by the courts for serious errors. The cost of the client/family suffering is not calculable.

This chapter describes selected, essential content related to the administration of medications, a multifaceted activity. Selected content areas include the "rights" of drug administration, factors that modify drug response, guidelines for various routes of administration, and related nursing implications.

The "Five-Plus-Five Rights" of Drug Administration

The rights of medication administration are well known in health. Nurses' rights about safe medication administration may be less well known. The nurses' six rights include: Right to a complete and clear order; right to have the correct drug, route (form), and dose dispensed; right to have access to information; right to have policies to guide safe medication administration; right to administer medications safely and to identify system problems; and right to stop, think, and be vigilant when administering medications. Discussions of these rights can assist in increasing the safety of medication administration.

To provide safe drug administration, the nurse should practice the "rights" of drug administration. The traditional five rights are (1) the right client, (2) the right drug, (3) the right dose, (4) the right time, and (5) the right route. Experience indicates that five additional rights are essential to professional nursing practice: (1) the right assessment, (2) the right documentation, (3) the client's right to education, (4) the right evaluation, and (5) the client's right to refuse.

The **right client** determination is essential. The Joint Commission requires two forms of identification prior to the administration of the medication. Some clients answer to any name or are unable to respond, so client identification should be verified each time a medication is administered.

Nursing implications include the following:
- Verify client by checking the identification bracelet. Some facilities put the client's photo on his or her health record.
- Distinguish between two clients with the same last name; have warnings highlighted in a bright color on identification (ID) tools such as med cards, bracelet, or Kardex.
- Some institutions have ID bracelets coded for allergy status. Be aware of this policy.
- When clients do not wear ID bands (e.g., schools, occupational health departments, outpatient departments, health care provider offices), the nurse also has the responsibility of accurately identifying the individual when administering a medication.

The **right drug** means that the client receives the drug that was prescribed. Medication orders may be prescribed by a physician (MD), dentist (DDS), podiatrist (DPM), or licensed health care provider such as an advanced practice registered nurse (APRN) with authority from the state to order medications. Prescriptions may be written on a prescription pad and filled by a pharmacist at a drug store or hospital pharmacy (Figure 3–1). For institutionalized clients, the drug orders may be written on "order sheets" and signed by the duly authorized person (Figure 3–2). A telephone order (TO) or verbal order (VO) for medication must be cosigned by the prescribing health care provider within 24 hours. The nurse must comply with the institution's policy regarding a TO, which sometimes requires that two licensed practitioners listen to and sign the order.

The use of computerized order systems has added speed and a safety feature to the order process. Orders can be written from virtually any location and sent via modem. The computer will not process the order unless all the information is included. Also, there is no need to worry about illegible orders or signatures. The same benefits are available for nurses to record the medications given or refused. In general, the same information is documented in both written and computerized systems.

FIGURE 3–1   Example of prescription pad medication order.

FIGURE 3–2   Example of client's order form.

The components of a drug order are as follows:
- Date and time the order is written
- Drug name (generic preferred)
- Drug dosage
- Route of administration
- Frequency and duration of administration (e.g., × 7 days, × 3 doses)
- Any special instructions for withholding or adjusting dosage based on nursing assessment, drug effectiveness, or laboratory results
- Physician or other health care provider's signature or name if TO or VO
- Signatures of licensed practitioners taking TO or VO

Although the nurse's responsibility is to follow an appropriate order, if any one of the components is missing, the drug order is incomplete and the drug should not be administered. Clarification of the order must be done in a timely manner; the health care provider is usually contacted and the conversation content documented. The following is an example of a drug order and its interpretation:

6/4/08 10:10A Lasix 40 mg, PO, daily (signature). (Give 40 mg of Lasix by mouth daily.)

To avoid drug error, the drug label should be read three times: (1) at the time of contact with the drug bottle or container, (2) before pouring the drug, and (3) after pouring the drug. The first dose, one-time, and "as needed" (PRN) medication orders should be checked against original orders. Nurses should be aware that certain drug names sound alike and are spelled similarly. Examples are digoxin and digitoxin; quinidine and quinine; Keflex and Kantrex; Demerol and dicumarol; and Percocet and Percodan. More specifically, Percocet contains oxycodone and acetaminophen, whereas Percodan contains oxycodone and aspirin. A client may be allergic to aspirin, so it is important that this client receive Percocet. Read the labels carefully.

Nursing implications include the following:
- Check that the medication order is complete and legible. If the order is not complete or legible, notify the nurse manager and health care provider.
- Know the reason the client is to receive the medication.
- Check the drug label three times before administration of the medication.
- Know the date the medication was ordered and any ending date (e.g., for controlled substances and antibiotics and for limited or a specific number of doses). Some agencies have "automatic stop orders" which are generally facility specific. Examples of such orders include controlled drugs that need to be renewed every 48 hours, anticoagulants and antibiotics to be renewed after 7 days, and cancellation of all medications when the client goes to surgery.

The following are the four main categories of drug orders:
1. Standing
2. One-time (single)
3. PRN
4. STAT (at once)

Table 3–1 summarizes the drug order categories with examples of each.

The **right dose** is the dose prescribed for a particular client. In most cases, this dose is within the recommended range for the particular drug. Nurses must calculate each drug dose accurately, considering the variables: drug availability and the prescribed drug dose. The client's weight is an important consideration in multiple contexts such as pediatrics and many medical, surgical, and critical care situations. Refer to the section on drug calculations in Chapter 4.

Before calculating a drug dose, the nurse should have a general idea of the answer based on knowledge of the basic formula or ratios and proportions. Calculation of drug doses should be rechecked if a fraction of a dose or an extremely large dose has been calculated. Consultation with a peer or a pharmacist should occur whenever doubt exists.

The stock drug method and unit dose method are the two most frequently used methods of drug distribution.

Table 3–2 describes these methods and the advantages and disadvantages of each.

In the traditional **stock drug method**, the drugs are dispensed to all clients from the same containers. In the **unit dose method**, drugs are individually wrapped and labeled for single doses. The unit dose method is popular in many institutions and community settings. Unit dosing has eliminated many drug dosage errors.

Automation of medication administration, introduced more than a decade ago, is promoted as saving time and decreasing costs associated with the administration of medications. Some features include a link to the pharmacy information system and current clinical client data. In addition, the ability to automatically collect information about charting and recording of medication is available. An activity report menu is a popular feature. Flexible dose modes are available, including single dose, multidose, and multiple medications. Pyxis is an example of automated medication-dispensing technology (Figure 3–3). It assists the nurse in correctly and quickly administering medications. This

Table 3–1

Categories of Drug Orders

Category	Description	Examples
Standing orders	May be an ongoing order or may be given for a specific number of doses or days	Digoxin 0.25 mg PO daily
		Colace 100 mg PO daily PRN
	May have special instructions to base administration on laboratory values	Digoxin, maintain blood level of 0.5-2 ng/ml
	May include PRN orders	
One-time or single orders	Given once and usually at a specific time	Versed 2 mg IM at 7 AM on 10/5/05
PRN orders	Given at the client's request and nurse's judgment concerning need and safety	Tylenol 650 mg q3 to 4h PRN for headache
STAT orders	Given once, immediately	Morphine sulfate 2 mg IV STAT

IM, Intramuscular; *IV*, intravenous; *PO*, by mouth; *PRN*, as needed; *STAT*, immediately.

Table 3–2

Drug Distribution Methods

Stock Method	Unit Dose Method
Description	
Drugs are stored on unit and dispensed to all clients from the same container	Drugs are packaged in doses for 24 h by the pharmacy
Advantages	
Always available	Saves time for nurse; no dose calculation required
Cost-efficiency of large quantities	Billed for specific doses
	More accountability
	Less chance for contamination and error
Disadvantages	
Drug errors are more prevalent with multiple "pourers"	Potential delay in receiving drug
More risk of abuse by health care workers	Not immediately replaceable if contaminated
Less accountability for amount used; unable to track usage	More expensive
Increased opportunity for contamination (multiple pourers challenge aseptic/sterile status)	

FIGURE 3–3 Computerized medication management system. (Courtesy Pyxis Corp., San Diego, California)

FIGURE 3–4 Military time.

technology has the potential to improve client care by promoting accurate and quick access to medications.

The nursing implications include the following:

- Calculate the drug dose correctly. When in doubt, the drug dose should be recalculated and checked by another nurse. In many settings, the first nurse to administer the particular drug to the client must calculate the dose according to the stated formulary doses and sign in the nurse's signature space once the safety parameter has been established. In some settings, two registered nurses (RNs) are required to check dosage for specific medications such as insulin and heparin.
- Check the PDR, American Hospital Formulary, drug package insert, or other drug references for recommended range of specific drug doses

The **right time** is the time at which the prescribed dose should be administered. Daily drug dosages are given at specified times during a day, such as twice a day (b.i.d.), three times a day (t.i.d.), four times a day (q.i.d.), or every 6 hours (q6h), so that the plasma level of the drug is maintained. When the drug has a long half-life ($t^{1}/_2$), the drug is given once a day. Drugs with a short half-life are given several times a day at specified intervals. (This topic is covered in Chapter 1.) Some drugs are given before meals, and others are given with meals or with food.

Many nursing settings currently use military time (a 24-hour clock). For example, 2 AM is 0200, 2 PM is 1400, 6:10 AM is 0610, and 5:30 PM is 1730. AM hours correlate with the traditional clock; 12 hours are added for the PM hours (Figure 3–4). Military time has the advantage of reducing administration errors and decreasing documentation.

Nursing implications include the following:

- Administer drugs at the specified times. Drugs may be given 0.5 hour before or after the time prescribed if the

administration interval is >2 hours. Refer to agency policy.
- Administer drugs that are affected by foods (e.g., tetracycline) before meals.
- Administer drugs that can irritate the stomach (gastric mucosa), for example, potassium and aspirin, with food.
- The drug administration schedule may sometimes be adjusted to fit the schedule of the client's lifestyle, activities, tolerances, or preferences.
- It is the nurse's responsibility to check whether the client is scheduled for any diagnostic procedures such as endoscopy or fasting blood tests that would contraindicate the administration of medications. Determine per policy whether the medication should be given after the test is completed.
- Check the expiration date. Discard the medication or return it to the pharmacy (depending on policy) if the date has passed.
- Antibiotics should be administered at even intervals (e.g., q8h rather than t.i.d.) throughout a 24-hour period so therapeutic blood levels are maintained.

The **right route** is necessary for adequate or appropriate absorption. The more common routes of absorption include oral (by mouth): liquid, elixir, suspension, pill, tablet, or capsule; **sublingual** (under tongue for venous absorption); **buccal** (between gum and cheek); via feeding tube; topical (applied to the skin); **inhalation** (aerosol sprays); instillation (in nose, eye, ear); **suppository** (rectal, vaginal); and four **parenteral** routes: intradermal, subcutaneous (subQ), intramuscular (IM), and intravenous (IV).

Nursing implications include the following:

- Assess the client's ability to swallow before the administration of oral medications.
- Do not crush or mix medications in other substances before consultation with a pharmacist. Do not mix medications with sweet substance to "trick" children into taking medications. Do not mix medications in an infant's formula feeding.

- Use aseptic technique when administering drugs. Sterile technique is required with the parenteral routes.
- Administer the drugs at the appropriate sites.
- Stay with the client until oral drugs have been swallowed.
- If it is necessary to combine medication with another substance, explain this to the client.

The **right assessment** requires that appropriate data be collected before administration of the drug. Examples of assessment data may include measuring the apical heart rate before the administration of digitalis preparations or serum blood sugar levels before the administration of insulin.

The **right documentation** requires that the nurse immediately record the appropriate information about the drug administered. This includes (1) the name of the drug, (2) the dose, (3) the route (injection site if applicable), (4) the time and date, and (5) the nurse's initials or signature. Documentation of the client's response to the medication is required with a variety of medications: (1) narcotics (How effective was the pain relief?), (2) nonnarcotic analgesics, (3) sedatives, (4) antiemetics, and (5) unexpected reactions to the medication, such as gastrointestinal (GI) irritation or signs of skin sensitivity. A delay in charting could result in forgetting to chart the medication or in another nurse's administration of the drug because it was assumed the drug was not given. It is never appropriate to sign medications off prior to administration.

To assist in the accurate and timely recording of drugs administered, many health care facilities use a graphic format or computerized systems (Figure 3–5).

The **right to education** requires that clients receive accurate and thorough information about the medication and how it relates to their particular situation. Client teaching also includes therapeutic purpose, possible side effects of the drug, any dietary restrictions or requirements, skill of administration, and laboratory monitoring. This right is a principle of **informed consent**, which is based on the individual having the knowledge necessary to make a decision. An informed client/family is critical to preventing medication errors.

The **right evaluation** requires that the effectiveness of the medication be determined by the client's response to the medication. Evaluation in this context asks, "Did the medication do for the client what it was supposed to do?" It is also appropriate to determine the extent of side effects and adverse reactions, if any.

The client has the **right to refuse** the medication. Clients can and do refuse to take a medication. It is the nurse's responsibility to determine, when possible, the reason for the refusal and to take reasonable measures to facilitate the client's taking the medication. Explain to the client the risk of refusing to take the medication, and reinforce the reason for the medication. When a medication is refused, this refusal must be documented immediately. The nurse manager, primary nurse, or health care provider should be informed when the omission may pose a specific threat to the client, such as with insulin. Follow-up is also required when a

A

B

FIGURE 3–5 Medication record. A, Computerized. B, Written format.

change is expected in the laboratory test values, such as with insulin and warfarin (Coumadin).

All medication errors are serious or potentially serious. A medication error may involve one or more of the following: administration of the wrong medication or IV fluid; the incorrect dose or rate; administration to the wrong client, by the incorrect route, at the incorrect schedule interval; administration of a known allergenic drug or IV fluid; omission of a dose or discontinuation of medication or IV fluid that was not discontinued.

The Institute of Medicine (IOM) report of 1999, *To Err is Human: Building A Safer Health Care System*, spurred work on identifying system changes to decrease errors. More than 100,000 medication errors were reported by hospitals nationwide in 2001. A medication error may be defined as "any preventable event that may cause or lead to inappropriate medication use or harm to a patient." Medication errors may occur throughout the cycle; one national report included 39% related to ordering, 12% transcribing, 11% preparing, and 38% administering.

A major factor affecting medication errors is the increase in the number of drugs: from 3000 in 1990 to more than

30,000 in 2008. Other contributing causes include violation of "10 rights"; lack of drug knowledge; memory lapses; transcription, dispensing, or delivery problems; inadequate monitoring; distractions; staff being overworked; lack of standardization; confusing packaging prescription; equipment failures; inadequate client history; and poor interdepartmental communication.

In response to the escalating number of medication errors causing human deaths and costing billions of dollars, in 2002 the Food and Drug Administration (FDA) proposed a rule titled *Bar Code Label Requirements for Human Drug Products and Blood* which has increased the prominence of this coding. At a minimum the bar code would contain the drug's national drug code that "uniquely identifies the drug, its strength, and its dosage form." A revision to this rule eliminates blood and blood products that have had bar codes since 1985. Once the rule is published in the Federal Registry, companies have 3 years to comply. The FDA reports that in hospitals with bar coding, a 71% to 86% decrease in the rate of medication errors has resulted. Most staff embraces bar coding once they are proficient with its use. They note, however, that bar coding is a tool but not a substitute for critical thinking.

Computerized prescriber order entry (CPOE) systems interact with laboratory, pharmacy, and client data. This integrated system of client data is the basis for the success of bar coding. The FDA posits that the bar coding rule will have hospitals act on investing in the required technologies. With bar coding, the client's medication administration record (MAR), a part of the database that is encoded in the client's wristband, is accessible to the nurse using a handheld device. After scanning the client's wristband, the nurse would see the individual's MAR on the device. To administer a medication, nurses would first scan the drug's bar code, then the number of the client's medical record, and finally their own ID badge code. The client's MAR would then be updated accordingly. Figure 3–6 shows a nurse scanning a client's wristband. The nurse receives verification on the handheld device of "5 rights," warnings, and clinical alerts (e.g., drug is discontinued or not ordered for client). As part of their 2004 National Patient Safety Goals, The Joint Commission on Accreditation of Healthcare Or-

ganizations (currently The Joint Commission [TJC]) announced that all accredited organizations may no longer use the following abbreviations, acronyms, and symbols:
- U, u (for unit)
- IU (for International Unit)
- QD, Q.D., qd, q.d. (for every day)
- QOD, Q.O.D., qod, q.o.d. (for every other day)
- Trailing zero and lack of leading zero; never write a zero by itself after a decimal point (e.g., 5.0 mg), and always use a zero before a decimal point (e.g., 0.5 mg).
- MS, MSO_4, MgSO4

Please see Table 3–3 for a comprehensive list of accepted abbreviations. Visit The Joint Commission website at *www.jointcommission.org* and the Institute for Safe Medication Practices at *www.ismp.org* for detailed safety information.

An additional safety feature is the "black box" warning, the FDA's strongest labeling requirement, warning health care providers of risks associated with certain drugs. A recent study reported frequent failure to comply with laboratory monitoring.

2007 National Patient Safety Goals

Six of the eight goals relate to medication safety:
1. *Improve the accuracy of patient identification.*
   - Use at least 2 patient identifiers when providing care, treatment, or services.
2. *Improve the effectiveness of communication among caregivers.*
   - For verbal or telephone orders or for telephonic reporting of critical care test results, verify the complete order or test result by having the person receiving the information record and "reread back" the complete order or test result.
   - Standardize a list of abbreviations, acronyms, symbols, and dose designations that are not to be used throughout the organization.
   - Implement a standardized approach to "hand off" communications, including an opportunity to ask and respond to questions.
3. *Improve the safety of using medications.*
   - Standardize and limit the number of drug concentrations used in the organization.
   - Identify and, at a minimum, annually review a list of look-alike/sound-alike drugs used in the organization, and take action to prevent errors involving the interchange of these drugs.
   - Label all medications, medication containers (for example, syringes, medicine cups, basins), or other solutions on and off the sterile fields.
4. *Accurately and completely reconcile medications across the continuum of care.*
   - There is a process for comparing the patient's current medications with those ordered for the patient while under the care of the organization.
   - A complete list of the patient's medications is communicated to the next provider of service when a pa-

FIGURE 3–6 Bar code reader used to scan the client's wristband. (From Kee JL, Marshall SM: Clinical calculations: with applications to general and specialty areas, ed 6, St. Louis, 2009, Saunders.)

Table 3-3

Abbreviations

In 2005, The Joint Commission (TJC) (formerly known as the Joint Commission on Accreditation of Healthcare Organization [JCAHO]) issued a new list of abbreviations that should not be used but written out to avoid misinterpretation. Below is the "Do Not Use" abbreviation list, followed by a list of abbreviations that could possibly be included in future "Do Not Use" lists.

Abbreviation	Preferred
q.d., Q.D.	Write "daily" or "every day."
q.o.d., Q.O.D.	Write "every other day."
U	Write "unit."
IU	Write "International Unit."
MS, MSO4	Write "morphine sulfate."
MgSO4	Write "magnesium sulfate."
.5 mg	Use zero before a decimal point when the dose is less than a whole (write 0.X mg).
1.0 mg	Do not use a decimal point or zero after a whole number (write X mg).

The following abbreviations could possibly be included in future Joint Commission "Do Not Use" lists.

Abbreviation	Preferred
c.c.	Use "ml" (milliliter).
μg	Use "mcg."
>	Write "greater than."
<	Write "less than."
Drug name abbreviations	Write out the full name of the drug.
Apothecary units	Use metric units instead.
@	Write "at."

Lists of acceptable abbreviations follow the TJC lists in three categories: drug measurements and drug forms, routes of drug administration, and times of administration. Selected abbreviations are listed here. These are frequently used in drug therapy and must be known by the nurse.

Drug Measurements and Drug Forms

Abbreviation	Meaning
cap	capsule
dr	dram
elix	elixir
g, gm, G, GM	gram
gr	grain
gtt	drops
kg	kilogram
l, L	liter
m2	square meter
mcg	microgram
mEq	milliequivalent
mg	milligram
mL, ml	milliliter
m, min	minim
oz	ounce
pt	pint
qt	quart
SR	sustained release
ss., s̄s̄	one half
supp	suppository
susp	suspension
T.O.	telephone order
T, tbsp	tablespoon
t, tsp	teaspoon
V.O.	verbal order

Routes of Drug Administration

Abbreviation	Meaning
A.D., ad	right ear
A.S., as	left ear
A.U., au	both ears
ID	intradermal
IM	intramuscular
IV	intravenous
IVPB	intravenous piggyback
KVO	keep vein open
L	left
NGT	nasogastric tube
O.D., od	right eye
O.S., os	left eye
O.U., ou	both eyes
PO, po, os	by mouth
®	right
SC, subc, sc, SQ, subQ	subcutaneous
SL, sl, subl	sublingual
TKO	to keep open
Vag	vaginal

Times of Administration

Abbreviation	Meaning
AC, ac	before meals
ad lib	as desired
B.i.d., b.i.d.	twice a day
c̄	with
hs	hour of sleep
NPO	nothing by mouth
PC, pc	after meals
PRN, p.r.n.	whenever necessary, as needed
q	every
qAM	every morning
qh	every hour
q2h	every 2 hours
q4h	every 4 hours
q6h	every 6 hours
q8h	every 8 hours
s̄	without
SOS	once if necessary: if there is a need
Stat	immediately
T.i.d., t.i.d.	three times a day

Please refer to The Joint Commission website at *www.jointcommission.org* and Institute for Safe Medication practices at *www.ismp.org* for more detailed safety information.

tient is referred or transferred to another setting, service, practitioner, or level of care within or outside the organization. The complete list of medications is also provided to the patient on discharge from the facility.

5. *Encourage the patient's active involvement in their own care as a patient safety strategy.*
   - Define and communicate the means for patients and their families to report concerns about safety and encourage them to do so.

6. *The organization identifies safety risks inherent in the patient population.*

   Refer to the full text of the 2007 goals and requirements at *www.jointcommission.org.*

Disposal of Medications

Do not throw medications "down the toilet" where they will pollute the environment and may be a danger to others and animals. It is recommended that you add kitty liter to the drugs and put in a sealed bag.

Watch for Preventing Medication Errors boxes throughout the text.

The nurse must be ever vigilant about safety in medication administration. Actions to create a culture of safety include:

- Use drug references and visit *www.ismp.org* regularly.
- Contact the health care provider; do not guess about the order. Document clarification.
- Double-check all calculated doses.
- Use leading zero (0.5); do not use trailing zero (5.0).
- Avoid verbal orders; if you must take them, repeat out loud to confirm.
- Scan bar code at the point-of-care.
- Include the pharmacist on client rounds.
- Use a computerized prescriber order entry (CPOE).
- Avoid dangerous abbreviations (e.g., HCT: hydrocortisone or hydrochlorothiazide?).
- Consistently think critically.

Additional Safety Risks for Safe Medicine Administration

It is estimated that for every 100 medication administrations there are 5 medication errors. Several reports indicate the majority of medication errors occur during administration of the drug (41%), followed by documenting (21%), dispensing (17%), prescribing (11%), monitoring (1%), and other (10%).

Additional risks to safety include:

- Pill splitting. In an effort to counteract the steeply rising drug costs, some clients are cutting their pills in half. In the Half Tablet Program, with physician approval, copays are cut in half. However splits can be unsafe and dangerous. A small dose change (from uneven splitting) can cause a big effect on the client. Client attributes such as diminished vision, cognitive problems, and hand coordination problems can all contribute to the risk.
- Buying drugs on the internet. The FDA reports that consumers wanted sleep aids and actually received powerful antipsychotics that caused them to seek treatment at the emergency room.
- Counterfeit drugs (copies or fake medicines) look like the regular drug but may have no active ingredient, the wrong active ingredient, or the wrong amount of active ingredient. Improper packaging or contamination can also be problems. Counterfeit drugs may look remarkably like the real drug!

To reduce your risk of exposure to counterfeit drugs:

1. Purchase drugs only from licensed pharmacies. Refer to National Association of Boards of Pharmacy at *www. nabp.net* for information. The NABP reviews internet pharmacies also. After site review, the NABP grants the Verified Internet Pharmacy Practice Sites Accreditation Program (VIPPS) seal.

2. When refilling a prescription always check the color, texture, shape, and taste of the drug. Check with the pharmacist if you notice any changes.

3. Legislation is in process to promote safe handling of drugs after they leave the authorized wholesaler by introducing "pedigree" requirements at federal and state levels.

Several resources address medication errors and their prevention; two of these resources follow. A current database of medication errors and "near misses" will assist all health care personnel to identify, implement, and evaluate strategies to prevent medication errors. It is strongly suggested that one report list errors or "near misses" to the FDA at (800) 23-ERROR. (The report will be held confidential.) The National Coordinating Council for Medication Error Reporting and Prevention (NCCMERP) specializes in medication errors from an interdisciplinary perspective; contact them at (800) 822-8772.

Medication Self-Administration

Self-administration (SAM) of medication is a common practice in the home and in many community-based settings such as the workplace. However, SAM is relatively new to clients and staff in institutional settings. In practical terms, SAM means that the nurse gives the client a packet of appropriate medications and instructions that are kept at the bedside and go home with the client on discharge. Clients are responsible for taking their medication according to instructions when they feel they need it. The client has a key role in his or her care and exercises control associated with taking selected medications. SAM helps clients to manage medications during the hospital stay and prepares them to keep as comfortable as possible at home. For example, see Chapter 52, Female Reproductive Cycle I: Pregnancy and Preterm Labor Drugs, and Chapter 53, Female Reproductive Cycle II: Labor, Delivery, and Preterm Neonatal Drugs, for a detailed description of SAM for the maternity client.

Special Considerations: Factors That Modify Drug Response

The pharmacologic response to a drug is complex. Nurses must be mindful of the number and variety of factors that influence an individual's response to a drug. Examples of factors that modify drug responses include the following:

- *Absorption.* A major variable in absorption is the route of administration of the drug. Oral absorption takes place as drug particles move from the GI tract (stomach and small intestine) to body fluids. Any GI disturbances (e.g., vomiting or diarrhea) affect drug absorption.
- *Distribution.* Protein binding is a major modifier of drug distribution in the body. Propranolol (Inderal) is 90% protein-bound. Another factor is the blood-brain barrier, which allows only lipid-soluble drugs (e.g., general anesthetics, barbiturates) to enter into the brain and cerebrospinal fluid. Compounds that are strongly ionized and poorly soluble in fat are barred from entry into the brain. Neoplastic agents are examples of drugs that do not cross the blood-brain barrier. The placental barrier is a membrane that, for the most part, keeps the blood of the mother and fetus separate. However, both lipid-soluble and lipid-insoluble drugs can diffuse across the placenta. Some drugs have teratogenic effects if taken during the first trimester of pregnancy; that is, they may induce aberrant development of fetal organs or body systems. This is especially true if the drugs are taken during the fourth through eighth weeks of gestation.
- *Metabolism (biotransformation).* The liver is the primary organ for drug metabolism. All infants, especially neonates and low-birth-weight infants, have immature liver and kidney function. Influences on liver function such as the aging process and chronic liver disease also affect the metabolism of a medication.
  - *Excretion.* The main route of drug excretion is via the kidney. Through the normal aging process and chronic disease or kidney failure, there is a decrease in the functioning cells of the kidney, resulting in decreased excretion of drugs. Bile, feces, respiration, saliva, and sweat are also routes of drug excretion.
  - *Age.* Infants and the elderly are more sensitive to drugs. The elderly are hypersensitive to barbiturates and central nervous system (CNS) depressants. Such clients have poor absorption through the GI tract because of decreased gastric secretion. Infant doses are calculated based on weight in kilograms rather than on biologic or gestational age.
  - *Body weight.* Drug doses (e.g., of antineoplastics) may be ordered according to body weight. Obese persons may need increased drug doses, and very thin persons may need decreased doses.
- *Toxicity.* This term refers to the first adverse symptoms that occur at a particular dose. Toxicity is more prevalent in persons with liver or renal impairment and in the very young and old.

- *Pharmacogenetics.* This term refers to the influence of genetic factors on drug response. If a parent has an adverse reaction to a drug, the child may also. Some genetic factors are associated with ethnicity.
  - *Route of administration.* Drugs administered by IV act more rapidly than those administered by mouth.
  - *Time of administration.* The presence or absence of food in the stomach can affect the action of some drugs.
  - *Emotional factors.* Suggestive comments about the drug and its side effects may influence its effects.
  - *Preexisting disease state.* Liver, kidney, heart, circulatory, and GI disorders are examples of preexisting states that can affect a response to a drug. For example, persons with diabetes should not be given elixirs or syrups that contain sugar.
  - *Drug history.* Be aware that past use of the same or different drugs may reduce or intensify the effects of the drug.
- *Tolerance.* The ability of a client to respond to a particular dose of a certain drug may diminish after days or weeks of repeated administration. A combination of drugs may be given to decrease or delay the development of tolerance for a specific drug.
- *Cumulative effect.* This occurs when the drug is metabolized or excreted more slowly than the rate at which it is being administered.
  - *Drug-drug interaction.* The effects of a combination of drugs may be greater than, equal to, or less than the effects of a single drug. Some drugs may compete for the same receptor sites. An adverse reaction may lead to toxicity or complications such as anaphylaxis.
  - *Food-drug interaction.* The effects of selected foods may speed, delay, or prevent absorption of specific drugs.

Discussions of factors that modify drug response may also be found in Chapters 1, 7, 10, and 11.

Guidelines for Drug Administration

General guidelines for drug administration are listed in Boxes 3–1 and 3–2. These guidelines are summarized as the *do's* and *don'ts* of drug administration. Nurses should follow these guidelines to enhance safety when administering medications. Application of the nursing process to medication administration is presented later in this chapter.

Forms and Routes for Drug Administration

A variety of forms and routes are used for the administration of medications, including sublingual, buccal, oral (tablets, capsules, liquids, suspensions, elixirs), transdermal, topical, instillation (drops and sprays), inhalations, nasogastric and gastrostomy tubes, suppositories, and parenteral (Figure 3–7). A brief description of each follows.

Box 3–1

Guidelines for Correct Administration of Medications

Preparation

1. Wash hands before preparing medications.
2. Check for drug allergies; check the assessment history and Kardex.
3. Check medication order with health care provider's orders, Kardex, medicine sheet, and medicine card.
4. Check label on drug container three times.
5. Check expiration date on drug label, card, Kardex; use only if date is current.
6. Recheck drug calculation of drug dose with another nurse as needed or by policy.
7. Verify doses of drugs that are potentially toxic with another nurse or pharmacist.
8. Pour tablet or capsule into the cap of the drug container. With unit dose, open packet at bedside after verifying client identification.
9. Pour liquid at eye level. Meniscus, the lower curve of the liquid, should be at the line of desired dose (see Figure 3–8).
10. Dilute drugs that irritate gastric mucosa (e.g., potassium, aspirin) or give with meals.

Administration

11. Administer only drugs that you have prepared. Do not prepare medications to be administered by another.
12. Identify the client by ID band or ID photo.
13. Offer ice chips to numb taste buds when giving bad tasting drugs.
14. When possible, give bad-tasting medications first, followed by pleasant-tasting liquids.
15. Assist the client to an appropriate position, depending on the route of administration.
16. Provide only liquids allowed on the diet.
17. Stay with the client until the medications are taken.
18. Administer no more than 2.5 to 3 ml of solution intramuscularly at one site. Infants receive no more than 1 ml of solution intramuscularly at one site and no more than 1 ml subcutaneously. Never recap needles (universal precautions).

19. When administering drugs to a group of clients, give drugs last to clients who need extra assistance.
20. Discard needles and syringes in appropriate containers.
21. Drug disposal is dependent on agency policy and state law. For example, discard drugs in the sink or toilet, not in the trash can. Controlled substances must be returned to the pharmacy. Some disposals need signatures of witnesses.
22. Discard unused solutions from ampules.
23. Appropriately store (some require refrigeration) unused stable solutions from open vials.
24. Write date and time opened and your initials on label.
25. Keep narcotics in a double-locked drawer or closet. Medication carts must be locked at all times when a nurse is not in attendance.
26. Keys to the narcotics drawer must be kept by the nurse and not stored in a drawer or closet.
27. Keep narcotics in a safe place, out of reach of children and others in the home.
28. Avoid contamination of one's own skin or inhalation to minimize chances of allergy or sensitivity development.

Recording

29. Report drug error immediately to client's health care provider and to the nurse manager.
30. Complete an incident report.
31. Charting: record drug given, dose, time, route, and your initials.
32. Record drugs promptly after given, especially STAT doses.
33. Record effectiveness and results of medication administered, especially PRN medications.
34. Report to health care provider and record drugs that were refused with reason for refusal.
35. Record amount of fluid taken with medications on input and output chart.

ID, Identification; *PRN*, as needed; *STAT*, immediately.

Tablets and Capsules

- Oral medications are not given to clients who are vomiting, lack a gag reflex, or who are comatose. Clients who gag may need a brief rest before proceeding with further intake of medications.
- Do not mix with a large amount of food or beverage or with contraindicated food. Clients may not be able to eat all the food and will not get the full dose of medication. Do not mix in infant formula.
- Enteric-coated and timed-release capsules must be swallowed whole to be effective.
- Administer irritating drugs with food to decrease GI discomfort.

- Administer drugs on an empty stomach if food interferes with medication absorption.
- Drugs given sublingually (placed under tongue) or buccally (placed between cheek and gum) remain in place until fully absorbed. No food or fluids should be taken while the medication is in place.
- Encourage the use of child-resistant caps. The Consumer Public Safety Commission has ordered a redesign of these caps because the current caps are difficult for elderly clients to use. This has contributed to a safety hazard for children and others because many people, in an effort to have easy access to their medications, leave the caps off. The new design requires a person to lightly

squeeze the two side bottle tabs and turn the cap. Non–child-resistant caps are available on request.

Liquids

- There are several forms of liquid medication, including elixirs (sweetened, hydroalcoholic liquid used in preparation of oral liquid medications), emulsions (mixture of two liquids that are not mutually soluble), and suspensions (particles are mixed with but not dissolved in another fluid.
- Read the labels to determine whether dilution or shaking is required.
- The **meniscus** is at the line of desired dose (Figure 3–8).
- Many liquids require refrigeration once reconstituted.

Transdermal

- **Transdermal** medication is stored in a patch placed on the skin and absorbed through skin, thereby having systemic effect. Widespread use of such patches began in the 1980s. Patches for cardiovascular drugs, neoplastic drugs, hormones, drugs to treat allergic reactions, and insulin are in production or being developed. Transdermal drugs provide more consistent blood levels than oral and injection forms and avoid GI absorption problems associated with oral products. Transdermal patches should be rotated to different sites and not reapplied over the exact same area when changed. Additionally, the area should be thoroughly cleaned prior to administration of a new transdermal patch. This practice will prevent errors in overdosing the client (Figure 3–9).
- A common question is whether to cut the patches in half. A nurse might suggest the purchase of patches with a lower dosage rather than cutting the patch and guessing the dose the client will receive. However, depending on the client's situation and the type of patch, it may be appropriate to cut the patch. If the drug is embedded in a matrix patch and diffuses into the skin (e.g., Climara, Vivelle, Nicotrol, Nitro-Dur, and Testoderm), the drug is spread over the entire surface of the patch and probably may be cut. Clients must be alert for underdosing or overdosing. The drug is pooled in a reservoir patch and is released via a semipermeable membrane (e.g., Catapres-TTS, Duragesic, Estraderm, Transderm Scōp, Transderm-Nitro, Androderm). These patches should not be cut because too much drug may be released.

Box 3–2

Behaviors to Avoid During Medication Administration

- Do not be distracted when preparing medications.
- Do not give drugs poured by others.
- Do not pour drugs from containers with labels that are difficult to read or whose labels are partially removed or have fallen off.
- Do not transfer drugs from one container to another.
- Do not pour drugs into the hand.
- Do not give medications for which the expiration date has passed.
- Do not guess about drugs and drug doses. Ask when in doubt.
- Do not use drugs that have sediment, are discolored, or are cloudy (and should not be).
- Do not leave medications by the bedside or with visitors.
- Do not leave prepared medications out of sight.
- Do not give drugs if the client says he or she has allergies to the drug or drug group.
- Do not call the client's name as the sole means of identification.
- Do not give drug if the client states the drug is different from the drug he or she has been receiving. Check the order.
- Do not recap needles. Use universal precautions.
- Do not mix with large amount of food or beverage or foods that are contraindicated.

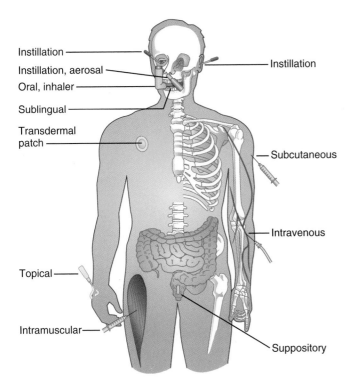

FIGURE 3–7 Some routes for medication administration.

FIGURE 3–8 To read the meniscus, locate the lowest fluid mark.

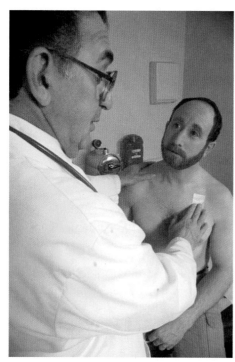

FIGURE 3–9 Example of a transdermal patch. © 2007 JupiterImages Corporation.

However, it is possible to peel back the protective layer halfway. Advise clients to secure the patch with tape, being careful not to apply it too tightly, which could alter the drug delivery. For legal and financial reasons, manufacturers do not recommend cutting the patches. To avoid skin burns remember to remove temporarily a patch with any metallic component before magnetic resonance imaging (MRI) is performed. Many patches have a foil backing to prevent leakage.

Topical

- **Topical** medications can be applied to the skin in a number of ways, such as with a glove, tongue blade, or cotton-tipped applicator. Nurses should never apply a topical medication without first protecting their own skin.
- Use appropriate technique to remove the medication from the container and apply it to clean, dry skin, when

Preventing MEDICATION ERRORS
Safety alert:

- To prevent burns, remember to remove foil-backed patches before magnetic resonance imaging (MRI) is performed.

- Observe sterile technique when the skin is broken. Take precautions to avoid medication stains.

- Use firm strokes if the medication is to be rubbed in.

possible. Do not contaminate the medication in a container; instead use gloves or an applicator.

- Do not "double dip." Gloves and applicators that come in contact with a client should not be reinserted into the container. Estimate the amount needed and remove it from the container or use a fresh sterile applicator each time the container is entered.

Instillations

Instillations are liquid medications usually administered as drops, ointment, or sprays in the following forms:

- Eyedrops (Box 3–3, Figure 3–10)
- Eye ointment (Box 3–4, Figure 3–11)

Box 3–3

Administration of Eye Drops

1. WASH HANDS.
2. Instruct client to lie or sit down and to look up toward ceiling.
3. Remove any discharge by gently wiping out from inner canthus. Use separate cloth for each eye.
4. Gently draw skin down below the affected eye to expose the conjunctival sac.
5. Administer the prescribed number of drops into the center of the sac. Medication placed directly on the cornea can cause discomfort or damage. Do not touch eyelids or eyelashes with dropper. Self-administration of drops is enhanced with the use of Drop-eze, a cup-like device that holds the eyelids open.
6. Gently press on the lacrimal duct with sterile cotton ball or tissue for 1 to 2 min after instillation to prevent systemic absorption through lacrimal canal.
7. Client should keep eyes closed for 1 to 2 minutes following application to promote absorption.

FIGURE 3–10 To administer eye drops, gently pull down the skin below the eye to expose the conjunctival sac.

Box 3-4

Administration of Eye Ointment

1. WASH HANDS.
2. Instruct client to lie or sit down and to look up toward ceiling.
3. Remove any discharge by gently wiping out from inner canthus. Use separate cloth for each eye.
4. Gently draw skin down below the affected eye to expose the conjunctival sac.
5. Squeeze strip of ointment (about ¼ inch unless stated otherwise) onto conjunctival sac. Medication placed directly on cornea can cause discomfort or damage.
6. Instruct client to close eyes for 2 to 3 minutes.
7. Instruct client to expect blurred vision for a short time. Apply at bedtime if possible.

Box 3-5

Administration of Eardrops

1. WASH HANDS.
2. Medication should be at room temperature.
3. Client should sit up with head tilted slightly toward the unaffected side. To straighten the external ear canal for better visualization and to facilitate drops reaching the affected area, see Figure 3–12.
4. Child: pull down and back on auricle. After 3 years of age, same as adult. Adult: pull up and back on auricle.
5. Instill prescribed number of drops.
6. Take care not to contaminate dropper.
7. Have client maintain position for 2 to 3 minutes.

FIGURE 3–11 To administer eye ointment, squeeze a ¼-inch-wide strip of ointment onto the conjunctival sac.

- Eardrops (Box 3–5, Figure 3–12)
- Nose drops and sprays (Box 3–6, Figures 3–13 and 3–14)

Inhalations

- Handheld nebulizers deliver a very fine-sized particle spray of medication.
- Handheld metered-dose devices are a convenient method of administration for these medications (Figure 3–15).
- **Spacers** are devices used to enhance the delivery of medications from the **metered-dose inhaler (MDI)**. Figure 3–15 illustrates the distribution of medication with and without a spacer. Aero Chamber (distributed by Forest Pharmaceuticals, St. Louis) and InspirEase (distributed by Key Pharmaceuticals, Kenilworth, NJ) are examples of available spacers.
- The preferred client position is semi- or high Fowler's.
- Teach the client correct use of equipment.
- Nebulizer (aerosol) changes a liquid medication into a fine mist.

FIGURE 3–12 To administer eardrops, straighten the external ear canal by pulling down on the auricle in children (A) or pulling back on the auricle in adults (B).

Box 3-6

Administration of Nose Drops and Sprays

1. Have client blow nose.
2. Have client tilt head back for drops to reach frontal sinus and tilt head to affected side to reach ethmoid sinus.
3. Administer the prescribed number of drops or sprays. Some sprays have instructions to close one nostril, tilt head to closed side, and hold breath or breathe through nose for 1 minute.
4. Have client keep head tilted backward for 5 minutes after instillation of drops.

FIGURE 3–13 Administering nose drops.

FIGURE 3–14 Administering nasal spray.

- MDIs are hand-held devices that deliver medications to oropharyngeal and lower respiratory tracts. See Box 3–7 for the correct use of an inhaler and Figure 3–16 to monitor the amount of medication in the **canister**. Monitoring the number of doses in the canister is challenging to most clients. Ideally, the most accurate way is for the client to count and record (e.g., on box or calendar) the number of inhalations used; however, this is often not practical. A technique to estimate the amount of medication remaining in the canister is to put the canister in water. The client may overestimate the amount of medication due to the inhalant when using this method. Combination products have counter for the number of inhalations used. Research is in process on the counter functionality for all inhalation products; it will be a most welcome addition. Every effort should be made to have the client know how much medication is in the canister and to anticipate/obtain refills in a timely manner.

Nasogastric and Gastrostomy Tubes
- Check for proper placement of tube.
- Pour drug into syringe without plunger or bulb, release clamp, and allow medication to flow in properly, usually by gravity.
- Flush tubing with 50 ml of water or prescribed amount. (Refer to agency policy for exact amount.)
- Clamp tube and remove syringe.

Suppositories
Rectal Suppositories
- Medications administered as suppositories or enemas can be given rectally for local and systemic absorption. The numerous small capillaries in the rectal area promote absorption.
- The foil around the suppository is removed, and the suppository may be lubricated before insertion. When medications such as antipyretics and bronchodilators are given, the client must be reminded to retain the medication and not to expel it.

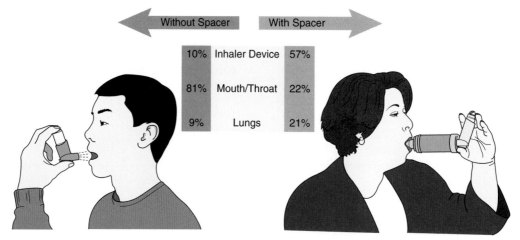

FIGURE 3–15 Distribution of medication with and without a spacer.

Box 3-7

Correct Use of Metered-Dose Inhaler

1. Insert the medication canister into the plastic holder.
2. Shake the inhaler well before using. Remove cap from mouthpiece.
3. Breathe out through the mouth. Open mouth wide and hold the mouthpiece 1 to 2 inches from the mouth. Do not put mouthpiece in the mouth unless using a spacer. Discuss techniques with the health care provider.
4. With mouth open, take slow, deep breath through mouth and at same time push the top of the medication canister once. Autohalers (e.g., Maxair) do not require coordination of pushing down top of canister and taking deep breath. With the autohaler in upright position, raise lever and shake. Inhale deeply through mouthpiece with steady, moderate force, which triggers the release of medicine, making a "click" sound and puffing out the medicine. Continue to take deep breaths.
5. Hold breath for 10 seconds; exhale slowly through pursed lips.
6. If a second dose is required, wait 1-2 minutes and repeat the procedure by first shaking the canister in the plastic holder with the cap on.
7. If the inhaler has not been used recently or when it is first used, "test spray" before administering the metered dose.
8. If a glucocorticoid inhalant is to be used with a bronchodilator, wait 5 minutes before using the inhaler containing the steroid.
9. Teach client to monitor pulse rate.
10. Caution against overuse, because side effects and tolerance may result.
11. Teach client to monitor amount of medication remaining in the canister (see Figure 3–15). Advise the client to ask his or her health care provider or pharmacist to estimate when a new inhaler will be needed based on dosing schedule. A common practice of placing the canister in water to determine the amount of drug remaining is not appropriate for all inhalers; ask health care provider or pharmacist.
12. Teach client to rinse mouth out after using metered dose inhaler. This is especially important when using a steroid drug. Rinsing mouth helps prevent irritation and secondary infection to the oral mucosa.
13. Instruct client to avoid smoking.
14. Teach client to do daily cleaning of the equipment, including (1) wash hands; (2) take apart all washable parts of equipment and wash with warm water; (3) rinse; (4) place on clean towel and cover with another clean towel to air dry; and (5) store in a clean plastic bag when completely dry. It is a good idea to have two sets of washable equipment to make this process easier.

FIGURE 3–16 Measure the amount of medication remaining in an inhaler canister by immersion in water. (From Lilley L, Harrington S, Snyder J: *Pharmacology and the nursing process*, ed 4, St. Louis, 2005, Mosby.)

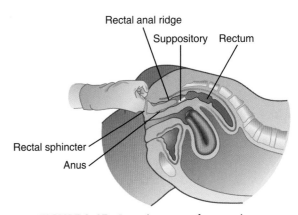

FIGURE 3–17 Inserting a rectal suppository.

- Suppositories tend to soften at room temperature and therefore need to be refrigerated.
- Explain the procedure to the client and provide privacy.
- Use a glove for insertion.
- Instruct client to lie on left side and breathe through the mouth to relax the anal sphincter.
- Apply a small amount of water-soluble lubricant to the tip of the unwrapped suppository, and gently insert the suppository beyond the internal sphincter (Figure 3–17).
- Have client remain lying on side for 20 minutes after insertion.
- If indicated, teach clients how to self-administer suppositories, and observe a return demonstration for effectiveness.

Vaginal Suppositories

Vaginal suppositories are similar to rectal suppositories. They are generally inserted into the vagina with an applicator (Figure 3–18). Wear gloves. The client should be in the lithotomy position. After insertion of the medication, provide the client with a sanitary pad.

FIGURE 3–18 Inserting a vaginal suppository.

Parenteral

Safety is always a special concern with parenteral medication. Thus manufacturers have responded with safety features in an effort to decrease or eliminate needlestick injuries and the possible transfer of blood-borne diseases such as hepatitis and human immunodeficiency virus (HIV). (Figure 3–19 shows examples of safety needles.) Nursing implications for administration of parenteral medications are at the end of this section.

There are multiple types of parenteral routes, including **intradermal**, **subcutaneous**, **intramuscular**, **Z-track technique**, and **intravenous**. A description of each follows with special considerations noted for the pediatric client.

Intradermal

Action

- Local effect
- A small amount is injected so that volume does not interfere with wheal formation or cause a systemic reaction.

- Used for observation of an inflammatory (allergic) reaction to foreign proteins. Examples include tuberculin testing, testing for drug and other allergic sensitivities, and some immunotherapy for cancer.

Sites

Locations are chosen so that an inflammatory reaction can be observed. Preferred areas are lightly pigmented, thinly keratinized, and hairless, such as the ventral midforearm, clavicular area of the chest, and scapular area of the back (Figure 3–20).

Equipment

- Needle: 25 to 27 gauge; $3/8$ to $5/8$ inches in length
- Syringe: 1 ml calibrated in 0.01-ml increments (usually 0.01 to 0.1 ml injected)

Technique

- Cleanse the area using a circular motion; observe sterile technique.
- Hold the skin taut.
- Insert the needle, bevel up, at a 10- to 15-degree angle; the outline of the needle under the skin should be visible (Figure 3–21).
- Inject the medication slowly to form a wheal (blister or bleb).
- Remove the needle slowly; do not recap.
- Do not massage the area; also instruct the client not to do so.
- Mark the area with a pen, and ask the client not to wash it off until read by a health care provider.
- Assess for allergic reaction in 24 to 72 hours; measure the diameter of local reaction. For tuberculin, measure only the indurated area; do not include redness in the measurement.

FIGURE 3–19 Safety needles. (Courtesy Becton Dickinson and Company, Franklin Lakes, NJ.)

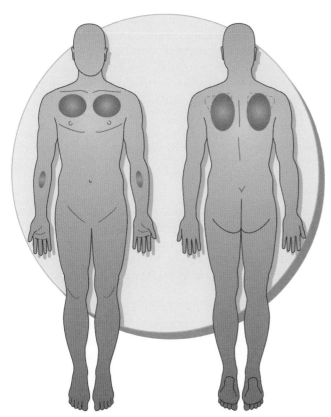

FIGURE 3–20 Common sites for intradermal injection.

Subcutaneous

Action

- Systemic effect
- Sustained effect; absorbed mainly through capillaries; usually slower in onset than with the IM route
- Used for small doses of nonirritating, water-soluble drugs

Sites

Locations for subQ injection are chosen for adequate fat-pad size and include the abdomen, upper hips, upper back, lateral upper arms, and lateral thighs (Figure 3–22). Sites should be rotated with subcutaneous injections such as insulin and heparin.

Equipment

- Needle: 25 to 27 gauge, ½ to ⅝ inches in length
- Syringe: 1 to 3 ml (usually 0.5 to 1.5 ml injected)
- Insulin syringe measured in units for use with insulin only

Technique

- Cleanse the area with a circular motion using sterile technique.
- Pinch the skin.
- Insert the needle at an angle appropriate to body size: 45 to 90 degrees (45 degrees for those with little subQ tissue) (see Figure 3–21).
- Release the skin.

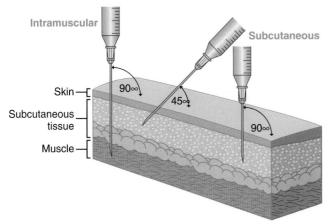

FIGURE 3–21 Needle-skin angle for intradermal, subcutaneous, and intramuscular injections.

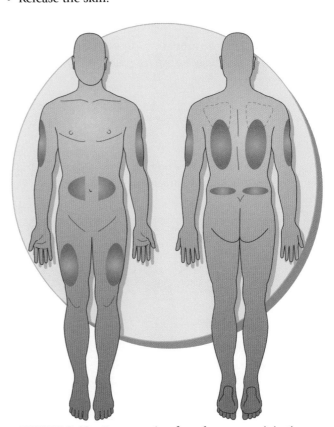

FIGURE 3–22 Common sites for subcutaneous injections.

- Aspirate except heparin, LMWH, and insulin.
- Inject the medication slowly.
- Remove the needle quickly; do not recap.
- Gently massage the area unless contraindicated, as with heparin and LMWH.
- Apply gentle pressure to the injection site to prevent bleeding or oozing into the tissue and subsequent bruising and tissue damage, especially if the client is on anticoagulant therapy.
- Apply bandage if needed.

Intramuscular

Action

- Systemic effect
- Usually more rapid effect of drug than with the subQ route
- Used for irritating drugs, aqueous suspensions, and solutions in oils

Sites

Locations are chosen for adequate muscle size and minimal major nerves and blood vessels in the area. Locations include ventrogluteal, dorsogluteal, deltoid, and vastus lateralis (pediatrics). A section on each site is shown in the diagrams of the sites (Figures 3–23 through 3–26) and includes the volume of drug administered, needle size, angle of injection, client position, site location, advantages and disadvantages of site, and additional considerations, if any. Clients with low weight should be evaluated for sites with adequate muscle. The ventrogluteal is the preferred site for adults and infants older than 7 months.

Equipment

- Needle: 20 to 23 gauge; 18 gauge for blood products; 1 to 1.5 inches in length

Technique

- Same as for subQ injection, with two exceptions: flatten the skin area using the thumb and index finger and inject between them; insert the needle at a 90-degree angle into the muscle (see Figure 3–21)
- Syringe: 1 to 3 ml (usually 0.5 to 1.5 ml injected)

Preferred Intramuscular Injection Sites

Table 3–4 presents the four sites, client position, advantages, and disadvantages of each injection site. Diagrams of each injection site with associated landmarks are presented in Figures 3–23 through 3–26.

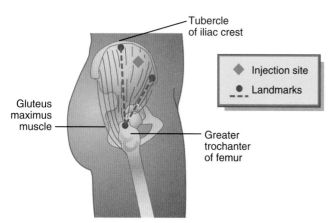

FIGURE 3–23   Ventrogluteal injection site.

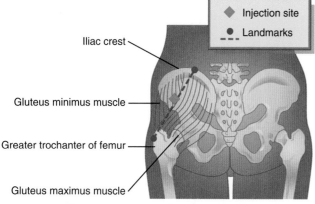

FIGURE 3–24   Dorsogluteal injection site.

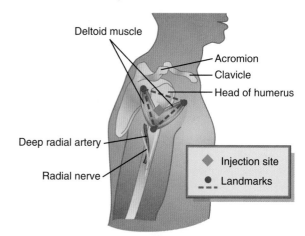

FIGURE 3–25   Deltoid injection site.

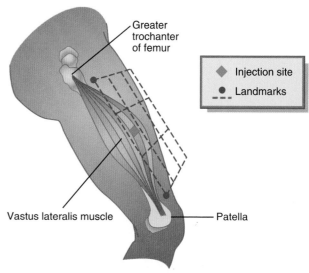

FIGURE 3–26   Vastus lateralis injection site in children.

Table 3–4

Intramuscular Injection Sites: Client Position, Advantages, and Disadvantages

Site	Client Position	Advantages	Disadvantages
Ventrogluteal	Supine, lateral	Anatomic landmarks well defined Muscle mass suited for deep IM or Z-track injections Free of major nerves	In the event of hypersensitivity reaction, medication absorption can be delayed by tourniquet
Dorsogluteal	Prone	Muscle mass suited for deep IM or Z-track injections	Requires correct/accurate site and technique to avoid injury to major nerves and vascular structures In the event of hypersensitivity reaction, medication absorption cannot be delayed by tourniquet
Deltoid	Lateral, prone, sitting, supine	Readily accessible In the event of hypersensitivity reaction, medication absorption cannot be delayed by tourniquet	Small muscle mass; limited to small volume doses Close to nerves; requires accurate technique
Vastus lateralis	Sitting, supine	Good site for infants Size acceptable for multiple injections Free of major nerves	Special attention required to avoid sciatic nerve or femoral structures if long needle is used

IM, Intramuscular.

- *Ventrogluteal* (see Figure 3–23). Volume of drug administered is 1 to 3 ml, with a 20- to 23-gauge, 1.25- to 2.5-inch needle. Slightly angle the needle toward the iliac crest.
- *Dorsogluteal* (see Figure 3–24). Volume of drug administered is 1 to 3 ml; 5 ml gamma globulin with 18- to 23-gauge, 1.25- to 3-inch needle. Place the needle at a 90-degree angle to the skin with the client prone.
- *Deltoid* (see Figure 3–25). Volume of drug administered is 0.5 to 1 ml, with a 23- to 25-gauge, $^{5}/_{8}$ to 1.5-inch needle. Place the needle at a 90-degree angle to the skin or slightly toward acromion.
- *Vastus lateralis* (see Figure 3–26). Volume of drug administered is < 0.5 ml in infants (max = 1 ml), 1 ml pediatrics, 1 to 1.5 ml adults (max = 2 ml). Direct the needle at the knee at a 45- to 60-degree angle to the frontal, sagittal, and horizontal planes of the thigh.

Z-Track Injection Technique

The Z-track technique prevents medication from leaking back into the subQ tissue. It is frequently advised for medications that cause visible and permanent skin discolorations (e.g., iron dextran). The gluteal site is preferred. While following the medication's order policy and aseptic technique, draw up the medication. Replace the first needle with a second needle of appropriate gauge and length to penetrate muscle tissue and deliver the medication to the selected site. Removal of the first needle prevents the medication that is adhering to the needle shaft from being taken into the subQ tissue. If removal is not possible, gently wipe the needle with a sterile source; this does present a chance for contamination and also for "self-sticks." Consider having the medication prepared in the pharmacy.

The Z-track injection technique is presented in Figure 3–27.

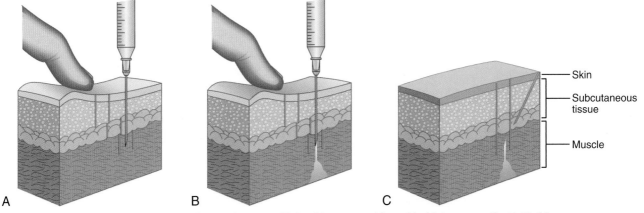

FIGURE 3–27 Z-track injection. A, Pull the skin to one side and hold; insert needle. B, Holding skin to side, inject medication. C, Withdraw needle and release skin. This technique prevents medication from entering subcutaneous tissue.

Intravenous

Action

- Systemic effect
- More rapid than the IM or subQ routes

Sites

Accessible peripheral veins (e.g., cephalic or cubital vein of arm; dorsal vein of hand) are preferred (Figure 3–28). When possible, ask the client about preference. Avoid needless body restriction. In newborns, the veins of the feet, lower legs, and head may also be used after the previous sites have been exhausted.

Equipment

- Needle
- Adults: 20 to 21 gauge (16 to 21 gauge in ER, etc.); 1 to 1.5 inches
- Infants: 24 gauge; 1 inch
- Children: 22 gauge; 1 inch
- Larger bore for viscous drugs, whole blood or fractions; large volume for rapid infusion
- Electronic IV delivery device, an infusion controller, or pump
- Patient-controlled analgesia (PCA) system, if ordered
- Eutectic mixture of local anesthetics (EMLA), if appropriate

Technique

- Apply a tourniquet.
- Cleanse the area using aseptic technique.
- Insert butterfly or a catheter and feed up into the vein until blood returns. Remove tourniquet.
- Stabilize the needle and dress site.
- Monitor the flow rate, distal pulses, skin color and temperature, and insertion site.
- Consult agency policy regarding the addition of medications to bottle or bag, piggyback technique, and IV push. Be alert that all tubing is connected correctly.

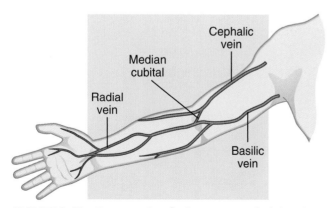

FIGURE 3–28 Common sites for intravenous administration.

Nursing Implications for Administration of Parenteral Medications

Sites

- Ventrogluteal site is preferred for IM injections in adults and infants older than 7 months.
- Do not use the dorsogluteal site for IM injections in children. For infants younger than 7 months, the vastus lateralis is preferred.

Equipment

- Use a needle size and syringe appropriate to the client's needs.
- The syringe size should approximate the volume of medication to be administered.
- Use the tuberculin syringe for amounts <0.5 ml.
- Use the filter needle to draw up the medication from a glass vial or ampule. Change the needle before administration to prevent tissue irritation from any medication left on the needle.

Technique

- Explain to the client what is going to be done. Gain the client's cooperation. Allow the client time to cooperate, if possible.
- Demonstrate empathy and concern for every client and his or her family, as well as using proper technique.
- Allay anxiety. Encourage expression of feelings.
- Position the client.
- Administer medication only via the ordered route.
- Inspect the skin before each injection.
- Inject medication slowly to minimize tissue damage.
- Stabilize skin during needle removal to reduce pain.
- Do not administer injections if sites are inflamed, edematous, or lesioned (e.g., moles, birth marks, scars).
- Rotate the injection site to enhance absorption of the drug (e.g., insulin). Document the injection site.
- Observe the client for drug effectiveness. Report any untoward reactions immediately.
- Multiple products are available to reduce pain of parenteral medication administration. Examples of these products include: EMLA, lidocaine, and tetracaine in topical patch, and "shot buster"—a mechanical device based on gate control theory of pain management.

Developmental Needs of Pediatric Clients

Anticipate developmental needs. Examples of needs associated with administration of medications include the following (refer to Chapter 10 for additional examples):

- Stranger anxiety (infant): Maintain a nonthreatening approach and move slowly.

FIGURE 3–29 A patient-controlled analgesia system. (Courtesy Smiths Medical MD, Inc., St. Paul, Minnesota.)

- Hospitalization, illness, or injury may be viewed as punishment (3 to 6 years old): Allow control where appropriate; obtain child's view of situation; encourage positive relationships and expression of feelings in acceptable manner and activities. Include the family or a support person if appropriate.
- Fear of mutilation (3 to 6 years old): Explain the procedures carefully; use less intrusive routes whenever possible, such as the oral route; allow children to give "play injections" to a doll or stuffed animal.

Technologic Advances

Advances in drug administration therapy continue to enhance safety, increase accessibility to sites, promote client mobility, and improve client adherence. Examples of these advances include the following:

- Robotic medication dispensing systems
- Pain-free delivery of insulin through patch
- PCA infusion machine that scans Abbott drugs (Figure 3–29). Drug name and concentration are automatically entered when syringe is inserted (Abbott Laboratories).
- Data from medication administration record (MAR) are displayed on handheld device that is updated with each prescriber's medication entry. This device, compatible with most computerized documentation systems, signals when a new medication order is received, is linked to infusion pump, and the nurse is alerted about future doses (Baxter Health Care Corps).
- An infusion pump with a scanner is used so that after reading the IV bag label the nurse scans the medication; then the nurse and client ID band and information regarding infusion are programmed into the pump (B. Braun Medical Inc.).

Nursing Process

Overview of Medication Administration

ASSESSMENT

- Obtain appropriate vital signs and relevant laboratory test results for future comparisons and evaluation of the therapeutic response.
- Obtain drug history, including drug allergies.
- Identify high-risk clients for reactions.
- Assess client's capability to follow therapeutic regimen.

POTENTIAL NURSING DIAGNOSES

- Risk for injury related to possible adverse reaction
- Ineffective individual/family therapeutic regimen management related to knowledge deficit, economic difficulties, or complexities of the regimen
- Knowledge, readiness for enhanced management of medication regimen
- Effective therapeutic regimen management related to medication administration

PLANNING

- Identify goals.
- Promote therapeutic response and prevent or minimize adverse reactions.
- Identify strategies to promote adherence.
- Identify interventions.

NURSING INTERVENTIONS

- Prepare equipment and environment; wash hands.
- Check for allergies and other assessment data.
- Check drug label three times; check expiration date.
- Be certain of drug calculation; verify dose with another RN as necessary.
- Pour liquids at eye level on flat surface.
- Keep all drugs stored properly, especially related to temperature, light, and moisture.
- Avoid contact with topical and inhalation preparations.
- Verify client identification.
- Administer only drugs that you have prepared.
- Assist client to desired position.
- Discard needles and syringes in "sharps" container.
- Follow policy related to discarding drugs and controlled substances.
- Report drug errors immediately.
- Document all appropriate information in a timely manner.
- Record effectiveness of drugs administered and reason for any drugs refused.

Client Teaching

General
- Emphasize safety.
- Monitor client's physical abilities regularly as needed.
- Keep or store medications in original labeled containers with child-resistant caps when needed.
- Provide client or family with written instructions (or audio instructions if visually impaired) about the drug regimen.
- Advise client or family about the expected therapeutic effect and length of time to achieve a therapeutic response from the medication and the expected duration of treatment.
- Instruct client or family about possible drug-laboratory test interaction.
- Advise client of nonpharmacologic measures to promote therapeutic response.
- Encourage client or family to have adequate supply of necessary medications available.
- Caution against the use of OTC preparations including herbal remedies without *first* contacting the health care provider.
- Reinforce the importance of follow-up appointments with health care providers.
- Encourage client to wear Medic-Alert band with medications or allergies indicated.
- Reinforce that community resources are available and need to be mobilized according to the client or family needs.

Diet
- Advise client or family about possible drug-food interactions.
- Advise client or family what foods are contraindicated.
- Instruct regarding alcohol use.

Self-Administration
- Instruct client or family regarding drug dose and dosing schedule.
- Instruct client or family on all psychomotor skills related to the drug regimen.
- Provide client or family with contact person and telephone number for questions and concerns.

Side Effects
- Instruct client or family about general side effects and adverse reactions of the medications.
- Advise client or family when and how to notify health care provider.

Cultural Considerations ❖
- Assess personal beliefs of clients and family.
- Modify communications to meet cultural needs of client and family.
- Communicate respect for culture and cultural practices of client and family.

EVALUATION

- Evaluate effectiveness of medications administered.
- Identify expected time frame of desired drug response; consider modification of therapy as needed.
- Determine client satisfaction with regimen.

KEY WEBSITES

The Institute for Safe Medication Practice: www.ismp.org
U.S. Food and Drug Administration (FDA): www.fda.gov/loc/initiatives/barcode.html (The FDA issues bar code regulations)
National Coordinating Council for Medication Error Reporting and Prevention (NCC MERP): www.nccmerp.org

NCLEX Study Questions

1. "Digoxin to maintain blood level at 0.5-2 ng/ml." This is an example of what category of drug order?
   a. standing
   b. single
   c. PRN
   d. STAT

2. An advantage of the unit dose method of drug distribution is:
   a. more expensive
   b. cost efficiency
   c. always available
   d. increased accountability

3. Your 9-month-old client has a medication ordered via the IM route. The preferred site for this is:
   a. ventrogluteal
   b. dorsogluteal
   c. vastus lateralis
   d. deltoid

4. According to The Joint Commission, which of the following is NOT an acceptable abbreviation for ordering or documenting medications?
   a. QD
   b. h.s.
   c. T.I.W.
   d. b.i.d.

5. Your client refuses to take his prescribed medications. The nurse's best response is to:
   a. explain benefits and side effects of drug
   b. leave medication at bedside to be taken later
   c. coerce client into taking medication
   d. explain risks of not taking medication

6. JW, your 3-year-old client, has an IM medication ordered. What is the most appropriate approach to gain JW's cooperation?
   a. engage in fantasy play
   b. give injection to bear
   c. restrain upper extremities
   d. ask family members to leave room

Answers: 1. a; 2. d; 3. c; 4. a; 5. d.

TWO

Medications and Calculations

Unit Two (Chapter 4) provides practice in the calculation of drug dosages. The chapter is divided into six sections: (A) systems of measurement, (B) four general methods for calculating drug dosages and two individualized methods, (C) calculations of oral dosages, (D) calculations of injectable dosages, (E) calculations of intravenous fluids, and (F) pediatric drug calculations. Though the sections in Chapter 4 are condensed, there are many practice problems.

This unit is thorough and could be used by students in place of the purchase of a drug calculation text. It may also serve as a review of drug calculation in preparing for state boards or for nurses in practice settings.

Extra practice problems are available on the companion CD.

4
Medications and Calculations

Overview

This chapter on medications and calculations is subdivided into six sections: (A) systems of measurement with conversion, (B) methods for calculation, (C) calculations of oral dosages, (D) calculations of injectable dosages, (E) calculations of intravenous (IV) fluids, and (F) pediatric drug calculations. The nurse may proceed independently through Sections A to F to practice and master calculation of drug dosages during the fundamental nursing or pharmacology course. This chapter also serves as a review of drug calculation for nurses in practice settings.

Numerous drug labels are used in the drug calculation problems to familiarize the nurse with important information on a drug label. That information is then used in correctly calculating the drug dose.

Six calculation methods are explained. Four are general methods: (1) basic formula, (2) ratio and proportion, (3) fractional equation, and (4) dimensional analysis. The nurse should select one of these general methods for the calculation of drug dosages. The other two methods are used to individualize drug dosing by body weight and body surface area. Each of the calculation methods has a color-coded icon that identifies the method used in the chapters.

The drug calculation charts in Tables 4A–4 and 4B–1 may be used in the clinical setting. The nurse might find it helpful to review Chapter 3, Principles of Drug Administration.

Keeping in mind that the goal is to prepare and administer medications in a safe and correct manner, the following recommendations are offered:

- **Think**. Focus on each step of the problem. This applies to simple and difficult problems.
- **Read accurately**. Pay particular attention to the location of the decimal point and to the operation to be done, such as conversion from one system of measurement to another.
- **Picture the problem.**
- **Identify an expected range for the answer.**
- **Seek to understand the problem**. Do not merely master the mechanics of how to do it. Ask for help when unsure of the calculation.

Section 4A   SYSTEMS OF MEASUREMENT WITH CONVERSION

Outline . . . .

Objectives

- Discuss the three systems of measurement.
- Convert measurement within the metric system, larger units to smaller units, and smaller units to larger units.
- Convert measurements within the apothecary system, larger units to smaller units, and smaller units to larger units.
- Convert measurements within the household system, larger units to smaller units, and smaller units to larger units.
- Convert metric, apothecary, and household measurements among the three systems of measurement as appropriate.

Terms

apothecary system, p. 48
dram, p. 48
grain, p. 48

gram, p. 47
household measurement,
　p. 49

liter, p. 47
meter, p. 47
metric system, p. 47

minim, p. 48
ounce, p. 48

Three systems of measurement—metric, apothecary, and household—are used to measure drugs and solutions. The metric system, developed in the late eighteenth century, is the internationally accepted system of measure. It is replacing the apothecary system, which dates back to the Middle Ages and had been used in England since the seventeenth century. Household measurement is commonly used in community and home settings in the United States.

Metric System

The **metric system** is a decimal system based on the power of 10. The basic units of measure are **gram** (g, gm, G, Gm) for weight; **liter** (l, L) for volume; and **meter** (m, M) for linear measurement, or length. Prefixes indicate the size of the units in multiples of 10. Table 4A–1 gives the metric units of measure in weight (gram), volume (liter), and length (meter) in larger and smaller units that are commonly used.

Kilo is the prefix used for larger units (e.g., kilometer), and *milli, centi, micro,* and *nano* are the prefixes for smaller units (e.g., millimeter). The prefix stands for a specific degree of magnitude; for instance, *kilo* stands for thousands, *milli* for one thousandth, *centi* for one hundredth, and so on. Because the difference between degrees of magnitude is always a multiple of 10, converting from one magnitude to another is relatively easy.

Table 4A–1

Metric Units of Measurement

Unit	Names and Abbreviations	Measurements
Gram (weight)	1 kilogram (kg, Kg)	1000 g
	1 gram (g, gm, G, Gm)	1 g
	1 milligram (mg)	0.001 g
	1 microgram (mcg)	0.000001 g
	1 nanogram (ng)	0.000000001 g
Liter (volume)	1 iloliter (kl, KL)	1000 L (l)
	1 liter (L, l)	1 L (l)
	1 milliliter (ml)	0.001 L (l)
Meter (length)	1 kilometer (km)	1000 m
	1 meter (m, M)	1 m
	1 centimeter (cm)	0.01 m
	1 millimeter (mm)	0.001 m

NOTE: 1 ml (milliliter) = 1 cc (cubic centimeter). Values are the same in drug and fluid therapy. 1 mg (milligram) = 1000 mcg (micrograms).

Conversion within the Metric System

The metric units most frequently used in drug notation are the following:

$$1 \text{ g} = 1000 \text{ mg}$$
$$1 \text{ L} = 1000 \text{ ml}$$
$$1 \text{ mg} = 1000 \text{ mcg}$$

To be able to convert a quantity, one of the values must be known, such as gram or milligrams, liter or milliliters, and milligrams or micrograms. Gram, liter, and meter are larger units; milligram, milliliter, and millimeter are smaller units.

Metric Conversion

A. When converting *larger* units to smaller units in the metric system, move the decimal point one space to the *right* for each degree of magnitude change.
   Note: This does *not* apply to micro and nano units.

EXAMPLE   Change 1 gram to milligrams.
   Grams are three degrees of magnitude *greater* than milligrams (see Table 4A-1). Move the decimal point three spaces to the right.

$$1 \text{ g} = 1.000 \text{ mg} \quad \text{or} \quad 1 \text{ g} = 1000 \text{ mg}$$

B. When converting *smaller* units to larger units in the metric system, move the decimal point one space to the *left* for each degree of magnitude of change.

EXAMPLE   Change 1000 milligrams to grams.
   Milligrams are three degrees of magnitude *smaller* than grams. Move the decimal point three spaces to the left.

$$1000 \text{ mg} = 1\,000.\text{ g} \quad \text{or} \quad 1000 \text{ mg} = 1 \text{ g}$$

REMEMBER: When changing *larger* units to smaller units, move the decimal point to the *right*, and when changing *smaller* units to larger units, move the decimal point to the *left*.

PRACTICE
PROBLEM I

METRIC CONVERSION	
Larger to Smaller Units	**Smaller to Larger Units**
1. Change 2 g to mg	4. Change 1500 mg to g
2. Change 0.5 ($^1/_2$) g to mg	5. Change 3 g to kg
3. Change 2.5 L to ml	6. Change 500 ml to L

Apothecary System

The **apothecary system** of measurement was the common system used by most practitioners before the universal acceptance of the International Metric System. Now all pharmaceuticals are manufactured using the metric system, and the apothecary system is no longer included on any drug labels. All medication should be prescribed and calculated using metric measures, but occasionally the use of the fluid ounce or grains is found. For those rare circumstances, nurses should have a general understanding of the apothecary system.

The apothecary system uses Roman numerals instead of Arabic numbers to express the quantity. The Roman numeral is placed after the symbol or abbreviation for the unit of measure. The Roman numerals are written in lowercase letters; for example, gr x stands for 10 grains. The letters s̄s̄ indicate one half; for example, gr s̄s̄ stands for $^1/_2$ grain.

In the apothecary system, the unit of weight is the **grain** (gr), and the units of fluid volume are the **ounce** (fluidounce), the **dram** (fluidram), and the **minim** (min, or ♏). Drams and minims are used infrequently.

In clinical practice, ounce and dram are more frequently used for measurement of fluid volume than for dry weights. Therefore, when writing fluid volume, the word fluid (f) in front of an ounce or dram is usually dropped. Table 4A–2 gives the apothecary equivalent of larger and smaller units of measure in dry weight and fluid volume.

Your nursing program may have you omit the apothecary system. If so, study only the metric system and the household system in this section and the following sections of the Unit.

Apothecary Conversion

A. When converting a *larger* unit to a smaller unit, *multiply* the measurement that is requested by the basic equivalent value.

EXAMPLE

1. 3 Fluidounces (fl oz) = _____ fluid dram (fl dr).
   The equivalent value is   1 fl oz = 8 fl dr

   $$3 \text{ fl oz} \times 8 \text{ fl dr} = \underline{24} \text{ fl dr}$$

B. When converting a *smaller* unit to a larger unit, *divide* the requested number by the basic equivalent value.

EXAMPLE

1. 8 fluidounces (fl oz) = _____ pint (pt).
   The equivalent value is 1 pt = 16 fl oz

   $$8 \text{ fl oz} \div 16 \text{ fl oz} = \tfrac{1}{2} \text{ pt}$$

Table 4A–2

Apothecary Equivalents in Weights and Fluid Volume

Dry Weight			Fluid Volume*		
Larger Units		**Smaller Units**	**Larger Units**		**Smaller Units**
1 ounce (oz)	=	480 grains (gr)	1 quart (qt)	=	2 pints (pt)
1 ounce (oz)	=	8 drams (dr)	1 pint (pt)	=	16 fluid ounces (fl oz)
1 dram (dr)	=	60 grains (gr)	1 fluid ounce	=	8 fluid dram (fl dr)
1 scruple	=	20 grains (gr)	1 fluid dram	=	60 minims (min, or m)
			1 minim	=	1 drop (gt)

*Fluid volume units are more commonly used than dry weight units and thus should be remembered.

PRACTICE
PROBLEM 2

APOTHECARY CONVERSION

Larger to Smaller Units	Smaller to Larger Units
1. Change 3 qt to pt	3. Change 3 pt to qt
2. Change 1.5 pt to fl oz	4. Change 32 fl oz to qt

Household System

Household measurement is not as accurate as the metric system because of the lack of standardization of spoons, cups, and glasses. The measurements are approximate. A teaspoon (t) is considered to be equivalent to 5 ml according to the official *United States Pharmacopeia*. Milliliters (ml) is the same as cubic centimeters (cc) in value. Three teaspoons equal 1 tablespoon (T). Ounces (oz) are fluid ounces in the household measurement system; the word "fluid" in front of ounce is usually not used. One milliliter of water fills a cubic centimeter exactly.

Table 4A–3 gives the household equivalents in fluid volume. The measurements with asterisks are frequently used in drug therapy and should be remembered.

Household Conversion

A. When converting *larger* units to smaller units within the household system, *multiply* the requested number by the basic equivalent value.

EXAMPLE

Change 2 glasses of water to ounces.
   The equivalent value is 1 medium-sized glass = 8 oz (fl oz)
   2 glasses × 8 oz = <u>16</u> oz (fl oz)

Table 4A–3

Household Equivalents in Fluid Volume

1 measuring cup	=	8 ounces (oz)
1 medium-size glass (tumbler size)	=	8 ounces (oz)
1 coffee cup (c)	=	6 ounces (oz) (varies with cup size)
1 ounce (oz)	=	2 tablespoons (T)
1 tablespoon (T)	=	3 teaspoons (t)
1 teaspoon (t)	=	60 drops (gtt)*
1 drop (gt)*	=	1 minim (min, or m)

*Varies with viscosity of liquid and dropper opening.

PRACTICE PROBLEM 3

HOUSEHOLD CONVERSION

REMEMBER: To change *larger* units to smaller units, *multiply* the requested number of units by the basic equivalent value. To change *smaller* units to larger units, *divide* the requested number of units by the basic equivalent value. Refer to Table 4A-3 as needed.

Larger to Smaller Units

1. Change 3 oz to T
2. Change 5 T to t
3. Change 3 coffee cups to oz

Smaller to Larger Units

4. Change 3 T to oz
5. Change 16 oz to a measuring cup
6. Change 12 t to T

Conversion among the Metric, Apothecary, and Household Systems

Drug doses are usually ordered in metric units (grams, milligrams, liters, or milliliters), but some health care providers still use the apothecary units of measurement (grain) when prescribing medication. To calculate drug doses, the same unit of measure (grams, milligrams, or grains) must be used. The nurse needs to be familiar with the three systems of measure and their equivalents (Table 4A–4). Note that the metric and apothecary equivalents are approximate; thus the equivalents should be rounded off to a whole number, for example, 1 g = 15.432 gr, or 1 g = 15 gr.

Some authorities indicate that it is easier to convert to the unit used on the bottle or container. The answer is in the system of the drug to be dispensed. If the label on the bottle reads in milligrams and the order is in grains, the conversion should be from grains to milligrams.

EXAMPLE   Order: Compazine spansule gr $1/4$.

Available: Compazine spansule 15 mg. Convert grains to milligrams, gr $1/4$ = 15 mg.

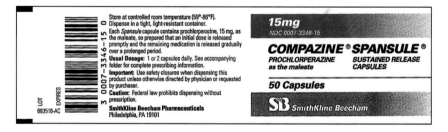

Metric, Apothecary, and Household Equivalents

Conversion to one unit of measure is essential in the administration of drugs. With discharge teaching for a client who requires liquid medication(s) at home, the nurse may find it necessary to convert metric to household measurements. Table 4A–4 gives the metric and apothecary equivalents by weight, and the metric, apothecary, and household equivalents by volume.

Table 4A–4

Approximate Metric, Apothecary, and Household Equivalents

	Metric System		Apothecary System	Household System
Weight	1 kg;	1000 g	2.2 lb	2.2 lb
	*1 g;	1000 mg	15 (16) gr	
	0.5 g;	500 mg	7$^1/_2$ gr	
	0.3 g;	300 (325) mg	5 gr	
	0.1 g;	100 mg	1$^1/_2$ gr	
	*0.06 g;	60 (65) mg	1 gr	
	0.03 g;	30 (32) mg	$^1/_2$ gr	
	0.01g	10 mg	$^1/_6$ gr	
		0.6 mg	$^1/_{100}$ gr	
		0.4 mg	$^1/_{150}$ gr	
		0.3 mg	$^1/_{200}$ gr	
Volume	1 L; 1000 ml		1 qt; 32 oz (fl oz)	
	0.5 L; 500 ml		1 pt; 16 oz (fl oz)	
	0.24 L; 240 ml		8 fl oz	1 glass
	0.18 L; 180 ml		6 fl oz	1 c
	*30 ml		1 fl oz; 8 fl dr	2 T; 6 t
	15 ml		½ fl oz; 4 fl dr	1 T; 3 t
	†5 ml			1 t
	4 ml		1 fl oz; 60 ℥ (min)	1 t
	1 ml		15 (16) ℥	15-16 gtt
Height/Distance	2.54 cm		1 in	1 in
	25.4 mm		1 in	1 in

*Equivalents commonly used for computing conversion problems by ratio.
†5 ml = 1 t (teaspoon); official United States Pharmacopeia measurement.
fl dr, Fluid dram; *fl oz*, fluid ounce; ℥, minim; *cm*, centimeter; *g*, gram; *gr*, grain; *gtt*, drops; *in*, inch; *kg*, kilogram; *L*, liter; *lb*, pound; *mg*, milligram; *ml*, milliliter; *mm*, millimeter; *pt*, pint; *qt*, quart; *T*, tablespoon; *t*, teaspoon; *c*, coffee cup.

PRACTICE PROBLEM 4

SUMMARY: METRIC, APOTHECARY, AND HOUSEHOLD MEASUREMENTS

Metric System: Refer to Table 4A-1 as needed.

1. 2 g = _____ mg   5. 500 mg = _____ g

2. 1.2 kg = _____ g   6. 10,000 mcg = _____ mg

3. 5 mg = _____ mcg   7. 2400 mg = _____ g

4. 2.5 L = _____ ml   8. 1500 ml = _____ L

Apothecary System: Refer to Table 4A-2 as needed.

1. 5 qt = _____ pt   5. 8 fl oz = _____ pt

2. 2 pt = _____ fl oz   6. 3 pt = _____ qt

3. fl oz v = _____ fl dr   7. 12 fl dr = _____ fl oz

4. 1.5 pt = _____ fl oz   8. 32 fl oz = _____ qt

Household System: Refer to Table 4A-3 as needed.

1. 5 glasses = _____ oz   4. 4 oz = _____ T

2. 3 T = _____ t   5. 15 t = _____ T

3. 2 c = _____ oz   6. 5 T = _____ oz

ANSWERS TO PRACTICE PROBLEMS

I METRIC CONVERSION

1. 2.0 g = 2. 000 mg   or   2.0 g = 2000 mg

The gram is three degrees of magnitude greater than the milligram, so the decimal point is moved three spaces to the right.

2. 0.5 g = 0. 500 mg   or   0.5 g = 500 mg

The gram is three degrees of magnitude greater than the milligram, so the decimal point is moved three spaces to the right.

3. 2.5 L = 2. 500 ml   or   2.5 L = 2500 ml

The liter is three degrees of magnitude greater than the milliliter, so the decimal point is moved three spaces to the right.

4. 1500 mg = 1 500. g   or   1500 mg = 1.5 g

The milligram is three degrees of magnitude smaller (less) than the gram, so the decimal point is moved three spaces to the left.

5. 3 g = 003. kg   or   3 g = .003 kg

The gram is three degrees of magnitude smaller than the kilogram, so the decimal point is moved three spaces to the left.

6. 500 ml = 500. L   or   500 ml = 0.5 L

The milliliter is three degrees of magnitude smaller than the liter, so the decimal point is moved three spaces to the left.

2 APOTHECARY CONVERSION

1. 3 qt × 2 pt = 6 pt;
   the equivalent value is 1 qt = 2 pt

2. 1.5 pt × 16 = 24 fl oz;
   the equivalent value is 1 pt = 16 fl oz

3. 3 pt = 1.5 qt;
   the equivalent value is 1 qt = 2 pt; 3 pt ÷ 2 = 1.5 qt

4. 32 fl oz = 2 pt or 1 qt;
   the equivalent values are 1 pt = 16 fl oz or 1 qt = 2 pt

3 HOUSEHOLD CONVERSION

1. 3 oz = 6 T;
   the equivalent value is 3 oz × 2 = 6 T

2. 5 T = 15 t;
   the equivalent value is 1 T = 3 t

3. 3 c = 18 oz;
   the equivalent value is 1 c = 6 oz

4. 3 T = $1\frac{1}{2}$ oz;
   the equivalent value is 3 T ÷ 2 or $1\frac{1}{2}$ oz

5. 16 oz = 2 c;
   the equivalent value is 1 measuring cup= 8 oz

6. 12 t = 4 T;
   the equivalent value is 1 T = 3 t

4 SUMMARY: METRIC, APOTHECARY, AND HOUSEHOLD MEASUREMENTS

Metric

1. 2000 mg (1 g = 1000 mg)
   2 × 1000 mg = 2000 mg
   or 2.000 mg

   (three spaces to the right)

2. 1200 g

3. 5000 mcg (1 mg = 1000 mcg)

4. 2500 ml

5. 0.5 g (1000 mg = 1 g)
   500 ÷ 1000 = 0.5
   or 500. g = 0.5 g

   (three spaces to the left)

6. 10 mg

7. 2.4 g

8. 1.5 L

Apothecary

1. 10 pt

2. 32 fl oz

3. 40 fl oz (v = 5 [Roman numeral])

4. 24 fl oz

5. $\frac{1}{2}$ pt

6. $1\frac{1}{2}$ qt

7. $1\frac{1}{2}$ fl oz

8. 1 qt

Household

1. 40 oz

2. 9 t

3. 12 oz

4. 8 T

5. 5 T

6. $2\frac{1}{2}$ oz

Section 4B METHODS FOR CALCULATION

SECTION A

Objectives..................

- Select a formula—the basic formula, the ratio-and-proportion method, fractional equation, or dimensional analysis—for calculating drug dosages.
- Convert all measures to the same system and same unit of measure within the system before calculating drug dosage.
- Calculate drug dosage using one of the general formulas.
- Calculate drug dosage according to body weight and body surface area.
- Discuss meanings for abbreviations used in drug therapy.

Terms..................

The four general methods for the calculation of drug doses are the (1) basic formula, (2) ratio and proportion, (3) fractional equation, (4) and dimensional analysis. These methods are used to calculate oral and injectable drug doses. The nurse should select one of the methods to calculate drug doses and use that method consistently.

For drugs that require individualized dosing, calculation by body weight (BW) or by body surface area (BSA) may be necessary. In the past, these two methods (5) and (6) have been used for the calculation of pediatric dosage and for drugs used in the treatment of cancer (antineoplastic drugs). BW and BSA methods of calculation are especially useful for individuals whose BW is low, who are obese, or who are older adults.

Before calculating drug doses, all units of measure must be converted to a single system (see Section 4A). It is most helpful to convert to the system used on the drug label. If the drug is ordered in grains (gr) and the drug label gives the dose in milligrams (mg), then convert grains to milligrams (the measurement on the drug label) and proceed with the drug calculation. Table 4B–1 gives the metric and apothecary conversions most frequently used for dry and liquid measurements.

Again, if your nursing program prefers to use only the metric system for drug calculations, it will not be necessary for you to learn the conversion between metric and apothecary; however, conversion within the metric system—grams and milligrams—should be studied and remembered.

Interpreting Oral and Injectable Drug Labels

Pharmaceutical companies usually label their drugs with the brand name of the drug in large letters and the generic name in smaller letters. The dose per tablet, capsule, or liquid (for oral and injectable doses) is printed on the drug label. Two examples of drug labels are given below, the first for an oral drug and the second for an injectable drug.

Table 4B-1

Metric and Apothecary Conversions

Metric		Apothecary
Grams (g)	**Milligrams (mg)**	**Grains (gr)**
1	1000	15
0.5	500	$7\frac{1}{2}$
0.3	300 (325)	5
0.1	100	$1\frac{1}{2}$
0.06	60 (64)	1
0.03	30 (32)	$\frac{1}{2}$
0.015	15 (16)	$\frac{1}{4}$
0.010	10	$\frac{1}{8}$
0.0006	0.6	$\frac{1}{100}$
0.0004	0.4	$\frac{1}{150}$
0.0003	0.3	$\frac{1}{200}$
Liquid (Approximate)		
30 ml	=	1 oz (fl oz) = 2 tbsp (T) = 6 tsp (t)
15 ml	=	0.5 oz = 1 T = 3 t
1000 ml	=	1 quart (qt) = 1 liter (L)
500 ml	=	1 pint (pt)
5 ml	=	1 tsp (t)
4 ml	=	1 fl dr
1 ml	=	15 minims (♏) = 15 drops (gtt)

fl dr, Fluid dram; *fl oz*, fluid ounce; *ml*, milliliter; *tbsp*, tablespoon; *tsp*, teaspoon.

EXAMPLE 1
ORAL DRUG

Tagamet is the brand (trade) name, cimetidine is the generic name, and the dose is 200 mg/tablet.

EXAMPLE 2
INJECTABLE DRUG

Compazine is the brand (trade) name, prochlorperazine is the generic name, and the dose is 5 mg/ml injectable.

Method 1: Basic Formula (BF)

The **basic formula** is easy to recall and is most frequently used in calculating drug dosages. The basic formula is the following:

$$\frac{D}{H} \times V = A$$

where D is the desired dose (i.e., drug dose ordered by the health care provider),
H is the on-hand dose (i.e., drug dose on label of container [bottle, vial]),
V is the vehicle (i.e., drug form in which the drug comes [tablet, capsule, liquid]), and
A is the amount calculated to be given to the client.

EXAMPLES

1. Order: cefaclor (Ceclor) 0.5 g PO b.i.d.
   Available:

   a. The unit of measure that is ordered (grams) and the unit on the bottle (milligrams) are from the same system of measurement, the metric system. Conversion to the same unit is necessary to work the problem. Because the bottle is in milligrams, convert grams to milligrams.

   To convert grams (large value) to milligrams (smaller value), move the decimal point three spaces to the right (see Section 4A: Conversion Within the Metric System).

$$0.5 \text{ g} = 0.500 \text{ mg or } 500 \text{ mg}$$

   b. $\dfrac{D}{H} \times V = \dfrac{500 \text{ mg}}{250 \text{ mg}} \times 1 \text{ capsule} = \dfrac{500}{250} = 2 \text{ capsules}$

2. Order: codeine gr i (1) PO STAT
   Available:

   a. Grains must be converted to milligrams before the drug dose can be calculated (see Table 4A–4 or 4B–1). 1 gr = 60 mg

   b. $\dfrac{D}{H} \times V = \dfrac{60 \text{ mg}}{30 \text{ mg}} \times 1 \text{ tablet} = \dfrac{60}{30} = 2 \text{ tablets}$

SECTION B

Method 2: Ratio and Proportion (RP)

The **ratio-and-proportion** method is the oldest method currently used in the calculation of drug dosages. The formula is the following:

$$H \ : \ V \ :: \ D \ : \ x$$

Known   Desired

where *H* is the drug on hand (available),
V is the vehicle or drug form (tablet, capsule, liquid),
D is the desired dose (as ordered),
x is the unknown amount to give, and
:: stands for "as" or "equal to."

Multiply the means and the extremes. Solve for x; x is the divisor.

EXAMPLES

1. Order: amoxicillin (Amoxil) 100 mg PO q.i.d.
   Available:

   a. Conversion is not needed because both are expressed in the same unit of measure.

   b.
$$H \ : \ V \ :: \ D \ : \ x$$
   250 mg : 5 ml :: 100 mg : x ml

$$250x = 500$$
$$x = 2 \text{ ml}$$
   Answer: amoxicillin 100 mg = 2 ml

2. Order: aspirin/ASA gr *x* q4h PRN
   Available: aspirin 325 mg/tablet
   a. Convert to one system and unit of measure. Change grains to milligrams (see Table 4A-4 or 4B-1).

   b.
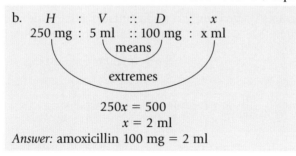

$$H \ : \ V \ :: \ D \ : \ x$$
   325 mg : 1 tab :: 600 (650) mg : x

$$325x = 600 \ (650)$$
$$x = 1.8 \text{ tablets or 2 tablets}$$
   (round off or use 650 instead of 600)
   Answer: Aspirin gr *x* = 2 tablets

Method 3: Fractional Equation (FE)

The **fractional equation** method is similar to ratio and proportion except it is written as a fraction.

$$\frac{H}{V} = \frac{D}{X} \qquad \frac{H}{V} \ \text{dosage on hand} = \frac{D}{X} \ \text{desired dosage}$$
Vehicle   unknown

Cross-multiply and solve for *x*.

EXAMPLES   Order: ciprofloxacin (Cipro) 500 mg PO q12h
               Available:

How many tablet(s) should the client receive per dose?
Answer:

$$\frac{H}{V} = \frac{D}{X} \qquad \frac{250 \text{ mg}}{1 \text{ ml}} = \frac{500 \text{ mg}}{X \text{ ml}}$$

Cross-multiply and solve for x.
$250x = 500$
$\qquad x = 2$ tablets of Cipro per dose

Method 4: Dimensional Analysis (DA)

Dimensional analysis (DA) is a calculation method known as units and conversions. The advantage of DA is that it decreases a number of steps required to calculate a drug dosage. It is set up as one equation.

1. Identify the unit/form (tablet, capsule, ml) of the drug to be calculated. If the drug comes in tablet, then tablet = (equal sign)
2. The known dose and unit/form from the **drug label** follows the equal sign.
   Order: Amoxicillin 500 mg
   On the drug label: 250 mg per 1 capsule

$$\text{capsule} = \frac{1 \text{ cap}}{250 \text{ mg}}$$

3. The mg (250 mg) is the *denominator* and it must match the next *numerator*, which is 500 mg (desired dose or order). The NEXT denominator would be 1 (one) or blank.

$$\text{capsule} = \frac{1 \text{ cap} \times 500 \text{ mg}}{250 \text{ mg} \times 1} =$$

4. Cancel out the mg, 250 and 500. What remains is the capsule and 2. Answer: 2 capsules.

   When conversion is needed between milligrams (drug label) and grams (order), then a conversion factor is needed, which appears *between* the drug dose on hand (drug label) and the desired dose (order). You should REMEMBER or CHECK the Metric and Apothecary Tables 4A–4 and 4B–1.

Metric Equivalent	Metric-Apothecary Equivalent
1 g = 1000 mg	1 g = 15 gr
1 mg = 1000 mcg	1000 mg = 15 gr
	1 gr = 60 mg

EXAMPLES   Order: Amoxicillin 0.5 g, PO, q8h

Available: 250 mg = 1 capsule (drug label). A conversion is needed between g and mg. Remember 250 mg is the denominator; therefore 1000 mg (conversion factor which is 1000 mg = 1 g) is the NEXT numerator and 1 g becomes the NEXT denominator. The third numerator is 0.5 g and the denominator is 1 (one) or blank.

$$\text{capsule} = \frac{1\ \text{cap} \times 1000\ \cancel{\text{mg}} \times 0.5\ \cancel{\text{g}}}{250\ \cancel{\text{mg}} \times 1\ \cancel{\text{g}} \times 1\ (\text{or blank})}$$
(Drug label) (Conversion) (Drug order)

If conversion from grams to milligrams is not needed, the middle step can be omitted. The following are formulas for dimensional analysis (DA):

$$\text{V (form of drug)} = \frac{\text{V (drug form)} \times \text{D (desired dose)}}{\text{H (on hand)} \times 1\ \text{or blank}}$$
(Drug label)   (Drug order)

$$\text{For conversion: V (form of drug)} = \frac{\text{V (drug form)} \times \text{C (H)} \times \text{D (desired dose)}}{\text{H (on hand)} \times \text{C (D)} \times 1\ \text{or blank}}$$
(Drug label) (Conversion factor) (Drug order)

As with other methods for calculation, the three components are D, H, and V. With dimensional analysis, the conversion factor is built into the equation and is included when the units of measurement of the drug order and the drug container differ. If the two are of the same units of measurement, the conversion factor is eliminated from the equation.

EXAMPLES   Order: acetaminophen (Tylenol) gr xv, PO, PRN
Available:

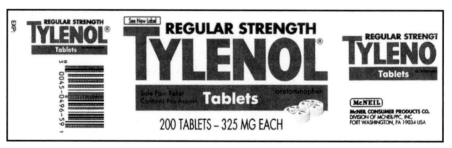

Factors: 325 mg = 1 tablet (from drug label)

15 gr/1 (from drug order)

Conversion factor: 1000 mg = 15 gr

How many tablet(s) should be given? _____

$$\text{tab} = \frac{1\ \text{tab} \times 1000\ \cancel{\text{mg}} \times \cancel{15}\ \cancel{\text{gr}}}{325\ \cancel{\text{mg}} \times \cancel{15}\ \cancel{\text{gr}} \times 1} = \frac{1000}{325} = 3.07\ \text{tab or 3 tab}$$

Method 5: Body Weight (BW)

The **body weight (BW)** method of calculation allows for the individualization of the drug dose and involves the following three steps:

1. Convert pounds to kilograms if necessary (lb ÷ 2.2 = kg).

2. Determine drug dose per BW by multiplying as follows:

   drug dose × body weight = client's dose per day

3. Follow the basic formula, ratio and proportion, fractional equation, or dimensional analysis method to calculate the drug dosage.

EXAMPLES

1. Order: fluorouracil (5-FU), 12 mg/kg/day IV, not to exceed 800 mg/day. The adult weighs 132 lb.

   a. Convert pounds to kilograms by dividing the number of pounds by 2.2 (1 kg = 2.2 lb).

      132 ÷ 2.2 = 60 kg

   b. mg × kg = client's dose

      12 × 60 = 720 mg IV/day

   Answer: fluorouracil 12 mg/kg/day = 720 mg

2. Order: cefaclor (Ceclor) 20 mg/kg/day in three divided doses. The child weighs 31 lb.

   Available:

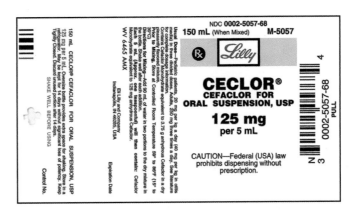

   a. Convert pounds to kilograms.

      31 ÷ 2.2 = 14 kg

   b. 20 mg × 14 kg = 280 mg/day

      280 mg ÷ 3 divided doses = 93 mg/dose

   c. BF: $\dfrac{D}{H} \times V' = \dfrac{93}{125} \times 5 = \dfrac{465}{125} = 3.7$ ml $\quad$ or $\quad$ DA: ml $\dfrac{5 \text{ ml} \times 93 \text{ mg}}{125 \text{ mg} \times 1} =$

   $\dfrac{465}{125} = 3.7$ ml

   or RP: $\quad \dot{H} \;:\; V \;::\; D \;:\; x$ $\qquad$ or $\qquad$ FE: $\dfrac{H}{V} = \dfrac{D}{x} \quad \dfrac{125}{5} = \dfrac{93}{X} =$

   $\qquad$ 125 mg : 5 ml :: 93 mg : x ml $\qquad\qquad$ cross-multiply $125x = 465$

   $\qquad\qquad 125x = 465$ $\qquad\qquad\qquad\qquad\qquad\qquad x = 3.7$ ml

   $\qquad\qquad x = \dfrac{465}{125} = 3.7$ ml

   Answer: cefaclor 20 mg/kg/day = 3.7 ml per dose

Method 6: Body Surface Area (BSA)

The **body surface area (BSA)** method is considered the most accurate way to calculate the drug dose for infants, children, older adults, and clients who are on antineoplastic agents or whose BW is low. The BSA, in square meters (m^2), is determined by where the person's height and weight intersect the nomogram scale (Figures 4B–1 [children] and 4B–2 [adults]). To calculate the drug dosage using the BSA method, multiply the drug dose ordered by the number of square meters.

$$100 \text{ mg} \times 1.8 \text{ m}^2 \text{ (BSA)} = 180 \text{ mg/day}$$

FIGURE 4B–1 West nomogram for infants and children. Directions: *(1)* Find height. *(2)* Find weight. *(3)* Draw a straight line that connects the height and weight. *(4)* Where the line intersects on the surface area column is the body surface area (m²). (Modified from data by Boyd E, West CD. In Behrman RE, Kliegman RM, Jensen HB: *Nelson textbook of pediatrics*, ed 18, Philadelphia, 2007, Saunders.)

EXAMPLES

1. Order: cyclophosphamide (Cytoxan) 100 mg/m²/day, IV
   Available:

HEIGHT **BODY SURFACE AREA** **WEIGHT**

FIGURE 4B–2 Nomogram of body surface area for adults. Directions: *(1)* Find height. *(2)* Find weight. *(3)* Draw a straight line that connects the height and weight. *(4)* Where the line intersects on the body surface area column is the body surface area (m²). (From Deglin JH, Vallerand AH, Russin A: *Davis's drug guide for nurses*, ed 2, Philadelphia, 1991, FA Davis; Lentner C, editor: *Geigy scientific tables*, ed 8, vol 1, Basel, Switzerland, 1981, Ciba-Geigy, pp. 226-227.)

Client is 70 inches tall and weighs 160 lb.
a. 70 inches and 160 lb intersect the nomogram scale at 1.97 m² (BSA).
b. 100 mg × 1.97 = 197 mg.
Answer: Administer cyclophosphamide 197 mg or 200 mg/day.
2. Order: mephenytoin (Mesantoin) 200 mg/m² PO in three divided doses. Child is 42 inches tall and weighs 44 lb.
a. 42 inches and 44 lb intersect the nomogram scale at 0.8 m².
b. 200 mg × 0.8 = 160 mg/day or 50 mg (53) t.i.d.
Answer: Administer mephenytoin 50 mg t.i.d.

BSA with the Square Root

BSA can be calculated by using the square root and a fractional formula of height and weight divided by a constant. Now that calculators are readily available, research has shown that this method results in fewer errors than drawing intersecting lines on a nomogram.

The formula for BSA using the square root is

$$BSA = \sqrt{\frac{\text{height (inches)} \times \text{wt (lb)}}{3131 \text{ (constant)}}}$$

EXAMPLE Order: melphalan (Alkeran) 16 mg/m² q 2 weeks. Client is 68 inches tall and weighs 172 lb. Use the BSA inches and pounds formula.

a. $BSA = \sqrt{\dfrac{68 \text{ in} \times 172 \text{ lb}}{3131}}$

$BSA = \sqrt{\dfrac{11696}{3131}}$

$BSA = \sqrt{3.73}$

$BSA = 1.9 \text{ m}^2$

b. 16 mg 3 1.9 m² 5 30.4 mg/m² or 30 mg/m². Client should receive 30 mg every 2 weeks.

PRACTICE PROBLEM I

DRUG DOSAGE USING BASIC FORMULA, RATIO AND PROPORTION, OR FRACTIONAL EQUATION

Solve the problem and determine the drug dose given the following:

1. Order: cimetidine (Tagamet) 0.4 g PO, q6h
   Available:

   How many tablet(s) of Tagamet should the client receive? _____

2. Order: doxycycline hyclate (Vibra-Tab), PO, initially 200 mg; then 50 mg, PO, b.i.d.
   Drug available:

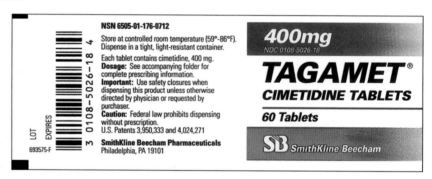

   a. How many tablet(s) would you give as the initial dose? _____
   b. How many tablets would you give for each dose after the initial dose? _____

3. Order: phenobarbital gr ½ PO, t.i.d.
   Available: phenobarbital 15-mg tablet
   How many tablet(s) should the client receive? _____

4. Order: hydrochlorothiazide (HydroDIURIL) 25 mg PO, daily
   Available:

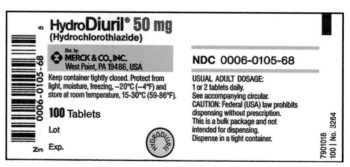

   How many tablet(s) should the client receive? _____

5. Order: cefadroxil (Duricef) 500 mg PO, b.i.d.
   Available:

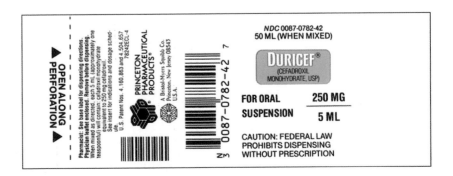

How many milliliters should the client receive? _____

6. Order: dicloxacillin 100 mg PO, q8h
   Available: dicloxacillin 62.5 mg/5 ml
   How many milliliters should the client receive? _____

7. Order: meperidine (Demerol) 35 mg IM STAT
   Available:

How many milliliters should the client receive? _____

8. Order: atropine sulfate gr $\frac{1}{200}$ SC on call
   Available: atropine sulfate 0.4 mg/1 ml

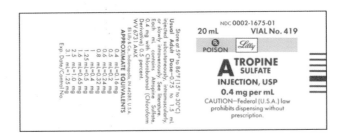

How many milliliters should the client receive? _____

DRUG DOSAGE USING DIMENSIONAL ANALYSIS

9. Order: ampicillin (Principen) 50 mg/kg/day PO in four divided doses (q6h). Client weighs 88 pounds, or 40 kg (88 ÷ 2.2 = 40 kg).
   Available:

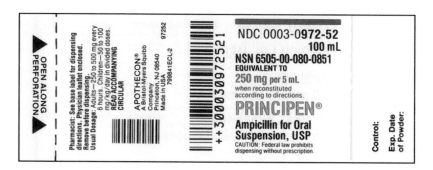

Factors: 250 mg = 5 ml (drug label)
Conversion factor: none (both are in milligrams)
a. How many milligrams per day should the client receive? _____
b. How many milligrams per dose should the client receive? _____
c. How many milliliters should the client receive per dose? _____

10. Order: Codeine gr i (1) PO, STAT
    Available:

Factors: 30 mg = 1 tablet (drug label)
Conversion factor: 1 gr = 60 mg
How many tablet(s) should be given? _____

11. Order: Ciprofloxacin (Cipro) 0.5 g, PO, b.i.d.
    Available:

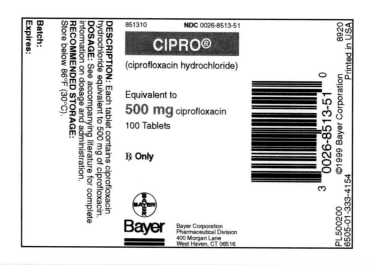

How many tablets should the client receive per dose? _____

PRACTICE PROBLEM 3

DRUG DOSAGE USING BODY WEIGHT

12. Order: sulfisoxazole (Gantrisin) 50 mg/kg/day PO in four divided doses (q6h). Child weighs 44 lb.
    How many mg should the client receive per day? _____ Per dose? _____

13. Order: albuterol (Proventil) 0.1 mg/kg/day PO in four divided doses. Client weighs 86 lb.
    How many mg should the client receive per dose? _____

14. Order: cefprozil (Cefzil) 15 mg/kg/day PO in two divided doses. Child weighs 33 lb.
    Available:

    a. How many milligrams should be given per day? _____
    b. How many milliliters should the child receive per dose? _____

PRACTICE PROBLEM 4

DRUG DOSAGE USING BODY SURFACE AREA

15. Client is 62 inches tall and weighs 130 lb. What is the BSA? _____

16. Order: bleomycin sulfate 20 units/m² IV. Client is 70 inches tall and weighs 160 lb.
    How many unit(s) should the client receive? ___

17. Order: sulfisoxazole (Gantrisin) 2 g/m² in four divided doses. Child is 50 inches tall and weighs 60 lb.
    Available: sulfisoxazole 500 mg/5 ml
    a. What is the child's BSA? _____
    b. How many gram(s) should the child receive per day? _____
    c. How many milliliters should the child receive per dose? _____

ANSWERS TO PRACTICE PROBLEMS

I **DRUG DOSAGE USING BASIC FORMULA, RATIO AND PROPORTION, OR FRACTIONAL EQUATION**

1. **a.** Convert grams to milligrams by moving the decimal point three spaces to the right.

   $0.4 \text{ g} = 0.400 \text{ mg}$

   b. BF: $\dfrac{D}{H} \times V = \dfrac{400 \text{ mg}}{400 \text{ mg}} \times 1 \text{ tablet} = 1 \text{ tablet}$

2. **a.** Initially:

   BF: $\dfrac{D}{H} \times V = \dfrac{\overset{2}{200}}{\underset{1}{100}} \times 1 = 2 \text{ tablets}$

   or

   RP: $H \quad : \quad V \quad :: \quad D \quad : \quad x$

   $\quad$ 100 mg : 1 tab :: 200 mg : x

   $\quad\quad\quad 100x = 200$

   $\quad\quad\quad\quad\quad x = 2 \text{ tablets}$

   or

   FE (cross-multiply):

   $\dfrac{100}{1} = \dfrac{200}{x} =$

   $\quad 100x = 200$

   $\quad\quad\quad x = 2 \text{ tablets}$

   or

   DA: No conversion factor

   Tablet(s) $= \dfrac{1 \times \overset{2}{200}}{\underset{1}{100} \times 1} = 2 \text{ tablets}$

   b. Daily: RP: $\quad H \quad : \quad V \quad :: \quad D \quad : \quad x$

   $\quad\quad$ 100 mg : 1 tab :: 50 mg : x

   $\quad\quad\quad\quad 100x = 50$

   $\quad\quad\quad\quad\quad\quad x = \frac{1}{2} \text{ tablet}$

   or

   DA: No conversion factor

   Tablet(s) $= \dfrac{1 \text{ tab} \times \overset{1}{50} \text{ mg}}{\underset{1}{100} \text{ mg} \times 1} = \frac{1}{2} \text{ tablet}$

3. **a.** Covert grains to milligrams. Table 4A-4 or 4B-1 gives 30 mg = ½ gr, or 60 mg = 1 gr

   $\quad$ 60 mg : 1 gr :: x mg : ½ gr

   $\quad\quad\quad 100x = 60 \times 0.5 \ (\frac{1}{2})$

   $\quad\quad\quad\quad\quad x = 30 \text{ mg}$

   b. RP: $\quad H \quad : V \quad :: \quad D \quad : \quad x$

   $\quad\quad$ 15 mg : 1 :: 30 mg : x

   $\quad\quad\quad\quad 15x = 30$

   $\quad\quad\quad\quad\quad x = 2 \text{ tablets}$

4. ½ tablet

5. 10 ml

6. FE: $\dfrac{H}{V} = \dfrac{D}{x} \quad \dfrac{62.5 \text{ mg}}{5 \text{ ml}} = \dfrac{100 \text{ mg}}{x \text{ ml}}$

   $62.5x = 500$

   $x = 8 \text{ ml}$

7. 0.7 ml

8. **a.** The drug level shows 0.4 mg = 1 ml. Change $^1/_{200}$ gr to milligrams (see Table 4A-4 or 4B-1). $^1/_{200}$ gr = 0.3 mg

   b. BF: $\dfrac{D}{H} \times V = \dfrac{0.3}{0.4} \times 1 \text{ ml} = 0.4\overline{)0.3.0}^{\,0.75} = 0.75 \text{ ml}$

   or

   RP: $\quad H \quad : \quad V \quad :: \quad D \quad : x$

   $\quad\quad$ 0.4 mg : 1 ml :: 0.3 mg : x

   $\quad\quad\quad\quad 0.4x = 0.3 = 0.75 \text{ ml}$

2 **DRUG DOSAGE USING DIMENSIONAL ANALYSIS**

9. **a.** 50 mg/kg/day = 50 × 40 = 2000 mg

   b. 2000 mg ÷ 4 = 500 mg per dose

   c. ml $= \dfrac{5 \text{ ml} \times \overset{2}{500} \text{ mg}}{\underset{1}{250} \text{ mg} \times 1} = \dfrac{10}{1} = 10 \text{ ml}$

10. Tablets $= \dfrac{1 \text{ tab} \times \overset{2}{60} \text{ mg} \times 1 \text{ gr}}{\underset{1}{30} \text{ mg} \times 1 \text{ gr} \times 1} = 2 \text{ tablets}$

11. tab $= \dfrac{1 \text{ tab} \times \overset{2}{1000} \text{ mg} \times 0.5 \text{ g}}{\underset{1}{500} \text{ mg} \times 1 \text{ g} \times 1} = 1 \text{ tablet}$

3 **DRUG DOSAGE USING BODY WEIGHT**

12. **a.** 44 lb ÷ 2.2 kg = 20 kg

   b. 50 mg × 20 kg = 1000 mg/day

   $\quad$ 1000 ÷ 4 times a day = 250 mg q.i.d., or q6h

13. **a.** 86 ÷ 2.2 = 39 kg

   b. 0.1 mg × 39 = 3.9 mg, or 4 mg

   $\quad$ 4 ÷ 4 = 1 mg q6h

14. 33 ÷ 2.2 = 15 kg

   15 mg × 15 = 225 mg/day

   225 ÷ 2 times a day = 112.5 mg, q12h per dose

   $\dfrac{D}{H} \times V = \dfrac{112.5}{125} \times 5 \text{ ml} = \dfrac{562.5}{125} = 4.5 \text{ ml q12}$

   a. Administer cefprozil 225 mg/day

   b. Administer 112.5 mg = 4.5 ml, q12h

4 DRUG DOSAGE USING BODY SURFACE AREA

15. 1.65 m²

16. a. Client's height and weight intersect the nomogram scale at 1.97 m².

    b. 20 Unit × 1.97 = 39.4 or 39 Unit

17. a. Height and weight intersect the nomogram scale at 0.98 m².

    b. 2 g × 0.98 = 1.96 g, or 2 g/day

    c. 5 ml (convert grams to milligrams.

        0.5 g = 0.500 mg

Section 4C   CALCULATIONS OF ORAL DOSAGES

Outline

Objectives

Terms

Tablets, Capsules, and Liquids

Interpreting Oral Drug Labels

Drug Differentiation
Preventing Medication Errors

Calculation for Tablet, Capsule, and Liquid Doses

Body Weight and Body Surface Area

Drugs Administered via Nasogastric Tube

Objectives

- Calculate oral dosages from tablets, capsules, and liquids with selected formula.
- Calculate oral medications according to body weight and body surface area.
- Calculate the amount of tube feeding solution needed for dilution according to the percentage ordered.

Terms

Eighty percent of all drugs consumed are given orally. Oral drugs are available in tablet, capsule, powder, and liquid form. The written abbreviation for drugs given orally is P.O. or PO (per *os*, or *by mouth*). Oral medications are absorbed by the gastrointestinal (GI) tract, mainly from the small intestine.

Oral medications have the following advantages: (1) the client frequently can take oral medications without assistance, (2) the cost of oral medications is usually less than when given via other routes (e.g., parenteral), and (3) oral medications are easy to store. The disadvantages include (1) variation in absorption as a result of food in the GI tract and pH variation of GI secretions, (2) irritation of the gastric mucosa by certain drugs (e.g., potassium chloride), and (3) destruction or partial inactivation of the drugs by liver enzymes. This section discusses oral dosages for adults; Section 4F discusses oral dosages for children.

Tablets, Capsules, and Liquids

Tablets come in different forms and drug strengths. Most tablets are scored and thus can be readily broken when half of the drug amount is needed. **Capsules** are gelatin shells that contain powder or time-release pellets (beads). **Sustained-release** (pellet) capsules and controlled-release capsules *should not* be crushed and diluted, because the medication will be absorbed at a much faster rate than indicated by the manufacturer. Many medications that are in tablet form are also available in liquid form. When the client has difficulty taking tablets, the liquid form of the medication is given. The liquid form can be in a suspension, syrup, elixir, or tincture. Some liquid medications that irritate the stomach, such as potassium chloride, are diluted. The tincture form is always diluted.

Enteric-coated (hard shell) tablets *must* not be crushed, because the medication could irritate the gastric mucosa. Enteric-coated drugs pass through the stomach into the small intestine where the drug's coating dissolves and then absorption occurs. Oral drugs (tablets, capsules, liquids) that irritate the gastric mucosa should be taken with 5 to 8 ounces of fluids or taken with food. Figure 4C–1 shows the different forms of tablets and capsules.

Liquid medications are poured into a medicine cup that is calibrated in ounces, teaspoons, tablespoons, and milliliters. Figure 4C–2 shows the markings on a medicine cup.

Interpreting Oral Drug Labels

Pharmaceutical companies usually label their drugs with the brand (trade) name of the drug in large letters and the generic name in smaller letters. The dose per tablet, capsule, or liquid is often printed under the drug name.

EXAMPLES   Ceftin is the brand (trade) name, and cefuroxime axetil is the generic name. The dose is 125 mg/5 ml (oral suspension).

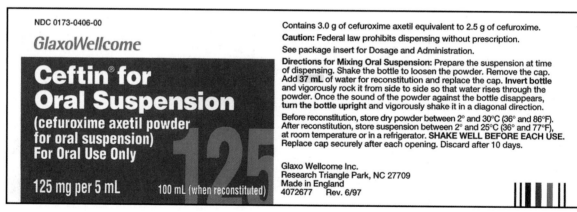

NDC 0173-0406-00

GlaxoWellcome

Ceftin® for Oral Suspension
(cefuroxime axetil powder for oral suspension)
For Oral Use Only

125 mg per 5 mL   100 mL (when reconstituted)

Contains 3.0 g of cefuroxime axetil equivalent to 2.5 g of cefuroxime.
Caution: Federal law prohibits dispensing without prescription.
See package insert for Dosage and Administration.
Directions for Mixing Oral Suspension: Prepare the suspension at time of dispensing. Shake the bottle to loosen the powder. Remove the cap. Add **37 mL** of water for reconstitution and replace the cap. **Invert bottle and vigorously rock it from side to side** so that water rises through the powder. Once the sound of the powder against the bottle disappears, turn the bottle upright and vigorously shake it in a diagonal direction.
Before reconstitution, store dry powder between 2° and 30°C (36° and 86°F). After reconstitution, store suspension between 2° and 25°C (36° and 77°F), at room temperature or in a refrigerator. **SHAKE WELL BEFORE EACH USE.** Replace cap securely after each opening. Discard after 10 days.

Glaxo Wellcome Inc.
Research Triangle Park, NC 27709
Made in England
4072677   Rev. 6/97

FIGURE 4C–1   Shapes of tablets and capsules. A and B, Tablets; C and D, capsules.

FIGURE 4C–2   Medicine cup for liquid measurement. (From Kee JL, Marshall SM: *Clinical calculations,* ed 6, St. Louis, 2009, Saunders.)

Drug Differentiation

Preventing Medication Errors

Some drugs' spellings look alike or sound alike but have different chemical drug structures and are prescribed for different health problems. When ordering drugs, make sure the spelling of the drug is correct, and be extremely careful when administering drugs whose names look alike. Caution: Physicians' handwriting of drug names.

EXAMPLE 1
QUINIDINE AND QUININE

Quinidine is an antiarrhythmic drug, and quinine is an antimalarial drug. Read drug label three times before pouring the drug.

EXAMPLE 2
CELEBREX, CELEXA, AND CEREBYX

All three drugs are brand drugs and have a similar spelling. Celebrex (celecoxib) is an analgesic, a cyclo-oxygenase 2 (COX-2) inhibitor; Celexa (citalopram) is an antidepressant, a selective serotonin reuptake (SSR) inhibitor; and Cerebyx (fosphenytoin sodium) is an anticonvulsant.

EXAMPLE 3
PERCODAN AND PERCOCET

Percodan contains oxycodone and aspirin, and Percocet contains oxycodone and acetaminophen. A client may be allergic to aspirin or should not take aspirin because of a stomach ulcer; therefore it is important that the client take Percocet. *Read the drug labels carefully.*

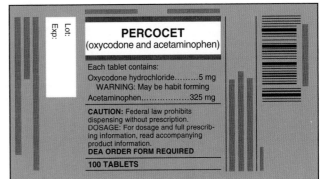

SECTION C

EXAMPLE 4
HYDROXYZINE AND HYDRALAZINE

Hydroxyzine is an antianxiety drug, and hydralazine is an antihypertensive drug.

Calculation for Tablet, Capsule, and Liquid Doses

When calculating oral dosages, choose one of the methods for calculation from Section 4B.

1. Order: diltiazem (Cardizem) 60 mg PO, b.i.d.
   Available:

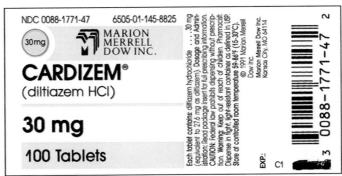

How many tablets would you give? ____

a. BF: $\dfrac{D}{H} \times V = \dfrac{60}{30} \times 1 = 2$ tablets

b. RP:

H	:	V	::	D	:	x
30 mg	:	1 tab	::	60 mg	:	x tab

$$30x = 60$$
$$x = 2 \text{ tablets}$$

Answer: diltiazem (Cardizem) 60 mg = 2 tablets

c. FE: $\dfrac{H}{V} = \dfrac{D}{x}$ $\dfrac{30}{1} \times \dfrac{60}{x}$ (cross multiply) = $30x = 60$
                                 $x = 2$ tablets

d. DA: $\text{tab} = \dfrac{1 \text{ tab} \times \overset{2}{60} \text{ mg}}{\underset{1}{30} \text{ mg} \times 1} = 2$ tablets

Conversion is not needed.

2. Order: codeine phosphate 1 gr PO, STAT
   Available: See the conversion Tables 4A-4 or 4B-1.

How many tablets would you give? _____

a. BF: gr 1 = 60 mg

$$\dfrac{D}{H} \times V = \dfrac{60}{30} \times 1 = 2 \text{ tablets}$$

b. FE: $\dfrac{H}{v} = \dfrac{D}{x}$ $\dfrac{30}{1} = \dfrac{60}{x} =$

$$30x = 60$$
$$x = 2 \text{ tablets}$$

c. DA: $\text{tablet} = \dfrac{1 \times \overset{2}{60} \text{ mg} \times 1 \text{ gr}}{\underset{1}{30} \text{ mg} \times 1 \text{ gr} \times 1} = 2$ tablets

Answer: codeine 1 gr = 2 tablets

3. Order: clarithromycin (Biaxin) 100 mg, PO q6h
   Available:

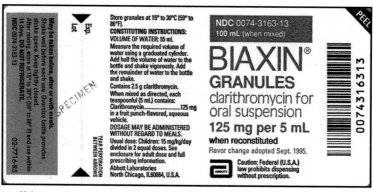

How many milliliters should the client receive per dose? _____

a. BF: $\dfrac{D}{H} \times V = \dfrac{100}{\overset{}{\underset{25}{125}}} = \dfrac{\overset{1}{\cancel{5}}}{} = 4 \text{ ml}$

or

b. RP: H : V :: D : V
125 : 5 :: 100 : x
125x = 500
x = 4 ml

or

c. DA: ml $\dfrac{5 \text{ ml} \times \overset{4}{\cancel{100}} \text{ mg}}{\underset{5}{\cancel{125}} \text{ mg} \times 1} = \dfrac{20}{5} = 4 \text{ ml}$

PRACTICE PROBLEM 1

ORAL MEDICATIONS

Solve the drug problems for x, the unknown amount of drug to be given. See Sections 4A and 4B for the conversion tables, methods of conversion, and the method chosen to solve the drug problems.

1. Order: doxepin HCl (Sinequan) 30 mg PO, at bedtime.
   Available:

   How many capsule(s) should the client receive? _____
2. Order: lisinopril (Zestril) 5 mg PO, daily.
   Available:

   How many tablets should the client receive? _____
3. Order: aspirin gr *x* STAT
   Available: aspirin 325 mg tablet
   How many tablet(s) of aspirin should the nurse give? _____
4. Order: digoxin (Lanoxin) 0.5 mg PO, daily.
   Available:

   How many tablet(s) should the nurse administer? _____

5. Order: nitroglycerin (Nitrostat) $^1/_{150}$ gr sublingual STAT
   Available:

   How many sublingual tablet(s) should the client take? _____

6. Order: bethanechol Cl (Urecholine) 20 mg PO, t.i.d.
   Available:

   a. Which Urecholine bottle should the nurse select? _____
   b. How many tablet(s) should the client receive per dose? _____

7. Order: amoxicillin clavulanate (Augmentin) 500 mg PO, b.i.d.
   Available:

   How many milliliters should the client receive per dose? _____

8. Order: cefadroxil (Duricef) 500 mg PO, b.i.d.
    Available:

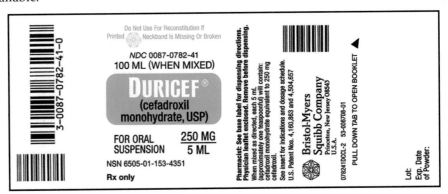

How many milliliters should the client receive per dose? _____

9. Order: prazosin (Minipress) 10 mg PO, daily.
    Available: prazosin 1-mg, 2-mg, and 5-mg tablets
    Which tablet should be selected and how much should be given? _____

10. Order: carbidopa-levodopa (Sinemet) 12.5-125 mg PO, b.i.d.
    Available: Sinemet 25- to 100-, 25- to 250-, 10- to 100-mg tablets
    Which tablet should be selected and how much should be given? _____

Additional Dimensional Analysis

11. Order: omeprazole (Prilosec) 20 mg PO, daily.
    Available:

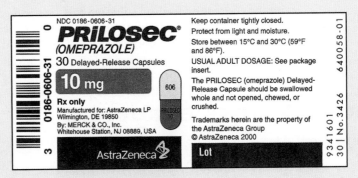

Factors: 10 mg = 1 capsule (drug label)
Conversion factor: none (both are in milligrams)
How many capsule(s) should the client receive? _____

12. Order: amoxicillin (Amoxil) 0.1 g PO, q8h
    Available:

Factors: 200 mg = 5 ml (drug label)
Conversion factor: 1000 mg = 1 g
How many milliliters should the client receive per dose? _____

Body Weight and Body Surface Area

Calculating the drug dosage for adults by body weight (BW) and body surface area (BSA) is used mostly when administering drugs to treat cancer (antineoplastic drugs). These two individualized methods are also used frequently to calculate drug dosages for children. Examples and practice problems for pediatrics are given in Section 4F.

To use the body weight method, convert the person's weight in pounds to kilograms (kg). To convert, divide pounds by 2.2 to equal kilograms. To use the **body surface area (BSA)** method, the person's weight and height and a nomogram are needed. (See Sections 4B and 4F). Daily requirements are usually divided into two to four doses per day.

EXAMPLE

1. Order: cyclophosphamide (Cytoxan) 2 mg/kg PO daily. Client weighs 143 lb.
How much does the client weigh in kilograms? _____ How many milligrams (mg) should the client receive? _____
Answer: 143 lb ÷ 2.2 = 65 kg
2 mg × 65 = 130 mg of cyclophosphamide daily

PRACTICE PROBLEM 2

BODY WEIGHT

1. Order: valproic acid (Depakene) 8 mg/kg/day in four divided doses. Client weighs 165 lb.
How much Depakene should be administered per dose? _____
2. Order: cyclophosphamide (Cytoxan) 4 mg/kg/day. Client weighs 176 lb.
How much Cytoxan should the client receive per day? _____

Drugs Administered via Nasogastric Tube

Oral medications can be administered through a nasogastric tube but should not be mixed with the entire **tube feeding** solution. Mixing the medications in a large volume of tube feeding solution decreases the amount of drug the client receives for a specific time. The medication (NOT time-released or sustained-release capsules and psyllium hydrophilic mucilloid [Metamucil]) should be diluted in 1 ounce (30 ml) of warm water *unless otherwise instructed*, administered through the tube, and followed with extra water to ensure that the drug reaches the stomach and is not left in the tube.

ANSWERS TO PRACTICE PROBLEMS

I **ORAL MEDICATIONS USING BASIC FORMULA, RATIO AND PROPORTION, FRACTIONAL EQUATION, OR DIMENSIONAL ANALYSIS**

1. 3 capsules of Sinequan
2. 2 tablets of Zestril
3. Convert grains to milligrams. See Tables 4A-4 or 4B-1.

5 gr = 300, or 325 mg; thus 10 gr = 650 mg (approximate value)

a. BF: $\dfrac{D}{H} \times V = \dfrac{650}{325} \times 1 = 2$ tablets

or

b. RP: $H \quad : \quad V \quad :: \quad D \quad : \quad x$
325 mg : 1 tab :: 650 mg : x tab
$325x = 650$
$x = 2$ tablets

c. DA: $\text{tab} = \dfrac{1 \quad \times 1000\ \cancel{mg} \times \overset{2}{\cancel{10}}\ \cancel{gr}}{325\ \cancel{mg} \times \underset{3}{\cancel{15}}\ \cancel{gr} \times 1}$

$\dfrac{2000}{975} = 2.05$ or tab

4. 2 tablets

a. BF: $\dfrac{D}{H} \times V = \dfrac{0.5}{0.25} \times 1 = 0.25\overline{)0.50\,0}^{\,2.0} = 2$ tablets

or

b. RP: $H \quad : \quad V \quad :: \quad D \quad : \quad x$
0.25 mg : 1 tab :: 0.5 mg : x tab
$0.25x = 0.5 = 2$ tablets

c. DA: $\text{tab} = \dfrac{1 \quad \times 0.5\ \cancel{mg}}{0.25\ \cancel{mg} \times 1} := 2$ tablets

5. 1 sublingual tablet
Convert grains to milligrams. $^1/_{150}$ gr = 0.4 mg

6. a. Select Urecholine 10 mg bottle.

b. BF: $\dfrac{D}{H} \times V = \dfrac{20\ \cancel{mg}}{10\ \cancel{mg}} \times 1\ \text{tab} = \dfrac{20}{10} = 2$ tablets

or

DA: $\text{tab} = \dfrac{1 \quad \times 20 \ \cancel{mg}}{10 \ \cancel{mg} \times \quad 1} = 2 \text{ tablets}$

no conversion needed

7. 20 ml of Augmentin suspension

8. 10 ml of cefadroxil

    a. BF: $\dfrac{D}{H} \times V = \dfrac{500}{250} \times 5 = \dfrac{2500}{250} = 10 \text{ ml}$

    b. FE: $\dfrac{H}{V} = \dfrac{D}{x} = \dfrac{250 \text{ mg}}{5 \text{ ml}} = \dfrac{500 \text{ mg}}{x \text{ ml}}$

                       $250x = 2500$

                          $x = 10 \text{ ml}$

    c. DA: $\text{ml} = \dfrac{5 \text{ ml} \quad \times \overset{2}{\cancel{500}} \ \cancel{mg}}{\underset{1}{\cancel{250}} \ \cancel{mg} \times \quad 1} = 10 \text{ ml}$

9. Select 5 mg tablets. Give two tablets.

10. Select 25–250 mg strength. Give half a tablet.

11. 2 capsules

    $\text{capsules} = \dfrac{1 \text{ cap} \ \times \overset{2}{20} \ \cancel{mg}}{\underset{1}{\cancel{10}} \ \cancel{mg} \times \quad 1} = 2 \text{ capsules}$

12. 2.5 ml per dose

    $\text{ml} = \dfrac{5 \text{ ml} \times \overset{5}{\cancel{1000}} \ \cancel{mg} \times 0.1 \ \cancel{g}}{\underset{1}{\cancel{200}} \ \cancel{mg} \times \quad 1 \ \cancel{g} \quad \times 1}$

    $= 2.5 \text{ ml per dose}$

---

2   BODY WEIGHT

1. 75 kg; 150 mg/dose; 600 mg/day

2. 80 kg; 320 mg/day

Section 4D   CALCULATIONS OF INJECTABLE DOSAGES

Outline

Objectives

Terms

Injectable Preparations

Vials and Ampules

Syringes
Prefilled Drug Cartridges and Syringes

Needles

Interpreting Injectable Drug Labels

Intradermal Injections

Subcutaneous Injections
Calculations: Subcutaneous Injections

Insulin Injections
Types of Insulins
Mixing Insulins

Intramuscular Injections
Drug Solutions for Injection
Powdered Drug Reconstitution
Mixing Injectable Drugs

Objectives

- Describe the difference between vials and ampules.
- Describe the types of syringes and needles and their uses.
- Explain how to administer intradermal, subcutaneous, and intramuscular injections.
- Calculate dosage of drugs for subcutaneous and intramuscular injections.
- Identify the amount of insulin dosage with the use of an insulin syringe.
- Explain the methods for mixing two insulins in one insulin syringe and for mixing two injectable drugs in one syringe.
- Describe the procedure for the preparation and calculation of medications in powdered form for injectable use.

Terms..

....

When medications cannot be taken by mouth because of (1) an inability to swallow, (2) a decreased level of consciousness, (3) an inactivation of the drug by gastric juices, or (4) a desire to increase the effectiveness of the drug, the parenteral route may be the route of choice. **Parenteral** medications are administered intradermally (under the skin), subcutaneously (into the fatty tissue), intramuscularly (IM, within the muscle), and intravenously (IV, in the vein). IV injectables are discussed in Section 4E. The injectables in this section include intradermal, subQ (including insulin and heparin), and IM from prepared liquid and reconstituted powder in vials and ampules. Prefilled drug cartridges (syringes) are also discussed.

This section is divided into five parts: (1) injectable preparations, (2) intradermal injections, (3) subQ injections, (4) insulin injections, and (5) IM injections. Examples and practice problems to solve for the correct dosage are provided.

Injectable Preparations

The appropriate drug container (vial or ampule) and the correct selection of needle and syringe are essential in the preparation of the prescribed drug dose. The route of administration is part of the medication order.

Vials and Ampules

A **vial** is usually a small glass container with a self-sealing rubber top. Some are multiple-dose vials, and when properly stored, they can be used over time. An **ampule** is a glass container with a tapered neck for snapping open and using only once. Drugs that deteriorate readily in liquid form are packaged in powder form in vials and ampules for storage. Once the dry form of the drug is reconstituted (usually with sterile water, bacteriostatic water, or saline), the drug is used immediately or must be refrigerated. Check the accompanying drug circular for specific storage length and other instructions. The person reconstituting the drug should write on the label when the drug is to be discarded and include her or his initials. Usually a vial should be used within 96 hours.

Drug labels on vials and ampules provide the following information: (1) generic and brand name of the drug, (2) drug dose in weight (milligrams, grams, milliequivalents) and amount (milliliters), (3) expiration date, and (4) directions about administration. If the drug is in powdered form, mixing instructions and dose equivalents (e.g., milligrams equal milliliters) may be given. Figure 4D–1 is a diagram of a vial and ampule.

Syringes

The syringe is composed of a barrel (outer shell), plunger (inner part), and the tip where the needle joins the syringe (Figure 4D–2). Syringes are available in various types and sizes, the most common of which are the 3-ml and 5-ml tuberculin, insulin, and metal and plastic syringes for prefilled cartridges. Glass syringes may be used in the operating room and on special instrument trays. The tip of the syringe and inside of the plunger should remain sterile.

The 3-ml syringe is calibrated in tenths (0.1 ml) and minims. The amount of fluid in the syringe is determined by the black rubber end of the plunger (the inner end of the plunger) that is closest to the tip (Figure 4D–3). REMEMBER: Milliliter (ml) and cubic centimeter (cc) may be used interchangeably, but milliliter (ml) is preferred. An advance in safety needle technology is

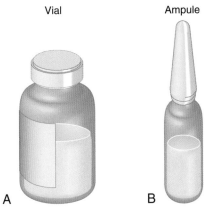

FIGURE 4D–1 A, Vial. B, Ampule. (From Kee JL, Marshall SM: *Clinical calculations*, ed 6, Philadelphia, 2009, Saunders.)

FIGURE 4D–2 Parts of a syringe. (From Kee JL, Marshall SM: *Clinical calculations*, ed 6, Philadelphia, 2009, Saunders.)

FIGURE 4D–3 A 3-ml syringe. (From Kee JL, Marshall SM: *Clinical calculations*, ed 6, Philadelphia, 2009, Saunders.)

the SafetyGlide shielding hypodermic needle (Figure 4D–4). This type of needle reduces needlestick injuries.

The 5-ml syringe is calibrated in 0.2-ml marks. A 5-ml syringe is usually used when the fluid needed is more than 2.5 ml. It is frequently used when reconstituting the dry drug form with sterile bacteriostatic water or saline. The needleless syringes are used primarily for intermittent infusion therapy to irrigate the intermittent infusion device for maintaining patency and to administer IV medication through the IV tubing device. See intermittent infusion adapters/devices in Section E. Figure 4D–5 shows the 5-ml syringe and 5-ml needleless syringe.

The **tuberculin syringe** is a 1-ml slender syringe with markings in tenths (0.1) and hundredths (0.01). It is also marked in minims (Figure 4D–6). This syringe is used when the amount of drug solution to be administered is less than 1 ml and for pediatric and heparin dosages. The tuberculin syringe is also available in a 0.5-ml syringe. Figure 4D–7 illustrates the 0.5-ml and 1-ml tuberculin syringes.

The **insulin syringe** has the capacity of 1 ml; however, insulin is measured in units, and insulin dosage *must not* be calculated in milliliters. Insulin syringes are calibrated as 2-unit marks, and 100 units equal 1 ml (Figure 4D–8). *Insulin syringes must be used for the administration of insulin.*

Insulin syringes are available as low-dose insulin syringes. The 1-ml insulin syringe may be purchased with a permanent attached needle or a detachable needle (Figure 4D–9).

Prefilled Drug Cartridges and Syringes

Many injectable drugs are packaged in prefilled, disposable cartridges. The disposable cartridge is placed into a Tubex injector or a reusable metal or plastic holder. Usually the prefilled cartridge contains 0.1 to 0.2 ml of excess drug solution. Based on the amount of drug to be administered, the excess solution must be expelled before administration. Figure 4D–10, *A*, illustrates the Carpuject syringe; Figure 4D–10, *B*, shows the Tubex syringe.

Needles

Needle size has two components: **gauge** (diameter of the lumen) and length. The larger the gauge number, the smaller the diameter of the **lumen**, and the smaller the gauge, the larger the diameter of the lumen. The most common gauge numbers of needles range from 18 to 26. Needle length varies from $^3/_8$ inch to 2 inches. Table 4D–1 lists the needle gauges and lengths for use in subcutaneous and IM injections.

FIGURE 4D–4   SafetyGlide needle. (Courtesy Becton-Dickinson Division, Franklin Lakes, NJ.)

FIVE-MILLILITER SYRINGE

FIGURE 4D–5   Five-milliliter syringes: A, 5-ml syringe with 0.2-ml markings; B, needleless 5-ml BD syringe that can penetrate a rubber-top vial.

FIGURE 4D–6   Tuberculin syringe. (From Kee JL, Marshall SM: *Clinical calculations,* ed 6, Philadelphia, 2009, Saunders.)

FIGURE 4D–7   Two types of tuberculin syringes. (Courtesy Becton-Dickinson Division, Franklin Lakes, NJ.)

FIGURE 4D–8 Insulin syringe. (From Kee JL, Marshall SM: *Clinical calculations*, ed 6, Philadelphia, 2009, Saunders.)

FIGURE 4D–9 Various types of insulin syringes. (Courtesy Becton-Dickinson Division, Franklin Lakes, NJ.)

FIGURE 4D–10 A, Carpuject syringe. B, Tubex syringe.

Table 4D–1

Needle Size and Length

Type of Injection	Needle Gauge	Needle Lengths (Inches)
Intradermal	25, 26	$3/8$, $1/2$, $5/8$
Subcutaneous	23, 25, 26	$3/8$, $1/2$, $5/8$
Intramuscular	19, 20, 21, 22	1, $1\frac{1}{2}$, 2

FIGURE 4D–11 Parts of a needle.

When choosing the needle length for an IM injection, the size of the client and the amount of fatty tissue must be considered. A client with minimal fatty (subQ) tissue may need a needle length of 1 inch. For an obese client, the length of the needle for an IM injection would be 1.5 to 2 inches.

Many insulin syringes and prefilled cartridges have permanently attached needles. With other syringes, the needle can be changed to the desired needle size. Needle gauge and length are indicated on the syringe package or on the top cover of the syringe. It appears as gauge/length; for example, 20 g/1$^{1}/_{2}$.

Figure 4D–11 illustrates the parts of a needle.

Angles for Injections

For injections, the needle enters the skin at different angles. Intradermal injections are given at a 10- to 15-degree angle, subQ injections at a 45- to 90-degree angle, and IM injections at a 90-degree angle. Figure 3–21 illustrates the angles for intradermal, subQ, and IM injections.

PRACTICE PROBLEM I

SYRINGES AND NEEDLES

Think through and answer each question. Correct answers are given at the end of the section.

1. To mix 4 ml of bacteriostatic water in a vial with a powdered drug, which size syringe should be used?

2. To give 0.4 ml of drug solution subQ, what type of syringe should be used?

3. Meperidine (Demerol) is available in a prefilled cartridge. Half of the drug solution is used. Should the remaining solution in the cartridge be saved for future use?

4. Which has the larger needle lumen, a 21-gauge needle or a 26-gauge needle?

5. Which needle has a length of $^{5}/_{8}$ inch, a 21-gauge needle or a 25-gauge needle?

6. Which needle is used for an IM injection, a 20-gauge needle with a 1.5-inch length or a 25-gauge needle with a $^{5}/_{8}$-inch length?

Interpreting Injectable Drug Labels

Drugs for injections are stored in liquid and powder form in vials and ampules. If the drug is in liquid form, the drug dose with its equivalent in milliliters is printed on the drug label. However, drugs in powder form must be reconstituted (i.e., changed to liquid form before use). Usually the instructions for reconstitution are given on the drug label and drug instructions. If this is not the case, consult a pharmacist or the drug circular.

EXAMPLE

Nafcillin sodium is the generic name; there is no brand (trade) name. The drug is for IM or IV administration. Instructions on the drug label read: "When reconstituted with 6.6 ml of diluent, each vial contains 8 ml of solution."

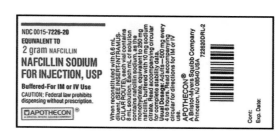

Intradermal Injections

An **intradermal** injection is usually used for skin testing to diagnose the cause of an allergy or to determine the presence of a microorganism. The choice of syringe for intradermal testing is the tuberculin syringe with a 25-gauge needle.

The inner portion of the forearm is frequently used for diagnostic testing because there is less hair in the area and the test results are more visible. The upper back may also be used as a testing site. The needle is inserted with the **bevel** pointing upward at a 10- to 15-degree angle. Do not aspirate. Test results are read 48 to 72 hours after the intradermal injection. A reddened or raised area is a positive reaction.

Subcutaneous Injections

Drugs injected into the **subcutaneous (subQ)** or fatty tissue are absorbed slowly because there are fewer blood vessels in fatty tissue. The amount of drug solution administered subQ is generally 0.5 to 1 ml at a 45-, 60-, or 90-degree angle. Drug solutions that irritate fatty tissues are given IM because they can cause sloughing of the subQ tissue.

The two types of syringes used for subQ injections are the tuberculin syringe (1 ml), calibrated in 0.1 ml and 0.01 ml, and the 3-ml syringe, calibrated in 0.1 ml. The needle gauge commonly used is 25 or 26, and the length is $^3/_8$ to $^5/_8$ inch. Insulin is also administered subQ and is discussed later in this section.

Calculations: Subcutaneous Injections

To calculate dosages for subQ injections, use the basic formula of $D/H \times V$, the ratio-and-proportion method, fractional equation, or dimensional analysis (see Section 4B). Heparin is a drug frequently administered subQ. It can be given at a 60- to 90-degree angle, depending on the amount of fatty tissue. The skin is lifted, and the heparin solution is injected into the subQ tissue. Do not aspirate or massage the injected site, because massage could cause small-vessel damage and bleeding.

Units should be written out as a word and not abbreviated as "U" only. When U is written, it may appear as O, and thus the client could receive a higher dose of the drug.

EXAMPLE

Order: heparin 2500 units subQ
Available: heparin 10,000 Units/ml in multiple-dose vial (10 ml)

Basic Formula:

$$\frac{D}{H} \times V = \frac{2500 \text{ units}}{10,000 \text{ units}} \times 1 \text{ ml} = \frac{25}{100} = 0.25 \text{ ml}$$

Ratio-and-Proportion Method:

$$H \quad : \quad V \quad :: \quad D \quad : \quad x$$
$$10,000 \text{ units} \quad : \quad 1 \text{ ml} \quad :: \quad 2500 \text{ units} \quad : \quad x \text{ ml}$$

$$10,000x = 2500$$
$$x = \frac{25}{100} = 0.25 \text{ ml}$$

Fractional Equation:

$$\frac{H}{V} = \frac{D}{x} = \frac{10,000 \text{ units}}{1 \text{ ml}} = \frac{2500 \text{ units}}{x \text{ ml}}$$
$$10,000x = 2500$$
(cross multiply) $\qquad x = 0.25 \text{ ml}$

Answer: Heparin 2500 units = 0.25 ml

Dimensional Analysis:

$$ml = \frac{1 \text{ ml} \times 2500 \text{ units}}{10,000 \text{ units} \times 1} = {}^1/_4 \text{ or } 0.25 \text{ ml}$$

PRACTICE PROBLEM 2

SUBCUTANEOUS INJECTIONS

Use the formula chosen for the calculation of drug dosages from Section 4B. The same formula should be used when calculating oral, subQ, IM, insulin, and IV dosages. Refer to conversion Tables 4A-4 or 4B-1 as needed.

EXAMPLES

1. Order: heparin 7500 units subQ
   Available:

   How many milliliters should the client receive? _____
2. Order: Lovenox (enoxaparin) 20 mg, SubQ, q12h. Lovenox is a low–molecular weight heparin (LMWH).
   Available:

   How many milliliters (ml) would you give per dose? _____
3. Order: atropine sulfate 0.5 mg subQ
   Available:

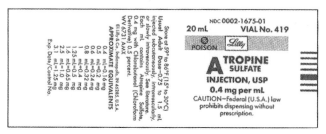

   How many milliliters should the client receive? _____
4. Order: epinephrine (Adrenalin) 0.2 mg subQ, STAT
   Available: epinephrine 1 mg/ml (1:1000) in ampule
   What type of syringe should be used? _____

Insulin Injections

Insulin is prescribed and measured in United States Pharmacopeia (USP) units. Most insulins are produced in concentrations of 100 units/ml. Insulin should be administered with an insulin syringe, which is calibrated to correspond with the 100 units of insulin. Insulin bottles and syringes are color-coded to avoid error. The 100 units/ml (or U-100) insulin bottle and the 100 units/ml syringe are coded orange. Administering insulin with a tuberculin syringe *should be avoided*.

Administration of medication requires attention to detail, and insulin is no exception. Insulin is ordered in units. For example, if the prescribed insulin dosage is 30 units, withdraw 30 units from a bottle of 100 units of insulin using a 100-unit calibrated insulin syringe (Figure 4D–12).

Insulin is administered subQ at a 45-, 60-, or 90-degree angle into the subQ tissue. The subQ absorption rate of insulin is slower because there are fewer blood vessels in the fatty tissue than in muscular tissue. The angle for administering insulin depends on the amount of fatty tissue. For an obese person, the angle may be 90 degrees; for a very thin person, the angle may be 45 to 60 degrees.

FIGURE 4D–12   Bottle of U 100 insulin and a U 100 calibrated insulin syringe. (From Kee JL, Marshall SM: *Clinical calculations*, ed 6, St. Louis, 2009, Saunders.)

Types of Insulins

Insulins are clear (regular or crystalline insulin) and cloudy (NPH) because of the substance protamine, which is used to prolong the action of insulin in the body. Only clear (regular) insulin can be given IV as well as subQ. The source of insulin is human (Humulin).

Insulin is categorized as (1) fast-acting (regular and lispro [Humalog]), (2) intermediate-acting (Humulin N), and (3) long-acting (Lantus). Commercially premixed combination insulins, Humulin 70/30 and Humulin 50/50, are popular for the client with diabetes who mixes fast-acting and intermediate-acting insulins. Humulin 70/30 and Humalog 75/25 come in pre-filled disposable pens. Chapter 51, Antidiabetics, discusses the various types of insulins and preparations and their peak and duration times.

The new long-acting insulin is Lantus, and insulin glargine that is an analog of human insulin. Lantus is the first long-acting recombinant DNA (rDNA) human insulin for clients with type 1 and 2 diabetes mellitus. It is a clear color insulin that is to be given subcutaneously only and NOT intravenously. It can NOT be missed with other insulins. The Lantus vial is taller and narrower than the other types of insulin. It has a purple top and purple writing on the label. It is usually administered at bedtime; incidence of nocturnal hypoglycemia is not as common as with other insulins. Some clients complain of more pain at the site when Lantus is used as compared to Humulin N insulin.

The use of commercially premixed combination insulins has become popular for the client with diabetes who mixes fast-acting and intermediate-acting insulins. Examples of combination insulins are Humulin 70/30, Novolin 70/30, and Humulin 50/50. The Humulin 70/30 vial contains 70% human insulin isophane and 30% human (regular) insulin, and the Humulin 50/50 vial contains 50% human insulin isophane and 50% human (regular) insulin. Humulin 70/30 may come in vials or prefilled cartridge pens (see Figures 4D–13 and Figure 4D–14). Some people need less than 30% regular (Humulin R) insulin and more isophane (Humulin N) insulin; they will need to mix the two insulins together.

Many individuals have been allergic to beef insulin, so in 1998, beef insulin was no longer manufactured. Pork insulin was frequently prescribed because it has biologic properties similar to those of human insulin. Since December 2005, pork insulin is NO longer available in the United States. Some clients may be importing it. Lente insulins have been discontinued. Combinations of Humulin R and N (isophane) may be prescribed for use with an insulin syringe or an insulin pen.

Fast-acting insulins

Intermediate-acting insulins

Long-acting insulins

Combinations of insulins

Insulins for pen injections

FIGURE 4D–13 Selected insulins.

Mixing Insulins

Regular insulin is frequently mixed with insulin containing protamine (NPH). The following is an example of a method for mixing insulin.

EXAMPLE   Order: regular insulin 10 units and NPH insulin 35 units subQ every day at 7:00 AM
Available: regular insulin 100 units/ml and NPH insulin 100 units/ml. Insulin syringe: 100 units/ml

FIGURE 4D–14   Insulin pens. (From Eli Lilly and Company, Indianapolis, Indiana.)

Method

1. Clean the rubber tops of the insulin bottles.
2. Draw up 35 units of air and inject into the NPH insulin bottle. Avoid letting the needle contact the NPH insulin solution. Withdraw the needle.
3. Draw up 10 units of air and inject into the regular insulin bottle.
4. First, withdraw 10 units of regular insulin. Regular insulin is always drawn up first.
5. Insert needle into NPH bottle and withdraw 35 units of NPH insulin. The total is 45 units.
6. Administer the two insulins immediately after mixing. Do *not* allow the insulin mixture to stand, because unpredicted physical changes may occur.

PRACTICE PROBLEM 3

INSULINS

Indicate on the insulin syringe the amount of insulin that should be withdrawn for each type of insulin.

1. Order: NPH insulin 45 units subQ
   Available: NPH insulin 100 units/ml and insulin syringe 100 units/ml

2. Order: regular insulin 15 units and Humulin N insulin 25 units subQ
   Available: regular insulin 100 units/ml and NPH insulin 100 units/ml, and insulin syringe 100 units/ml

3. Order: regular insulin 6 units and Humulin N insulin 40 units
   Available: regular insulin 100 units/ml and Humlin N insulin 100 units/ml, and insulin syringe 100 units/ml

Intramuscular Injections

Muscle has more blood vessels than fatty tissue, so medications given by **intramuscular (IM)** injection are absorbed more rapidly than those given by subQ injection. The volume of solution for an IM injection is 0.5 to 3 ml, with the average being 1 to 2 ml. A volume of drug solution greater than 3 ml causes increased muscle tissue displacement and possible tissue damage. Occasionally 5 ml of selected drugs, such as magnesium sulfate, may be injected into a large muscle, such as the dorsogluteal. A dose greater than 3 ml is usually divided and given at two different sites.

The needle gauges for IM injections that contain thick solutions are 19 and 20, and 20 and 21 for thin solutions. IM injections are administered at a 90-degree angle. The needle length depends on the amount of adipose (fat) and muscle tissues; the average needle length is 1.5 inches.

The discussion on IM injections is divided into three subsections: (1) drug solutions for injection, (2) powdered drug reconstitution, and (3) mixing injectable drugs. An example is given for each subsection, and practice problems follow.

Sites of IM injections are shown in Chapter 3, Principles of Drug Administration.

Drug Solutions for Injection

Commercially premixed drug solutions are stored in vials and ampules for ready use. The drug label on the container gives the drug dose by weight and its equivalent in milliliters.

EXAMPLE

Order: gentamicin (Garamycin) 50 mg IM
Available: gentamicin 80 mg/2 ml in a vial

a. BF: $\dfrac{D}{H} \times V = \dfrac{50}{80} \times 2 = \dfrac{100}{80} = 1.25$ ml

b. RP:

$$H \quad : \quad V \quad :: \quad D \quad : \quad x$$
$$80 \text{ mg} \quad : \quad 2 \text{ ml} \quad :: \quad 50 \text{ mg} \quad : \quad x \text{ ml}$$

$$80x = 100$$
$$x = \dfrac{100}{80} = 1.25 \text{ ml}$$

c. FE: $\dfrac{H}{V} = \dfrac{D}{x} \qquad \dfrac{80 \text{ mg}}{2 \text{ ml}} = \dfrac{50 \text{ mg}}{x}$

(cross multiply) $\qquad 80x = 100$
$\qquad\qquad\qquad\quad x = 1.25$ ml

d. DA: $\text{ml} = \dfrac{2 \text{ ml} \times 50 \text{ mg}}{80 \text{ mg} \times 1} = \dfrac{100}{80} = 1.25$ ml

Powdered Drug Reconstitution

Certain drugs lose their potency in liquid form; therefore manufacturers package these drugs in powdered form. They are reconstituted using a **diluent** (bacteriostatic water or saline) before administration. The drug label or the instructional insert (accompanying pamphlet) frequently gives the type and amount of diluent to use. If the type and amount of diluent are not on the drug label or in the instructional insert, contact the pharmacist.

Usually manufacturers determine the amount of diluent to mix with the drug powder to yield 1 to 2 ml/dose. The powdered drug occupies space; therefore the volume of the drug solution is increased. Once the powdered drug has been reconstituted, the unused drug solution should be dated and initialed on the drug label. Unused drug solutions in vials are refrigerated and may be used for 48 hours to 1 week according to the manufacturer's recommendation. Unused drug solutions in ampules are discarded.

EXAMPLE

Order: cefotetan disodium (Cefotan) 0.5 g IM, q12h

Available (NOTE: Circular states to add 2.6 ml of diluent to yield 3 ml of drug.):

Add 2.6 ml of diluent; 1 g of cefotetan disodium = 3 ml

BF: $\dfrac{D}{H} \times V = \dfrac{0.5}{1} \times 3 \text{ ml} = 1.5 \text{ ml} = 0.5 \text{ g of cefotetan disodium}$

DA: $\text{ml} = \dfrac{3 \text{ ml} \times 0.5 \text{ g}}{1 \text{ g} \times 1} = 1.5 \text{ ml}$

No conversion is needed.

Mixing Injectable Drugs

Drugs mixed together in the same syringe must be compatible to prevent precipitation. To determine drug compatibility, check drug reference texts or with a pharmacist. When in doubt about compatibility, do *not* mix drugs.

The three methods used for mixing drugs are (1) mixing two drugs in the same syringe from two vials, (2) mixing two drugs in the same syringe from one vial and one ampule, and (3) mixing two drugs in a prefilled cartridge from a vial.

Method 1: Mixing Two Drugs in the Same Syringe from Two Vials

1. Draw air into the syringe to equal the amount of solution to be withdrawn from the first vial, and inject the air into the first vial. Do *not* allow the needle to come into contact with the solution. Remove the needle.
2. Draw air into the syringe to equal the amount of solution to be withdrawn from the second vial. Invert the second vial, and inject the air. Withdraw the desired amount of solution from the second vial.
3. Change the needle, unless the entire volume in the first vial will be used.
4. Invert the first vial, and withdraw the desired amount of solution.

Method 2: Mixing Two Drugs in the Same Syringe from One Vial and One Ampule

1. Inject air into the vial.
2. Remove the desired amount of solution from the vial.
3. Withdraw the desired amount of solution from the ampule.

Method 3: Mixing Two Drugs in a Prefilled Cartridge from a Vial

1. Check the drug dose and the amount of solution in the prefilled cartridge. If a smaller dose is needed, expel the excess solution.
2. Draw air into the cartridge to equal the amount of solution to be withdrawn from the vial. Invert the vial, and inject the air.
3. Withdraw desired amount of solution from the vial. Be sure that the needle remains in the fluid, and do *not* take more solution than needed.

EXAMPLE
MIXING
DRUGS IN THE
SAME SYRINGE

Order: meperidine (Demerol) 25 mg and atropine sulfate 0.4 mg IM

Available: meperidine in a Tubex cartridge labeled 50 mg/ml

Atropine sulfate in a multidose vial labeled 0.4 mg/ml

How many milliliters of each drug should be given, and how are they mixed? _____

1. Meperidine dose

a. $\dfrac{D}{H} \times V = \dfrac{25}{50} \times 1 = \dfrac{25}{50} = 0.5$ ml

b.
$$H \quad : \quad V \quad :: \quad D \quad : \quad x$$
$$50 \text{ mg} \quad : \quad 1 \text{ ml} \quad :: \quad 25 \text{ mg} \quad : \quad x \text{ ml}$$

$$50x = 25$$
$$x = \frac{1}{2} = 0.5 \text{ ml}$$

2. Atropine dose:
   The label indicates 0.4 mg = 1 ml.

   Answer: Give meperidine 0.5 ml and atropine 1 ml.

Procedure

Mix two drugs in the cartridge with one drug from a vial and the other drug in the prefilled cartridge.

1. Check the drug dose and volume on the prefilled cartridge.
2. Expel 0.5 ml and any excess drug solution (meperidine) from the cartridge (0.5 ml remains in the cartridge). Have another nurse witness the waste of a narcotic.
3. Draw 1 ml of air into the cartridge, and inject the air into the vial that contains the atropine.
4. Withdraw 1 ml of atropine from the vial into the meperidine solution in the cartridge.

PRACTICE PROBLEM 4

INTRAMUSCULAR INJECTIONS

1. Order: cefazolin (Ancef) 500 mg IM, q6h
   Available:

   How many milliliters should be given? _____

2. Order: atropine sulfate 0.3 mg IM, STAT
   Available: atropine sulfate

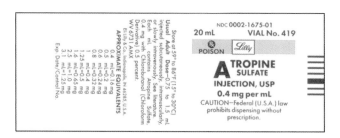

How many milliliters (ml) of atropine should be given? _____

3. Order: oxacillin 250 mg IM q6h
   Available: (Drug label states to add 2.7 ml of diluent = 3 ml of drug solution)

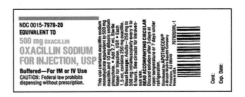

How many milliliters should be given? _____ After the drug is reconstituted, how long can it be refrigerated? _____

4. Order: digoxin 0.25 mg IM q.d.
   Available: digoxin 0.5 mg/2 ml

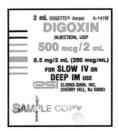

How many milliliters should be given? _____What should be done with the excess digoxin solution? _____ (Usually parenteral digoxin is administered IV.)

5. Order: chlorpromazine (Thorazine) 50 mg IM, STAT
   Available:

How many milliliters should be given? _____ Can the vial be used again? _____

6. Order: meperidine 60 mg and hydroxyzine (Vistaril) 25 mg, IM. These two drugs are compatible.
   Available: Hydroxyzine 100 mg/2 ml in vial

How many milliliters of meperidine and how many of hydroxyzine should be given? _____
Explain how the two drugs would be mixed.

7. Order: morphine SO₄ 6 mg IM q4h, PRN
   Available:

a. Which morphine vial should be selected? _____
   Explain _____

b. How many milliliters of morphine should be administered per dose? _____
   Explain _____

8. Order: ampicillin 250 mg q6h IM
   Available:

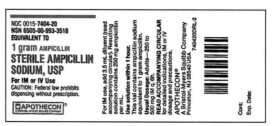

a. How many milliliters of diluent should be added to the ampicillin vial? _____
b. How many milliliters of ampicillin should the client receive per dose? _____
c. How many milligrams should the client receive per day? _____

9. Order: diazepam (Valium) 6 mg, IM, STAT and repeat in 4 hours if necessary.
   Available:

a. Which ampule or vial of diazepam would you select? _____
b. How many milliliters (ml) of diazepam should the client receive? _____

Additional Dimensional Analysis (Refer to Section 4B as needed.)

10. Order: tobramycin 60 mg IM q8h. The adult client weighs 180 pounds.
    Dose parameter: 3 mg/kg/day in three divided doses
    Available:

1 box • 25 vials • 2 mL   NDC 0003-2725-10

Equivalent to **80** mg TOBRAMYCIN/**2** mL (40 mg/mL)

TOBRAMYCIN
Sulfate Injection USP

For INTRAMUSCULAR or INTRAVENOUS use
Must dilute for IV use

TOBRAMYCIN Sulfate Injection USP
Each mL contains 40 mg tobramycin (as sulfate), 0.1 mg edetate disodium, 3.2 mg
sodium metabisulfite, and 5 mg phenol, as a preservative, in Water for Injection.
pH 3.0-6.5; sulfuric acid and, if necessary, sodium hydroxide have been added for
pH adjustment. Sealed under nitrogen.
Usual Dosage: Read accompanying package insert for dosage and IV dilution.
Store at controlled room temperature 15°-30° C (59°-86° F).
Caution: Federal law prohibits dispensing without prescription.

APOTHECON®
A Bristol-Myers Squibb Co.
Princeton, NJ 08540
Made in USA   C1640 / P2510

Factors: 80 mg = 2 ml (drug label)
Conversion factor: none (both are in milligrams)
 a. How many kilograms does the client weigh? _____
 b. How many milligrams should the client receive per day? _____
 c. Is the drug dose within safe parameters? _____
 d. How many milliliters should the client receive per dose? _____

11. Order: Cefobid 500 mg IM, q12h
 Available (NOTE: Instructions state to add 1.6 ml of diluent to the vial; drug liquids in 1 g = 2 ml.):

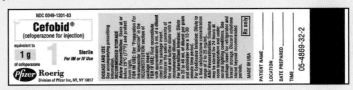

 Factors: 1 g = 2 ml (drug label and after reconstitution)
 Conversion factor: 1000 mg = 1 g
 How many milliliters should the client receive per dose? _____

12. Order: meperidine (Demerol) 35 mg and promethazine (Phenergan) 10 mg, IM
 Drugs available: meperidine 50 mg/ml in an ampule; promethazine 25 mg/ml in an ampule

 a. How many milliliters of meperidine would you give? _____
 b. How many milliliters of promethazine would you give? _____
 c. Explain how the two drugs would be mixed.

ANSWERS TO PRACTICE PROBLEMS

I   **SYRINGES AND NEEDLES**

1. 5-ml syringe
2. Tuberculin syringe (1 ml)
3. No, it should be discarded in the sink or toilet and witnessed by another RN or LPN, according to policy.

4. 21-gauge needle
5. 25-gauge needle
6. 20-gauge needle 1.5 (1½) inches in length

2   SUBCUTANEOUS INJECTIONS

1. 0.75 ml

2. Lovenox 0.2 ml for 20 mg

3. The drug label reads: 1.25 ml = 0.5 mg of atropine. Also, under the word "atropine," it reads 0.4 mg/ml

   a. BF: $\dfrac{D}{H} \times V = \dfrac{0.5}{0.4} \times 1 = 1.25$ ml

   b. RP: H : V :: D : x
   $$0.4 \text{ mg} : 1 \text{ ml} :: 0.5 \text{ mg} : x \text{ ml}$$
   $$0.4x = 0.5$$
   $$x = \dfrac{0.5}{0.4} = 1.25 \text{ ml}$$

   c. DA: $\text{ml} = \dfrac{1 \text{ ml} \times 0.5 \cancel{\text{mg}}}{0.4 \cancel{\text{mg}} \times 1} = 1.25 \text{ ml}$

   Answer: atropine sulfate 0.5 mg = 1.25 ml

4. A tuberculin syringe should be used.

   a. $\dfrac{D}{H} \times V = \dfrac{0.2}{1.0} \times 1 = 1.0\sqrt{0.20} = 0.2 \text{ ml}$

   b. H : V :: D : x
   $$1.0 \text{ mg} : 1 \text{ ml} :: 0.2 \text{ mg} : x \text{ ml}$$
   $$1.0x = 0.2$$
   $$x = \dfrac{0.2}{1.0} = 0.2 \text{ ml}$$

   Answer: epinephrine 0.2 mg = 0.2 ml

3   INSULINS

4   INTRAMUSCULAR INJECTIONS USING BASIC FORMULA, RATIO AND PROPORTION, FRACTIONAL EQUATION, OR DIMENSIONAL ANALYSIS

1. Instructions on the drug label read: add 2.5 ml of sterile water. The drug solution equals 3.0 ml (drug powder is equal to 0.5 ml).

   Change 1 g to mg. 1 g = 1000 mg or
   Change 500 mg to g. .500 mg = 0.500 g (0.5 g)

   a. BF: $\dfrac{D}{H} \times V = \dfrac{0.5}{1 \text{ g}} \times 3 \text{ ml} = 1.5 \text{ ml}$

   b. RP: H : V :: D : x
   $$1000 \text{ mg} : 3 \text{ ml} :: 500 \text{ mg} : x \text{ ml}$$
   $$1000x = 1500$$
   $$x = 1.5 \text{ ml}$$

   c. DA: $\text{ml} = \dfrac{3 \text{ ml} \times 1 \cancel{\text{g}} \times \overset{1}{\cancel{500}} \text{ mg}}{1 \cancel{\text{g}} \times \underset{2}{\cancel{1000}} \text{ mg} \times 1} = \dfrac{3}{2}$
   $$= 1.5 \text{ ml}$$

   Answer: cefazolin 500 mg = 1.5 ml

2. The atropine drug label is marked as 0.4 mg/ml. The approximate equivalent of 0.3 mg is 0.8 ml as marked on the label. If the 0.3 mg = 0.8 ml is unknown, the problem may be calculated using 0.4 mg = 1 ml

   BF: $\dfrac{D}{H} \times V = \dfrac{0.3}{0.4} \times 1 = \dfrac{0.3}{0.4} = 0.75$, or 0.8 ml

3. For oxacillin sodium, the drug label indicates that 2.7 ml of sterile water should be added to the vial containing 500 mg of drug. The total volume would be 3 ml.

   a. BF: $\dfrac{D}{H} \times V = \dfrac{250}{500} \times 3.0 = \dfrac{750}{500} = 1.5$ ml

   b. FE: $\dfrac{H}{V} = \dfrac{D}{x}$ $\dfrac{500 \text{ mg}}{3 \text{ ml}} = \dfrac{250 \text{ mg}}{x \text{ ml}}$

   $$500\,x = 750$$
   $$x = 1.5 \text{ ml}$$

   c. DA: ml $= \dfrac{3 \text{ ml} \times \overset{1}{250} \text{ mg}}{\underset{2}{500} \text{ mg} \times 1} = 1.5$ ml

   No conversion is needed.
   Answer: Oxacillin 250 mg = 1.5 ml. It can be refrigerated for 96 hr after it has been reconstituted.

4. BF: $\dfrac{D}{H} \times V = \dfrac{0.25}{0.50} \times 2 = \dfrac{0.50}{0.50} = 1$ ml

   Withdraw 1 ml from the ampule. Discard the remaining 1 ml of digoxin solution.

5. Thorazine 50 mg = 2 ml. Yes, the vial can be used for multiple doses.

6. Meperidine 60 mg = 0.6 ml; hydroxyzine 25 mg = 0.5 ml

   Meperidine
   BF: $\dfrac{D}{H} \times V = \dfrac{60}{100} \times 1 = \dfrac{60}{100} = 0.6$ ml

   Hydroxyzine
   BF: $\dfrac{D}{H} \times V = \dfrac{25}{100} \times 2 = \dfrac{50}{100} = 0.5$ ml

   Procedure
   a. Withdraw 0.5 ml of hydroxyzine from the vial.
   b. Meperidine is in a dosette ampule. Withdraw 0.6 ml of meperidine solution into the syringe containing hydroxyzine.
   c. Total amount of the two drug solutions is 1.1 ml. Administer IM.

7. a. Morphine vials 8 mg/ml and 10 mg/ml. Morphine 5 mg/ml vial could not be used because it is a single-vial dose.

   b. *Morphine 8 mg/ml*
   BF: $\dfrac{D}{H} \times V = \dfrac{6 \text{ mg}}{8 \text{ mg}} \times 1 \text{ ml} = \dfrac{6}{8} = 0.75$ ml

Morphine 10 mg/ml
   BF: $\dfrac{D}{H} \times V = \dfrac{6 \text{ mg}}{10 \text{ mg}} \times 1 \text{ ml} = \dfrac{6}{10} = 0.6$ ml

8. a. 3.5 ml of diluent (3.5 ml diluent + 0.5 ml of powdered drug = 4 ml of 1 g of ampicillin)
   b. 1 ml = 250 mg (1 g or 1000 mg = 4 ml)
   c. 250 mg × 4 (q6h) = 1000 mg or 1 g/day

9. a. Either the ampule or the vial could be used. The diazepam 5 mg/ml is a multiple-dose vial that contains 10 ml of drug solution. The 10 mg/2 ml ampule is to be used one time; if not entirely used, it has to be discarded.

   b. Vial: BF: $\dfrac{D}{H} \times V = \dfrac{6 \text{ mg}}{5 \text{ mg}} \times 1 \text{ ml} = 1.2$ ml

   or
   Ampule: RP: H : V :: D : x
   10 mg : 2 ml :: 6 mg : x ml
   $$10\,x = 12$$
   $$x = 1.2 \text{ ml}$$

   or
   Vial: DA: ml $= \dfrac{1 \text{ ml} \times 6 \text{ mg}}{5 \text{ mg} \times 1} = \dfrac{6}{5} = 1.2$ ml

   or
   Ampule: FE: $\dfrac{H}{V} = \dfrac{D}{x}$
   $= \dfrac{10 \text{ mg}}{2 \text{ ml}} \times \dfrac{6 \text{ mg}}{x} = 1.2$ ml
   (cross-multiply)

10. a. The client weighs 180 pounds, or 81.8 kg.
    b. 245.4 mg per day
    c. The dose is safe, 180 mg per day, which is below the dose parameters for the client's weight.
    d. 1.5 ml per dose

    DA: ml $= \dfrac{2 \text{ ml} \times \overset{3}{60} \text{ mg}}{\underset{4}{80} \text{ mg} \times 1} = \dfrac{6}{4} = 1.5$ ml

11. 1 ml per dose

    DA: ml $= \dfrac{2 \text{ ml} \times 1 \text{ g} \times \overset{1}{500} \text{ mg}}{1 \text{ g} \times \underset{2}{1000} \text{ mg} \times 1} = \dfrac{2}{2} = 1$

12. a. *meperidine:*

    DA: ml $= \dfrac{1 \text{ ml} \times \overset{7}{35} \text{ mg}}{\underset{10}{50} \text{ mg} \times 1} = \dfrac{7}{10} = 0.7$ ml

    b. *promethazine*

    DA: ml $= \dfrac{1 \text{ ml} \times \overset{2}{10} \text{ mg}}{\underset{5}{25} \text{ mg} \times 1} = \dfrac{2}{5} = 0.4$ ml

    c. Procedure:
    1. Obtain 0.7 ml of meperidine from the ampule and 0.4 ml of promethazine from the ampule.
    2. Discard the remaining solutions within the ampules.

Section 4E CALCULATIONS OF INTRAVENOUS FLUIDS

Outline . . . .

Objectives

Terms

Continuous Intravenous Administration
Intravenous Sets
Calculating Intravenous Flow Rate
Mixing Drugs for Continuous Intra-
venous Administration

Intermittent Intravenous Administration

Secondary Intravenous Sets without IV Pumps

Intermittent Infusion Adapters/Devices

Direct Intravenous Injections

Electronic Intravenous Regulators

Patient-Controlled Analgesia
Client Teaching

Calculating Flow Rates for Intravenous Drugs

Objectives . . . .

- Describe the differences between continuous intravenous infusion and intermittent intravenous infusion.
- Define macrodrip and microdrip sets, keep vein open (KVO), and to keep open (TKO).
- Calculate intravenous flow rate using one of the given formulas.
- Explain how intravenous drug solutions administered by secondary set are calculated.
- Differentiate between volumetric and nonvolumetric intravenous regulators and pump electronic regulators.

Terms . . . .

bolus, p. 94
drop factor, p. 95
electronic intravenous (IV)
    regulators, p. 100
IV piggyback (IVPB),
    p. 98

keep vein open (KVO),
    p. 95
macrodrip set, p. 95
microdrip (minidrip) set,
    p. 95

nonvolumetric regulator,
    p. 100
patient-controlled analge-
    sia (PCA), p. 101
primary IV line set, p. 98

secondary IV line set,
    p. 98
to keep open (TKO),
    p. 95
volumetric regulator,
    p. 100

Intravenous (IV) fluid therapy is used to administer fluids that contain water, dextrose, vitamins, electrolytes, and drugs. Today an increasing number of drugs are administered by the IV route for direct absorption and fast action. Some drugs are given by IV push (**bolus**). Many drugs administered IV irritate the veins, so these drugs are diluted in 50 to 100 ml of fluid. Other drugs are delivered in a large volume of fluid over a specific period, such as 4 to 8 hours.

Two methods are used to administer IV fluids and drugs: continuous IV infusion and intermittent IV infusion. Continuous IV infusion replaces fluid loss, maintains fluid balance, and serves as a vehicle for drug administration. Intermittent IV infusion is used primarily to give IV drugs.

Nurses have an important role in the preparation and administration of IV solutions and IV drugs. The nursing functions and responsibilities during drug preparation include the following:
- Knowing IV sets and their drop factors
- Calculating IV flow rates
- Mixing and diluting drugs in IV fluids
- Gathering equipment
- Knowing the drugs and the expected and untoward reactions

Nursing responsibilities continue with assessment of the client for effectiveness and untoward effects of the therapy and assessment of the IV site.

Continuous Intravenous Administration

When IV solutions are required, the health care provider orders the type and amount of IV solution in liters over a 24-hour period or in milliliters per hour. The nurse calculates the IV flow rate according to the drop factor, the amount of fluids to be administered, and the time period.

Intravenous Sets

Various IV infusion sets are marketed by Abbott, Cutter, McGaw, and Travenol. The **drop factor,** the number of drops per milliliter, is normally printed on the packaging cover of the IV set. A set that delivers large drops per milliliter (10 to 20 gtt/ml) is called a **macrodrip set,** and one with small drops per milliliter (60 gtt/ml) is called a **microdrip (minidrip) set.** Examples of drop factors, macrodrip sets, and microdrip sets are listed in Table 4E–1.

In most instances, the nurse has the choice of using either the macrodrip or microdrip set. If the IV rate is to infuse at 100 ml/hr or more, the macrodrip set is usually used. If the infusion rate is less than (<) 100 ml/hr or the client is a child, the microdrip set is preferred. Slow drip rates of <100 ml/hr make macrodrip adjustment difficult.

At times, IV fluids are given at a slow rate to **keep vein open (KVO),** also called to **keep open (TKO).** The reasons for ordering KVO include a suspected or potential emergency situation for rapid administration of fluids and drugs and the need for an open line to give IV drugs at specified hours. For KVO, a microdrip set (60 gtt/ml) and a 250-ml IV bag may be used. KVO is usually regulated to deliver 10 ml/hr.

Calculating Intravenous Flow Rate

Three different methods may be used to calculate IV flow rate (drops per minute, gtt/min). The nurse should select one method, memorize it, and consistently use it to calculate IV flow rate. Method II is usually the preferred method.

Method I: Three-Step

1. $\dfrac{\text{Amount of solution}}{\text{Hours to administer}} = \text{milliliters/hour (ml/h)}$

2. $\dfrac{\text{Milliliters per hour}}{60 \text{ minutes}} = \text{milliliters/minute (ml/min)}$

3. Milliliters per minute × drops per milliliter of IV set = drops/minute (gtt/min)

Method II: Two-Step

1. $\dfrac{\text{Amount of fluid}}{\text{Hours to administer}} = \text{milliliters/hour (ml/h)}$

2. $\dfrac{\text{Milliliters per hour} \times \text{Drops per milliliter (IV set)}}{60 \text{ minutes}} = \text{drops/minute (gtt/min)}$

If the milliliters per hour is known, then use Step 2 to determine the drops per minute.

Method III: One-Step

1. $\dfrac{\text{Amount of fluid} \times \text{Drops per milliliter (IV set)}}{\text{Hours to administer} \times \text{Minutes per hour (60)}} = \text{drops/minute (gtt/min)}$

SECTION E

Table 4E–I		
Intravenous Sets		
	Manufacturer	**Drops (gtt/ml)**
	Macrodrip Sets	
	Abbott	15
	Cutter	20
	McGaw	15
	Travenol	10
	Microdrip Sets	
	Travenol	60
	Minidrip sets	60

Mixing Drugs for Continuous Intravenous Administration

Drugs such as potassium chloride and vitamins are frequently added to the IV solution bag for continuous IV infusion. Drugs should be added to the bag or bottle immediately before administering the IV fluid. Inject the drug into the rubber stopper on the IV bag or bottle and rotate the bag several times to ensure that the drug is dispersed throughout the solution (Figure 4E–1). *Do not add the drug while the infusion is running unless the bag is rotated.* A drug solution injected into an upright infusing IV solution concentrates the drug into the lower portion of the IV bag, preventing it from dispersing evenly. The client receives a concentrated drug solution, which may be harmful, for example, if the drug is potassium chloride. If drugs are injected into the IV bag before use, the bag should be refrigerated to maintain drug potency.

There are various nutrients (e.g., dextrose) and electrolytes in commercially prepared IV solutions. The commonly used solutions are 5% dextrose in water (D_5W), normal saline (NSS), one-half normal saline ($\frac{1}{2}$ NSS), and lactated Ringer's (LR). Abbreviations for these types of solutions are listed in Table 4E–2.

FIGURE 4E–1 Intravenous bag. (From Kee JL, Marshall SM: *Clinical calculations*, ed 6, St. Louis, 2009, Saunders.)

Table 4E–2	
Abbreviations of Solutions	
Intravenous Solutions	**Abbreviations**
5% Dextrose in water	D_5W, 5% D/W
10% Dextrose in water	$D_{10}W$, 10% D/W
0.9% Sodium chloride, normal saline solution	0.9% NaCl, NSS
0.45% Sodium chloride, $\frac{1}{2}$ normal saline solution	0.45% NaCl, $\frac{1}{2}$ NSS
5% Dextrose in 0.9% sodium chloride	D_5NSS, 5% D/NSS, 5% D/0.9% NaCl
5% Dextrose in 0.45% sodium chloride or 5% Dextrose in $\frac{1}{2}$ normal saline solution	$D_5/\frac{1}{2}$ NSS, 5% D/$\frac{1}{2}$ NSS
Lactated Ringer's solution	LR

EXAMPLE Order: 1000 ml of 5% dextrose in water (D$_5$W) with potassium chloride (KCl) 20 mEq in 8 h

    Available: 1000 ml of 5% dextrose in water

                    Potassium chloride 40 mEq/20 ml ampule

                    IV set labeled 10 gtt/ml

Drug calculation: Use the basic formula, the ratio-and-proportion method, fractional equation, or dimensional analysis (refer to Section 4B if needed).

a. BF: $\dfrac{D}{H} \times V = \dfrac{20}{40} \times 20 = \dfrac{400}{40} = 10$ ml of KCl

b. RP:

$$
\begin{array}{ccccccc}
H & : & V & :: & D & : & x \\
40 \text{ mEq} & : & 20 \text{ ml} & :: & 20 \text{ mEq} & : & x \text{ ml}
\end{array}
$$

$$40x = 400$$
$$x = 10 \text{ ml of KCl}$$

c. DA: $ml = \dfrac{20 \text{ ml} \times \overset{1}{\cancel{20}} \text{ mEq}}{\underset{2}{\cancel{40}} \text{ mEq} \times 1} = 10$ ml of KCl

The calculation of IV flow rate is described using the three methods outlined previously. However, it is strongly recommended that only one method be selected to determine IV flow rate.

Method I

1. $\dfrac{1000 \text{ ml}}{8 \text{ h}} = 125$ ml/h

2. $\dfrac{125 \text{ ml}}{60 \text{ min}} = 2.0\text{–}2.1$ ml/min

3. $2.1 \times 10 = 21$ gtt/min

Method II

1. $1000 \div 8 = 125$ ml/h

2. $\dfrac{125 \text{ ml/h} \times \overset{1}{\cancel{10}} \text{ gtt/ml}}{\underset{6}{\cancel{60}} \text{ min}} = \dfrac{125}{6} = 20\text{–}21$ gtt/min

Method III

1. $\dfrac{1000 \text{ ml} \times \overset{1}{\cancel{10}} \text{ gtt/ml}}{8 \text{ h} \times \underset{6}{\cancel{60}} \text{ min}} = \dfrac{1000}{48} = 20$ or 21 gtt/min

PRACTICE
PROBLEM 1

CONTINUOUS INTRAVENOUS FLOW RATES

Select one of the three methods to calculate IV flow rate.

1. Order: 1000 ml of D$_5$/$^1\!/_2$ NSS to infuse over 12 h
   Available: macrodrip set with 10 gtt/ml and a microdrip set with 60 gtt/ml
   a. Should a macrodrip or microdrip IV set be used? _____
   b. Calculate the IV flow rate in drops per minute according to the IV set that was selected. _____

2. Order: 3 L of IV solutions to infuse over 24 h
   1 liter of D$_5$W and 2 liters of D$_5$/$^1\!/_2$ NSS
   a. One liter is equal to how many milliliters? _____
   b. Each liter should infuse for how many hours? _____
   c. The institution uses a set with a drop factor of 15 gtt/ml. How many drops per minute should the client receive? _____

3. Order: 250 ml of D$_5$W to KVO
   a. What type of IV set should be used? _____
   b. Determine how many drops per minute the client should receive. _____

4. Order: 1000 ml of D$_5$/$^1\!/_2$ NSS, 1 vial of multiple vitamin (MVI), and 10 mEq of KCl (potassium chloride) in 10 h
   Available: 1000 ml of D$_5$/$^1\!/_2$ NSS
   Macrodrip set: 15 gtt/ml; microdrip set: 60 gtt/ml

MVI: 5 ml vial

KCl: 20 mEq/20 ml vial

a. How many milliliters of KCl should be injected into the IV bag? _____

b. How many drops per minute should the client receive using the macrodrip set and microdrip set? _____

Intermittent Intravenous Administration

Some IV drugs are prescribed to be administered three to six times a day in a small volume of IV fluid (50 to 100 ml of D₅W or NSS 0.9% sodium chloride). The drug solution is usually infused over a period of 15 minutes to 1 hour. Separate tubing for IV drugs, the **secondary IV line set,** is inserted into a port (rubber stopper) of the IV connector on the continuous, or **primary IV line set.** This type of IV administration is called *intermittent IV therapy.*

Secondary Intravenous Sets without IV Pumps

Two IV sets available to administer IV drugs are (1) the calibrated cylinder (chamber) with tubing, such as the Buretrol, Volutrol, and Soluset; and (2) the secondary IV set, which is similar to a regular IV set except the tubing is shorter (Figure 4E–2). The secondary IV line set is used mostly to infuse small volumes—50, 100, 250 ml and for children's IV solution. The chamber of the Buretrol, Volutrol, and Soluset holds 150 ml of solution. Medication is injected into the chamber and then diluted with solution. These methods of administering IV drugs are referred to as **IV piggyback (IVPB).**

Drugs for IV infusion are diluted before infusion. Clinical agencies frequently have their own protocols for dilutions; the pharmacist and the drug circular are also resources for infusion guidelines. Guidelines and protocols help to prevent drug and fluid incompatibility.

The current trend to IV medication administration is the use of premixed IV drugs in 50- to 500-ml bags. These premixed IV medications can be prepared by the manufacturer or by the

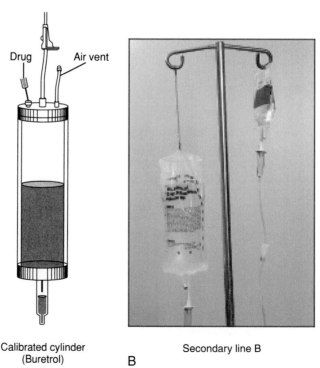

Calibrated cylinder
(Buretrol)
A   Secondary line **B**

FIGURE 4E–2   A, The calibrated cylinder (Buretrol) is an example of a secondary intravenous (IV) device. B, An example of a secondary line containing medication. The primary IV bag is 6 inches below the secondary IV bag. (A, From Kee JL, Marshall SM: *Clinical calculations,* ed 6, St. Louis, 2009, Saunders. B, From Leahy JM, Kizilay PE: *Foundations of nursing practice: a nursing process approach,* Philadelphia, 1998, Saunders.)

hospital pharmacy. The problems of contamination and drug errors are decreased with the use of premixed IV medication. Each IV drug bag has separate tubing to prevent admixture. Cost is higher but risk is lower with the use of premixed IV drug bags. Because not all medication can be premixed in the solution, nurses will continue to prepare some drugs for IV administration.

Note: When using a calibrated cylinder such as the Buretrol, add 15 ml of IV solution to flush the drug out of the IV line after the drug infusion is completed. The flush volume is added to the client's intake.

Intermittent Infusion Adapters/Devices

When continuous IV fluid infusion is to be discontinued and intermittent drug therapy is to begin, an adapter is attached to the IV catheter or needle where the IV tubing was disconnected. Adapters have ports (stoppers) where needles, needleless, or IV tubing can be inserted as needed to continue drug therapy. The use of adapters increases the client's mobility by not having an IV line "tagging along" and is cost-effective because less IV tubing, solution, and equipment are needed. See Figure 4E–3 for examples of needleless infusion devices.

Direct Intravenous Injections

Medications that are given by the IV injection route are calculated in the same manner as medications for intramuscular (IM) injection. This route is often referred to as *IV push*. Clinically, it is the preferred route for clients with poor muscle mass or decreased circulation or for a drug that is poorly absorbed from the tissues. Medications administered by this route have a rapid onset of action, and calculation errors can have serious, even fatal, consequences. Drug information inserts must be read carefully, and attention must be given to the amount of drug that can be given per minute. If the drug is pushed into the bloodstream at a faster rate than specified in the drug literature, adverse reactions to the medication are likely to occur.

EXAMPLE   Order: Lasix 80 mg, IV, STAT.

Drug available: Lasix 10 mg/ml. IV infusion not to exceed 40 mg/min

a. RP: H : V :: D : x

10 mg : 1 ml :: 80 mg : x

$10x = 80$

$x = 8$ ml of Lasix

or

DA: $ml = \dfrac{1\ ml \times \overset{8}{\cancel{80\ mg}}}{\underset{1}{\cancel{10\ mg}} \times 1} = 8$ ml of Lasix

FIGURE 4E–3   Needleless infusion devices. Medication in a needleless syringe can be inserted into a needleless infusion device. (From Kee JL, Marshall SM: *Clinical calculations*, ed 6, St. Louis, 2009, Saunders.)

b. known drug : known minutes :: desired drug : desired minutes

40 mg   :   1 min   ::   80 mg   : x

$40x = 80$

$x = 2$ min

DIRECT IV INJECTION

1. Order: protamine sulfate 40 mg IV, STAT
   Available:

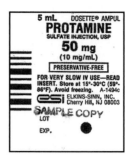

   IV infusion NOT to exceed 5 mg/min
   a. How many milliliters (ml) should the client receive? _____
   b. For how many minutes should protamine be administered? _____
2. Order: morphine sulfate 5 mg, IV, q3h, PRN
   Available:

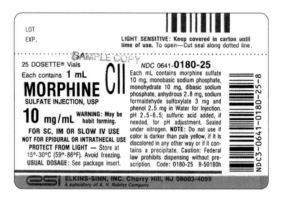

   IV infusion NOT to exceed 10 mg/4 minutes
   a. How many milliliters (ml) should the client receive? _____
   b. For how many minutes should morphine be administered? _____
   Note: When giving drugs by direct IV infusion, always verify the compatibility of the IV solution and the drug, or precipitation can result. Incompatibility can be avoided if the IV tubing is flushed with compatible solution of either normal saline or sterile water before and after administration.

Electronic Intravenous Regulators

Pumps are **electronic intravenous (IV) regulators** used in hospitals and some community settings. The electronic IV regulators are set to deliver a prescribed rate of IV solution. If the flow rate is obstructed, an alarm sounds.

IV pumps deliver IV solution against resistance. The flow rate is set in milliliters per hour. Pumps do not recognize infiltration. The alarm does not sound until the pump has exerted its maximum pressure to overcome resistance.

IV pumps are recommended for use with all central lines, such as femoral and subclavian sites, and peripheral lines. Ongoing nursing assessment is essential when using electronic IV regulators.

There are two types of flow control for electronic IV regulators: volumetric and nonvolumetric regulators. A **volumetric regulator** delivers a specific volume of fluid at a specific rate, in milliliters per hour. A **nonvolumetric regulator** is designed to infuse at a drop rate in drops per minute. To determine whether the machine is volumetric or nonvolumetric, check to see whether the panel display is calibrated for ml/hr or gtt/min. Figure 4E–4 shows double pump regulator. There are various electronic IV regulators for the administration of IV fluids and drugs (Figure 4E–5).

FIGURE 4E-4   Double intravenous Baxter pump.

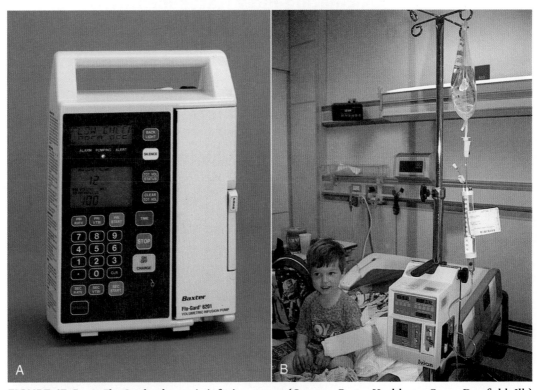

FIGURE 4E-5   A, Flo-Gard volumetric infusion pump. (Courtesy Baxter Healthcare Corp., Deerfield, Ill.) B, Buretrol with an electronic IV regulator for IV drug administration. (From Bowden VR, Dickey SB, Greenberg CS: *Children and their families: a continuum of care,* Philadelphia, 1998, Saunders.)

Patient-Controlled Analgesia

Patient-controlled analgesia (PCA) is another method used to administer drugs IV. The objective of PCA is to provide a uniform serum concentration of drug(s), thus avoiding drug peaks and valleys. This method is designed to meet the needs of clients who require at least 24 to 48 hours of regular IM narcotic injections.

Several reasons for the use of PCA include (1) effective pain control without the client feeling over-sedated, (2) considerable reduction in the amount of narcotic used (approximately one half that of IM delivery), and (3) clients' feelings of having greater control over their pain.

There are choices available in the delivery of PCA. The pump is programmed to administer the prescribed medication (1) at client demand, (2) continuously, and (3) continuously and supplemented by client demand (see Figure 3-29, p. 43).

The health care provider's order must include the following:
- Drug ordered
- Loading dose: administered by the health care provider to obtain baseline serum concentration of analgesic
- PCA dose: amount to be administered each time client activates the button
- Lockout interval: time during which PCA cannot be administered
- Dose limit: the maximum amount the client can receive during a specified time

Client Teaching

- Inform the client that the pain should be tolerable, not necessarily absent.
- Advise the client of the pump's safety features, including the alarms.
- Instruct the client in the use of the control button (medication administered when button is *released*).
- Instruct the client to report any side effects or adverse reactions to the medication.
- Have naloxone (Narcan) easily accessible.

Calculating Flow Rates for Intravenous Drugs

IV drug infusion rates depend on the drug dosing instructions, which indicate the amount of solution for dilution, and the length of infusion time. The nurse must first calculate the drug dose from the health care provider's order, then calculate the flow rate.

1. *Secondary Sets:* To find drops per minute for IV drugs, use calibrated cylinders (Buretrol, Volutrol), 50- to 250-ml bag (Add-A-Line), or any nonvolumetric regulator.

$$\frac{\text{Amount of solution} \times \text{Drops per milliliter of the set}}{\text{Minutes to administer}} = \text{Drops/minute (gtt/min)}$$

2. *Volumetric Regulators:* To find milliliters per hour (Infusion rate)

$$\text{Amount of solution} \div \frac{\text{Minutes to administer}}{60 \text{ min/hr}} = \text{Milliliters/hour (ml/hr)}$$

Problems for calculating IV drug dosage and IV flow rate in drops per minute and in milliliters per hour are given below.

EXAMPLE   Order: ceftazidime (Fortaz) 1.5 g IV q6h
Available:

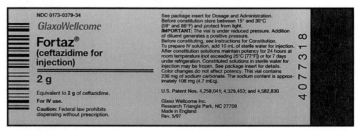

Set and solution: Cylinder set with drop factor of 60 gtt/ml; 500 ml of D₅W.
Instruction: Dilute ceftazidime 1.5 g in 100 ml of D₅W and infuse over 30 minutes.

1. Calculate drug dosage according to drug label.
2. Calculate drops per minute for drug solution.
3. Calculate milliliters per hour using volumetric infusion pump rate (ml/hr).

Answer

1. Drug Calculation
Drug label states to add 10 ml of sterile water (2 g = 10 ml)

BF: $\dfrac{D}{H} \times V = \dfrac{1.5 \text{ g}}{2 \text{ g}} \times 10 \text{ ml} = \dfrac{15}{2} = 7.5 \text{ ml of ceftazidime}$

DA: $\text{ml} = \dfrac{10 \text{ ml} \times 1.5 \text{ g}}{2 \text{ g} \times 1} = \dfrac{15}{2} = 7.5 \text{ ml}$

2. Secondary Set

$$\frac{\text{Amount of solution} \times \text{Drops per milliliter (set)}}{\text{Minutes to administer}} = \frac{100 \text{ ml} \times \overset{2}{\cancel{60}} \text{ gtt}}{\underset{1}{\cancel{30}} \text{ min}} = 200 \text{ gtt/min}$$

Inject 7.5 ml of ceftazidime in 100 ml of D$_5$W in the cylinder chamber.

Regulate IV flow rate to 200 gtt/min. It may be impossible to count 200 gtt/min. Instead of using the cylinder chamber, the nurse may use a secondary set that has a larger drop factor or a regulator. If the cylinder set is the only available secondary IV set, then the 200 gtt/min may be approximated.

3. Volumetric Infusion Pump Rate

$$\text{Amount of solution} \div \frac{\text{Minutes to administer}}{60 \text{ minutes per hour}} = 100 \text{ ml} + 7.5 \text{ ml (drug)} \div \frac{30 \text{ min}}{60 \text{ min}}$$

$$(\text{invert the divisor and multiply}) \qquad = 107.5 \text{ ml} \times \frac{\overset{2}{\cancel{60}}}{\underset{1}{\cancel{30}}} = 215 \text{ ml/h}$$

Set volumetric infusion rate at 215 ml/hr to deliver drug in 30 min.

PRACTICE PROBLEM 3

INTERMITTENT INTRAVENOUS SET

Solve the IV drug problems by (1) calculating the drug dosage according to the drug label or information given and (2) calculating drops per minute for the drug solution.

1. Order: kanamycin (Kantrex) 15 mg/kg/day in three divided doses (q8h) IV. Client weighs 50 kg.
   Available:

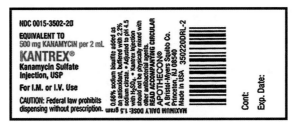

   How many milliliters of kanamycin should the client receive per dose? _____
   Set and solution: Cylinder set with a drop factor of 60 gtt/ml; 500 ml D$_5$W.
   Instruction: Dilute the drug in 75 ml of D$_5$W and infuse over 30 min.
   a. Drug dosage per day should be _____.
   b. Drug dosage per 8 hours _____.
   c. How many drops per minute should the client recieve? _____

2. Order: cefamandole (Mandol) 500 mg IV q6h
   Available: cefamandole (Mandol) is in powdered form in a vial

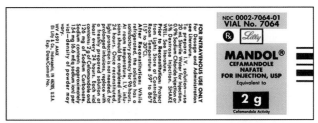

   For reconstitution: Add 6.6 ml of diluent = 8 ml of drug solution (2 g = 8 ml).
   Set and solution: Secondary set with 100 ml D$_5$W. Drop factor is 15 gtt/ml.
   Instruction: Dilute drug solution in 100 ml of D$_5$W and infuse over 30 min.
   a. How many mg should the client receive per dose? _____
   b. How many gtt/min _____.

3. Order: tobramycin (Nebcin) 50 mg IV q8h
Drug parameters: 3 mg/kg/day in three divided doses. Client weighs 65 kg.
Available:

Set and solution: Cylinder IV set with drop factor of 60 gtt/ml; 500 ml D₅W.
Instruction: Dilute tobramycin in 100 ml of D₅W and infuse over 40 min.
a. How many ml should the client receive per dose? _____
b. How many gtt/min _____.
c. Is the tobramycin dose within safe parameters? _____ Explain.

4. Order: ampicillin 500 mg IVq6h
Available: Add 4.5 ml of diluent = 5 ml (2 g = 5 ml)

Convert grams to milligrams.
Set and solution: Cylinder set with drop factor of 60 gtt/ml; 500 ml of D₅W.
Instruction: Dilute ampicillin in 50 ml of D₅W and infuse over 15 min.
a. How many ml should the client receive per dose? _____
b. How many gtt/min using the cylinder set? _____
c. Determine the volumetric infusion rate. _____

5. Order: ticarcillin (Ticar) 750 mg IV g6h
Available:

Set and solution: Cylinder IV set with drop factor of 60 gtt/ml; 500 ml D₅W.
Instruction: Dilute ticarcillin in 20 ml of D₅W and infuse over 30 min.
a. How many milliliters (ml) should the client receive per dose? _____
b. How many gtt/min should the client receive? _____
c. Determine the volumetric infusion rate. _____

6. Order: ciprofloxacin (Cipro) 0.1 g, IV, q12 h
Available:

Set and solution: Secondary set with drip factor 15 gtt/ml; 100 ml of D₅W

Instruction: Dilute drug in 100 ml of D_5W and infuse in 60 minutes

a. Change grams to milligrams

b. How many milliliters (ml) of Cipro should be given per dose? _____

c. What is the IV flow rate in drops per minute? _____

d. Determine the volumetric infusion rate. _____

7. Order: gentamicin 100 mg, IV q8h

Client weighs 165 pounds

Drug parameters: 3-5 mg/kg/day in 3 divided doses

Available: gentamicin 80 mg/2 ml vial

Set and solution: Cylinder IV set with drop factor 60 gtt/ml; 250 ml of D_5W

Instruction: Dilute gentamicin in 75 ml of D_5W and infuse over 40 minutes.

a. How many kg does the client weigh? _____

b. Is the gentamicin dose within safe parameters? _____

c. How many milliliters (ml) of gentamicin should the client receive per dose? _____

d. What is the IV flow rate? _____

e. Determine the volumetric infusion rate _____

8. Order: etoposide (VePesid) 75 mg/m²/day for 5 consecutive days q3-4wk. Client's weight is 134 lb and height is 66 inches.

Use the nomogram to determine body surface areas (BSA, m²) (Figure 4E–6).

FIGURE 4E–6 Nomogram of body surface area for adults. Directions: (1) Find height. (2) Find weight. (3) Draw a straight line that connects the height and weight. (4) Where the line intersects on the body surface area column is the body surface area (m²). (Sources: Deglin, Vallerand, Russin A: *Davis's drug guide for nurses*, ed 2, Philadelphia, 1991, FA Davis; Lentner C, editor: *Geigy scientific tables*, ed 8, vol 1, Basle, Switzerland, 1981, Ciba-Geigy, pp. 226-227.)

Available:

a. What is the client's BSA? _____
b. How many milligrams should the client receive? _____
c. How many milliliters of drug solution should the client receive? _____

Set and solution: Secondary set with 250 ml of D_5W to run for 60 min. Drop factor is 15 gtt/ml.

Determine the volumetric pump for this problem in addition to the drug and IV flow calculations.

ANSWERS TO PRACTICE PROBLEMS

1   CONTINUOUS INTRAVENOUS FLOW RATES

1. a. Microdrip set because the client is to receive 83 ml/h

   b. Two-step method: for continuous IV flow rate

   Step 1. $\dfrac{1000}{12} = 83$ ml/h

   Step 2. $\dfrac{83 \text{ ml/h} \times \overset{1}{\cancel{60}} \text{ drops}}{\underset{1}{\cancel{60}} \text{ min}} = 83$ gtt/min

2. a. 1000 ml

   b. 8 h

   c. Step 1. $\dfrac{1000}{8} = 125$ ml/h

   Step 2. $\dfrac{125 \text{ ml/h} \times \overset{1}{\cancel{15}} \text{ gtt}}{\underset{4}{\cancel{60}} \text{ min}} = \dfrac{125}{4} = 31$ gtt/min

3. a. Microdrip set

   b. Step 1. $\dfrac{250}{24} = 10$ ml/hr

   Step 2. $\dfrac{10 \text{ ml/h} \times \overset{1}{\cancel{60}} \text{ gtt}}{\underset{1}{\cancel{60}} \text{ min}} = 10$ gtt/min

4. a. BF: $\dfrac{D}{H} \times V = \dfrac{10}{20} \times 20 = \dfrac{200}{20} = 10$ ml KCl

   b. $\dfrac{1000}{10} = 100$ ml/hr

   Macrodrip set $\dfrac{100 \times \overset{1}{\cancel{15}}}{\underset{4}{\cancel{60}} \text{ min}} = 25$ gtt/min

   Microdrip set $\dfrac{100 \times \overset{1}{\cancel{60}}}{\underset{1}{\cancel{60}} \text{ min}} = 100$ gtt/min

2   DIRECT IV INJECTION

1. a. BF: $\dfrac{D}{H} \times V = \dfrac{40 \text{ m\cancel{g}}}{10 \text{ m\cancel{g}}} \times 1 \text{ ml} = 4$ ml

   $\dfrac{1 \text{ ml} \times 40 \text{ m\cancel{g}}}{10 \text{ m\cancel{g}} \times 1} = \dfrac{40}{10} = 4$ ml

   b. DA:
   known drug : known min :: desired drug : desired min
   5 mg   :   1 min   ::   40 mg   :   x
   $5x = 40$
   $x = 8$ min

2. a. RP: H : V :: D : x
   10 mg : 1 ml :: 5 mg : x
   $10x = 5$
   $x = \dfrac{5}{10} = \frac{1}{2}$ or 0.5 ml drug

   b.
   known drug : known min :: desired drug : desired min
   10 mg   :   4 min   ::   5 mg   :   x
   $10x = 20$
   $x = 2$ min

3 **INTERMITTENT INTRAVENOUS SET**

1. a. 750 mg per day

  b. Drug calculation for q8h

$$\text{BF: } \frac{D}{H} \times V = \frac{250 \text{ mg}}{500 \text{ mg}} \times 2 = \frac{500}{500}$$
$$= 1 \text{ ml of kanamycin}$$

  or

  RP: H : V :: D : x

    500 mg : 2 ml :: 250 mg : x ml

          $500x = 500$

            $x = 1$ ml of kanamycin

  c. IV flow calculation: $\dfrac{75 \text{ ml} \times 60 \text{ (set)}}{30 \text{ min}} = \dfrac{4500}{30}$
$$= 150 \text{ gtt/min}$$

2. a. Drug calculation: Change 2 g to milligrams.

  2 g = 2.000 mg

$$\text{BF: } \frac{D}{H} \times V = \frac{500}{2000} \times 8 \text{ ml} = \frac{4000}{2000} = 2 \text{ ml Mandol}$$

  or

$$\text{DA: ml} = \frac{8 \text{ ml} \times \quad 1 \cancel{g} \quad \times \overset{1}{\cancel{500}} \text{ mg}}{2 \cancel{g} \times \underset{2}{\cancel{1000}} \text{ mg} \times \quad 1} = \frac{8}{4}$$
$$= 2 \text{ ml of Mandol}$$

  b. IV flow calculation: $\dfrac{100 \text{ ml} \times \overset{1}{\cancel{15}} \text{ gtt (set)}}{\underset{2}{\cancel{30}} \text{ min}}$
$$= \frac{100}{2} = 50 \text{ gtt/min}$$

3. a. Drug calculation: BF: $\dfrac{D}{H} \times V = \dfrac{50}{80} \times 2 = \dfrac{100}{80}$
$$= 1.25 \text{ ml of tobramycin}$$

  b. IV flow calculation: $\dfrac{100 \text{ ml} \times \overset{3}{\cancel{60}} \text{ gtt (set)}}{\underset{2}{\cancel{40}} \text{ min}}$
$$= \frac{300}{2} = 150 \text{ gtt/min}$$

  c. Drug parameter: It is within safe parameters
(3 kg × 65 = 195 mg/day)
Client is receiving 50 mg × 3 = 150 mg/day.

4. a. Drug calculation: Convert to milligrams.

  2 g = 2.000 mg

$$\text{BF: } \frac{D}{H} \times V = \frac{500}{2000} \times 5 = \frac{5}{4} = 1.25 \text{ ml of}$$
$$\text{ampicillin}$$

  or

  RP: H : V :: D : x

    2000 mg : 5 ml :: 500 mg : x ml

          $2000x = 2500$

            $x = 1.25$ ml of ampicillin

  b. IV flow calculation:

$$\frac{50 \text{ ml} \times \overset{4}{\cancel{60}} \text{ gtt (set)}}{\underset{1}{\cancel{15}} \text{ min}} = \frac{200}{1} = 200 \text{ gtt/min}$$

  c. Volumetric infusion pump rate:

$$50 \text{ ml} + 1.25 \text{ ml} \div \frac{15}{60} = 51.25 \text{ ml} \times \frac{\overset{4}{\cancel{60}}}{\underset{1}{\cancel{15}}}$$
$$= 205 \text{ ml/hr}$$

5. a. $\text{BF: } \dfrac{D}{H} \times V = \dfrac{750 \text{ mg}}{1000 \text{ mg}} \times 4 \text{ ml} = \dfrac{3000}{1000}$
$$= 3 \text{ ml of Ticar}$$

  or

$$\text{DA: ml} = \frac{4 \text{ ml} \times \quad 1 \cancel{g} \quad \times \overset{3}{\cancel{750}} \text{ mg}}{1 \cancel{g} \times \underset{4}{\cancel{1000}} \text{ mg} \times \quad 1} = \frac{12}{4}$$
$$= 3 \text{ ml of Ticar}$$

  b. IV flow calculation: $\dfrac{20 \text{ ml} \times \overset{2}{\cancel{60}} \text{ gtt (set)}}{\underset{1}{\cancel{30}} \text{ min}} = \dfrac{40}{1}$
$$= 40 \text{ gtt/min}$$

  c. Volumetric infusion pump rate:

$$20 \text{ ml} + 3 \text{ ml} \div \frac{30}{60} = 23 \text{ ml} \times \frac{\overset{2}{\cancel{60}}}{\underset{1}{\cancel{30}}} = 46 \text{ ml/h}$$

(Increase in D_5W solution may be desired)

6. a. 0.1 g = 0.100 mg = 100 mg

  b. $\text{BF: } \dfrac{D}{H} \times V = \dfrac{\overset{1}{\cancel{100}} \text{ mg}}{\underset{2}{\cancel{200}} \text{ mg}} \times 20 \text{ ml} = \dfrac{20}{2} = 10 \text{ ml}$

$$\text{DA: ml} = \frac{20 \text{ ml} \times \overset{1}{\cancel{100}} \text{ mg}}{\cancel{200} \text{ mg} \times \quad 1} = \frac{20}{2} = 10 \text{ ı}$$

  c. $\dfrac{10 \text{ ml} + 100 \text{ ml} \times 15 \text{ gtt/ml (set)}}{60 \text{ min to admin}} = \dfrac{110 \times 15}{60} =$
27.5 or 28 gtt/min

  d. $10 \text{ ml} + 100 \text{ ml} \div \dfrac{\overset{1}{\cancel{60}} \text{ min to admin}}{\underset{1}{\cancel{60}} \text{ min/hr}} = 110 \text{ ml/hr}$

7. a. 165 pounds ÷ 2.2 = 75 kg

  b. Yes, dose is within safe parameters.

  3 mg × 75 kg = 225 mg divided by 3 doses = 75 mg

  5 mg × 75 kg = 375 mg divided by 3 doses = 125 mg

  c. $\text{BF: } \dfrac{D}{H} \times V = \dfrac{100 \text{ mg}}{80 \text{ mg}} \times 2 \text{ ml} = \dfrac{200}{80} = 2.5 \text{ ml}$

$$\text{DA: ml} = \frac{2 \text{ ml} \times \overset{5}{\cancel{100}} \text{ mg}}{\underset{4}{\cancel{80}} \text{ mg} \times 1} = \frac{10}{4} = 2.5 \text{ ml}$$

d. $\dfrac{75 \text{ ml} \times \overset{3}{\cancel{60}} \text{ gtt/ml (set)}}{\underset{2}{\cancel{40}} \text{ min to admin}} = \dfrac{225}{2} =$

112.5 gtt/min

e. $75 \text{ ml} \div \dfrac{40 \text{ min to admin}}{60 \text{ min/hr}} =$

invert divisor and multiple $\quad 75 \times \dfrac{\overset{3}{\cancel{60}}}{\underset{2}{\cancel{40}}} = \dfrac{225}{2} =$

112.5 or 113 ml/hour

8. a. Client's BSA is 1.75.

b. 75 mg × 1.75 (BSA) = 131.25 or 131 mg

c. $\dfrac{D}{H} \times V = \dfrac{131}{150} \times 7.5 \text{ ml} = \dfrac{982.5}{150} = 6.55 \text{ or } 6.6 \text{ ml}$

IV flow calculation with secondary set:

$\dfrac{250 \text{ ml} \times 15 \text{ gtt (set)}}{60 \text{ min}} = \dfrac{3750}{60} = 62.5 \text{ gtt/min}$

Volumetric pump rate: 250 ml + 6.6 ml

$(256.6 \text{ or } 257 \text{ ml}) \div \dfrac{60}{60} = 257 \text{ ml} \times \dfrac{\overset{1}{\cancel{60}}}{\underset{1}{\cancel{60}}}$

$= 257 \text{ ml/hr}$

Section 4F   PEDIATRIC DRUG CALCULATIONS

Outline

Objectives

Terms

Oral

Intramuscular

Pediatric Dosage per Body Weight

Pediatric Dosage per Body Surface Area

Pediatric Calculations for Injectables

Objectives

- Use one of the two primary methods to determine pediatric drug dosage.
- Describe the dosage inaccuracies that may occur with pediatric drug formulas.
- Identify the steps used to determine body surface area from a pediatric nomogram.
- Calculate the drug dosages correctly in the practice problems.

Terms

body surface area (BSA), or m², p. 109

body weight (BW), p. 109

Pediatric drug dosages differ greatly from those for adults because of the physiologic differences between the two. Neonates and infants have immature kidney and liver function, which delays metabolism and elimination of many drugs. In neonates, drug absorption is different as a result of slow gastric emptying time. Decreased gastric acid secretion in children younger than 3 years contributes to altered drug absorption. Neonates and infants have a lower concentration of plasma proteins, which can cause toxicity with drugs that are highly bound to proteins. Young children have less total body fat and more body water; therefore lipid-soluble drugs require smaller doses when less-than-normal fat is present. Water-soluble drugs can require large doses because of a greater percentage of body water. It is the nurse's responsibility to ensure that a safe drug dosage is given and to closely monitor signs and symptoms of side effects and adverse drug reactions.

The purpose of learning how to calculate pediatric drug dosages is to ensure that children receive the correct dose within the approved therapeutic range. The two methods that are considered safe in the administration of drugs to children are the **body weight (BW)** (kg) and **body surface area (BSA, or m²)** methods. Many manufacturers supply information in their literature concerning drug doses for children according to BW. Also, manufacturers frequently give drug parameters for safe dose ranges. It is the nurse's responsibility to check the dose ranges given by the pharmaceutical manufacturers to be certain that the prescribed dose is within the parameters.

Oral

Oral pediatric drug delivery usually requires the use of a calibrated measuring device because most drugs for small children are in liquid form. The measuring device can be a small plastic cup, an oral dropper, a measuring spoon, or an oral syringe (Figure 4F–1). Some liquid medications come with their own calibrated droppers. The type of measuring device chosen depends on the age or the developmental level of the child. For infants and toddlers, the oral syringe and dropper can provide better drug delivery than a small cup. A young child who is cooperative is able to use a small cup or measuring spoon. The cup or spoon may be rinsed with water or juice to ensure that the child has received all of the drug. Avoid giving oral medications to a crying child or infant because the drug could be easily aspirated or the child could "spit out" the drug. For the older child, some drugs are available in chewable form. Children should be told not to chew drugs that are enteric-coated or in time-release form.

Intramuscular

Intramuscular (IM) sites for drug administration are chosen on the basis of the age and muscle development of the child (Table 4F–1). All injections should be given in a manner that minimizes physical and psychosocial trauma. Explanations of injection administration should be given to children who can comprehend. With the very young child, distraction or brief restraint may be necessary. Comfort measures should immediately follow the injection.

FIGURE 4F–1 Calibrated measuring devices. (From Kee JL, Marshall SM: *Clinical calculations,* ed 6, Philadelphia, 2009, Saunders.)

Table 4F–1

Pediatric Guidelines for Intramuscular Injections According to Muscle Group*

	Amount by Muscle Group (ml)					
	Vastus Lateralis	Rectus Femoris	Ventrogluteal	Dorsal Gluteal	Gluteus Maximus	Deltoid
Neonates	0.5 ml	Not safe	Not safe	Not safe	Not safe	Not safe
Infants 1-12 months	0.5-1 ml	Not safe	Not safe	Not safe	Not safe	Not safe
Toddlers 1-2 years	0.5-2 ml	0.5-1 ml	Not safe	Not safe	Not safe	0.5-1 ml
Preschool to child 3-12 years	2 ml	2 ml	0.5-3 ml	0.5-2 ml	0.5-2 ml	0.5-1 ml
Adolescent 12-18 years	2 ml	2 ml	2-3 ml	2-3 ml	2 ml	1-1.5 ml

*The safe use of all sites is based on normal muscle development and size of the child. Follow institutional policies and procedures. (From Kee JL, Marshall SM: *Clinical calculations*, ed 6, St. Louis, 2009, Elsevier.)

Pediatric Dosage per Body Weight

EXAMPLE   Order: cefaclor (Ceclor) 50 mg q.i.d. Child weighs 15 lb or 6.8 kg (15 ÷ 2.2 = 6.8)
Child's drug dosage: 20-40 mg/kg/day in three divided doses
Available:

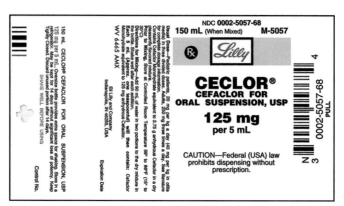

Is the prescribed dose safe? _____

Answer:

Drug parameters: 20 mg × 6.8 kg = 136 mg/day
                   40 mg × 6.8 kg = 272 mg/day

Dosage order: 50 mg × 4 = 200 mg/day

Dosage is within safe drug parameters.

a. BF: $\dfrac{D}{H} \times V = \dfrac{50}{125} \times 5 = \dfrac{250}{125} = 2$ ml

b. RP:

$$H \quad : \quad V \quad :: \quad D \quad : \quad x$$
$$125\ \text{mg} \quad : \quad 5\ \text{ml} \quad :: \quad 50\ \text{mg} \quad : \quad x\ \text{ml}$$

$$125x = 250$$
$$x = 2\ \text{ml (cc)}$$

Cross-multiply:

c. FE: $\dfrac{H}{V} = \dfrac{D}{X}$ $\dfrac{125 \text{ mg}}{5 \text{ ml}} = \dfrac{50 \text{ mg}}{x \text{ ml}}$

$$125x = 250$$
$$x = 2 \text{ ml}$$

d. DA: ml $= \dfrac{5 \text{ ml} \times \overset{2}{\cancel{50}} \text{ mg}}{\underset{5}{\cancel{125}} \text{ mg} \times 1} = \dfrac{10}{5} = 2 \text{ ml}$

Cefaclor 50 mg = 2 ml. Give 2 ml four times a day.

Pediatric Dosage per Body Surface Area

To calculate pediatric dose by BSA, the child's height and weight are needed. Figure 4F-2 is the nomogram used to determine the BSA for infants and children.

FIGURE 4F–2 Nomogram of body surface area for infants and children. Directions: (1) Find height. (2) Find weight. (3) Draw a straight line that connects the height and weight. (4) Where the line intersects on the body surface area column is the body surface area (m²). (Sources: Deglin, Vallerand, Russin A: *Davis's drug guide for nurses*, ed 2, Philadelphia, 1991, FA Davis; Lentner C, editor: *Geigy scientific tables*, ed 8, vol 1, Basle, Switzerland, 1981, Ciba-Geigy, pp. 226-227.)

SECTION F

EXAMPLE

Order: methotrexate (Mexate) 50 mg weekly. Child's height is 54 inches and weight is 90 lb (41 kg).

Child's drug dosage: 25-75 mg/m²/week
Child's height and weight intersect at 1.3 m² (BSA).
Is the prescribed dose safe? _____
Answer:
Multiply the BSA, 1.3 m², by the minimum and maximum doses.
25 mg × 1.3 m² = 32.5 mg
75 mg × 1.3 m² = 97.5 mg

Dosage is considered safe within the parameters according to the child's BSA.

PRACTICE
PROBLEM I

PEDIATRIC DOSING (ORAL)

Solve the following problems using the BW or BSA method. The safe dosage is given in drug reference books.

1. Order: dicloxacillin sodium 100 mg q6h. Child weighs 55 lb (_____ kg).
   Child's drug dosage range: less than 40 kg, 12.5-25 mg/kg/day
   Available: dicloxacillin 62.5 mg per 5 ml
   a. Is the prescribed dose safe? _____
   b. How many milliliters should be given for each dose? _____

2. Order: digoxin (Lanoxin), 35 mcg/kg/loading dose, PO.
   Child weighs 10 kg.
   Available: Lanoxin 50 mcg/ml (0.05 mg/ml)
   a. How many micrograms or milligrams should the child receive? _____
   b. How many milliliters should be given for the loading dose? _____

3. Order: amoxicillin (Amoxil) 200 mg PO q8h. Child weighs 26 lb (12 kg).
   Child's drug dosage: 20-40 mg/kg/day in three divided doses
   Available:

   a. Is the prescribed dose safe? _____
   b. How many milliliters should be given every 8 hr? _____

4. Order: azithromycin (Zithromax), PO. First day: 10 mg/kg/day; next 4 days; 5 mg/kg/day.
   Client weighs 44 pounds.
   Available:

   a. How much does the child weigh in kilograms? _____

b. How many milliliters should the child receive for the first day? _____

c. How many milliliters should the child receive each day for the next 4 days (second to fifth days)? _____

5. Order: amoxicillin and clavulanate potassium (Augmentin) 100 mg PO q8h.

Child weighs 28 lb.

Child's drug dosage: 20-40 mg/kg/day

Available:

a. Is the prescribed drug dose within safe drug parameters? _____

b. How many milliliters should the child receive per dose? _____

6. Order: doxycycline (Vibramycin) 50 mg PO q12h.

Child is 10 years old and weighs 88 lb.

Child's drug dosage: 2.2-4.4 mg/kg/day in one to two doses

Available:

a. What would be the dosage parameter range for this child? _____

b. Is the prescribed drug dose within safe drug parameters? _____

c. How many milliliters should the child receive per dose? _____

7. Order: ampicillin 200 mg PO q6h.

Child weighs 27 kg.

Child's drug dosage: 25-50 mg/kg/day

Available:

Is the prescribed dose safe? _____

How many milliliters should the child receive per dose? _____

8. Order: vinblastine (Velsar)

Child's BSA is 1.2 m².

Child's drug dosage: 2.5 mg/m²

How many milligrams should the child receive? _____

Pediatric Calculations for Injectables

The same methods used to calculate oral dosages for children are used to calculate injectable dosages. They are calculated from (1) BW (kg) and (2) BSA (m^2). Use the nomogram for BSA.

PRACTICE PROBLEM 2

PEDIATRIC INJECTABLES

Solve the following drug problems and indicate whether the drug dose is within the safe drug parameters.

1. Order: tobramycin (Nebcin) 10 mg IM q8h.
   Child weighs 10 kg.
   Child's drug dosage: 3 mg/kg/day in three divided doses
   Available:

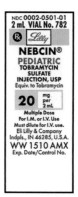

   a. Is the dose within safe drug parameters? _____
   b. How many milliliters should the child receive per dose? _____

2. Order: promethazine (Phenergan) 20 mg IM q6h.
   Child weighs 45 kg.
   Child's drug dosage: 0.25-0.5 mg/kg/dose; repeat every 4 to 6 hr
   Available: Phenergan 25 mg/ml
   a. Is the dose within safe drug parameters? _____
   b. How many milliliters should the child receive per dose? _____

3. Order: oxacillin sodium 250 mg IM q6h.
   Child weighs 15 kg.
   Child's drug dosage: 50-100 mg/kg/day in divided doses
   Available: 2.7 ml of diluent = 3 ml

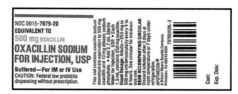

   a. How many milligrams should the child receive per day? _____
   b. How much diluent should be added? _____
   c. How many milliliters should the child receive per dose? _____
   d. Is the dose within safe drug parameters? _____

4. Order: nafcillin sodium 200 mg IM q6h.
   Child weighs 10 kg.
   Child's drug dosage: 100-300 mg/kg/day in divided doses
   Available: 1.8 ml of diluent = 2 ml

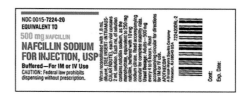

a. How many milligrams will the child receive per day? _____
b. Is the drug dosage per day within safe drug parameters? _____
c. How many milliliters should the child receive per dose? _____

5. Order: The newborn is to receive AquaMEPHYTON (vitamin K) 0.5 mg immediately after delivery.
   Available:

a. Which AquaMEPHYTON container should be selected? _____
b. How many milliliters should the newborn receive? _____

6. Order: cefazolin (Ancef) 125 mg IM q6h.
   Child weighs 22 kg.
   Child's drug dosage: 25-50 mg/kg/day in three to four divided doses (up to 100 mg/kg/day)
   Available:

a. How many milligrams should the child receive per day? _____
b. Is the dose within safe drug parameters? _____
c. The drug label does not give the amount of diluent to add to the Ancef powder. Check the pamphlet insert. With 3.4 ml of diluent added, it is equivalent to 4 ml of drug solution.
d. How many milliliters of cefazolin should the child receive per dose? _____

7. Order: hydroxyzine (Vistaril) 50 mg IM.
   Child's height is 47 inches and weight is 45 lb.
   Child's drug dosage: 30 mg/m²
   Available: Vistaril 25 mg/ml
   a. Is the dose within safe drug parameters? _____

8. Order: methotrexate (Mexate) 50 mg IM weekly.
   Child's height is 56 inches and weight is 100 lb.
   Child's drug dosage: 25-75 mg/m²/wk
   Available: methotrexate 2.5 mg/ml; 25 mg/ml; 100 mg/ml
   a. Is the dose within safe drug parameters? _____
   b. Which methotrexate should be selected? _____

ANSWERS TO PRACTICE PROBLEMS

I	PEDIATRIC DOSING (ORAL) USING BASIC FORMULA, RATIO AND PROPORTION, OR DIMENSIONAL ANALYSIS

1. a. Child weighs 25 kg (55 lb ÷ 2.2 = 25 kg)
  Drug parameters:
  12.5 mg × 25 kg = 312.5 mg/day
  25 mg × 25 kg = 625 mg/day
  Dosage order: 100 mg × 4 times a day (q6h) = 400 mg/day
  Dosage is within safe drug parameters.

b. BF: $\dfrac{D}{H} \times V = \dfrac{100}{62.5} \times 5\ ml = \dfrac{500}{62.5}$

RP: H : V :: D : x
  62.5 mg : 5 ml :: 100 mg : x ml
  $62.5x = 500$
  $x = 8$ ml of dicloxacillin

SECTION F

2. Child's drug dosage:

   a. 35 mcg × 10 kg = 350 mcg, or 0.35 mg

      350 mcg = 0.350 mg

   b. $\dfrac{D}{H} \times V = \dfrac{350 \text{ mcg}}{50 \text{ mcg}} \times 1 \text{ ml} = 7 \text{ ml loading dose}$

      or

      $\dfrac{0.35 \text{ mg}}{0.05 \text{ mg}} \times 1 \text{ ml} = 7 \text{ ml loading dose}$

3. Drug parameters:

   20 mg × 12 kg = 240 mg/day

   40 mg × 12 kg = 480 mg/day

   Dosage order: 200 mg × 3 (q8h) = 600 mg/day

   Dosage is *not* within safe drug parameters. Dose exceeds the drug parameters.

   Health care provider must be contacted.

4. **a.** 20 kg

   b. First day: 10 mg × 20 kg = 200 mg

      BF: $\dfrac{D}{H} \times V = \dfrac{\overset{1}{\cancel{200 \text{ mg}}}}{\underset{1}{\cancel{200 \text{ mg}}}} \times 5 \text{ ml} = 5 \text{ ml}$

      or

      RP: H : V :: D : x

        200 mg : 5 ml :: 200 mg : x

                $200x = 1000$

                   $x = 5 \text{ ml}$

      or

      DA: $\text{ml} = \dfrac{5 \text{ ml} \times \overset{1}{\cancel{200 \text{ mg}}}}{\underset{1}{\cancel{200 \text{ mg}}} \times 1} = 5 \text{ ml}$

      First day give 5 ml.

---

   c. Second to fifth days (next 4 days):

      5 mg × 20 kg = 100 mg

      Give 2.5 ml/day. Same answer worked out by BF, RP, and DA.

5. **a.** Drug parameters: (28 lb ÷ 2.2 = 12.7 kg)

      20 mg × 12.7 kg = 254 mg/day

      40 mg × 2.7 kg = 508 mg/day

      Dosage order: 100 mg × 3 (q8h) = 300 mg/day

      Dosage is within safe drug parameters.

   b. 4 ml of Augmentin

6. **a.** Drug parameters: 88 mg to 176 mg per day

   b. Dose is within safe drug parameters.

   c. 10 ml per dose of Vibramycin

7. Drug parameters:

   25 mg × 27 kg = 675 mg/day

   50 mg × 27 kg = 1350 mg/day

   Dosage order: 200 mg × 4 (q6h) = 800 mg/day

   Dosage is within safe drug parameters.

   $\dfrac{D}{H} \times V = \dfrac{200}{250} \times 5 = \dfrac{1000}{250} = 4 \text{ ml of ampicillin}$

8. Drug dosage: 2.5 mg × 1.2 m² = 3 mg

   Administer 3 mg vinblastine.

---

2   PEDIATRIC INJECTABLES

1. **a.** Tobramycin parameter: 3 mg/kg/day × 10 kg = 30 mg/day in three divided doses

      Drug order: 10 mg × 3 (q8h) = 30 mg/day

      Dosage is within safe drug parameters.

   b. 10 mg = 1 ml/dose

      Child should receive 1 ml per dose.

2. **a.** Phenergan parameters:

      0.25 mg/kg/dose × 45 kg = 11.25 mg/dose

      0.50 mg/kg/dose × 45 kg = 22.5 mg/dose

      Drug order: Phenergan 20 mg IM per dose

      Dosage is within safe drug parameters.

   b. Phenergan 20 mg = 0.8 ml

3. **a.** 250 mg × 4 (q6h) = 1000 mg/day

   b. Add 2.7 ml of diluent = 3 ml of drug solution

   c. 1.5 ml

   d. Dosage is within safe drug parameters.

4. **a.** 200 mg × 4 (q6h) = 800 mg/day

   b. Dose per day is safe but not in therapeutic range. Notify health care provider.

      100 mg × 10 kg × 1000 mg

      300 mg × 10 kg = 3000 mg

   c. Add 1.8 ml diluent = 2 ml (500 mg = 2 ml)

      Nafcillin 200 mg = 0.8 ml

5. **a.** Preferred selection is AquaMEPHYTON 1 mg = 0.5 ml.

   b. *AquaMEPHYTON 1 mg = 0.5 ml*

      $\dfrac{D}{H} \times V = \dfrac{0.5 \text{ mg}}{1.0 \text{ mg}} \times 0.5 \text{ ml} = \dfrac{0.25}{1.0} = 0.25 \text{ ml}$

AquaMEPHYTON 10 mg = 1 ml

$$\frac{D}{H} \times V = \frac{0.5 \text{ mg}}{10 \text{ mg}} \times 1.0 \text{ ml} = \frac{0.5}{10} = 0.05 \text{ ml}$$

For AquaMEPHYTON 1 mg = 0.5 ml. Give 0.25 ml. (Use a tuberculin syringe.)

For AquaMEPHYTON 10 mg = 1 ml. Give 0.05 ml. (Use a tuberculin syringe; however, it would be difficult to give this small amount.)

6. **a.** 125 mg × 4 (q6h) = 500 mg

   b. Drug parameters: 22 kg × 25 mg/kg/day = 550 mg

   22 kg × 50 mg/kg/day = 1100 mg

   22 kg × 100 mg/kg/day = 2200 mg maximum (range: 550-2200 mg)

   Drug dose per day is below the suggested child's drug dose range. The nurse should contact the health care provider. The daily drug dose may need to be increased.

   c. Add 3.4 ml of diluent yielding 4 ml of drug solution.

   d. Give 1 ml of cefazolin (Ancef) per dose.

7. Height and weight intersect at 0.82 m².

   Hydroxyzine parameter: 30 mg/m² × 0.82 m² = 24.6 mg, or 25 mg

   Drug order: hydroxyzine 50 mg IM

   Dosage ordered is *not* within safe parameters. Dosage exceeds the drug parameters. *Do not* give the medication. Notify the health care provider.

8. Height and weight intersect at 1.38 m².

   Methotrexate parameters:

   25 mg/m²/wk × 1.38 m² = 34.5 mg/wk

   75 mg/m²/wk × 1.38 m² = 103.5 mg/wk

   Drug order: methotrexate 50 mg/wk IM

   Dosage is within safe drug parameters.

   (1) If methotrexate 25 mg/ml is used, give 2 ml (50 mg) **or**

   (2) If methotrexate 100 mg/ml is used, give 0.5 ml. Because of the amount of solution, it may be more desirable to give 0.5 ml of the 100 mg/ml solution.

THREE

Contemporary Issues in Pharmacology

This unit comprises nine chapters that cover a range of issues affecting drug therapy and nursing. Chapter 5, The Drug Approval Process, discusses drug standards and federal legislation for American and Canadian drugs that establish safety guidelines for drug use, drug names, and drug resources. Ethical considerations in the pharmacotherapeutic regimen are also addressed.

Chapter 6, Transcultural and Genetic Considerations, helps the nurse understand and respond to unique cultural and genetic factors that may influence drug therapy for a particular client. Factors such as heritage, communication styles, family organization, spirituality and religion, health beliefs and practices, biocultural ecology, and complementary, alternative, and traditional medicine are discussed.

Chapter 7, Drug Interaction and Over-the-Counter Drugs, and Chapter 8, Drugs of Abuse, cover drug interactions and drug abuse, two areas of special interest to nurses. Assessing drug interaction has always been and remains an ongoing function of the nurse. Because drug abuse is a national problem from which no portion of the population is immune—including health professionals—it is a topic of great concern to nurses.

Chapter 9, Herbal Therapy with Nursing Implications, explores the increasingly popular herbal-based preparations that are available over-the-counter. It covers the most commonly used herbs and discusses their indications, preparation, dosages, potential hazards, and tips for safe and effective use.

Chapter 10, Pediatric Pharmacology, and Chapter 11, Geriatric Pharmacology, cover pharmacokinetic and pharmacodynamic effects specific to these age groups. It also discusses the special attention required when administering drugs to these age groups. Specific recommendations are described.

With the increasing movement of health care into the community, nurses, above all other health care providers, are gaining more responsibilities and opportunities to guide clients in safe medication administration. Chapter 12, Medication Administration in Community Settings, focuses on aspects of drug therapy unique to the home, school, workplace, and other alternative care settings.

Chapter 13, The Role of the Nurse in Drug Research, discusses the nurse's challenges regarding drug research. In general practice the nurse identifies specific needs that may be met by medications. When part of clinical drug trials, the nurse needs to be aware of informed consent and the client's response to drugs.

5

The Drug Approval Process

ELECTRONIC RESOURCES

evolve

Evolve website (http://evolve.elsevier.com/KeeHayes/pharmacology/):
- *Case Studies*
- *Content Updates*
- *Frequently Asked Questions*
- *Student Review Activities*
- *WebLinks*
- *Additional Reference Material*

Companion CD-ROM:
- *NCLEX Examination Review Questions*
- *Pharmacology Animations*
- *IV Therapy Checklists*
- *Medication Error Checklists*
- *Drug Calculation Problems*
- *Electronic Calculators*
- *Top 200 Drugs with Pronunciations*
- *References from the Textbook*

Outline

Objectives

Terms

Drug Standards and Legislation
Drug Standards
Federal Legislation

Nurse Practice Acts

Canadian Drug Regulation

Initiatives to Combat Drug Counterfeiting

Drug Names

Drug Resources

Food and Drug Administration

Pregnancy Categories

Poison Control Centers

Ethical Considerations

International Issues

Key Websites

NCLEX Study Questions

Objectives

- Discuss the various federal legislation acts related to Food and Drug Administration drug approvals.
- Explain the three Canadian schedules for drugs sold in Canada.
- Describe the function of nurse practice acts.
- Differentiate between chemical, generic, and brand names of drugs.
- Describe two drug resource (reference) books.
- Explain various ethical values that the nurse should consider in relation to health care.

Terms

American Hospital Formulary Service (AHFS) Drug Information, p. 125
brand (trade) name, p. 124
chemical name, p. 124
controlled substances, p. 122

Drug Enforcement Administration (DEA), p. 122
Drug Facts and Comparisons (F & C), p. 125
Food and Drug Administration (FDA), p. 121
generic name, p. 124

malfeasance, p. 123
misfeasance, p. 123
nonfeasance, p. 123
Physicians' Desk Reference (PDR), p. 125
pharmacology, p. 121

United States Pharmacopeia—Drug Information (USP-DI), p. 125
United States Pharmacopeia National Formulary (USP-NF), p. 121

Pharmacology is the study of the effects of chemical substances on living tissues. Early drugs were derived from plants, animals, and minerals. Records of drug use date back to 2700 BC in the Middle East and China. The drugs most commonly used then were laxatives and emetics to induce vomiting.

In 1550 BC the Egyptians wrote their empirical observations of drug therapy on what has come to be known as the Ebers Medical Papyrus. They suggested castor oil for a laxative and opium for pain. They also suggested that moldy bread be applied to wounds and bruises—3500 years before Alexander Fleming's discovery of penicillin.

The Roman physician and writer Galen (131-201 AD) was considered an authority in medicine and pharmacy for hundreds of years. He initiated the common use of prescriptions and used several ingredients to treat a specific illness.

After the fall of the Roman Empire, medicine and pharmacy returned to the realms of folklore and tradition. During this time, however, Christian monks kept information on medicine and pharmacy in their monasteries and tended the sick and needy. The medicines used by the monks were derived from plants and herbs grown in monastery gardens.

Around 1240 AD, Arabic doctors formulated the first set of drug standards and measurements (grains, drams, minims), known as the *apothecary system*. (Currently the units of the metric system are used internationally to measure drugs; the apothecary system is being phased out.) In fifteenth-century England, apothecary shops were owned by barber-surgeons, physicians, and independent merchants dispensing herbal and chemical remedies.

In the eighteenth century, the following breakthrough drugs were introduced: the vaccine for smallpox, digitalis (from the foxglove plant) for strengthening and slowing the heartbeat, and vitamin C from citrus fruit. In the nineteenth century, morphine and codeine were extracted from opium; atropine, bromides, and iodine were introduced; amyl nitrite was used to relieve the pain of angina; and the anesthetics ether and nitrous oxide were discovered.

In the early twentieth century, aspirin was derived from salicylic acid, and phenobarbital, insulin, and the sulfonamides were introduced. A vast majority of modern drugs date back to the early 1940s. Antibiotics (penicillin, tetracycline, streptomycin), antihistamines, and cortisone were marketed in the 1940s. In the 1950s, antipsychotic drugs, antihypertensives, oral contraceptives, and the polio vaccine were introduced. The year 2006 brought FDA approval for 18 new drugs. The annual average of newly approved drugs for the prior six years was 26 drugs. Pharmaceutical companies are now spending more on research, yet experiencing decreased approvals. This decrement coincides with a focus on "hard to treat" disorders.

Drug Standards and Legislation

Drug Standards

The set of drug standards used in the United States is the *United States Pharmacopeia* of 1820. The **United States Pharmacopeia National Formulary** (USP-NF), the current authoritative source for drug standards, is revised every 5 years by a group of experts in nursing, pharmaceutics, pharmacology, chemistry, and microbiology. Drugs included in the USP-NF have met high standards for therapeutic use, client safety, quality, purity, strength, packaging safety, and dosage form. Drugs that meet these standards have the initials *USP* following their official name.

The *International Pharmacopeia*, first published in 1951 by the World Health Organization (WHO), provides a basis for standards in strength and composition of drugs for use throughout the world. The book is published in English, Spanish, and French and, like the USP-NF, is revised every 5 years.

Federal Legislation

Through federal legislation, the public is protected from drugs that are impure, toxic, ineffective, or not tested before public sale. The primary purpose of this federal legislation is to ensure safety. America's first law to regulate drugs was the Federal Pure Food and Drug Act of 1906, which did not include drug effectiveness and drug safety.

1938: Food, Drug, and Cosmetic Act

The Food, Drug, and Cosmetic Act of 1938 empowered a governing body, the **Food and Drug Administration (FDA)**, to monitor and regulate the manufacture and marketing of drugs. It is the FDA's responsibility to ensure that all drugs are tested for harmful effects, have labels with accurate information, and enclose with the drug packaging detailed literature that explains adverse effects. The FDA can prevent the marketing of any drug it judges to be incompletely tested or dangerous. Only drugs considered safe by the FDA are approved for marketing.

1952: Durham-Humphrey Amendment to the 1938 Act

The Durham-Humphrey amendment to the Food, Drug, and Cosmetic Act of 1938 distinguished between drugs that can be sold with or without prescription and those that should not be refilled without a new prescription. Those drugs that should not be refilled without a new prescription, such as narcotics, hypnotics, or tranquilizers, must be so labeled.

1962: Kefauver-Harris Amendment to the 1938 Act

The Kefauver-Harris amendment to the Food, Drug, and Cosmetic Act of 1938 resulted from the widely publicized thalidomide tragedy of the 1950s in which pregnant European women who took the sedative-hypnotic thalidomide during the first trimester of pregnancy gave birth to infants with extreme limb deformities. The Kefauver-Harris amendment tightened controls on drug safety, especially experimental drugs, and required that adverse reactions and contraindications must be labeled and included in the literature. Also included in the amendment were provisions for the evaluation of testing methods used by manufacturers, the process for withdrawal of approved drugs when safety and effectiveness were in doubt, and the establishment of the effectiveness of new drugs before marketing.

1970: The Controlled Substances Act

In 1970 the Controlled Substances Act (CSA) of the Comprehensive Drug Abuse Prevention and Control Act, Title II, was passed by Congress. This act, designed to remedy the escalating problem of drug abuse, included several provisions: (1) the promotion of drug education and research into the prevention and treatment of drug dependence; (2) the strengthening of enforcement authority; (3) the establishment of treatment and rehabilitation facilities; and (4) the designation of schedules, or categories, for controlled substances according to abuse liability.

Controlled substances are described in five schedules, or categories, which are listed in Table 5-1. Schedule I drugs are not approved for medical use; schedule II through V drugs have accepted medical use. In addition, the abuse potential and extent of physical and psychologic dependence are greatest with schedule I drugs. This dependency decreases as one moves through the schedule, with schedule V drugs having only limited abuse potential. Some drugs might be listed in more than one schedule category. Codeine is a schedule II drug, but when it is added to acetaminophen, it becomes a schedule III drug, and when it is used in combination as a cough preparation, it becomes a schedule V drug.

Nursing Interventions: Controlled Substances

- Account for all controlled drugs.
- Keep a special controlled-substance record for required information.
- Countersign all discarded or wasted medication.
- Ensure that records and drugs on hand match.
- Keep all controlled drugs locked up; narcotics must be kept under double lock.
- Be certain that only authorized persons have access to the keys.

In 1983 the **Drug Enforcement Administration (DEA)** of the Department of Justice was charged with the role of being the nation's sole legal drug enforcement agency. The Bureau of Narcotics and Dangerous Drugs, which preceded the DEA, is defunct.

1978: Drug Regulation Reform Act

This reform act shortened the time in which new drugs could be developed and marketed.

1992: Drug Relations Act

The regulations were changed to increase the approval rate of drugs used to treat acquired immunodeficiency syndrome (AIDS) and cancer. The pharmaceutical companies pay a user fee at the time they file the application for the new drug. The fee is for the FDA drug approval process.

1997: The Food and Drug Administration Modernization Act

There are five provisions in this act: (1) review and use of new drugs is accelerated; (2) drugs can be tested in children before marketing; (3) clinical trial data are necessary for experimental drug use for serious or life-threatening health conditions; (4) drug companies are required to give information on "off-label" drugs (non-FDA approved drugs) and their uses and costs; and (5) drug companies that plan to discontinue drugs must inform health professionals and clients at least 6 months before stopping drug production.

2003: Health Insurance Portability and Accountability Act (HIPAA)

This act sets the standards for the privacy of individually identifiable health information as of 2003. This rule gives clients more control over their health information, including boundaries on the use and release of health records. Visit *www.hhs.gov/ocr/hipaa* for details.

Implications of HIPAA related to the individual's therapeutic regimen includes limitation on access to informa-

Table 5-1		
Schedule Categories of Controlled Substances		
Schedule	**Examples of Substances**	**Description**
I	heroin, hallucinogenics (LSD, marijuana [except when prescribed with cancer treatment], mescaline, peyote, psilocybin)	Drugs with high abuse potential. No accepted medical use. Labeled C-I.
II	meperidine (Demerol), morphine, hydrocodone, hydromorphone, methadone, oxycodone, codeine, amphetamines, secobarbital, pentobarbital	High potential for drug abuse. Accepted medical use. Can lead to strong physical and psychologic dependency. Labeled C-II.
III	codeine preparations, paregoric, nonnarcotic drugs (pentazocine, propoxyphene)	Medically accepted drugs. Potential abuse is less than that for schedules I and II. May cause dependence. Labeled C-III.
IV	phenobarbital, benzodiazepines (diazepam, oxazepam, lorazepam, chlordiazepoxide), chloral hydrate, meprobamate	Medically accepted drugs. May cause dependence. Labeled C-IV.
V	opioid-controlled substances for diarrhea and cough (e.g., codeine in cough preparations)	Medically accepted drugs. Very limited potential for dependence. Labeled C-V

C, Control; *LSD*, lysergic acid diethylamide.

tion from the pharmacy. For example, the client history can be released only to the client. In addition, the pharmacist must provide a private area for consultation with the client and have all clients sign a statement that they have received a copy of the privacy statement.

2003: Pediatric Research Equity Act

The FDA is authorized to require testing by drug manufacturers of drugs and biologic products for their safety and effectiveness in children. One must not assume that children are small adults.

2003: Medicare Prescription Drug Improvement and Modernization Act (MMA)

The Medicare Prescription Drug Improvement and Modernization Act serves to provide financial assistance to seniors to purchase needed prescription medications. This Act became effective January 1, 2006. According to the MMA, as of 2006 the client is responsible for a monthly premium of $35 and a $250 annual deductible. This benefit will pay 75% of the total cost of the prescription drugs up to a maximum of $2250. There is no drug coverage between $2250 and $5100; Medicare will pay 95% of the drug costs beyond $5100. Between $2250 and $5100, the senior will pay full price for the drugs. Medicare seniors may have supplemental insurance coverage for prescription medications; they must choose whether to continue this policy or sign up for the Medicare drug benefit. Double coverage is not an option.

Nurse Practice Acts

Every state has its own laws regarding drug administration by nurses. Generally, nurses cannot prescribe or administer drugs without a health care provider's order, but state laws vary. Practicing nurses should request a copy and be knowledgeable about the nurse practice act in the state in which they are licensed. In some states nurses who administer a drug without a physician's order are in violation of the nurse practice act and could have their licenses revoked.

In a civil court, the nurse can be prosecuted for giving the wrong drug or dosage, omitting a drug dose, or giving the drug by the wrong route. The legal terms for these offenses are the following:

- *Misfeasance.* Negligence; giving the wrong drug or drug dose that results in the client's death
- *Nonfeasance.* Omission; omitting a drug dose that results in the client's death
- *Malfeasance.* Giving the correct drug but by the wrong route that results in the client's death

Canadian Drug Regulation

In Canada, the Health Protection Branch, Department of National Health and Welfare, is responsible for the administration of the two acts that are the foundation of national drug laws. The manufacture, distribution, and sale of drugs (except narcotics) are controlled by the Canadian Food and Drug Act, amended in 1953. The manufacture, distribution, and sale of narcotic drugs are controlled by the 1996 Controlled Drugs and Substances Act. Like the U.S. Controlled Substances Act, the Canadian act requires prescriptions and strict record keeping for all narcotics.

Drugs sold in Canada are assigned to one of the following schedules:

1. Schedule F Prescription Drugs. All prescription drugs except for narcotics and controlled substances are available only with a prescription (written or verbal); thus these drugs have essentially no potential for abuse. Manufacturing labels are required to include $\boxed{\text{Pr}}$.
2. The Controlled Drug and Substance Act (CDSA) (control and sale of narcotics controlled and abuse substances) identifies eight schedules (schedules V through VIII in process of development) based on potential for abuse. Record keeping and degree of control are specified for each. Labels must include $\Diamond$ for controlled agents and $\langle N \rangle$ for all narcotic agents. Since 2000, benzodiazepines are "targeted substances" with t/c on all labels.

Schedule I: opium poppy and its derivatives (e.g., morphine, heroin); methadone; coca and its derivates (e.g., cocaine)

Schedule II: cannabis and its derivatives (e.g., marijuana, hashish)

Schedule III: amphetamines, methylphenidate, lysergic acid diethylamide (LSD), methaqualone, psilocybin, mescaline

Schedule IV: sedative-hypnotic agents (e.g., barbiturates, benzodiazepines); anabolic steroids

This Act covers select codeine preparations. Low-dose codeine (20 mg/30 ml and 8 mg tablets) is an exception and can be sold only by a pharmacist. Two additional medicinal ingredients, usually caffeine and acetylsalicylic acid, must be part of this codeine preparation.

Nonprescription drugs are administered by the Pharmacy Acts of the respective Canadian provinces which identify the place and conditions of sale. These drugs are assigned to one of three categories:

1. Nonprescription drugs sold at any retailer; no requirement for professional supervision. Labeling provides information for client to make informed choice for safe use. An example of this category is antiulcer medications.
2. Pharmacy Only Nonprescription Drugs. Pharmacist must be available for requested advice. Client self-selects medication which may have risks for certain populations. An example of this category is antihistamines.
3. Restricted Access Nonprescription Drugs are available from pharmacist only. Consultation with pharmacist required and referral to health care provided, if necessary. An example in this category is insulin.

To address the proliferation of a variety of provincial schedules and regulations, the National Association of Pharmacy Regulatory Authorities (NAPRA) has proposed to "harmonize" regulations nationwide by creating a three-schedule national drug schedule using the same nomenclature and numbering as the controlled substances schedule system:

Schedule I: All prescription drugs, including narcotics and controlled substances

Schedule II: Restricted Access of Pharmacist Only Nonprescription Drugs

Schedule III: Pharmacy Only Nonprescription Drugs

Unscheduled Drugs: drugs available at retail outlet not placed in the above categories

The NAPRA website, *www.napra.ca*, provides detailed information on schedules.

In Canada, therapeutic and toxic levels are monitored according to the International System of Units (SI); this is also true in many European countries. The mole (mol) was adopted to express drug concentration in body fluid in molar units, such as millimoles per liter (mmol/L), instead of the traditional expression of mass units, milligrams per liter (mg/L). Some institutions in the United States use the SI units; however, the traditional use of mass units in the United States continues.

Initiatives to Combat Drug Counterfeiting

The numbers of counterfeit and adulterated prescription drugs are on the rise. Contributing reasons for this are lack of mandatory reporting of counterfeit incidents and that counterfeiting has features of a "perfect crime" (medicine taken, evidence is gone). The FDA and consumer groups are working on strategies to combat this problem, including tougher oversight of distributors, a rapid alert system, and better-informed consumers. The role of the nurse is critical in consumer education. Both the nurse and the client must be ever vigilant. Strategies include being alert to slight variations in packaging or labeling (e.g., color, package seal); advising clients to report any differences in taste or in the appearance of drug or packaging; noting any unexpected side effects; buying drugs from a reputable source. Reputable online pharmacies have an approval seal—VIPPS—Verified Internet Pharmacy Practice Site. If any suspicion of counterfeit arises, the nurse should contact the FDA at *www.fda.gov/medwatch* or call (800) FDA-1088.

Drug Names

Each drug may have several names. The **chemical name** describes the drug's chemical structure. The **generic name** is the official or nonproprietary name for the drug. This name is not owned by any pharmaceutical (drug) company and is universally accepted. Most drugs are ordered by generic name. The **brand (trade) name**, also known as the proprietary name, is chosen by the drug company and is usually a registered trademark owned by that specific manufacturer. Drug companies market a compound using their given

name (brand name). For example, *Narcan* is the brand (proprietary) name registered with the manufacturer, and *naloxone HCl* is the generic name recognized by the USP.

There are pros and cons to using generic drugs (Figure 5–1). Today generic drugs must be approved by the FDA before they can be marketed. If the generic drug is found to be bioequivalent to the brand or trade drug, then the generic drug is considered to be therapeutically equivalent and is given an "A" rating. If the peak serum concentration (C_{max}) and the plasma-concentration curve (AUC) of the generic drug fall within 80% to 125% of the brand drug, it is considered equivalent to the brand drug.

Generic approved drugs can be checked on the Internet at *www.fda.gov/cder/ob/default.htm*. The FDA also publishes a list of approved generic drugs that are bioequivalent to brand-name drugs. Generic drugs are usually cheaper and have the same active ingredients as brand-name, or tradename, drugs. However, some generic drugs have inert fillers and binders that may result in variations of drug effectiveness. Generic drugs are less expensive because manufacturers do not have to do extensive testing; these drugs were clinically tested for safety and efficacy by the pharmaceutical company that first formulated the drug.

The health care provider and client must exercise care in choosing generic drugs, because there may be some variation in the action of or response to them. Brand-name drugs are preferred when ordering anticonvulsants for seizures, anticoagulants (e.g., Coumadin), medication for heart failure (e.g., Lanoxin), and aspirin when used in large doses for rheumatoid arthritis. A study showed that 23 seizure-free epileptic clients who switched to the generic drug experienced renewed seizure activity. The nurse should check with the health care provider or pharmacist when generic drugs are prescribed. The health care provider must note on the prescription (computerized or paper) whether the pharmacist may substitute the generic drug when the brand name is prescribed.

Throughout this text, both generic and brand names are given for drugs. Because many brand names may exist for a single generic name, the generic name is given first in lower-case letters, followed by the most commonly used brand name in parentheses. With generic drugs, the name may be long and difficult to pronounce. Brand names always begin with a capital letter. An example of a generic and brand-name drug listing is "furosemide (Lasix)."

FIGURE 5–1 There is a $5 difference between the brand-name and generic-name vitamins.

Drug Resources

There are many resource reference books on drugs, including nursing texts that identify related nursing interventions and areas for health teaching.

The *American Hospital Formulary Services* (AHFS), *Physicians' Desk Reference* (PDR), *Drug Facts and Comparisons* (F & C), and the *United States Pharmacopeia—Drug Information* (USP-DI) are resources that provide valuable information for approved drugs. The method for presentation of the drugs varies.

American Hospital Formulary Service (AHFS) Drug Information is published yearly by the American Society of Health-System Pharmacists in Bethesda, Maryland. It is an excellent reference that provides accurate and complete drug information on nearly all prescription drugs marketed in the United States. This reference text contains drugs listed according to therapeutic drug classification. The information given for each drug includes chemistry and stability, pharmacologic actions, pharmacokinetics, uses, cautions per body system, precautions, contraindications, acute toxicity, drug interactions, dosage and administration, and preparations.

This reference book is updated yearly and with monthly supplements. The supplementary editions contain new marketed drugs with their dosage forms and strengths, uses, and cautions. This text is unbiased in that it does not contain information about the drug from only a pharmaceutical company. Many drug handbooks are available as quick drug references, and most of these include nursing implications. When more information is needed about a drug, the PDR or the AHFS is frequently suggested.

The Physicians' Desk Reference (PDR) lists several thousand drugs with complete drug information given by pharmaceutical companies. The PDR is published yearly. It contains seven sections, two of which are the most useful to nurses: the second (pink) section, which is the drug name index; and the sixth (white) section, which gives information about the drugs. The PDR is a useful drug resource, but it does not provide complete pharmacologic and therapeutic information and does not include nursing interventions. The drug information is reprinted from drug package inserts supplied by pharmaceutical companies which pay to have their drugs listed in the PDR.

Drug Facts and Comparisons (F & C) contains information on almost all drugs marketed in the United States. The reference consists of drug actions, indications, warnings and precautions, dosage and route for administration, adverse reactions, client information, overdosage, drug interactions, contraindications, and comparison charts and tables.

The United States Pharmacopeia—Drug Information (USP-DI) is a three-volume set that is available in most hospitals and pharmacies. Monthly supplements are available. Volumes IA and IB provide drug information for the health care provider. The sections in these volumes include pharmacology, precautions to consider, side and adverse effects, client consultation, general dosing information, and dosage forms. Volume II gives drug information for the client. It is a client-oriented volume that explains information in an understandable way for the client. The sections included in Volume II are administration of drug, drug effects, indications, adverse reactions, dosage guidelines, and what to do for missed doses.

The Medical Letter on drugs and therapeutics is published biweekly by the Medical Letter, Inc., in New Rochelle, New York. This is a nonprofit publication for physicians, nurse practitioners, and other health professionals. Biweekly issues cover one of two themes, such as (1) drugs for the treatment of disease entities (e.g., human immunodeficiency virus [HIV], peptic ulcers) or (2) two to four new drugs that have been approved by the FDA. The following information is included with each new drug: pharmacokinetics, clinical studies, dosage, adverse effects, interactions, and a conclusion.

Prescriber's Letter is published monthly by the Therapeutic Research Center in Stockton, California, and addresses new FDA-approved drugs, the various uses of older drugs, and FDA warnings. This is primarily a newsletter.

The Handbook on Injectable Drugs by Lawrence A. Trissel is published by the American Society of Hospital Pharmacists. It is an excellent reference for injectable medications and lists drug compatibility with other drugs, base fluids, and drugs available in large-volume parenterals. Also, it includes the pH of each drug and gives some dosing administration guidelines.

Numerous nursing drug reference books are updated yearly. Examples include the *Saunders' Nursing Drug Handbook* (W.B. Saunders), *Nursing Drug Guide* (Prentice Hall), and *NDR* (Delmar).

The Internet is also a source for drug information. Several drug-related Internet sites are listed in the WebLinks for this textbook's companion website (*http://evolve.elsevier.com/KeeHayes/pharmacology/*). NOTE: Drug information can be posted by anyone, so information may not always be accurate and comprehensive.

Food and Drug Administration Pregnancy Categories

The FDA developed a classification system related to the effects of drugs on the unborn child (fetus). In the drug literature and drug reference books, a pregnancy category is indicated for most drugs. Categories A and B are considered to be within safe limits for drug use in pregnancy, especially in the first trimester. Table 5–2 lists the FDA pregnancy categories and describes each category's effect on the fetus.

Poison Control Centers

Poison control centers (PCCs) are present in almost all cities. The website is *www.nlu.edu/aapcc*. Telephone numbers for PCCs are listed in the front pages of most telephone books. The centers provide information about the drug or toxic chemical compounds and the immediate action that

Table 5–2

FDA Pregnancy Categories

Pregnancy Category	Description
A	No risk to fetus. Studies have not shown evidence of fetal harm.
B	No risk in animal studies, and well-controlled studies in pregnant women are not available. It is assumed there is little to no risk in pregnant women.
C	Animal studies indicate a risk to the fetus. Controlled studies on pregnant women are not available. Risk versus benefit of the drug must be determined.
D	A risk to the human fetus has been proved. Risk versus benefit of the drug must be determined. It could be used in life-threatening conditions.
X	A risk to the human fetus has been proved. Risk outweighs the benefit, and drug should be avoided during pregnancy.

FDA, Food and Drug Administration.

should be taken to prevent injury or death. Client education about PCCs is a function of the nurse. Refer to Appendix F for listings of contact information for PCCs nationwide.

Each year, PCCs respond to more than 1.5 million cases related to a possible ingested drug or chemical toxic compound. About 90% of these cases are in children younger than 3 years and occur at home. Iron tablets, chocolate-covered laxatives, flavored acetaminophen, and flavored liquid medicines are common drugs that children ingest; in large doses they can be toxic to the child. Consumption of most household cleaning chemicals and insecticides can pose additional threats.

The mortality rate from poisoning in the United States is about 28,000 deaths per year, of which 70% are from accidental causes and 30% are from suicides. Immediate reporting of an excess drug or chemical ingestion followed by a proper action may prevent a death or more serious injury from the toxic agent.

Ethical Considerations

Ethical values related to drug administration and client care are an ongoing consideration for nurses. Nurses should be morally and ethically responsible for the client's total care. Drug administration should be correctly prepared and administered.

The American Nurses Association (ANA) and the Canadian Nurses Association (CNA) have a "Code of Ethics for Nurses." Both the ANA and CNA have developed similar standards for ethical practice in nursing. Box 5–1 lists the nine standards of the ANA Code of Ethics for Nurses.

Nurses need to respect the rights, dignity, and wishes of clients. Clients have the right to know about their drugs, drug actions, and any side effects. They have the right to refuse drugs even after a thorough explanation of the drugs and desired effects are given. According to the ANA Code of Ethics for Nurses, the nurse safeguards client's rights, safety, dignity, and health care. The nurse seeks consultation, accepts responsibility, and demonstrates competency in nursing care. The nurse's primary obligation is to the client.

International Issues

Two examples of international issues are the reduced prices of many drugs available to be bought directly from Canada and the availability of expensive drugs for AIDS sufferers in Africa. First, many drugs can be bought from Canada at a

Box 5–1

American Nurses Association Code of Ethics for Nurses

1. The nurse, in all professional relationships, practices with compassion and respect for the inherent dignity, worth, and uniqueness of every individual, unrestricted by considerations of social or economic status, personal attributes, or the nature of health problems.
2. The nurse's primary commitment is to the patient, whether an individual, family, group, or community.
3. The nurse promotes, advocates for, and strives to protect the health, safety, and rights of the patient.
4. The nurse is responsible and accountable for individual nursing practice and determines the appropriate delegation of tasks consistent with the nurse's obligation to provide optimum patient care.
5. The nurse owes the same duties to self as to others, including the responsibility to preserve integrity and safety, to maintain competence, and to continue personal and professional growth.

6. The nurse participates in establishing, maintaining, and improving health care environments and conditions of employment conducive to the provision of quality health care and consistent with the values of the profession through individual and collective action.
7. The nurse participates in the advancement of the profession through contributions to practice, education, administration, and knowledge development.
8. The nurse collaborates with other health professionals and the public in promoting community, national, and international efforts to meet health needs.
9. The profession of nursing, as represented by associations and their members, is responsible for articulating nursing values, for maintaining the integrity of the profession and its practice, and for shaping social policy.

From American Nurses Association, Washington, DC (revised 2001). Available at www.nursingworld.org/ethics/chcode.htm.

reduced rate compared with those in the United States. There are claims that drugs available on the Canadian websites may be counterfeit drugs from unregulated sources. The second issue is that the cost of AIDS drugs is prohibitive for impoverished individuals in Africa. Recently there has been a change in the World Trade Organization (WTO) Accord that now permits manufacture of the generic version of these (without regard to patents) in emergency situations, such as for people with AIDS in Africa.

KEY WEBSITES

Internet Drug Index: www.rxlist.com
Food and Drug Administration: www.fda.gov/medwatch
Nursing Ethics Resources: www.nursingethics.ca

NCLEX Study Questions

1. What legislation increased controls on drug safety and required that adverse reactions and contraindications must be included on the label?
   a. Kefauver-Harris Amendment to 1938 Act
   b. Controlled Substances Act
   c. Food, Drug, and Cosmetic Act
   d. Durham-Humphrey Amendment to 1938 Act

2. According to U.S. standards, the highest potential for drug abuse is found in drugs included in schedule:
   a. II
   b. III
   c. IV
   d. V

3. The Food and Drug Administration Modernization Act of 1997 contains all the following provisions except:
   a. review of new drugs is accelerated
   b. drug companies to give information on "off label" drugs

   c. privacy of individually identifiable health information
   d. drug companies to notify of plan to discontinue drugs

4. Factors that alert the client or nurse that a drug is counterfeit or adulterated include all the following except:
   a. variations in packaging
   b. unexpected side effects
   c. different taste
   d. different chemical components

5. Your pregnant client asks you what "category C" drugs are. The most appropriate response is:
   a. no risk to fetus
   b. no risk in animal studies
   c. risk to human fetus proven
   d. animal studies indicate risk to fetus

6. Most drugs are ordered by what name format?
   a. generic
   b. brand
   c. trade
   d. chemical

Answers: 1, a; 2, a; 3, c; 4, d; 5, d; 6, a.

6

Transcultural and Genetic Considerations

Michelle M. Byrne

ELECTRONIC RESOURCES

Evolve website (http://evolve.elsevier.com/KeeHayes/pharmacology/):
- *Case Studies*
- *Content Updates*
- *Frequently Asked Questions*

- *Student Review Activities*
- *WebLinks*
- *Additional Reference Material*

Companion CD-ROM:
- *NCLEX Examination Review Questions*
- *Pharmacology Animations*
- *IV Therapy Checklists*
- *Medication Error Checklists*

- *Drug Calculation Problems*
- *Electronic Calculators*
- *Top 200 Drugs with Pronunciations*
- *References from the Textbook*

Outline

Objectives

- Recognize verbal and nonverbal communication practices used by various ethnocultural individuals and groups.
- Anticipate client's individual response to drugs based on genetic, biological marker, and ethnic variations.
- Assess clients for use of traditional and folk therapies.
- Assess clients in the context of biocultural ecology.
- Collaborate with traditional and folk practitioners.
- Facilitate client's understanding and adherence with prescriptive therapies.

Terms

biocultural ecology, p. 132
ethnocultural, p. 129

ethnopharmacology,
    p. 128

spatial distancing, p. 131

temporality, p. 131

Ethnopharmacology is a relatively new domain that integrates pharmacodynamics (drug concentrations and its effects on the body) and pharmacokinetics (drug movement through the body) with genetic and ethnic variations. As the field of genetics evolves, we will increase our understanding of biochemical variants. Historically, most research addressing drugs has focused on European Americans, whereas current trends support a need for broader sampling and reporting of drug information. There is already some published information available about differential drug response by race (Donovan 2005, Shah 2004, Overfield 1995,). Racial, hereditary, and genetic influences have a profound effect on the way clients metabolize drugs as well as experience and tolerate side effects of medications (Matthews 1997; Soo-Jin Lee, Mountain, Koenig 2001; Twedell 2003). Differences in the pharmacokinetics of drugs support processes that are biologically or chemically mediated. These processes are related to the bioavailability of drugs, protein binding, volume distribution, hepatic metabolism, and renal tubular absorption (Johnson 1997). Specific pharmacodynamic variations linked with ethnic diversity include ethanol, isoniazid, phenylthiocarbamide, and succinylcholine. Factors affecting the efficacy and compliance with drug therapy include environment and culture (Finn 1994). **Ethnocultural** (combination of ethnic and cultural variables) perceptions and beliefs of illness play an important role in the client's acceptance and adherence to prescriptive therapy and understanding of medical treatment (Hines 2000, Levy 1993).

Gender, age, diurnal rhythms, dietary practices, living conditions, and high-risk behaviors also affect drug metabolism, efficacy, and client adherence to prescriptive therapy (Donovan 2005). To meet the needs of diverse ethnic and cultural groups, health care professionals need to have an understanding of the variables that influence medication usage, differences in physiologic responses to medications, and the client's beliefs regarding medication (Purnell 2003a). Immigration is altering the landscape of clients in North America. According to Burchard et al (2005) Latinos are the largest minority group in the United States. Further, this group is extremely heterogeneous as persons originate from many different regions and cultural backgrounds. Therefore nurses cannot overgeneralize cultural patterns, languages, or disease prevalence among these persons, yet they must be cognizant of individual and group differences.

Understanding clients' beliefs related to their desire and willingness to take medications can improve the health care provider's cultural competence in designing strategies to increase usage among diverse ethnocultural populations (Katz 2004; Levy 1995). This is especially important when the cultural beliefs of the nurse differ from or even conflict with the cultural beliefs of a client, family, or group.

The Purnell Model for Cultural Competence

This chapter uses selected domains and concepts from the Purnell Model for Cultural Competence to provide essential information in the context of some ethnic, racial, and cultural responses to medication administration and compliance. The Purnell Model for Cultural Competence (Figure 6–1) is a circle with an outlying rim that represents global society, a second rim that represents community, a third rim that represents family, and an inner rim that represents the person; these are the macroaspects of the model.

The interior of the circle is divided into 12 pie-shaped wedges that depict cultural domains and their concepts.

The domains have bidirectional arrows indicating that each domain relates to and is affected by all other domains; these are the microaspects of the model.

The center of the model is empty and represents unknown aspects about the cultural group. Along the bottom of the model is an erose (jagged) line that represents the nonlinear concept of cultural competence. This nonlinear line represents the degree of cultural competence attained by the health care provider or organization. Culturally competent nursing care requires that providers understand their culture and the client's culture and negotiate and integrate folk practices with allopathic care.

The Domains of Culture

Overview/Heritage

Overview/heritage includes concepts related to origins, topography, economics, and education. Racial origin affects responses to some drugs. It is important for students to understand that racial categories and labels are more socially-culturally applied than concise genetic markers. Definitions of race and ethnicity and their relationship are unclear and ambiguous (Munoz 2006, Burchard et al 2005). Genetic relationships to biologic markers for ethnic groups demonstrate different distributions of gene frequencies. Assumptions may be made that different racial groups or racial characteristics have relationships with disease prevalence and body-drug interactions. Therefore one's ethnic group may become a marker for underlying genetic or environmental differences (McDowell 2006). There are different prevalence rates for different diseases for different ethnic groups. One example is an increased incidence of diabetes in African Americans, Hispanics, and those living in all Western countries (Carulli, Rondienlla, Lombardidni et al 2005). Asian Americans have increased sensitivity to beta-blockers, whereas African Americans respond better to monotherapy for hypertension than do their European-American cohort groups (Jamerson, DeQuattro 1996; Levy 1993).

Topography, the landscape and surface configuration of terrain, may affect clients physiologically. For example, clients coming from high-altitude mountainous climates normally have increased red blood cell counts because of the lowered oxygen tension in the high-altitude climate. Clients coming from low-lying, swampy terrain are at an increased risk for dengue fever, malaria, and sickle cell anemia (Overfield 1995).

A client's socioeconomic status has an impact on his or her ability to afford expensive prescription drugs. Poverty is also a cultural characteristic that crosses all racial and ethnic groups. A client's lack of access to resources will impact their ability to purchase prescriptive drugs. Impoverished patients often cannot afford preventive services and oftentimes enter the health care system when their pathology is in advanced stages (Byrne 2006). Nurses must assess the socioeconomic status of their clients and help them access necessary drugs. In some cases the nurse can

FIGURE 6–1 The Purnell Model for Cultural Competence. (Courtesy Larry Purnell, Newark, Delaware.)

recommend a generic equivalent or other acceptable drug that is more affordable.

The educational status of clients may determine how the nurse provides information to the client. For clients who are unable to read or do not have English-language skills, the nurse may need to devise pictures to teach medication schedules. Non-English speaking clients may lack trust and understanding of the health care system. Directions should be provided to clients in their preferred language and at a level they can understand.

Communication

Communication includes concepts related to language, dialect, contextual use of the language, volume, and tone. Spatial distancing, touch, use of eye contact, preferred greetings, temporality, time, and format for names are also key concepts to understand for the nurse who wishes to be effective in the assessment and counsel of clients. It is imperative that culturally competent nurses care for clients of difference with awareness for the following communication variations and cultural mores.

Language

Given that 16% (Minnesota) to 62.9% (California) of people speak another language besides English at home (Language Spoken at Home, U.S. Census 2000); there are increased challenges for nurses to teach clients about their medication schedules and the side effects of medications. Because dialects may differ significantly, the nurse should attempt to identify a dialect-specific interpreter. Clients may be able to read English but not speak or understand it; therefore detailed written instructions are helpful.

The nurse needs to be aware of the contextual use of languages to better understand and communicate with culturally diverse clients. English and the Romance languages—Italian, Spanish, French, Portuguese, and Romanian—are low-contexted languages with the majority of the message in the explicit verbal mode. In low-contextual languages, many words are used to express a thought, and verbal skills are considered important. People may be uncomfortable with silence. However, in high-contexted languages, such as American Indian dialects, Chinese, and Vietnamese, the majority of the message is in the nonverbal mode. Few words are used to convey thoughts. Silence is considered important. In high-contexted languages, to interrupt someone or give a hasty response may be considered rude.

Not all languages have the numerous verb tenses that occur in the English language. For example, Finnish and Chinese only have the present tense; one must interpret the statement within its context. For example, the person may say, "I go to doctor today, I go to doctor tomorrow," or "I go to doctor yesterday." The nurse must give very precise instructions, such as "take one pill at 9 PM." Sometimes there is no future tense, therefore the nurse should not say, "You will/should take one pill at bedtime." The English language is the only language that uses contractions such as "don't" or "can't," so the nurse should remember to say "do not" or "cannot" to prevent confusion and improve understanding among culturally diverse clients.

Paralanguage

Some cultural groups, such as African Americans, European Americans, and Arabs, speak in a voice volume that may carry to those nearby. Asians and American Indians usually speak in a lower-volume voice. Because clients speak in a loud voice volume does not mean that they are angry, nor does speaking in a soft voice tone indicate that the person is reticent or not interested in the discussion. Likewise, the use of eye contact may vary among cultural groups and individuals. In general, European Americans maintain eye contact without staring when conversing, which signals that the person is listening. Arabs and Greeks usually maintain intense eye contact in conversations, which should not be interpreted as aggression. Because many Asians/Pacific Islanders do not maintain eye contact with people in a perceived higher social status, this does not mean that they are not interested or not listening to the conversation. They are demonstrating respect for the person's status.

Spatial Distancing

Spatial distancing, defined as the physical proximity between people conversing, varies between and among cultural groups. Most European Americans maintain approximately 18 to 24 inches when engaged in conversation with the health care provider. However, traditional Germans may see this as a violation of personal space, preferring to stand at a distance greater than 2 feet (Steckler 2003). Traditional Arabs and some Hispanics may stand very close to each other with less than 18 inches between them. The nurse may be uncomfortable with this close personal space but should not take offense, accepting it as a cultural variation.

Temporality

Temporality, or the perspective of time, determines whether the client stresses a past, present, or future orientation, and needs to be considered when the nurse cares for clients from diverse cultures. For example, many Portuguese, Haitians, and Hispanics are primarily present-oriented; whatever occurs at the moment is more important than what may occur later. With present-oriented clients, the nurse may need to take extra time and stress the importance of taking the medication, especially those used for prevention, and implement a follow-up protocol to investigate client medication usage. Future-oriented individuals are usually more likely to comply with prescription regimens.

Client orientation to clock time may also affect how the nurse perceives them. Mexican Americans (Zoucha, Purnell 2003) and Brazilians (Purnell 2003b) have a more relaxed perception of time than do European Americans and the dominant U.S. health care system. For Mexican Americans and American Indians (Still, Hodgins 1998), appointments are flexible, adherence to medication schedules is more fluid, and clients expect to be seen regardless of how late they arrive. If the provider does not see them, it may be interpreted as a noncaring behavior. However, in the dominant European American health care system, a client with an appointment for 10 AM is expected to arrive before that time to ensure that he or she is ready for the appointment. For a client with a present-orientation that stresses flexibility, the nurse may need to adjust medication schedules to be congruent with the client's lifestyle. Therefore, nurses need to gain information about daily routines and habits and perhaps link medication scheduling with meal and bedtimes rather than insist upon adherence to the clock.

Greetings

Culturally appropriate greetings demonstrate respect and enhance the therapeutic relationship between nurse and client. The more informal style practiced by many Americans may not be acceptable to all cultural groups. Many traditional Asians, Hispanics, and Germans prefer to be addressed formally, using Mr., Mrs., Miss, or their title. To address them informally may be perceived as insolence or disrespectful behavior. Therefore the nurse should always greet the client formally until told otherwise.

The format for names may cause confusion for nurses unfamiliar with diverse cultures. Among Hispanics, extended family names are common and may include a woman's married name and the last names of both parents. For example, Rosa Nunez Arosemina would indicate a single woman whose father's last name is Nunez and whose mother's maiden name is Arosemina. If Rosa marries Jorge Sanchez, her complete name becomes Senora (depicting a married woman) Rosa Sanchez de Nunez Arosemina. She would be called Mrs. Sanchez in a formal setting and Rosa by her family and close friends. The traditional Korean woman does not take her husband's last name when she marries. However, because many Koreans know this causes confusion for health care providers in the United States, many are beginning to take their husband's name (Purnell, Kim 2003). Thus the nurse needs to specifically ask the client his or her family name and given name.

Family Organization

Family organization with the concepts of head of household and gender roles must be considered when the nurse assesses and intervenes with clients. The nurse must recognize that not all individuals adhere to the common U.S. value of egalitarian decision making between men and women. Among traditional Central American Indian groups, men are expected to provide for their families in terms of outside resources and protect them from harm. When a family travels from its village, the procession may look something like this: The husband (or other adult male) leads the way, followed by the children who are old enough to walk. An older child may carry a smaller child. Bringing up the rear is the wife, who may be pregnant or breastfeeding an infant. In this order, the wife can watch all of the children and the man is in a better position to protect the family from harm.

In many cultures, women take care of the home and provide the majority of child care (Figure 6–2). Men may work at a distance from the house or sometimes in another village, mixing more with the outside world. Therefore they have a greater sphere of knowledge from which to make decisions. In cultures in which men are expected to make most decisions, the nurse may be expected to direct questions to the man, even though the woman may provide the answers with the man being the spokesperson, a culturally prescribed role. When traditional women work outside the home, family dynamics may change. Men may feel guilt for being unable to provide for their families, and women feel they are abandoning their children because they are working, especially if extended family members are not available for childcare.

Biocultural Ecology

Biocultural ecology includes concepts related to biologic variations, heredity, genetics, endemics, and drug metabolism. Genetic background can affect a client's response to drugs. For example, African Americans have high rates of hypertension and respond better to monotherapy because their hypertension is usually related to volume expansion, decreased renin, and increased intracellular concentration of sodium and calcium (McDowell 2006; Munoz, Hilgenberg 2006, Seeman 2004). For people of Greek and Chinese Heritage with glucose-6-phosphate dehydrogenase deficiency, life-threatening hemolytic crises may occur if oxidating drugs such as quinine and chloramphenicol are prescribed (Purnell, Papadopoulos 2003; Wang 2003). Many Asians/Pacific Islanders experience increased side effects of alcohol with facial flushing, tachycardia, and palpitations (Pacquiao 2003; Purnell, Kim 2003; Wang 2003). Additional biochemical variations exist with isoniazid, a drug to treat tuberculosis, which can be inactivated rapidly or slowly depending on a specific phenotype. Slow inactivation of isoniazid occurs in approximately 60% of European and African Americans, 10% to 40% of Native Americans and 10% to 20% of Asians (Overfield 1995). Perioperative nurses need to be aware that the enzyme pseudocholinesterase inactivates succinylcholine, a commonly used muscle relaxant used in surgery. Succinylcholine is rapidly inactivated by most individuals, however some individuals, especially Alaskan Eskimos, are at a considerably greater risk for having an atypical form of pseudocholinesterase and thereby suffer from prolonged muscular paralysis and inability to spontaneously breathe after receiving this drug (Overfield 1995).

FIGURE 6–2 Women may be responsible for taking care of the home and providing child care. (Copyright 2007 JupiterImages Corporation.)

High-Risk Behaviors

The domain *high-risk behaviors* includes the use of tobacco, alcohol, sex practices, and recreational drugs. Oftentimes tobacco use causes more rapid elimination of medicines from the body; thus the prescribed drug does not have its full therapeutic effect. There is some evidence tobacco decreases serum levels of traditional antipsychotic medications (Munoz, Hildgenberg 2006). Alcohol interferes with some psychotropic medications and enhances the effects of analgesics. Recreational use of drugs such as marijuana, antihistamine combinations, and cocaine may potentiate the effects of medications, resulting in increased side effects, an enhanced therapeutic response, or an overdose. It is incumbent upon the nurse to establish a trusting client relationship and to ask open-ended, nonjudgmental questions regarding these issues.

Nutrition

The domain *nutrition* includes concepts related to common foods, eating rituals, limitations in obtaining nutritious foods, enzyme deficiencies, and how foods are used for health promotion and wellness. Each ethnocultural group has preferred foods and rituals that are passed on through the generations. Traditional Appalachian people frequently use extra lard to prepare fried foods. The diets of many Asians/Pacific Islanders are high in sodium. Some African Americans use fatback to add extra flavor to vegetables. The proportion of fats, carbohydrates, and proteins may have an effect on how some drugs are absorbed or metabolized. Dietary consideration must be taken into account when prescriptions are given. Newer immigrants may have difficulty finding preferred native foods and may not be aware of which foods to substitute to provide a nutritious diet. Asians/Pacific Islanders, Hispanics, and African Americans have higher incidences of lactose intolerance, resulting in maldigestion and bloating,

All societies have "prescriptions" for what is considered a "normal" diet, although these prescriptions have great variability within each ethnocultural group. Among conservative Jews, a kosher diet demands that dairy and meat should not be eaten at the same meal. Among some Haitians (Colin, Paperwalla 2003), Hispanics/Latinos (Zoucha, Purnell 2003; Purnell 2003c), Vietnamese (Nowak 2003), Greeks and Greek Cypriots (Purnell, Papadopoulos 2003), and Iranians (Hafizi, Lipson 2003), foods may be classified as "hot" or "cold" and a balance of these foods are consumed at each meal. Some believe that if this is not followed then illness may result. Drugs may also classify as hot or cold. Antibiotics can be considered hot and therefore should not be taken with cold water because their effect would be negated; use room temperature or tap water instead. Because hot and cold foods and conditions vary within each group interpretation, the nurse must specifically ask clients their food preferences. Clients should be questioned for determining whether they perceive if their diet interferes with drug absorption or interactions.

Spirituality

Spirituality includes concepts related to religious preference, meaning of life, and individual sources of strength. Clients' religious practices may prescribe what is acceptable in terms of diet (e.g., Islamic and orthodox Jewish), acceptability for genetic counseling, and use and choice of contraceptive methods. Muslims who celebrate the holiday Ramadan fast from sunup to sundown. Fasting may also include not taking medications. If medications are to be taken on a full or empty stomach, then eating behaviors and fasting rituals should be determined. However, in times of illness, clients may be permitted to take their prescribed medications. The nurse can improve medication usage by working with the client to determine an acceptable medication schedule during religious holidays. Because clients may not eat on a regular daytime schedule, insulin administration must be adjusted accordingly. Times of food abstinence must be determined to understand blood glucose fluctuations. Empty or full stomachs can influence drug absorption and gastric irritation. In addition, some cultural groups may believe that illness results from past sins and is punishment from a higher being. A belief similar to this may inhibit a person from taking medication to alleviate pain or illness because it could be perceived as interfering with God's will.

Meaning of Life

Spirituality and meaning of life are culturally embedded. Holistic health beliefs may inhibit a person from taking medication that could be perceived as "artificial" or altering a higher order's life plan. Among some people of Mexican, Guatemalan, and Panamanian ancestry, family may be the most important aspect of their lives and gives meaning to life (Purnell 1998; Purnell 2000; Zoucha, Purnell 2003). Thus it can be especially important to include the family in teaching strategies. Illness is considered a family affair and should be treated accordingly.

Health Care Practices

Health care practices include the focus of health care, traditional medical practices, self-medicating practices, barriers to accessing health care, the sick role, and perceptions of mental illness. Health care in the United States is undergoing a paradigm shift from acute care to wellness, with health promotion and maintenance and disease and illness prevention the current focus. Whereas this concept is congruent with many ethnocultural groups, for some, prevention activities are unknown. For example, some Western health practices such as breast exams, pelvic exams, mammograms, and colonoscopies could be interpreted as extremely personally invasive and embarrassing. Personal questions addressing sexual practices are taboo in many cultural groups.

Complementary, Alternative, and Traditional Medicine

Many people may prefer their traditional medical practices either as complementary to or as an alternative to allopathic medicine (Figure 6–3; Herbal Alert 6–1). Traditional Chinese medicine, Ayurvedic medicine, herbal and naturopathic medicine, and a host of other therapies may be preferred by some or used in conjunction with other therapies. Therefore nurses must obtain a thorough health history to ascertain what types of herbs, remedies, or medications have already been taken. Many ethnic people, accustomed to taking medications for only 2 or 3 days in their home countries, may believe that Western medicine is too strong, is supposed to only relieve symptoms, or has too many side effects. Thus they may stop taking the medication when symptoms disappear.

Self-Medicating Practices

All clients self-medicate to some degree. Many use over-the-counter medications or folk remedies for the initial symptoms of an illness. Some ethnic groups may have family or friends bring medication from their home country that may not be available in the United States. For example, in Panama and throughout Central America, clients can purchase a wide variety of antibiotics, injectable vitamins, and even intravenous fluids without a prescription. To prevent contraindications in medication administration, the nurse must ask clients in a nonjudgmental manner whether they take any prescription medications, nonprescription medications, or herbal therapies (Figure 6–4). The internet is an avenue for many people to access prescriptive-only drugs, and these drugs may be unknown to the health care provider.

Sick Role

In some Hispanic and Arabic cultures, clients can enter the sick role without feelings of guilt or attached stigma. Any reason is acceptable for being ill, and the person is relieved of normal responsibilities (Kulwicki 2003; Zoucha, Purnell 2003). However, among some German and Polish people, clients may be expected to carry out their obligations unless they are severely ill (From 2003, Steckler 2003). This is one area in which the nurse can hasten the client's recovery with culturally appropriate counseling.

Pain

Pain—the primary reason most people see a health professional—is expressed differently among ethnocultural groups. For example, among some Asians/Pacific Islanders, clients are reluctant to express pain because they believe it is God's will or a punishment for past sins (Pacquiao 2003, Nowak 2003, Sharts-Hopko 2003). Among some Arabic peoples, clients are expected to express their pain openly and expect immediate relief, preferably through injectable or intravenous medication (Purnell 2003d).

Mental Illness

Mental illness is a culture-bound phenomenon. What is perceived as a mental illness in one culture may be seen as normal in another; for example, having visions and hallucinations about God is an expected behavior among some Hispanic groups (Dossey 1998). Although the "evil eye" occurs in numerous cultures, someone from a culture who does not believe in the evil eye may see those who do believe in it as having a mental health problem. Thus nurses must interpret a client's behavior within cultural boundaries. In addition, there is evidence that there

FIGURE 6–3 In some cultures people may rely on traditional nonprescription drugs.

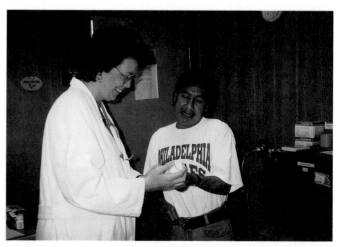

FIGURE 6–4 The nurse needs to ask the client about all medications and remedies taken so that any potential interactions with the prescribed medication regimen can be identified.

Herbal ALERT 6–1

Gender-Specific Herb Protocols

Women have traditionally sought substitutes for hormonal replacement therapy, especially if there are adverse side effects. With increased media attention given to natural hormone replacement therapies, more women are using phytoestrogens such as those found in flaxseed, licorice, black cohosh, and soybeans. Health care providers need to query their clients regarding their use of these naturally occurring phytoestrogens because they are contraindicated in women with a history or risk for hormonally mediated cancers and benign tumors.

are gender differences in antipsychotic drug therapy. The differences in disease processes and gender may be related to hormones, differing amounts of body fat, and co-morbidity problems (Seeman 2004).

Health Care Practitioners

The domain *health care* practitioners includes concepts related to the status of health care providers, folk practitioners, gender, and the health care system. For some Arabs and Arab-Americans, the most respected health care provider is an experienced middle-aged to elderly male physician with several degrees (Hafizi, Lipson 2003). Among some Appalachian people, foreign-educated physicians may have difficulty being accepted because they are considered outsiders, not because of their ethnocultural background (Purnell 2003e). In many Arab countries nursing is not seen as a desirable profession, because it requires contact between the genders (Kulwicki 2003).

Folk Practitioners

Folk practitioners may be preferred over allopathic educated physicians because treatments are less invasive. Folk practitioners are often better known to the client. Usually they do not treat the symptoms of an illness, they remove the cause of the illness. Allopathic physicians can only treat the symptoms. Health care providers should elicit information about folk practices that impact a client's health and illness status.

Gender and Health Care

As evidence-based nursing and medical practice evolves, researchers may determine more gender-related issues pertinent to disease manifestation, symptom management, pharmacodynamics, and prescriptive therapy (Donovan 2005, Seeman 2004). Some Islamic women prefer health care providers of the same gender and may refuse treatment from male health care providers. However, the nurse should remind them that the *Koran* sanctions the use of male health care providers if female providers are not available. If only a male is available, physical examination should be performed through one layer of clothes or by the health care provider using gloves to prevent direct skin contact. Most European-American and African-American men and women generally accept care from either gender. More traditional and younger clients may prefer a same-gender provider for intimate care. This should be accommodated whenever possible.

Transcultural Considerations

ASSESSMENT

- Assess ethnocultural and racial background.

- Assess socioeconomic resources and ability to access and pay for pharmaceutical therapy.
- Assess length of time away from country of origin.
- Assess travel history, both within and outside the country.
- Assess language ability and preferred language for instruction.
- Assess nonverbal communication practices such as spatial distancing, temporality, use of touch, and eye contact.
- Assess high-risk health behaviors.
- Assess preferred foods, preparation practices, and eating patterns.
- Assess for illness and disease patterns commonly found in client's family and cultural group.
- Assess use of traditional and folk practices.
- Assess use of traditional health care practitioners.

PLANNING

- Collaborate with client to reduce high-risk health behaviors.
- Develop a culturally congruent dietary plan that helps client understand his or her dietary practices in relation to drug interactions.

NURSING INTERVENTIONS

- Incorporate nonharmful traditional and folk practices with biomedical prescriptions.
- Collaborate with traditional and folk practitioners.
- Maintain culturally congruent communication practices to develop a trusting relationship with client and family.
- Incorporate cultural beliefs and practices into the plan of care.

Client Teaching

- Involve family in teaching about prescriptive therapies.
- Provide explanation for all prescriptions, treatments, and procedures.
- Provide written instruction (or videos) in client's preferred language.

EVALUATION

- Client correctly demonstrates understanding of prescriptive therapies and treatments.
- Client integrates prescriptive therapies in their treatment plan.
- Family members are involved in client's overall health plan.
- Client eliminates or decreases high-risk health behaviors.
- Client selects food choices congruent with prescriptive therapies.

KEY WEBSITES

American Medical Association: http://www.ama-assn.org/ama/pub/category/4848.html

Center for Cross-Cultural Health: http://www.crosshealth.com/

The Center for Cross Cultural Research: http://www.wwu.edu/.culture

Center for Healthy Families and Cultural Diversity: http://www2.umdnj.edu/fmedweb/chfcd/

Culturally and Linguistically Appropriate Services (CLAS) in Health Care—CLAS Standards: http://www.omhrc.gov/clas/

Cross Cultural Health Care Program: http://www.xculture.org/

Ethnicity and Health: http://www.tandf.co.uk/journals/carfax/13557858.html

Management Sciences for Health: The Provider's Guide to Quality and Culture: http://erc.msh.org/quality&culture

National Center for Cultural Competence: http://www.georgetown.edu/research/gucdc/nccc/

New York University School of Medicine Center for Immigrant Health: http://www.med.nyu.edu/cih/

Transcultural and Multicultural Health Links: http://www.iun.edu/.libemb/trannurs/trannurs.htm

Diversity Rx: www.diversityrx.org

The Office of Minority Health: www.omhrc.gov

Transcultural Nursing Society: www.tcns.org

Critical Thinking Case Study

Ana Maria de Navarro, age 63 years, is a migrant worker on a large farm. She has been recently diagnosed with hypertension and is 45 pounds overweight. She speaks minimal English, eats a traditional Mexican diet, and is the primary cook for the family. She takes furosemide, 40 mg daily. Twice within the last month, she fainted while picking vegetables. Each time, her family took her to a shaded area, where she regained consciousness within a few minutes. She admits to feeling dizzy when she awakes each morning but is glad that she no longer has headaches since she started taking her medicine. Her skin is dry and has decreased turgor. You are the public health nurse responsible for the employees in the migrant worker camp. You want her to keep a diary of her blood pressure and pulse four times a day for the next week. You speak minimal Spanish.

1. What type of medicine is furosemide?
2. Is the dose within therapeutic range?
3. Why is Ana Maria experiencing dizziness?
4. Why did Ana Maria faint twice in the last month?
5. How might you teach her family to take and record Ana Maria's blood pressure and pulse?
6. At what times each day do you recommend her vital signs be taken?
7. How will you communicate this with her and with her family?
8. What recommendation do you have for Ana Maria to combat her morning dizziness?
9. What recommendations do you have for her medication regimen?
10. If Ana Maria wanted to see a traditional healer, which one(s) might you recommend?
11. What culturally congruent goals might you collaborate on with Ana Maria?
12. What evaluation measures would you include in terms of nutrition and hydration?

NCLEX Study Questions

1. African Americans have a higher rate of hypertension because of (select all that apply):
   a. increased renin
   b. decreased renin
   c. Increased intracellular concentration of Ca++
   d. Glucose 6 phosphate dehydrogenase deficiency
   e. Increase in lactic acid production

2. Which menu item would not be found on a kosher diet?
   a. cereal and milk
   b. salmon
   c. milkshake
   d. cheeseburger

3. Your diabetic 57-year-old Muslim client is celebrating Ramadan. What should the nurse encourage related to the usual insulin dose?
   a. Double your insulin dosage.
   b. Stop taking your insulin.
   c. Check your blood glucose more often to determine your sliding scale dosage.
   d. You should see your physician.

4. You suspect your client is impoverished. Which of the following questions would provide you the most insight during a history?
   a. Describe the foods that you ate yesterday.
   b. How much money do you make a year?
   c. Are you employed?
   d. Where did you go to college?

Answers: 1, b, c; 2, d; 3, c; 4, a.

7

Drug Interactions and Over-the-Counter Drugs

ELECTRONIC RESOURCES

Evolve website (http://evolve.elsevier.com/KeeHayes/pharmacology/):
- *Case Studies*
- *Content Updates*
- *Frequently Asked Questions*
- *Student Review Activities*
- *WebLinks*
- *Additional Reference Material*

Companion CD-ROM:
- *NCLEX Examination Review Questions*
- *Pharmacology Animations*
- *IV Therapy Checklists*
- *Medication Error Checklists*
- *Drug Calculation Problems*
- *Electronic Calculators*
- *Top 200 Drugs with Pronunciations*
- *References from the Textbook*

Outline

Objectives

Terms

Drug Interaction
Pharmacokinetic Interactions
Pharmacodynamic Interactions

Drug-Food Interactions

Drug-Laboratory Interactions

Drug-Induced Photosensitivity

Over-the-Counter Drugs
Cough and Cold Remedies
Sleep Aids

Weight-Control Drugs
Nursing Process: Drug Interactions

Key Websites

Critical Thinking Case Study

NCLEX Study Questions

Objectives

- Define the term drug interaction.
- Differentiate the four pharmacokinetic processes related to drug interaction.
- Explain the three effects associated with pharmacodynamic interactions.
- Explain the effects of drug-food interactions.
- Explain the meaning of drug-induced photosensitivity.
- Discuss the nursing implications related to clients' use of over-the-counter (OTC) drugs.

Terms

additive effect, p. 140
adverse drug reaction, p. 138

antagonistic effects, p. 141
drug incompatibility, p. 138

drug interaction, p. 138
over-the-counter (OTC) drugs, p. 144

photosensitivity, p. 142
synergistic effect, p. 141

Drug therapy has become complex because of the increasing number of drugs available. Drug-drug, drug-food, and drug-laboratory interactions have also become an increasing problem. Because of the possibility of numerous interactions, the nurse should be knowledgeable about drug interactions and should closely monitor client responses. Thorough and timely communication among members of the health team is essential. Clients at high risk for interactions include those who have chronic health conditions, take multiple medications, see more than one health care provider, and use multiple pharmacies. Older adults—75% take prescription drugs and 82% take OTC preparations—are at high risk for drug interactions.

Drug Interaction

A **drug interaction** is defined as an altered or modified action or effect of a drug as a result of interaction with one or more other drugs. It should not be confused with adverse drug reaction or drug incompatibility. An **adverse drug reaction** is an undesirable drug effect that ranges from mild untoward effects to severe toxic effects, including hypersensitivity reaction and anaphylaxis. **Drug incompatibility** is a chemical or physical reaction that occurs among two or more drugs in vitro. In other words, the reaction occurs between two or more drugs within a syringe, IV bag, or any other artificial environment outside of the body.

Drug interactions can be divided into two categories: (1) pharmacokinetic interactions and (2) pharmacodynamic interactions. These two categories of drug interaction are discussed individually.

Pharmacokinetic Interactions

Pharmacokinetic interactions are changes that occur in the absorption, distribution, metabolism or biotransformation, and excretion of one or more drugs.

Absorption

When a person takes two drugs at the same time, the rate of absorption of one or both drugs can change. One drug can block, decrease, or increase the absorption rate of another drug. It can do this in one of three ways:

- By decreasing or increasing gastric emptying time
- By changing the gastric pH
- By forming drug complexes

Drugs that increase the speed of gastric emptying (e.g., laxatives or metoclopramide) may lead to an increase in gastric and intestinal motility and cause a decrease in drug absorption. Most drugs are absorbed primarily in the small intestines; exceptions include barbiturates, salicylates, and theophylline. Narcotics and anticholinergic drugs (e.g., atropine) decrease gastric emptying time and gastrointestinal (GI) motility, thus causing an increase in absorption rate. For those drugs that undergo gastric absorption, the amount or extent of absorption increases the longer the drug remains in the stomach.

When the gastric pH is decreased, a weakly acidic drug such as aspirin is less ionized and more rapidly absorbed. Drugs that increase the pH of gastric juices decrease absorption of weak-acid drugs. Antacids such as Maalox and Amphojel raise the gastric pH and block or slow absorption. Some drugs may react chemically. For example, tetracycline and the heavy-metal ions (calcium, magnesium, aluminum, iron) found in antacids or iron may lead to the formation of a drug complex and thereby prevent the absorption of tetracycline. This phenomenon may also be observed when products that contain divalent cations are ingested with fluoroquinolone antibiotics such as ciprofloxacin. Consequently, dairy products, multivitamins, and antacids should be avoided 1 hour before and 2 hours after tetracycline or ciprofloxacin consumption.

Other drugs besides antacids that can form complexes with drugs include certain cholesterol-lowering drugs such as cholestyramine and colestipol. Because of the formed complexes, the drugs are less soluble, which results in less drug absorption.

There exist situations in which drug complexation may be desired. For example, activated charcoal may be administered after a toxic ingestion of a medication to decrease its absorption and, consequently, any untoward effects associated with the overdose.

Alteration of bacteria normally found in the GI tract may impact the pharmacokinetics of a medication. For example, intestinal microflora have the ability to metabolize digoxin. Digoxin is a digitalis preparation that is used to treat heart failure and arrhythmias. Metabolism of this drug by gut bacteria serves to decrease its bioavailability. Erythromycin, a macrolide antibiotic, and tetracycline are broad-spectrum antibiotics which destroy or inhibit the growth of these GI microflora. Consequently, the administration of one of these drugs to a client on digoxin therapy may lead to an increase in the absorption of digoxin and, ultimately, to toxicity. Another example of this phenomenon occurs in the case of oral contraceptives. Gut bacteria are necessary to hydrolyze estrogen conjugates into free estrogens so that they may be optimally absorbed to exert their contraceptive effect. Concurrent antibiotic administration may alter these intestinal bacteria thereby impairing this process and preventing the optimal absorption and effectiveness of the oral contraceptive. A woman who is taking oral birth control to prevent pregnancy should utilize a barrier form of protection during sex when she begins a course of antibiotics.

Distribution

A drug's distribution to tissues can be affected by its binding to plasma/serum protein. Only drugs unbound to protein are free active agents and can enter body tissues. Two drugs that are highly protein-bound and administered simultaneously can result in drug displacements. Factors that influence displacement of drugs are (1) the drug concentration in the blood, (2) protein-binding power of the drugs, and (3) volume of distribution (Vd).

Two drugs that are highly bound to protein or albumin will compete for binding sites in the plasma. The result is a decrease in protein binding of one or both drugs; therefore more free drug circulates in the plasma and is available for drug action. This effect can lead to drug toxicity. When two highly protein-bound drugs need to be taken concurrently, the drug dosage of one or both drugs may need to be decreased to avoid drug toxicity.

Examples of drugs that are highly protein-bound include the anticoagulant warfarin, anticonvulsants such as phenytoin and valproic acid, gemfibrozil, most nonsteroidal antiinflammatory drugs (NSAIDs), sulfisoxazole, glyburide, and quinidine. Warfarin is 99% protein-bound, allowing only 1% to be free drug. If 2% to 3% of warfarin is displaced from albumin binding sites, the amount of free warfarin would be 3% to 4% instead of 1%. This action has the potential to increase the anticoagulant effect of warfarin, and excess bleeding may result.

A significant decrease in the serum albumin level because of liver disease or poor nutritional status can increase the free amount of highly protein-bound drugs such as phenytoin and warfarin, making more drug available to exert its pharmacological effect.

Metabolism or Biotransformation

Many drug interactions of metabolism occur with the induction or inhibition of the hepatic microsomal system. A drug can increase the metabolism of another drug by stimulating liver enzymes. Drugs that promote induction of enzymes are called *enzyme inducers*. Barbiturates such as phenobarbital are enzyme inducers. Phenobarbital increases the metabolism of most antipsychotics and theophylline. Increased metabolism promotes drug elimination and decreases plasma concentration of the drug. The result is a decrease in drug action. Sometimes liver enzymes convert drugs to active or passive metabolites. The drug metabolites may be excreted or may produce an active pharmacologic response.

The anticonvulsant drugs phenytoin and carbamazepine and the antimicrobial medication rifampin are hepatic enzyme inducers that can increase drug metabolism, for example, for the anticoagulant drug warfarin. A larger dose of warfarin is usually needed while the client takes a hepatic inducer, because metabolism aids in decreasing the amount of drug. If the drug inducer is withdrawn, warfarin dosages need to be decreased, because less drug is eliminated by hepatic metabolism. Usually interaction occurs after 1 week of drug therapy and can continue for 1 week after the drug inducer is discontinued. Drugs with narrow therapeutic ranges should be closely monitored.

Cigarette smoking increases hepatic enzyme activity and can increase theophylline clearance. For smokers who take theophylline, the theophylline dose should be increased. With chronic alcohol use, hepatic enzyme activities are increased; with acute alcohol use, metabolism is inhibited.

Some drugs are also enzyme inhibitors. The antiulcer drug cimetidine is an enzyme inhibitor that decreases the metabolism of certain drugs such as theophylline. As the result of decreasing theophylline metabolism, there is an increase in the plasma concentration of theophylline. The theophylline dose needs to be decreased to avoid toxicity. If cimetidine or any enzyme drug inhibitor is discontinued, the theophylline dosage should be adjusted. Other well-known hepatic enzyme inhibitors are erythromycin and itraconazole, an antifungal medication.

The use of tobacco and alcohol may have variable effects on drug biotransformation. Polycyclic aromatic hydrocarbons found in cigarette smoke induce production of the specific family of enzymes responsible for theophylline metabolism. Chronic cigarette smoking leads to an increase in hepatic enzyme activity and can increase theophylline clearance. Asthmatics who smoke and take theophylline to manage their disease may require an increase in theophylline dosage.

Table 7–1

Drugs: Enzyme Inducer or Enzyme Inhibitor

Drug Category	Drug Effect
Drug enzyme inducer	Onset and termination of drug effect is slow, approximately 1 week.
	Drug dosage may need to be increased with use of drug inducer.
	Drug dosage should be adjusted after termination of drug inducer.
	Monitor serum drug levels, especially if the drug has a narrow therapeutic drug range.
Drug enzyme inhibitor	Onset of drug effect usually occurs rapidly.
	Half-life ($t^{1/2}$) of the second drug may be increased, causing a prolonged drug effect.
	Interaction may occur related to the dosage prescribed.
	Disease entities affect drug dosing.
	Monitor serum drug levels, especially if the drug has a narrow therapeutic range.

The ingestion of alcohol may have variable effects on biotransformation. With chronic alcohol use, hepatic enzyme activities are increased; with acute alcohol use, metabolism is inhibited.

Natural or herbal products may also have an impact on metabolism. St. John's wort, an OTC herbal product to manage symptoms of depression, induces the metabolism of certain drugs such as warfarin, digoxin, and theophylline. This action potentially decreases the effectiveness of these medications, possibly necessitating a dose increase to sustain efficacy. Flavonoids, a group of naturally-occurring compounds found in the juice and pulp of citrus fruits, are potent inhibitors of the metabolism of certain drugs. Clients who are stabilized on therapeutic doses of carbamazepine, diazepam, or a statin may subject themselves to adverse effects from greater-than-expected drug levels if they eat or drink grapefruit products concurrently with the drug.

Certain drugs alter hepatic blood flow, causing a decrease in liver metabolism. Table 7–1 describes the effects of drug enzyme inducers and inhibitors.

Excretion

Most drugs are filtered through the glomeruli and excreted in the urine. With some drugs, excretion occurs in the bile, which passes into the intestinal tract. Drugs can increase or decrease renal excretion and have an effect on the excretion of other drugs. Drugs that decrease cardiac output, decrease blood flow to the kidneys, and decrease glomerular filtration can also decrease or delay drug excretion. The antiarrhythmic drug quinidine decreases the excretion of digoxin; therefore the plasma concentration of digoxin is increased and digitalis toxicity can occur.

Diuretics promote water and sodium excretion from the renal tubules. Furosemide (Lasix) acts on the loop of Henle, and hydrochlorothiazide (HydroDIURIL) acts on the distal tubules. Both diuretics decrease reabsorption of water, sodium, and potassium. A renal loss of potassium, which may lead to a condition known as hypokalemia, can enhance the action of digoxin and digitalis toxicity could occur (see Drug-Laboratory Interactions).

Two or more drugs which undergo the same route of excretion may compete with one another for elimination from the body. Probenecid (Benemid), a drug for gout, decreases penicillin excretion by inhibiting the secretion of penicillin in the renal tubules of the kidneys. In some cases this effect may be desirable to increase or maintain the plasma concentration of penicillin (which has a short half-life) for a prolonged period of time.

Changing urine pH affects drug excretion. The antacid sodium bicarbonate causes the urine to be alkaline. Alkaline urine promotes the excretion of drugs that are weak acids (e.g., aspirin and barbiturates). Alkaline urine also promotes reabsorption of weak base drugs. Acid urine promotes the excretion of drugs such as quinidine that are weak bases.

With clients who have decreased renal or hepatic function, there is usually an increase in free drug concentration. It is essential to closely monitor such a client for drug toxicity when the individual takes multiple drugs. Checking serum drug levels, a practice also known as *therapeutic drug monitoring* (TDM), is especially important for drugs that have a narrow therapeutic range and are highly protein-bound. Digoxin and phenytoin are two such drugs that require therapeutic drug monitoring. Table 7–2 summarizes the drug interactions that affect pharmacokinetics.

Pharmacodynamic Interactions

Pharmacodynamic interactions are those that result in additive, synergistic or antagonistic drug effects.

Additive Drug Effect

When two drugs with similar action are administered, the drug interaction is called an **additive effect** and is the sum of the effects of the two drugs. Additive effects can be desirable or undesirable. For example, a desirable additive drug effect occurs when a diuretic and a beta blocker are administered for the treatment of hypertension; used in combination, these two drugs utilize different mechanisms to

Table 7–2

Pharmacokinetic Interactions of Drugs

Process	Drug	Effect
Absorption	Laxatives	Speeds gastric emptying time Increases gastric motility Decreases drug absorption
	Narcotics	Slows gastric emptying time
	Anticholinergics	Decreases gastric motility Increases drug absorption or decreases absorption depending on where the drug is delayed (gastric vs. intestinal)
	Aspirin	Decreases gastric pH Increases drug absorption
	Antacids	Increases gastric pH Slows absorption of acid drugs
	Antacids and tetracycline	Forms drug complexes Blocks drug absorption
Distribution	Anticoagulant and anti-inflammatory (sulindac)	Competes for protein-binding sites Increases free drug (e.g., increases anticoagulant)
Metabolism or biotransformation	Barbiturates	Promotes induction of liver enzymes Increases drug metabolism Decreases drug plasma concentration of second drug
	Antiulcer (cimetidine)	Inhibits liver enzyme release Decreases drug metabolism of diazepam (Valium), phenytoin (Dilantin), morphine, etc. Increases drug plasma concentration of second drug
Excretion	Antiarrhythmic (quinidine)	Decreases renal excretion of second drug (e.g., digoxin) Increases digoxin concentration
	Antigout (probenecid)	Decreases excretion of penicillin by competing for renal tubular secretion Increases penicillin concentration
	Antacid (sodium bicarbonate)	Promotes excretion of weak acid drug (e.g., aspirin, barbiturates, sulfonamides)
Other: Decrease cardiac output and renal blood flow	Aspirin, ammonium chloride	Promotes excretion of weak base drugs (e.g., quinidine, theophylline)
	Most drug categories	Decreases drug excretion, increases drug plasma concentration

have a more pronounced blood pressure lowering effect. As another example, aspirin and codeine are two analgesics that work by different mechanisms but can be given together for increased pain relief.

An example of an undesirable additive effect is that from two vasodilators: hydralazine (Apresoline) prescribed for hypertension and nitroglycerin prescribed for angina. The result could be a severe hypotensive response. Another example is the interaction of aspirin and alcohol. Aspirin is directly irritating to the stomach, causes platelet dysfunction, and inhibits prostaglandin-mediated mucus production of the gastric mucosa, which protects the underlying tissues of the stomach. Alcohol disrupts the gastric mucosal barrier and suppresses platelet production. Both aspirin and alcohol can prolong bleeding time and when taken together may result in gastric bleeding.

Synergistic Drug Effect or Potentiation

When two or more drugs are given together, one drug can potentiate or have a **synergistic effect** on another. In other words, the clinical effect is substantially greater than the combined effect of the two. An example of this is the combination of meperidine (Demerol, a narcotic analgesic) and promethazine (Phenergan, an antihistamine). One of the major side effects of promethazine is sedation. When used with meperidine in post-surgery clients, promethazine enhances or potentiates the drowsiness effect of meperidine. Less meperidine is required when it is combined with promethazine, which can be a desirable effect. An example of an undesirable effect occurs when alcohol and a sedative-hypnotic drug such as chlordiazepoxide (Librium) or diazepam (Valium) are combined; central nervous system (CNS) depression increases as a result.

Some antibacterials (antibiotics) have an enzyme inhibitor added to the drug to potentiate the therapeutic effect. Examples are ampicillin with sulbactam and amoxicillin with clavulanate, in which sulbactam and clavulanate potassium are bacterial enzyme inhibitors. Ampicillin and amoxicillin can be given without these inhibitors; however, the desired therapeutic effect may not occur because of the bacterial beta-lactamase which inactivates the drugs and causes bacterial resistance. The combination of the antibiotic with either sulbactam or clavulanate inhibits bacterial enzyme activity and enhances the effect or broadens the spectrum of activity of the antibacterial agent.

Antagonistic Drug Effect

When two drugs that have opposite effects, or **antagonistic effects,** are administered together, each drug cancels the effect of the other. In other words, the actions of both drugs are nullified. An example of an antagonistic effect occurs when the adrenergic beta stimulant isoproterenol (Isuprel) and the adrenergic beta blocker propranolol (Inderal) are given together. Isoproterenol is a drug that is used in emergency situations to treat bradycardia, which is defined as a heart rate of less than 60 beats per minute. If

given to a client receiving a drug that decreases blood pressure and heart rate, the action of each drug is cancelled. Neither delivers the expected therapeutic effect.

There are some situations in which the antagonistic effect is desirable. In the case of morphine overdose, naloxone is given as an antagonist (antidote) to block the narcotic response. This is a beneficial drug interaction of an antagonist.

The use of two prescription drugs can have an additive, synergistic, antagonistic, or no effect. This is especially true of warfarin. When taken with another drug, the effects of the second drug can increase, decrease, or have no effect on the anticoagulant. Table 7–3 lists the drugs that may be taken with an anticoagulant and the effects that the second drug has on the anticoagulant.

Table 7–4 summarizes the drug responses associated with pharmacodynamic interactions. Refer to Table 7–5 for a list of selected drug-drug interactions.

Common symptoms of drug-drug interactions include nausea, GI upset, headache, and dizziness. The client needs to contact the pharmacist or health care provider if they experience any unusual reaction. The most feared interactions are those that result in a dramatic drop in blood pressure or cause a rapid or irregular heart rate. Equally as concerning are those drug interactions that produce toxins that may damage vital organs such as the heart or liver. Fortunately, most interactions are not severe or life threatening. Clients need to be alert that both prescription and OTC drugs can interact with each other. It is a myth that interactions occur only with prescription medications.

Drug-Food Interactions

Food is known to increase, decrease, or delay drug absorption. Food can bind with drugs, causing less or slower drug absorption. An example of food binding with a drug is the interaction of tetracycline and dairy products. The result is a decrease in the plasma concentration of tetracycline. Because of the binding effect, tetracycline should be taken 1 hour before or 2 hours after meals and *should not* be taken with dairy products. The absorption of levothyroxine, which is used to treat hypothyroidism, is erratic in the presence of food.

Food may also have an impact on the absorption of different dosage forms of the same drug. Itraconazole solution is best absorbed on an empty stomach. Amazingly, itraconazole capsules, which require an acidic environment for absorption, have a higher availability when administered with food. Other examples in which food increases drug absorption include the antibiotic nitrofurantoin (Macrodantin), the beta blocker metoprolol (Lopressor), and the cholesterol-lowering lovastatin (Mevacor). These drugs should be taken at mealtime or with food.

The composition of a meal may also influence drug absorption. For example, the absorption of levodopa, one of the components of the antiparkinsonism drug Sinemet,

Table 7–3

Drug Interaction with Anticoagulants and Prescription Drugs

Prescription Drugs	Anticoagulant Effects
Selected Antilipidemics	
Fibrate group	Increased effect; may cause increase in bleeding
Statin group	
lovastatin	Increased effect
pravastatin	No known effects
Angiotensin-Converting Enzyme Inhibitors	No known effects
Aminoglycosides	No known effects
Aspirin	Strong effects; can cause bleeding
Antineoplastic Drugs	
Cytoxan, 5-fluorouracil, methotrexate, doxorubicin, vincristine	Increased effects; can cause bleeding
Cytoxan, mercaptopurine, mitotane	Decreased effects; Cytoxan may cause increased or decreased effects
Barbiturates	Reduced effect of anticoagulants
Benzodiazepines	No known effects
Beta Blockers	No known effects
Selected Cephalosporins	
Cefamandole	Increased effects; may cause bleeding
Nonsteroidal Antiinflammatory Drugs (NSAIDs)	
ibuprofen	Normal doses; no effects
diclofenac, ketoprofen, tolmetin	May increase effects
Quinolone Antibiotics	Usually no effects
ciprofloxacin, norfloxacin, ofloxacin	Increased effects in isolated cases
Sulfonamides	
Bactrim-cotrimoxazole	Increased effects in 35% of persons
Tricyclic Antidepressants	No known effects
Vitamin K	Decreased effects of anticoagulants
Food	
Aspartame (artificial sweetener)	Increased effects
Green vegetables (spinach, broccoli, Brussels sprouts)	Decreased effects; vegetables are rich in vitamin K
Alcohol	
Mild to moderate drinking	No effects unless heavy drinking
Heavy drinking	Increased effects if liver function is impaired

Table 7–4

Pharmacodynamic Interactions of Drugs

Interaction	Effect
Additive	In the same drug category, the drug effect is the sum of both drug effects.
Synergistic or potentiation	One drug potentiates or enhances the effect of the other drug (greater than effect of each alone).
Antagonistic	Two drugs in opposing drug categories cancel drug effects of both drugs.

such as cheese, wine, organ meats, beer, yogurt, sour cream, or bananas. More norepinephrine is released, and the result could be a hypertensive crisis. These foods must be avoided when taking monoamine oxidase inhibitors.

Drug-Laboratory Interactions

Abnormal plasma or serum electrolyte concentrations can affect certain drug therapies. If the client takes digoxin and there are decreased serum potassium and serum magnesium levels or an increased serum calcium level, digitalis toxicity may result. Certain drugs, such as those from the thiazide diuretic group, can cause abnormal electrolyte concentrations. An example is hydrochlorothiazide (HydroDIURIL), which can decrease serum potassium, magnesium, and sodium levels and can increase the serum calcium level. Hydrochlorothiazide promotes potassium loss, and low serum potassium results in an increase in the uptake of digoxin by myocardial tissue. This sensitization of the myocardium to digoxin increases the risk of digitalis-induced arrhythmias. When digoxin and hydrochlorothiazide are taken together, the nurse should observe the client for digitalis toxicity. Symptoms are nausea, vomiting, bradycardia, and stated visual problems. Clients on long-term therapy should have regular digoxin levels drawn to detect early toxicity.

Drug-Induced Photosensitivity

A drug-induced **photosensitivity** reaction is a skin reaction that is caused by exposure to sunlight. It is caused by the interaction of a drug and exposure to ultraviolet A (UVA) light, which can cause cellular damage. Usually the skin area that is exposed is affected.

There are two types of photosensitivity reactions: photoallergy and phototoxicity. Photoallergy occurs when a drug (e.g., sulfonamide) undergoes activation in the skin by ultraviolet light to a compound that is more allergenic than the parent compound. Because it takes time to develop antibodies, photoallergenic reactions are a type of delayed hypersensitivity reaction. With phototoxocity, photosensitive drug undergoes photochemical reactions within the skin to cause damage. This type of reaction is different from photoallergy in that it is not immune-mediated. The onset of phototoxicity with erythema can

is significantly reduced when it is taken with high protein meals.

The classic drug-food interaction occurs when an antidepressant of the monoamine oxidase (MAO) inhibitor type (e.g., phenelzine) is taken with tyramine-rich foods

Table 7–5

Selected Drug-Drug Interactions

Drugs and Drug Categories	Interacting Effects with Drugs
Acyclovir	IV incompatible with dobutamine, dopamine, and morphine.
Alteplase	IV incompatible with dobutamine, dopamine, heparin, morphine, and nitroglycerin.
Aminoglycosides	Cephalosporins, ethacrynic acid, furosemide, polymyxin, and vancomycin can increase the risk of nephrotoxicity and ototoxicity. This is especially true with the young and older adults.
Aminophylline	IV incompatible with dobutamine, dopamine, meperidine, and ondansetron.
Angiotensin-converting enzyme (ACE) inhibitors example: captopril	Antacids will decrease absorption of ACE inhibitors. Potassium-sparing diuretics will decrease potassium excretion, and lithium use will decrease lithium excretion. Antihypertensives, nitrates, and diuretics enhance hypotensive effects.
Anticoagulants example: warfarin (Coumadin)	Drugs that may enhance anticoagulant effects include acetaminophen (high doses), alcohol, antiplatelet drugs, aspirin, aminoglycosides, cephalosporins, erythromycins, furosemide, fluoroquinolones, isoniazid, NSAIDs, sulfonamides, thiazides, tricyclic antidepressants, and vitamin E.
Anticonvulsants example: phenytoin (Dilantin)	Alcohol decreases phenytoin effect. Warfarin absorption may be decreased. Oral contraceptives' and corticosteroids' effectiveness may be decreased. Isoniazid increases phenytoin levels.
Antipsychotic agents example: phenothiazides	Alcohol increases CNS depression. Antacids and antidiarrheals decrease drug absorption. Tricyclic antidepressants may increase the risk of hypotension. Anticonvulsant dose may need to be increased because phenothiazides can decrease seizure threshold.
Antitubercular agents example: isoniazid	Alcohol increases risk of hepatotoxicity. Antacids decrease absorption of isoniazid. Phenytoin levels can increase and could result in phenytoin toxicity.
Aspirin (salicylates)	Anticoagulants can increase the risk of bleeding when taken with aspirin. Oral antidiabetic agents may increase the risk of hypoglycemia.
Benzodiazepines example: diazepam, lorazepam	Alcohol, narcotics, and anticonvulsants can increase CNS depression. Cimetidine can increase diazepam and lorazepam toxicity. Levodopa effects may be decreased. Phenytoin serum levels may be increased.
Beta (adrenergic) blockers example: propranolol (Inderal)	Diuretics, antihypertensives, and phenothiazines can increase the state of hypotension. Atropine can correct bradycardia. Antacids decrease propranolol absorption. Cimetidine decreases drug clearance and increases beta blocker effects.
Calcium channel blockers example: nifedipine (Procardia)	Digoxin levels may be increased. Beta blockers have an additive effect and can cause bradycardia. H2 blockers decrease drug clearance, thus calcium blocker levels could be elevated.
Cardiac glycosides example: digoxin (Lanoxin)	Thiazide and loop diuretics, corticosteroids, laxatives, and amphotericin B can cause hypokalemia, which could cause digitalis toxicity. Antacids, antidiarrheals, and colestipol decrease absorption of digoxin. Quinidine, verapamil, and erythromycin increase digoxin levels.
Diazepam	IV incompatible with dobutamine, heparin, meperidine, and potassium in D5W.
Diuretics (potassium-wasting) (thiazide and loop)	Digoxin toxicity may result from hypokalemia because of loop or thiazide diuretics. Corticosteroids increase potassium loss. Lithium levels may be increased.
Fluoroquinolones example: ciprofloxacin (Cipro)	Theophylline levels and warfarin (Coumadin) levels may be increased. Antacids and iron products can decrease ciprofloxacin absorption.
Furosemide	IV incompatible with dobutamine, meperidine, morphine, and ondansetron.
Lithium carbonate	Diuretics, NSAIDs, tetracyclines, and methyldopa can increase lithium toxicity. Theophylline, sodium bicarbonate, and potassium or sodium citrate can promote lithium excretion.
Narcotics examples: morphine and meperidine (Demerol)	Alcohol, sedatives, benzodiazepines, barbiturates, and tricyclic antidepressants can increase CNS depression. Monoamine oxidase inhibitors (MAOIs) may cause a hypertensive crisis.
Nonsteroidal antiinflammatory drugs (NSAIDs) example: ibuprofen (Motrin)	Warfarin, heparin, and alcohol may prolong bleeding time. Lithium and methotrexate levels may increase; lithium toxicity may result. Corticosteroids may cause a peptic ulcer.
Penicillins	Warfarin effects may be decreased. NSAIDs prolong the effects of penicillin. Diuretics with penicillin G-K may cause hyperkalemia. Oral contraceptives' effectiveness may be decreased. Rifampin inhibits the action of penicillin.
Phenytoin	IV incompatible with dobutamine, heparin, meperidine, morphine, nitroglycerin, and potassium in D5W.
Sulfonylureas	Alcohol, aspirin, anticoagulants, some NSAIDs, anticonvulsants, sulfonamides, and oral contraceptives may increase the risk of hypoglycemia. Corticosteroids, thiazide diuretics, estrogen, calcium channel blockers, phenytoin, and thyroid drugs may increase the blood sugar level.
Tetracyclines	Milk, antacids, and iron supplements decrease tetracycline absorption. Oral contraceptive effects can be decreased.
Theophylline	Erythromycins, fluoroquinolones, and tacrine can increase theophylline levels. Lithium excretion may be increased. Cigarette smoking decreases theophylline levels.
Tricyclic antidepressants example: amitriptyline	Warfarin's anticoagulant effects can be increased. Alcohol, narcotics, and sedatives increase CNS depression. MAOIs should not be taken with tricyclics. Antihypertensive drug effects may be reduced. Cimetidine may increase tricyclic serum levels.

be rapid, occurring within 2 to 6 hours of sunlight exposure.

Both types of reactions are the result of light exposure, but differ according to the wavelength of light and the photosensitive drug. Phototoxicity may be the result of the drug dose, whereas photoallergenic reactions are not and only require previous exposure, or sensitization, to the offending agent. Examples of drugs that can induce photosensitivity are listed in Table 7–6.

Most photosensitive reactions can be avoided by using sunscreen with a protection factor (SPF) greater than 15, avoiding excessive sunlight, and wearing protective clothing. The higher the drug dose administered, the more likely that drug photosensitivity will occur. Decreasing drug dose may decrease the risk of photosensitivity if treatment is required. It may be necessary, however, to discontinue use of the offending drug altogether.

Over-the-Counter Drugs

Over-the-counter (OTC) drugs, drugs that are attainable without a prescription, are found in most households (Figure 7–1). The Food and Drug Administration (FDA) finds that OTC preparations do not require that you be in the care of a health care provider to have access to these products. More than 90% of all illnesses are initially treated with OTC drugs, and their use is unknown to many health care providers. A study of 7 resident physicians and 414 adult clients revealed that more than half the clients reported OTC use, and physicians questioned OTC use in one third of the visits. Almost 60% of those reporting OTC use did not tell physician, and at the same time only 14% of the clients indicated it was not important to report OTC use to physician.

Be alert to internet drug purchases and the mass solicitations received daily on our computers. In their desire to save money, people can be tempted to buy these drugs and to self-medicate. Refer to Chapter 5 for more information on purchasing drugs via the internet.

Over-the-counter drugs include vitamin supplements, cold and cough remedies, analgesics for pain, antacids, laxatives, antihistamines, sleep aids, nasal sprays, weight-control drugs, and herbal products. Some clients do not consider herbal products to be OTC drugs. More than $4 billion is spent annually on herbal products, nutraceuticals, and dietary supplements; most of these products are minimally regulated by the FDA. Refer to Chapter 9 for more discussion of herbal therapy.

Today many drugs which were previously available only by prescription are available over the counter. Examples of recent prescription-to-OTC switches include proton pump inhibitors (e.g., Prilosec-OTC) and Plan B® emergency contraception.

Multiple factors contribute to the increase in the number and use of OTC products. Mass-media marketing surrounds us. These remedies are used by family and friends,

Table 7–6

Drug-Induced Photosensitivity

Drug-Induced	Occurrence
Amantadine	Confirmed by positive photopatch testing
Amiodarone	Frequency may be 10% to 75%. Sunscreen lotion with UVA can help reduce incidence of photosensitivity
benzodiazepines	Has been reported with drugs alprazolam and chlordiazepoxide
carbamazepine	Frequency is less than 1%; however, photocopy machines can trigger photosensitivity
corticosteroids	Was reported with positive photopatch testing and with use of hydrocortisone
Fluorouracil	Avoid sunlight with topical or intravenous use; erythema and hyperpigmentation could occur
NSAIDs	Aspirin, ibuprofen, and indomethacin have been reported to have low phototoxic effect; however, there is a possibility for photosensitive effect with ibuprofen (dose related)
Methotrexate	Avoid sunlight to prevent severe photosensitive reaction (sunburn)
calcium blockers	diltiazem: possible phototoxic reaction nifedipine: may cause phototoxicity with high drug doses
phenothiazines	Reported cases of phototoxic reaction with chlorpromazine and other phenothiazines at high drug doses
Piroxicam	Was confirmed with positive photopatch testing; photosensitive reaction occurs after a few days of piroxicam and exposure to sunlight
Pyrazinamide	Skin color may change to reddish brown; usually occurrence is dose-related
Quinolones (fluoroquinolones)	Phototoxicity occurs with lomefloxacin, enoxacin, ofloxacin, and nalidixic acid; ciprofloxacin causes less photosensitivity
Sulfonamides	Photosensitive reaction has been reported
Sulfonylureas	Photosensitive reaction has been reported
Tetracyclines	Highly photosensitive; demeclocycline and doxycycline have a higher degree of photosensitive reaction than minocycline
Thiazides	Thiazide-induced photosensitivity has been reported; hydrochlorothiazide has a greater photosensitivity than bendroflumethiazide
Trimethoprim	Photosensitivity has been reported
Vinblastine	Photosensitivity has been reported

NSAIDs, Nonsteroidal antiinflammatory drugs; UVA, ultraviolet A.

FIGURE 7–1 Commonly used over-the-counter preparations.

and many people now are into "self-treatment." It is one of the nurse's responsibilities to advocate for the client making educated choices.

The FDA has been working to standardize OTC labeling. OTC labeling is designed to provide consumers with better information and describe the benefits and risks associated with taking over-the-counter medications. ALERT: Multiple OTC drugs may have the same active ingredients; avoid taking an excess amount of an ingredient.

Nurses need to be aware of OTC products and the implications of their use for their clients' drug therapy. OTC drugs provide both advantages and potential serious complications for the consumer. The nurse needs to emphasize that many of these drugs are potent medications and can cause moderate to severe side effects, especially when taken with other drugs. Self-diagnosing and self-prescribing OTC drugs may mask the seriousness of the clinical condition. Based on an increase in serious adverse reactions and deaths of infants and toddlers, the FDA (2007) recalled all OTC medications with directions/dosages for children 2 years and younger.

In 1952 Congress enacted the Durham-Humphrey amendment to the Food, Drug, and Cosmetic Act of 1938, allowing FDA-approved drugs considered safe for consumption to be sold as nonprescription or OTC drugs. In 1962 the Kefauver-Harris amendment required proof of efficacy and safety of drugs; the catalyst for this amendment was the number of thalidomide-induced birth defects found in Europe during the 1950s. Though thalidomide had not yet been approved by the FDA or marketed in the United States, the amendment was passed as a proactive approach to ensure client safety.

The FDA has the responsibility for monitoring the safety of drug therapy. This group of professionals is charged with identifying standards for known active ingredients and establishing mandatory labeling to assist the consumer in the proper use of the drug. The FDA OTC drug categories are listed in Box 7–1.

As a result of the review by the FDA panel, drugs are placed in one of three categories:

Category I: Drugs judged to be both safe and effective

Box 7–1

FDA Over-the-Counter Drug Categories

- Allergy treatment products (internal)
- Analgesics—antipyretics (internal)
- Antacids and antiflatulents
- Antidiarrheal products
- Antimicrobials
- Antiperspirants
- Antirheumatic products
- Antitussives
- Bronchodilators and antiasthmatic products
- Cold remedies and decongestants
- Contraceptive products
- Dandruff products
- Dentifrices and other dental products
- Dermatologic products
- Emetics and antiemetics
- Hematinics
- Hemorrhoidal products
- Herbal products
- Laxatives and cathartics
- Nicotine gum or transdermal patches
- Ophthalmic products
- Oral-hygiene drug products
- Sedatives and sleep aids
- Stimulants
- Sunburn prevention and treatment products
- Vitamin–mineral supplements
- Weight-loss aids
- Miscellaneous products (OTC products not covered in above categories)

FDA, Food and Drug Administration; *OTC,* over-the-counter.

Category II: Drugs judged to be either unsafe or ineffective; these drugs should not be included in nonprescription products

Category III: Drugs for which there are insufficient data to judge safety or efficacy

The FDA has recommended that drugs in category II be reformulated to be included in category I or removed from the market. (Note: Manufacturers can maintain the brand name after changing the components of an OTC product.)

The FDA has also recommended that selected prescription drugs be reclassified so they can be sold over the counter. The prescription drug Motrin became available as the OTC drug ibuprofen in 1984. Tagamet, another prescription drug, was made available as the OTC drug cimetidine. Because of the process, more than 700,000 OTC products have ingredients or dose strengths that were available only by prescription three decades ago. As a result, it is vitally important that nurses be aware of current drug information, any changes in FDA recommendations, and the implications of this information for an informed client population. The following cautions may be of assistance when OTC preparations are considered:

- Delay in professional diagnosis and treatment of serious or potentially serious conditions may occur if the client self-prescribes OTC drugs.

- Symptoms may be masked, thereby making diagnosis more complicated.
- Labels and instructions should be followed carefully.
- The client's health care provider or pharmacist should be consulted before OTC preparations are taken.
- Ingredients in OTC products may interact with medications that are prescribed by the health care provider or are self-prescribed by the client.
- Inactive ingredients (e.g., alcohol, dyes, preservatives) may result in adverse reactions.
- Potential for overdose exists because of the use of several preparations with similar active ingredients. A double dose does not translate into a quicker recovery.
- The risk for adverse drug reactions and drug-drug interactions will increase as more medications, whether prescription or OTC, are added to drug therapy regimens.
- Interactions of selected prescription medications and OTC preparations are potentially dangerous. Many individuals routinely reach for aspirin, acetaminophen, and ibuprofen to relieve a discomfort or pain without being aware of these interactions. For example, ibuprofen increases fluid retention, which could worsen the condition of a client with heart failure; use of ibuprofen on a long-term basis may decrease the effectiveness of antihypertensive drugs.

Several OTC drugs, such as cough and cold preparations, are composed of two to four compounds. For those clients who are already taking maintenance medicine, it is conceivable that there could be a drug-drug interaction with a cough medicine and one of the medications prescribed by the client's health care provider.

Clients with asthma need to be aware that aspirin can trigger an acute asthma episode. Aspirin is not recommended for children with flu symptoms or chickenpox, because it has been associated with Reye syndrome.

Clients with impaired renal function should avoid aspirin, acetaminophen, and ibuprofen because each can further decrease renal function, especially with long-term use. Also, clients taking moderate to high doses of aspirin, ibuprofen, or naproxen concurrently with an oral anticoagulant may be at increased risk for bleeding.

The aforementioned examples are not all-inclusive. Caution is advised before using any OTC preparations, including antacids, decongestants, laxatives, and cough syrup (Figure 7–2). Clients should check with their health care providers and read drug labels before taking OTC medications so they are aware of possible contraindications and adverse reactions. Always read OTC labels and look for product name, active ingredients, purpose, uses, warnings, directions, storage information, and inactive ingredients (e.g., color, flavors). It is a good idea to check your supply of medications at least once a year and to properly dispose of those medications that have expired. Store medications in their original container in a cool, dry place or as directed on the label. A medicine cabinet located in the bathroom is probably not an ideal location to store medications, because of the increased moisture. If

FIGURE 7–2 Consumers often have questions when choosing an over-the-counter preparation.

you are pregnant or breast-feeding, consult your health care provider or pharmacist before taking any medicine.

Polypharmacy is a real problem in the U.S., and the elderly are especially at risk. Elders commonly have multiple prescribers and many use multiple pharmacies. In response to this need, some university medical centers have hired PhD-prepared pharmacists to assist health care providers with medication regimens by identifying incompatibilities and dangerous combinations. Many elders lack support systems and insurance and can experience neurosensory impairments, thus making them a vulnerable group. Refer to Chapter 11 for more information.

A good source for OTC drug information is *The Handbook of Nonprescription Drugs*, published by the American Pharmacists Association in Washington, DC (1-800-237-2742). The Internet is another great resource.

Cough and Cold Remedies

Most OTC cough and cold remedies are used to relieve coughs and nasal and sinus congestion. These products contain ingredients such as guaifenesin, dextromethorphan, pseudoephedrine, an analgesic, and an antihistamine.

The majority of ingredients to treat nasal congestion are sympathomimetic (i.e., they stimulate the sympathetic nervous system). Examples include phenylephrine, phenylpropanolamine, and pseudoephedrine. The FDA has ordered removal of phenylpropanolamine from OTC cold remedies and weight-control drugs because of the increased risk of hemorrhagic stroke in young women who take the drug. It has been reported that phenylpropanolamine may also cause psychosis, hypertension, renal failure, and cardiac dysrhythmias.

OTC cough and cold remedies are primarily safe for children older than 6 years. For children ages 2 to 6, consult with a health care provider. The use of medications in children less than 2 is not recommended. In fact, in the January 2007 issue of *Morbidity and Mortality Weekly Report*, researchers from the Centers for Disease Control and Prevention (CDC) reported that cough and cold medications can be harmful and should be used with caution in children under 2 years of age. This statement was issued in response to the discovery of 3 infant deaths in 2005 from the toxic effects of these medications. The report stated that more than 1500 emergency room visits in 2004 and 2005 were due to adverse effects associated with cough and cold medication use in children less than 2 years old.

Clients with heart disease, hypertension, or thyroid disease should not take these OTC preparations without approval from their health care provider. Side effects of cough and cold OTC drugs that contain a sympathomimetic include headache, nervousness, increased blood pressure, and insomnia. The most common side effect of the antihistamine is drowsiness.

Health professionals should discuss the pros and cons of taking cough and cold remedies with their client and read labels carefully. The recommended dose should not be exceeded for either adults or children. Iatrogenic conditions (treatment-induced disorders) are another concern. In situations with limited choices in pharmacotherapy, the client and health care provider at times have to deal with a second condition resulting from the treatment with a particular drug. An example of an iatrogenic condition is when a person medicated with antiinflammatory steroids develops a Cushing's appearance. People on long-term ASA therapy are prone to develop ulcers.

Sleep Aids

The FDA restricts the number of OTC sleep aids. Before 1979 most of the OTC sleep aids contained bromides, scopolamine, or a combination of antihistamines. Most OTC sleep aids currently contain an antihistamine with or without an analgesic such as aspirin or acetaminophen. The side effect of an antihistamine is drowsiness, which is useful as a sleep aid. If the client has night pain that causes sleeplessness, an analgesic with antihistamine is helpful. In small children or older adults, these sleep aids may cause CNS stimulation instead of sedation. These drugs should not be taken with a depressant because they can have an additive depressive effect on the CNS.

Weight-Control Drugs

For years most weight-control drugs contained amphetamines. The amphetamines were prescription drugs prescribed to suppress the appetite. The effectiveness of the amphetamines was short-term because they were effective only as long as the therapeutic blood level of the drug was maintained. Drug dependence was a problem associated with amphetamines. Side effects included nervousness, heart palpitations, increased blood pressure, and insomnia.

Currently many OTC weight-control drugs are on the market. The weight-control drugs are contraindicated for clients with heart disease, hypertension, diabetes mellitus, and thyroid disease.

On February 7, 2007, the FDA approved the marketing of orlistat as an OTC weight control medication. As such,

orlistat-OTC became the first FDA-approved weight loss medication to be sold in the U.S. without a prescription. Marketed under the brand name *Alli*, orlistat works by inhibiting lipase enzymes within the GI tract. The drug blocks the dietary absorption of fat by about 30%. It is to be used as part of a weight loss program that includes a reduced calorie, low-fat diet and exercise program. The drug has been approved for use in adults age 18 or older. A daily multivitamin should be taken when Alli is used as part of a weight control program. The most common side effects of orlistat include oily spotting on underwear, flatulence, urgent bowel movements, and fatty or oily stools.

The nonpharmacologic measures of consuming fewer calories and exercising more are the foundation of any weight loss program. If the client continues to eat large meals and snacks while taking weight-control drugs, little to no weight loss occurs.

Drug Interactions

ASSESSMENT

- Obtain a medication history on your client. Include questions regarding OTC drugs and herbal product use. There could be a drug interaction with the prescribed drug.
- Review all literature provided by drug companies and pharmacy.
- Assess for drug reaction when two highly protein-bound drugs are taken together daily. For example, the anticoagulant warfarin (Coumadin) and the antiinflammatory sulindac (Clinoril) have a high affinity to protein. When warfarin is displaced from the plasma protein binding sites, this leads to more free warfarin and a possible increase in bleeding risk.
- Determine if there is potential for drug interaction problems related to an increased or decreased absorption rate of two drugs. Drug enzyme inducers that increase the metabolism of an affected drug may result in a decrease in effect of that drug.
- Assess the client for drug toxicity when a drug enzyme inducer has been discontinued or when a drug enzyme inhibitor is taken concurrently with other drugs.
- Determine whether the client is a cigarette smoker. Tobacco is an enzyme inducer and can increase the metabolic rate of drugs. If client is taking a drug such as theophylline to control asthma and also smokes, the drug dosage may need to be increased. For nonsmokers, the theophylline dosage should be within the suggested drug dosing range.
- Determine renal function by checking for adequate urine output; it should be greater than 600 ml daily. The guideline is 30 ml/h for adults.

NURSING DIAGNOSES

■ Knowledge-deficient related to lack of information about drug interactions and OTC drugs
■ Risk of tissue injury related to adverse reaction to drug interaction

PLANNING

■ Client will be aware of drug interactions, will avoid drugs that may cause a severe reaction, and will know what to report immediately to health care provider.
■ Client will not take any OTC drugs without consultation with health care provider.

NURSING INTERVENTIONS

■ Contact the health care provider to assess the need for a drug dose adjustment if one has not been ordered after a drug enzyme inducer has been discontinued.
■ Recognize drugs of the same category that might have an additive effect. The additive drug effect might be undesirable and could cause a severe physiologic response.
■ Notify the health care provider of drugs ordered that have antagonistic or opposite effects, such as beta stimulants and beta blockers.
■ Consult a pharmacist about use of a drug interaction computer program.
■ Encourage the client to use one pharmacy.

Client Teaching

• Advise clients not to take OTC drugs with prescribed drugs without first notifying the health care provider.
• Remind clients to be cautious about taking herbal products, especially if taking OTC or prescription medications; check with health care provider first.

EVALUATION

■ Evaluate the effectiveness of the drugs and determine that client is free of side effects.

KEY WEBSITES

Facts and Comparisons' Guide to Popular Natural Products: www.drugfacts.com
National Library of Medicine fact sheets on supplements: www.nlm.nih/gov/medlineplus/vitaminandmineralsupplements.htm
PubMed: www.ncbi/nlm.nih.gov/PubMed

Critical Thinking Case Study

Your client is taking phenytoin, warfarin, Phenergan, meperidine, and valium. What general teaching is appropriate for this client? Be certain to include specifics about probable drug interactions. During your teaching session, the client shares that he plans to start taking OTC products to boost his energy. What is the nurse's best response (including rationale) to the client comment?

NCLEX Study Questions

1. The rate of absorption of drugs can change when two drugs are taken at the same time. As the nurse you are aware that the rate of absorption can be changed by all the following except:
   a. modifying gastric emptying time
   b. changing gastric pH
   c. decreasing inflammation
   d. forming drug complexes

2. The drug(s) least likely to cause photosensitivity is/are:
   a. phenytoin
   b. benzodiazepines
   c. quinolones
   d. NSAIDs

3. A category of preparations that is NOT included for OTC products is:
   a. drugs judged to be both safe and effective
   b. drugs judged to be either unsafe or ineffective
   c. drugs with insufficient data to judge safety or efficacy
   d. drugs in clinical trials

4. Clients at high risk for drug interactions include:
   a. elderly
   b. those with chronic health conditions
   c. those taking three or more drugs
   d. all of the above

5. When a client takes a hepatic enzyme inducer, the dose of the warfarin is usually:
   a. tripled
   b. halved
   c. remains the same
   d. doubled

6. Your client has alkaline urine which promotes excretion of drugs that are weak acids such as:
   a. phenytoin
   b. aspirin
   c. quinidine
   d. none of the above

7. Which of the following statements is correct about synergistic drug effects?
   a. antagonistic effects
   b. action of drugs nullified
   c. acts like antidote
   d. greater effect when drugs combined

8. Which of the following is not a caution associated with use of OTC medications?
   a. delay in professional diagnosis
   b. symptoms may be masked
   c. diagnosis is easier to make
   d. inactive ingredients may result in adverse reactions

Answers: 1, c; 2, a; 3, d; 4, d; 5, a; 6, b; 7, d; 8, c.

8

Drugs of Abuse

ELECTRONIC RESOURCES

Evolve website (http://evolve.elsevier.com/KeeHayes/pharmacology/):
- *Case Studies*
- *Content Updates*
- *Frequently Asked Questions*
- *Student Review Activities*
- *WebLinks*
- *Additional Reference Material*

Companion CD-ROM:
- *NCLEX Examination Review Questions*
- *Pharmacology Animations*
- *IV Therapy Checklists*
- *Medication Error Checklists*
- *Drug Calculation Problems*
- *Electronic Calculators*
- *Top 200 Drugs with Pronunciations*
- *References from the Textbook*

Outline

Objectives

- Define and differentiate among drug (substance) abuse, drug (substance) misuse, addiction, dependence, tolerance, detoxification, withdrawal, and abstinence.
- Describe the short-term and long-term effects of the relationships among brain structures and neurotransmitters involved in the neurobiology of addictive drugs.
- Identify the physical and psychologic assessment findings associated with the use of commonly abused central nervous system stimulants and depressants, cannabis, psychedelic agents, and inhalants.
- Explain the rationale for the use of pharmacologic treatments during toxicity, withdrawal, and maintenance of abstinence of commonly abused drugs.
- Prioritize appropriate nursing interventions to use during treatment of clients with substance toxicity and withdrawal.
- Identify nursing interventions appropriate during management of surgical experiences and pain in clients who abuse drugs.
- Describe the nurse's role in recognizing and promoting treatment of chemical impairment among nurses.
- Implement the nursing process in the care of clients who abuse drugs.

Terms

Most drugs are used safely and within prescribed guidelines, but it is possible for all drugs to be misused or abused. Drug abuse and **addiction** are serious and complex social and health problems that nurses address in all areas of practice. However, the focuses of this chapter are primarily the physiologic effects of abused drugs and the pharmacologic treatment of abuse.

The Context of Drug Abuse

Cultural Considerations

Describing what constitutes drug misuse and abuse is difficult because culture and social expectations influence the definitions and perception of drug abuse. In Moslem Middle Eastern populations, any use of alcohol or mind-altering drugs would be considered abuse. The same would be true in the United States among Mormon and some conservative Christian groups. Yet in many European cultures, alcohol use is expected and present in all family and social gatherings. In some subcultures in the United States, occasional use of marijuana is not considered abuse, nor is the use of psychedelic agents in some Native American religious rites. Cigarette smoking, which was glamorized in the past, is now less socially acceptable than moderate alcohol use.

Rates of drug abuse and addiction are similar among white, African American, and Hispanic populations in the United States. Native Americans, however, have much higher rates of alcoholism. White American populations tend to abuse alcohol and amphetamines, whereas African Americans and Hispanics prefer to use heroin and cocaine, respectively. Sociocultural factors arising from unemployment, poverty, or adverse social conditions also affect the incidence of drug abuse. A major responsibility of nurses in addressing drug abuse in ethnic and cultural groups is to assess and treat the client within his or her cultural perspective as described in detail in Chapter 6.

Definitions

Although small differences exist in their definitions, the terms drug, substance, and chemical are often used interchangeably within the context of drug abuse. **Drug misuse** generally refers to indiscriminate use of a chemical substance or its use for purposes other than those for which it is intended. **Drug abuse** is culturally defined and may be considered drug use inconsistent with medical or social norms. It generally refers to an overindulgence of a chemical substance that results in a negative impact on the psychologic, physical, or social functioning of an individual. Chronic abuse of a drug may lead to addiction. **Drug addiction** should be considered a complex disease of the central nervous system (CNS) characterized by a compulsive, uncontrolled craving for and **dependence** on a substance to such a degree that cessation causes severe emotional, mental, or physiologic reactions. **Physical dependence** is not necessary or sufficient for addiction to occur. These and additional terms used in describing drug abuse are presented in Table 8–1.

The drugs that are abused most often are psychoactive agents that result in pleasure or modify thinking and perception. They include legal substances such as alcohol and tobacco and drugs with therapeutic value such as analgesics, sedative-hypnotics, tranquilizers, and amphetamines. Common illegal substances that are abused include, in descending prevalence, marijuana and hashish, cocaine, hallucinogens, inhalants, and heroin.

Neurobiology of Addictive Drugs

Current research indicates that most addictive drugs increase the availability of dopamine and other neurotransmitters in the "pleasure" area of the mesolimbic system of the brain. This area has been identified as the **brain reward system**, an ancient system that creates the sensation of pleasure for certain behaviors necessary for survival, such as eating and sexual behavior.

Normally dopamine is released at a slow rate in the mesolimbic system, producing a normal mood. However, certain drugs such as opioids and cocaine increase the release of dopamine or decrease its reuptake at the synapse. Nicotine, alcohol, marijuana, amphetamines, and caffeine are also believed to increase dopamine activity at the synapse. The resulting increase in dopamine in the system leads to mood elevation or euphoria, factors that provide strong motivation to repeat the experience. Many addictive drugs also increase the availability of other neurotransmitters such as serotonin and gamma-aminobutyric acid (GABA), but dopamine's effect on the reward system appears to be pivotal to the addictive process.

Table 8–1	
Terminology of Drug Abuse	
Term	**Definition**
Abstinence	Avoidance of substance use.
Addiction	A compulsive, uncontrollable craving for and dependence on a substance to such a degree that cessation causes severe emotional, mental, or physiologic reactions.
Chemical impairment	A term used by health professionals to describe behaviors related to the effects of drugs or substances on performance
Craving	Subjective need for a substance, usually experienced after decreased use or abstinence. Cue-induced craving is stimulated in the presence of situations previously associated with drug-taking.
Dependence	Reliance on a substance that has reached the level that its absence will cause an impairment in function.
Psychologic	Compulsive need to experience pleasurable response from the substance.
Physical	Altered physiologic state from prolonged substance use; regular use is necessary to prevent withdrawal syndrome.
Drug abuse	Overindulgence in and dependence on a substance that has a negative impact on psychologic, physiologic, and social functioning of an individual; synonymous with chemical dependence.
Drug misuse	Indiscriminate use of a drug for purposes other than those for which it is intended.
Relapse	Return to substance use during abstinence.
Substance	Drug, chemical, or biologic entity.
Tolerance	Decreased effect of a substance that results from repeated exposure. It is possible to develop cross-tolerance to other substances in same category.
Withdrawal syndrome	Constellation of physiologic and psychologic responses that occur when there is abrupt cessation or reduced intake of a substance on which an individual is dependent or when the effect is counteracted by a specific antagonist.

Addiction results from the prolonged effects of addictive drugs on the brain. Repeated use of addictive drugs remodels the neural circuitry of the brain cells and reduces the responsiveness of receptors. This decreased responsiveness leads to **tolerance**, the need for a larger dose of a drug to obtain the original euphoria, and also reduces the sense of pleasure from experiences that previously resulted in positive feelings. Without the drug, the individual experiences depression, anxiety, and irritability. Even to feel normal, the individual must take the drug. Drug **craving** is another characteristic of addiction. An important type of craving experienced by addicts, **cue-induced craving**, occurs in the presence of people, places, or things they have previously associated with drug taking. New studies indicate that these encounters produce surges in dopamine levels, and these surges push the individual toward active drug seeking and drug taking. Cue-induced craving may occur after long periods of **abstinence** and is a common cause of **relapse**.

Continued research into the biologic and genetic basis of addictions is of crucial importance in the development of drugs to treat addiction. There is increasing evidence that genetics play a significant role in alcoholism and nicotine use and that there are significant gender differences in drug abuse risk. A natural genetic mutation that inhibits nicotine metabolism in the brain has been identified. Men with the mutation are less likely to become addicted to nicotine and find it easier to quit smoking. However, the presence or absence of the defective gene does not affect women's smoking. Women also have less stomach metabolism of alcohol, resulting in higher blood alcohol levels than men after the same amount of alcohol intake. A genetic differ-

ence in the activity of a liver enzyme in African Americans results in slower metabolism of nicotine, resulting in the consumption of fewer cigarettes per day than Whites.

Biologic and genetic research has led to the development of drugs to treat opioid, nicotine, and alcohol addiction. However, currently no medications are approved by the Food and Drug Administration (FDA) for treating addiction to cocaine, lysergic acid diethylamide (LSD), phencyclidine hydrochloride (PCP), marijuana, methamphetamine and other stimulants, or inhalants.

Overview of Addictive States

Intoxication

Intoxication is a state of being poisoned by a drug or other toxic substance. In the client who abuses a drug, intoxication is commonly caused by a drug overdose. The signs and symptoms seen are the toxic effects of the drug when taken in excessive doses.

Detoxification

Detoxification involves treating an intoxicated client to diminish or remove drugs or their effects from the body. Treatments may involve administration of antagonistic drugs, promotion of metabolism and elimination of the drug, or intensive supportive care until the drug is naturally eliminated.

Withdrawal Syndrome

Withdrawal syndrome is a group of signs and symptoms that occurs in physically dependent persons when drug use is stopped. The symptoms are often opposite the effects the drug produced before it was withdrawn. Opioids, alcohol, barbiturates, and anxiolytics cause relatively strong physical dependence and withdrawal syndrome. Cannabinoids and amphetamines cause weaker physical dependence. Hallucinogens such as LSD do not cause physical dependence or abstinence signs. Withdrawal syndrome is treated by slow weaning of the drugs, administration of drugs to control symptoms, and supportive care.

Cessation and Maintenance of Abstinence

To promote cessation and abstinence of the abused drug, treatment with other drugs may be used to decrease craving and prevent withdrawal syndrome. Specific receptor blockers, less potent drugs of the same class, or nonaddicting substitutes are treatment options. In addition to the use of drugs to maintain abstinence, cognitive-behavioral therapies enhance the effectiveness of medications and are recommended for treatment of all drug abuse and addiction.

Stimulants

Nicotine

Nicotine is the alkaloid in tobacco that causes dependence and is the most rapidly addicting of the drugs of abuse. Smoking cigarettes is the most damaging method of nicotine use. Cigarette smoke contains more than 4000 chemicals and gases, including at least 45 cancer-causing or tumor-promoting agents and a number of hydrocarbons or solvents. Although nicotine is not believed to be carcinogenic, it is the addictive substance and has no therapeutic value.

Pharmacodynamics

In low doses, such as those obtained through cigarettes, nicotine activates nicotinic receptors. Most effects occur from activated receptors in autonomic ganglia and the adrenal medulla. In the CNS, nicotine rapidly acts on the mesolimbic reward system of the brain, promoting the release of dopamine and mimicking the effects of cocaine and other highly addictive substances.

Pharmacokinetics

Nicotine is rapidly absorbed into the blood through the lungs in smoking and more slowly through the buccal mucosa in chewing and the nasal mucosa in snuffing. It crosses membranes easily and is widely distributed throughout the body. Nicotine passes freely into breast milk and may be toxic to the nursing infant. Plasma protein binding of nicotine is <5%. The liver is the major site of nicotine metabolism. Nicotine and its more than 20 metabolites are eliminated in the urine. The elimination half-life of nicotine is 1 to 2 hours.

Side Effects and Adverse Reactions

Stimulation of nicotinic receptors in the sympathetic ganglia and the adrenal medulla result in marked cardiovascular stimulation and increased myocardial oxygen consumption. In the brain the action of nicotine causes general CNS stimulation. Physical effects include increased respiratory rate and tremors. Psychologic effects include increased alertness and arousal. In the gastrointestinal (GI) tract, nicotine increases GI secretions and smooth-muscle tone. Many abusers of nicotine report that nicotine has a depressant effect, promoting relaxation and relief of anxiety. However, it is thought that these effects actually occur when periodic nicotine withdrawal is relieved by further nicotine.

Nicotine causes a very strong **psychologic dependence**. In addition, physiologic dependence occurs with regular heavy use. Withdrawal symptoms may occur within the first few hours after stopping smoking, peak in 24 to 48 hours, and last from a few weeks to several months. After withdrawal subsides, cue-induced craving may cause smoking relapse. The effects of nicotine and symptoms of withdrawal are presented in Table 8–2.

Treatment

Treatment of nicotine addiction has received considerable attention in the past few years because of its association with preventable illness and death. Chronic smoking can affect nearly every organ of the body. In addition to cardiovascular disease, chronic lung disease, and cancers of the larynx, lung, esophagus, oral cavity, and bladder, smoking is now associated with leukemia, cataracts, abdominal aortic aneurysm, and cancers of the cervix, kidney, pancreas, and stomach. To help end thousands of these unnecessary health problems, nurses must be proactive, identifying and talking with tobacco users and providing them with information on ways to stop the use of tobacco.

Nine drug products are now available to aid smoking cessation. Except in special circumstances, nicotine replacement therapy (NRT) or other smoking cessation agents are recommended for all tobacco users in addition to behavioral and support therapies. Five NRTs in the form of gum, lozenges, transdermal patches, nasal spray, and inhalers have been approved by the FDA to reduce the craving and withdrawal symptoms associated with tobacco cessation. These agents enable a smoker to reduce nicotine previously obtained from cigarettes with a system that provides slower delivery of the drug and eliminates the carcinogens and gases associated with tobacco smoke. Table 8–3 describes the various nicotine replacement products.

Bupropion is an atypical (heterocyclic) antidepressant unrelated to nicotine that has been approved by the FDA for smoking cessation. The mechanism of action of bupropion is unknown. It is a weak inhibitor of neuronal uptake of norepinephrine, serotonin, and dopamine that reduces the urge to smoke and reduces some symptoms of nicotine withdrawal. Bupropion may be combined with NRT to provide additional benefit. Bupropion is marketed as Zyban for smoking cessation; it is available as Wellbutrin for use as an antidepressant. Refer to Chapter 27 for more information on antidepressants.

Varenicline (Chantix) is a new drug approved for smoking cessation that is an alternative to NRT and bupropion. It is a nicotinic receptor partial agonist that reduces cravings for nicotine and decreases the pleasurable effects of cigarettes and other tobacco products if tobacco is used. The approved course of varenicline treatment is 12 weeks,

Table 8–2

Effects of Frequently Abused Drugs

Substance	Physiologic and Psychologic Effects	Toxicity	Withdrawal Syndrome
Stimulants			
Nicotine	Increased arousal and alertness; performance enhancement; increased heart rate, cardiac output, and blood pressure; cutaneous vasoconstriction; fine tremor, decreased appetite; antidiuretic effect; increased gastric motility	Rare: Nausea, abdominal pain, diarrhea, vomiting, dizziness, weakness, confusion, decreased respirations, seizures, death from respiratory failure	Craving, restlessness, depression, hyperirritability, headache, insomnia, decreased blood pressure and heart rate, increased appetite
Cocaine/amphetamines amphetamine (Benzedrine) benzphetamine (Didrex) dextroamphetamine (Dexedrine) methamphetamine (Desoxyn) methylphenidate (Ritalin) pemoline (Cylert) phenmetrazine (Preludin)	Euphoria, grandiosity, mood swings, hyperactivity, hyperalertness, restlessness, anorexia, insomnia, hypertension, tachycardia, marked vasoconstriction, tremor, dysrhythmias, seizures, sexual arousal, dilated pupils, diaphoresis	Agitation; increased temperature, pulse, respiratory rate, blood pressure; cardiac dysrhythmias; myocardial infarction; hallucinations; seizures; possible death	Severe craving, severely depressed mood, exhaustion, prolonged sleep, apathy, irritability, disorientation
Caffeine	Mood elevation, increased alertness, nervousness, jitteriness, irritability, insomnia, increased respirations, increased heart rate and force of myocardial contraction, relaxation of smooth muscle, diuresis	Rare: Nervousness, confusion, psychomotor agitation, anxiety, dizziness, tinnitus, muscle twitching, elevated blood pressure, tachycardia, extrasystoles, increased respiratory rate	Headache, irritability, drowsiness, fatigue
Depressants			
Alcohol			
Sedative-hypnotics Barbiturates secobarbital (Seconal) pentobarbital (Nembutal) amobarbital (Amytal) Benzodiazepines diazepam (Valium) chlordiazepoxide (Librium) alprazolam (Xanax) Nonbarbiturates/nonbenzodiazepines methaqualone (Quaalude) chloral hydrate (Noctec)	Initial relaxation, emotional lability, decreased inhibitions, drowsiness, lack of coordination, impaired judgment, slurred speech, hypotension, bradycardia, bradypnea, constricted pupils	Shallow respirations; cold, clammy skin; weak, rapid pulse; hyporeflexia; coma; possible death	Anxiety, agitation, insomnia, diaphoresis, tremors, delirium, seizures, possible death
Opioids heroin morphine opium codeine fentanyl (Sublimaze) meperidine (Demerol) hydromorphone (Dilaudid) propoxyphene (Darvon) oxycodone (OxyContin, Percocet) methadone (Dolophine)	Analgesia, euphoria, drowsiness, detachment from environment, relaxation, constricted pupils, constipation, nausea, decreased respiratory rate, slurred speech, impaired judgment, decreased sexual and aggressive drives	Slow, shallow respirations; clammy skin; constricted pupils; coma; possible death	Watery eyes, dilated pupils, runny nose, yawning, tremors, pain, chills, fever, diaphoresis, nausea, vomiting, diarrhea, abdominal cramps

Continued

Table 8–2

Effects of Frequently Abused Drugs—cont'd

Substance	Physiologic and Psychologic Effects	Toxicity	Withdrawal Syndrome
Cannabis Marijuana Hashish	Relaxation, euphoria, amotivation, slowed time sensation, sexual arousal, abrupt mood changes, impaired memory and attention, impaired judgment, reddened eyes, dry mouth, lack of coordination, tachycardia, increased appetite	Fatigue, paranoia, panic reactions, hallucinogen-like psychotic states	With heavy use: insomnia, restlessness, irritability, tremor, weight loss, hyperthermia, chills
Psychedelics lysergic acid diethylamide (LSD) psilocybin (mushrooms) dimethyltryptamine (DMT) diethyltryptamine (DET) 3,4-methylendioxy-amphetamine (MDMA, Ecstasy) mescaline (peyote) phencyclidine (PCP)	Perceptual distortions, hallucinations, delusions (PCP), depersonalization, heightened sensory perception, euphoria, mood swings, suspiciousness, panic, impaired judgment, increased body temperature, hypertension, flushed face, tremor, dilated pupils, constricted pupils (PCP), nystagmus (PCP), violence (PCP)	Prolonged effects and episodes, anxiety, panic, confusion, blurred vision, increases in blood pressure and temperature	No physical withdrawal, but psychologic desire may occur
Inhalants Aerosol propellants fluorinated hydrocarbons Nitrous oxide (in deodorants, hair spray, pesticide, whipped cream spray, spray paint, cookware coating products) Solvents Gasoline, kerosene, nail polish remover, typewriter correction fluid, cleaning solutions, lighter fluid, paint, paint thinner, glue Anesthetic agents Nitrous oxide, chloroform Nitrites amyl nitrite, butyl nitrite	Euphoria, decreased inhibitions, giddiness, slurred speech, illusions, drowsiness, clouded sensorium, tinnitus, nystagmus, dysrhythmias, cough, nausea, vomiting, diarrhea, irritation to eyes, nose, mouth	Anxiety, respiratory depression, cardiac dysrhythmias, loss of consciousness, sudden death	None

and those who successfully quit smoking during treatment may continue with an additional 12 weeks to increase long-term cessation. In clinical trials the most common adverse effects were nausea, headache, vomiting, flatulence, insomnia, abnormal dreams, and a change in taste perception.

Nortriptyline (Aventyl, Pamelor) and clonidine (Catapres) are used as second-line drugs to reduce nicotine withdrawal symptoms and promote cessation. These drugs are not approved by the FDA for this purpose, and their action in nicotine addiction is not clearly understood. Nortriptyline is a tricyclic antidepressant (see Chapter 27). Clonidine is a centrally acting alpha$_2$-agonist used to treat hypertension. Refer to Chapter 43 for more information on antihypertensives.

Research related to the development of new agents and new uses of approved drugs in smoking cessation is a priority of the National Institute for Drug Abuse. Clinical trials are currently in progress to examine the effects of various combinations of nicotine-replacement agents, combinations of nicotine-replacement agents with antidepressants, neurotransmitter modulators, nicotine vaccines that produce antibodies that bind in the blood with nicotine, and nicotine receptor-blocking agents. More information on nicotine abuse and its effects can be found in the discussion of lower respiratory disorders in Chapter 40.

Table 8–3

Nicotine-Replacement Agents

General Considerations for Nicotine Replacement Therapy (NRT):
- NRT should not be used by pregnant or nursing women.
- Smoking while using NRT may cause nicotine overdose.
- Tapering of all agents except transdermal patches is required.
- Replacement agents used are usually a matter of personal preference.
- The stronger doses of agents should be used by heavy smokers.
- Using more than one agent at the same time should be discussed with the health care provider.
- Generic preparations are available for some of the agents.

Agents	Absorption	Side Effects	Considerations
Gum (OTC) Nicorette 2 mg, 4 mg	Buccal mucosa	Hiccups, mouth ulcers, indigestion, jaw pain	Specific 30-min chewing regimen with periods of holding the gum between cheek and teeth; food and drink should be avoided 15 min before or during use.
Lozenge (OTC) Commit 2 mg, 4 mg	Buccal mucosa	Nausea and indigestion, hiccups, headache, cough, mouth soreness, flatulence	Dissolves in the mouth in 20-30 min; chewing and swallowing the lozenge increases GI side effects.
Patch (OTC) NicoDerm CQ Nicotine transdermal system 18 hr, 24 hr doses	Skin	Skin rash at patch site, headache, dizziness, weakness, indigestion, diarrhea, sleep disturbances with 24-hr patch	Differs from other agents, in that it helps prevent craving; cannot be used by those with adhesive allergies.
Nasal Spray Nicotrol NS	Nasal mucosa	Nose and throat irritation, sneezing, rhinitis, watery eyes, cough	Requires a prescription; nasal irritation may limit use; affects airways and not a good choice for those with asthma, allergies, or sinus problems.
Inhaler Nicotrol nicotine inhalation system, delivers 4 mg	Oral mucosa	Cough; nose, mouth, and throat irritation; heartburn and nausea	Requires a prescription; simulates smoking with mouthpiece and nicotine cartridge; may not be advisable for those with asthma or pulmonary disease.

GI, Gastrointestinal; *OTC*, over-the-counter.
Additional information and client instructions are available from the American Lung Association at *http://www.lungusa.org*.

Cocaine

Cocaine is the most potent of the abused stimulants. It is an alkaloid that was originally obtained from the leaves of the coca plant, but today it can be prepared synthetically. Historically cocaine was used as a local anesthetic, but it has been largely replaced by synthetic agents with no abuse potential. Cocaine is a Schedule II drug under the Controlled Substances Act. Illicit cocaine is available as a white powder (cocaine hydrochloride) and as cocaine base (alkaloidal cocaine, freebase), a crystalline substance. "Crack," a cocaine base that gets its name from the popping sound the crystals make when heated, is popular because it is less expensive, readily available, easy to use, and has increased purity over cocaine hydrochloride.

Pharmacodynamics

Cocaine inhibits the neuronal uptake of dopamine in the brain and increases the activation of dopamine receptors in the brain reward system. This action magnifies pleasures and leads to rapid dependence.

Cocaine also increases norepinephrine at postsynaptic receptor sites, producing intense vasoconstriction and cardiovascular stimulation. Drug interactions with cocaine are identified in Table 8–8.

Pharmacokinetics

Absorption rates of cocaine depend on the route of administration. Cocaine hydrochloride is usually "snorted" intranasally. Cocaine can also be smoked as "crack" cocaine or in "freebase" form, injected intravenously (IV), taken orally, or absorbed through mucous membranes. Smoking and IV methods result in the fastest absorption and the highest "rush" (Figure 8–1). Peak blood levels develop within 5 to 30 minutes with most methods of administration. The longest effects occur following intranasal use because absorption is delayed by vasoconstriction of the nasal vessels. Cocaine is rapidly metabolized by the liver. Elimination half-lives by oral, intranasal, and IV routes are 50, 80, and 60 minutes, respectively. Tolerance appears to occur with long-term use, but users can also become more sensitive to the drug's anesthetic and convulsant effects. Cocaine readily crosses the placenta in pregnant women and accumulates in the fetal circulation. Conflicting research exists about the effect of prenatal cocaine exposure on the development of the child.

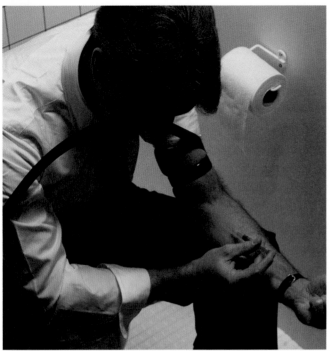

FIGURE 8–1 Drug abuse often includes the intravenous use of cocaine, opioids, and central nervous system depressants. (Copyright 2007 JupiterImages Corporation.)

Side Effects and Adverse Reactions

At usual doses cocaine produces euphoria and increased energy and alertness. In addition to stimulation of the CNS, effects include peripheral adrenaline-like actions (Table 8–2). Chronic use may lead to impairment of concentration and memory, irritability and mood swings, paranoia, and depression.

A stimulant psychosis may occur with the chronic use of any stimulant. A cocaine psychosis usually progresses from paranoid delusions to visual hallucinations of "snow lights," (colored lights when cocaine is administered) and tactile hallucinations of bugs crawling under the skin. Skin excoriations from scratching; needle marks; and elevated blood pressure, heart rate, and temperature are findings that help differentiate a stimulant psychosis from schizophrenia.

Acute cocaine toxicity may be manifested by cardiac palpitations, tachycardia, increased respiratory rate, and fever. At high levels of overdose, grand mal seizures, hypertension, and dysrhythmias or myocardial ischemia can occur. The client experiences restlessness, paranoia, agitated delirium, and confusion. Bizarre, erratic, and violent behavior may occur. Death is often related to a cerebrovascular accident, fatal dysrhythmias, or myocardial infarction.

The degree of physical dependence produced by cocaine appears to vary among individuals. Some users report little or no evidence of physical withdrawal with abstinence, but others report symptoms similar to those associated with amphetamine withdrawal: dysphoria, fatigue, depression, and a need to sleep. In the first 9 hours to 14 days of abstinence, many users experience an intense psychologic response characterized by intense craving and cocaine-seeking behavior (Table 8–2). Eventually, mood becomes more normal, but a desire to return to the drug, especially prompted by cue-induced craving, remains for an indefinite period. In rare instances withdrawal can be prolonged and difficult.

Treatment

Emergency management of cocaine toxicity depends on the client findings at the time of treatment. Treatment may be complicated by the possibility that the client has combined the use of cocaine with heroin, alcohol, or PCP. There is no specific antidote for cocaine toxicity, but during an overdose most symptoms can be controlled with a variety of drugs. Emergency interventions for assessment findings in cocaine toxicity are presented in Table 8–4.

Cognitive-behavioral therapies are often the only effective approach to cocaine addiction, but maintenance of cocaine abstinence with behavioral therapies has been difficult to achieve in most users. No drugs are currently approved to promote cocaine abstinence, and most that have been tried have had little effect. However, recent studies indicate that disulfiram (Antabuse), a well-established medication for the treatment of alcoholism, has helped nonalcoholic people addicted to cocaine reduce drug use from 2.5 days a week to 0.5 days a week on average. It has also been found that when modafinil (Provigil), a CNS stimulant used for treatment of narcolepsy, is combined with behavioral therapy the likelihood of cocaine abstinence is increased. Also under study as potential cocaine treatment agents are the anticonvulsant topiramate (Topamax) and the central-acting muscle relaxant baclofen (Lioresal).

Amphetamines

Amphetamine is a synthetic drug and, with its derivatives and similar stimulants, is strictly regulated today as a Schedule II drug of the Controlled Substance Act. Specific drugs classified as amphetamines are identified in Table 8–2 and Chapter 19. Because amphetamines may be used therapeutically as CNS stimulants, abuse may rise out of slow escalation of a prescribed dose. However, they are more often initially used as the "poor man's cocaine." Methamphetamine (crank) and methamphetamine crystals (crystal meth, ice) can be made easily in clandestine settings with relatively inexpensive over-the-counter ingredients. Traditionally associated with rural, lower-income men and women, methamphetamine abuse is now a growing problem in all segments of the population and geographic regions.

Pharmacodynamics

Amphetamines act similarly to cocaine, stimulating the release of dopamine and norepinephrine in the brain and the sympathetic nervous system. The dopamine release in the brain reward system produces euphoria and an increase in self-confidence. Drug interactions with amphetamines are identified in Table 8–8.

Pharmacokinetics

Amphetamines are usually taken orally, with peak effects occurring within 60 to 90 minutes and lasting 2 to 4 hours. More rapid effects are obtained by smoking, snorting, or IV injection (Figure 8–1). Amphetamines have a longer half-life than cocaine and, because they are more often taken orally, have a longer effect. Additional information regarding the pharmacodynamics and pharmacokinetics of amphetamines can be found in Chapter 19.

Side Effects and Adverse Reactions

Initial use of amphetamines results in increased alertness, improved performance, relief of fatigue, and anorexia. Stimulation of the sympathetic nervous system leads to cardiovascular stimulation with increased heart rate and blood pressure. Amphetamines used over time may lead to irritability, anxiety, paranoia, and hostile and violent behaviors.

Toxic reactions to amphetamines are similar to those of cocaine. Increased levels of stimulation, sometimes described as "overamping," may result in amphetamine psychosis, paranoia, seizures, and death (Table 8–2). Without medical intervention, death may occur as a result of dysrhythmias, myocardial infarction, hyperthermia, and cerebral hemorrhage.

Withdrawal symptoms of amphetamines are similar to those of cocaine use and are presented in Table 8–2. Amphetamines usually cause only mild physical dependence, but craving can be intense during abstinence. IV use will cause the onset of withdrawal symptoms in approximately 2 hours, whereas oral use results in withdrawal symptoms in 8 to 10 hours.

Treatment

Clients often seek treatment for complications of amphetamine abuse such as panic reactions or temporary psychosis related to intoxication, overdose, or withdrawal. Emergency management of amphetamine toxicity is the same as that for cocaine. Elevated blood pressure and tachycardia can be controlled with vasodilators and adrenergic β-blockers. Drug elimination can be enhanced by administering agents such as ammonium chloride that acidify the urine. Emergency treatment of amphetamine toxicity is presented in Table 8–4.

Cessation and maintenance of abstinence are difficult in amphetamine abuse. Like cocaine, withdrawal causes more psychologic symptoms than physical symptoms. Depression can last for months and is a common cause of relapse. No specific drug therapy is recommended to help maintain abstinence. It is possible that agents being tested to promote cocaine abstinence may also be effective for amphetamine abuse.

Caffeine

Caffeine is the most widely used psychoactive substance in the world. Its use to promote alertness and to alleviate fatigue is safe in most people. However, of growing concern to health professionals is the recent explosion in the marketing of caffeine-laden energy drinks—500 new products worldwide in 2006. Used by about 30 percent of 18-to-24-year-olds in the United States, these products provide a "buzz" to fight fatigue, brighten mood, and increase physical and mental performance. The demand for the buzz is so high that caffeine is now added to alcoholic drinks [e.g., Budweiser B^e (B-to-the-e)] or energy drinks are used as mixers for alcoholic drinks. Caffeine with alcohol appears to improve response time but does not reduce the errors in judgment caused by alcohol. Although weaker than other stimulant drugs, caffeine shares characteristics of intoxication, tolerance, and withdrawal symptoms in some individuals, especially when high doses are used.

Table 8–4

Drug Therapy for Cocaine and Amphetamine Toxicity

Assessment Findings	Drug Therapy
Cardiovascular	
Palpitations	Establish IV access and initiate fluid replacement as appropriate.
Tachycardia	Anticipate the need for propranolol (Inderal) or labetalol (Normodyne) for hypertension
Hypertension	and tachycardia.
Dysrhythmias	Severe hypertension may require administration of nitroprusside (Nipride) or phentolamine
Myocardial ischemia or infarction	(Regitine).
	Treat ventricular dysrhythmias as appropriate with lidocaine, bretylium (Bretylol), or procainamide (Pronestyl).
	Aspirin may be administered to lower the risk of myocardial infarction.
Central Nervous System (CNS)	
Feeling of impending doom	Naloxone (Narcan) IV should be given if CNS depression is present and concurrent opiate
Euphoria	use is suspected.
Agitation	Administer diazepam (Valium) or lorazepam (Ativan) IV for agitation and seizures.
Combativeness	Administer chlorpromazine (Thorazine) or haloperidol (Haldol) IV for psychosis and hallucinations.
Seizures	
Hallucinations	
Confusion	
Paranoia	
Fever	

IV, Intravenous.

Pharmacodynamics

Caffeine is a methylxanthine that stimulates the CNS, especially the medullary respiratory center. It also is a diuretic and myocardial stimulant. Caffeine relaxes smooth muscles and promotes peripheral vasodilation and cerebral vasoconstriction.

Pharmacokinetics

Caffeine is readily absorbed from the GI tract and reaches peak plasma levels in about 1 hour. Additional information regarding the pharmacodynamics and pharmacokinetics of caffeine is presented in Chapter 19.

Side Effects and Adverse Reactions

Oral doses of 200 mg (two cups of coffee) can elevate mood, produce insomnia, increase irritability, cause anxiety, and offset fatigue. Heavy intake of 500 mg or more per day is known to cause intoxication manifested by nervousness, insomnia, gastric hyperacidity, muscle twitching, confusion, chest pain, tachycardia, and cardiac dysrhythmias. In toxic doses, caffeine influences behavior patterns and may precipitate panic states. Until the advent of caffeine pills and highly caffeinated energy drinks, caffeine overdoses were very rare because people developed undesirable symptoms before they could take enough. Now toxicity can result when several cans of energy drinks or caffeine supplements are taken at a time or if smaller doses of caffeine are taken by young children. Although the government does not require food and drink manufacturers to list caffeine content, public concern about children's access to energy drinks have induced soft drink manufacturers to start labeling caffeine content on drinks.

Physical and psychologic dependence on caffeine have been found with chronic use of more than 500 mg daily. However, dependence may occur in some individuals at lower doses. The most commonly reported withdrawal symptoms are headache, irritability, drowsiness, and fatigue occurring within 12 to 24 hours following abstinence. Caffeine withdrawal may be responsible for some cases of headache that occur after general anesthesia. It is thought that weekend headaches may also be related to caffeine withdrawal, because caffeine consumption in many individuals is higher at work than at home. The effects of caffeine are presented in Table 8–2.

Treatment

Toxic reactions to caffeine and lethal doses of caffeine are managed symptomatically. Attention is given to controlling hypertension, dysrhythmias, and seizures as with other CNS stimulants. Management of the client with symptoms of caffeine dependence includes assisting the client to reduce gradually or to stop the intake of caffeine. A list of caffeinated products with their dosages may help the client avoid caffeine intake. Substituting decaffeinated beverages may also help. Decaffeinated coffee and tea contain 2 to 4 mg of caffeine per cup.

Depressants

Drugs classified as depressants have common physiologic and psychologic effects. Drugs in this category include alcohol, sedative-hypnotics, anxiolytics, and opioid narcotics. With the exception of alcohol and some federally regulated drugs, most CNS depressants are medically useful. These drugs are also widely recognized for their abuse potential, which leads to rapid tolerance, dependence, and medical emergencies involving overdose and withdrawal.

Alcohol

Alcohol is the most widely consumed substance of abuse in the United States. Most people use alcohol in moderation, with some positive cardiovascular and cognitive benefits. Abuse of alcohol, however, can lead to dependence and significant health, social, legal, and interpersonal problems. Alcoholism, or alcohol dependency, is currently viewed as a chronic, progressive, potentially fatal disease if left untreated.

Pharmacodynamics

Alcohol affects almost all cells of the body and has complex effects on the neurons in the CNS. Alcohol is a general CNS depressant. In addition, alcohol binds with receptors in the brain reward system, promoting the release of dopamine and the addictive process.

Pharmacokinetics

Alcohol is absorbed directly from the stomach and small intestine. Absorption from the stomach is slower in the presence of water or food, especially proteins and fats. Faster absorption occurs when alcohol is mixed with carbonated liquids. Alcohol is distributed to all body tissues and fluids. It crosses the placenta and can affect fetal development. Alcohol is primarily metabolized in the liver, although a small amount is metabolized in the stomach. Unlike most other drugs in which the metabolic rate increases as plasma drug levels rise, alcohol is usually metabolized at a relatively constant rate. In an occasional or moderate drinker, that metabolic rate is approximately one drink (7 g of alcohol) per hour. One drink is equal to 12 ounces of beer, 5 ounces of wine, or 1 ounce of distilled spirits. However, regular or heavy use of alcohol increases the rate of liver metabolism of alcohol and other drugs. Because women have significantly lower rates of stomach metabolism, they have higher blood alcohol levels than men after the same amount of alcohol intake.

The concentration of alcohol in the body can be determined by assessing the blood alcohol concentration (BAC). For the nondependent drinker, the BAC is fairly predictable of alcohol's effects and is presented in Table 8–5. The relationship between BAC and behavior is different in a person who has developed tolerance to alcohol and its effects. This individual is commonly able to drink large amounts without obvious impairment at BAC levels several times higher than those that would produce obvious impairment in the nontolerant drinker. However, little tolerance develops to respiratory depression. Chronic heavy alcohol users reach the lethal BAC at almost the same level as nonusers.

Alcohol interacts with many commonly prescribed or over-the-counter medications (Table 8–8). Potentiation

Table 8–5

Blood Alcohol Concentration and Related Effects

BAC* (mg%)	Physical and Psychologic Effects
20 (0.02)	Light and moderate drinkers begin to feel some effects after one drink.
40 (0.04)	Most people begin to feel relaxed.
60 (0.06)	Judgment is mildly impaired. People are less able to make rational decisions about their capabilities (e.g., driving skills).
80 (0.08)	Definite impairment of muscle coordination and driving skills occurs. Person is legally intoxicated in some states.
100 (0.10)	Clear deterioration of reaction time and control is observed. Person is legally intoxicated in most states.
120 (0.12)	Vomiting occurs unless this level is reached slowly.
150 (0.15)	Balance and movement are impaired. Equivalent of one half pint of whiskey is circulating in the bloodstream.
300 (0.30)	Many people lose consciousness.
400 (0.40)	Most people lose consciousness, and some die.
450 (0.45)	Breathing stops; person eventually dies.

*Blood alcohol concentration (BAC) is generally recorded in milligrams of alcohol per deciliter (mg/dl) of blood or milligrams percent (mg%). Percentage is used for legal definitions of intoxication. BAC is dependent on how much alcohol is consumed, how fast it is consumed, and the individual's weight.

and cross-tolerance with other CNS depressants also may occur. **Potentiation** occurs when an additional CNS depressant is taken with alcohol, increasing the effect. **Cross-tolerance**, the need for an increased dose of other drugs, also develops to general anesthetics, barbiturates, and other general CNS depressants. No cross-tolerance develops to opioids.

Side Effects and Adverse Reactions

Alcohol intoxication is evidenced with an increasing BAC and results in behavioral and physical changes described in Tables 8–2 and 8–5. Acute overdose produces vomiting, coma, and respiratory depression. Alcohol-induced hypotension may lead to renal failure and cardiogenic shock, common causes of alcohol-related death.

The effects of chronic alcohol use are numerous. One condition that can be prevented is **Wernicke's encephalopathy**, an inflammatory, hemorrhagic, degenerative condition of the brain resulting from a deficiency of thiamine. Untreated or progressive Wernicke's encephalopathy may lead to **Korsakoff's psychosis**, a form of amnesia characterized by loss of short-term memory and an inability to learn.

After excessive drinking, nondependent individuals experience hangovers manifested by malaise, nausea, headache, thirst, and a general feeling of fatigue. In alcoholics,

sudden withdrawal may have life-threatening effects. Withdrawal syndrome should be anticipated if the individual reports consumption of more than 10 drinks every day for a period of 2 weeks. Four characteristic signs of withdrawal are gross tremors, seizures, hallucinations, and alcohol withdrawal delirium.

The onset of withdrawal symptoms is variable, depending on the person's drinking pattern. Symptoms may occur the first 4 to 6 hours after the last drink, peak at 24 to 28 hours, and last up to 5 days. Anticipation of withdrawal syndrome should always include assessment of the time of the last alcohol intake. Characteristic symptoms are presented in Table 8–2. Seizures are most likely to occur 7 to 48 hours after the last drink. Alcohol withdrawal delirium is a serious complication that may occur from 30 to 120 hours after the last drink. Delirium components include disorientation, visual or auditory hallucinations, and increased hyperactivity without seizures. Death may be caused by hyperthermia, peripheral vascular collapse, or cardiac failure.

Treatment

Initial treatment of acute alcohol intoxication or overdose requires implementation of the basic principles of airway, breathing, and circulation (ABCs). No antidote for alcohol is available, and stimulants should not be given. Alcohol-induced hypotension cannot be corrected with vasoconstrictors. Alcohol may be removed from the body by gastric lavage and dialysis. Because symptoms of Wernicke's encephalopathy may be difficult to distinguish from those of intoxication, and because Wernicke's is potentially reversible, IV thiamine at a dose of 300 mg daily is often administered to intoxicated clients. Clients with alcohol intoxication may also be hypoglycemic because of a lack of food intake. Glucose solutions may precipitate Wernicke's encephalopathy in a previously unaffected client. For this reason, thiamine should be started before treatment with IV glucose solution in all clients with alcoholism and continued until the client resumes a normal diet.

Although specific drugs are not indicated for acute alcohol toxicity, drugs are available to facilitate alcohol withdrawal and help maintain abstinence. Management of alcohol withdrawal frequently includes the use of a variety of drugs. Anticipating withdrawal syndrome in clients is important because alcohol withdrawal delirium can usually be prevented by administration of benzodiazepines such as lorazepam (Ativan), discussed further in Chapter 20. Benzodiazepines with long half-lives are the most effective drugs in alcohol withdrawal to stabilize vital signs, reduce symptoms, and decrease the risk of seizures and delirium. Additional drugs used as adjuncts to benzodiazepines are included in Table 8–6.

Rehabilitation and sustained abstinence are the primary long-term goals of alcohol treatment. Drugs approved to maintain abstinence may be used in addition to cognitive-behavioral therapy for long-term treatment. These include disulfiram (Antabuse), which prevents drinking by causing

Table 8-6

Drug Therapy for Alcohol Withdrawal

Clinical Manifestations	Medications
Minor Withdrawal Syndrome	
Tremulousness, anxiety	Long-acting benzodiazepines (e.g., lorazepam [Ativan], chlordiazepoxide [Librium]) to
Insomnia	stabilize vital signs, reduce anxiety, and prevent seizures and delirium
Increased heart rate	Thiamine to prevent Wernicke's encephalopathy
Increased blood pressure	Multivitamins (folic acid, B vitamins) for nutritional support
Sweating	Magnesium sulfate if serum magnesium is low
Nausea	Glucose solutions IV if hypoglycemia present (after thiamine)
Hyperreflexia	
Major Withdrawal Syndrome	
Disorientation	Continue use of benzodiazepines and add:
Visual/auditory hallucinations	Antipsychotic drugs (e.g., haloperidol [Haldol]) for hallucinations and delirium
Increased hyperactivity without seizures	Carbamazepine (Tegretol) or phenytoin (Dilantin) to prevent or treat seizures
Gross tremors	
Seizures	
Alcohol withdrawal delirium	

IV, Intravenous.

an unpleasant reaction if alcohol is consumed, and naltrexone, which blocks the desired effects of alcohol. Disulfiram disrupts alcohol metabolism, causing accumulation of acetaldehyde when alcohol is ingested. An adverse reaction to the accumulated acetaldehyde begins with flushing in the face and develops into intense vasodilation of the face, neck, and upper part of the body. Hyperventilation and palpitations may occur. Nausea occurs in 30 to 60 minutes with copious vomiting. Headache, sweating, thirst, chest pain, weakness, blurred vision, and hypotension follow. Blood pressure may decline to shock levels. The reaction lasts from 30 minutes to several hours and can be brought on by ingesting as little as 7 ml of alcohol. In its most severe form, it can be life threatening. In the absence of alcohol, disulfiram may cause drowsiness and skin eruptions that diminish over time. Disulfiram is metabolized by the liver, and excretion of metabolites occurs through the kidneys and lungs. Up to 20% of the drug is excreted unchanged in the feces. Effects may persist for up to 2 weeks after the last dose is taken. Client education regarding disulfiram therapy is extremely important. Clients must be made aware that consumption of any alcohol while taking disulfiram can cause a severe, potentially fatal reaction. All food and liquid medication labels must be checked for the presence of alcohol, and alcohol must not be used on the skin. Because disulfiram is self-administered, clients must be highly motivated to abstain from alcohol for it to be effective.

Naltrexone is a pure opioid antagonist that decreases craving for alcohol and blocks the "high" of alcohol use. It was originally approved for treatment of opioid addiction but was also approved for alcohol dependency when clinical trials found that it reduced alcohol relapse rates by 50% when combined with extensive counseling. Naltrexone (ReVia, Depade) 50 mg once a day by mouth is the usual dose

for alcohol dependency. Naltrexone is also available in an injectable extended-release form (Vivitrol) that is given intramuscularly once a month. This drug is indicated for alcohol-dependent clients who are able to abstain from drinking in an outpatient setting and are not actively drinking when starting treatment. Naltrexone is discussed further with opioid abuse later in this chapter and in Chapter 24.

Acamprosate (Campral) was recently approved to decrease unpleasant feelings such as tension, dysphoria, and anxiety brought about by abstinence from alcohol. It is thought to act on the brain pathways related to alcohol abuse. Dosing should start immediately after detoxification and continue even if relapse occurs. Acamprosate is not addicting but somewhat less effective than naltrexone. Combining acamprosate with naltrexone is more effective than acamprosate alone but no better than naltrexone alone. The most common adverse effects reported include headache, diarrhea, flatulence, and nausea.

Two marketed drugs are currently being studied for their use in long-term alcohol abstinence. Ondansetron (Zofran), an antagonist of receptors in the brain reward system, decreases motivation for drinking in early onset alcoholism; and topiramate (Topamax), an anticonvulsant, may be helpful in decreasing craving for alcohol as well as cocaine.

Sedative-Hypnotics

Commonly abused sedative-hypnotic agents include barbiturates, benzodiazepines, and barbiturate-like drugs. Benzodiazepines have largely replaced barbiturates as therapeutic agents for anxiety and insomnia, because they have less risk of toxicity, tolerance, and dependence. The short-acting barbiturates are preferred as recreational drugs because they more frequently produce euphoric effects. Chapter 20 covers the topic of CNS depressants in greater detail.

Pharmacodynamics and Pharmacokinetics

Sedative-hypnotic drugs act primarily on the CNS. Benzodiazepines enhance the effects of gamma-aminobutyric acid (GABA), an inhibitory neurotransmitter in the brain. Barbiturates not only enhance the inhibitory effect of GABA, but they can directly mimic the actions of GABA. Barbiturates are powerful respiratory depressants and can readily cause death by overdose. For more on the pharmacodynamics and pharmacokinetics of these drugs, see Chapter 20.

Side Effects and Adverse Reactions

The abuse potential is much greater for barbiturates than benzodiazepines. The drugs are usually taken orally, but both may be injected intravenously (Figure 8–1). Excessive doses produce an initial euphoria and intoxication similar to that of alcohol. The effects of sedative-hypnotics are presented in Table 8–2.

Tolerance develops rapidly to the sedative effects of barbiturates, requiring higher doses to achieve euphoria. Little tolerance develops to respiratory depression, however, and increasing doses may trigger hypotension and respiratory depression, resulting in death. Cross-tolerance also develops between barbiturates and other CNS depressants such as alcohol, benzodiazepines, and general anesthetics. Little cross-tolerance occurs with opioids, however. In addition, many drug interactions are associated with barbiturates and benzodiazepines (Table 8–8). An overdose of a sedative-hypnotic produces respiratory depression and coma. Other symptoms of overdose are listed in Table 8–2.

Withdrawal from sedative-hypnotics can be very serious. In the first 12 to 16 hours following the last dose, the client may develop anxiety, tremors, weakness, nausea, vomiting, muscle cramps, and increased reflexes. After 24 hours the client is craving the drug and may experience delirium, grand mal seizures, and respiratory and cardiac arrest (Table 8–2). Symptoms of withdrawal peak on the second or third day for short-acting drugs (e.g., alprazolam, secobarbital, pentobarbital) and on the seventh or eighth day for long-acting drugs (e.g., diazepam, chlordiazepoxide, phenobarbital).

Treatment

Overdoses of benzodiazepines are treated with flumazenil (Romazicon), a specific benzodiazepine antagonist. No antagonists are known to counteract the effects of barbiturates or other sedative-hypnotic drugs. Emergency life support measures must be taken in cases of overdose. Gastric lavage may be used if the drug was taken orally within 4 to 6 hours. Dialysis may be required to decrease the drug level. Gradual withdrawal of the drug is required during withdrawal syndrome. Phenobarbital, a long-acting barbiturate, may be used to control withdrawal symptoms in a client dependent on barbiturates. Phenobarbital is then gradually withdrawn when the client is stable. To manage their symptoms safely, hospitalization is recommended during drug withdrawal for individuals who have been abusing large amounts of barbiturates.

Opioids

Opioids include the naturally occurring opiates derived from opium, in addition to the many semisynthetic and synthetic narcotic agents used as analgesics (Table 8–2). Individuals who abuse opioids include those who use illegal drugs sold on the street and individuals who misuse opioids in a medical setting. Those who begin drug use illegally constitute the largest group of abusers. Street use usually involves the use of heroin. In a medical setting, some people misuse prescribed analgesics. A significant group in the medical setting includes health care professionals, who may have the highest rate of opioid abuse and dependence of any middle-class population. Ready access to drugs, stresses of the workplace environment, and long hours that interfere with family life are considered contributing factors in health care professionals. Drug abuse and chemical dependency in nurses are discussed later in this chapter.

Pharmacodynamics and Pharmacokinetics

The pharmacodynamics and pharmacokinetics of opioids are presented in Chapter 24. Important to the abuse potential of opioids is their ability to activate the brain reward system, reinforcing their addictive effect. As drugs of abuse, opioids are taken orally, sniffed, smoked, or injected subcutaneously ("skin-popping") or intravenously ("mainlining"). IV use will produce effects in seconds (Figure 8–1). Smoking or sniffing produces a longer onset and effect. Drug interactions with opioids are identified in Table 8–8.

Side Effects and Adverse Reactions

The primary effects of opioids include analgesia, drowsiness, slurred speech, and detachment from the environment. IV use usually causes a "rush" of feelings in the lower abdomen, along with warm skin flushing and a strong sense of euphoria (Table 8–2). Opioid use leads to rapid tolerance and physical dependence after short-term use. Cross-tolerance among the opioids is common, but cross-tolerance to other CNS depressants does not occur. However, additive effects of other CNS depressants may lead to increased CNS depression.

Signs of overdose of opioids include pinpoint pupils, clammy skin, depressed respiration, coma, and death, if not treated. Unintentional overdose frequently occurs with recreational use of the drugs because of the unpredictability in potency and purity. Signs of toxicity are presented in Table 8–2. Withdrawal symptoms occur with decreased amounts or cessation of the drug after prolonged moderate to heavy use. The administration of a narcotic antagonist such as naloxone (Narcan) will cause withdrawal symptoms in dependent individuals. Symptoms may include craving, abdominal cramps, diarrhea, nausea, and vomiting. Additional symptoms are presented in Table 8–2. Symptoms appear about 8 to 10 hours after the last dose, peak within 36 to 48 hours, and usually subside in 96 hours. Although opioid withdrawal is acutely uncomfortable, it is not usually life threatening, as is withdrawal from other CNS depressants.

Treatment

Overdose of opioids can precipitate a medical emergency. A narcotic antagonist such as naloxone (Narcan) should be given as soon as life support is instituted. The use of naloxone and other narcotic antagonists is discussed in Chapter 24. Treatment of withdrawal syndrome is symptom-based and does not always require the use of medication. Methadone (Dolophine) in decreasing doses over 10 to 14 days is the drug most often used to decrease symptoms during opioid detoxification. Some clients obtain relief from withdrawal symptoms with the use of clonidine (Catapres), a centrally acting alpha$_2$-adrenergic agonist that may also be used for nicotine addiction (see Chapter 43). It is most effective against GI hyperactivity, but it does not decrease craving. The action of clonidine in nicotine and opioid addiction is not fully understood.

Long-term management of opioid addiction involves the use of opioid agonists, opioid antagonists, and mixed opioid agonist-antagonists (Table 8–7 and Chapter 24). Methadone is the most commonly used opioid agonist. By substituting oral methadone for the abused opioid, withdrawal syndrome can be avoided, and the euphoria that leads to craving can be prevented. Methadone is an addictive drug, but its use in maintenance programs alters the

drug-using lifestyle, reduces exposure to infectious disease, and controls drug use. To prevent methadone abuse, it is available for addiction treatment only through agencies approved by the FDA and state authorities.

Buprenorphine is an agonist-antagonist opioid that may be used for detoxification and maintenance therapy. Because of its action on specific opiate receptors, it can decrease the symptoms of withdrawal and suppress drug craving, yet it has a low potential for abuse. For treatment of withdrawal symptoms, it is available in a sublingual tablet marketed as Subutex. For long-term maintenance it is combined with naloxone in a sublingual tablet marketed as Suboxone. In this preparation, naloxone is added to the buprenorphine to prevent addicts from injecting the tablets intravenously, which has happened with tablets containing only buprenorphine. Because it contains naloxone, Suboxone can produce intense withdrawal symptoms if it is used intravenously by opioid-addicted individuals, but the risk of withdrawal is low when Suboxone is taken as prescribed, because little naloxone is absorbed with sublingual administration. Buprenorphine in other forms (e.g., Buprenex) is not approved for treatment of opioid addiction and is used only as a Schedule III analgesic.

Naltrexone (oral ReVia, injectable Vivitrol) is an opioid antagonist that blocks euphoria and all other opioid effects.

Table 8–7

Drugs Used in Opioid Addiction

State with Signs and Symptoms	Drugs

Toxicity
    Respiratory depression
    Coma
	Opioid antagonists:
	    naloxone (Narcan): Short acting and may need to be repeated until opioid levels decrease; too much will cause withdrawal symptoms.
	    Nalmefene (Revex): Long acting; may cause prolonged withdrawal if dose is excessive

Detoxification/withdrawal
    Nausea, vomiting, diarrhea
    Abdominal cramping
    Bone and muscle pain
    Muscle spasms
    Tremor, chills, diaphoresis
	Opioid substitution:
	    methadone (Dolophine): An opioid agonist that may be used to prevent withdrawal syndrome; when used for withdrawal, it is given in decreasing oral doses over 10 to 14 days after the client is stabilized.
	    buprenorphine (Subutex): an opioid agonist-antagonist that can be substituted for abused opioids to prevent withdrawal syndrome but can cause withdrawal if an opioid agonist is in the bloodstream; for treatment of withdrawal, it must be given after withdrawal symptoms begin.
	Centrally acting alpha$_2$-adrenergic agonist:
	    clonidine (Catapres): effective in decreasing GI hyperactivity and some other symptoms of withdrawal; does not reduce craving for the drug.

Maintenance of abstinence
    Craving, cue-induced craving
	Opioid agonists:
	    methadone (Dolophine): substitution for abused opioids may be used for long-term treatment of dependency. Addiction is maintained with this method and withdrawal occurs if methadone is stopped, but drug use can be controlled and drug-using lifestyles changed with methadone maintenance.
	Opioid antagonists:
	    naltrexone (ReVia, Depade): blocks opioid receptors, preventing the desired effects if opioids are used; long-acting oral preparation that must be used voluntarily.
	Mixed opioid agonist/antagonists:
	    buprenorphine (Subutex), a sublingual tablet, can be used instead of methadone for maintenance therapy. To prevent abuse of buprenorphine itself, it is also marketed in combination with naltrexone as Suboxone. If this preparation is crushed and injected, opioid withdrawal will occur in an opioid-addicted individual. When Suboxone is used sublingually, the opioid agonist effect predominates.

Like naloxone, it will precipitate withdrawal symptoms when administered to opioid-dependent individuals. When naltrexone is used, administration of an opioid produces no effect, eliminating the reinforcing properties of drug use. It does not prevent craving, however. Naltrexone is used rather than naloxone for maintenance treatment, because it is longer acting and can be taken orally. Usual dosing is orally once a day or alternate days, or intramuscularly once a month.

Other Drugs of Abuse

Cannabis

In North America, cannabis is usually sold as marijuana or hashish. Tetrahydrocannabinol (THC) is the active ingredient in cannabis responsible for most of the psychoactive effects. Although a number of potential benefits of THC have been reported, the only approved THC preparation is dronabinol (Marinol), used to control nausea and vomiting resulting from cancer chemotherapy. Dronabinol is also used to simulate appetite in clients with acquired immunodeficiency syndrome (AIDS).

Pharmacodynamics

At low to moderate doses, THC produces fewer physiologic and psychologic alterations than do other classes of psychoactive drugs, including alcohol. Although its mechanism of action is uncertain, THC affects cannabinoid receptors in the brain and may act in part through the same reward system as opioids and cocaine.

Pharmacokinetics

When marijuana is smoked, effects usually occur in 20 to 30 minutes and may last up to 7 hours. Because THC is stored in body fat, it is eliminated slowly, resulting in a half-life of 2 to 7 days. When taken orally, it is almost completely absorbed but undergoes extensive first-pass metabolism.

Side Effects and Adverse Reactions

Marijuana and hashish are usually smoked as a cigarette. Usual effects include euphoria, sedation, and hallucinations. Responses are varied and depend on dose, expectations of the user, and the setting of drug use. Low to moderate doses result in euphoria and relaxation, enhanced sensory perception, and distortion of time perception. Undesirable responses include short-term memory loss, decreased ability to perform multi-step tasks, and temporal disintegration. High doses may cause serious psychologic effects. Intense anxiety, delusion, paranoia, and a state of toxic psychosis can occur. Effects vary among individuals. Some individuals experience ill effects only at extremely high doses, while others routinely experience adverse effects at moderate doses. Physiologic effects are seen most commonly in the cardiovascular and respiratory systems. Decreased sperm production and decreased reproductive hormones in both men and women may occur. Signs of intoxication are presented in Table 8–2. Problems of chronic heavy use include impaired short-term memory, decreased motor coordination, tremors, and increased heart and respiratory rates. A condition known as *amotiva-tional syndrome*, characterized by apathy, dullness, and disinterest, may also occur.

Acute reactions, including intoxication and withdrawal, are usually mild and time-limited. Marijuana has low toxicity, and there is no known level of lethal dose. Complications may result when marijuana is used with other drugs such as heroin and cocaine (Table 8–8). When taken in extremely high doses, marijuana can produce tolerance and physical dependence. Abrupt cessation of high-dose marijuana may cause irritability, restlessness, nervousness, insomnia, and tremor. In rare instances withdrawal can be prolonged and difficult.

Treatment

Individuals using marijuana may seek treatment for panic reactions or may be treated for toxic reactions to a combination of drugs that includes marijuana. Treatment is directed toward relief of symptoms, and the administration of drugs is avoided if possible. There is no antidote or substitution therapy for cannabis at this time.

Psychedelic Agents

Psychedelic drugs are often referred to as hallucinogens. These drugs produce a change in level of consciousness and induce hallucinations and mental states that resemble psychosis. Primarily they bring about alterations in thoughts, perceptions, and feelings that normally only occur in dreams. Common agents and their effects are identified in Table 8–2. Although LSD originally was thought to provide a model for the study of psychosis, this idea was found to be incorrect. As a result, the drugs have no recognized medical use. Currently Ecstasy (3,4-methylenediosymethamphetamine or MDMA) is the most commonly used psychedelic. Among adolescents and young adults, it is a popular drug at nightclubs and all-night dance parties known as "raves." Ecstasy also may be abused as a "date-rape" drug.

The effects of psychedelic drug use are primarily psychologic, but cardiovascular and neurologic toxicity may occur. Little or no physical dependence develops, but acute panic reactions are common with toxicity. Panic attacks may be treated with an antianxiety agent such as diazepam (Valium) and by providing a nonthreatening environment. Although a toxic reaction may mimic psychosis, the use of antipsychotic agents such as phenothiazines (e.g., haloperidol, chlorpromazine) can intensify rather than ameliorate the experience.

Inhalants

Inhalation is the major route of ingestion for a number of common household and industrial volatile substances. Forms of use include sniffing, huffing, bagging, or spraying. Because inhalants are readily accessible, inexpensive, and produce a rapid high, they are more often used by preadolescents and adolescents.

The four main classes of inhalants are volatile solvents, aerosols, anesthetic agents, and nitrites. They act as CNS

Table 8–8

Drug Interactions: Drugs of Abuse

Drug of Abuse	Interacting Drugs	Effects
Nicotine/smoking*	isoproterenol (Isuprel) phenylephrine (Neo-Synephrine)	Increased effects with use of nicotine/smoking (After smoking cessation, dosages may need to be increased.)
	pentazocine (Talwin) propoxyphene (Darvon) benzodiazepines (e.g., diazepam [Valium]) Tricyclic antidepressants propranolol (Inderal) theophylline heparin insulin	Decreased effects with use of nicotine/smoking (After smoking cessation, dosages may need to be reduced.)
Cocaine	Sympathomimetics/adrenomimetics CNS stimulants Cholinesterase inhibitors (e.g., neostigmine)	May increase CNS and cardiac effects of cocaine
	Tricyclic antidepressants, digoxin, methyldopa	May increase cocaine-induced dysrhythmias
	Adrenergic beta-blockers	Cocaine may decrease effects
Amphetamines	Tricyclic antidepressants Sympathomimetics/adrenomimetics CNS stimulants	Increased effect of tricyclics and sympathomimetics; increased effect of amphetamines
	GI antacids/urinary alkalinizing agents MAO inhibitors	Increased amphetamine effect
	meperidine (Demerol)	Amphetamines increase analgesic effect; meperidine increases risk of seizures and vascular collapse
	thyroid hormone	Reciprocal increase in effects
	Adrenergic blockers Antihistamines Antihypertensives	Amphetamines may decrease effects.

Alcohol	Other CNS depressants:
	  Sedative-hypnotics
	  Opioids
	  General anesthetics
		Increased CNS depression with increased risk of death from respiratory depression

	Nonsteroidal antiinflammatory drugs	Combined effect increases risk of gastric bleeding
	acetaminophen (e.g., Tylenol)	Increased risk of liver injury
	Antihypertensives	Decreased effect of antihypertensives

Barbiturates	Other CNS depressants:
	  alcohol
	  Opioids
	  General anesthetics
	  Other sedative/hypnotics
	  MAO inhibitors
	  valproic acid (Depakene)
		Increased CNS depression

	Oral anticoagulants Cortico- and other steroid hormones griseofulvin doxycycline	Effect decreased by barbiturates

Benzodiazepines	Other CNS depressants:
	  alcohol
	  Opioids
	  General anesthetics
	  Other sedative/hypnotics
	Herbs:
	  kava kava, valerian
		Increased CNS depression

Opioids	Other CNS depressants:
	  alcohol
	  General anesthetics
	  Sedative/hypnotics
	  Phenothiazines
	  Antiemetics
		Increased CNS depression

	Mixed agonist/antagonist opioids	Reduces the effect of pure opioid agonists and may precipitate withdrawal syndrome
	MAO inhibitors	May cause severe fatal reaction
	Diuretics	Opioids may decrease effect
Marijuana/hashish	CNS stimulants/sympathomimetics Anticholinergic agents Tricyclic antidepressants	Additive hypertension, tachycardia, drowsiness
	CNS depressants	Additive drowsiness and CNS depression
	theophylline	Decreased effect of theophylline

depressants but are also extremely damaging to the cardio-vascular and respiratory systems. Common agents and their effects are presented in Table 8–2. Users may develop peripheral neuropathies and exhibit tremors and weakness. Sudden death may occur from direct toxic effects, aspiration of gastric contents, trauma, and suffocation. No antidotes are available for these substances, and treatment of toxicity is symptomatic.

Special Needs of Drug-Abusing Clients

Surgical Clients

An individual who abuses drugs is at high risk for drug interactions, complications, and death when surgery is required. Preoperative assessment of all clients must include an assessment of drug use. Respiratory changes in smokers make introduction of endotracheal and suction tubes more difficult and increase the risk for postoperative respiratory problems. Postoperative headaches may be caused by caffeine withdrawal in heavy users. During the client's postoperative period, the nurse should be alert for signs and symptoms of drug interactions with pain medications or anesthesia and for signs of drug withdrawal. Reactions that should be considered in surgical clients who abuse drugs are presented in Box 8–1.

Special precautions must be taken for the client who is intoxicated or alcohol dependent and requires surgery. Alcohol use may be overlooked in an accident victim if there are injuries that cause CNS depression. In addition, many persons are undiagnosed as alcoholics at the time of admission for elective surgery. The client who is alcohol dependent but is not currently drinking usually requires an increased level of anesthesia because of cross-tolerance. The intoxicated individual needs a decreased level of anesthesia because of the synergistic effect of alcohol. Whenever possible, surgery is postponed in alcohol-intoxicated individuals until the BAC is less than 200 mg%. Synergistic effects occur with anesthesia when the BAC is >150 mg%, and a client with a BAC >250 mg% has a significantly increased surgical risk and mortality rate. Alcohol-withdrawal delirium may be triggered by surgery and the cessation of alcohol consumption. Anesthetics and pain medications used in the acute period can delay withdrawal syndrome for up to 5 days postoperatively.

Pain Management

Although nurses and physicians may be reluctant to administer opioids to drug-dependent clients for fear of promoting or enhancing addictions, there is no evidence that providing opioid analgesia to these clients in any way worsens their addictive disease. When addicted clients experience any type of acute pain, the goal is to treat the pain. Addiction treatment is not the priority while the client is in pain.

If the client acknowledges opioid use, it is important to determine the types and amounts of drugs used. It is best to avoid exposing the client to the drug of abuse, and effective equianalgesic doses of other opioids can be determined if daily drug doses are known. If a history of drug abuse is unknown, or if the client does not acknowledge drug abuse, the nurse should suspect abuse when normal doses of analgesics do not relieve the client's pain or signs of withdrawal occur. Withdrawal symptoms can exacerbate pain and lead to drug-seeking behavior or illicit drug use. Toxicology screens may be helpful in determining recently used drugs.

Severe pain should be treated with opioids, but at much higher doses than those used with drug-naïve clients. The use of one opioid is preferred. Mixed opioid agonist-antagonists such as butorphanol (Stadol) or buprenorphine (Buprenex) should be avoided because these may precipitate withdrawal symptoms. Nonopioid and adjuvant analgesics and nonpharmacologic pain relief measures may also be used. To maintain opioid blood levels and prevent withdrawal symptoms, analgesics should be provided around the clock. Supplemental doses should be used to treat breakthrough pain. Although patient-controlled analgesia (PCA) is controversial for treating addicted clients, its use may improve pain control and reduce drug-seeking behavior.

A written agreement or treatment plan that describes the pain management should be developed with the client. The plan should assure that pain will be treated based on the client's perception and report of pain but also clearly outline the gradual tapering of the analgesic dose and eventual substitution of long-acting oral preparations for parenteral analgesics.

Chemical Impairment in Nurses

Chemical impairment is a term used by health professionals to indicate impaired performance as a result of drug use. Drug use and abuse is a serious concern in the nursing

---

Box 8–1

Surgical Considerations: Clients with Drug Abuse

- Standard amounts of anesthetic and analgesic medication may not be sufficient because of cross-tolerance.
- Anesthetic agents may have a prolonged sedative effect if the client has liver dysfunction.
- Increased doses of pain medication may be required if the client is dependent on opioids.
- Dosage of pain medications must be reduced gradually.
- Clients have an increased susceptibility to cardiac and respiratory depression.
- Clients have an increased risk for bleeding, postoperative complications, and infection.
- Withdrawal symptoms from central nervous system (CNS) depressants may be delayed for up to 5 days because of effects of anesthetics and pain medications.

profession. It is estimated that 10% to 20% of nurses (i.e., 300,000 to 600,000) have substance-abuse problems and that 3% to 6% (i.e., 90,000 to 180,000) demonstrate impaired practice resulting from the use of drugs (chemicals). Alcohol is the most commonly abused drug among nurses. Other drugs include meperidine (Demerol), oxycodone (Percodan), diazepam (Valium), and alprazolam (Xanax).

Contributing Factors

Factors contributing to drug abuse among nurses have been identified. Specific stressors that are commonly thought to contribute to this problem include chronic fatigue, illness, responsibility for clients' responses to illness and dying, professional dissatisfaction, access to drugs, marital and child care problems, and downsizing. Other factors include nurses' false beliefs that drugs can relieve problems or that knowledge of drugs provides immunity to drug problems. The issue has become less of a priority within the nursing community over the past several years, partly because the nursing shortage and workplace hazards have received more attention. Yet these current trends lead to increasing stressful working conditions that put nurses at even greater risk for substance-related disorders.

Characteristics

Evidence of chemical dependence may be seen by changes in personality and behavior, job performance, and attendance. Behaviors related to the influence of the drug or signs of withdrawal may also be present. Poor judgment, errors, inappropriate behavior, and illogical documentation are common in the chemically impaired nurse. Discrepancies in controlled-drug handling and records may indicate *drug diversion*, the deliberate redirecting of a drug from a client or facility to the employee for his or her own or others use. Nurses often enable substance abuse to continue among co-workers by covering their mistakes or tardiness, excusing their behavior, or simply ignoring obvious signs and symptoms. When it is recognized that a nurse is impaired, help for the nurse requires sharing observations and concerns with the nurse and supervisor to provide the means for rehabilitation.

Management

Management of drug abuse in nurses largely depends on the state in which the nurse practices and the policies of the employing facility. Sometimes employment is simply terminated, allowing the nurse to work elsewhere with no resolution of the problem. Some states or facilities require that management report the nurse to regulatory agencies that may revoke licensure to practice or refer the case to the criminal justice system. These approaches are disciplinary and contribute to the reluctance by nurses to report impaired co-workers.

The tragedy of allowing a treatable disease to go untreated is costly in both human and economic terms. In an effort to help impaired nurses, the American Nurses Association, the National Student Nurse Organization, and other nursing organizations and nurse substance-abuse experts strongly advocate rehabilitation for nurses who are chemically dependent. Alternatives to discipline have developed in most states. Alternatives include diversion programs associated with the state board of nursing that allow nurses to maintain their licenses while being monitored through recovery; state nurses' association peer assistance programs; and employee assistance programs. The goals of these programs are to protect the safety of the public, to maintain the integrity of the profession, and to ensure that the nurse is offered the possibility of treatment and rehabilitation before the license to practice is revoked or the job is terminated. Other efforts are under way to prevent chemical dependency in nurses through substance abuse educational programs, both for nursing students and nurse employees.

Summary

All nurses care for clients dependent on drugs, whether they are identified as dependent or not, simply because of the prevalence of drug abuse. It is important for nurses to suspect, identify, and intervene with clients who are abusing drugs. Knowledge of the commonly abused drugs and treatment during intoxication, overdose, withdrawal, and cessation are critical to maintaining life and promoting healthy, drug-free lifestyles.

Nursing Process

Smoking (Nicotine) Cessation

ASSESSMENT

- Assess current smoking status and smoking history.
- Identify the cultural context of client's smoking pattern.
- Determine the willingness of client to attempt to quit.
- Have client identify negative consequences of smoking and the potential benefits of quitting.
- Ask client to identify any barriers or impediments to quitting.
- Identify what rewards for quitting are most important to client.

NURSING DIAGNOSES

- Health-seeking behavior: Smoking cessation, as manifested by a stated desire to quit smoking and a request for professional assistance

PLANNING

- Client will eliminate tobacco use.

NURSING INTERVENTIONS

- Set a quit date with client, ideally within 2 weeks.
- Teach client about the nicotine-replacement systems and other agents available to assist in smoking cessation.
- Help client choose the best method to quit smoking based on client preferences and anticipated benefits.
- Refer client to support groups or quit-tobacco programs available in the community.
- Teach client to anticipate withdrawal symptoms and challenges of quitting.
- Teach client to keep a list of "slips" and near-slips to learn to avoid their causes.
- Teach client to avoid environments and activities previously associated with smoking.
- Schedule frequent follow-up contacts with client to offer encouragement; help client deal with lapses.

EVALUATION

- Evaluate effectiveness of the cessation plan, including use of drugs and support systems to avoid relapses.
- Determine the smoking status of client.

KEY WEBSITES

American Society of Addiction Medicine: www.asam.org

National Clearinghouse for Alcohol and Drug Information: www.health.org/about/

National Institute on Drug Abuse: www.drugabuse.gov

Critical Thinking Case Study

LM, a 57-year-old farmer, is admitted to the surgical unit in preparation for back surgery, after conservative treatment for a recent back injury has not relieved his pain. His wife tells the nurse she hopes the surgery will be successful. She confides that her husband has just been sitting around the house drinking more beer than usual, because he has not been able to work. LM appears relaxed and unconcerned about his anticipated surgery. He jokes with the nurse, telling her that his back would be cured if "a cute young thing" like her "would only rub his back."

1. What assessments of LM's alcohol use should the nurse make and communicate to the surgeon and anesthesiologist before he is further prepared for surgery?
2. How would the nurse's approximation of LM's BAC affect his surgical experience?
3. During LM's postoperative period, when would the nurse expect signs of withdrawal syndrome to occur and why?
4. What early signs and symptoms would alert the nurse to the development of withdrawal syndrome?
5. What drug regimens might be used during LM's postoperative period to manage problems associated with his alcohol use?

NCLEX Study Questions

1. When caring for a client recovering from an episode of opioid toxicity, the nurse determines that the client has an addiction to the drug based on a finding of:
   a. physical withdrawal signs
   b. a history of daily use
   c. craving that results in drug-seeking behaviors
   d. intravenous use of the drug rather than oral use

2. While teaching the parents of an adolescent who has been using marijuana, the nurse explains that the euphoria that results from the use of abused psychoactive substances is believed to be caused by:
   a. blockade of opioid receptors in the mesolimbic system of the brain
   b. stimulation of the dopamine pathways in the pleasure areas of the brain
   c. an increased release of serotonin in all areas of the brain
   d. a reduction in the responsiveness of brain receptors

3. A client hospitalized with a fractured femur following an automobile accident develops diarrhea and vomiting with abdominal cramps, chills with goose bumps, and dilated pupils. The nurse suspects the client is experiencing:
   a. opioid withdrawal
   b. alcohol toxicity
   c. flashbacks from psychedelic abuse
   d. barbiturate withdrawal

4. Drugs that the nurse would anticipate administering to a client who has been admitted with acute alcohol intoxication include (select all that apply):
   a. naloxone (Narcan)
   b. thiamine
   c. lorazepam (Ativan)
   d. naltrexone (ReVia)
   e. intravenous glucose solution
   f. flumazenil (Romazicon)

5. A client is admitted to the emergency department with acute cocaine toxicity. The most important intervention by the nurse is to:
   a. institute cardiac monitoring and obtain frequent blood pressures
   b. monitor the client for decreasing respiratory function and level of consciousness

   c. provide reality orientation with a calm, quiet approach
   d. administer oral fluids with caffeine to prevent withdrawal symptoms

6. A client scheduled for elective gallbladder surgery is addicted to heroin and is in a methadone treatment program. Postoperatively the nurse would expect the client's surgical pain to be treated with:
   a. a saline placebo and nonpharmacologic pain relief measures
   b. increased doses of methadone
   c. combination buprenorphine/naltrexone (Suboxone)
   d. morphine or other opioids

7. A nurse observes a colleague taking oral opioids from the medication room at the hospital. The best action by the nurse is to:
   a. report the finding to the nursing supervisor to enable the colleague's participation in a diversion program
   b. ignore the situation to protect the colleague from dismissal and possible loss of licensure
   c. confront the colleague and demand that the drugs be returned before someone notices their absence
   d. ask the colleague to request pain medications from a physician rather than stealing them from the hospital

8. A client who smokes tells the nurse that he sees no reason to stop smoking, because it keeps his stress levels down and not everyone who smokes develops lung cancer. An appropriate nursing diagnosis for the client is:
   a. ineffective coping related to use of smoking as an emotional crutch
   b. ineffective denial related to inability to personalize risks of smoking
   c. health-seeking behavior related to need to be convinced of smoking risk
   d. defensive coping related to false positive self-evaluation

Answers: 1, c; 2, b; 3, a; 4, b, c, e; 5, a; 6, d; 7, a; 8, b.

9

Herbal Therapy with Nursing Implications

ELECTRONIC RESOURCES

Evolve website (http://evolve.elsevier.com/KeeHayes/pharmacology/):
- *Case Studies*
- *Content Updates*
- *Frequently Asked Questions*
- *Student Review Activities*
- *WebLinks*
- *Additional Reference Material*

Companion CD-ROM:
- *NCLEX Examination Review Questions*
- *Pharmacology Animations*
- *IV Therapy Checklists*
- *Medication Error Checklists*
- *Drug Calculation Problems*
- *Electronic Calculators*
- *Top 200 Drugs with Pronunciations*
- *References from the Textbook*

Outline

Objectives

- Discuss at least four important points associated with consumer and health care provider education.
- Compare at least four common herbs and their associated toxicity.
- Differentiate at least eight of the most common herbal therapies and at least one situation in which they seem to be helpful.
- Describe the recommendations for labels on herbal therapy.
- Discuss the nursing implications, including client teaching, related to herbal products.

Terms. . . . .

The purpose of this chapter is to inform nurses about herbal therapy and the herbal products that clients may use. It is critical for nurses to know about herbs and include herbal preparations as part of their assessment. Herbal products can have both positive and negative effects and important interactions with prescription and OTC medications. Nurses are in an excellent position to educate clients about these interactions.

An **herb**, according to *Webster's New Collegiate Dictionary*, is a "plant or plant part valued for its medicinal, savory, or aromatic qualities." Herbs have strong roots in Judeo-Christianity (e.g., the "tree of life"). Herbs have long been and continue to be sources of old and new drugs: foxglove (source of digitalis), snakeroot (source of reserpine), willow bark (source of aspirin), and Pacific yew tree (source of Taxol) to name just a few. The therapeutic value of **phytomedicine** (medicine derived from plants) relates to several factors including dosage, potency, and purity. Research into the effects of herbal medicine is increasing.

Many Americans are using herbal products for therapeutic or preventive reasons. Herbs are the earliest form of medicine, and many cultural groups continue to routinely use herbs as medicine. Herbal therapy has surged in popularity in recent years. Marketing and the media have fueled the demand. Magazines, newspapers, billboards, and displays in grocery and drug stores are ablaze with products and advertisements. It is estimated that herbal products are used by greater than 60 million Americans. Herbal therapy has grown into a multimillion-dollar business as a result of the "back to nature" movement of the 1970s and the more health-conscious modern citizenry. Worldwide annual sales of herbal products represent greater than 60 billion US dollars, and the strong market is expected to continue. In addition, herbal therapy is now being addressed in the professional literature with increasing frequency and seriousness. Health care providers and consumers are asking questions about herbal therapy such as, "How effective is it?," "Are herbs toxic?," and "In what ways do herbs mix with current medications?" What do these questions mean for consumers and their health? Consumers should be skeptical of potentially dangerous TV, radio, and other advertisements that imply that herbs will cure anything. Herbs can be useful, but they can also be useless or even dangerous (Herbal Alert 9–1).

Herbs were the original medicines and are still in wide use throughout the world. It is estimated that phytomedi-

Herbal ALERT 9–1

Client Responsibility

To optimize the therapeutic regimen, the client has the responsibility to (1) consult with the health care provider before taking any herbal preparation, (2) report all herbal preparations taken to all health care providers, and (3) inform health care providers of any allergy or sensitivity to any herbal products.

cines are prescribed by the majority of physicians in Germany. This practice is promoted because the government's health insurance pays for botanical remedies. Americans have long used botanicals, but outside the mainstream. In China, herbs are generally combined with drugs as they are believed to increase the effectiveness of drugs by decreasing side effects and fortifying the effects of the drugs. The United States exports significant quantities of herbs to Europe. Few pharmacy schools in the United States offer courses in botanical remedies.

In 1992, Congress instructed the National Institutes of Health to develop an Office of Alternative Medicine to support studies of alternative therapies. This office is now called the National Center for Complementary and Alternative Medicine (NCCAM). NCCAM lists current clinical trials with herbal products *(www. nccam.nih.gov/clinicaltrials)*. The Natural Standard Research Collaboration also reviews global literature on herbal studies by clinicians and researchers. A reported caution is that many studies were conducted on a small number of women over a limited time period.

It is reasonable to expect an associated expense of $350 million to bring a new drug to market. A botanical remedy cannot be patented; thus manufacturers generally cannot justify this expense in an already booming conventional medicine economy.

This chapter describes selected aspects of herbal therapy including (1) herbal monographs, (2) the Dietary Supplement Health and Education Act of 1994, (3) varieties of herbal preparations, (4) the most commonly used herbs, (5) herbs used to treat selected common ailments, (6) potential hazards of herbs, (7) tips for consumers and health care providers, and (8) herbal resources.

Herbal Monographs

The two primary types of **herbal monographs** are therapeutic and qualitative. Therapeutic monographs contain information on use, dosage, side effects, and contraindications. Qualitative monographs have information on areas such as compliance with compounding guidelines and standards of purity. Integrating herbs into the American health care system requires both types of monographs, which the United States currently does not have.

Work to develop these monographs is in progress by several organizations including the United States Pharmacopeia (USP), World Health Organization (WHO), American Herbal Pharmacopeia (AHP), European Scientific Cooperative of Phytomedicines (ESCOP), and German Commission E.

The American Botanical Council has translated the German Commission E monographs into English in an effort to bring more information to the American public. Much work remains to be done related to the effects of preparations and the improvement of manufacturing and marketing processes.

The German Commission E, an oversight commission in Germany, works to determine the safety of an herbal product with "reasonable certainty." In addition "standardized" is an important feature within herbal products. *Standardization* is movement toward consistency and comparison. A standardized herbal extract has one or multiple ingredients whose levels are guaranteed in the sold product. Examples of standardized herbal products are presented in Table 9-1.

Dietary Supplement Health and Education Act of 1994

The **Dietary Supplement Health and Education Act of 1994 (DSHEA)** clarified marketing regulations for herbal remedies. DSHEA reclassified herbals as "dietary supplements" distinct from food or drugs. Herbal supplements can be marketed with suggested dosages. Consumers are reminded that premarket testing for safety and efficacy is

not required, and manufacturing is not standardized. The physiologic effects of the product can be noted, but no claims can be made about preventing or curing specific conditions. For example, a claim cannot say the agent "prevents heart disease," but it can say that the agent "helps to increase blood flow to the heart." In addition, there is need for a disclaimer that indicates that the herb is not approved by the Food and Drug Administration (FDA) and that it is not meant to be used as a drug.

In January 2000 the FDA finalized rules for claims on dietary supplements noting that supplements may make structure and function claims without FDA approval. However, it may not be claimed that the supplement can prevent, treat, cure, mitigate, or diagnose diseases. This ruling may cause label changes on products but is not expected to affect product availability or consumer access. Health maintenance claims (e.g., "maintain a healthy immune system") and claims for relief of minor symptoms related to life stages (e.g., "alleviates hot flashes") are acceptable because they do not relate to disease. Herbal products using a "may be beneficial" disclaimer rather than claims of definite benefit are appropriate legally. Dietary supplement manufacturers are still required to substantiate any claims they make.

Proposed Standards

The FDA proposed standards for marketing and labeling for dietary supplements in 2003. Known as the **Current Good Manufacturing Practices (CGMPs)**, these standards are multifaceted and require that package labels give quality and strength of all contents and that products be free of contaminants and impurities. Manufacturing quality control procedures are part of the CGMPs.

Herbal Preparations

Herbal remedies are available in a variety of preparations and forms. Examples include fresh aloe, dried ginger, peppermint oil, elderberry syrup, and chamomile tea. Following is a description of selected preparations and forms of herbs including dried kelp extracts, fresh oils, salves, teas, tinctures, syrups, capsules, and tablets. The consumer and health care provider also need to be knowledgeable about the differences in dosages between extracts and powders as well as issues associated with standardization.

Dried herbs are fresh herbs that have had the moisture removed by sun or heat. They can be stored for about 6 months. **Extracts** are made by isolating certain components, resulting in more reliable dosing. Dissolving the herb in a solvent such as alcohol or water is a common way to prepare an extract, which may or may not be standardized. **Fresh herbs** may decay after a few days because of enzyme activity; hence they have a short life. Drying is a means of preservation. **Oils** are made by soaking dried herb in olive or vegetable oil and then heating for an extended time. The vegetable oil promotes the concentration

Table 9-1

Selected Herbal Products with Standardized Concentrations

Herb	Standardized Concentration of Active Ingredient
Bilberry	25% anthanocyanosides
Feverfew	0.2% parthenolide
Ginkgo biloba	24% flavone glycosides; 6% terpene lactones
Goldenseal	8%-12% alkaloid
Hawthorn	20% procyanidins
St. John's wort	0.13%-0.30% hypericin
Saw palmetto	85%-95% fatty acids

of some of the active components, and it may last for months if stored correctly. These infused oils are not "essential oils" (volatile oils extracted from plants that produce an odor and stimulate taste sensations). **Salves,** semisolid fatty preparations, are made by melting a wax in oil and allowing it to cool and harden. If stored correctly, they last for several months as balms, creams, and ointments. **Teas** are made by steeping fresh or dried herbs in boiling water. Tea made from bark and roots is often simmered. It is recommended that only a 2- to 3-day supply be prepared at one time and that it be stored in the refrigerator. Teas may be used as a drink, added to baths, and applied topically in a compress. **Tinctures** are commonly made by soaking fresh or dried herbs in solvent such as water or alcohol. Both water- and fat-soluble components are concentrated in the final form. Alcohol promotes preservation, yielding a shelf life of 1 year. Alcohol-free, glycerin-based tinctures are available for people who do not consume alcohol. **Syrups** are made by adding a sweetener, usually honey or sugar, to the herb and then cooking it. Syrups are used to treat colds, coughs, and sore throats.

Capsules are commonly a powdered form of dried supplement, but they may hold juices or oils. They have a slower effect than liquids because of decreased absorption. They store and travel well. Tablets are similar to capsules; they are a powder compressed with stabilizers and binders.

Commonly Used Herbal Remedies

Most herbal therapies are used for chronic conditions, are unlikely to cause harm, and may provide some relief in selected situations (Figure 9–1). This section discusses some of the more commonly used herbs.

FIGURE 9–1 Commonly used herbal preparations.

Aloe Vera (Aloe barbadensis)

The juice is used externally for treatment of minor burns, insect bites, and sunburn. There has been some success with the treatment of dandruff, oily skin, and psoriasis. Taken internally, aloe vera is a powerful laxative. Menstrual flow is increased with small doses.

Chamomile (Matricaria recutita)

Dried flower heads of *Matricaria recutita* are ingredients of a popular tea for relief of digestive and gastrointestinal (GI) complaints. Chamomile tea's antispasmodic and antiinflammatory effects on the GI tract make it useful for relief of irritable bowel syndrome and infant colic. In addition, chamomile may have sedative effects.

Chamomile tea is prepared by steeping one teaspoon of flower heads for 10 to 15 minutes in boiling water; suggested use is three to four times per day. An extremely rare allergic reaction of urticaria and bronchoconstriction may occur in an individual allergic to daisy or ragweed-type plants. Pharmacokinetics and pharmacodynamics are not known.

Dong Quai (Angelica sinensis)

Dong quai, an all-purpose woman's tonic herb, has long been popular in China and Japan for the treatment of menstrual cramps and to regulate the menstrual cycle. This herb has not been well studied, and preparations are frequently mixed with fillers. Dong quai contains vitamin B_{12}, which may promote manufacture of blood cells. Rare side effects include fever and excessive menstrual bleeding. Pharmacokinetics and pharmacodynamics are not known. The recommendation is to avoid the use of this herb.

Echinacea (Echinacea angustifolia)

Echinacea, a popular supplement, is used as an immune enhancer; it acts by furthering phagocytosis by means of increasing leukocytes and spleen cells and activating granulocytes. In addition, echinacea inhibits hyaluronidase activity and increases the release of tumor necrosis factor. The leaf preparation is given for respiratory and urinary tract infections. The root extract is used to treat flulike symptoms. German Commission E recommends that echinacea preparations be avoided by persons with autoimmune diseases and those with abnormal T-cell functioning (e.g., human immunodeficiency virus [HIV], acquired immunodeficiency syndrome [AIDS], tuberculosis). Echinacea is used by Native Americans to treat snakebites and has many other uses.

Echinacea should be purchased only from reliable sources. There are many reports of fraudulent substitution with other plants and varying potency. Recommendations for duration of treatment are inconsistent. German Commission E recommends use of echinacea up to 8 weeks; others recommend a week's "drug holiday" (i.e., not taking the preparation for a specific time period) before continuing therapy. Pharmacokinetics is unknown. Immunosuppression may occur after extended therapy.

Feverfew (Chrysanthemum parthenium)

The plant compound parthenolide is believed to inhibit platelet aggregation and act as a serotonin antagonist in mediating vascular headaches. Feverfew is popular for the relief of migraine headaches and their accompanying nausea and vomiting.

Only standardized extracts should be used. Wide variation in the amount of active compound in plants and commercial capsules is a potential dosing problem. Pharmacokinetics and pharmacodynamics are not known.

Garlic (Allium sativum)

Garlic, frequently called the "herb of endurance," is reported to lower cholesterol and triglyceride levels, decrease blood pressure, and reduce the clotting capability of blood. It also acts as an antibiotic to treat infections and wounds both internally and externally. Warm garlic oil is used in the ear for treatment of earache. Garlic may be used for some types of heavy-metal poisoning. Pharmacokinetics and pharmacodynamics are not known.

Ginger (Zingiber officinale)

Ginger boosts the immune system. It is used to treat migraine headache, stomach problems, and digestive disorders, including motion sickness. Long-time use for relief from nausea is validated by modern research. In addition, it may provide relief from pain, swelling, and stiffness of both osteoarthritis and rheumatoid arthritis (dosage is 500 to 4000 mg daily). Pharmacokinetics and pharmacodynamics are limited. Metabolites are excreted via urine within 24 hours, and it is 90% protein-bound.

Ginkgo (Ginkgo biloba)

Ginkgo biloba, extract of one of the oldest plant species, is the most commonly prescribed herbal remedy worldwide. When it crosses the blood-brain barrier, ginkgo has central nervous system (CNS) effects, increasing both cerebral arterial dilation and uptake of oxygen and glucose. It assists cells during periods of hypoxia (e.g., during transient ischemic attacks) and decreases free-radical damage to neurons. In addition, there is inhibition of platelet adhesion and degranulation. German Commission E monograph #55 lists the use of ginkgo for dementia syndromes, intermittent claudication, vertigo, and tinnitus when these symptoms are secondary to diminished blood flow. There is some evidence that ginkgo improves cognition and may be helpful in Alzheimer's disease, early stroke, and Raynaud's phenomenon.

Ginkgo biloba is generally given as 120 to 240 mg daily in two to three divided doses for up to 90 days. Rare side effects include headache and GI disturbances. Limited information is available on pharmacokinetics and pharmacodynamics. Bioavailability is not affected by food; urinary excretion is less than 30% metabolites.

Ginseng (Panax ginseng)

Preparations of ginseng are taken for short-term relief of stress, to boost energy, and to give digestive support. Ginseng tends to support the immune system and assist in the prevention of chronic infections. Red Korean or Chinese ginseng may be overstimulating in chronic inflammatory conditions such as arthritis. Pharmacokinetics and pharmacodynamics are not known.

Goldenseal (Hydrastis canadensis)

Goldenseal is frequently used with echinacea to ward off infection and promote wound healing. Common uses include treatment of GI ulcers, mouth ulcers, bladder infection, and postpartum hemorrhage. It is used to treat congestion associated with the common cold. In addition, it is used as a tonic and astringent. Active ingredients are deactivated in the stomach. Goldenseal is expensive and scarce; thus it is frequently adulterated with fillers. Its ability to stimulate the immune system has been questioned, and it can be toxic if overused. Pharmacokinetics and pharmacodynamics are not known.

Kava (Piper methysticum)

Kava has practical and ceremonial roles in the Pacific Island cultures. The root promotes sleep and muscle relaxation and is an antiepileptic, antidepressant, and antipsychotic; it also promotes wound healing. Tea can help with urinary tract infections. Kava may be used in combination with other herbs, such as valerian and St. John's wort, for relaxation. Kava may cross the placenta and be present in breast milk. Little is known about its pharmacokinetics and pharmacodynamics.

Licorice (Glycyrrhiza glabra)

Licorice may have physiologic effects similar to aldosterone and corticosteroids related to glycyrrhizin, a major ingredient. Licorice may help with chronic fatigue syndrome. The deglycyrrhizinated form is used to treat ulcers. It relieves heartburn and indigestion by decreasing stomach acid; it also has a laxative effect. Side effects from excessive use of licorice include increased blood pressure, headache, lethargy, water retention, increased potassium excretion, and, rarely, heart failure. Licorice root is considered safe in dosages of 5 to 15 mg when taken as tea. Its recommended use is limited to 6 weeks. Pharmacokinetics and pharmacodynamics are not known.

Milk Thistle (Silybum marianum)

This herbal extract has the remarkable ability to prevent damage to liver cells and stimulate regeneration of liver cells. Milk thistle is widely used in Europe to treat hepatitis, cirrhosis, and fatty liver associated with drugs and alcohol. Pharmacokinetics and pharmacodynamics are not known.

Peppermint (Mentha piperita)

Peppermint stimulates appetite and aids in digestion when taken internally. The digestive tract is protected by the tannins, and peppermint is used in treatment of bowel disorders. Hot peppermint tea stimulates circulation, reduces fever, clears congestion, and helps restore energy. Peppermint oil is an effective treatment for tension headache when rubbed on the forehead. In research in Germany, peppermint has been shown to be comparable with acetaminophen (extra-strength Tylenol) in relieving headache. Pharmacokinetics and pharmacodynamics are not known.

St. John's Wort (Hypericum perforatum)

Current research suggests St. John's wort is not effective when used by individuals with moderate to severe depression. Botanical experts indicate it is to be used for mild depression. St. John's wort has at least 10 pharmacologically active components. The compound used for standardization is hypericin. Researchers recommend that prospective trials be conducted to compare St. John's wort with standard antidepressant medication and to identify dosages, effectiveness in different stages of depression, and implications of long-term use. St. John's wort has been nicknamed "herbal Prozac" because of its great popularity in the United States and its use as a "tonic" for the nervous system. St. John's wort is used in combination with yarrow to treat enuresis. When taken concomitantly with a prescription antidepressant, an adverse effect of St. John's wort may be suicidal ideations. This herbal remedy is considered a dietary supplement in the United States and has not been FDA approved. In Germany it is licensed for relief of anxiety, depression, and insomnia. The 1984 German Commission E monograph on hypericin indicated the agent was an experimental monoamine oxidase (MAO) inhibitor for use in depression, anxiety, and psychogenic disturbances. The mechanism of action is unknown.

The usual dose of St. John's wort is 300 mg t.i.d. of extract (standardized to 0.3% hypericin). A tea can be prepared from 1 to 2 teaspoonsful of herb steeped for 10 minutes. One to two cups of tea per day for 4 to 6 weeks is recommended. Users need to apply sunscreen freely when outdoors, although phototoxicity has not been reported in humans. Users of St. John's wort do not need to avoid tyramine-rich foods. St. John's wort crosses blood-brain and placental barriers and may enter breast milk. Minimal information is known about the pharmacokinetics and pharmacodynamics.

Saw Palmetto (Serenoa repens)

Double-blind studies indicate that the herb saw palmetto relieves symptoms of benign prostatic hypertrophy and urinary conditions. Saw palmetto has earned the name "plant catheter." Other indications for this herb include use as an expectorant and treatment for colds, asthma, bronchitis, and thyroid deficiency. The recommended dose is 160 mg of standardized extract twice a day. Pharmacokinetics and pharmacodynamics are not known.

Valerian (Valeriana officinalis)

Valerian, a mild sedative and sleep-inducing agent, has an effect similar to benzodiazepines. It is popularly known as "herbal Valium." Most researchers report no hangover effect. A "dirty socks" odor is related to the dried plant, resulting in no risk of overdose. Preparations from fresh root are reported to be better relaxants and have a sweet aroma. There have been no reports of habituation and addiction. Drowsiness may occur, as with any relaxant. The dosage depends on the symptoms, such as insomnia and anxiety. To treat insomnia 400 mg of tincture extract or 2.5 to 5 mg of solid extract is recommended at bedtime. For anxiety a tea steeped with 1 teaspoonful of dried herb is taken several times a day. About 5% to 10% of users report a stimulant effect. Pharmacokinetics and pharmacodynamics are not known.

Summary of Commonly Used Herbal Remedies

A summary of the actions/uses, dosage, interactions, and side/adverse effects of selected herbs is given in Table 9–2. Vitamins and elements commonly used in conjunction with herbal therapy are vitamins B_6, A, C, and E; selenium; and zinc. The American Herbal Products Association has categorized herbal products based on "reasonable use" of the herb into four classes. Refer to the note at the end of Table 9–2 for a description of the classes.

Using Herbs to Treat Selected Common Ailments

Herbs often seem helpful for conditions such as cough, sore throat, cuts, and as "cholesterol chasers." For example, oil of eucalyptus is found in many cough medicines. Breathing and respiratory ailments are frequently eased with eucalyptus tea. The effectiveness of the aloe vera plant is known to many; gel from a broken leaf of the potted aloe houseplant can be spread directly on minor cuts and burns to relieve pain. The fresh plant, easily grown in pots or a garden, is superior to commercial preparations. In the case of garlic and onions, lowering cholesterol levels may be the most documented values.

Potential Hazards of Herbs

Both consumers and health care providers need to remember that although herbs are natural substances, they are not necessarily safe. No preparations are safe in all situations, and herbs are no exception. Consumers and health care providers need to be alert to potential hazards with herbal therapy. It is essential that the health care provider get a complete list of all the herbal preparations the client

Text continued on p. 180

Table 9–2

Summary Table of Selected Herbs

Herb	Actions and Uses	Dosage	Interactions/Precautions	Side/Adverse Effects
Common and *botanical* names Class and part used				
Aloe/aloe Vera *Aloe barbadensis* Class 1 Leaf gel Class 2b/2d Dried, juice Class 2d Topical Bladelike leaf	Uses: Internal for constipation; externally to relieve pain and promote healing of burns, wounds, sunburn, psoriasis	Internal: Tincture/ extract: 50-300 mg External: t.i.d. or PRN	Internal use contraindicated if pregnant, lactating, children <12 y Consult with HCP before taking if have ulcerative colitis or Crohn's disease, taking cardiac glycosides, antiarrhythmics, thiazide diuretics, licorice, or corticosteroids Monitoring of electrolytes	Internal: Overdose/ long-term may cause arrhythmias, neuropathies, edemas, albuminuria, hematuria (side effects are rare)
Bilberry *Vaccinium myrtillus L.* Class 4 Extract of dried fruit and leaf	Uses: Fruit may promote healthy vision, increase visual pigment regeneration; decrease diarrhea in children Leaf used for diabetes, arthritis, dermatitis, gout	Fruit extract: 80-160 mg t.i.d. (St: 25% anthocyanosides) Leaf: no information	Avoid with pregnancy, lactation, children No reported significant interaction with fruit Leaf: May decrease blood sugar and triglyceride levels; may increase action of anticoagulants and NSAIDs; monitor for dose adjustments	Leaf: Long-term higher doses (in animals) anemia, icterus, excitation, death
Black cohosh (bugwort, snakeroot, squaw root) *Cimicifuga racemosa* Class 2b/2c Root	Suppresses luteinizing hormone, optimizes estrogen levels Uses: Antispasmodic, astringent, diuretic, vasodilator, PMS, dysmenorrhea, infertility, menopausal symptoms	Cap/tab: 20 mg b.i.d. Tincture: 2-5 mg b.i.d.	Avoid with pregnancy, lactation, children Limit use to 6 mo; no data on long-term use Under supervision of qualified herbalist, increases action of antihypertensives; may alter effects of HRT May decrease iron absorption	Higher doses: dizziness, headache, nausea, change in heart rate
Chamomile (green chamomile) *Matricaria recutita* Class 2b Dried flower tops	Stimulates normal digestion, antiinflammatory, antispasmodic, mild sedative, mild diuretic, mild antibacterial with topical use Uses: Anxiety, insomnia, indigestion, inflammatory skin conditions	Between meals: Cap/tab: 2-3 g t.i.d., Tea: 1-4 c/d Tincture: max: 1 tsp t.i.d.	Avoid if allergic to daisy family (e.g., ragweed, asters, chrysanthemums) May increase effects of sedatives and interfere with action of anticoagulants. H/F, H/H: None known.	None known
Cranberry *Vaccinium macrocarpon Ait.* Class 4 Berries	Prophylaxis (not treatment) of urinary tract infections; to treat kidney stones	Extract: 300-400 mg concentrated juice b.i.d. Cocktail: 300 ml/d commercial cranberry juice	Caution: avoid use with oliguria and anuria. Clients with DM should use sugar-free cranberry juice; lactating clients, children <12 y, and clients with history of oxalate kidney stones limit to 1 L/day. H/D, H/F, H/H: None known	Doses of >3 L/day may produce diarrhea

b.i.d., Twice a day; *c*, cup; *cap*, capsule; *d*, day; *DM*, diabetes mellitus; *HCP*, health care provider; *H/D*, herb-drug interaction; *H/F*, herb-food interaction; *H/H*, herb-herb interaction; *HRT*, hormone replacement therapy; *max*, maximum; *NSAIDs*, nonsteroidal antiinflammatory drugs; *PMS*, premenstrual syndrome; *PRN*, as needed; *St*, standardized to; *tab*, tablet; *t.i.d.*, three times a day; *y*, year.

Continued

Table 9–2

Summary Table of Selected Herbs—cont'd

Herb	Actions and Uses	Dosage	Interactions/Precautions	Side/Adverse Effects
Dong Quai *Angelica Sinensis* Class 2b (root) Roots, rhizomes	Phytoestrogen activity; vasodilation, small muscle relaxation Decreased IgE antibody production Uses: PMS, menopausal symptoms, cardiovascular support	Tea: 1-4 c/d (equivalent 1-2 g dried herb) Tincture: ½-4 ml, Max: 6×/d	AVOID USE OF THIS HERB Avoid use with prescription anticoagulants, history of bleeding disorders, pregnancy, if at risk for breast cancer Herb-Drug Interaction: additive bleeding effect with anticoagulants, aspirin, NSAIDs	Rash and photosensitivity; fever, bleeding
Echinacea (purple coneflower) *E. purpura; E. angustifolia, E. pallida* Class 1 (root/seed) Aerial parts of E. pallida; root of E. pallida and angustifolia	Stimulates immune system; antibacterial, antiviral, antipyretic Antifungal as topical Uses: Prevention and early treatment of colds and flu; recurrent respiratory, ear, and urinary tract infections Topical: Canker sores, fungal infections Investigational use: Stimulate immune system of HIV/AIDS clients.	Tab: 500 mg-1 g t.i.d. Tea: 1-5 c/d Tincture: max: 2 tsp t.i.d.	Short-term use: 2 wk; 8 wk if low dose; may be hepatotoxic if taken continuously Avoid use with immunosuppressants such as corticosteroids (may counteract); persons with chronic systemic disease of immune system (e.g., SLE, HIV, TB, MS) Safety not determined in pregnancy lactation, and in children <2 y	Lozenge/tincture: Temporary numbness or tingling of tongue Cross-sensitivity in clients allergic to daisy family, GI upset, diarrhea
Evening primrose *Oenothera biennis* Class 4 Oil of seed	Natural estrogen promoter Uses: PMS, problems with synthesis of fatty acids, abnormal prostaglandin production, diabetic neuropathies, chronic inflammatory conditions (eczema), overactive immune systems	Take with meals (increases absorption): Oil: PMS: 3-6 g/d for 6 mo, 14 days before menses Inflammatory conditions: 4-8 g/d for 3-4 mo MS: 500 mg/d for 3 wk with exacerbation	Avoid use during pregnancy and lactation May lower seizure threshold if taken with anticonvulsants; anticonvulsant dose may need modification or do not use concurrently. H/F, H/H: None known	GI upset, nausea, headache, rash. Immunosuppression with long-term use
Feverfew *Tanacetum parthenium; chrysanthemum parthenium* Class 2b (whole herb) Leaves, flowering tops	Interferes with platelet aggregation, inhibits release of serotonin from platelets, blocks proinflammatory mediators, digestive relaxant Uses: Prevention and long-term management of migraine headaches; rheumatoid arthritis; menstrual problems; allergies	Cap/tab (at least 2% parthenolide) 125 mg/d; increase to 1-2 g with acute attack	May be 4-6 wk before effect; continuous use for best outcome Cross sensitivity to plants in daisy family Avoid with pregnancy, lactation, with prescription anticoagulants, and in children <2 y Consult HCP before using herb if taking prescription NSAIDs (decreases effectiveness) May interfere with SSRI antidepressants (e.g., Prozac)	Possible gastric distress or mouth sores if using raw leaves; muscle stiffness; may have rebound headache if discontinued abruptly

AIDS, Acquired immunodeficiency syndrome; *GI,* gastrointestinal; *HIV,* human immunodeficiency virus; *mo,* month; *MS,* multiple sclerosis; *SLE,* systemic lupus erythematosus; *SSRI,* selective serotonin reuptake inhibitor; *TB,* tuberculosis; *wk,* week.

Table 9–2

Summary Table of Selected Herbs—cont'd

Herb	Actions and Uses	Dosage	Interactions/Precautions	Side/Adverse Effects
Garlic *Allium sativum* Class 2c Bulb	Detoxifies body and increases immune function; decreases platelet aggregation; increases HDL and decreases cholesterol and triglycerides, broad antimicrobial activity, mild antihypertensive; hypoglycemia Uses: Hypercholesterolemia, mild HTN, colds and flu	Caps (enteric coated): (ED of 5000 mcg of allicin/d in divided doses) Raw garlic clove is best source; minimum: 1/d	Avoid use during pregnancy and lactation (may stimulate labor or cause infant colic) and hypothyroidism Blood pressure may decrease in 30 min and return to baseline in about 2 hr Caution: Use with anticoagulants because of increased fibrinolysis and decreased platelet aggregation; modify antidiabetic doses. H/F: None; H/H: Acidophilus deceases absorption of garlic	Heartburn, flatulence, gastric irritation, decreased RBCs; dizziness, diaphoresis
Ginger *Zingiber officinale* Class 1 (fresh root) Class 2b/2d Dried root Rhizome	Stimulates digestion, increases bile and motility; antispasmodic; decreased platelet aggregation; decreases absorption and increases excretion of cholesterol; antioxidant Uses: Nausea, pregnancy morning sickness (short term, low dose ONLY); motion sickness; gastric protection with NSAIDs	Take with food Cap/tab/tea: 2-4 g in 2-3 divided doses For motion sickness start 2 d to 2 hr before travel Inflammatory joint disease: 4 g in 2-3 divided doses Nausea (pregnancy related): 1 g in divided doses for 1-4 d Tincture: 1.5-3 ml in 8 oz juice q.i.d., PRN	Avoid long-term use with pregnancy, thrombocytopenia (abortifacient in large amounts) Caution: With prescription anticoagulants (additive effect) Consult with HCP before use if have gallstones May increase absorption of all PO medications H/F, H/H: None known	May cause gastric discomfort if not taken with food; anorexia
Ginkgo biloba *Gingko folium* Class 1 (leaf) Leaves	Antioxidant; peripheral vasodilation and increased blood flow to CNS, reduces platelet aggregation Uses: Allergic rhinitis, Alzheimer's disease, anxiety/stress, dementia, Raynaud's disease, tinnitus, vertigo, impotence, poor circulation; altitude sickness	Cap/tab: 120-240 mg/d in 2-3 divided doses (standardized to at least 24% ginkgo flavone glycosides and 6% Terpene lactones) Tincture: 5-10 ml b.i.d., t.i.d. Circulation/memory: 120 mg/d in 2-3 divided doses Alzheimer's dementia, tinnitus: up to 240 mg/d in 2-3 divided doses	Effects seen in 2-3 wk; 12-wk course recommended Avoid use in pregnancy, lactation, children, and with MAOIs Caution: With prescription anticoagulants monitor bleeding and prothrombin times. Extra caution if using ginger, garlic, or feverfew May increase BP if used with thiazide diuretics Discontinue 2 wk before surgery Ginkgo fruit may result in severe rash; seeds are toxic. H/F, H/H: None known	Initially, mild transient headache that usually stops in 2 d; mild gastric distress Toxicity: vomiting, diarrhea, dermitis, irritability

BP, Blood pressure; *CNS*, central nervous system; *ED*, effective dose; *HDL*, high density lipoprotein; *HTN*, hypertension; *MAOIs*, monoamine oxidase inhibitors; *PO*, orally; *RBCs*, red blood cells.

Continued

Table 9–2

Summary Table of Selected Herbs—cont'd

Herb	Actions and Uses	Dosage	Interactions/Precautions	Side/Adverse Effects
Ginseng, eleuthera or Siberian *Eleutherococcus senticosus, Acanthopanax senticosus* Class 2b/2c/2d Root	Supports adrenal glands, enhances energy levels by inhibiting alarm phase SNS response, stimulates RBC production, decreases blood sugar levels, protects from cellular mutation from carcinogens Uses: Cold and flu prevention, adaptation to stress, chronic fatigue syndrome, SLE, HIV, mental fatigue and physical exhaustion, following chemotherapy or radiation treatments, recovery from chronic or long-term illness	Cap/tab: 2-3 g/d in 3-4 divided doses Tea: 1-4 c/d Tincture: 5-20 ml/d in 3-4 divided doses	Take for 6-8 wk; then 1 wk drug holiday, and resume for total of 3 mo Avoid with BP >170/90, pregnancy, lactation, children, bipolar or psychic disorders, DM, may increase or decrease anticoagulants (dependent on species), anticoagulants May increase effects of caffeine and HRT, falsely elevate digoxin levels, interact with antipsychotic drugs. H/F: Overstimulation may occur with caffeinated coffee, cola, and tea. H/H: None	Hypertension, palpitations, occasional diarrhea, possible insomnia if taken at bedtime Ginseng abuse syndrome: Edema, insomnia, hypertonia; may be life threatening
Goldenseal *Hydrastis canadensis* Class 2b Root, rhizome	Stimulates immune system and bile secretion, antipyretic, broad spectrum antibiotic activity Uses: For infection: respiratory, digestive, urinary tract, mucous membranes, cholecystitis, cirrhosis	Cap/tab: 2-4 g/d in divided doses (standardized to 8%-12% alkaloid content)	Avoid with pregnancy, lactation, children, HTN Dosing >5-7 d of higher doses may increase liver enzymes or malabsorption of B vitamins May decrease effect of heparin, anticoagulants, cardiac glycosides; increased effect of antiarrhythmics, antihypertensives, beta-blockers, and CNS depressants Caution: In clients with cardiovascular disease, DM, or glaucoma	In higher doses may be hepatotoxic Toxicity: CNS depression, restlessness, seizures, cardiovascular collapse Endangered plant species
Hawthorn *Crataegus laevigata, C. oxycantha, C. monogyna* Class 1 Ripe fruit, leaves, flowers	Peripheral dilation and increased coronary circulation, improves cardiac oxygenation, antioxidants, mild diuretic, decreases proinflammatory substances Uses: Mild HTN, early HF, stable angina	Cap/tab: 100-900 mg/d in divided doses (standardized to 20% procyanidins) Average/dose: 100-250 mg t.i.d. Tea: 2.5-5 ml t.i.d. Tea: 1 c t.i.d. (4-5 g dried/day)	May need to modify doses of beta blockers, digitalis, and ACE inhibitors Increased effects of digitalis, beta blockage, ACE inhibitors, CNS depressants High doses contraindicated with chronic atrial fibrillation and hypotension from dysfunction of valve: IH/F None known; H/H increases action of Lily of the Valley	Hypotension, fatigue Sedation, nausea, vomiting, anorexia

ACE, Angiotensin-converting enzyme; *HF,* heart failure; *SNS,* sympathetic nervous system.

Table 9–2

Summary Table of Selected Herbs—cont'd

Herb	Actions and Uses	Dosage	Interactions/Precautions	Side/Adverse Effects
Kava *Piper methysticum* Class 2b/2c/2d Dried rhizome, roots	CNS sedation without loss of mental acuity or memory Uses: Anxiety, insomnia, skeletal muscle spasm Good with psychotic disorders, no risk of tolerance	Cap/tab: Anxiety: 50-100 mg up to t.i.d. Insomnia: 180-210 mg at bedtime (standardized to 70% kavalactones) Max: 300 g/wk	Avoid with pregnancy, lactation, parkinsonism, and if taking levodopa; not for young children Avoid alcohol use and if need to be alert or operate machinery Increases CNS sedating drugs, especially benzodiazepines Fat soluble, so may have delayed effects. H/F increased absorption when taken with food; H/H: None known Unstable gait, numb tongue, mild GI upset	Leaf: Long-term higher doses (in animals) anemia, icterus, excitation, death High doses may cause loss of balance, pulmonary hypertension May cause liver toxicity Banned in several European countries Use >3 mo may turn skin yellow: discontinue drug HTN, headache, weakness
Licorice *Glycyrrhiza glabra* Class 2b/2c/2d (root) Root, leaf	Antiinflammatory, antibacterial, antiviral, hepato and gastric protective, antidepressant, estrogenic, laxative Uses: Viral infection, upper respiratory infection, inflammation, Addison's disease, depression, ulcers Topically: Herpes, psoriasis, eczema DCL: IBS, mouth ulcers	Cap/tab: 200-600 mg glycyrrhizin in 3 divided doses; max: 4-6 wk Tea: 3 c/d (equivalent to 1-2 g/d) Tincture: 2.5-5 ml t.i.d. DGL: 300-380 mg; max: 1200 mg/d in chewable form 20 min before meals for 8-16 wk	Avoid with pregnancy, lactation, children, HTN, kidney or liver disorders, or if at risk for hypokalemia Caution with DM Increased aldosterone effect with increasing dose and duration Antagonizes antihypertensive meds and spirolactone Potentiates corticosteroids and digitalis. H/F none known; H/H may cause hypokalemia with aloe	Doses >5000 mg/d results in aldosterone-like syndrome that reverses when herb discontinued
Milk thistle (Mary thistle wild artichoke) *Silybum marianum* Class 1 Seeds of dried flowers	Increased regeneration of liver cells; increases antioxidant activity Uses: Liver disease (hepatitis), cholecystitis, psoriasis	Cap/tab: Initially: 500 mg/d in 3 divided doses for 6-8 wk With improvement: 120-240 mg/d in divided doses; may take 7-10 d for effect; 4-8 wk if liver diseased with alcohol Tincture: 1 ml t.i.d. (avoid ETOH-based tinctures)	Avoid use in pregnancy, lactation, in children, with drugs metabolized by P-450 enzyme Herb does not reverse cirrhotic liver changes but disease may be slowed with increased quality of life. H/F, H/H: None known	Diarrhea first days of therapy, nausea, vomiting, menstrual changes
Peppermint *Mentha piperita, var. officinalis or vulgaris* Class 4 Aerial parts	Antispasmodic, increase bile flow, carminative, external analgesic Uses: IBS, indigestion, cholecystitis, infant colic, nasal decongestant Topically: Musculoskeletal pain, itching, colds	Cap/tab: enteric coated: 1-2 t.i.d. between meals Tea: 2-3 c/d (equivalent 3-6 g dried herb) Tincture/oil: 6-12 gtts/d diluted in divided doses	Consult HCP before taking if have cholecystitis or obstructed bile duct No known drug interactions; may interfere with iron absorption	None known

DCL, Deglycyrrhizinated licorice; *Eq*, equivalent to; *ETOH*, alcohol; *IBS*, irritable bowel syndrome.

Continued

Table 9–2

Summary Table of Selected Herbs—cont'd

Herb	Actions and Uses	Dosage	Interactions/Precautions	Side/Adverse Effects
Psyllium *Plantago psyllium* Class 4	Uses: Laxative, treatment of hemorrhoids, colitis, Crohn's disease, IBS Herb of longevity, poultice: wound healing effects	½ t soaked in water for 15-60 min at bedtime with at least 8 oz water PO extract: 1-4 ml t.i.d.	Major ingredient in Metamucil May decrease lithium absorption Avoid use during pregnancy, lactation, in children	None known
Sage *Salvia officinalis* Class 2b/2d (leaf) Whole plant	Gargle tea for sore throat, dries up mother's milk, decreases hot flashes Antidepressant and antiviral activity	Take with food Cap/tab: (standardized to at least 0.1% hypericin) 300 mg t.i.d.	Limit use to 2 wk to avoid toxic effects of tannins Caution clients with DM and seizure disorders	Nausea, vomiting, anorexia, oral irritation
St. John's wort *Hypericum perforatum* Class 2d Flowers	Uses: Mood swings, mild to moderate depression, anxiety, sleep disorders Topically: Burns/wounds	Tea: 1-2 c/d for 4-6 wk Tincture: 1-2 ml t.i.d.	Long-term use recommended; effects seen in 4-8 wk Avoid with pregnancy, lactation, prescription antidepressants, MAOIs, indinavir, children <2 y May decrease effect of digoxin related to bioavailability Monitor serum digoxin levels Use with amphetamines, trazodone, tricyclics may cause serotonin syndrome Interferes with absorption of iron and other minerals; high doses may increase liver enzymes	Skin photosensitivity, headache, occasional GI upset, dry mouth, dizziness, confusion
Saw palmetto *Serenoa repens, Sabal serrulata* Class 4 Berries	Decreases size of prostate; increases breakdown of estrogen, progesterone, and prolactin: antiandrogenic Diuretic Uses: BPH, chronic cystitis; sexual potency	Cap/tab: 230 mg/d in 1-2 doses (standardized to 85%-95% fatty acids) Tea: 1 c t.i.d. (equivalent dose 1-2 g/d) Liquid extract: 5-6 ml daily	Recommend 45-90 d of treatment; effects seen after 30 d. If effective, may take long term Avoid in pregnancy, lactation, in children, in clients with breast cancer Effectiveness of prophylactic treatment not shown May interfere with PSA test; discontinue herb 1-2 wk before test May increase or decrease effects of antiinflammatories and immunostimulants; may antagonize hormone therapy	Headache, dysuria, back pain Gastric disturbance (rare)

BPH, Benign prostatic hypertrophy.

takes, the reason they are taken, and their perceived effectiveness. This assessment needs to be updated regularly along with information on clients' prescription and over-the-counter (OTC) drug use.

Clients may choose not to disclose use of herbal products to health care providers for a variety of reasons, including the sense that the health care provider is biased against and not knowledgeable about herbal products and that these products are not considered medications.

Contamination is one area of concern, most likely resulting from lack of standards in manufacture and regulation of herbs. It is the responsibility of consumers to educate themselves about herbs before use and to purchase products only from reputable dealers. Determination of the purity and concentration of a particular product can be done only through assays, a costly process; thus most products have not had appropriate human toxicologic analysis.

Table 9–2

Summary Table of Selected Herbs—cont'd

Herb	Actions and Uses	Dosage	Interactions/Precautions	Side/Adverse Effects
Valerian *Valeriana officinalis* Class 1 Root	Sedative/hypnotic, antispasmodic, increases deep sleep Uses: Insomnia, stress headaches, mild anxiety, muscle cramps and spasms	Cap/tab: (standardized to 0.5% essential oils, equivalent to 2-3 g up to b.i.d.) Tea: 1-3 c/d or at bedtime Tincture: 1-3 ml; may repeat 2-3 × over 6 h	Effects may take several doses For long-term use; monitor liver function if elevated, discontinue herb Avoid in pregnancy, lactation, children, with prescription sedative/hypnotics, MAOIs, anticoagulants Increased sedative effect with barbiturates; negates effects of phenytoin Foul smell; no dependence or tolerance	Anxiety, headache, occasional GI upset and hang-over effect with high doses, CNS depression

MAOIs, Monoamine oxidase inhibitors.
Note: The American Herbal Products Association (described in the Botanical Safety Handbook) has categorized herbal products based on "reasonable use" of the herb into the following four classes:
Class 1
Herbs that can be safely consumed when used appropriately
Class 2
Herbs for which the following use restrictions apply unless otherwise directed by an expert qualified in the use of the described substance:
2a: For external use only
2b: Not to be used during pregnancy
2c: Not to be used while nursing
2d: Other specific use restrictions as noted
Class 3
Herbs for which significant data exist to recommend the following labeling: "To be used only under the supervision of an expert qualified in the appropriate use of this substance." Labeling must include proper use information as follows: Dosage, contraindications, potential adverse effects and drug interactions, and any other relevant information related to safe use of the substance
Class 4
Herbs for which insufficient data are available for classification

Interaction with conventional drugs is another area in which health care providers should be alert. For example, an additive effect of digoxin can result from the use of the laxative herbs cascara and senna. Also, elevation of the blood level of lithium may result from juniper, dandelion, and other herbs with diuretic properties. Clients at high risk for interactions include the elderly and those taking three or more drugs for chronic conditions. Refer to Table 9–3 for selected herbal ingredients and drug interactions.

Herbal products can also impact laboratory test results. One significant interaction is the effect of herbal products on blood coagulation as measured by the International Normalized Ratio (INR) system. Examples of herbs that that may decrease INR include St. John's wort, yarrow, and green tea (dose dependent). Herbs that may increase INR include bilberry, black cohosh, chamomile, dong quai, feverfew, garlic, kava kava, and milk thistle.

Not all compounds are safe via all routes. For example, comfrey *(Symphytum officinale)* has both internal and external preparations. Internal use is discouraged because hepatic damage may be fatal. For external use, comfrey is used as an ointment for relief of swelling associated with abrasions and sprains.

In 1997 the FDA proposed controls on dietary supplements containing ephedra, also known as *ma huang*, which is used for weight loss and to boost energy. Use of this supplement has markedly declined since reports of adverse effects came to light (e.g., palpitations, stroke). Ephedrine and pseudoephedrine, components of ephedra, have stimulant and bronchodilation effects. Ephedra is currently banned from the market (Herbal Alert 9–2).

All the herbal products listed in Herbal Alert 9–3 have significance for clients facing surgery. Many products may interfere with the absorption, breakdown, and excretion of anesthetics, anticoagulants, and other surgery-related medications. For example, valerian may increase or prolong the sedative effects of anesthetic agents. Echinacea and St. John's wort have the potential of immunosuppression required for transplant surgeries. Consult the health care provider about the length of herb-free "washout" before surgery. Guidelines reflective of the complexities of surgery related to herbal products are needed.

Herbal product advocates have petitioned the FDA to reconsider herbal dietary supplement classification and change to a drug model consistent with European herbal regulation. The FDA is currently formulating rules that set

Table 9–3

Selected Herb-Drug Interactions*

Herbal Ingredient Common Name (Botanical Name)	Documented Drug Interaction	Comment	Potential Drug Interaction	Comment
Alfalfa *(Medicago sativa)*	—	—	Anticoagulants	⇓ Drug effect
			Oral contraceptives	⇓ Drug effect
Aloe *(Aloe vera)*	—	—	Antidiabetics	⇑ Drug effect
			Antiplatelets	⇑ Drug effect
			digoxin	⇑ Drug effect
			Diuretics	⇑ Hypokalemia
Angelica root *(Angelica sp)*	—	—	warfarin	⇑ Drug effect
Arnica flower *(Arnica montana)*	—	—	warfarin	⇑ Drug effect
Astragalus *(Astragalus membranaceus)*	—	—	cyclophosphamide	⇓ Drug effect
Betel nut *(Areca catechu)*	fluphenazine	⇑ Drug toxicity	—	—
Bilberry *(Vaccinium myrtillus)*	—	—	Anticoagulants	⇑ Drug effect
			Antidiabetics	⇑ Drug effect
Black cohosh *(Cimicifuga racemosa)*	—	—	Antihypertensives	⇑ Drug effect
			digoxin	⇑ Drug absorption
			Iron salts	⇓ Drug absorption
Bladderwrack *(Fucus vesiculosus)*	—	—	lithium	⇑ Drug effect
			thyroxine	⇑ Drug effect
Boldo *(Peumus boldus)*	warfarin	⇑ Drug effect	—	—
Cascara *(Rhamnus purshiana)*	—	—	Corticosteroids	⇑ Hypokalemia
			digoxin	⇑ Drug effect
Cat's claw *(Uncaria tomentosa)*	—	—	cyclosporine	⇑ Drug effect
			Protease inhibitors	⇑ Drug effect
Cayenne *(Capsicum annuum)*	theophylline	⇑ Drug absorption	Antiplatelets	⇑ Drug effect
Chamomile *(Matricaria chamomilla)*	—	—	Sedatives	⇑ Drug effect
	simvastatin			⇑ Drug effect
	warfarin			⇑ Drug effect
Chasteberry *(Vitex agnus-castus)*	—	—	Prolactin inhibitors	⇑ Drug effect
Cocoa *(Theobroma cacao)*	—	—	Antidiabetics	⇓ Drug effect
Cranberry *(Vaccinium macrocarpon)*	—	—	warfarin	⇑ Drug effect
Dandelion *(Taraxacum officinale)*	—	—	Antidiabetics	⇑ Drug effect
			Diuretics	⇑ Drug effect
			lithium	⇑ Drug levels
Danshen *(Salvia bowelyana; Saliva miltorrhiza)*	warfarin	⇑ Drug effect	Antiplatelets	⇑ Drug effect
Devil's claw *(Harpago-phytum procumbens)*	warfarin	⇑ Drug effect	Antiplatelets	⇑ Drug effect
Dong quai *(Angelica sinensis)*	warfarin	⇑ Drug effect	Antiplatelets	⇑ Drug effect
Echinacea *(Echinacea spp.)*	—	—	Immunomodulators	Altered drug effect
			Protease inhibitors	⇑ Drug effect
Elder *(Sambucus nigra)*	—	—	Antidiabetics	⇑ Drug effect
Evening primrose *(Oenothera biennis)*	—	—	Anticoagulants	⇑ Drug effect
			Antiplatelets	⇑ Drug effect
			phenothiazines	⇑ Seizure risk
Fennel *(Foeniculum vulgare)*	—	—	fluoroquinolones	⇓ Drug absorption
Fenugreek *(Trigonella sp.)*	warfarin	⇑ Drug effect	Iron	⇓ Drug absorption
Feverfew *(Tanacetum parthenium)*	—	—	Antiplatelets	⇑ Drug effect
Flaxseed *(Linum usitatissium)*	—	—	warfarin	⇑ Drug effect
Garcinia *(Garcinia cambogia)*	—	—	warfarin	⇓ Drug effect
Garlic *(Allium sativum)*	Protease inhibitors	⇓ Drug levels	Anticoagulants	⇑ Drug effect
	warfarin	⇑ Drug effect	Antidiabetics	⇑ Drug effect
			Antiplatelets	⇑ Drug effect
			cyclosporine	⇑ Drug effect
			Non-nucleoside RTIs	⇑ Drug effect
Ginger *(Zingiber officinale)*	phenprocoumon	⇑ Bleeding risk	Anticoagulants	⇑ Drug effect
			Antiplatelets	⇑ Drug effect
Ginkgo *(Ginkgo biloba)*	trazodone	⇑ Drug effect	Anticoagulants	⇑ Drug effect
	Antiplatelet agents	⇑ Bleeding risk	Antiepileptics	⇓ Drug effect
	nifedipine	⇑ Drug effect	cyclosporine	⇓ Drug absorption
	omeprazole	⇑ Drug effect	Ca^{++} channel blockers	⇓ Drug effect
			MAO inhibitors	⇑ Drug effect

*Updated information in this table provided by Joseph I. Boullata, PharmD, BCNSP.

Table 9–3

Selected Herb-Drug Interactions—cont'd

Herbal Ingredient Common Name (Botanical Name)	Documented Drug Interaction	Comment	Potential Drug Interaction	Comment
Ginseng (Panax ginseng, Panax quin-quefolia)	warfarin phenelzine	⇓ Drug effect ⇑ Drug effect	Anticoagulants Antidiabetics Antiplatelets Immunomodulators MAO inhibitors	Altered drug effect ⇑ Drug effect Altered drug effect Altered drug effect ⇑ Drug effect
Goldenseal (Hydrastis canadensis)	—	—	Anticoagulants Antihypertensives Immunomodulators	⇓ Drug effect ⇓ Drug effect Altered drug effect
Green tea (Camellia sinensis)	warfarin	⇓ Drug effect	—	—
Guggul (Commiphora mukul)	—	—	Anticoagulants Antiplatelets diltiazem	⇑ Drug effect ⇑ Drug effect ⇓ Drug effect
Hawthorn (Crataegus laevigata)	—	—	CNS depressants Antiarrhythmics digoxin	⇑ Drug effect Altered drug effect ⇑ Drug effect
Hibiscus (Hibiscus sabdarifa)	—	—	chloroquine	⇓ Drug absorption
Juniper (Juniperus communis)	—	—	Antidiabetics Diuretics lithium	⇓ Drug effect ⇑ Drug effect ⇑ Drug levels
Kava (Piper methysticum)	alprazolam levodopa	⇑ Drug effect ⇓ Drug effect	Antiepileptics CNS depressants	⇑ Drug effect ⇑ Drug effect
Lemon balm (Melissa officinalis)	—	—	CNS depressants	⇑ Drug effect
Licorice (Glycyrrhiza glabra)	spironolactone	⇓ Drug effect	Antihypertensives Antiplatelets Corticosteroids digoxin Diuretics warfarin	⇓ Drug effect ⇑ Drug effect ⇑ Drug effect ⇑ Drug effect ⇑ Hypokalemia ⇑ Drug effect
Meadowsweet (Filipendula ulmaria)	—	—		
Milk thistle (Silybum marianum)	indinavir	⇓ Drug concentration	CYP3A substrate	Altered drug effect
Oleander (Nerium oleander)	—	—	digoxin	⇑ Drug effect
Papaya (Carica papaya)	warfarin	⇑ Drug effect	—	—
Passionflower (Passiflora incarnate)	—	—	Antiepileptics CNS depressants warfarin	⇑ Drug effect ⇑ Drug effect ⇑ Drug effect
Peppermint (Mentha piperita)	—	—	Iron salts	⇓ Drug absorption
Psyllium (Plantago spp.)	Lithium	⇓ Drug absorption	digoxin	⇓ Drug effect
Red clover (Trifolium pretense)	—	—	warfarin	⇑ Drug effect
Rosemary (Rosmarinus officinalis)	—	—	Antidiabetics	⇓ Drug effect
St. John's wort (Hypericum perforatum)	alprazolam amitriptyline cyclosporine digoxin imatinib indinavir irinotecan midazolam nifedipine Oral contraceptives SSRIs simvastatin tacrolimus talinolol theophylline warfarin	⇓ Drug effect ⇓ Drug level & effect ⇓ Drug level & effect ⇓ Drug level & effect ⇓ Drug level ⇓ Drug level & effect ⇓ Drug level ⇓ Drug level ⇓ Drug level ⇓ Drug effect Serotonin syndrome ⇓ Drug level ⇓ Drug level & effect ⇓ Drug level ⇓ Drug level ⇓ Drug effect	amiodarone amsacrine carbamazepine diltiazem etoposide omeprazole Protease inhibitors Triptans verapamil Other CYP3A4 or P-gp substrate	⇓ Drug level & effect ⇓ Drug effect ⇓ Drug level & effect ⇓ Drug level & effect ⇓ Drug effect ⇑ Photosensitivity risk ⇓ Drug level & effect Serotonin syndrome ⇓ Drug level & effect ⇓ Drug level & effect

Continued

Table 9–3

Selected Herb-Drug Interactions—cont'd

Herbal Ingredient Common Name (Botanical Name)	Documented Drug Interaction	Comment	Potential Drug Interaction	Comment
Saw Palmetto (*Serenoa repens*)	—	—	Hormone therapy warfarin	⇓ Drug effect ⇑ Drug effect
Senna (*Cassia senna*)	—	—	Corticosteroids digoxin	⇑ Hypokalemia ⇑ Drug effect
Soy (*Glycine max*)	warfarin	⇓ Drug effect	—	—
Uva ursi (*Arctostaphylos uva ursi*)	—	—	Iron	⇓ Drug absorption
Valerian (*Valeriana officinalis*)	Barbiturates	⇑ Drug effect	Antiepileptics CNS depressants	⇑ Drug effect ⇑ Drug effect
Willow bark (*Salix spp.*)	—	—	warfarin	⇑ Drug effect
Yohimbe (*Pausinystalia yohimbe*)	—	—	Antihypertensives MAO inhibitors	⇓ Drug effect ⇑ Hypertension

Interaction risk will depend on patient age, gender, genotype, and comorbid conditions as well as herb or drug dosage form, composition, quality, and duration of use.

standards for preparing and labeling dietary supplements to enable the consumer to make more informed choices, for example, the appropriate dosage.

Tips for Consumers and Health Care Providers

The following are guidelines about prudent use of herbs:
- Do not take herbs if pregnant or attempting to become pregnant.
- Do not take herbs if nursing.
- Do not give herbs to infants or young children.
- Do not take a large quantity of any one herbal preparation.
- Buy only preparations that have the plant and their quantities listed on the packet; there is no guarantee of safety.
- Contact a health care provider before stopping use of a prescription medication.
- Store herbal remedy in a cool, dry, dark place; dark glass containers are preferred.

Herbal ALERT 9–2

Ephedra

On December 31, 2003, the FDA banned ephedra based on links to heart problems, strokes, and death.

Herbal ALERT 9–3

Anticoagulants

The following commonly used herbal products have been reported to interfere with anticoagulants: bilberry, cat's claw, chamomile (German), dong quai, feverfew, garlic, ginger, ginkgo, and licorice.

- Use only herbs that are bought currently and are fresh.
- Do not delay in seeking care from the health care provider for persisting or severe symptoms.
- Advise against belief in unsubstantiated claims of "miracle cures."

It is essential that both consumers and health care providers become aware of several crucial factors before trying the herbal therapy approach. Alschuler et al (1997) identified these as the following:
- Consumers need to think of herbs as medicines; more is not necessarily better.
- Herbs are not placebos.
- Most herbal remedies are less potent than conventional drugs. However, when prescription and OTC drugs and herbs with similar actions are combined, there is an increased risk of adverse reactions.
- Results from conventional medicine may come faster.
- Safety, efficacy, and dosage are important; thus multiple reliable sources should be consulted.

Labeling of herbal products is an important aspect. The following recommended information should be on the label of herbal products:
- Scientific name of product and parts of the plant used in preparation
- Manufacturer's name and address
- Batch and lot number
- Dates of manufacture and expiration; many products have a short shelf life

Herbal Resources

Multiple herbal resources are available on the Web. Of course, the reader needs to evaluate the website and decide if the information is appropriate. Following are a few examples of the many Internet resources that provide herbal information.

Nursing Process

Herbal Preparations

ASSESSMENT

■ Obtain baseline information about client's use of nonconventional therapeutic agents and all prescription and OTC products used.

■ Determine product name, brand, dosage, frequency, side effects, and client's perception of effectiveness.

■ Identify all prescription and over-the-counter (OTC) medications taken by client; include dosage, frequency, side effects, and perceived effectiveness.

NURSING DIAGNOSES

■ Deficient knowledge about therapeutic regimen related to use of herbal products

PLANNING

Client/family will verbalize understanding of:
■ herbal therapy
■ prescription and OTC medications
■ interaction between herbal therapy and prescription and OTC medications
■ strategies for optimal participation in their therapeutic regimen

NURSING INTERVENTIONS

■ Check client's response to herbal therapy.
■ Monitor client's response to prescription and OTC medications.
■ Consult dietitian and other specialists as necessary.
■ Continue with same brand of herbal therapy; notify health care provider if considering changing brands/preparations.

Client Teaching

General

• Explain rationale for herbal therapy (Herbal Alert 9–1).
• Instruct client to first notify health care provider before substituting herbal product for prescription or OTC medication.
• Encourage client to read labels and heed the recommended information displayed on the label.
• Advise client of portion of plant used in preparation (e.g., flower or root).
• Inform client about optimal storage conditions of the herbal remedy.

Diet

• Teach client about foods that enhance or diminish the action of specific herbs.
• Advise client about foods to avoid, if any, while taking herbs.

Side Effects

• Advise client of potential side effects of herbal therapy.
• Instruct client about symptoms that require prompt reporting to the health care provider.

Self-Administration

• Instruct client about preparation of special remedies (e.g., steeping of specific teas).

Cultural Considerations ❖

• Assess personal beliefs of clients from different cultures.
• Modify communication to meet client/family cultural needs.
• Communicate respect for client/family culture.
• Evaluate effectiveness of cultural competence in interactions.
• Do not criticize folk practices; it deters clients from seeking follow-up care and decreases trust and confidence.
• Inquire about nutritional practices and incorporate harmless or non-conflicting practices into diet.
• Refrain from making prejudicial comments that may inhibit collaboration with folk healers.
• Obtain an interpreter when necessary; try not to rely on family members, who may not fully disclose because of honor or guilt.

EVALUATION

■ Evaluate the effectiveness of herbal remedies for alleviating symptoms.
■ Evaluate client's use of resources.

Organizations

American Botanical Council
P.O. Box 201660
Austin, TX 78720
www.herbalgram.org

NCCAM Clearinghouse provides information on complementary and alternative medicine (CAM) and NCCAM, including publications and searches of federal databases of scientific and medical literature. The Clearinghouse does not provide medical advice, treatment recommendations, or referrals to practitioners.
USA toll-free: 1-888-644-6226
www.nccam.nih.gov
Email: info@nccam.nih.gov

U.S. Food and Drug Administration (FDA)
USA toll-free: 1-888-463-6332
www.fda.gov

Office of Dietary Supplements (ODS), NIH
www.ods.nih.gov
Email: ods@nih.gov

CAM on PubMed: a service of the National Library of Medicine (NLM). PubMed contains publication information and (in most cases) brief summaries of articles from scientific and medical journals.
www.nccam.nih.gov/camonpubmed

The Cochrane Database of Systematic Reviews: a collection of evidence-based reviews produced by the Cochrane Library, an international nonprofit organization. Reviews summarize the results of clinical trials on health care interventions. Not copyrighted; duplication is encouraged.
www.cochrane.org/reviews/

United States Pharmacopeia
12601 Twinbrook Parkway
Rockville, MD 20852
(301) 816-8250
www.usp.org

Research Databases

Herbnet: *www.herbnet.com*
Herb Research Foundation: *www.herbs.org*

Summary

Herbal medicine is the most widely used and oldest form of medicine in the world. Currently there is no pressure from the U.S. government to enforce quality control of herbal products. Buyers need to be informed before purchasing herbal products and should deal only with reputable dealers. It is important for clients to share with the health care provider their use or anticipated use of herbal products so an optimal therapeutic plan can be implemented.

KEY WEBSITES

Herb Research Foundation: <u>www.herbs.org</u>
American Herbal Pharmacopoeia: <u>www.herbal-ahp.org</u>
The Mayo Clinic: <u>www.mayoclinic.com</u>

Critical Thinking Case Study

AB, a 49-year-old female accountant, reports periods of feeling tired that are increasing in frequency and intensity. On her health history she lists "no medications on a regular basis." During the nursing history, you learn that she has been taking ginseng 2 g, b.i.d., ginkgo biloba 300 mg b.i.d., and licorice root 2 mg b.i.d. for the past 6 months. Occasionally she takes 300 mg t.i.d. of St. John's wort extract.

- Is AB taking the recommended dose of ginseng and ginkgo biloba? If not, what modifications would you suggest that she consider?
- AB tells you that she has arthritis. What modifications would be appropriate based on this new information?
- What specific client teaching is appropriate for AB at this time?

NCLEX Study Questions

1. The Dietary Supplement Health and Education Act of 1994 (DHSEA) addressed all the following except:
   a. clarified marketing regulations
   b. reclassified herbs as dietary supplements
   c. herbal products can be marketed with suggested dosages
   d. required that package labels give quality and strength of all contents

2. The nurse discovers that her client has recently decided to take four herbal preparations. The best nursing intervention is:
   a. discuss cost of herbal products
   b. instruct client to inform health care provider of all products taken
   c. suggest client stop taking all herbal products now
   d. suggest client taper off use of products over next 2 weeks

3. Which of the following is an appropriate claim for an herbal product to make?
   a. prevents diabetes
   b. helps increase blood flow to extremities
   c. cures Alzheimer's disease
   d. is safe for all

4. Which of the following herbal products does NOT interfere with the action of anticoagulants?
   a. feverfew and dong quai   c. gingko and licorice
   b. garlic and ginger   d. aloe and cranberry

5. Which is a serotonin antagonist for relief of migraine headache?
   a. valerian   c. milk thistle
   b. feverfew   d. ginkgo

6. Which is the "herb of endurance" reported to decrease cholesterol, triglycerides, blood pressure, and blood clotting capability?
   a. ginger   c. ginseng
   b. ginkgo   d. garlic

7. Which herbal preparation has at least ten pharmacologically active components for relief of depression and anxiety?
   a. St. John's wort   c. saw palmetto
   b. licorice   d. goldenseal

Answers: 1, d; 2, b; 3, b; 4, d; 5, b; 6, d; 7, a.

10
Pediatric Pharmacology
Judith W. Herrman

ELECTRONIC RESOURCES

evolve

Evolve website (http://evolve.elsevier.com/KeeHayes/pharmacology/):
- *Case Studies*
- *Content Updates*
- *Frequently Asked Questions*
- *Student Review Activities*
- *WebLinks*
- *Additional Reference Material*

Companion CD-ROM:
- *NCLEX Examination Review Questions*
- *Pharmacology Animations*
- *IV Therapy Checklists*
- *Medication Error Checklists*
- *Drug Calculation Problems*
- *Electronic Calculators*
- *Top 200 Drugs with Pronunciations*
- *References from the Textbook*

Objectives

- Apply the principles of pharmacokinetics and pharmacodynamics to pediatric medication administration.
- Differentiate components of pharmacology unique to pediatric clients.
- Synthesize knowledge about pediatric medication safety and administration to current or potential nursing practice.

Terms

chronologic age, p. 191
developmental age, p. 191

pharmacodynamics, p. 190

pharmacokinetics, p. 188

A nurse who provides care to children must make certain adaptations in assessments, treatments, and evaluations of nursing care because of the physiologic, psychologic, and developmental differences inherent in this population. This is especially true in the science of pharmacology, both in the administration of medications to children and in the evaluation of the therapeutic and adverse effects of a medication. This chapter addresses pediatric nursing adaptations and discusses the impact a child's growth and development have on the many aspects of pharmacology: pharmacokinetics, pharmacodynamics, dosing and monitoring, methods of medication administration, and nursing implications.

Pharmacology as it relates to the nursing care of infants, children, and adolescents is limited by the research available in providing protocols of recommend dosages, safe practices, key assessments, and important nursing implications. Most information available about medications is concluded from studies that use adult samples, small sample sizes, or samples with healthy children. Few studies have been conducted to determine the effectiveness of medication for target populations of children diagnosed as having applicable illnesses. Generalizing results of adult studies to pediatric populations (as in applying principles of adult pharmacology to dictate pediatric nursing practice) may result in serious errors and

Preventing **MEDICATION ERRORS**

- Because of developmental factors and their smaller body size, infants and young children may receive very small dosages of medications. Careful calculations, double checking math, and checking with another registered nurse may prevent medication errors.

- Ensure families understand the units of measurement for a medication. Confusion may occur with the discussion of metric, household, and other measurement systems.

- For safety when administering injectable medications to children, use the smallest syringe that will ensure the most exact measurement of the medication.

- Make sure the correct medication and procedure are used to ensure safe dosing. Dilutions, different concentrations, and different solutions of a prescribed medication can complicate giving appropriate pediatric dosages.

- Infants and children may not be able to confirm identity, allergies, or medications. This means the nurse must be positive of such information prior to medication administration.

- Nurses must be vigilant for severe side effects or adverse reactions to medication, because information related to pediatric responses to medication is limited.

- According to *Research Activities* (2007), 11 medication classes are associated with one third of the medication errors in hospitalized children: morphine, fentanyl, vancomycin, ceftriaxone, gentamycin, insulin, potassium chloride, total parenteral nutrition (TPN), albuterol, dopamine, and heparin (Agency for Healthcare Quality and Research 2007). Nurses must exercise additional caution with the dosing and administration of these medications.

ignore the impact of growth and development on pharmacology.

Research related to pediatric clients is limited because of several factors. Research risks and obtaining informed consent make it difficult to establish a pediatric sample. Parents and guardians are reluctant to provide consent for children to participate in research studies because of the risk involved and the potentially invasive nature of data gathering. Pharmaceutical companies tend to put fewer resources into pediatric drug research because of the smaller market share afforded to pediatric medications. Many perceive pediatric pharmacologic research as unethical if it involves profit-margin factors. Others contend that the lack of pediatric data reflects a lack of due diligence,

especially when medications are administered to pediatric clients without supporting research data on which to base safe practices. As a result, less is known about the effects, uses, and dosages of pediatric medications, and nurses need to investigate pediatric medications carefully to provide knowledgeable nursing care for children.

Closely aligned with the conflicts that impact pediatric pharmacologic research are those associated with medication labeling and dosing instructions. Because many drugs have not undergone the clinical trials required for federal approval, they have not been approved for pediatric use. Safe use for children may be guided by small studies or the judgment of the clinician and may be based on anecdotal rather than scientific study. These conflicts have generated new legislation designed to protect the pediatric client and provide health care professionals with better information and resources.

In the United States approximately one quarter of all medications carry federally approved indications for use in children, but almost three quarters of drugs marketed for adults are also prescribed for children. As a result of legislation presented in 1992 and 1994, the Food and Drug Administration (FDA) now requires many medications to include known dosages, adverse effects, precautions, and effectiveness to provide health care professionals and the public some level of security when using medications. In 2003 a law known as the *Pediatric Research Equity Act* joined the Best Pharmaceuticals Act of 2002 to require drug manufacturers to study pediatric medication use and offer incentives for pediatric pharmacology research. Current research agendas continue to reinforce the need for pediatric medication research and the establishment of safe guidelines for pediatric medication dosing, administration, and evaluation. Even with increasing data, many drugs are prescribed based on off-label instructions, expert opinions, small clinical trials, or practitioners' personal experiences with the medication.

Pharmacokinetics

Significant differences exist in drug pharmacokinetics when discussing the pediatric population. These distinctions stem from differences in body composition and organ maturity and appear to be more pronounced in neonates and younger infants but less significant in older school-age and adolescent children. **Pharmacokinetics** may be defined as the study of the time course of drug absorption, distribution, metabolism, and excretion.

Absorption

The degree and rate of absorption are based on many factors such as the child's age, health status, and the route of administration. As children grow and develop, the absorption of medications generally becomes more effective; therefore less developed absorption in neonates and infants must be considered in dosage and administration. A contradiction occurs in the adolescent years, during which poor nutritional habits, changes in physical maturity, and hormonal differences may provide for poorer medication absorption. Hydration status, the presence of underlying disease, and gastrointestinal (GI) disorders in the child may be significant factors in the absorption of medications.

Drug absorption is initially influenced by the route of administration. For oral medication, conditions in the stomach and intestine such as gastric acidity, gastric emptying, gastric motility, gastrointestinal (GI) surface area, enzyme levels, and intestinal flora all mediate drug absorption. The lack of maturation of the GI tract is most pronounced in infancy, making the neonatal and infancy periods those most affected by changes in absorption physiology. Gastric pH is alkaline at birth, and acid production begins in the neonatal period. Gastric pH may not reach adult acidity until between 1 and 3 years of age. A low pH or acidic environment favors acidic drug absorption, whereas a high pH or alkaline environment favors basic drug formulations; therefore differences in pH may hinder or enhance the absorption of medications. Gastric emptying is generally prolonged in neonates and infants but increases as the child grows. Nurses should be aware that delayed emptying in children reduces the peak serum concentrations of medications.

Varying transit times through the GI system may also hinder or enhance absorption of oral medications, depending on the usual site of chemical absorption. In line with this issue, feeding methods may impact infant absorption; for example, breastfed infants have longer GI transit times than formula-fed infants. Frequent infant feedings also affect GI transit times. The more frequent the feedings, the less time the food is in contact with the gastric or intestinal lining.

Irregular peristalsis associated with immaturity or with symptoms of vomiting or diarrhea decreases the absorption time available for medications. In contrast, many pediatric medications actually cause diarrhea, which again bears on absorption rates. In younger infants and children, the GI surface area is greater than in adults, allowing for more absorptive area in the stomach and intestines. This difference in pediatric anatomy and physiology may affect the speed and effectiveness of absorption, especially in the small intestine. Immature enzyme function may also effect drug absorption; for example, low lipase levels deter the absorption of lipid-soluble medications. Microorganism colonization of the intestine, as it changes with pH and flora, creates different environments that are available to change medication absorption. All these factors should be considered when assessing the effectiveness of medications administered by the oral route (Figure 10–1).

For medications administered via the subcutaneous (subQ) or intramuscular (IM) routes, absorption occurs at the tissue level. The level of peripheral perfusion and effectiveness of circulation has an effect on the ability of medications to be absorbed. Conditions that alter perfusion (e.g., dehydration, cold temperatures, alterations in

FIGURE 10–1 An important nursing role is assessing effectiveness of medication on each child.

cardiac status) may impede absorption of medications at the tissue level. Intravenous (IV) medications are administered directly into the bloodstream.

Topical medications, or those absorbed through the skin, may be altered by the condition of the skin tissue. Because the skin of children is thinner and more porous, absorption may be enhanced. Because the skin surface area for children is proportionately higher than for adults, many medications are more readily absorbed, and the child may not only have the expected topical effect but also unwanted systemic effects.

Distribution

The distribution of a medication throughout the body of a child is impacted by factors such as body fluid composition, body tissue composition, protein-binding capability, and effectiveness of various barriers to medication transport. In neonates and young infants, the human body is about 70% water. (As the child grows, this percentage decreases to 50% to 60%.) This increased body fluid proportion for weight in the very young allows for a greater volume of fluid in which to distribute medication and a decreasing concentration of the drug. Until about 2 years of age, the pediatric client requires higher doses of water-soluble medications to achieve therapeutic levels. Younger clients also have higher levels of extracellular fluids, which increases the tendency for children to become dehydrated and changes the distribution of water-soluble medications.

Neonates and young infants tend to have less body fat than older children. The difference causes this age group to require less fat-soluble medications relative to adult populations, because fat-soluble drugs saturate fat tissue before acting on body tissues. Less fat available for saturation creates a need for less medication.

Drugs become bound to circulating plasma proteins in the body. Only drugs that are free, or unbound, are available to cross the cell membrane and exert an effect. Infants and neonates have less albumin than older clients and fewer protein receptor sites available for binding with medication. This allows medication to be more available for use and dictates a decrease in the dosage needed in young clients to produce the same therapeutic effect. Greater quantities of circulating drugs caused by reduced plasma proteins increase the propensity for adverse or toxic reactions in infants less than 1 year of age. In neonates, high bilirubin levels may pose a health risk with regard to the administration of medications. Bilirubin molecules may bind with plasma protein sites, making the sites unavailable to medications and allowing large amounts of drug to remain free and available for effect. If neonatal medications are prescribed, dosage needs to be decreased and closely monitored to both ensure therapeutic effectiveness and avoid adverse effects.

Anatomic barriers to medication distribution such as the skin or the blood-brain barrier (BBB) must be considered when drugs are administered to the pediatric client. The skin is more absorptive in young children, as previously described, and provides for rapid distribution of medication. Infants' blood-brain barriers are relatively immature, allowing medications to pass easily into nervous system tissue and increasing the likelihood for toxicity in young infants. As a child matures, both of these barriers become more impervious to medication, and dosages need to be titrated accordingly.

Metabolism

The metabolism of medications depends greatly upon the maturation level of the pediatric client and varies from child to child. Metabolism is carried out primarily in the liver, with the kidneys and lungs playing a small part in the metabolic stage. For most infants, until about 2 years of age, sustained decreases in levels of hepatic enzymes result in slower metabolism of medications. Hepatic metabolic activity is lower in neonates; infant hepatic function matures at 1 to 2 months of age. This issue, as with other pharmacokinetic factors, reinforces the importance for the nurse to evaluate therapeutic effects and monitor adverse effects of medications.

Children inherently have higher metabolic rates than adults, causing metabolism to occur more rapidly. This may necessitate a higher medication requirement than for adults. For example, pain medication for children may require increased dosages or decreased durations between dosages. After oral medications are absorbed, they are subject to metabolism in the liver. This phenomenon, called the *first-pass effect*, provides that drugs administered by the oral route and absorbed via the GI tract undergo some metabolism in the hepatocytes in the liver before they are made available to the body tissues. For select medications, when the oral route is ordered, the first-pass effect must be considered in the calculation of dosages. Some medications are administered by the rectal route to avoid the hepatic first-pass effect.

Excretion

The excretion of medications occurs in the kidneys, intestines, lungs, sweat glands, salivary glands, and mammary glands, with the kidneys providing the most elimination.

Before about 9 months of age, infants experience a reduction in the elimination capacity of the kidneys because of decreases in renal blood flow, decreases in glomerular filtration rate, and reductions in renal tubular function. (At the onset of adolescence, renal tubular function is again decreased.) Because medications are excreted more slowly as a result of this decreased renal function, they can accumulate and may reach toxic levels. Water is needed for the effective excretion of medication, and clients need to be evaluated for dehydration, which could lead to toxic drug levels. Nurses need to carefully monitor renal function, urine flow, and medication effectiveness to evaluate the impact of medication excretion on client status.

Pharmacodynamics

Pharmacodynamics have also been used to describe differences in pediatric pharmacology. **Pharmacodynamics** refers to the mechanisms of action and effect of a drug on the body and includes the onset, peak, and duration of effect of a medication. It can also be described as the intensity and time course of therapeutic and adverse effects of medications. The variables of pharmacokinetics—absorption, distribution, metabolism, and excretion—all affect the parameters of pharmacodynamics. These processes determine the time a medication begins to function, reaches its peak, and sustains its length of action. The half-life of a medication may be different in children than in adults. Pediatric variables such as organ function, developmental implications, and administration issues impact drug pharmacodynamics and require nurses to knowledgeably evaluate the action and effectiveness of pediatric medications.

Nursing Implications
Pediatric Medication Dosing and Monitoring

Because of the changes in pharmacokinetics and pharmacodynamics inherent in pediatric clients, a key nursing role is to monitor the client for therapeutic effect and adverse reactions. The processes described earlier may be measured using plasma or serum drug levels, which indicate the amount of medication in a client's body. Close monitoring of serum drug levels can assist in establishing appropriate dosages, schedules, and routes of administration. Monitoring can also assist in indicating when the dose is too high (toxic) or too low (not therapeutic). The ranges established for many drug levels are based on adult studies, so it is important for the nurse to assess pediatric clients in conjunction with monitoring blood levels. Serum blood levels are not available for all medications because of the lack of methods available to measure medications. As a result, client clinical responses to medication are especially important in the monitoring of drug effects (Figure 10–2).

The calculation of pediatric dosages, as discussed earlier, is based in part on FDA recommendations, approved

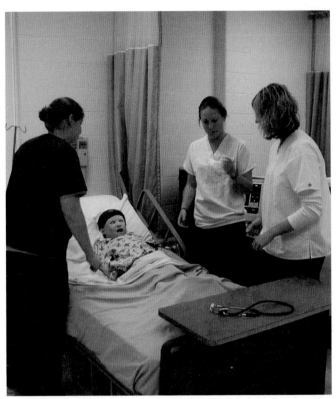

FIGURE 10–2 Nursing laboratory resource centers with pediatric simulators help students learn about the effects of medications on pediatric clients.

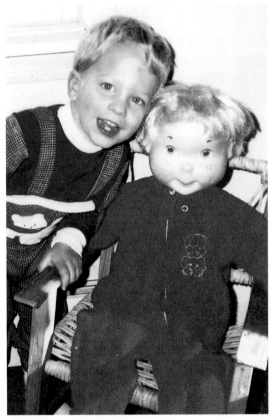

FIGURE 10–3 Many children's medication dosages are calculated based on the child's weight.

protocols, research studies, and provider experience. Most medications are ordered based on the child's weight in kilograms; therefore a "dose per unit of weight" calculation is required. In caring for obese children, there are times when dosages should be calculated on lean body mass to ensure an appropriate dose (Adcock 2006). Some medications such as chemotherapies are prescribed based on body surface area (BSA, or mg/m^2). BSA provides parameters for assessing the distribution, metabolism, and excretion of medications.

When recommended pediatric dosages are not available, medication dose may be extrapolated based on the adult dose. Using a nomogram (see Chapter 4, Section F), the BSA for the child is determined (Figure 10–3). The following equation then may be used to find the pediatric dosage for the child:

$$\text{child's dose} = \text{m}^2 \text{ (body surface area)}/ \\ 1.73 \text{ m}^2 \times \text{adult dose}$$

Although this is not the recommended method to calculate pediatric medication dosages, it can be used when medication ranges based on the child's weight are not easily accessible. BSA calculators have been developed to reduce errors that may occur when using the nomogram. Dosing must also consider the individual child's status, including age, organ function, health, and the route of administration.

Pediatric Medication Administration

A key issue with pediatric medication administration is confirming the identification of the client who is to receive the dose. Using the client's identification wristband in inpatient settings is the most effective method to ensure client identity; outpatient and other settings pose a greater challenge. A child may not be able to communicate or want to divulge their name. To ensure safe medication administration, a reliable method to identify clients for each setting must be created.

Developmental and cognitive differences must always be considered when administering medication to children. It is important for the nurse to differentiate the child's **developmental age** from the **chronologic age,** because this has an impact on the child's response and responsiveness to medication. The pediatric client's ability to understand the process, the reasons for medication, and the need to cooperate with the procedure must always figure prominently in the pediatric nurse's plan of care. The child's temperament may influence understanding and level of cooperation. When possible, family members or caregivers should be solicited to assist in medication administration, taught how to administer the medications, and instructed on methods to evaluate effectiveness. These significant persons in the child's life, individuals who know the child on a day-to-day basis, are usually in the best position to evaluate the effectiveness of a medication and observe for adverse reactions. Some adverse reactions of medication in a child (e.g., ringing in the ears or nausea) may be difficult to evaluate; those closest to the child may be in the best position to assess for these responses. In contrast, parents or other family members may request not to participate in invasive procedures. This request should be respected and the parent or guardian encouraged to provide comfort to the child after medication is administered. Caregivers should always be supported in their caring function so that the child feels safe and secure.

Cognitive issues such as the ability to understand (1) the reason for the medication, (2) the need for the medication despite unpleasant taste or method of administration, and (3) the need to complete all doses and courses of medication must be addressed. When the family is taught about pediatric drug administration, education for the child—at a developmentally appropriate level—must also be included. Communication with the child and family must always consider the level of knowledge, developmental age, cultural factors, and levels of anxiety. The nurse should use optimal interpersonal skills to ensure the best outcome in the administration of medications to pediatric clients.

The primary concerns in administering medications to infants are maintaining safety with the minimum restraint necessary, administering the correct dosage, and providing care with as much comforting as possible. Toddlers may react violently and negatively to medication administration. Simple explanations, a firm approach, and enlisting the imagination of a toddler through play may enhance success with medication administration. Preschoolers are fairly cooperative and respond well to age-appropriate explanations. Allowing some level of choice and control may enlist success with preschool children. School-age children, though cooperative, may fear bodily injury and need to be permitted even more control, involvement in the process, and information. Age-appropriate fears related to pain, changes in body image, and injury are prevalent among older school-age and adolescent clients. The nurse should establish a positive rapport with the client, contract with the adolescent related to the plan of care, and ensure privacy in all aspects of medication administration.

Most pediatric medications are administered via the oral route. This route is the least invasive, the easiest to use, and can be used by family and home caregivers. Topical, rectal, and parenteral routes—subcutaneous (subQ), IM, IV—are also used to deliver medications to pediatric clients for whom the oral route is contraindicated. Because of tissue differences among children, the IV route is more predictable than other routes.

Most oral medications are administered to a child using an oral syringe. Oral syringes ensure more exact dosing of medication and are relatively easy to use. Syringes may be marked to ensure correct dosages. The syringe is inserted into either side of the mouth and pointed toward the buccal mucosa. Depositing the medication too close to the

front of the mouth increases the likelihood that medication will be spit out. Pointing the syringe directly toward the back of the mouth may increase the risk for gagging or choking. Infants may suck medication from a bottle nipple into which the measured medication has been "squirted" from the oral syringe. Gently blowing into a young infant's face may stimulate the natural swallow reflex and facilitate medication administration. Preschool and school-age children are usually able to inject oral medication into their own mouths, enhancing their sense of control over what can be an anxiety-provoking situation.

Nurses may need to crush pills or dissolve capsules in fluid for administration to pediatric clients. It is the nurse's responsibility to access information on the advisability of crushing or dissolving a medication before administration; some medications such as time-release and enteric-coated medications should NOT be crushed or dissolved. Some medications may be made more palatable by adding jelly, syrup, or honey (infants less than 1 year old should not be given honey because of the risk of botulism). Small volumes should be used to dilute medications so that the client is ensured the full dose. As pediatric medication research increases, more medication will be available in stable liquid pediatric forms. Until then, the nurse should work closely with the pharmacist and hospital policies to ensure safe administration of oral medications to children. So that future food aversions are avoided, medications should not be added to infant formula. For children who refuse to take medication by mouth or for children who require tube feeding, oral medications can be administered via nasogastric, orogastric, or gastrostomy tubes. Precautions required when giving medications via this route are similar to those implemented when administering feedings.

The administration of subcutaneous, IM, and IV medications to children includes many of the same principles as adults, with some additional considerations. Safe restraint and atraumatic care principles should be used when possible. Hockenberry (2007) defines *atraumatic care* as the delivery of therapeutic care through the implementation of interventions that "eliminate or minimize the psychologic and physical distress experienced by children and their families in the health care system." Depending on developmental age, the child may have incorrect interpretations about the need for medication, believing that the medication is a punishment or a result of wrongdoing. The nurse should provide preparation for the procedure at the appropriate level for the child and involve caregivers in all aspects of care. One method to ensure atraumatic care is through the use of topical analgesics on the site before IM, subQ, or IV injections. Eutectic mixture of local anesthetics (EMLA), a topical cream, anesthetizes the site of injection if applied 1 to 2.5 hours before injection (Hockenberry 2007; Weise, Nahata 2005). After EMLA is applied to the injection site, the site is covered with a transparent dressing for containment. Also available are iontophoresis (Numby Stuff), a vasocoolant spray, or buffered lidocaine injections (Hockenberry, 2007). Based on the cognitive level of the child, distraction and other nonpharmacologic methods of pain and anxiety control can also be used to decrease the perception of pain. The use of creative imagery and hypnosis with toddlers and preschool children has been explored as a pain-management strategy (Butler et al. 2005). Injections should NEVER be given to a sleeping child with the intent to surprise the child with a quick procedure. The child may subsequently experience a lack of trust and be reluctant to sleep in the future.

IV infusion sites must be protected, especially in infants and toddlers, who do not understand the rationale or importance of maintaining the IV site. The patency of an IV site should be checked before each medication administration to avoid infiltration and extravasation. Any injection site on a preschooler should be covered with a bandage, preferably a decorated one, so that the young child does not fear "leakage" from the area. Selection of injection and IV sites are made based on developmental variables, site of preference, and access to administration sites. IM injections should not be given in the gluteal muscle until children have been ambulating for a full year. The ventrogluteal or the vastus lateralis are the preferred sites for pediatric IM injections (Hockenberry 2007). The length of the needle depends on the child's muscle mass, subQ tissue, and the site of injection. The child may prefer subQ injections in the leg or upper arm rather than in the abdomen. IV sites may be difficult to find in children. Amount of fat tissue, hydration status of the child, and ability to isolate and immobilize veins are all mitigating factors.

When administering medications to children, the basic principles to follow are: honesty, respect, age-appropriate teaching and explanations, attention to safety, atraumatic care, using the least amount of restraint necessary, providing positive reinforcement for age-appropriate cooperation, refraining from use of negative messages or behaviors, and upholding family-centered principles. These standards may be used throughout the pediatric life span and highlight the need for nursing intervention that is sensitive, individualized, and caring.

Nursing Process

In working with pediatric clients, key developmental differences need to be considered when administering and monitoring medications. The nursing process provides the framework to guide nursing practice in administering medications, planning and evaluating nursing care, providing client and family teaching, and incorporating the family into all aspects of treatment.

Teaching is a key component for the family and client. Much of the information the nurse has knowledge of should be passed on to the client and family as well. Issues such as the indications for the medication, the side effects, the dose, how to measure the dose, how to administer the dose, the therapeutic effect of the medication, any adverse effects to be monitored, the duration, and the frequency are all important information needed by the family or caregiver. Specifics such as the need for refrigeration, the need to shake the medicine, the difference between household and prescriptive teaspoons, and other issues should be addressed to ensure client safety. Adherence to the medication regimen is of paramount importance with children and families; providing written instructions or a medication calendar may facilitate this through concrete reminders. Nurses should also be aware of the tendency for parents to liberally treat infants and children with over-the-counter analgesics. One study indicated that one half to two thirds of parents provide frequent analgesia to their children and that parents are largely unaware of the potential for misuse and overuse in the pediatric population (Dlugocz, Chater, Engle 2006).

Considerations for the Adolescent

Nursing care of the adolescent client warrants individualized care specific for this developmental stage. These age-oriented developmental considerations include physical changes, cognitive level and abilities, emotional factors, and the impact of chronic illness.

Physically, adolescence is a highly diverse period of growth and development. Growth rates during the teen years may be affected by nutrition, factors within the environment, genetics and heredity, and gender. A group of adolescents of similar ages may manifest very different sizes, height-to-weight proportions, secondary sex characteristics, and other indicators of physical maturity. These differences may warrant individualization of dosages based on weight or body surface area, even when the adolescent meets or exceeds the size of standard adults. For example, an adjustment may be required in the dosage of a lipid-soluble medication, because changes in lean-to-fat body mass, especially in young adolescent males, coincide with physical maturation. Hormonal changes and growth spurts may necessitate changes in medication dosages; many children with chronic illness require dosage adjustments in the early teen years as a result of these transitions. Sleep requirements and metabolic rates may greatly increase during the teen years, along with appetites and food consumption, which may affect their scheduling of and response to medications. Although adolescents resemble the physical appearance and organ structure and function of adults, their bodies continue to grow and change, requiring increased vigilance in monitoring therapeutic and toxic drug levels.

The cognitive level and abilities of the adolescent may pose even greater challenges to the pediatric nurse. Cognitive theorists have posited that adolescents progress from concrete to abstract reasoning (Hockenberry 2007). Individuals who are still in the concrete operational stage may have difficulty comprehending how a medication exerts its effects on the body and the importance of meticulous dosing and administration. Teens may also have difficulty understanding such concepts as drug interactions, side effects, adverse reactions, and therapeutic levels. For example, the client taking birth control pills may or may not be able to comprehend the potential implications and extra precautions necessary when taking an antagonistic antibiotic during an acute infection. Client teaching must consider the cognitive level of the individual; as adolescents learn to reason in an abstract manner, teaching may be based on more complex information.

The common teen perception of invulnerability and their difficulty in relating future consequences to current actions may dictate that the nurse adapt teaching to address specific adolescent thought processes. The adolescent who is told that an insulin injection schedule must be adhered to in order to avoid long-term complications may not understand the rationales for treatment if they are only substantiated by abstract, future-oriented risks. That same teen may find the relationship between using insulin to maintain normoglycemia and the ability to participate in sports more immediate and relevant. Although teens may physically resemble soon-to-be adults, the nurse must continue to assess clients' cognitive levels as they relate to medications.

Emotional development of the teen also occurs on an individual basis. The teen years are characterized by sensation seeking, risk taking, questioning, formation of identity, and increasing influences exerted by peer groups. The nurse should assess for high-risk behaviors, including use of alcohol, tobacco, and recreational drugs, to avoid potential drug interactions. Other issues including sexual practices, stressful family and social situations, and lifestyle behaviors may impact the client's response to medications. Nurses must be respectful of the emotional needs of adolescence while attending to the mental health issues that may surface during the teen years. A comprehensive history must be solicited from the teen client to ensure appropriate medication administration.

The nurse is often positioned in a key role for establishing a productive working relationship with the client and providing the client with appropriate levels of privacy. Allowing the adolescent to verbalize concerns about the medication and regimen may offer opportunities for clarifying misconceptions and learning new concepts. The nurse must also be conscious of the need to exercise care in offering confidentiality in the event that information needs to be divulged to other health care providers, parents, or caregivers to ensure client safety.

As adolescents attain greater levels of independence from their parents, self-care can be increased. The nurse should assess the teen's abilities to self-administer medication and self-monitor therapeutic and adverse reactions. Teens who spend less time with parents and caregivers may need increased instruction about their medication regimen and the key observations that are needed. Although during the teen years young people frequently display "breaking away" behaviors in response to parental bonds, teens often continue to use parent or caregiver medication habits as role models for their own medication behaviors.

For the child with chronic illness, issues may change throughout the teen years. Engaging peers in the medica-

tion plan of care, allowing the teen to have safe choices and flexibility within that plan, setting up mutual medication contracts with adolescent clients, and permitting the teen to design his or her own adult-monitored medication regimen may facilitate compliance. The family's key role in management of chronic illness changes during adolescence. Such issues as rebellion against rules, refusal to take medications, and participation in high-risk behaviors may need to be dealt with. The nurse can facilitate required adaptations and support both the client and family during these trying times.

Teens needing to receive medications may require assistance with decision making, organization of a medication schedule, and understanding the key physical, cognitive, and emotional changes characteristic of this stage. Nurses' levels of knowledge and caring support may offer a great contribution to adolescent clients and their families.

Herbal ALERT 10–1

Pediatric

Herbal preparations are generally not recommended for use in children.

Nursing Process

Pediatrics

ASSESSMENT

■ Record the age, weight, and height of the child. Drug calculations are based on these three factors.
■ Assess developmental age, health status, nutritional status, and hydration status.
■ Assess history of drug use (prescriptions, over-the-counter [OTC], herbal).
■ Assess family understanding and child's cognitive level.

NURSING DIAGNOSES

■ Delayed growth and development related to physiological, congenital, or environmental factors
■ Ineffective tissue perfusion related to decreased fluid volume, decreased cardiac output, or developmental physiologic differences
■ Impaired urinary elimination related to decreased fluid volume, renal immaturity, congenital anomalies, or decreased renal perfusion
■ Deficient knowledge related to new parenting role, lack of exposure to children and adolescents, language barrier, cognitive discrepancy, or new diagnosis
■ Risk for injury related to developmental, cognitive, and environmental factors

PLANNING

■ The child receives drug dosage based on age, weight, and height. Most drug calculations for children are related to weight in kilograms or body surface area (BSA) (see Chapter 4, Section F).

NURSING INTERVENTIONS

■ Use appropriate drug references to obtain the drug parameters or ranges, side effects, and contraindications for use when administering drugs to children.
■ Monitor infants closely for side effects of drugs because of their immature liver and kidneys. Because infants and young children have limited communication skills, changes in their usual behavior pattern may be indicative of side effects.
■ Communicate with health care provider about drug dosages that are questionable for infants because of the drug's prolonged half-life and the infant's decreased drug excretion.
■ Calculate the child's drug dose according to weight in kilograms or BSA.

Client Teaching

• Teaching clients and families about medications, dosages, therapeutic effects, side effects, and precautions is key in the pediatric population, especially with nonverbal, young, or at-risk children.
• Instruct the responsible family member not to give OTC drugs to children without asking the health care provider.
• Instruct the family member to immediately report side effects of the medication to the health care provider.
• Advise mothers who are breastfeeding their newborn or infant to avoid taking OTC drugs or another person's medication, because a portion of most drugs is excreted in breast milk.
• Nurses should be aware that parents and families frequently perceive that all pediatric infections should be treated with an antibiotic. The nurse is key in raising awareness about avoiding the overuse of antibiotics for viral infections and allergic responses to ensure that resistance to antibiotics does not occur across the lifespan (Sagraves 2002).
• Advise the family member to keep medications out of reach of children.
• Instruct the family member to use child-resistant medication containers.

Cultural Considerations ❖

• Consider parenting, caregiving, and cultural differences when providing care and teaching about medications to children and families. This may include such areas as eye contact, personal space, time orientation, parenting roles/beliefs, the value of children, and communication styles.
• Some cultures may adhere to folk and other health practices, including using herbal preparations for their children and family. Nurses should ensure that families understand the contraindications and precautions associated with giving herbs to children.
• When soliciting adolescent health histories, consider issues related to sexual practices, risk behaviors, recreational drug use, and other lifestyles that may impact medication administration and safety.

EVALUATION

■ Evaluate the family member's knowledge about the drug, drug dosage, schedule for drug administration, and side effects.
■ Evaluate the child's physiologic and psychologic response to the drug regimen.
■ Evaluate the therapeutic and adverse effects of the medication(s).

KEY WEBSITES

General information about medications:
http://pediatrics.about.com/ce/childhoodmedications
American Academy of Pediatrics: www.aap.org
General pediatric information: www.keepkidshealthy.com

 Critical Thinking Case Study

AJ is a 9-month-old infant admitted for heart failure secondary to an unrepaired congenital heart defect. Several medications are ordered to be administered by mouth. You are providing discharge teaching to the family.

1. How does a nurse adapt teaching methods when the client is an infant?
2. AJ does not readily take the medications by mouth. What suggestions could you offer this family to enhance medication administration?
3. The mother is concerned with the child's current diarrhea. With your knowledge of absorption, distribution, metabolism, and excretion, what impact may this symptom have on the effectiveness of the medications?

CC is a 12-year-old boy receiving daily injections of growth hormone. He is extremely afraid of injections.

1. What advice could you offer his caregivers to facilitate injection technique?
2. The family is considering using topical anesthetic to ease the administration of injections. Why may this be an effective strategy?
3. Based on CC's developmental level, how could the nurse enlist the 12-year-old's cooperation?

NCLEX Study Questions

1. An 8-month-old child is discharged from the hospital with a plan of care to receive intramuscular (IM) injections each day. The parents have been taught how to administer IM injections. The nurse would reinforce using the following site for IM injections in an 8-month-old child:
   a. vastus lateralis
   b. dorsogluteal
   c. deltoid
   d. IM injections are contraindicated in the pediatric population

2. A 4-year-old client is to be discharged home on an oral liquid drug suspension of 4 cc per dose. Which of the following would ensure the highest level of accuracy in home administration of the medication?
   a. using a household teaspoon
   b. using a cooking measuring spoon
   c. using an oral syringe
   d. using a graduated medicine cup

3. A child is ordered to receive naloxone (Narcan) IV, STAT. The child's weight is 20 kg, and the recommended child's drug dosage is 0.01 mg/kg. Naloxone is available in 400 mcg/ml solution. The nurse should administer:

a. 0.25 ml
b. 0.5 ml
c. 0.75 ml
d. 1 ml

4. A pediatric client is ordered to receive 3 mg/kg of a medication. The client weighs 88 pounds. The medication is available in a 15 mg/ml elixir. How much medication should the client receive?
   a. 2 ml
   b. 4 ml
   c. 8 ml
   d. 16 ml

5. The nurse needs to understand the differences in drug excretion in children. The nurse bases decisions in medication administration on the knowledge that drug excretion in infants and children is usually:
   a. decreased
   b. increased
   c. the same as adults
   d. unaffected by developmental differences

6. A parent is learning to administer medication to a preschool child. Which of the following strategies would be most effective in achieving cooperation?
   a. enlisting physical restraint
   b. tolerating violent reactions
   c. providing age-appropriate explanations
   d. establishing medication contracts

Answers: 1, a; 2, c; 3, b; 4, c; 5, a; 6, c.

11

Geriatric Pharmacology

ELECTRONIC RESOURCES

Evolve website (http://evolve.elsevier.com/KeeHayes/pharmacology/):
- *Case Studies*
- *Content Updates*
- *Frequently Asked Questions*
- *Student Review Activities*
- *WebLinks*
- *Additional Reference Material*

Companion CD-ROM:
- *NCLEX Examination Review Questions*
- *Pharmacology Animations*
- *IV Therapy Checklists*
- *Medication Error Checklists*
- *Drug Calculation Problems*
- *Electronic Calculators*
- *Top 200 Drugs with Pronunciations*
- *References from the Textbook*

Objectives

- Explain the physiologic changes of the aging process that have a major effect on drug therapy.
- Explain the pharmacokinetics and pharmacodynamics of the older adult that relate to drug dosing.
- Differentiate the effects of two drug categories on the older adult.
- Discuss reasons for noncompliance to drug regimen by the older adult.
- Describe nursing implications related to drug therapy in the older adult.

Terms

Older Americans (Figure 11–1) constitute almost 20% of the population, and nurses will care for increasing numbers of elders representing the "core business" of health care. Geriatric pharmacology for the **older adult** (elderly client) requires special attention to the age-related factors of drug absorption, distribution, metabolism, and excretion. Drug dosages are adjusted according to the older adult's weight, adipose tissue, laboratory results (e.g., serum protein, electrolytes, liver enzymes, blood urea nitrogen [BUN], creatinine), and current health problems. Modifications in drug therapy for the older adult are frequently required. Because of declining organ functioning in the older adult, the effect of drug therapy must be closely monitored to prevent the risk of adverse reactions to drugs and possible drug toxicity.

About 12% of the U.S. population are persons older than 65 years of age; this age group consumes approximately 30% of all prescription medications and 40% of

FIGURE 11-1 Many elders live in community settings. (Copyright 2007 JupiterImages Corporation.)

FIGURE 11-2 Does the client know what the medications are for and whether they are all necessary?

over-the-counter (OTC) drugs. By 2030 it is expected that the number of older adults will be nearly twice the number in 2000, with a greater increase in the number of Hispanics, Asians, and African Americans than in whites. Women 65 years of age presently outnumber 65-year-old men by 134 to 100; in the 75-year-old age group, there are 100 women to 55 men. A fast-growing population is those 85 years and older, and their use of drug therapy will likely continue to grow. The cost of drugs in the United States reached more than $160 billion annually, much of it spent by elderly. However, medications may save money spent on hospitalizations and surgeries.

Approximately 70% of clients older than 65 take at least one or two prescribed drugs daily, and the other 30% take five or more. Older adults take pain, sleep, and laxative OTC drugs more frequently than the general population. At the time of hospital admission, about 15% of clients older than 65 years are not taking any medications prescribed or self medicated. During hospitalization older adults take an average of three to five drugs. One third of clients in nursing homes receive 6 to 12 drugs daily. Figure 11-2 shows a client with a "handful" of drugs.

The adverse reactions and drug interactions that occur in the older adult are three to seven times greater than those for middle-aged and young adults. Older adults consume numerous drugs because of chronic and multiple illnesses, therefore they are susceptible to adverse reactions and interactions. Additional problems that can cause adverse reactions from drugs include self-medicating with OTC drugs, taking drugs that were prescribed for other health problems, consuming drugs ordered by several different health care providers, overdosing when symptoms do not subside, using drugs that were prescribed for another person, and, of course, the ongoing physiologic aging process.

Drug toxicity may develop in the older adult for drug doses that are within therapeutic range for the average adult. These therapeutic drug ranges are usually safe for young and middle-aged adults but are not always within safe range for older adults. It has been suggested that the drug dose for older adults should initially be prescribed at a low to low-average therapeutic range and then gradually increased according to tolerance and lack of adverse reactions; start low and go slow. This approach prevents a toxic reaction to the drug in older adults. Older adults at risk of problems with medication administration frequently have common characteristics such as lack of coordinated care, recent discharge from the hospital, self treatment, multiple diagnoses, and cognitive impairment.

Physiologic Changes

The physiologic changes associated with the aging process have a major effect on drug therapy. Table 11-1 describes the physiologic changes that occur in the gastrointestinal (GI), cardiac and circulatory, hepatic (liver), and renal (kidney) systems of the older adult and how these changes can affect pharmacologic response to drug therapy.

Polypharmacy

Polypharmacy (administration of many drugs together) is more common in older adults because of the use of (1) multiple health care providers, (2) herbal therapy, (3) OTC drugs, and (4) discontinued prescription drugs. Polypharmacy can cause confusion, falls, malnutrition, renal and liver dysfunction, and nonadherence. The nurse needs to coordinate the health care for older adults, including drug therapy, to avoid duplication of drugs from various health care providers and misuse of OTC and herbal supplements. For example, an older client may take a prescribed drug, ranitidine (Zantac), with an OTC drug, famotidine (Pepcid AC), for GI discomfort; this drug combination causes duplication to occur. Some older adults do not think herbal drugs are actually drugs that could cause adverse reactions when taken with other prescription or OTC drugs. Older adults should be encouraged to use the same pharmacy and give the pharmacist a list of all drugs they take, both prescribed and OTC. Pharmacists conduct clinical reviews of medications that focus primarily on drug interactions.

Pharmacokinetics

Parameters of **pharmacokinetics** for the older adult are described in Table 11–2.

Absorption

Drug absorption from the GI tract is slowed in the older adult because of decreases in both blood flow and GI motility. In this age group, acidic drugs are poorly absorbed because of increased alkaline gastric secretions, but enteric-coated tablets dissolved in alkaline fluid can break down more rapidly. Drugs remain in the GI tract longer, because there is a decrease in gastric motility. Iron and calcium tablets may not be absorbed as readily, but generally, the amount of an oral dose that is absorbed is not affected by age.

Distribution

Older adults have a loss of protein-binding sites for drugs which causes increased circulation of free drug and increased chance for adverse drug reaction. During the aging process there is a loss of body water, and water-soluble drugs become more concentrated in the body. Because of an increase in body fat in the older adult, the lipid-soluble drugs are absorbed into the fat, causing a decrease in desired drug effects.

Table 11–1

Physiologic Changes in the Older Adult

System	Physiologic Change	Effect on Drug Administration
Gastrointestinal	↑ pH (alkaline) gastric secretions ↓ peristalsis with delayed intestinal emptying time ↓ motility ↓ first-pass effect	Slower absorption of oral drugs
Cardiac and circulatory	↓ cardiac output ↓ blood flow	Impaired circulation can delay transportation of drugs to the tissues
Hepatic	↓ enzyme function ↓ blood flow	Drugs metabolized more slowly and less completely
Renal	↓ blood flow ↓ functioning nephrons (kidney cells) ↓ glomerular filtration rate	Drugs excreted less completely

↓, Decrease; ↑, increase.

Table 11–2

Pharmacokinetics in Geriatric Pharmacology

Phases	Body Effects and Possible Drug Responses
Absorption	Decrease in gastric acidity (increased gastric pH) alters absorption of weak acid drugs such as aspirin. Decrease in blood flow to the GI tract (40% to 50% less) is caused by decrease in cardiac output. Because of reduced blood flow, absorption is slowed but not decreased. Reduction in GI motility rate (peristalsis) may delay onset of action. Reduction in gastric emptying time occurs.
Distribution	Because of a decrease in body water, water-soluble drugs are more concentrated. Increase in fat-to-water ratio in older adult; fat-soluble drugs are stored and likely to accumulate. Decrease in circulating serum protein. Two most common proteins are albumin and alpha-1 acid glycoprotein. Acidic drugs (e.g., nonsteroidal antiinflammatory drugs [NSAIDs], aspirin, benzodiazepines, phenytoin, and warfarin) bind to albumin; basic drugs (e.g., beta-adrenergic blockers, tricyclic antidepressants, lidocaine) bind to alpha-1 acid glycoprotein. With fewer protein-binding sites, there is more free drug available to body tissue at receptor sites. Drugs with a high affinity for protein (>90%) compete for protein-binding sites with other drugs. Drug interactions result because of lack of protein sites and increase in free drugs.
Metabolism	Decrease in hepatic enzyme production, hepatic blood flow, and total liver function. These decreases cause a reduction in drug metabolism. With reduction in metabolic rate, $t^{1/2}$ of drugs increases; drug accumulation can result. Metabolism of a drug inactivates drug/drug metabolite and prepares it for elimination via the kidneys. When drug clearance by liver is decreased, drug $t^{1/2}$ is prolonged; when drug clearance is increased, drug $t^{1/2}$ is shortened. With prolonged $t^{1/2}$, drug accumulation can result and drug toxicity could occur.
Excretion	Decrease in renal blood flow and decrease in glomerular filtration rate of 40% to 50%. With decrease in renal function comes decrease in drug excretion; drug accumulation results. Drug toxicity should be assessed continually while client takes drug.

GI, Gastrointestinal; $t^{1/2}$, half-life.

Metabolism or Biotransformation

Hepatic blood flow in the older adult may be decreased by 40% to 45%. Also, aging causes a decrease in liver size. Drug clearance by hepatic metabolism is affected more in older male adults than in females.

Liver dysfunction caused by the aging process decreases enzyme function, which decreases the liver's ability to metabolize and detoxify drugs, thereby increasing the risk of drug toxicity.

The liver and kidneys are the major organs responsible for drug clearance from the body. *Biotransformation* refers to drug metabolism that occurs in the liver (hepatic cells) and contributes to the clearance of drugs. Biotransformation during hepatic metabolism can occur either in phase I by oxidation reaction or in phase II by conjugation reaction. Hepatic microsomal enzymes are responsible for phase I, oxidation reaction. The hepatic microsomal oxidation can be impaired by the aging process, liver diseases (e.g., cirrhosis, hepatitis), and drugs that reduce oxidation capability. Drug clearance by the liver is then reduced. An example of a drug that undergoes a phase I biotransformation oxidation reaction is diazepam (Valium). Diazepam is biotransformed to its active metabolite, desmethyldiazepam. In the older adult, the plasma-serum diazepam level would remain high because of an impaired phase I oxidation reaction. Other drugs that are biotransformed by phase I include barbiturates, codeine, ibuprofen, phenytoin, meperidine, lidocaine, certain benzodiazepines (alprazolam, flurazepam, midazolam, prazepam), and warfarin (Coumadin).

Phase II of biotransformation involves the conjugation or attachment of the drug to an inactive state. Hepatic conjugation is usually not influenced by older age, liver diseases, or drug interaction, so the drug is inactivated and excreted in the urine. Examples of drugs that are biotransformed or metabolized by phase II are aspirin, acetaminophen, certain benzodiazepines (lorazepam, oxazepam, temazepam), procainamide, and sulfanilamide. The benzodiazepines lorazepam, oxazepam, and temazepam that undergo conjugation reaction do not have active metabolites. The drug metabolic process, phase I or II, for drug clearance for the older adult client is an important consideration with drug selection.

To assess liver function, liver enzymes need to be checked. Elevated levels indicate possible liver dysfunction. However, normal liver enzyme results may not indicate normal drug metabolism. The older adult could have normal liver function test (LFT) results and still have impaired hepatic microsomal enzyme-drug oxidation reactions.

Excretion

Cardiac output and blood flow throughout the circulatory system are decreased in older adults, affecting blood flow to the liver and kidneys. After the age of 65, nephron function may be decreased by 35%; after 70, blood flow to the kidneys may be decreased by 40%.

Kidney function is assessed by monitoring urine output, laboratory values of BUN and serum creatinine (Cr), and the creatinine clearance (CLcr or CrCl) test (estimated). Creatinine clearance is an indicator of glomerular filtration rate (GFR). To evaluate renal function based on serum creatinine alone may not be accurate for the older adult because of the decrease in muscle mass. A decrease in muscle mass can cause a decrease in serum creatinine. Creatinine is a byproduct of muscle catabolism; however, creatinine is primarily excreted by the kidneys. With older clients, serum creatinine may be within normal values because of a lack of muscle mass, but there still could be a decrease in renal function. With the young or middle-aged adult, serum creatinine would be increased with a decrease in renal function.

The 24-hour creatinine clearance test and the serum creatinine level should be used to evaluate renal function. If a 24-hour creatinine clearance test is not feasible, the following formulas can be used to estimate creatinine clearance:

$$CLcr \text{ (males)} = (140\text{-age}) \times kg/72 \times \text{ serum Cr level}$$
$$= ml/min$$
$$CLcr \text{ (females)} = \text{value of males} \times 0.85 = ml/min$$

The normal creatinine clearance value for an adult is 80 to 130 ml/min.

With liver and kidney dysfunction, the efficacy of a drug dose is usually reduced. Multiple drug use may intensify drug effect in the older adult. When the efficiency of the hepatic and renal systems is reduced, the half-life of the drug is prolonged and drug toxicity is probable.

Factors contributing to adverse reactions in the older adult include (1) a loss of protein-binding sites, which increases the amount of free circulating drug; (2) a decline in hepatic first-pass metabolism; and (3) a prolonged half-life of the drug because of decreased liver and kidney function. As a result of these factors, the time interval between doses of a drug may need to be increased for the geriatric client.

Pharmacodynamics

Pharmacodynamics refers to how a drug interacts at the receptor site or at the target organ. Because there is a lack of affinity to receptor sites throughout the body in the older adult, the pharmacodynamic response may be altered. The older adult could be more or less sensitive to drug action because of age-related changes in the central nervous system (CNS), changes in the number of drug receptors, and changes in the affinity of receptors to drugs. Frequently the drug dose needs to be lowered. Consideration of changes in organ function are important in drug dosing.

In the geriatric client the compensatory response to physiologic changes is decreased. When a drug with vasodilator properties is administered and the sympathetic feedback does not occur quickly, orthostatic hypotension (i.e., rapid decrease in blood pressure when standing up quickly) could result. In the younger adult, the sympathetic response of vasoconstriction works to avert a severe hypotensive effect.

Effects of Selected Drug Groups on Older Adults

Hypnotics, diuretics and antihypertensives, cardiac glycosides, anticoagulants, antibacterials (antibiotics), GI drugs (antiulcer, laxatives), antidepressants, and narcotic analgesics are drug categories for which drug effects on the older adult are possible. The number of drugs taken, drug interactions (see Chapter 7), and physical health of the older adult (cardiac, renal, and hepatic function) are factors associated with drug effects in the older adult population. Drug selection is extremely important. Drugs with a shorter half-life are less likely to cause problems as a result of drug accumulation than drugs with a long half-life. If severe side effects occur, the drug with a shorter half-life is eliminated more quickly than the drug with a longer half-life.

Drugs that are classified as phase II (conjugation) are tolerated and eliminated more quickly than are those from phase I (oxidation). If phase I drugs are used, drug selection should be from those agents that have fewer active metabolites. Evaluation of hepatic and renal function is imperative, especially if the older adult takes multiple drugs. When side effects and adverse reactions occur, prescription and nonprescription drugs should be assessed (Herbal Alert 11–1).

Hypnotics

Insomnia is a frequent problem in the geriatric population. Sedatives and hypnotics are the second most common group of drugs prescribed or taken OTC. Insomnia may be described as having difficulty in falling asleep, frequently awakening during the night, or awakening early in the morning with difficulty falling back to sleep. Types of hypnotics differ according to the cause of insomnia. Five benzodiazepine hypnotics (flurazepam, quazepam, temazepam, triazolam, and estazolam) have been approved by the U.S. Food and Drug Administration (FDA) as hypnotics to control insomnia. For the older client, low doses of benzodiazepines with short or intermediate half-lives are usually prescribed. Short-term therapy is suggested. Usually benzodiazepines are prescribed at higher doses for sedative and hypnotic effects and at lower doses for anti-

Herbal ALERT 11-1

Older Adults
Advise clients to consult with health care provider before starting herbal products. Common herbal preparations interact with many drugs (e.g., anticoagulants) that elderly clients take to treat chronic health disorders.

anxiety effects. About 35% of the older adult population takes a hypnotic.

Flurazepam HCl (Dalmane), the first benzodiazepine hypnotic, was introduced in 1970. It has three metabolites and is considered to be both a short- and long-acting hypnotic. Its principal metabolite is desalkylflurazepam, which is long-acting, has a long half-life, and is slowly eliminated. This drug is not suggested for persons older than age 65. Drug hangover is a problem. Quazepam (Doral) has effects similar to flurazepam. It is a precursor of desalkylflurazepam and has a prolonged half-life.

Temazepam (Restoril) was introduced in 1981. Because it is biotransformed in the liver by conjugation and not by oxidation, it is prescribed frequently for the older adult client. Temazepam's principal metabolite, glucuronide, is conjugated with no pharmacologic effects and excreted in the urine. Temazepam is slowly absorbed, so it should be taken 1 to 2 hours before bedtime. It is classified as an intermediate-acting benzodiazepine. Food delays its action. Temazepam is more effective for frequent awakenings during the night than for problems falling asleep.

Triazolam (Halcion) is an intermediate-acting benzodiazepine. It has a short half-life and at low doses (0.0625 to 0.125 mg) is considered safe for the older adult. It is metabolized by hepatic microsomal oxidation, although the drug doses differ from oxidized benzodiazepines. Triazolam helps with problems falling asleep, and it also decreases frequent awakenings during the night. To avoid rebound insomnia when the drug is discontinued, doses should be tapered rather than abruptly stopped.

Estazolam, a new benzodiazepine, is an intermediate- to long-acting drug. It is metabolized in the liver to two metabolites that are not highly potent.

The benzodiazepines lorazepam and oxazepam can be used for insomnia. These agents have an intermediate half-life and should be taken 1 hour before bedtime. Other benzodiazepines are more effective as anxiolytics (antianxiety drugs) than as hypnotics.

Diuretics and Antihypertensives

Diuretics are frequently prescribed for treatment of hypertension or heart failure (HF). For the older adult, the dose is usually reduced because of dose-related side effects. Hydrochlorothiazide (HydroDIURIL) is generally prescribed in low doses of 12.5 mg daily. Higher doses of 25 to 50 mg daily with chronic use can cause electrolyte imbalances (e.g., hypokalemia, hyponatremia, hypomagnesemia, hypercalcemia), hyperglycemia, hyperuricemia, and hypercholesterolemia.

Many geriatric clients are hypertensive (blood pressure >140/90 mmHg). Nonpharmacologic methods to reduce blood pressure such as exercise, weight reduction if obese, reduction of salt and alcohol intake, and adequate rest are suggested. These actions can reduce the systolic and diastolic pressure by 8 to 10 mmHg. Drugs such as diuretics, beta-adrenergic blockers or antagonists, calcium channel blockers, angiotensin-converting (ACE) inhibitors, angiotensin II receptor antagonists (A-II blockers), and centrally acting alpha-2 agonists are used as antihypertensive drugs. Calcium blockers, angiotension-converting inhibitors, and A-II blockers are frequently the agents of choice because of their low incidence of electrolyte imbalance and CNS side effects (see Chapter 43). Usually antihypertensive dosing for older adults begins with reduced doses that are gradually increased according to need, tolerance, and adverse reactions. Because of adverse reactions such as orthostatic hypotension, alpha-1 blockers or antagonists (prazosin, terazosin) and centrally acting alpha-2 agonists (methyldopa, clonidine, guanabenz, guanfacine) are infrequently prescribed for geriatric clients.

Cardiac Glycosides

Digoxin is commonly prescribed for older adults; however, long-term use of the drug should be carefully monitored because of its narrow therapeutic range (0.5 to 2 ng/ml) and the possibility of digitalis toxicity. Digoxin is given for left ventricular heart failure, chronic atrial fibrillation, and atrial tachycardia. Its half-life is doubled (70 hours) in clients older than 80 years of age. Most of the digoxin is eliminated by the kidneys, so a decline in kidney function (decreased GFR) could cause digoxin accumulation. With close monitoring of serum digoxin levels, creatinine clearance tests, and vital signs (pulse should not be <60 beats per minute), digoxin is considered safe for the older adult.

Anticoagulants

Bleeding may occur with chronic use of anticoagulants in older adult clients. Warfarin (Coumadin) is 99% protein bound; with a decrease in serum albumin, which is common among older adults, there is an increase in free, unbound circulating warfarin and a potential risk for bleeding. Geriatric clients should have their prothrombin time (PT) or international normalized ratio (INR) checked periodically, and the nurse should check for signs of bleeding.

Antibacterials

Penicillins, cephalosporins, tetracyclines, and sulfonamides are normally considered safe for the older adult. If renal drug clearance is decreased and the drug has a prolonged half-life, the drug dose should be reduced. Aminoglycosides, fluoroquinolones (quinolones), and vancomycin are excreted in the urine. These drug agents are not frequently prescribed for clients older than 75 years, and if they are prescribed, the drug dose is usually reduced.

Gastrointestinal Drugs

Histamine (H2) blockers and sucralfate are safer drugs than other antiulcer agents for the treatment of peptic ulcers. Cimetidine (Tagamet) was the first histamine blocker or antagonist and is not suggested for the older adult because of its side effects and multiple potential drug interactions. Ranitidine, famotidine, and nizatidine may be prescribed for the geriatric client instead of cimetidine.

Laxatives are frequently taken by the older adult. In long-term facilities such as nursing homes, 75% of residents take laxatives on a daily basis. Fluid and electrolyte imbalances may occur with excessive use. Increased GI motility with laxative use could decrease other drug absorptions. Nonpharmacologic measures such as increasing fluid intake, consuming high-fiber foods such as prunes, and exercising should be encouraged.

Antidepressants

An antidepressant drug dose for the older adult is normally 30% to 50% of the dose for young and middle-aged adults. Drug dose should be gradually increased according to the client's tolerance and the desired therapeutic effect. Close monitoring for possible adverse reactions is important.

Tricyclic antidepressants are generally effective in the geriatric population, but they do have anticholinergic properties that can cause side effects: dry mouth, tachycardia, constipation, and urinary retention. Tricyclic antidepressants can also contribute to narrow-angle glaucoma. Fluoxetine (Prozac), a bicyclic antidepressant, has fewer side effects than the tricyclics, and the side effects are mostly dose-related. The monoamine oxidase (MAO) inhibitors are not often prescribed for older adults because of adverse reactions such as drug-food interactions which could result in hypertensive crisis and severe orthostatic hypotension. Further discussion of antidepressants can be found in Chapter 27.

Narcotic Analgesics

Narcotics can cause dose-related adverse reactions when taken by the older adult. Hypotension and respiratory depression may result from narcotic use. Close monitoring of vital signs is essential when providing nursing care and support to the geriatric client on narcotic analgesics.

Table 11–3 presents a list of drugs not generally recommended for use in the elderly. The list includes drawbacks and alternatives.

Noncompliance/Nonadherence

Nonadherence with a drug regimen can be a problem in all client age groups, but it is especially troublesome in the elderly. Frequently the older adult fails to ask questions during interactions with health care providers; therefore the drug regimen may not be fully understood or precisely followed. Nonadherence can cause underdosing or overdosing that could be harmful to the client's health. Some barriers to effective medication use by older adults are listed in Table 11–4.

Working with the geriatric client is an ongoing nursing responsibility. The nurse should plan strategies with the client and family or friends to encourage **compliance** with prescribed regimens. Daily contact may be necessary at first. Mere ordering of medication does not mean that the client is able to get the drugs or is taking them correctly. Figure 11–3 shows the different medications to be taken by

Table 11-3

Drugs not Generally Recommended For Use in the Elderly

Drugs	Drawbacks	Alternatives
Analgesics		
ketorolac (Toradol and others)	Serious GI toxicity	
meperidine (Demerol and others)	Confusion, convulsions	Morphine preferred
propoxyphene (Darvon and others)	Convulsions, limited effectiveness	
Antidepressants, Tricyclic		
amitriptyline (Elavil and others)	Anticholinergic effects (constipation, uri-	Selective serotonin reuptake
doxepin (Sinequan and others)	nary retention, blurred vision, confu-	inhibitors (SSRIs) other than
	sion), orthostatic hypotension, sedation,	daily fluoxetine; other anti-
	and cardiac arrhythmias	depressants preferred
Antihistamines, First Generation		
chlorpheniramine (Chlor-Trimeton and others)	Anticholinergic effects; some such as di-	Second-generation antihista-
diphenhydramine (Benadryl and others)	phenhydramine and promethazine are	mines such as fexofenadine
hydroxyzine (Vistaril and others)	highly sedating	(Allegra) or loratadine (Clar-
promethazine (Phenergan and others)		itin and others) preferred
Antispasmodics		
belladonna alkaloids (Donnatal and others)	Anticholinergic effects	
dicyclomine (Bentyl and others)		
hyoscyamine (Levsin and others)		
propantheline (Pro-Banthine and others)		
Muscle Relaxants		
carisoprodol (Soma and others)	Anticholinergic effects, sedation, limited ef-	
cyclobenzaprine (Flexeril and others)	fectiveness at tolerated doses	
methocarbamol (Robaxin and others)		
metaxalone (Skelaxin and others)		
Sedatives		
Barbiturates	Sedation, addiction	
benzodiazepines, long-acting	Prolonged sedation	Low doses of shorter-acting
chlordiazepoxide (Librium and others)		benzodiazepines such as lo-
diazepam (Valium and others)		razepam (Ativan and others)
flurazepam (Dalmane and others)		preferred
meprobamate (Equanil and others)	Sedation, addiction	
Other		
chlorpropamide (Diabinese and others)	Long half-life may cause prolonged hypo-	Shorter-acting sulfonylureas
	glycemia	are preferred
cimetidine (Tagamet and others)	Confusion, many drug interactions	Other H2-agonists preferred
nitrofurantoin (Macrobid and others)	Limited efficacy in renal impairment	Other antibiotics preferred
trimethobenzamide (Tigan and others)	Extrapyramidal effects, limited effectiveness	

From *The Medical Letter*, 48:7, 2006.

Table 11-4

Barriers to Effective Medication Use by Older Adults

Causes	Nursing Actions
Taking too many medications at different times (Figure 11-2)	Develop a chart indicating times to take drugs. Provide space to place a mark for each drug taken. Use an organizer device to mark days and weeks.
Failure to understand purpose or reason for drug	Explain purpose, drug action, and importance of medication. Provide time for questions and reinforcement. Reinforce with written information.
Impaired memory	Encourage family members or friends to monitor drug regimen.
Decreased mobility and dexterity	Advise family members or friends to have drugs and water or other fluid accessible. Assist older adult as needed.
Visual and hearing disturbances	Suggest eye and ear examinations (glasses or hearing aids).
High cost of prescriptions	Contact the social services department of your institution; contact "compassionate care programs" as appropriate.
Childproof drug bottles	Suggest that client request non-childproof bottle caps.
Side effects or adverse reactions from the drug	Educate client and family about side effects to report to health care provider.

FIGURE 11–3 A possible cause of noncompliance in an older adult client is the need to take many different medications at different times.

a client at different times. Such a complicated array of drugs can cause confusion and **noncompliance**. Older adults often do not have insurance that includes prescription drug coverage, so they choose to buy food and other necessities before medication. Some delay purchasing or never purchase the drugs prescribed. The older adult is more apt to experience serious side effects from drug administration than the young or middle-aged adult. If a drug such as ibuprofen (Advil, Motrin) irritates the GI tract, the older adult frequently will not take it, unaware that another drug such as magnesium hydroxide (Maalox) taken before the ibuprofen dose will decrease this side effect. He or she may not know that food can also decrease gastric irritation from ibuprofen.

Health Teaching with the Older Adult

A comprehensive discussion of health teaching in the nursing process is presented in Chapter 2. Specific guidelines for health teaching with the geriatric client include:
- If needed, be sure client is wearing clear, clean eyeglasses and has working hearing aids in place.
- Speak in tone of voice that client can hear; sit facing client.
- Treat client with respect; never infantilize; expect that he or she can learn.
- Use large print and bright colors in teaching aids.
- Review all medications at each client visit.
- Encourage a simple dosing schedule when possible.
- With onset of new confusion or disorientation, suspect recently prescribed medication(s).
- Encourage client to report that a drug is not improving the condition for which it was prescribed.

The NIH websites on aging are excellent resources for both health care providers and older adults and their families. The website for health care providers is *www.nia.nih.gov*

and has sections on health information, research, grants, training, news, and events. The website for the older adult is *http://nihseniorhealth.gov*.

Geriatrics

ASSESSMENT

- Assess the older adult's sensorium, mental awareness, and visual and auditory acuity. Is the person confused or disoriented? Is this state transitory? Does client live alone with or without social support?
- Obtain a history of kidney, liver, or GI disorders and determine whether eyesight is failing. Kidney or liver disorders can cause a decrease in the function of these organs and increase the half-life of drugs. Longer drug half-life and frequent drug dosing can result in drug toxicity. Assess client's use of eyeglasses, and check the date of the last eye examination.
- Determine whether client takes OTC drugs, including herbal preparations, how often, and for what length of time. Specifically ask about laxatives and antacids, which can affect gastric pH, electrolyte balance, and GI motility. Many people do not think of these agents as drugs. Remind client and/or family to tell the pharmacist about prescribed drugs when contemplating the purchase of OTC preparations.
- Assess compliance with taking drugs correctly and reasons for noncompliance. Does client have problems opening drug containers?

NURSING DIAGNOSES

- Risk for constipation related to analgesics
- Urinary retention related to drug therapy
- Imbalanced nutrition: less than body requirements related to metabolism of drugs
- Ineffective health maintenance related to lack of transportation
- Deficient knowledge related to lack of understanding about reason for taking medication
- Noncompliance/nonadherence related to lack of insurance with prescription drug coverage
- Effective therapeutic regimen management related to medication administration

PLANNING

- Client will take prescribed medications as ordered.
- Drug therapy will be effective with no or few side effects.

NURSING INTERVENTIONS

■ Monitor client's laboratory results in relation to kidney and liver function. Are blood urea nitrogen (BUN), serum creatinine, and creatinine clearance levels within normal range (reference values)? Are liver enzymes (LFTs) within normal range? Discuss findings with health care provider.

■ Check client's serum drug level as ordered and report abnormal findings to nurse manager or health care provider. Remember: Older adults who take water-soluble drugs such as digoxin are likely to have higher blood levels because of reduced body water.

■ Communicate with pharmacist or health care provider when drug dose is in question. Check drug reference books for recommended drug doses for older adults.

■ Observe client for adverse reactions when multiple drugs are being taken. An older adult with hypertension and heart failure might take a diuretic (e.g., hydrochlorothiazide [HydroDIURIL]) and digoxin. The diuretic may cause potassium loss and if potassium replacement is not ordered, digitalis toxicity may occur. Hypokalemia (low serum potassium) enhances action of digoxin, causing toxicity. Symptoms of digitalis toxicity may be a slow (bradycardia, <60 beats/min) or irregular pulse rate, nausea and vomiting, and blurred vision.

■ Recognize a change in usual behavior or an increase in confusion. One of the first signs of drug toxicity is confusion. Report changes to the health care provider.

■ Ascertain whether financial problems are preventing client from purchasing prescribed drugs. Assistance programs are available.

Client Teaching

General

• Review medications with client and family, including reason for medication, route of administration, how often it is to be taken, common side effects, and when to notify health care provider.

• Explain to client/family the importance of adherence to the drug regimen. Emphasize taking drug as prescribed, discarding unused or old drugs, and keeping a record of medication taken. REMEMBER: Drugs are the property of client and may not be disposed of without his or her permission.

• Be available to answer client's questions. Be supportive of the older adult and the family. Discuss problems related to the medications.

• Instruct client not to share prescribed medications with others or to take medications prescribed for another person.

• Inform client to use one pharmacy to fill prescriptions. Tell client to inform pharmacist of all OTC and herbal drugs taken.

• If client has arthritis in the hand joint or difficulty opening childproof bottle caps, have client/family request a non-childproof cap from pharmacy. Client may need to sign permission at pharmacy.

Self-Administration

• Instruct client to keep a medication record of drugs and when they are to be taken. This removes barriers, increases drug adherence, and avoids drug errors.

Diet

• Instruct clients controlling hypertension with a potassium-wasting diuretic (e.g., hydrochlorothiazide [HydroDIURIL]) to eat foods rich in potassium (bran cereal, tomatoes, raisins, potatoes, bananas, avocados) and to take potassium supplements if recommended by health care provider.

• Inform client about how to maintain a generally well-balanced diet and give examples.

Side Effects

• Advise client/family to immediately report mental and physiologic changes (confusion, GI bleeding) to health care provider.

Cultural Considerations ❖

• Recognize that language difficulties for older adults in various cultural groups may interfere with understanding the prescribed drug regimen. Many do not speak English.

• Provide additional time for verbal and written explanation to ensure that the older adult will take drugs as prescribed.

• The more traditional and older individuals in some cultures do not maintain eye contact. Do not assume that lack of eye contact means the client is not listening or does not care; it might indicate respect.

EVALUATION

■ Evaluate compliance with the drug regimen and answer any questions the older adult may have.

■ Evaluate drug effect and ascertain side effects or adverse reactions.

KEY WEBSITES

Beers' Criteria for Potentially Inappropriate Medication use in the Elderly: www.hartfordign.org

Senior Care Pharmacist: www.seniorcarepharmacist.com

American Society of Consultant Pharmacists: www.ascp.com

Critical Thinking Case Study

RT, a 72-year-old woman, has osteoarthritis. She had taken aspirin and later was prescribed naproxen (Naprosyn). Both drugs caused her GI distress. The health care provider discontinued the naproxen and prescribed celecoxib (Celebrex) 100 mg twice a day. Celecoxib is a nonnarcotic, cyclooxygenase-2 (COX-2) inhibitor.

1. How does celecoxib differ from naproxen? (NOTE: Refer to Chapters 24 and 25.)
2. Describe the advantages and disadvantages of RT taking celecoxib.
3. What is the rationale for checking RT's renal and liver function before prescribing celecoxib? Explain.

4. What should be included in the nursing assessment in regard to RT's physical and drug histories?

RT states that her arthritic pain is not relieved with this new drug. She wants to take naproxen with the celecoxib.

5. Explain the effects of these two medications when taken together.
6. What is the most appropriate response by the nurse to RT's request? Explain.
7. Develop a teaching plan for RT that includes medication use and nursing measures to relieve pain.

NCLEX Study Questions

1. Persons over 65 years of age consume what percentage of all prescription medications?
   a. 10
   b. 20
   c. 30
   d. 40

2. Common reasons for nonadherence to the drug regimen in the older adult include all the following except:
   a. taking multiple drugs at one time
   b. impaired memory
   c. decreased integrity
   d. increased mobility

3. You know that your 88-year-old client's slower absorption of oral meds is due to:
   a. decreased cardiac output
   b. decreased blood flow
   c. decreased enzyme function
   d. increased pH of gastric secretions

4. Drugs are metabolized more slowly in the elderly due to decreased:
   a. first-pass effect
   b. enzyme function
   c. glomerular filtration rate
   d. motility

5. Your geriatric client has loss of protein-binding sites that influences:
   a. increased circulation of free drug
   b. decreased hepatic blood flow
   c. decreased calcium absorption
   d. increased motility

Answers: 1, c; 2, d; 3, b; 4, a; 5, a.

12
Medication Administration in Community Settings

Outline

Objectives	Cultural Considerations	**Summary**
Client Teaching	**Community-Based Settings**	Nursing Process: Overview of Medication Administration
General	Home Setting	**Key Websites**
Diet	School Setting	**Critical Thinking Case Study**
Self-Administration	Work Setting	**NCLEX Study Questions**
Side Effects		

Objectives

- Describe common elements of client teaching about medication administration in community settings.
- Explain specific points related to administration of medications in the home.
- Discuss specific points related to administration of medications in the school.
- Describe specific points related to administration of medications in the work site.
- Explain the application of the nursing process to medication administration in community settings.

Health and illness care has shifted from traditional institutions to community settings. The faces of a community are many, varied, and ever-changing (Figure 12–1). With the movement of health care into the community, nurses—more than any other health care provider—have the opportunity to shape the health care of society. This chapter describes selected aspects of medication administration of prescription, over-the-counter (OTC), and herbal preparations within each of the major community settings: home, school, and work. In all settings, client safety is the primary concern. Chapter 3 of this book provides a detailed presentation on medication administration.

The process of medication administration in the home, school, and work site must be consistent with professional, legal, and regulatory requirements. In each setting it must first be determined what the nursing personnel will teach clients about medications and then the routes by which the medications can be administered. Once these decisions have been made, criteria for administration, instruction and client teaching, and ongoing supervision need to be developed, implemented, and evaluated. Mechanisms for communication and "paper tracking" must be in place to promote efficacy of the medication and avoidance of untoward responses and medication errors.

With the skyrocketing costs of medications, the nurse in any community setting is likely to become aware of clients who need assistance paying for their prescriptions. Ready resources for the nurse and client are pharmaceutical companies' assistance programs.

The backbone of health promotion and disease prevention is the client knowledge base. The role of the nurse in establishing this base is critical. A comprehensive discus-

FIGURE 12–1 A community has many different faces. (A and B, Copyright 2007 JupiterImages Corporation.)

sion of client teaching is offered in Chapter 2. Assessment of learning needs and styles is another essential component to achieving the identified teaching goal (Figure 12–2).

Client Teaching

Regardless of the state and agency regulations related to medication administration in community settings, the following hints for client teaching are associated with medication administration. These hints are grouped into five categories: (1) general, (2) diet, (3) self-administration, (4) side effects, and (5) cultural considerations.

General

Within the general area, client safety is of primary concern, so a client's physical abilities require ongoing assessment. Capabilities of the client may be temporarily impaired with the use of certain drugs (e.g., narcotics, selected eye medications, psychotropics). It is essential that clients be advised not to operate hazardous machinery during such times and to use caution at all other times. It is appropriate to discuss with clients and families what situations in the

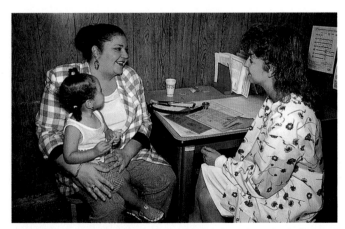

FIGURE 12–2 Effective client teaching is based on the individual client's learning needs. (From Potter PA, Perry AG: *Fundamentals of nursing*, ed 6, St. Louis, 2005, Mosby.)

daily routine require full alertness and cannot be influenced by medication for the sake of safety.

Numerous safety concerns are associated with the storage of medications. Medications should be kept in their original labeled containers, with childproof caps when needed.

The client or family should be provided with written instructions (audio instructions if client is sight impaired) about the drug regimen. Large print may be helpful or necessary. Another part of the teaching plan is to advise the client or family about any necessary laboratory tests to monitor the blood level of the medication and any possible drug-laboratory test interactions. This information should be included in the written instructions as well.

An important yet frequently misunderstood component of the written instructions is the expected therapeutic effect and the length of time required to achieve a therapeutic response from the medication. These vary widely among different medications (e.g., most narcotics act within 30 minutes; many antibiotics act within 24 hours; some psychotropics act within 6 weeks). Having clients understand the expected time frame for results can markedly diminish their concerns and promote adherence to the therapeutic plan.

The client or family must also be aware of the need to have an adequate supply of necessary medications available at all times—at home, school, work, and while traveling. It is best to order prescription refills in advance. If the pharmacy is local, at least 1 week should be allowed; several weeks should be allowed if drugs are ordered through the mail. It is a good idea to pack extra medication when going on trips, both short and extended. This is preferred at all times and is essential for foreign travel.

Impress on the client or family to first contact the health care provider before using OTC preparations. Common OTC preparations that may cause problems are laxatives, diet aids, cold and cough preparations, and overdose of fat-soluble vitamins. Reinforce with the client or family the importance of follow-up appointments with health care providers. Encourage wellness checkups, including preventive and restorative dental care, because the presence of other conditions may impact on the current therapeutic regimen. In addition, advise clients of the need to complete laboratory studies in a timely manner. Encourage clients to wear Medic-alert bands that indicate medications taken and any allergies (Herbal Alert 12–1)

When disposing of medications, remember to protect the environment. The White House Office of National Drug Control advises to "take unused, unneeded, or expired prescriptions out of their original containers and throw them in the trash". Prior to throwing in the trash, mix them in litter or used coffee grounds and place in empty cans or sealed bags. Flushing meds down the toilet

is not recommended; some drugs can kill helpful bacteria in the sewer/septic systems. The same procedure should be followed with OTC preparations.

Some pharmacies, health care providers, and governmental sites have programs providing for safe disposal of medications; contact your local resources. Refer to federal drug disposal guidelines at *www.whitehousedrugpolicy.gov/drugfact/proper_disposal.html.*

Reinforcement of the availability of community resources is important. Availability does not always equate with accessibility, so the client or family needs to know how to mobilize resources according to individual needs. Matching community resources and client needs is a prerequisite. While acknowledging the variability of each, the following are offered as examples:

- The telephone book is a frequently overlooked resource that can direct clients and families to contacts and addresses of associations of relevant health conditions (e.g., American Heart Association, American Cancer Society). Most agencies and associations have or can direct the caller to a wealth of health education resources available in a variety of media (e.g., written, audiocassettes, videotapes, occasionally braille).
- Churches may have outreach groups in which volunteers pick up prescriptions and deliver them to homebound clients.
- Pharmacists can frequently clarify a client's or family's concern over the telephone.
- Meals on Wheels enables clients to remain at home and adhere to taking medications with food.
- In a college town, students of the health professions may be motivated caregivers to assist clients or families in the community.

Clients or families need to be encouraged to have a contact person for their concerns and questions, frequently a nurse. Use of appropriate resources is likely to increase compliance with and effectiveness of the therapeutic regimen.

Diet

Diet is the second area that requires the nurse's attention. There is an overall need to advise clients or families about possible drug-food interactions, detailing which foods are to be avoided and which foods are encouraged for specific nutrient value. For example, tyramine-rich foods are contraindicated with monoamine oxidase (MAO) inhibitors, and potassium-rich foods are recommended for clients taking potassium-wasting diuretics. Alcohol may be contraindicated with selected medications. Lists of foods—and pictures when appropriate—may be helpful to clients and others involved with their diet.

Self-Administration

The third area of concern is self-administration of medications. Based on the level of the client's or family's knowledge, instructions should be given on all skills related to the drug regimen. Examples are: how to take the pulse for

---

Herbal ALERT 12–1

Community

🌿 Encourage client/family to consult the health care provider before taking herbal preparations; some products may interact with prescription or other over-the-counter (OTC) medications they are taking.

clients who take digitalis preparations, correct use and cleaning of inhalers, techniques for successful administration of parenteral medications, and how to decrease risks of infection for clients taking immunosuppressants. The nurse should allow time for instruction and questions, including demonstration of the skill and return demonstration. Clients should be given graphic illustrations for future reference as appropriate. It is essential that the nurse provide the client or family with the name of a contact person and telephone number for questions and concerns. It is not uncommon for a client or family member to return-demonstrate a skill (e.g., administration of insulin, use of inhaler) with relative ease and then forget information or become confused when trying self-administration of the drug when alone.

Side Effects

Side effects are the fourth area for client teaching. The client or family should be advised about general side effects of the medications. This is not done to scare clients but rather to inform them about the more commonly occurring side effects. Clients need to know when to notify their health care provider if they experience an adverse reaction.

Cultural Considerations

Cultural considerations are the fifth general area of concern. Initially the nurse assesses the client's personal beliefs (Figure 12–3). Based on these beliefs, the nurse then modifies communications to meet client or family cultural practices. The nurse needs to communicate respect for the client or family culture at all times. It is incumbent on the nurse to assess his or her own beliefs and biases related to cultural competence and diversity. Then one needs to evaluate the effectiveness of interactions and their acceptability within the cultural realm. For a comprehensive presentation of cultural considerations, see Chapter 6.

FIGURE 12–3 Providing culturally sensitive care starts with an assessment of the client's and family's particular beliefs, customs, and preferences. (From Harkreader H, Hogan MA, Thobaben M: *Fundamentals of nursing: caring and clinical judgment,* ed 3, St. Louis, 2007, Saunders.)

Culturally sensitive and competent health care promotes client or family compliance with the therapeutic regimen. Respect for cultural diversity may be demonstrated by inclusion of traditional and folk practices into the plans for improved communication, health promotion, and disease prevention. Although applicable to multiple settings, the following are some common cultural concerns presented as examples for illustrative purposes (Purnell 2003).

Home Care

Hispanics and Asians/Pacific Islanders frequently say they agree with the plan of care out of respect for health care providers, although they may not intend to follow it. This practice may have dangerous or life-threatening outcomes. Egyptians are accustomed to the oral tradition of communication and thus may not keep reliable written records for medication schedules and glucose monitoring results. A call from an Amish family is probably a true emergency because of their religious and cultural obligations to care for themselves first before seeking outside resources. Food rituals are important to the Appalachian, Jewish, Muslim, and Asian/Pacific Island people and must be incorporated into the plan of care if a prescription is to be followed. Self-medication and self-diagnosis are common among Asians.

School

African-American grandmothers play a significant role in dealing with health care concerns and must be included in the plans for care. Because being overweight is seen as positive to many African Americans, the health care provider may need to reeducate clients (children and families) in this cultural group frequently and carefully explain the health risks associated with obesity.

Work Site

African Americans have increased risk for development of hypertension. They prefer to be addressed formally. For Asians/Pacific Islanders, confidentiality is especially important, and they may not provide needed information if they perceive that the information might be shared and other community members may obtain knowledge about their health problems. It may be difficult for outsiders to develop rapport with Appalachian people because of past inequities from government agencies.

A summary of these guidelines is presented in Box 12–1.

Community-Based Settings

Home Setting

The home setting provides nurses with many challenges related to medication administration. A major question that quickly arises is, "Who can administer medications in the home setting?" The response does not develop so quickly.

In general, medications are administered by licensed nurses in the home setting according to the order of the health care provider. Drugs that are administered by

Box 12–1

Summary of Client Teaching Hints About Medication Use and Administration in the Community

General

- Client safety is of primary concern.
- Client's physical abilities require ongoing assessment.
- Keep or store medications in original labeled containers with childproof caps when needed.
- Provide client or family with written instructions (audio instructions if sight impaired) about the drug regimen.
- Advise client or family about the expected therapeutic effect and length of time to achieve a therapeutic response from the medication; also inform clients of the expected duration of treatment.
- Advise client or family about possible drug-laboratory test interaction.
- Advise client of nonpharmacologic measures to promote therapeutic response.
- Advise client or family to have adequate supply of necessary medications available.
- Caution against the use of over-the-counter (OTC) preparations without first contacting the health care provider.
- Reinforce the importance of follow-up appointments with health care providers.
- Encourage clients to wear Medical-Alert band that indicates medications and allergies.
- Reinforce that community resources are available and need to be mobilized according to client or family needs.

Diet

- Advise client/family/student/employee about possible drug-food interactions.
- Advise client/family/student/employee what foods are contraindicated.
- Advise client/family/student/employee regarding alcohol use.

Self-Administration

- Instruct client/family/student/employee regarding drug dose and dosing schedule.
- Instruct client/family/student/employee on all psychomotor skills related to the drug regimen.
- Provide client/family/student/employee with contact person and telephone number for questions and concerns.

Side Effects

- Advise client/family/student/employee about general side effects and adverse reactions of the medications.
- Advise client/family/student/employee when to notify health care provider.

Cultural Considerations

- Assess personal beliefs of client/family/student/employee.
- Modify communications to meet cultural needs of client/family/student/employee.
- Communicate respect for client/family/student/employee culture.

nursing personnel in the home must be approved by the Food and Drug Administration (FDA). The nurse also initiates instructions about the medication to the client or family (Figure 12–4). The licensed nurse may also administer the medication on a short-term basis for a disease-related condition if a caregiver with an order from the health care provider is unable to do so.

The order from the health care provider must be current and complete (drug, dosage, frequency, route of administration, and signature). The medication must be labeled by the pharmacist or health care provider. The nurse should not administer any medication that is not properly labeled. It is the nurse's responsibility to contact the health care provider, pharmacist, or other group identified by the agency with any concerns about the medication for a specific client. The expiration date must be checked at the time of each administration. Storage and deterioration of the medication are also evaluated. Significant side effects, allergies, and adverse reactions are reported promptly to the health care provider. Each client is assessed for allergies before administering the drug.

The establishment of policy and procedures for medication administration promotes safety and consistency; however, errors do occur. When a medication error occurs, it is reported to the health care provider and nursing supervisor. The client and family are instructed when to notify the nurse or health care provider if an adverse drug reaction is suspected. Ultimately the health care provider should be notified of all adverse drug reactions.

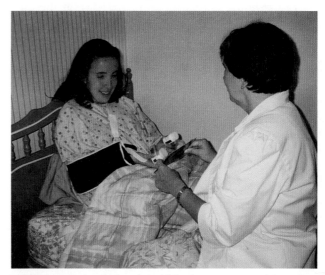

FIGURE 12–4 A vital aspect of home care is teaching clients about medications.

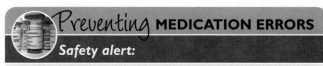

Preventing MEDICATION ERRORS

Safety alert:

- Do not give (or take) medications in the dark; proper lighting is important to avoid errors.
- Dispose of all medications in a safe manner.

An agency policy for medication administration generally addresses guidelines for specific medications. Examples of these specific agents include allergy vaccines, chemotherapy, gamma globulin, gold, experimental drugs, and narcotics. The guidelines are agency-specific and may include that the first dose of allergy vaccine be given by the health care provider in a controlled environment or that family members be taught how to administer narcotics to the client by the parenteral route if the order is so written by the health care provider. When the order is discontinued, the health care provider needs to be notified if any unused narcotics are in the home. Licensed practical nurses may not administer gamma globulin intravenously, and family members may not be taught to administer selected drugs (e.g., iron dextran [Imferon]). Chemotherapy for cancer commonly presents a special challenge. The client's blood work must be current before the administration of the chemotherapeutic drugs, the client must be under regular and ongoing care of a physician, and safety requirements may be identified (e.g., gloves and goggles may be used).

Certified home health aides work under the supervision of the registered nurse. Home health aides are commonly asked to administer medications to a client by the client, family, or friends. In the current health care environment, the home health aide may receive pressure to administer medications, but legally home health aides may only assist with medications the client customarily self-administers.

Additional challenges related to medication administration in the home setting include adherence to the therapeutic regimen, especially the right drug, right dose, and right time. Some clients need but do not have a primary caregiver to oversee follow-up with medications and other aspects of care. The quality and preparation of meals may also be a factor related to medication administration, such as what foods to avoid with certain medications and what foods complement a medication. In addition, it may be difficult for clients to get their medications and to get them in a timely manner. Coordinated skill may be required by the client or family, for example, with the use of an inhaler or administration of insulin. In all these situations, the nurse is frequently the person who coordinates the resources.

School Setting

Health and education are natural partners. The ability to learn is influenced by health factors.

The Centers for Disease Control and Prevention (CDC) summarized the benefits of care of chronic health conditions as: improved attendance, alertness, and physical stamina; fewer symptoms and restrictions on taking part in physical activities; and decreased numbers of emergencies.

Administration of medications in the school setting is of special concern. A recent study reports that in any given two-week time interval, about 13 million children in grades K-12 take medications. The most frequently taken medications were drugs for ADHD, OTC preparations, and medications for the treatment of asthma. In addition, there was a dramatic increase in the kinds of medications taken at school: from 58 in the late 1980s to 200 currently. School health services are not immune from the phenomenon of downsizing personnel, and many school systems are dealing with the questions "Where are the nurses?" and "Who is responsible for the administration of medication?"

In the absence of federal and state law, some school districts have elected not to employ school nurses. The average national caseload for a school nurse is an alarming 3098 students. This is a reality despite the long-standing recommendation of having one registered nurse for every 750 students. Coupled with this is the impact of a federal law that entitles children with handicaps to attend public schools in their residential areas. It is not unreasonable to assume that these children have special needs that may require professional nursing services (Figure 12-5).

In 1990 the Office of School Health Policy of the University of Colorado Health Sciences Center recognized that medication administration was a serious policy issue. Massachusetts developed its model with a goal "to develop regulations that provided minimum standards for the safe and proper administration of prescription medications in the Commonwealth schools" (Sheetz, Blum 1998). The development of this model has many strengths, including representation of professional associations, community groups, and regulatory bodies. Consistent consent forms were designed and adopted, and orientation and training programs were instituted for all personnel in school health positions. The established regulations apply to both public and nonpublic schools. This model appears to have applicability to other states that are grappling with the important child health issue of medication administration in schools.

The Minnesota Guidelines for Medication Administration in Schools (May 2005) are organized as follows: legal considerations; roles; staffing; delegation of medication administration by the licensed school nurse/registered nurse; general procedures for medication administration; education and training; policies and procedures; quality assur-

FIGURE 12-5 Many schoolchildren have special health needs. (From James SR, Ashwill J: *Nursing care of children: principles and practice,* ed 3, St. Louis, 2007, Saunders.)

ance, monitoring, and assessment; school and family relationships; and finances. Guideline #5, General Procedures for Medical Administration, is presented in Box 12–2.

It is essential that nurses be aware of the policies and procedures for medication administration in their own state, county, and school system. Standardized policies for medication administration are necessary for safe practice and should promote self-management programs for students with chronic conditions such as asthma and diabetes. Nurses must get actively involved in developing these policies and in ensuring that the needs of individual students are met.

In some states or school systems, persons who are not nurses may be responsible for medication administration. This presents additional concerns that need to be addressed, such as adherence to instructions and to the principle that medication administration is a process, more than merely "giving the student a pill." A major component of medication administration is assessment of the need for the medication and its effectiveness of action. The effectiveness of action includes being alert to side effects and adverse reactions that the client may experience.

While recognizing the variability among policies on medication administration, Igoe and Speer (1996) identified the following basic requirements for administration of medications in schools:

1. Medications are given only with parents' written permission.

2. Medications requiring a prescription are given only on the written authorization of a health care provider.
3. For medications requiring a prescription, there must be an individual pharmacy-labeled bottle for each student.
4. Medications must be recorded by the school personnel who administer them. This record states the student's name, medication, dosage, time, and the name of the person administering the medication.
5. Medications must be stored in a secure, locked, clean container or cabinet.

Child care and adult day care services have similar rules for the administration of medications. In general, these facilities administer medications or supervise self-administration within the Nurse Practice Act of the specific state. In addition, most facilities require labeling of medications in accordance with the Pharmacy Rules and Regulations of the specific state. Guidelines for safe storage of medications must be followed, including the rule that medications be accessible only to personnel responsible for their administration or for distribution of self-administered medications. Some states require that internal and external medications be stored separately. Care must be taken to ensure that prescription medications be used only for whom the medication was prescribed.

The National Association of School Nurses (*www.nasn.org*) is a good resource for information on the many-faceted aspects of school nursing.

> ## Box 12–2
>
> ### Guideline #5: General Procedures for Medication Administration
>
> Principle 1: Guarantee that medication administration is a clean procedure by washing hands.
> Principle 2: Give medication exactly as ordered by the health care provider or indicated on manufacturer's instructions.
> Principle 3: Everything should be done to avoid "no-shows," especially for seizure medications and antibiotics.
> Principle 4: Prevent errors! Do not allow yourself to be distracted. Do not use one student's medication for another.
> Principle 5: Keep individual student information private.
> Principle 6: Apply child development principles when working with students (e.g., students generally do not want to be considered unique).
> Principle 7: If there is an error or medication incident, it must be reported. Follow district procedure for notifying your school nurse, administration (WITHIN 24 HOURS), the student's parent/legal guardian, and physician. Complete documentation. It is important to act as soon as the error is discovered. The school administrator or supervisor should evaluate errors by all persons administering medications.

Data from Minnesota Guidelines for Medication Administration in Schools, May 2005. Retrieved April 11, 2008 from *http://www.health.state.mn.us/divs/cfh/shs/pubs/medadmin/guide5.html*.

Work Setting

Most adult Americans and many youth are employed and spend a significant amount of time at the work site on a regular basis; thus the work site is an ideal setting to promote personal health behaviors and decrease environmental hazards.

Healthy employees are more productive than unhealthy employees. This fact, coupled with the escalating costs of health care and insurance, has inspired many businesses to offer some type of health care at the work site. This care may range from emergency first aid and work-related health and safety problems to the provision of primary care and referral services.

Occupational and environmental health nursing is a specialty practice that provides for and delivers health care services to workers and worker populations. The practice is autonomous and focuses on the promotion, protection, and restoration of workers' health within the context of a safe and healthy work environment. According to the American Association of Occupational Health Nurses (AAOHN) occupational and environmental health nurses may function in a variety of roles, including (but not limited to) solo practitioner, manager, educator, consultant, nurse practitioner, case manager, and corporate director, and these nurses often work with the other members of an occupational health and safety team (e.g., medicine, safety, industrial hygiene) (AAOHN, 2001).

The nurse needs to be aware of the policies and procedures for administration of medication at the specific work site. There is great diversity in policy and procedure among settings. For example, the following are two of the many current practices at work sites:

- At one setting the registered nurse essentially follows protocols for selected employee complaints (e.g., back injuries: acute and chronic; burns: thermal, chemical, and electrical; eye emergencies; herpes; adult immunizations). Each protocol includes the following areas with relevant information for the specific complaint: assessment, treatment/medications, client education, referral, and follow-up. Medications are identified as appropriate and noted under the treatment/medications section with the stated drug, dosage, frequency, and route.
- Another work site has established self-care stations for minor illnesses and injuries. Each station has designated criteria for use. Examples include stations for colds, superficial cuts, and menstrual cramps. Employees are familiarized with this service as part of the orientation process. Upon arrival at the stations, employees note date, time, and signature on the sign-in sheet posted at each station. They indicate their chief complaint or reason for seeking medication and the specific OTC medications they have taken from the OTC preparations supplied at each station.

An excellent resource for care of clients in the work setting is the AAOHN website: *www.aaohn.org*.

Summary

This chapter discusses only a minute, but significant, portion of the nurse's role in a variety of community settings. Specifically the focus is on selected concerns associated with the administration of medications and the need to practice in accordance with the Nurse Practice Act of a specific state. The role of the nurse in drug administration is growing in complexity. The nurse in the twenty-first century must have a strong knowledge base.

Nursing Process

Overview of Medication Administration

ASSESSMENT

- Obtain appropriate vital signs and relevant laboratory test results for future comparisons and evaluation of the therapeutic response.
- Obtain drug history (prescription, over-the-counter, and herbal preparations), including drug allergies.
- Identify high-risk clients/students/employees for reactions.
- Assess client's/student's/employee's capability to follow therapeutic regimen.

- Determine client/student/employee learning needs.

NURSING DIAGNOSES

- Risk for injury related to possible adverse reaction
- Risk for ineffective therapeutic regimen management
- Deficient knowledge related to therapeutic regimen
- Effective therapeutic regimen management related to medication administration

PLANNING

- Identify goals.
- Promote therapeutic response and prevent or minimize adverse reactions.
- Identify strategies to promote adherence.
- Identify interventions.

NURSING INTERVENTIONS

- Prepare equipment and environment; wash hands.
- Determine allergies and other assessment data.
- Check drug label three times; check expiration date.
- Be certain of drug calculation; verify dose with another registered nurse as necessary.
- Pour liquids at eye level on flat surface.
- Keep all drugs stored properly, especially related to temperature, light, and moisture.
- Avoid contact with topical and inhalation preparations.
- Verify client/student/employee identification.
- Administer only drugs you have prepared.
- Assist the client to desired position.
- Discard needles and syringes in "sharps" container.
- Follow policy related to discarding drugs and controlled substances.
- Report drug errors immediately.
- Document all appropriate information in a timely manner.
- Record effectiveness of drugs administered and reason for any drugs refused.

Cultural Considerations ❖

- When language barriers are present, use literature and videos in client's preferred language and with pictures of that group to promote compliance with health interventions.
- Obtain an interpreter when necessary; do not rely on family members, who may not fully disclose because of honor and shame. Provide interpreter with the same ethnic background and gender if possible, especially with sensitive topics.
- When offering a prescription, instructions, or pamphlets to Asians and Pacific Islanders, use both hands to show respect.
- Include grandmothers when providing support and health teaching in the African American population.

• Encourage clients to disclose the use of folk healers and treatments prescribed. Incorporate harmless and nonconflicting practices into the therapeutic plan.

EVALUATION

■ Evaluate effectiveness of medication(s) administered.

■ Identify expected time frame of desired drug response; consider need for modification of therapy.

■ Determine client/student/employee satisfaction with regimen.

■ Determine client/student/employee knowledge of medication regimen.

KEY WEBSITES

Directory of Prescription Drug Patient Assistance Programs: www.phrma.org

American Association of Occupational Health Nurses (AAOHN): www.aaohn.org

National Association of School Nurses (NASN): www.nasn.org

 ## Critical Thinking Case Study

The Rivera family (José, age 30; wife, Maria, age 29, 7 months pregnant; children José Jr, age 11; Angel, age 8; Tony, age 7) recently moved into a new community. José is employed full time by a large credit card corporation, and Maria handles the child care and works part time as a cashier.

1. Give examples of culturally sensitive and competent care for the Rivera children in the school setting.
2. Identify culturally sensitive and competent care for the parents at the work sites.
3. What modifications would you suggest for a family of African-American heritage?

 ## NCLEX Study Questions

1. You are preparing for a health teaching session with your client. The most important information in the general area is:
   a. foods to avoid
   b. client safety
   c. storage of medication
   d. lab test results

2. Teaching related to OTC preparations in all settings includes the importance of contacting the health care provider:
   a. if using products
   b. if symptoms persist
   c. when meds "run out"
   d. when adding an herbal product

3. Grandmothers from what culture are known to play a significant role in dealing with health care issues?
   a. Pacific Islanders
   b. Asians
   c. African Americans
   d. Europeans

4. In general, who administers medications when working in the home care setting?
   a. neighbors
   b. nurses aides
   c. advanced practice nurses
   d. licensed nurses

5. Guidelines for use of interpreters do not include:
   a. do not rely on family members
   b. same ethnicity
   c. same gender
   d. do rely on family members

Answers: 1. b; 2. a; 3. c; 4. d; 5. d.

13

The Role of the Nurse in Drug Research

ELECTRONIC RESOURCES

Evolve website (http://evolve.elsevier.com/KeeHayes/pharmacology/):
- *Case Studies*
- *Content Updates*
- *Frequently Asked Questions*
- *Student Review Activities*
- *WebLinks*
- *Additional Reference Material*

Companion CD-ROM:
- *NCLEX Examination Review Questions*
- *Pharmacology Animations*
- *IV Therapy Checklists*
- *Medication Error Checklists*
- *Drug Calculation Problems*
- *Electronic Calculators*
- *Top 200 Drugs with Pronunciations*
- *References from the Textbook*

Outline

Objectives

- Discuss basic ethical principles.
- Relate three basic ethical principles governing informed consent and risk-to-benefit ratio.
- Describe the objectives of each phase of human clinical experimentation.
- Describe the role of the nurse in clinical drug trials using the nursing process.

Terms

News broadcasts or headlines often announce the release of a new drug for the treatment of acquired immunodeficiency syndrome (AIDS) or multiple sclerosis, an increase in a drug company's research and development budget, Food and Drug Administration (FDA) approval for promising drugs, or similar pharmacology-related news.

Such news items signal increasing awareness of the importance of drug research. Drug research involves risk and is also a "high-cost item," with the estimated average cost to develop each new drug being more than $800 million.

In the United States, all prescription drugs must be approved by the FDA prior to availability on the market.

Drug studies take place in a variety of inpatient and outpatient settings.

Drug research and development are complex processes that are of particular interest and importance to professional nursing practice. The nursing process facilitates the integration of cutting-edge research.

This chapter is devoted to a description of basic ethical principles governing informed consent and risk-to-benefit ratio, preclinical testing and human clinical experimentation, and the nurse's role and nursing process in clinical drug trials.

Basic Ethical Principles

Four basic ethical principles are relevant to research involving human subjects: (1) respect for persons, (2) beneficence, (3) justice, and (4) truth telling.

Respect for Person

Individuals undergoing treatment in any health care system should be treated as independent persons who are capable of making decisions in their own best interests. Individuals whose decision-making capability is diminished are entitled to protection. The nurse can determine this with consistent reassessment of the client's cognitive state. Clients should be made aware of the alternatives available to them in their health care, as well as the consequences that stem from those alternatives. Furthermore, the client's choice should be honored whenever possible. It is imperative that the nurse recognize when the client is not capable of rational decision making and therefore entitled to protection.

Autonomy is an integral component of *respect for persons*. **Autonomy** is the right of self-determination. In health care settings, health care personnel must respect the client's right to make decisions about themselves, even if the decision is not what the personnel wanted or thought was best for the client. Generally clients can refuse any and all treatments (*right of autonomy*) except when the decision poses a threat to others, such as with tuberculosis, when taking medications is legally mandated. Clients have the right to refuse to participate in a research study and may withdraw from the study at any time without penalty of any kind.

Beneficence

Beneficence is the duty to not harm others, to maximize possible benefits, and to minimize possible harm that might occur in research. It is often not possible to know whether something is beneficial unless it is tested and individuals have been exposed to the risks. A central question to this issue is Who makes this decision—the client or those caring for the client?

Justice

Justice requires that all people be treated fairly. Expansion of justice includes equal access to health care for all. Justice can be limited when it interferes with the rights of others.

The principle of justice, in the context of clinical drug trials means that social benefits and burdens can be allocated objectively and that those with equivalent circumstances should be treated equally. A challenge to the nurse is the allocation of scarce resources.

Truth telling (veracity) is a principle that requires health care personnel to tell the truth and the whole truth. When there is "bad news" to tell the client, the health care provider may be reluctant to tell the truth and answer questions honestly. The client has the right to know the truth, including the bad news. The principles of respect for person, beneficence, justice, and truth telling are integral to the issues of informed consent and risk-to-benefit ratio in research involving human subjects.

Informed Consent

Informed consent has its roots in the 1947 Nuremberg Code. The two most relevant aspects of this Code are the participant's right to be informed and that participation is voluntary, without coercion. If the nurse suspects that a client is being coerced to participate in a study, the nurse is obligated to report this promptly to the party named on the informed consent (the client should have copy of consent for reference). **Informed consent** has dimensions beyond protection of the individual client's choice and includes the following:

1. Promotion of individual autonomy
2. Protection of clients and subjects from harm
3. Avoidance of fraud and duress in health care
4. Encouragement for professionals to be thorough and clear in communicating information
5. Promotion of educated decision making among clients
6. Promotion of self-determination of the client

It is the role of the health care providers, *not* the nurse, to explain the study to the client (including the expectations of the client) and to respond to questions. During this time of giving written consent, the client must be alert and able to comprehend.

It is the nurse's role to protect clients from any anticipated harm. The nurse, in collaboration with the health care provider and pharmacist, must be knowledgeable about all aspects of the drug study, including all inclusion and exclusion criteria for participants (see Box 13–3 on p. 221).

Figure 13–1 shows an example of Permission for Clinical Investigation and Box 13–1 an Informed Consent Checklist form.

Risk-to-Benefit Ratio

The risk-to-benefit ratio is one of the most complex problems faced by the researcher. All possible consequences of a clinical study must be analyzed and balanced with the inherent risks and the anticipated benefits. Physical, psychological, and social risks must be identified and weighed against the benefits. A requirement of the Department of Health and Human Services (DHHS) is that institutional review boards (IRBs) determine that "risks to subjects are

Memorial Hospital
PERMISSION FOR CLINICAL INVESTIGATION

Completed by Client:

1. I hereby authorize Dr. _____ and/or such assistants as may be selected by him/her to conduct studies upon _____ for the following: _____

2. I further authorize Dr. _____ and/or such assistants as may be selected by him/her, to prescribe drugs or to perform certain procedures in connection with the diagnosis and treatment of my condition including the following drugs and/or extraordinary procedures: _____

3. I have (have not) been made aware of certain risks, possible consequences and discomfort associated with these drugs or extraordinary procedures which are: _____

4. I understand that no guarantee or assurance has been made as to the results that may be obtained although I have (have not) been advised of the possibility that certain benefits may be expected such as: _____

5. I have (have not) had explained to me alternative procedures/treatments/drugs that may be advantageous and they include the following: _____

6. I have (have not) received an offer to answer any inquiries concerning the procedures involved

7. I have (have not) had explained to me all medical terminology in connection with this study

8. I understand that it is in the intent of the principal investigator to maintain the confidentiality of records identifying subjects in this study. The Food and Drug Administration, however, may possibly inspect the records to monitor compliance with published federal regulations.

9. I understand that I may withdraw this consent and discontinue participation in this study at any time, without prejudice to my care, by informing Dr. _____ of my desire to withdraw. _____ Yes, I understand _____ No, I do not understand

10. I understand that Department of Health and Human Services regulations require the Memorial Hospital to inform me of any provisions to provide for medical treatment for any physical injury which may occur as a result of this study. In this connection, I understand that the Memorial Hospital does not have a formal plan or program to provide for the cost of medical treatment or compensation for any physical injury which occurs as a result of this study and for which they do not have legal liability. However, in the unlikely event that I am injured as a result of my participation, I understand that I should promptly inform Dr. _____

SIGNED _____

RELATIONSHIP _____

ADDRESS _____

DATED _____

Completed by witness:

I, the undersigned, hereby acknowledge that I was present during the explanation of the above consent for clinical investigation given by Dr. _____ to _____ during which the nature, purpose, risks, complications and consequences thereof were fully set forth and all questions answered and I was present while _____ signed the above consent.

Dated _____

_____
(witness)

_____
(address)

FIGURE 13–1 Example of informed consent.

Box 13–1

Informed Consent Checklist

- Participates voluntarily
- Identifies related drugs, treatments, and techniques
- Describes benefits and risks
- Describes other forms of treatment available
- Describes laboratory tests to monitor client's reactions
- Identifies extent of confidentiality of results
- Describes availability of emergency treatment for illness/injury, if any
- States compensation for study-related injury, if any
- States compensation for participation, if any
- Writes consent clearly and understands easily at the 10th-grade reading level
- Provides name and telephone number of contact person for client questions and concerns

Box 13–2

Basic Sequence of New Drug Development

1. Identification of potentially clinically useful chemical entity
2. Preclinical testing
3. Study designs
4. Human clinical experimentation
   - Phase I
   - Phase II
   - Phases III and IV

reasonable in relation to anticipated benefits, if any, to subjects" (DHHS, 1981). No matter how noble the intentions, the calculation of risks and benefits by the researcher cannot be totally accurate or comprehensive.

Varying amounts of time are required for the process of identifying a potentially useful chemical and having it become available to the general population; in many cases, 10 years may elapse. Only 1 in 10,000 potential drugs endures the research and development process and is used in a clinical situation. Box 13–2 lists the basic sequence of the development of a new drug.

Objectives and Phases of Human Clinical Experimentation

Good Clinical Practice (GCP): Consolidated Guideline, an international ethical and scientific standard for design, conduct, performance, monitoring, auditing, recording, analysis, and reporting, is the foundation of clinical trials. Guidance and information sheets are available from the FDA on multiple topics related to clinical trials. Examples include information sheets for IRBs and Clinical Investigators and Choice of Control Groups and Related Issues in Clinical Trials. Websites with this and expanded information are U.S. National Institutes of Health at *http://clinicaltrials.gov* and TrialsCentral at *http://trialscentral.org*. In addition, the World Medical Association **Declaration of Helsinki** has crafted ethical principles for medical research involving human subjects. This and other relevant websites are listed at the end of this chapter.

Preclinical Testing

Preclinical testing consists of in vitro and in vivo systems. In vitro experimentation is generally conducted in a test tube or other laboratory equipment, and in vivo testing is conducted with living organisms. This testing is followed by toxicity screening for the purposes of identifying (1) abnormal changes in animal organs related to drug administration and (2) the parameters of the safe therapeutic dose. Control and experimental groups of animals are compared. Participants in the **experimental group** receive the experimental intervention or treatment. Those in the **control group** do not receive the experimental intervention or treatment and provide a baseline against which to measure the effects of the treatment. Before initiating human studies, an assessment is made of the seriousness of the disease to be treated using this drug in relation to the drug's toxicity.

Human Clinical Experimentation

For every 5000 to 10,000 compounds screened as potential new medications, only five are entered into clinical trials. To bring a new drug to market takes an average of 9 to 12 years, and costs continue to rise. The cost is currently greater than $1.1 billion per drug. The **FDA Modernization Act of 1997** increased the minimum age for subjects of human clinical experimentation. The Act has five provisions, one of which requires pediatric evaluation of new products intended for use by children. The Act advocates for children and appropriate testing for drugs to be used by the pediatric population. The automatic universal exclusion of children from clinical trials is not justified. Refer to Chapter 5 for a listing of all the provisions of this act.

Clinical experimentation in drug research and development encompasses four phases, each with its own objectives. A multidisciplinary team approach (nurses, physicians, pharmacologists, statisticians, and research associates) is required to ensure throughout the phases that the data collected will answer the clinical questions. A brief description of each phase follows.

Phase I

Phase I trials are primarily designed to assess safety. The objectives of phase I are to determine the human dosage range based on response in healthy human subjects and to identify the pharmacokinetics (i.e., absorption, distribution, metabolism/biotransformation, excretion/elimination) of the drug. Progression to the next phase occurs if no serious adverse effects are demonstrated, the drug is eliminated in a reasonable amount of time, and the dose range is below that known to induce pathology in animals.

Phase II

The objective of phase II is to demonstrate the safety and efficacy of the drug in subjects ($n = 100$) who have the disease the drug is designed to treat. Phase III is initiated only when acceptable efficacy and safety data are generated and clearly documented in Phase II.

Phases III and IV

Phase III studies involve large numbers of subjects with the disease intended for treatment. The objectives of phases III and IV are to demonstrate the safety and efficacy of the drug for a wide client population and to include long-term data if a chronic regimen is under consideration. Phase IV studies may also examine potential new indications for approved drugs. The sponsor submits all relevant and analyzed data in a new drug application (NDA) to the FDA. In time the FDA decides to approve, reject, or recommend withdrawal or resubmission. After the NDA research has been approved, phase IV addresses the long-term use of the drug.

The pharmaceutical industry is eager to get new drugs to market. Delays in the FDA approval process were decreasing the valuable life of a drug's patent; therefore in 1992 Congress passed the **Prescription Drug User Fee Act,** which provided the FDA with funds to expedite the review process. As a result, the average drug approval time has decreased from 30 to 12 months.

Challenges and new directions await clinical trial programs of the future. Specifically, future trials are needed for certain populations at risk, such as profiling client and tumor for cancer-related trials.

Study Designs

An appropriate experimental design is important in being able to answer questions about drug safety and efficacy. The experimental design uses different groups of subjects (i.e., some groups who receive treatment and control groups who receive no treatment, an alternative treatment, or a combination of both), and assigns subjects randomly to treatment or control groups. Treatment groups and control groups do not differ in terms of baseline characteristics or demographics. If the subjects are different, variability is introduced and it becomes more difficult to determine a treatment effect. The following examples illustrate selected research designs:

A *quasi-experimental* design would be a comparison of intermittent intravenous (IV) device patency of those hospitalized clients who received heparin flushes and those who received saline flushes. This study would have a nonmatched comparison group but no random assignment to a treatment group. Such quasi-experimental designs may contribute valuable information but ultimately lack the power to ascribe *cause*, because the variables are uncontrolled and potentially influential. Ethical decisions do not permit the use of this experimental design in all situations. For example, an experimental study to determine whether nicotine causes cancer would be unethical because individuals would have to be exposed to a carcinogenic substance. However, it might be possible to use an already exposed group (smokers) as a comparator.

A researcher designs a study to show the effect of the independent variable (the drug) on the dependent variables (clinical responses or reactions). Intervening variables are specific to the research question and may include age, sex, weight, disease and its state of severity, diet, and the subject's social environment. It is important to control for as many of the intervening variables as possible to make it easier to determine whether there is a drug effect. Controlled treatment groups in drug research trials can receive no drug, a different drug, a **placebo** (pharmacologically inert substance), or the same drug with a different dose, route, or frequency of administration. A control group receiving a different drug is called an **active control.**

In some cases, such as cancer treatment, it would not be ethical to use a placebo as a control.

A *crossover* design uses each subject in several different situations. In the first instance, the experimental group receives the drug and the control group receives an alternative form of treatment or no treatment. Then both groups receive no therapy. Finally, the experimental group receives the control form of therapy and the control group receives the drug. In this design, the subject serves as his or her own control.

The researcher wants to generalize the findings from the sample of subjects to the larger target population, such as all women with breast cancer. A statistical method called *probability sampling* (subjects are randomly selected from the entire population) is typically used to provide relative confidence in the generalization of findings.

Various designs and techniques assist the researcher to reach valid, generalizable conclusions. In a *matched-pair* design, the researcher identifies several variables that may influence the outcome such as age, weight, or family history; then the subjects are matched for these variables. One of the pair is randomly assigned to the experimental group and the other to the control group. A less effective technique is nonrandom assignment to treatment group.

The **double-blind** technique is a powerful tool wherein neither the health care provider nor the subject knows whether the subject is receiving the experimental or control form of therapy. In **triple-blind** studies, a researcher other than the prescribing health care provider collects data and is also unaware of the subject's treatment group. In a **single-blind** study, only the subjects are unaware of which group to which they are assigned. An **open-label study** indicates that all parties—data collectors, prescribing health care provider, and subject—know the treatment group assignment. The double-blind and triple-blind techniques are preferred for drug research, because those involved in the study are not aware of the subject's treatment group, thereby removing a source of bias.

Nurse's Role

The nurse has a pivotal role in drug clinical trials. The research and development process for drug research requires the multifaceted roles of professional nursing practice. Nurses must first consider their own thoughts, feelings, and beliefs about clinical trials. The nurse is both the client and family advocate and the liaison between the client, health care provider, and research nurse responsible for the specific protocol. Communication that is both thorough and timely is essential in all aspects of the nurse's role. Nursing involvement is pivotal to the successful completion of clinical trials.

Asking relevant questions about informed consent and risk-to-benefit ratio is a major role of the nurse. Refer to the website for the Health Insurance Portability and Accountability Act (HIPAA) implications for clinical trials (e.g., consent and privacy issues). Awareness of initial indicators of change in the client and prediction of increased risk for adverse drug reaction are also dimensions of professional nursing practice.

Nursing responsibilities related to the specific research or clinical trial span the nursing process. Critical to the assessment phase are the recruitment and assessment of study subjects; a thorough understanding of the protocol, including inclusion and exclusion criteria for subjects; validity and reliability of measurement instruments; ongoing teamwork; and communication with the health care providers and sponsors.

Nursing input is important in the budget negotiations of the clinical trial as well as staff education on protocol requirements. Protocol guidelines are an essential component of staff education with special attention to ensuring that the subject's consent is "informed consent" obtained by the health care provider. The nurse is an ongoing resource when subject and family questions arise.

Protocol-based nursing implementations include comprehensive screening of subjects and monitoring parameters per protocol with relevant and timely communication with the entire health care team. Documentation on all predetermined components throughout the clinical trial is mandatory, including input from study subjects.

During the evaluation phase, the nurse's role involves examining the research statement or question. In addition, it considers elements such as Are the conclusions valid and data-based? Are the findings clinically significant?

Recent Developments and What Is on the Horizon

Tomorrow's anti–human immunodeficiency virus (HIV) drugs will block HIV from entering the cell; other compounds will promote plaque regression in individuals with Alzheimer's disease. There is expectation of more powerful drugs to supplement—and possibly replace—selected cardiac surgery. Anticancer drugs will attack only cells with abnormal growth (not healthy cells). In addition, there is major vaccine research for AIDS, Alzheimer's disease, and cancer. Highly lucrative drugs go "off patent." When a drug goes off patent, other companies are free to make their own form of the same drug, thus increasing competition among the pharmaceutical companies and resulting in lower drug costs.

Synthetic antibiotics, such as linezolid (Zyvox), are one of the first new classes of antibiotics in 30 years. Examples of drugs in the development pipeline include an injectable agent for non-small cell lung cancer with metastases to the brain, a product reformulation as disease-modifying therapy for multiple sclerosis, and an amphetamine derivative for treatment of ADHD. The FDA approves drugs based on safety and efficacy but does not address whether the drug is safer or more effective than other drugs. Objective, reliable data are needed about which drugs are most effective. Currently there is public outcry for these data because Medicare is about to spend greater than $400 billion over the next decade on new drug benefits.

Clinical Drug Trials

ASSESSMENT

- Explore own beliefs about clinical trials.
- Recruit subjects.
- Assess subjects.
- Assess protocol.
- Demonstrate thorough knowledge of all inclusion/exclusion criteria for subjects (Box 13–3).
- Articulate observations and concerns to health care providers and sponsors/pharmaceutical company.
- Communicate need for drug to address a specific need with the appropriate individuals.

PLANNING

- Develop fact sheet of protocol guidelines.
- Educate involved staff about protocol requirements.
- Provide input into budget negotiations.
- Coordinate personnel and budget, including office visits, special tests, and laboratory work.
- Ensure that subject consent is informed (see Box 13–1 and Figure 13–1).
- Respond to subject's questions.

NURSING INTERVENTIONS

- Screen subjects accurately and thoroughly based on established protocol.
- Adhere to protocol guidelines, including administration of drug.
- Monitor selected parameters. Observe and report toxicities promptly.
- Collect all data required by the sponsor (e.g., drug company).
- Communicate information in a complete, concise, accurate, and timely manner to the principal investigator and sponsor.
- Document data in a clear and timely manner.
- Record subjects' own evaluation; seemingly unrelated responses may be significant. At times, a drug is actually marketed for a different indication than the original testing.
- Report all deaths to physician, sponsor, Institutional Review Board, and FDA, whether or not the cause of death is drug related.

Cultural Considerations ❖

- Be alert to specific side effects in selected drug groups from clients of different ethnic backgrounds (e.g., African Americans and tricyclics and other psychotropic medications).

- Use an interpreter when necessary, preferably from the same ethnicity and gender, especially for sensitive and anxiety-raising topics.
- Depending on client's background, include the extended family in the teaching and support system.

EVALUATION

- Was the research design appropriate and maintained?
- Are the conclusions valid and based on data?
- Are the clinical findings significant?

Box 13–3

Inclusion/Exclusion Criteria for a Hypothetic Protocol for an Experimental Diuretic Medication

Inclusion

- Men and women between the ages of 18 and 65 years
- Weight between 50 and 100 kg
- Subjects receive cardiac medications only if dose has been stable for past 3 months
- Subjects on sodium-restricted diet

Exclusion

- Pregnant or nursing women
- All women of childbearing age who do not responsibly use oral contraceptives
- Persons with severe damage or disease of cardiac, hepatic, renal, neurologic, or musculoskeletal system
- Clinically significant laboratory values

KEY WEBSITES

Health Insurance Portability and Accountability Act (HIPAA): www.cms.hhs.gov/hipaa/

Good Practices: www.fda.gov/oc/gcp/default.htm

Declaration of Helsinki: Recommendation for Conduct of Clinical Research: www.bioscience.org/guides/dec/hels.htm

NCLEX Study Questions

1. The right of self determination is:
   a. beneficence
   b. autonomy
   c. justice
   d. informed consent

2. Your client plans to participate in a clinical trial. The responsibility to explain the study and respond to questions lies with the:
   a. registered nurse
   b. pharmacist
   c. research associate
   d. health care provider

3. A small proportion of drugs survive the research and development process; approximately one in how many potential drugs are actually used in clinical situations?
   a. 100
   b. 1000
   c. 10,000
   d. 100,000

4. Phase I clinical trials are primarily designed to:
   a. assess safety
   b. assess efficacy
   c. demonstrate side effects
   d. demonstrate cure

5. Double- and triple-blind techniques are preferred in clinical trials because they remove:
   a. knowledge
   b. conflicts
   c. prejudice
   d. bias

6. The foundation of clinical trials is:
   a. informed consent
   b. HIPAA
   c. GCP
   d. Declaration of Helsinki

7. Which of the following is not a dimension of informed consent?
   a. protection of subjects from harm
   b. assurance of cure of disease
   c. protection of client's self determination
   d. promotion of client's educated decision making

Answers: 1, b; 2, d; 3, c; 4, a; 5, d; 6, c; 7, b.

FOUR

Nutrition and Electrolytes

*T*he body requires vitamins, minerals, and electrolytes for cellular function. When there is a lack of these chemical components, replacement drug therapy is necessary. With regular nutritional dietary intake, vitamin, mineral, and electrolyte replacements are not needed.

Multiple vitamins have the highest sales volume of any over-the-counter (OTC) drugs. Usually vitamin replacements are not necessary, especially for those who maintain a nutritionally balanced daily diet.

The vitamins discussed in Chapter 14, Vitamin and Mineral Replacement, include the fat-soluble vitamins (vitamins A, D, E, and K) and the water-soluble vitamins (vitamin B complex [B_1, B_2, B_3, B_6, and B_{12}] and C). Iron is the primary mineral described. Other minerals discussed are copper, zinc, chromium, and selenium.

Body electrolytes are plentiful in extracellular and intracellular fluids and in the gastrointestinal mucosa. The cations (positively charged ions or electrolytes)—potassium (K), sodium (Na), calcium (Ca), and magnesium (Mg)—promote transmission and conduction of nerve impulses and contractility of muscles. Inadequate dietary intake and many disease entities contribute to electrolyte imbalances. Electrolyte replacements are discussed in Chapter 15, Fluid and Electrolyte Replacement, and nutritional support is discussed in Chapter 16, Nutritional Support.

14

Vitamin and Mineral Replacement

ELECTRONIC RESOURCES

Evolve website (http://evolve.elsevier.com/KeeHayes/pharmacology/):
- *Case Studies*
- *Content Updates*
- *Frequently Asked Questions*
- *Student Review Activities*
- *WebLinks*
- *Additional Reference Material*

Companion CD-ROM:
- *NCLEX Examination Review Questions*
- *Pharmacology Animations*
- *IV Therapy Checklists*
- *Medication Error Checklists*
- *Drug Calculation Problems*
- *Electronic Calculators*
- *Top 200 Drugs with Pronunciations*
- *References from the Textbook*

Outline

Objectives

- Discuss the four justifications for the use of vitamin supplements.
- Differentiate between water- and fat-soluble vitamins.
- Relate food sources and deficiency conditions associated with each vitamin.
- Explain the need for iron and foods that are high in iron content.
- Explain the uses for iron, copper, zinc, chromium, and selenium.
- Describe the nursing interventions, including client teaching, related to vitamin and mineral uses.

Terms

This chapter discusses two topics: vitamins and minerals. These substances are needed in correct portions for normal body function. Overuse of vitamins and minerals, particularly fat-soluble vitamins and iron, may lead to vitamin or iron toxicity.

Vitamins

Vitamins are organic chemicals that are necessary for normal metabolic functions and for tissue growth and healing. The body needs only a small amount of vitamins daily, which can be easily obtained through one's diet. A well-balanced diet has all the vitamins and minerals needed for body functioning. The intake of vitamins should be increased by those experiencing periods of rapid body growth, by those who are pregnant or breastfeeding, by those with a debilitating illness, and by those with inadequate diets (e.g., alcoholics, some geriatric clients). Children who have poor nutrient intake or are malnourished may need vitamin replacement. Persons on fad or restrictive diets frequently have vitamin deficiencies.

The sale of vitamins in the United States is a multibillion-dollar business (Figure 14–1). Some people take vitamins to relieve tiredness or to improve general overall health, both of which are inappropriate indications for vitamin therapy. Today numerous vitamins and herbal medications are available for various specialized needs such as cholesterol, memory, menopause, prostate, and others (Figure 14–2). Before purchasing these agents, the client should discuss with the health care provider the health value and use of multiple vitamins and herbal

medications. Vitamins are *not necessary* if the individual is healthy and consumes a well-balanced daily diet on a regular basis.

Vitamin deficiencies can cause cellular and organ dysfunction that may result in slow recovery from illness. Vitamin supplements are necessary for the vitamin deficiencies described in Table 14–1, but vitamins frequently are taken prophylactically rather than therapeutically.

The United States Department of Agriculture (USDA) provides *MyPyramid: Steps to a Healthier You* as a guide to daily food choices (Figure 14–3). Eating a variety of foods and getting the appropriate number of calories and grams of fat for a healthy weight are recommended. Visit the interactive website at *http://mypyramid.gov* to develop an individualized plan based on individual needs.

The National Academy of Sciences Food and Nutrition Board publishes the U.S. **recommended dietary allowance (RDA)** for daily dose requirements of each vitamin. The Food and Drug Administration (FDA) requires that all vitamin products be labeled according to the amount of vitamin content and the proportion of the RDA provided by the vitamin product. Individuals should be encouraged to check the RDA listed on a vitamin container to determine whether the product provides the RDA dose requirements. The RDA may need to be modified for clients who are ill.

FIGURE 14–1   Would a less expensive generic children's vitamin be just as good?

Table 14–1

Justification for Vitamin Supplements

Categories	Deficiencies
Inadequate absorption	Malabsorption, diarrhea, infectious and inflammatory diseases
Inability to use vitamins	Liver disease (cirrhosis, hepatitis), renal disease, certain hereditary deficiencies
Increased vitamin losses	Fever from infectious process, hyperthyroidism, hemodialysis, cancer, starvation, crash diets
Increased vitamin requirements	Early childhood, pregnancy, debilitating disease (cancer, alcoholism), gastrointestinal surgery, special diets

FIGURE 14–2   Drug companies offer vitamin and herbal supplements for specialized needs. Some of these agents have a combination of vitamins, minerals, and herbs.

MyPyramid
STEPS TO A HEALTHIER YOU
MyPyramid.gov

| GRAINS | VEGETABLES | FRUITS | MILK | MEAT & BEANS |

GRAINS	VEGETABLES	FRUITS	MILK	MEAT & BEANS
Make half your grains whole	Vary your veggies	Focus on fruits	Get your calcium-rich foods	Go lean with protein
Eat at least 3 oz. of whole-grain cereals, breads, crackers, rice, or pasta every day 1 oz. is about 1 slice of bread, about 1 cup of breakfast cereal, or ½ cup of cooked rice, cereal, or pasta	Eat more dark-green veggies like broccoli, spinach, and other dark leafy greens Eat more orange vegetables like carrots and sweetpotatoes Eat more dry beans and peas like pinto beans, kidney beans, and lentils	Eat a variety of fruit Choose fresh, frozen, canned, or dried fruit Go easy on fruit juices	Go low-fat or fat-free when you choose milk, yogurt, and other milk products If you don't or can't consume milk, choose lactose-free products or other calcium sources such as fortified foods and beverages	Choose low-fat or lean meats and poultry Bake it, broil it, or grill it Vary your protein routine — choose more fish, beans, peas, nuts, and seeds

For a 2,000-calorie diet, you need the amounts below from each food group. To find the amounts that are right for you, go to MyPyramid.gov.

| Eat 6 oz. every day | Eat 2½ cups every day | Eat 2 cups every day | Get 3 cups every day;
for kids aged 2 to 8, it's 2 | Eat 5½ oz. every day |

Find your balance between food and physical activity

- Be sure to stay within your daily calorie needs.
- Be physically active for at least 30 minutes most days of the week.
- About 60 minutes a day of physical activity may be needed to prevent weight gain.
- For sustaining weight loss, at least 60 to 90 minutes a day of physical activity may be required.
- Children and teenagers should be physically active for 60 minutes every day, or most days.

Know the limits on fats, sugars, and salt (sodium)

- Make most of your fat sources from fish, nuts, and vegetable oils.
- Limit solid fats like butter, stick margarine, shortening, and lard, as well as foods that contain these.
- Check the Nutrition Facts label to keep saturated fats, *trans* fats, and sodium low.
- Choose food and beverages low in added sugars. Added sugars contribute calories with few, if any, nutrients.

MyPyramid.gov
STEPS TO A HEALTHIER YOU

U.S. Department of Agriculture
Center for Nutrition Policy and Promotion
April 2005
CNPP-15

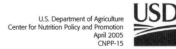

FIGURE 14–3 The U.S. Department of Agriculture food guide pyramid showing the MyPyramid Plan.

NOTE: Table 14–2 lists the fat- and water-soluble vitamins, their functions, suggested food sources, and selected deficiency conditions. Table 14–3 lists fat- and water-soluble vitamins, their RDA values, dosages for vitamin deficiencies, and therapeutic blood or urine ranges.

Fat-Soluble Vitamins

Vitamins fall into two general categories: fat-soluble and water-soluble. The **fat-soluble vitamins** are A, D, E, and K. They are metabolized slowly; can be stored in fatty tissue, liver, and muscle in significant amounts; and are excreted in the urine at a slow rate. Vitamins A and D are toxic if taken in excessive amounts over time. Vitamin A can be stored in the liver for up to 2 years. Vitamins E and K are less toxic than vitamins A and D. Foods rich in vitamin A are fruits, yellow and green vegetables, fish, and dairy products; foods rich in vitamin D are dairy products and nonhydrogenated margarine; foods rich in vitamin E are oils, nonhydrogenated margarine, milk, grains, and meats; and foods rich in vitamin K are green leafy vegetables, meats, eggs, and dairy products.

Table 14–2

Vitamins: Functions, Suggested Food Sources, and Selected Deficiency Conditions

Vitamin	Function	Food Sources	Deficiency Conditions
A	Required for development and maintenance of healthy eyes, gums, teeth, skin, hair, and selected glands. Needed for fat metabolism.	Whole milk, butter, eggs, leafy green and yellow vegetables and fruits* Natural vitamin A, found only in animal sources: cod, halibut, shark, tuna	Dry skin, poor tooth development, night blindness
B_1 (thiamine)	Promotes use of sugars (energy). Required for good function of nervous system and heart.	Enriched breads and cereals, yeast, liver, pork, fish, milk	Sensory disturbances, retarded growth, fatigue, anorexia
B_2 (riboflavin)	Promotes body's use of carbohydrates, proteins, and fats by releasing energy to cells. Required for tissue integrity.	Milk, enriched breads and cereals, liver, lean meat, eggs, leafy green vegetables†	Visual defects such as blurred vision and photophobia; cheilosis; rash on nose; numbness of extremities
B_6 (pyridoxine)	Important in metabolism, synthesis of proteins, and formation of red blood cells.	Lean meat, leafy green vegetables, whole-grain cereals, yeast, bananas	Neuritis, convulsions, dermatitis, anemia, lymphopenia
B_{12} (cobalamin)	Functions as a building block of nucleic acids and to form red blood cells. Facilitates functioning of nervous system.	Liver, kidney, fish, milk	Gastrointestinal disorders, poor growth, anemias
Folic acid (Folvite)	Helps in formation of genetic materials and proteins for the cell nucleus. Assists with intestinal functioning, prevents selected anemias.	Leafy green vegetables, yellow fruits and vegetables, yeast, organ meats	Decreased white blood cell count and clotting factors, anemias, intestinal disturbances, depression
pantothenic acid	Promotes body's use of carbohydrates, fats, and proteins. Essential for formation of specific hormones and nerve-regulating substances.	Eggs, leafy green vegetables, nuts, liver, kidney, skim milk	Natural deficiency unknown in man
niacin	In all body tissues. Necessary for energy-producing reactions. Assists nervous system.	Eggs, meat, liver, beans, peas, enriched bread, and cereals	Retarded growth, pellagra, headache, memory loss, anorexia, insomnia
biotin	Synthesis of fatty acids and energy production from glucose. Required by body chemical systems.	Eggs, milk, leafy green vegetables, liver, kidney	Natural deficiency unknown in man
C (ascorbic acid)	Helps tissue repair and growth. Required in formation of collagen.	Citrus fruits, tomatoes, leafy green vegetables, potatoes, strawberries	Poor wound healing, bleeding gums, scurvy, predisposition to infection
D (calciferol)	Promotes use of phosphorus and calcium. Important for strong teeth and bones.	Vitamin D–fortified milk, egg yolk, tuna, salmon	Rickets, deficit of phosphorus and calcium in blood
E	Protects fatty acids and promotes the formation and functioning of red blood cells, muscle, and other tissues.	Whole-grain cereals, wheat germ, vegetable oils, lettuce, sunflower seeds, milk, eggs, meat	Breakdown of red blood cells
K	Essential for blood clotting.	Leafy green vegetables, liver, cheese, egg yolk, vegetable oil, tomatoes	Increased clotting time, leading to increased bleeding and hemorrhage

*Yellow fruits and vegetables include apricots, cantaloupe, carrots, rutabaga, pumpkin, squash, and sweet potatoes.
†Leafy green vegetables include Brussels sprouts, chard, broccoli, kale, spinach, and turnip and mustard greens.

Table 14–3

Fat- and Water-Soluble Vitamins

Vitamin	RDA	Dosages for Vitamin Deficiencies	Therapeutic Ranges
Fat-Soluble			
A	Men: 1000 mcg or 5000 international units Women: 800 mcg or 4000 international units Preg: 1000 mcg, 5000 international units Lact: 1200 mcg, 6000 international units	10,000-20,000 international units or 3000-6000 mcg/dl	30-70 mcg/dl Deficit: <20 mcg/dl
D	Men and women: 40-80 mcg; 200-400 international units	Mild: 50-125 mcg/dl Moderate to severe: 2.5-7.5 mg/d; 2500-7500 mcg	Unknown
E	Men: 10 mg/d; 15 international units Women: 8 mg/d; 12 international units Preg: 10-12 mg/d	Malabsorption: 30-100 mg/d Severe deficit: 1-2 mg/kg/d or 50-200 international units/kg/d	0.5-0.7 mg/dl Deficit: <0.5 mg/dl
K	Men: 70-80 mcg/d Women: 60-65 mcg/d Taking broad-spectrum antibiotic: 140 mcg/d Preg: 65 mcg/d	5-15 mg/d	Based on prothrombin time (PT) results
Water-Soluble			
C	Men and women: 60 mg/d Preg: 70 mg/dl Lact: 95 mg/dl	150-300 mg Burns: 500-2000 mg/d	Serum: >1.30 mg/dl WBC: >15 mg/dl Deficit: Serum <0.2 mg/dl WBC: <7 mg/dl
B_1 (thiamine)	Men: 1.5 mg Women: 1.1 mg Preg: 1.5 mg Lact: 1.6 mg	30-60 mg/d	Urine: <50 mcg/d
B_2 (riboflavin)	Men: 1.4-1.7 mg Women: 1.2-1.3 mg Preg: 1.6 mg Lact: 1.8 mg	5-25 mg/d Prophylactic: 3 mg/d	Urine: <50 mcg/d
B_3 (nicotinic acid or niacin)	Men: 15-19 mg/d Women: 13-15 mg/d Preg: 18 mg/d Lact: 20 mg/d	Prevention: 5-20 mg/d Deficit: 50-100 mg/d Pellagra: 300-500 mg in 3 divided doses Hyperlipidemia: 1-2 g/d in 3 divided doses	Unknown
B_6 (pyridoxine)	Men: 2.0 mg/d Women: 1.6 mg/d Preg: 2.1 mg/d Lact: 2.2 mg/d	25-100 mg/d Isoniazid therapy prophylaxis: 25-50 mg/d Peripheral neuritis: 50-200 mg/d	Serum: >50 ng/ml Urine: <1 mg/d
Folic acid (folate)	Men and women: 400 mcg/d Preg: 600-800 mcg/d Lact: 600-800 mcg/d	1-2 mg/d	Serum folate: 6-20 ng/ml RBC: 160-600 ng/ml Deficit: Serum: <3-4 ng/ml RBC: <140 ng/ml
B_{12}	Men and women: 3 mcg/d Preg: 4 mcg/d	100 mg/dl 14 d Pernicious anemia: 50-100 mcg /d or 1000 mcg/wk × 3 wk	150-900 pg/ml Deficit: <100 pg/ml Schilling test >30% normal

d, Day; *lact*, lactation; *preg*, pregnancy; *RBC*, red blood cell; *WBC*, white blood cell; *wk*, week; >, greater than; <, less than.

Vitamin A

Vitamin A is essential for bone growth and the maintenance of epithelial tissues, skin, eyes, and hair. It has been used for the treatment of skin disorders such as acne; however, excess doses can be toxic. During pregnancy, excess amounts of vitamin A (>6000 international units) might have a teratogenic effect (birth defect) on the fetus. Prototype Drug Chart 14–1 describes the effects of vitamin A. The nursing process is applied as the drug data are obtained and the drug is administered. IM administration is

Prototype DRUG CHART 14–1

VITAMIN A

Drug Class

Fat-soluble vitamin
Trade names: Acon, Aquasol A
Pregnancy Category: A (X if doses are above RDA)

Dosage

Severe deficiency:
A & C >8 y: PO: 100,000-500,000 international units daily
  × 3 d; then 50,000 daily × 14 d
Maintenance:
10,000-20,000 international units daily × 60 d
1-8 y: PO/IM: 17,000-35,000 international units daily 3
  × 10 d
Dietary supplement:
4-8 y: PO: 15,000 international units daily
1-<4 y: PO: 10,000 international units daily

Contraindications

Hypervitaminosis A, pregnancy (massive doses)

Drug-Lab-Food Interactions

Drug: May decrease absorption of mineral oil,
  cholestyramine
Lab: May increase BUN, calcium, cholesterol
  triglycerides; may lower erythrocyte, leukocyte counts
Food: None known

Pharmacokinetics

Absorption: PO: 1 h
Distribution: PB: UK
Metabolism: t½: weeks-months
Excretion: Urine

Pharmacodynamics

PO: Onset: 1-2 h
Peak: 4-5 h
Duration: UK

Therapeutic Effects/Uses

To treat vitamin A deficiency (biliary tract or pancreatic disease, colitis, cirrhosis, celiac disease, sprue), prevent night
  blindness, treat skin disorders, promote bone development
Mode of Action: Essential for growth, bone and teeth development, vision, integrity of skin and mucous membranes, and reproduction

Side Effects

Headache, fatigue, drowsiness, irritability, anorexia,
  vomiting, diarrhea, dry skin, visual changes

Adverse Reactions

Evident only with toxicity: leukopenia, aplastic anemia,
  papilledema, increased intracranial pressure,
  hypervitaminosis A, bulging fontanelles in infants

A, Adult; *C,* child; *d,* day; *h,* hour; *IM,* intramuscular; *PB,* protein binding; *PO,* by mouth; *RDA,* recommended daily allowance; *t½,*
half life; *UK,* unknown; *y,* year; < less than; > greater than.

used only in the acutely ill or clients refractory to the oral route, such as those with gastrointestinal (GI) malabsorption syndrome.

Pharmacokinetics

When a person is deficient in vitamin A, the vitamin is absorbed faster than if there is no deficiency or intestinal obstruction. A portion of vitamin A is stored in the liver, and this function can be inhibited with liver disease. Massive doses of vitamin A may cause hypervitaminosis A, symptoms of which are hair loss and peeling skin.

The RDA for vitamin A supplementation is 5000 international units. Excess use of vitamin A should be avoided unless warranted because this vitamin is stored in the liver, kidneys, and fat and is slowly excreted from the body. Excess vitamin A is stored in the liver for up to 2 years. Vitamin A toxicity affects multiple organs, especially the liver.

To prevent the occurrence of vitamin A toxicity the dose for healthy clients should not be greater than 7500 international units.

Mineral oil, cholestyramine, alcohol, and antilipemic drugs decrease the absorption of vitamin A. Vitamin A is excreted through the kidneys and feces.

Pharmacodynamics

Vitamin A is necessary for many biochemical processes. It aids in the formation of the visual pigment needed for night vision, it is needed in bone growth and development, and it promotes the integrity of the mucosal and epithelial tissues. An early sign of vitamin A deficiency (hypovitaminosis A) is night blindness. This may progress to dryness and ulceration of the cornea and to blindness.

Vitamin A taken orally begins to take effect in 1 to 2 hours and peaks in 4 to 5 hours. Its duration of action is unknown. Because vitamin A is stored in the liver, the vitamin may be available to the body for days, weeks, or months.

Vitamin D

Vitamin D has a major role in regulating calcium and phosphorus metabolism and is needed for calcium absorption from the intestines. Dietary vitamin D is absorbed in the small intestine and requires bile salts for absorption. There are two compounds of vitamin D: vitamin D_2, ergocalciferol (a synthetic fortified vitamin D), and vitamin D_3, cholecalciferol (a natural form of vitamin D influenced by ultraviolet sunlight through the skin). Once absorbed, vitamin D is converted to calcifediol in the liver. Calcifediol is then converted to an active form, calcitriol, in the kidneys. Studies have suggested that Vitamin D, taken with calcium, can reduce fractures.

Calcitriol, the active form of vitamin D, functions as a hormone and, with parathyroid hormone (PTH) and calcitonin, regulates calcium and phosphorus metabolism. Calcitriol and PTH stimulate bone reabsorption of calcium and phosphorus. Excretion of vitamin D is primarily in bile; only a small amount is excreted in the urine. If serum calcium levels are low, more vitamin D is activated; when serum calcium levels are normal, activation of vitamin D is decreased.

Excess vitamin D ingestion (>40,000 international units) results in hypervitaminosis D and may cause hypercalcemia (an elevated serum calcium level). Anorexia, nausea, and vomiting are early symptoms of vitamin D toxicity.

Vitamin E

Vitamin E has antioxidant properties that protect cellular components from being oxidized and red blood cells from hemolysis. Vitamin E depends on bile salts, pancreatic secretion, and fat for its absorption. Vitamin E is stored in all tissues, especially the liver, muscle, and fatty tissue. About 75% is excreted in bile.

It has been reported that taking 400 to 800 international units of vitamin E per day reduces the number of nonfatal myocardial infarctions (MIs). Also, it has been stated that taking 200 international units a day for several years can reduce the risk of coronary artery disease (CAD). Today the use of vitamin E for CAD is being questioned. However, many still state that this vitamin protects the heart and arteries and aids in the prevention of macular degeneration because of its antioxidant effects (i.e., it inhibits the oxidation of other compounds by blocking a group of harmful chemicals called **free radicals**).

Side effects of large doses of vitamin E may include fatigue, weakness, nausea, GI upset, headache, and breast tenderness. Vitamin E may prolong the prothrombin time (PT). Persons taking warfarin should have their PT monitored closely. Iron and vitamin E should not be taken together because iron can interfere with the body's absorption and use of vitamin E.

Vitamin K

Vitamin K occurs in four forms: vitamin K_1 (phytonadione) is the most active form; vitamin K_2 (menaquinone) is synthesized by intestinal flora; and vitamin K_3 (menadione) and vitamin K_4 (menadiol) have been produced synthetically. Vitamin K_2 is not commercially available. Vitamins K_1 and K_2 are absorbed in the presence of bile salts. Vitamins K_3 and K_4 do not need bile salts for absorption. After vitamin K is absorbed, it is stored primarily in the liver and in other tissues. Half of vitamin K comes from the intestinal flora, and the remaining portion comes from one's diet.

Vitamin K is needed for synthesis of prothrombin and the clotting factors VII, IX, and X. For oral anticoagulant overdose, vitamin K_1 (phytonadione) is the only vitamin K form available for therapeutic use and is most effective in preventing hemorrhage. The commercial drugs for vitamin K_1 are Mephyton, AquaMEPHYTON, and Konakion, and the commercial drug for vitamin K_4 is Synkayvite. Vitamin K is used for two reasons: as an antidote for oral anticoagulant overdose, and to prevent and treat the hypoprothrombinemia of Vitamin K deficiency. Spontaneous hemorrhage may occur with vitamin K deficiency due to lack of bile salts and malabsorption syndromes that interfere with vitamin K uptake (e.g., celiac disease). Newborns are vitamin K deficient; thus a single dose of phytonadione is recommended immediately after delivery. This can elevate bilirubin level and cause hyperbilirubinemia with a risk of kernicterus. There are oral and parenteral forms of phytonadione; IV administration is dangerous and may cause death.

Water-Soluble Vitamins

Water-soluble vitamins are the B-complex vitamins and vitamin C. This group of vitamins is not usually toxic unless taken in extremely excessive amounts. Water-soluble vitamins are not stored by the body, so consistent, steady supplementation is required. Water-soluble vitamins are readily excreted in the urine. Protein binding of water-soluble vitamins is minimal. Foods that are high in vitamin B are grains, cereal, bread, and meats. Citrus fruits and green vegetables are high in vitamin C. If the fruits and vegetables are cut, washed, or cooked, a large amount of vitamin C is lost.

Vitamin B Complex

Vitamin B_1 (thiamine), vitamin B_2 (riboflavin), vitamin B_3 (nicotinic acid, or niacin), and vitamin B_6 (pyridoxine) are four of the vitamin B-complex members. This B-complex group is water-soluble.

Thiamine deficiency can lead to the polyneuritis and cardiac pathology seen in beriberi or to Wernicke encepha-

---

Preventing MEDICATION ERRORS

Do not confuse...

- **Aquasol A** or **Aquasol E** with **Anusol,** an antiinflammatory generally used to treat hemorrhoids lopathy that progresses to Korsakoff syndrome, conditions most commonly associated with alcohol abuse. Wernicke-Korsakoff syndrome is a significant central nervous system disorder characterized by confusion, nystagmus, diplopia, ataxia, and loss of recent memory. Unless treated it may cause irreversible brain damage. IV administration of thiamine is recommended for treatment of Wernicke-Korsakoff syndrome.

Riboflavin may be given to manage dermatologic problems such as scaly dermatitis, cracked corners of the mouth, and inflammation of the skin and tongue. To treat migraine headache, riboflavin is given in larger doses than for dermatologic concerns.

Niacin is given to alleviate pellagra and hyperlipidemia, for which large doses are required. Chapter 45 offers a discussion of niacin use to reduce cholesterol levels. However, large doses may cause GI irritation and vasodilation, resulting in a flushing sensation.

Pyridoxine is administered to correct vitamin B_6 deficiency. It may also help alleviate the symptoms of neuritis caused by isoniazid (INH) therapy for tuberculosis. Vitamin B_6 is an essential building block of nucleic acids, red blood cell formation, and synthesis of hemoglobin. Pyridoxine is used to treat vitamin B_6 deficiency caused by lack of adequate diet, inborn error of metabolism, or drug-induced deficiencies secondary to INH, penicillamine, or cyclosporine therapy. It is also used to treat neonates with seizures refractory to traditional therapy. Vitamin B_6 deficiencies may occur in alcoholics along with deficiencies of other B-complex vitamins. Alcoholics and diabetics may benefit from daily supplementation. Pyridoxine is readily absorbed in the jejunum and stored in the liver, muscle, and brain. It is metabolized in the liver and excreted in the urine.

Vitamin C

Vitamin C (ascorbic acid) is absorbed from the small intestine. Vitamin C aids in the absorption of iron and in the conversion of folic acid. Vitamin C is not stored in the body and is excreted readily in the urine. A high serum vitamin C level that results from excessive dosing of vitamin C is excreted by the kidneys unchanged.

The recommended daily dose of vitamin C for an adult is 50 to 100 mg per day. Some individuals take as much as 500 to 6000 mg a day to treat upper respiratory infections, cancer, or hypercholesterolemia. Massive doses of vitamin C can cause diarrhea and GI upset. Abrupt withdrawal can result in rebound deficiency, so vitamin C dosage should be reduced gradually. Prototype Drug Chart 14-2 gives drug information on vitamin C.

Pharmacokinetics

Vitamin C is absorbed readily through the GI tract and is distributed throughout the body fluids. The kidneys completely excrete vitamin C, mostly unchanged.

Pharmacodynamics

Vitamin C is needed for carbohydrate metabolism and protein and lipid synthesis. Collagen synthesis also requires vitamin C for capillary endothelium, connective tissue and tissue repair, and osteoid tissue of the bone.

Large doses of vitamin C may decrease the effect of oral anticoagulants. Oral contraceptives can decrease vitamin C concentration in the body. Smoking decreases serum vitamin C levels.

The use of **megavitamin therapy**, massive doses of vitamins, is questionable at best. Megadoses of vitamins can cause toxicity and might result in minimal desired effect. Most authorities believe that vitamin C does not cure or prevent the common cold; rather, they believe that vitamin C has a placebo effect. Moreover, megadoses of vitamin C taken with aspirin or sulfonamides may cause crystal formation in the urine (crystalluria). Excessive doses of vitamin C can cause a false-negative occult (blood) stool result and false-positive sugar result in the urine when tested by the Clinitest method. If large doses of megavitamins are to be discontinued, a gradual reduction of dosage is necessary to avoid vitamin deficiency. NOTE: There is danger of children overdosing on adult or children's multivitamins containing iron.

Folic Acid (Folate)

Folic acid is absorbed from the small intestine, and the active form of folic acid (folate) is circulated to all tissues. One third of folate is stored in the liver, and the rest is stored in tissues. Four fifths of folate is excreted in bile and one fifth in urine.

Folic acid is essential for body growth. It is needed for deoxyribonucleic acid (DNA) synthesis, and without folic acid there is a disruption in cellular division. Chronic alcoholism, poor nutritional intake, malabsorption syndromes, pregnancy, and drugs that cause inadequate absorption (phenytoin, barbiturates) or folic acid antagonists (methotrexate, triamterene, trimethoprim) are causes of folic acid deficiencies. Symptoms of folic acid deficiencies include anorexia, nausea, stomatitis, diarrhea, fatigue, alopecia, and blood dyscrasias (megaloblastic anemia, leukopenia, thrombocytopenia). These symptoms are usually not noted until 2 to 4 months after folic acid storage is depleted.

Folic acid deficiency during the first trimester of pregnancy can affect the development of the central nervous system (CNS) of the fetus. This may cause neural tube defects (NTDs) such as spina bifida (defective closure of the bony structure of the spinal cord) or anencephaly (lack of brain mass formation). The U.S. Public Health Services recommends that all women who may become pregnant consume 400 mcg of supplemental folic acid each day—in addition to the folate they get with food. Synthetic folate

Preventing MEDICATION ERRORS

Do not confuse...

pyridoxine (vitamin B₆) with:

- **paroxetine** (Paxil), an antidepressant

- **pralidoxime**, an antidote used to treat poisoning with organophosphate pesticides and chemicals that have anticholinesterase activity

- **phenazopyridine** (Pyridium), a urinary analgesic

Prototype DRUG CHART 14–2

VITAMIN C

Drug Class

Water-soluble vitamin
Trade names: Ascorbicap, Cecon, Cevalin, Solucap C,
♣Apo-C, Ce-Vi-Sol, Redoxon
Pregnancy Category: A (C if used in doses above RDA)

Dosage

Prophylactic:
A: PO: 45-60 mg/d
C: PO: 20-50 mg/D
Severe deficit: Scurvy
A: PO: IM: IV: 150-500 mg/d in 1 to 2 divided doses
C: PO: IM: IV: 150-300 mg/d in 1 to 2 divided doses
Pregnancy and lactation:
A: PO: 160-80 mg/d

Contraindications

Caution: Renal calculi, gout, anemia: sickle cell,
sideroblastic, thalassemia

Drug-Lab-Food Interactions

Decrease ascorbic acid uptake taken with salicylates;
may decrease effect of oral anticoagulants; may
decrease elimination of aspirins
Lab: May decrease bilirubin, urinary pH; may increase
uric acid, uric oxalate
Food: None known

Pharmacokinetics

Absorption: PO: quickly
Distribution: PB: 25%
Metabolism: t½: UK
Excretion: In the urine; unchanged with high doses

Pharmacodynamics

PO:
Onset: >2 d
Peak: UK
Duration: UK

Therapeutic Effects/Uses

To prevent and treat vitamin C deficiency (scurvy); to increase wound healing; for burns. Preserves integrity of blood
vessels.
Mode of Action: A water-soluble vitamin, essential for collagen formation and tissue repair (bones, skin, blood vessels). Synthesis of lipids, protein, carnithine.

Side Effects

Nausea, vomiting, diarrhea; increased urination with
dose >19.
Parenteral; flushing, headache, dizziness, soreness at
injection site

Adverse Reactions

Kidney stones, crystalluria, hyperuricemia
Life-threatening: Sickle cell crisis, deep vein thrombosis

A, Adult; *C,* child; *d,* day; *IM,* intramuscular; *IV,* intravenous; *PB,* protein binding; *PO,* by mouth; *t½,* half life; *UK,* unknown;
> greater than; ♣, Canadian drug name.

is more stable than food, bioavailability is >85% and
<59% respectively. There is some evidence that 400 to 800
mcg (0.4 to 0.8 mg) of folic acid per day can decrease the
incidence of CAD. It is thought that folic acid decreases the
amino acid homocysteine in the blood, which may contribute to heart disease. Folic acid may also offer some
protection from colorectal cancer.

Excessive doses of folic acid may mask signs of vitamin
B₁₂ deficiency, which is a risk in older adults. Clients taking

phenytoin (Dilantin) to control seizures should be cautious about taking folic acid. This vitamin can lower the
serum phenytoin level, which could increase the risk of
seizures. The phenytoin dose would need to be adjusted in
such clients.

Vitamin B₁₂

Vitamin B₁₂, like folic acid, is essential for DNA synthesis.
Vitamin B₁₂ aids in the conversion of folic acid to its active
form. With active folic acid, vitamin B₁₂ promotes cellular
division. It is also needed for normal hematopoiesis (development of red blood cells in bone marrow) and to
maintain nervous system integrity, especially the myelin.

The gastric parietal cells produce an intrinsic factor that
is necessary for the absorption of vitamin B₁₂ through the
intestinal wall. Without the intrinsic factor, little or no vitamin B₁₂ is absorbed. After absorption, vitamin B₁₂ binds

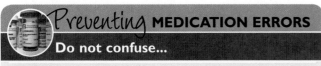

Preventing **MEDICATION ERRORS**

Do not confuse...

• **Folvite** with **Florvite,** a fluoride supplement put in
the water

to the protein transcobalamin II and is transferred to the tissues. Most vitamin B_{12} is stored in the liver. Vitamin B_{12} is slowly excreted, and it can take 2 to 3 years for stored vitamin B_{12} to be depleted and a deficit noticed.

Vitamin B_{12} deficiency is uncommon unless there is a disturbance of the intrinsic factor and intestinal absorption. Pernicious anemia (lack of the intrinsic factor) is the major cause of vitamin B_{12} deficiency. Vitamin B_{12} deficiency can also develop in strict vegetarians who do not consume meat, fish, or dairy products. Other possible causes of vitamin B_{12} deficiency include malabsorption syndromes (cancer, celiac disease, certain drugs), gastrectomy, Crohn's disease, and liver and kidney diseases. Symptoms may include numbness and tingling in the lower extremities, weakness, fatigue, anorexia, loss of taste, diarrhea, memory loss, mood changes, dementia, psychosis, megaloblastic anemia with macrocytes (overenlarged erythrocytes [red blood cells]) in blood, and megaloblasts (overenlarged erythroblasts) in the bone marrow.

To correct vitamin B_{12} deficiency, cyanocobalamin in crystalline form can be given intramuscularly for severe deficits. It cannot be given intravenously because of possible hypersensitive reactions. Cyanocobalamin can be given orally and is commonly found in multi-vitamin preparations.

Table 14–2 lists both the fat- and water-soluble vitamins with their functions, suggested food sources, and selected deficiency conditions. Table 14–3 lists fat- and water-soluble vitamins, their RDA values, dosages for vitamin deficiencies, and therapeutic serum blood or urine ranges.

Vitamins

ASSESSMENT

■ Check client for vitamin deficiency before start of therapy and regularly thereafter. Explore such areas as inadequate nutrient intake, debilitating disease, and GI disorders.
■ Obtain 24- and 48-hour diet history analysis.

NURSING DIAGNOSES

■ Risk for imbalanced nutrition; inadequate intake of food sources of vitamins
■ Deficient knowledge related to food sources of vitamins
■ Readiness for enhanced decision making related to food choices and vitamin supplementation

PLANNING

■ Client will eat a well-balanced diet that includes the foods and servings recommended in the food pyramid.

■ Client with vitamin deficiency will take vitamin supplements as prescribed.

NURSING INTERVENTIONS

■ Administer vitamins with food to promote absorption.
■ Store drug in light-resistant container.
■ When administering vitamins in drop form, use the supplied calibrated dropper for accurate dosing. Solution may be administered mixed with food or dropped into the mouth.
■ Administer IM primarily for clients unable to take by PO route (e.g., GI malabsorption syndrome).
■ To avoid risk of hemolytic anemia, recognize need for vitamin E supplements for infants receiving vitamin A.
■ Monitor for vitamin A therapeutic serum levels (80-300 international units/ml).

Client Teaching

General

• Instruct client to take prescribed amount of drug.
• Inform clients (adults and children) to read vitamin labels to determine which vitamin is most appropriate for them (Figure 14–4).
• Instruct client to consult with health care provider/pharmacist regarding interactions with prescription and OTC medications (e.g., vitamin B_6 interferes with action of levodopa).
• Discourage client from taking megavitamins over a long period unless these are prescribed for a specific purpose by health care provider. To discontinue long-term megavitamin therapy, a gradual decrease in vitamin intake is advised to avoid vitamin deficiency. Megadoses of vitamins can be toxic.
• Inform client that missing vitamins for 1 or 2 days is not a cause for concern, because deficiencies do not occur for some time.
• Advise client to check expiration dates on vitamin containers before purchasing and taking them home. Potency of the vitamin is reduced after the expiration date.
• Instruct client to avoid taking mineral oil with vitamin A on a regular basis, because it interferes with absorption of the vitamin. If needed, take mineral oil at bedtime.
• Explain to client that there is no scientific evidence that megadoses of vitamin C (ascorbic acid) will cure a cold.
• Alert client not to take megadoses of vitamin C with aspirin or sulfonamides because crystals may form in the kidneys and urine.
• Instruct client to avoid excessive intake of alcoholic beverages. Alcohol can cause vitamin B-complex deficiencies.

Diet

- Advise client to eat a well-balanced diet that includes the recommended amounts and types of food detailed in the food pyramid. Vitamin supplements are not necessary if the person is healthy and receives proper nutrition on a regular basis.
- Instruct client about foods rich in vitamin A, including whole milk, butter, eggs, leafy green and yellow vegetables, fruits, and liver. Foods rich in other vitamins are listed in Table 14–2.

Side Effects

- Instruct client that nausea, vomiting, headache, loss of hair, and cracked lips (symptoms of hypervitaminosis A) should be reported to the health care provider. Early symptoms of hypervitaminosis D are anorexia, nausea, and vomiting.

Cultural Considerations ❖

- Food and food choices have strong cultural roots. Determine the client's preferred and culturally meaningful foods, and incorporate them into food and supplement plan.
- Ask about folk practices and incorporate as appropriate.
- Use interpreters as appropriate.

EVALUATION

■ Evaluate the effectiveness of client's diet for the inclusion of the appropriate amounts and types of food from the food pyramid. Have client periodically keep a diet chart for a complete week.

■ Determine whether client with malnutrition is receiving appropriate vitamin therapy.

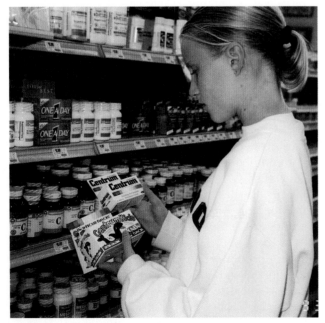

FIGURE 14–4 This 12-year-old is trying to decide whether an adult's or a children's vitamin is more appropriate for her needs.

Minerals

Various **minerals**, such as iron, copper, zinc, chromium, and selenium, are needed for body function.

Iron

Iron (ferrous sulfate, gluconate, or fumarate) is vital for hemoglobin regeneration. Sixty percent of the iron in the body is found in hemoglobin. One of the causes of anemia is iron deficiency. A normal diet contains 5 to 20 mg of iron per day. Foods rich in iron include liver, lean meats, egg yolks, dried beans, green vegetables (e.g., spinach), and fruit. Food and antacids slow the absorption of iron, and vitamin C increases iron absorption.

During pregnancy an increased amount of iron is needed, but during the first trimester of pregnancy megadoses of iron are contraindicated because of its possible teratogenic effect on the fetus. Larger doses of iron are required during the second and third trimesters of pregnancy.

The dose of iron for infants and children 6 months to 2 years of age is 1.5 mg per kilogram of body weight. For the adult, 50 mg daily is needed for hemoglobin regeneration. The ferrous sulfate tablet is 325 mg, of which 65 mg is elemental iron. Therefore one tablet of ferrous sulfate is sufficient as a daily iron dose when indicated. Prototype Drug Chart 14–3 describes the effects of iron preparations.

Pharmacokinetics

Iron is absorbed by the intestines and enters the plasma as heme, or it may be stored as ferritin. Although food decreases absorption by 25% to 50%, it may be necessary to take iron preparations with food to avoid GI discomfort. Vitamin C may slightly increase iron absorption, whereas tetracycline and antacids can decrease absorption (Herbal Alert 14–1).

Pharmacodynamics

Iron replacement is given primarily to correct or control iron-deficiency anemia, which is diagnosed by a laboratory blood smear. Positive findings for this anemia are microcytic (small), hypochromic (pale) erythrocytes (red blood cells [RBCs]). Clinical signs and symptoms include fatigue, weakness, shortness of breath, pallor, and, in cases of severe anemia, increased GI bleeding. The dosage of ferrous sulfate for prophylactic use is 300 to 325 mg daily; for therapeutic use, the dosage is 600 to 1200 mg daily in divided doses.

The onset of action for iron therapy takes days, and its peak action does not occur for days or weeks; therefore the client's symptoms are slow to improve. Increased hemoglobin and hematocrit levels occur within 3 to 7 days.

Iron toxicity is a serious cause of poisoning in children. As few as 10 tablets of ferrous sulfate (3 g) taken at one time can be fatal within 12 to 48 hours. Hemorrhage due to the ulcerogenic effects of unbound iron leads to shock. Parents should be cautioned against leaving iron tablets

---

Herbal **ALERT 14–1**

Iron

🌿 Chamomile, feverfew, peppermint, and St. John's wort interfere with the absorption of iron and other minerals.

Prototype **DRUG CHART 14–3**

IRON

Drug Class

Mineral for antianemia
Trade names:
ferrous sulfate (Feosol, Fer-Iron)
ferrous gluconate (Fergon, Fertinic)
ferrous fumarate (Feostat, Fumerin)
Pregnancy Category: A

Dosage

A: PO: 300-325 mg q.i.d.: increase to 650 mg q.i.d. as
  needed or tolerated
Pregnancy: PO: 300-600 mg/d
C: ≥2 y: PO: 8 mg/kg daily in divided doses

Contraindications

Hemolytic anemia, hemosiderosis, peptic ulcer,
  ulcerative colitis
Caution: Bronchial asthma, iron hypersensitivity

Drug-Lab-Food Interactions

Increased effect of iron with vitamin C; *decreased* effect
  of tetracycline, antacids, penicillamine
Lab: May increase bilirubin, may decrease calcium
Food: None known

Pharmacokinetics

Absorption: PO: 10%-30% intestines
Distribution: PB: UK
Metabolism: t½: 6 h
Excretion: Urine, feces, sweat

Pharmacodynamics

PO: Onset: 4 d
Peak: 7-14 d
Duration: 3-4 mo

Therapeutic Effects/Uses

To prevent and treat iron deficiency anemia
Mode of Action: Enables RBC development and oxygen transport via hemoglobin

Side Effects

Nausea, vomiting, diarrhea, constipation, epigastric
  pain; elixir may stain teeth

Adverse Reactions

Existing GI conditions may be aggravated Pallor,
  drowsiness
Life-threatening: Iron poisoning (mostly in children) and
  may result in cardiovascular collapse, metabolic
  acidosis

A, Adult; *C,* child; *d,* day; *GI,* gastrointestinal; *h,* hour; *mo,* month; *PB,* protein binding; *PO,* by mouth; *q.i.d.,* four times a day; *RBC,*
red blood cell; *t½,* half life; *UK,* unknown; ≥ greater than or equal to.

that look like candy (e.g., M&Ms) within a child's reach; most iron products are distributed in bubble packs. NOTE: There is also danger of children overdosing on adult or children's multivitamins containing iron.

Copper

Copper is needed for the formation of RBCs and connective tissues. Copper is a cofactor of many enzymes, and its function is in the production of the neurotransmitters norepinephrine and dopamine. Excess serum copper levels may be associated with Wilson's disease, which is an inborn error of metabolism that allows for large amounts of copper to accumulate in the liver, brain, cornea (brown or green Kayser-Fleischer rings), or kidneys.

A prolonged copper deficiency may result in anemia, which is not corrected by taking iron supplements. Abnormal blood and skin changes caused by a copper deficiency include a decrease in white blood cell count, glucose intolerance, and a decrease in skin and hair pigmentation. Mental retardation might also occur in the young.

The RDA for copper is 1.5 to 3 mg per day. Most adults consume about 1 mg per day. Foods rich in copper are shellfish (crab, oysters), liver, nuts, seeds (sunflower, sesame), legumes, and cocoa.

Zinc

Zinc is important to many enzymatic reactions and is essential for normal growth and tissue repair, wound healing, and taste and smell. The use of zinc has greatly increased in the past few years (Figure 14–5). Some believe zinc can alleviate symptoms of the common cold and shorten its duration. Individuals may take as much as 200 mg daily. The adult RDA is 12 to 19 mg. Foods rich in zinc include beef, lamb, eggs, and leafy and root vegetables.

Large doses, more than 150 mg, may cause a copper deficiency, a decrease in high-density lipoprotein (HDL) cholesterol ("good" cholesterol), and a weakened immune response. Zinc can inhibit tetracycline absorption. Clients taking zinc and an antibiotic should not take them to-

FIGURE 14–5 The use of zinc and other mineral supplements such as iron and selenium is on the rise.

gether; zinc should be taken at least 2 hours after taking an antibiotic. Clients on long-term parenteral nutrition are at risk for zinc deficiency. Serum zinc levels may not correlate with degree of deficiency.

Chromium

Chromium is said to be helpful in the control of type 2 diabetes (non–insulin-dependent diabetes). It is thought that this mineral helps to normalize blood glucose by increasing the effects of insulin on the cells. If a client is taking large doses of chromium and an oral hypoglycemic agent or insulin, the glucose level should be monitored closely for a hypoglycemic reaction. The dose of an oral hypoglycemic drug or insulin may need to be decreased. Some clients with an impaired glucose tolerance or clients who do not have diabetes may benefit by taking chromium. In addition, chromium claims to promote weight loss and muscle building. Multivitamin and mineral preparations contain chloride salt of chromium.

There is no RDA for chromium; however, 50 to 200 mcg per day is considered within the normal range for children older than 6 years and adults. Foods rich in chromium include meats, whole-grain cereals, and brewer's yeast.

Selenium

Selenium acts as a cofactor for an antioxidant enzyme that protects protein and nucleic acids from oxidative damage. Selenium works with vitamin E. It is thought that selenium has an anticarcinogenic effect, and doses greater than 200 mcg may reduce the risk of lung, prostate, and colorectal cancer. Excess doses of more than 200 mcg might cause weakness, a loss of hair, dermatitis, nausea, diarrhea, and abdominal pain. Also, there may be a garlic-like odor from the skin and breath.

The RDA for selenium is 40 to 75 mcg (lower dose for women, higher dose for men). Foods rich in selenium include meats (especially liver), seafood, eggs, and dairy products.

Nursing Process

Antianemia, Mineral: Iron

ASSESSMENT

■ Obtain a drug history of current drugs and herbs client is taking.
■ Obtain a history of anemia or health problems that may lead to anemia.
■ Assess client for signs and symptoms of iron deficiency anemia such as fatigue, malaise, pallor, shortness of breath, tachycardia, and cardiac dysrhythmia.
■ Assess client's RBC count, hemoglobin, hematocrit, iron level, and reticulocyte count before start of therapy and throughout thereafter.

NURSING DIAGNOSES

■ Fatigue, malaise, pallor, increased heart rate, altered oral mucous membranes (sore, swollen tongue; difficulty swallowing)
■ Risk for imbalanced nutrition; inadequate intake of food sources of iron
■ Deficient knowledge of food sources of iron
■ Readiness for enhanced decision making related to food choices and vitamin/mineral supplementation

PLANNING

■ Client will name six foods high in iron content.
■ Client will consume foods rich in iron.
■ Client with iron deficiency anemia or with low hemoglobin will take iron replacement as recommended by health care provider, resulting in laboratory results within the desired range.

NURSING INTERVENTIONS

■ Encourage client to eat a nutritious diet to obtain sufficient iron. Iron supplements are not needed unless the person is malnourished, pregnant, or has abnormal menses.
■ Store drug in light-resistant container.
■ Administer IM injection of iron by the Z-track method to avoid leakage of iron into the subQ tissue and skin, because it irritates and stains the skin.

Client Teaching

General
• Instruct client to take the tablet or capsule between meals with at least 8 ounces of juice or water to promote absorption. If gastric irritation occurs, instruct the client to take with food.

- Advise client to swallow the tablet or capsule whole.
- Instruct client to maintain upright position for 30 minutes to prevent esophageal corrosion from reflux.
- Do not administer the iron tablet within 1 hour of ingesting antacid, milk, ice cream, or other milk products such as pudding.
- Inform client that certain herbal drugs can decrease absorption of iron and other minerals (see Herbal Alert 14–1).
- Advise client to increase fluids, activity, and dietary bulk to avoid or relieve constipation. Slow-release iron capsules decrease constipation and gastric irritation.
- Instruct adults not to leave iron tablets within reach of children. If a child swallows many tablets, induce vomiting and immediately call the local poison control center; the telephone number is in the front of most telephone books (include this number on emergency reference list). Keep ipecac available; it is an OTC drug.
- Encourage client to take only prescribed amount of drug to avoid iron poisoning. **Be alert to iron in many multivitamin preparations.**
- Be alert that iron content varies among iron salts; therefore do not substitute one for another.
- Advise client that drug treatment for anemia is generally less than 6 months.

Diet
- Counsel client to include iron-rich foods in diet: liver, lean meats, egg yolk, dried beans, green vegetables, and fruit.

Side Effects
- Advise client taking the liquid iron preparation to use a straw to prevent discoloration of tooth enamel.
- Alert client that the drug turns stools a harmless black or dark green.
- Instruct client about signs and symptoms of toxicity, including nausea, vomiting, diarrhea, pallor, hematemesis, shock, and coma, and report occurrence to health care provider.

Cultural Considerations ❖
- Ask about folk practices, and incorporate as appropriate.
- Use interpreter as needed.

EVALUATION

■ Evaluate the effectiveness of iron therapy by determining that client is not fatigued or short of breath and that hemoglobin level is within desired range.

KEY WEBSITES
Center for Food Safety and Applied Nutrition:
www.cfsan.fda.gov
MyPyramid Plan: www.mypyramid.gov
National Library of Medicine: www.nlm.nih.gov

Critical Thinking Case Study

AP is pregnant and is taking two tablets of 325 mg of ferrous sulfate. She has a 2-year-old daughter.

1. What precautions should AP take in regard to the container of ferrous sulfate? Explain.
2. If AP asks whether she should take more than two tablets of iron a day, how should you respond?
3. AP states that she is constipated and wonders if iron is the cause. How can this problem be alleviated? What would be an appropriate response?
4. Develop a safety plan with AP related to medication safety in the home with children.

NCLEX Study Questions

1. You note that your client's prothrombin time is prolonged. What vitamin might be contributing to this?
   a. vitamin A   c. vitamin D
   b. vitamin B   d. vitamin E

2. Your client is experiencing hair loss and peeling skin. This may be caused by excess of what vitamin?
   a. vitamin A   c. vitamin C
   b. vitamin B   d. vitamin D

3. Vitamin D has a major role in:
   a. night vision
   b. regulating calcium and phosphorous metabolism
   c. body growth
   d. DNA synthesis

4. Folic acid is known to prevent CNS anomalies and may offer protection from:
   a. colorectal cancer   c. celiac disease
   b. diabetes mellitus   d. migraine headaches

5. Megadoses of what mineral may cause teratogenic effects during the first trimester?
   a. selenium   c. iron
   b. chromium   d. zinc

6. Fat soluble vitamins:
   a. are metabolized rapidly
   b. cannot be stored in liver
   c. are excreted slowly in urine
   d. cannot be toxic

7. An early sign of vitamin A deficiency is:
   a. muscle twitching   c. peeling skin
   b. night blindness   d. celiac disease

8. The most common cause of vitamin B_{12} deficiency is:
   a. coronary artery disease c. diabetes mellitus
   b. multiple sclerosis   d. alcoholism

Answers: 1. d; 2. a; 3. b; 4. a; 5. c; 6. c; 7. b; 8. d.

15

Fluid and Electrolyte Replacement

ELECTRONIC RESOURCES

evolve

Evolve website (http://evolve.elsevier.com/KeeHayes/pharmacology/):
- *Case Studies*
- *Content Updates*
- *Frequently Asked Questions*
- *Student Review Activities*
- *WebLinks*
- *Additional Reference Material*

Companion CD-ROM:
- *NCLEX Examination Review Questions*
- *Pharmacology Animations*
- *IV Therapy Checklists*
- *Medication Error Checklists*
- *Drug Calculation Problems*
- *Electronic Calculators*
- *Top 200 Drugs with Pronunciations*
- *References from the Textbook*

Outline

Objectives

- Describe osmolality and tonicity.
- Discuss the iso-osmolality range for serum and isotonicity of intravenous solutions.
- Describe the four classifications of intravenous fluids.
- Differentiate between cations and anions of electrolytes.
- Explain the major functions of cations.
- Discuss examples of potassium, calcium, and magnesium supplements.
- Explain the methods used to correct potassium, calcium, and magnesium excess.
- Describe several signs and symptoms of hypokalemia, hyperkalemia, hyponatremia, hypernatremia, hypocalcemia, hypercalcemia, hypochloremia, hyperchloremia, hypophosphatemia, and hyperphosphatemia.
- Explain the pharmacokinetics and pharmacodynamics of oral and intravenous potassium chloride and calcium salts.
- Describe the assessments, nursing interventions, and client teaching for fluid, potassium, sodium, calcium, and magnesium imbalances.

Terms

Fluid replacement is based on body fluid needs. The adult body is approximately 60% water, the human embryo is 97% water, and the newborn infant is 77% water. Of the 60% adult body water (fluid), 40% is intracellular fluid (ICF; cells), and 20% is extracellular fluid (ECF), of which 15% is interstitial (tissue) fluid and 5% is intravascular or vascular fluid (Table 15–1).

Electrolytes in the body are substances that carry either a positive charge **(cation)** or a negative charge **(anion).** Cations and anions are described in Table 15–2. The functions of cations are to transmit nerve impulses to muscles and to contract skeletal and smooth muscles.

The cations of the electrolytes are most plentiful in the cells (potassium, magnesium, and some calcium), in the ECF that is within the blood vessels and tissue spaces (sodium and some calcium), and in the gastrointestinal (GI) tract. Anions are attached to cations. Figure 15–1 illustrates those electrolytes that are plentiful in the stomach and intestines.

This chapter describes fluid and electrolyte replacements based on fluid and specific electrolyte deficits and excesses.

Body Fluids

The concentration of body fluid is described as osmolality and osmolarity; these terms are frequently used interchangeably. **Osmolality** is the osmotic pull exerted by all particles (solutes) per unit of water, expressed as osmoles or milliosmoles per kilogram (mOsm/kg) of water. Three types of fluid concentration are based on the osmolality of body fluids:

1. **Iso-osmolar** fluid, which has the same proportion of weight of particles (e.g., sodium, glucose, urea, protein) and water

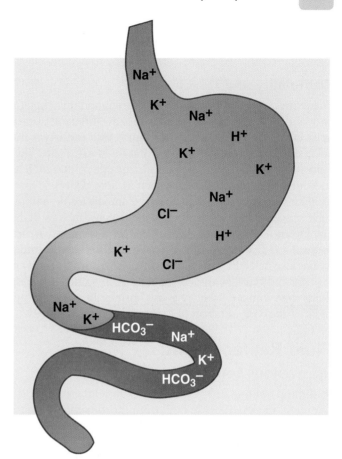

FIGURE 15–1 Plentiful electrolytes in the gastrointestinal tract include potassium (K^+), sodium (Na^+), hydrogen (H^+), bicarbonate (HCO_3^-), and chloride (Cl^-).

2. **Hypo-osmolar** fluid, which has fewer particles than water
3. **Hyperosmolar** fluid, which has more particles than water. The plasma/serum osmolality (concentration of circulating body fluids) can be calculated if the serum sodium level is known or the sodium, glucose, and blood urea nitrogen (BUN) levels are known. Sodium is the main extracellular electrolyte, and its major function is to regulate body fluids. The two formulas used to estimate serum osmolality are the following:

Double the serum sodium (Na) = serum osmolality

$$2 \times \text{serum Na} + \frac{\text{BUN}}{3} + \frac{\text{Glucose}}{18} = \text{serum osmolality}$$

The second formula is more accurate in estimating the correct serum osmolality.

Normal serum osmolality is 275 to 295 mOsm/kg. If the serum osmolality is less than 275 mOsm/kg, the body fluid is hypo-osmolar (fewer particles than water); if the serum osmolality is greater than 295 mOsm/kg, the body fluid is hyperosmolar (more particles, less water). Hypo-osmolality of body fluid may be the result of excess water intake or fluid overload (edema) caused by an inability to excrete excess water. Hyperosmolality of body fluid could

Table 15–1

Adult Body Fluid Volume

Fluid Compartment	Percentage
Intracellular (cellular) fluid (ICF)	40%
Extracellular fluid (ECF)	20%
Interstitial fluid (tissue spaces)	15%
Intravascular fluid (vascular fluid)	5%
Total body fluid	60%

Table 15–2

Cations and Anions

Cations	Anions
Potassium (K^+)	Chloride (Cl^-)
Sodium (Na^+)	Bicarbonate (HCO_3^-)
Calcium (Ca^{2+})	Phosphate (PO_4^-)
Magnesium (Mg^{2+})	Sulfate (SO_4^-)

be caused by severe diarrhea, increased salt and solutes (protein) intake, inadequate water intake, diabetes, ketoacidosis, or sweating.

Osmolality and Tonicity

The terms *osmolality* and *tonicity* have been used interchangeably, and although they are similar, they are different. Osmolality is the concentration of body fluids, and **tonicity** is the effect of fluid on cellular volume. Increased osmolality (hyperosmolality) can result from impermeable solutes such as sodium and permeable solutes such as urea (BUN). Hypertonicity results from an increase of impermeable solutes such as sodium but not of permeable solutes such as BUN. Hyperosmolality of body fluid occurs with increased serum sodium and BUN levels; however, it may also cause isotonicity because BUN does not affect tonicity. Serum osmolality is a better indicator of the concentration of solutes in body fluids than tonicity. Tonicity is used primarily as a measurement of the concentration of intravenous (IV) solutions.

Fluid Replacement

Intravenous Solutions

With fluid volume deficit from the extracellular body compartment, there is a loss of fluid from the interstitial (tissue) spaces and from the vascular (blood vessel) spaces. IV fluids in various concentrations are available to replace body fluid loss. The tonicities of many IV fluids are similar to serum osmolality, with the exception that the tonicity of solutions is wider. The average serum osmolality is 290 mOsm/kg water. For an IV solution, the isotonicity range is 240 to 340 mOsm/L. This is determined by using a factor of 50: subtract 50 from 290 mOsm to equal 240, and add 50 to 290 to equal 340. If the tonicity of the IV solution is less than 240 mOsm, it is a hypotonic solution; if it is greater than 340 mOsm, it is a hypertonic solution. Isotonic solutions include dextrose 5% in water (D_5W), which has 250 mOsm; normal saline solution or 0.9% sodium chloride (NaCl), which has 310 mOsm; lactated Ringer's solution, which has 275 mOsm; and Ringer's solution, which has 310 mOsm. These isotonic solutions have osmolalities similar to the ECFs and intracellular fluids. With fluid volume loss, isotonic IV solutions are usually indicated.

Dextrose in water, when used continuously or administered rapidly, becomes a hypotonic solution instead of an isotonic solution. The dextrose is rapidly metabolized to water and carbon dioxide (CO_2). Five percent dextrose in water (D_5W) should only be given IV and never subcutaneously (subQ). Normal saline solution or an isotonic solution of dextrose and saline may be administered subcutaneously.

The following are the four classifications of IV solutions used for fluid replacements:
- Crystalloids
- Colloids
- Blood and blood products
- Lipids

Crystalloids include dextrose, saline, and lactated Ringer's solutions. This group of solutions is used for replacement and maintenance fluid therapy.

Colloids are volume expanders that include dextran solutions, amino acids, hetastarch, and Plasmanate. Dextran is not a substitute for whole blood because it does not have any products that can carry oxygen. Dextran 40 tends to interfere with platelet function and can prolong bleeding time. Hetastarch is a nonantigenic volume expander and lasts for more than 24 hours, but it may persist for weeks in the body. Hetastarch is an isotonic solution (310 mOsm/L) that can decrease platelet and hematocrit counts and is contraindicated for clients with bleeding disorders, heart failure (HF), and renal dysfunction. Plasmanate is a commercially prepared protein product that is used instead of plasma or albumin to replace body protein.

Blood and blood products are whole blood, packed red blood cells (RBCs), plasma, and albumin. A unit of packed RBCs contains whole blood without plasma. The advantages of using packed cells instead of whole blood are (1) a decreased chance for causing circulatory overload, (2) a smaller risk of a reaction to plasma antigens, and (3) a possible reduction in the risk of transmitting serum hepatitis. Whole blood should not be used to correct anemia unless the anemia is severe. A unit of whole blood elevates the hemoglobin by 0.5 to 1 g, and a unit of packed RBCs elevates the hematocrit by three points.

Lipids are administered as fat emulsion solution and are usually indicated when IV therapy lasts longer than 5 days. Lipids add to balancing the client's nutritional needs. Total parenteral nutrition (TPN) or hyperalimentation (HA) is normally implemented for clients who require long-term IV therapy. TPN is discussed in Chapter 16.

Visit *http://evolve.elsevier.com/KeeHayes/pharmacology/* for a table of various IV solutions in the four classifications listed according to their tonicity, caloric and electrolyte compositions, and general comments.

Daily water requirements differ according to age and medical problems. The approximate daily water need for a client weighing 70 kg is 30 ml per kg of body weight, or 2000 ml per day. In pounds, the calculation is 15 ml per pound. A client weighing 150 pounds should receive 2250 ml of water daily. If the client has a fever, water needs increase by 15%. A client loses water daily: 400 to 500 ml through skin by normal evaporation, 400 to 500 ml from breathing, 100 to 200 ml in feces, and 1000 to 1200 ml in urine.

When IV fluids are prescribed for 24 hours, the total amount ordered is usually 2000 to 3000 ml. Normally, there is more than one type of solution used. Three liters of D_5W per day causes a hypo-osmolar body fluid state, and water intoxication (intracellular fluid volume excess) can result. If only hypertonic IV solutions such as dextrose in normal saline solution are used, dehydration can occur as a result of hyperosmolality, which pulls fluid from the cells and promotes fluid excretion. Usually one or two isotonic solutions (this could include D_5W) and one or two hypertonic solutions are administered per day.

Nursing Process

Fluid Replacement

ASSESSMENT

■ Assess vital signs and use for future baseline values. Report abnormal findings.

■ Check client's laboratory findings, especially hematocrit and blood urea nitrogen (BUN). If both values are elevated, may be because of fluid volume deficit (dehydration). If BUN is >60 mg/dl, renal impairment is most likely the cause.

■ Determine urine output. Report if urine output is <25 ml/h or 600 ml/day. Normal urine output should be >35 ml/hr or 1000 to 1200 ml/day.

■ Obtain urine specific gravity (SG). Normal range is 1.005 to 1.030. If urine specific gravity is >1.030, hypovolemia or dehydration may be the cause.

■ Check the types of IV fluid ordered per day. Report to health care provider if there is continuous use of one type of IV fluid such as 5% dextrose in water (D_5W). This could cause hypo-osmolality of body fluid.

■ Record client's weight for a baseline level.

NURSING DIAGNOSES

■ Risk for fluid volume excess related to excess volume infused, rapidly infused IV fluids, or volume infused too great for client's physical size or condition

■ Risk for deficient fluid volume related to inadequate fluid intake

■ Ineffective tissue perfusion (vascular) related to decreased blood circulation or inadequate fluid replacement

■ Deficient knowledge related to signs and symptoms of dehydration or fluid overload

PLANNING

■ Client will not develop fluid volume deficit or excess as the result of IV fluid replacement.

■ Client will be hydrated; vital signs and urine output will be within normal ranges.

NURSING INTERVENTIONS

■ Monitor vital signs and report abnormal findings. Rapid pulse rate could be indicative of hypovolemia (decrease in body fluids). Blood pressure changes should be reported. Decrease in blood pressure occurs when hypovolemia is severe and shock is occurring.

■ Monitor urine output. Report if urine output is less than 600 ml/day. Could be caused by fluid volume deficit or heart failure from fluid overload.

■ Measure weight daily. A gain of 2.2 to 2.5 pounds is equivalent to 1 L of fluid. If client gained 5 pounds in one day, it may indicate that client is retaining 2 L of fluid. This could be a sign of fluid overload.

■ Check for signs and symptoms of fluid volume deficit (dehydration) such as excess thirst (mild dehydration). Marked thirst, dry mucous membranes, poor skin turgor, decrease in urine output, tachycardia, and slight decrease in systolic blood pressure are indicators of marked dehydration.

■ Observe for signs and symptoms of fluid volume excess (fluid overload) such as constant, irritated cough; dyspnea; neck vein engorgement; hand vein engorgement; and moist rales in the lung.

■ Monitor laboratory results daily, especially BUN, hemoglobin, and hematocrit. Elevated values can indicate dehydration.

■ Monitor the types of fluids client is receiving. Report if only one type of IV fluid is being prescribed daily. This can cause fluid imbalance (hypo-osmolality or hyperosmolality).

■ Check IV injection site for infiltration or phlebitis.

Client Teaching

• Instruct client that thirst means there is a mild fluid deficit. Increasing fluid intake is important. Older clients' thirst mechanisms are frequently decreased. The nurse should offer fluids as needed to older adults.

• Advise client to report frequent vomiting or diarrhea. When vomiting and diarrhea occur constantly or over several days, severe fluid volume imbalance can result.

• Encourage client to monitor fluid intake and output. Inform client to report abnormal findings such as diuresis, weight gain or loss, peripheral edema, or tight shoes and rings to the health care provider.

Cultural Considerations ❖

• Use an interpreter as appropriate.

• Involve the extended family in health teaching and support.

• Incorporate wise food choices that are culturally acceptable.

EVALUATION

■ Evaluate that the IV therapy has replaced client's body fluids.

■ Evaluate that the IV therapy has not caused a deficit or an excess of client's body fluids.

Electrolytes

Potassium

Potassium (K^+), an important cellular cation, is 20 times more prevalent in the cells (ICF) than in the vessels (intravascular fluid, or plasma). The normal plasma or serum level (these terms are frequently used interchangeably) for potassium is 3.5 to 5.3 milliequivalents per liter (mEq/L). A serum potassium level less than 3.5 mEq/L is called **hypokalemia**, and a serum potassium level greater than 5.3 mEq/L is called **hyperkalemia**. Potassium has a narrow normal range. Too little potassium (hypokalemia), less than 2.5 mEq/L, or too much potassium (hyperkalemia), more than 7.0 mEq/L, may lead to cardiac arrest.

Potassium is poorly stored in the body, so daily potassium intake is necessary. The recommended potassium intake is approximately 40 to 60 mEq daily, consumed in such foods as fruits, fruit juices, and vegetables, or in the form of potassium supplements. Bananas and dried fruits are higher in potassium content than oranges and fruit juices.

Functions

Potassium is necessary for the transmission and conduction of nerve impulses and for the contraction of skeletal, cardiac, and smooth muscles. It is also needed for the enzyme action used to change carbohydrates to energy (glycolysis) and amino acids to protein. Potassium promotes glycogen (energy) storage in hepatic (liver) cells. It also helps in the regulation of osmolality (solute concentration) of cellular fluids.

Hypokalemia

Whenever cells are damaged from trauma, injury, surgery, or shock, potassium leaks from the cells into the intravascular fluid and is excreted by the kidneys. With cellular loss of potassium, potassium shifts from the blood plasma into the cell to restore the cellular potassium balance; thus hypokalemia usually results. Vomiting and diarrhea also decrease serum potassium levels. Between 80% and 90% of potassium in the body is excreted in the urine; 8% is excreted in the feces. If the kidneys shut down or are diseased, potassium accumulates in the intravascular fluid and hyperkalemia results.

When the serum potassium level is between 3.0 and 3.5 mEq/L, 100 to 200 mEq of potassium chloride (KCl) is needed to increase the serum potassium level 1 mEq (e.g., 3.0 to 4.0 mEq). If the serum potassium level is less than 3.0 mEq/L, then 200 to 400 mEq of KCl is needed to increase the serum potassium level 1 mEq. Administering potassium chloride cannot rapidly correct a severe potassium deficit.

Potassium can be given orally or IV and is combined with an anion such as chloride or bicarbonate. Oral potassium can be given as a liquid, powder, or tablet. Potassium is extremely irritating to the gastric and intestinal mucosa, so it must be given with at least a half glass or, preferably, a full glass of fluid (juice or water). Because cardiac arrest (standstill) results from excessive potassium, IV potassium must be diluted in IV fluids—it cannot be given as an IV push or IV bolus. Nurses must remember that when administering any type of potassium, it must be diluted. Table 15–3 lists the potassium preparations used to treat hypokalemia.

Table 15–3

Potassium Supplements

Preparation	Drug
Oral liquid	potassium chloride: 10% = 20 mEq/15 ml, 20% = 40 mEq/15 ml
	Kay Ciel (potassium chloride)
	Kaochlor 10% (potassium chloride)
	Kaon-Cl 20% (potassium chloride)
	potassium triplex: potassium acetate, bicarbonate, citrate. Rarely used.
Oral tablet or capsule	potassium chloride (enteric-coated tablet)
	Kaon (potassium gluconate)
	Kaon-Cl (potassium chloride)
	Slow-K (potassium chloride), 8 mEq
	Kaochlor (potassium chloride)
	K-Lyte (potassium bicarbonate), effervescent tablet
	K-Lyte/Cl (potassium chloride)
	K-Dur (potassium chloride)
	Micro-K (potassium chloride)
	Ten-K (potassium chloride)
	K-Tab (potassium chloride)
Intravenous potassium	potassium chloride in clear liquid in multidose vial or ampule (2 mEq/ml)

Signs and symptoms of hypokalemia include nausea and vomiting, dysrhythmias, abdominal distention, and soft, flabby muscles. If the serum potassium level is a low normal, foods high in potassium should be suggested: fruit juices, citrus fruits, dried fruits, bananas, nuts (peanut butter), some sodas and tea, and vegetables such as potatoes, broccoli, and green leafy vegetables.

Certain drugs such as potassium-wasting diuretics (hydrochlorothiazide [HydroDIURIL], furosemide [Lasix], ethacrynic acid [Edecrin]) and cortisone preparations promote potassium loss. Clients receiving these drugs should increase their potassium intake by consuming foods rich in potassium or by taking potassium supplements. Their serum potassium levels should be monitored for abnormal serum potassium levels. Potassium must be used cautiously in clients with renal insufficiency. If the urine output is less than 600 ml per day, the health care provider should be notified, especially if a potassium supplement is ordered.

Prototype Drug Chart 15–1 compares the pharmacokinetics and pharmacodynamics of oral and IV potassium preparations. The nursing process is based on the drug data.

Pharmacokinetics

Oral liquid potassium is absorbed faster than tablets or capsules; the pharmaceutic phase is decreased. Sustained-release capsules such as Micro-K, Slow-K, and K-tab release the potassium over a period of time. Plenty of water—no less than 4 ounces—must be taken with oral potassium preparations. The capsule may be taken with a meal or immediately after eating. IV potassium is immediately absorbed in the vascular fluids. IV potassium must be diluted in IV solutions and never given as a bolus or an IV push. REMEMBER: 80% to 90% of the potassium in body fluids is excreted in the urine; 8% is excreted in feces. Renal function should be monitored.

Prototype DRUG CHART 15–1

POTASSIUM

Drug Class

Electrolyte
Trade names: Kaochlor, Kaon Cl, Kay Ciel,
 Micro K, K Dur
Pregnancy Category: A

Contraindications

Renal insufficiency or failure, Addison's disease,
 hyperkalemia, severe dehydration, acidosis,
 potassium sparing diuretics
Caution: Cardiac disorders, burns

Dosage

Hypokalemia (maintenance):
A: PO: 20 mEq in 1 or 2 divided doses
Hypokalemia (correction):
PO: 40-80 mEq in 3 or 4 divided doses
A: IV: 20-40 mEq diluted in 1 L of IV solution

Drug-Lab-Food Interactions

Drug: Increase serum potassium level with ACE inhibitors, potassium-sparing diuretics, NSAIDs, beta
 adrenergic blockers, heparin, salt substitutes.
Lab: May increase serum potassium level (>5.5 mEq/L)
Food: None known

Pharmacokinetics

Absorption: PO: rapidly absorbed, 95% in body fluids
Distribution: PB: UK
Metabolism: t½: UK
Excretion: 80%-90% in urine; 10% in feces

Pharmacodynamics

PO: Onset: 30 min
 Peak: 1-2 h
 Duration: UK
IV: Onset: Rapid
 Peak: 1-1.5 h
 Duration: UK

Therapeutic Effects/Uses

To correct potassium deficit; strengthen cardiac and muscular activities; prevent hypokalemia in at-risk clients.
Mode of Action: Transmits and conducts nerve impulses; contracts skeletal, smooth, and cardiac muscles.

Side Effects

Nausea, vomiting, diarrhea, abdominal cramps, irritability, rash (rare); phlebitis with IV administration

Adverse Reactions

Hyperkalemia (elders with renal impairment); oliguria,
 ECG changes (peaked T waves, widened QRS complex,
 prolonged PR interval), GI ulceration
Life-threatening: Cardiac dysrhythmias, respiratory
 distress, cardiac arrest

A, Adult; *ACE*, angiotensin-converting enzyme; *ECG*, electrocardiogram; *GI*, gastrointestinal; *h*, hour; *IV*, intravenous; *PB*, protein-binding; *PO*, by mouth; *t½*, half life; *UK*, unknown; $>$ greater than.

Pharmacodynamics

Potassium maintains neuromuscular activity. Onset of action of oral potassium may be within 30 minutes; for IV potassium, it is immediate. Duration of action of potassium is not known; however, it may vary according to the dose taken. An electrocardiogram (ECG) and serum potassium levels should be closely monitored when large doses are administered.

Hyperkalemia

Hyperkalemia usually results from renal insufficiency or from the administration of large doses of potassium over time. For a mildly elevated serum potassium level such as 5.3 to 5.5 mEq/L, restricting foods rich in potassium may correct the excess potassium level. If renal insufficiency or failure is present, additional measures must be taken.

Drugs that might be ordered for hyperkalemia (serum potassium >5.3 mEq/L) are listed in Box 15–1. To immediately decrease a temporary potassium excess in the serum potassium level, sodium bicarbonate, calcium gluconate, or insulin and glucose may be prescribed. Sodium polystyrene sulfonate (Kayexalate) with sorbitol is ordered for severe hyperkalemia. This drug therapy exchanges a sodium ion for a potassium ion in the body and is a more permanent means of correcting hyperkalemia.

Signs and symptoms of hyperkalemia include nausea, abdominal cramps, oliguria (decreased urine output), tachycardia and later bradycardia, weakness, and numbness or tingling in the extremities. For mild hyperkalemia, foods rich in potassium are usually restricted.

Effect of Drugs on Potassium Balance

Potassium-wasting diuretics are a major cause of hypokalemia. Diuretics are divided into two categories: potassium-wasting and potassium-sparing drugs. Potassium-wasting diuretics excrete potassium and other electrolytes such as sodium and chloride in the urine. Potassium-sparing diuretics retain potassium but excrete sodium and chloride in the urine. Box 15–2 lists the trade and generic names of potassium-wasting and potassium-sparing diuretics and combined potassium-wasting/potassium-sparing diuretics.

Box 15–1

Potassium Excess (Hyperkalemia): Treatments and Rationales

Potassium Restriction

- Restriction of potassium intake will slowly lower serum level
- For mild hyperkalemia (slightly elevated K levels) (5.4-5.6 mEq/L, potassium restriction is normally effective)

Intravenous Sodium Bicarbonate (NaHCO₃)

- By elevating pH level, potassium moves back into cells and lowers serum level
- Temporary treatment

10% Calcium Gluconate

- Decreases irritability of myocardium resulting from hyperkalemia
- Temporary treatment; does not promote K loss
- *Caution:* administering to client on digitalis can cause digitalis toxicity

Insulin and Glucose (10%-50%)

- Moves potassium back into cells
- Temporary treatment; effective for approximately 6 hours and not always as effective when repeated

Kayexalate (Sodium Polystyrene) and Sorbitol 70%

- Kayexalate used as a cation exchange for severe hyperkalemia
- Can be administered orally or rectally
- Approximate dosages:
  Oral administration
  Kayexalate: 10-20 grams, 3 to 4 times daily
  Sorbitol 70%: 20 ml with each dose
  Rectal administration
  Kayexalate: 30-50 grams
  Sorbitol 70%: 50 ml; mix with 100-150 ml water
  (Note: Retention enema = 20-30 min)

Box 15–2

Potassium-Wasting and Potassium-Sparing Diuretics

Potassium-Wasting Diuretics
Thiazides
  chlorothiazide (Diuril)
  hydrochlorothiazide (HydroDIURIL)
Loop diuretics
  furosemide (Lasix)
  ethacrynic acid (Edecrin)
Carbonic anhydrase inhibitors
  acetazolamide (Diamox)
Osmotic diuretics
  mannitol

Potassium-Sparing Diuretics
Aldosterone antagonists
  spironolactone (Aldactone)
  triamterene (Dyrenium)
  amiloride (Midamor)

Combination: K-Wasting and K-Sparing Diuretics

Aldactazide
Spironazide
Dyazide
Moduretic

Nursing Process

Electrolyte: Potassium

ASSESSMENT

■ Assess for signs and symptoms of hypokalemia (decreased serum potassium) and hyperkalemia (elevated serum potassium). Symptoms of hypokalemia include nausea, vomiting, cardiac dysrhythmias, abdominal distention, and soft, flabby muscles. Symptoms of hyperkalemia include oliguria, nausea, abdominal cramps, tachycardia and, later, bradycardia, weakness, and numbness or tingling in the extremities.

■ Assess serum potassium level; normal serum potassium level is 3.5 to 5.3 mEq/L. Report serum potassium deficit or excess to the health care provider.

■ Obtain baseline vital sign (VS) and electrocardiograph (ECG) readings. Report abnormal findings. The VS and ECG results can be compared with future VS and ECG readings.

■ Check client for signs and symptoms of digitalis toxicity when receiving a digitalis preparation (digoxin) and a potassium-wasting diuretic (hydrochlorothiazide, furosemide) or a cortisone preparation (prednisone). A decreased serum potassium level enhances the action of digitalis. Signs and symptoms of digitalis toxicity are nausea, vomiting, anorexia, bradycardia (pulse rate <60 or markedly decreased), cardiac dysrhythmias, and visual disturbances.

NURSING DIAGNOSES

■ Imbalanced nutrition, less than body requirements related to anorexia
■ Impaired tissue integrity related to potassium imbalance
■ Deficient knowledge related to potassium-rich foods

PLANNING

■ Client's serum potassium level will be within normal range in 2 to 4 days.

■ Client with hypokalemia will eat foods rich in potassium such as fruits, fruit juices, and vegetables. Client with hyperkalemia will avoid potassium-rich foods.

NURSING INTERVENTIONS

■ Give oral potassium with sufficient amount of water or juice (at least 6 to 8 ounces) or at mealtime. Potassium is extremely irritating to the gastric mucosa.

■ Hang IV solutions containing potassium to be infused only on a pump or controlled infusion device.

■ Dilute IV potassium chloride in the IV bag and invert the bag several times to promote thorough mixing of potassium with IV fluids. Potassium cannot be given IM. Potassium should never be given as an IV bolus or push. Giving IV potassium directly into the vein causes cardiac dysrhythmias and cardiac arrest.

■ Check amount of urine output. If client is receiving potassium and the urine output is <25 ml/h or <600 ml/d, potassium accumulation occurs. REMEMBER: 80% to 90% of potassium is excreted in the urine. Report results to the health care provider.

■ Determine serum potassium level. Hypokalemia occurs if the serum potassium value is <3.5 mEq/L; hyperkalemia occurs when the serum potassium value is >5.3 mEq/L.

■ Monitor ECG. With hypokalemia, the T wave is flat or inverted, the ST segment is depressed, and the QT interval is prolonged. With hyperkalemia, the T wave is narrow and peaked, the QRS complex is spread, and the PR interval is prolonged.

■ Check IV site for infiltration if client is receiving potassium in the IV fluids. Potassium can cause tissue necrosis if it infiltrates into fatty tissue (subcutaneous tissue). The IV fluid with potassium should be discontinued when infiltration occurs.

■ Monitor clients receiving medications for hyperkalemia (e.g., sodium bicarbonate, calcium gluconate, insulin and glucose, sodium polystyrene sulfonate [Kayexalate], sorbitol) for signs and symptoms of continuing hyperkalemia or iatrogenic hypokalemia.

■ Prepare and administer sodium polystyrene sulfonate (Kayexalate) orally or by retention enema according to the drug circular. Client should have a cleansing enema before the retention enema. A suggested method for preparation and administration of sodium polystyrene sulfonate (Kayexalate) retention enema is as follows:

1. Use warm fluid to prepare (do not heat).
2. Mix with 20% dextrose in water or sorbitol.
3. Keep particles in suspension by stirring periodically and administer at body temperature by gravity.
4. Encourage client to try to retain the enema for a minimum of 30 to 60 minutes.
5. Flush tubing with 50 to 100 ml of fluid before clamping for retention.

6. After completion, irrigate the colon with 2 quarts of flushing liquid and drain the fluid contents.

Client Teaching

General

• Advise client to have serum potassium level checked at regular intervals when taking drugs that are potassium supplements or that decrease potassium levels.
• Instruct client to drink a full glass of water or juice when taking oral potassium supplements. Potassium preparations can be taken during or after a meal. Explain to client that potassium is very irritating to the stomach.
• Encourage client to comply with prescribed potassium dose, regular laboratory tests, and medical follow-up related to the health problem and drug regimen.

Diet

• Instruct client who is taking a potassium-wasting diuretic or a cortisone preparation to eat potassium-rich foods that include citrus juices, fruits (bananas, plums, oranges, cantaloupes, raisins), vegetables, and nuts.

Side Effects

• Instruct client to report signs and symptoms of hypokalemia and hyperkalemia (see ASSESSMENT for the list). When taking large amounts of potassium supplements, hyperkalemia could result.

Cultural Considerations ❖

• Use an interpreter as appropriate.
• Involve the extended family in health teaching and support.
• Incorporate wise food choices that are culturally acceptable.

EVALUATION

■ Evaluate client's serum potassium level and ECG. Report to the health care provider if the level remains abnormal. Potassium replacements and diet may need modification.

Laxatives, corticosteroids, antibiotics, and potassium-wasting diuretics are the major drug groups that can cause hypokalemia. The drug groups that may cause hyperkalemia include oral and IV potassium salts, central nervous system (CNS) agents, and potassium-sparing diuretics. Tables 15–4 and 15–5 list drugs that affect potassium balance.

Sodium

Sodium is the major cation in the ECF (vessels and tissue spaces). The normal serum or plasma sodium level is 135 to 145 mEq/L. A serum sodium level less than 135 mEq/L is called **hyponatremia**, and a serum sodium level greater than 145 mEq/L is called **hypernatremia**.

Table 15–4

Drugs Causing Hypokalemia (Serum Potassium Deficit)

Substances	Rationale
Laxatives	Abuse can cause potassium de-
Enemas (hyperosmolar)	pletion.
Corticosteroids	
cortisone	Ion-exchange agent.
prednisone	Steroids promote potassium loss and sodium retention.
Kayexalate	Exchange potassium ion for a sodium ion.
Licorice	Similar action to aldosterone, promoting K⁺ loss and Na⁺ retention.
levodopa/L-dopa	Increase potassium loss via
lithium	urine.
Antibiotic I	Have a toxic effect on renal tu-
amphotericin B	bules and thus decrease po-
polymyxin B	tassium reabsorption.
tetracycline (outdated)	
gentamicin	
neomycin	
amikacin	
tobramycin	
cisplatin	
Antibiotic II	Enhance potassium excretion is
penicillin	by the presence of nonreab-
ampicillin	sorbable anions.
carbenicillin	
ticarcillin	
nafcillin	
piperacillin	
azlocillin	
Alpha-adrenergic blockers	Promote movement of potas-
Insulin and glucose	sium into cells, thus lowering the serum potassium level.
Beta₂-agonists	Promote potassium loss.
terbutaline	
albuterol	
Estrogen	
Potassium-wasting	See Box 5–2.
diuretics	

Functions

Sodium is the major electrolyte that regulates body fluids. It promotes the transmission and conduction of nerve impulses. It is part of the sodium/potassium pump that causes cellular activity. Sodium constantly shifts into cells as potassium shifts out of cells to maintain water balance and neuromuscular activity. When sodium shifts into the cell, depolarization occurs; when sodium shifts out of the cell, potassium shifts back into the cell and repolarization occurs. Sodium combines readily with chloride (Cl^-) or bicarbonate (HCO_3^-) to promote acid-base balance.

Hyponatremia

Sodium loss can result from vomiting, diarrhea, surgery, and potent diuretics. Signs and symptoms of hyponatremia include muscular weakness, headaches, lethargy, con-

fusion, seizures, abdominal cramps, nausea, and vomiting; tachycardia and hypotension; pale skin and dry mucous membranes. The serum sodium level should be monitored as necessary.

For a serum sodium level between 125 and 135 mEq/L, normal saline (0.9% sodium chloride) may increase the sodium content in the vascular fluid. If the serum sodium level is 115 mEq/L, a hypertonic 3% saline solution may be necessary.

Hypernatremia

When the serum sodium level is elevated above 145 mEq/L, sodium restriction is indicated. Signs and symptoms of hypernatremia are flushed dry skin, agitation, elevated body temperature, elevated blood pressure, and rough, dry tongue; nausea, vomiting, anorexia; tachycardia, hypertension; muscular twitching, hyperreflexia. An increase in serum sodium can result from consuming certain drugs such as cortisone preparations, cough medications, and selected antibiotics.

The dietary requirement for sodium is 2-4 grams daily. Sodium-rich foods include bacon, beef cubes, catsup, corned beef, decaffeinated coffee, dill, ham, tomato juice, pickles, and soda crackers.

Nursing Process

Electrolyte: Sodium

ASSESSMENT

■ Assess client for signs and symptoms of hyponatremia and hypernatremia.
■ Check the serum sodium level. Report abnormally low sodium levels (<125 mEq/L), because prompt medical care is required.
■ Obtain history of health problems that may lead to sodium loss or excess.

NURSING DIAGNOSES

■ Risk for imbalanced (excess) fluid volume related to water retention
■ Deficient knowledge related to foods rich in sodium

PLANNING

■ Client's serum sodium level will be within normal range in 3 to 5 days.
■ Edema will be decreased in client with sodium retention.

NURSING INTERVENTIONS

■ Monitor prescribed medical regimen for correction of hyponatremia, example: water restriction, IV normal saline (0.9% sodium chloride), 3% saline solution to correct serum sodium levels <115 mEq/L.

■ Monitor serum sodium levels. Report abnormal level.

Client Teaching

- Instruct client with hypernatremia to avoid foods rich in sodium (canned foods, lunch meats, ham, pork, pickles, potato chips, pretzels). Instruct client to avoid using salt when cooking or adding salt to food at the table.
- Emphasize importance of reading labels on food products.

Cultural Considerations ❖

- Use interpreter as appropriate.
- Involve extended family in health teaching and support.
- Incorporate wise food choices that are culturally acceptable.

EVALUATION

■ Evaluate client's serum sodium level. Report if sodium imbalance continues.

Calcium

Calcium is found in approximately equal proportions in the ICF and ECF. The serum calcium range is 4.5 to 5.5 mEq/L, or 8.5 to 10.5 (9 to 11) mg/dl. A calcium deficit, less than 4.5 mEq/L, is called **hypocalcemia**, and a calcium excess, greater than 5.5 mEq/L, is called **hypercalcemia**. About half the calcium in body fluid is bound to protein. Calcium unbound to protein is free, ionized calcium and can cause a physiologic response. If serum protein (albumin) levels are decreased, there is more free circulating calcium, even when the serum calcium level is decreased.

Modern blood analyzers allow the ionized calcium (iCa) level to be measured. The normal serum iCa range is 2.2 to 2.5 mEq/L, or 4.25 to 5.25 mg/dl. Certain changes in blood composition can either increase or decrease the serum iCa level. When an individual is acidotic, calcium is released from serum protein and increases the serum iCa level. During alkalosis, calcium is bound to protein and there is less iCa.

Functions

Calcium promotes normal nerve and muscle activity. It increases contraction of the heart muscle (myocardium). This cation also maintains normal cellular permeability

Table 15–5

Drugs Causing Hyperkalemia (Serum Potassium Excess)

Substances	Rationale
potassium chloride (oral or IV) Potassium salt substitutes potassium penicillin (Pen-Vee K) KPO₄ enema	Excess ingestion or infusion can cause a potassium excess.
Angiotensin-converting enzyme (ACE) inhibitors captopril (Capoten) quinapril HCl (Accupril) ramipril (Altace and others)	Increase the state of hypoaldosteronism (decrease sodium and increase potassium) and impair renal potassium excretion.
Angiotensin II receptor antagonists losartan potassium (Cozaar)	Decrease adrenal synthesis of aldosterone; potassium is retained and sodium excreted.
Beta-adrenergic blockers propranolol (Inderal) nadolol (Corgard) and others	Decrease cellular uptake of potassium and decrease Na-K-ATPase function.
Digoxin	Therapeutic dose is not affected; however, with overdose, potassium excess may occur.
Heparin (>10,000 units/d)	Inhibits adrenal aldosterone production.
Low-molecular-weight heparin (LMWH)	Decreases potassium homeostasis; renal excretion of potassium is reduced.
Immunosuppressive drugs cyclosporine tacrolimus cyclophosphamide	Reduce potassium excretion by induction of hypoaldosteronism; loss of potassium from cells.
Nonsteroidal antiinflammatory drugs (NSAIDs) ibuprofen and others indomethacin	Impair potassium homeostasis and block cellular potassium uptake.
Succinylcholine: intravenous	Allows for leakage of potassium out of cells.
CNS agents Barbiturates Sedatives Narcotics heroin Amphetamines	Usually characterized by muscle necrosis and cellular shift of potassium from cells to serum.
Potassium-sparing diuretics	See Box 15–2.

and promotes blood clotting by converting prothrombin into thrombin. In addition, calcium is needed for the formation of bone and teeth.

Vitamin D is needed for calcium absorption from the GI tract. Aspirin and anticonvulsants can alter vitamin D, affecting calcium absorption. Loop or high-ceiling diuretics (furosemide [Lasix]; see Chapter 42), steroids (cortisone), magnesium preparations, and phosphate preparations promote calcium loss. Conversely, thiazide diuretics (hydrochlorothiazide [HydroDIURIL]) increase the serum calcium level.

Hypocalcemia

Inadequate calcium intake causes calcium to leave bone to maintain a normal serum calcium level. Because of calcium loss from bones (bone demineralization), fractures may occur if calcium deficit persists. Hypoparathyroidism, vitamin D deficiency, and multiple blood transfusions are common causes of hypocalcemia.

Signs and symptoms of hypocalcemia include anxiety, irritability, and tetany (twitching around the mouth, tingling and numbness of fingers, carpopedal spasm, spasmodic contractions, laryngeal spasm, and convulsions). If metabolic acidosis is present with hypocalcemia, tetany symptoms are absent because calcium leaves protein sites during an acidotic state; thus more ionized calcium is available. During an alkalotic state, more calcium binds with protein. There is less ionized calcium, and tetany symptoms usually result.

Many calcium preparations can be administered orally or IV. For treatment of calcium deficit, oral calcium tablets, capsules, or powder and IV calcium solutions may be given. Calcium preparations are combined with various salts such as chloride, carbonate, gluconate, gluceptate, and lactate. Calcium for IV use should be mixed with D₅W, NOT saline solution. Sodium encourages calcium loss. Prototype Drug Chart 15-2 compares the pharmacokinetics and pharmacodynamics of calcium preparations.

Pharmacokinetics

Vitamin D promotes calcium absorption from the GI tract; phosphorus inhibits calcium absorption. The pH affects the amount of circulating, free ionized calcium. When pH is decreased (acidic), there is more free calcium, because it has been released from protein-binding sites. With an increased pH (alkalosis) more calcium is bound to protein.

Pharmacodynamics

A calcium deficit causes tetany symptoms and, if severe, can be life-threatening. Rapid administration of IV calcium may cause tingling, warm sensations, and a metallic taste. Calcium needs to be administered at a moderate rate, and infiltration should be avoided. Calcium can be given undiluted IV in emergency situations.

Hypercalcemia

Elevated serum calcium may be a result of hyperparathyroidism, hypophosphatemia, tumors of the bone, prolonged immobilization, multiple fractures, and drugs such as thiazide diuretics. Pathologic fractures might occur because of thinning of the bone resulting from calcium loss

from the bony structure. Calcium leaves the bone and accumulates in the vascular fluid. Signs and symptoms of hypercalcemia are flabby muscles, pain over bony areas, and kidney stones of calcium composition.

Effect of Drugs on Calcium Balance

Phosphate preparations, corticosteroids, loop diuretics, aspirin, anticonvulsants, magnesium sulfate, and mithramycin are some of the groups of drugs that can lower the serum calcium level. Excess calcium salt ingestion or infusion and thiazide and chlorthalidone diuretics can all contribute to increasing serum calcium level. Table 15-6 lists drugs that affect calcium balance.

Clinical Management of Calcium Imbalance

Clinical management of hypocalcemia consists of oral supplements and IV calcium diluted in D₅W. Calcium should not be diluted in a normal saline solution (0.9%

Table 15-6

Drugs Affecting Calcium Balance

Substances	Rationale
Drugs Causing Hypocalcemia (Serum Calcium Deficit)	
magnesium sulfate propylthiouracil (Propacil) colchicine plicamycin (Mithracin) neomycin	Inhibit parathyroid hormone/PTH secretion and decrease serum calcium level.
Excessive sodium citrate acetazolamide aspirin Anticonvulsants glutethimide (Doriden) Estrogens Aminoglycosides gentamicin amikacin tobramycin	Can alter the vitamin D metabolism needed for calcium absorption.
Phosphate preparations: Oral, enema, intravenous sodium phosphate potassium phosphate	Can increase serum phosphorus level and decrease serum calcium level.
Corticosteroids cortisone prednisone	Decrease calcium mobilization and inhibit absorption of calcium.
Loop diuretics furosemide (Lasix)	Reduce calcium absorption from renal tubules.
Drugs Causing Hypercalcemia (Serum Calcium Excess)	
Calcium salts Vitamin D	Excess ingestion of calcium and vitamin D and infusion of calcium can increase the serum Ca level.
IV lipids	Can increase the calcium level.
Kayexalate, androgens Diuretics Thiazides chlorthalidone (Hygroton)	Can induce hypercalcemia.

Prototype DRUG CHART 15–2

CALCIUM

Drug Class

Electrolyte
Trade names:
calcium carbonate (Os-cal, Tums, Caltrate, Megacal)
calcium gluconate (Kalcinate)
Pregnancy Category: C
Drug forms: Tablet, capsule, liquid, injection

Contraindications

Hypercalcemia, renal calculi, digitalis toxicity,
  ventricular fibrillation
Caution: Renal or respiratory disorders, GI hypomotility

Dosage

Antacid use:
A: PO: 0.5 1 g q4 6h (dose varies according to the
  calcium salt)
Osteoporosis:
A: PO: 1200 mg/d
Tetany:
A: IV: 4-16 mEq
C: IV: 0.5-0.7 mEq/kg t.i.d., q.i.d.
Hypocalcemia:
A: PO: 500 mg/d in divided doses

Drug-Lab-Food Interactions

Drug: Increase digitalis toxicity: digoxin; decrease
  calcium channel blockers, verapamil; decrease absorption of tetracycline; increase serum calcium level:
  thiazide diuretics
Lab: May increase calcium gastrin, pH; may decrease
  phosphate, potassium
Food: None known

Pharmacokinetics

Absorption: PO: 35% absorbed, requires vitamin D
Distribution: PB: UK
Metabolism: t½: UK
Excretion: 20% in urine, 70% in feces, some in saliva

Pharmacodynamics

PO: Onset: UK
  Peak: UK
  Duration: 2-4 h
IV: Onset: Rapid
  Peak: UK
  Duration: 2-3 h

Therapeutic Effects/Uses

To correct calcim deficit or tetany symptoms, prevent osteoporosis
Mode of Action: Transmits nerve impulses, contracts skeletal and cardiac muscles, maintains cellular permeability;
  promotes strong bone and teeth growth

Side Effects

PO: Nausea, vomiting, constipation, pain, drowsiness,
  headache, muscle weakness

Adverse Reactions

Hypercalcemia, ECG changes (shortened QT interval),
  metabolic alkalosis, heart block, rebound hyperacidity
Life-threatening: Renal falure, cardiac dysrhythmias,
  cardiac arrest

A, Adult; *C*, child; *d*, day; *ECG*, electrocardiogram; *GI*, gastrointestinal; *h*, hour; *IV*, intravenous; *PB*, protein binding; *PO*, by mouth;
q.i.d., four times a day; *t½*, half life; *t.i.d.*, three times a day; *UK*, unknown.

NaCl), because sodium promotes calcium loss. Table 15–7 lists oral and IV preparations of calcium salts, their dosages, and drug form. Calcium carbonate can cause GI upset, because it produces carbon dioxide. For better calcium absorption, calcium supplements should contain vitamin D, and oral calcium should be taken 30 minutes before meals. Box 15–3 gives guidelines for the suggested clinical management of hypocalcemia.

The goal for managing hypercalcemia is to correct the underlying cause of serum calcium excess. Drugs such as calcitonin or IV saline solution administered rapidly and followed by a loop diuretic can be used to promote rapid urinary excretion of calcium.

 Nursing Process

Electrolyte: Calcium

ASSESSMENT

■ Assess client for signs and symptoms of hypocalcemia (decreased serum calcium) such as tetany (twitching of the mouth, tingling and numbness of the fingers, facial spasms, spasms of the larynx, and carpopedal spasm), muscle cramps, bleeding tendencies, and weak cardiac contractions.

■ Check serum calcium levels (normal, 4.5-5.5 mEq/L or 8.5-10.5 mg/dl) for hypocalcemia and hypercalcemia. Report abnormal test results. Serum ionized calcium (iCa: normal, 2.2-2.5 mEq/L, or 4.25-5.25 mg/dl) indicates free circulating calcium and is more accurate for determining calcium imbalance.

■ Obtain vital signs (VS) and electrocardiograph (ECG) readings. Report abnormal findings. VS and ECG results can be compared with future VS and ECG readings.

■ Gather current drug history for client. Calcium enhances the effect of digoxin. Elevated serum calcium level can cause digitalis toxicity. Signs and symptoms of digitalis toxicity include nausea, vomiting, anorexia, bradycardia (pulse rate <60 or markedly decreased), cardiac dysrhythmias, and visual disturbances. Thiazide diuretics can increase the serum calcium level. Drugs that decrease the effect of calcium are calcium channel blockers, tetracycline, and sodium chloride.

Table 15–7

Calcium Preparations

Calcium Name	Drug Form	Drug Dose
Orals		
calcium carbonate	650- to 1500-mg tablets	400 mg/g*
calcium citrate	950-mg tablet	211 mg/g*
calcium lactate	325- to 650-mg tablets	130 mg/g*
calcium gluconate	500- to 1000-mg tablets	90 mg/g*
Intravenous		
calcium chloride	10-ml size	272 mg/g*; 13.5 mEq
calcium gluceptate	5-ml size	90 mg/g*; 4.5 mEq
calcium gluconate	10-ml size	90 mg/g*; 4.5 mEq

*Elemental calcium is 1 g.

Box 15–3

Clinical Management of Hypocalcemia

Mild Calcium Deficit

Oral calcium salts with vitamin D, take twice daily. 10% IV calcium gluconate (10 ml) in D_5W solution. Administer slowly, 1-3 ml/min.

Moderate Calcium Deficit

10% IV calcium gluconate (10-20 ml) in D_5W solution. Administer slowly, 1-3 ml/min.

Severe Calcium Deficit

10% IV calcium gluconate (100 ml) in 1 L of D_5W. Administer over 4 h.

NURSING DIAGNOSES

■ Imbalanced nutrition, less than body requirements related to GI discomfort
■ Impaired tissue integrity related to numbness and tingling of hands
■ Deficient knowledge related to foods rich in calcium

PLANNING

■ Client's serum calcium level will be within normal range by 3 to 7 days.
■ Tetany symptoms will cease. Client will eat foods rich in calcium or take calcium supplements as ordered.
■ Client with hypercalcemia will avoid foods rich in calcium, such as milk products.

NURSING INTERVENTIONS

■ Monitor VS. Report abnormal findings. Compare with baseline VS. Monitor pulse rate if client is taking digoxin. Bradycardia is a sign of digitalis toxicity.

■ Administer IV fluids slowly with 10% calcium gluconate or chloride. Calcium should be administered with D_5W, not saline solution, because sodium promotes calcium loss. Calcium should not be added to solutions containing bicarbonate, because rapid precipitation occurs.

■ Check IV site for infiltration if client is receiving calcium in IV fluids. Calcium can cause tissue necrosis (sloughing of the tissue) if it infiltrates into subcutaneous tissue. Calcium gluceptate is the only calcium preparation that can be given IM.

■ Monitor serum calcium and iCa levels. Hypocalcemia occurs if serum calcium value is <4.5 mEq/L, or <8.5 mg/dl, or if iCa is <2.2 mEq/L. Hypercalcemia occurs if serum calcium value is >5.5 mEq/L, or >10.5 mg/dl, or if iCa is >2.5 mEq/L.

■ Monitor ECGs. With hypocalcemia, ST segment is lengthened and QT interval is prolonged. With hypercalcemia, ST segment is decreased and QT interval is shortened.

Client Teaching

General

• Instruct client to avoid overuse of antacids and the habit of chronic use of laxatives. Excessive use of certain antacids may cause alkalosis, decreasing calcium ionization. Chronic use of laxatives decreases calcium absorption from the GI tract. Suggest fruits and foods rich in fiber for improving bowel elimination.

• Encourage client taking calcium supplements to check that the calcium tablet is absorbable. To do this, put 1 tablet into 1 ounce of white vinegar. Stir every 3 minutes. The tablet should break up or dissolve within 30 minutes.

- Advise clients to take oral calcium supplements with meals or after meals to increase absorption.

Diet

- Suggest that client consume foods high in calcium such as milk, milk products, and protein-rich foods. Protein and vitamin D are needed to enhance calcium absorption.

Side Effects

- Instruct client to report symptoms related to calcium excess or hypercalcemia, including flabby muscles, pain over bony areas, ECG changes, and kidney (calcium form) stones.

Cultural Considerations ❖

- Use an interpreter as appropriate.
- Involve extended family in health teaching and support.
- Incorporate wise food choices that are culturally acceptable.

EVALUATION

- Evaluate client's serum calcium level. Report if calcium imbalance continues.
- Determine whether side effects caused by previous untreated hypocalcemia are absent.

Magnesium

Magnesium, a sister cation to potassium, is most plentiful in the ICF. When there is a loss of potassium, there is also a loss of magnesium. The normal serum magnesium level is 1.5 to 2.5 mEq/L or 1.8 to 3 mg/dl. A magnesium deficit is called **hypomagnesemia**, and a magnesium excess is called **hypermagnesemia**. Daily magnesium requirement is 8 to 20 mEq.

Functions

Magnesium promotes the transmission of neuromuscular activity; it is an important mediator of neural transmission in the CNS. Like potassium, it promotes contraction of the myocardium. It activates many enzymes for the metabolism of carbohydrates and protein. It is responsible for the transportation of sodium and potassium across cell membranes.

When there is a magnesium deficit, there frequently is a potassium or calcium deficit. A serum magnesium deficit increases the release of acetylcholine from the presynaptic membrane of the nerve fiber. This increases neuromuscular excitability. A serum magnesium excess has a sedative effect on the neuromuscular system, which can result in a loss of deep tendon reflexes. Cardiac (ventricular) dysrhythmias can occur as a result of hypomagnesemia. Hypotension and heart block may result from hypermagnesemia.

Hypomagnesemia is probably the most undiagnosed electrolyte deficiency. This is most likely because hypomagnesemia is asymptomatic until the serum magnesium level approaches 1 mEq/L. The total serum magnesium concentration is not representative of the cellular magnesium levels.

To correct severe hypomagnesemia, IV magnesium sulfate may be given. For hypermagnesemia, calcium gluconate may be given to decrease the serum magnesium level.

Effect of Drugs on Magnesium Balance

Sodium inhibits tubular absorption of magnesium and calcium. Long-term administration of saline infusions may result in losses of magnesium and calcium. Diuretics, certain antibiotics, laxatives, and steroids are drug groups that promote magnesium loss. Hypomagnesemia, like hypokalemia, enhances the action of digitalis and causes digitalis toxicity. Magnesium sulfate corrects hypomagnesemia and symptoms of digitalis toxicity. It is common practice after bypass surgery or myocardial infarctions for clients to be given magnesium sulfate orally, even when blood levels are normal, to prevent ventricular arrhythmias early in the post-op/post-event phase.

An excess intake of magnesium salts is the major cause of serum magnesium excess. Two drug groups that contain magnesium and could cause hypermagnesemia are laxatives (e.g., magnesium sulfate, milk of magnesia, magnesium citrate) and antacids (e.g., Maalox, Mylanta, Di-Gel). Table 15–8 lists drugs that affect magnesium balance.

Nursing Process

Electrolyte: Magnesium

ASSESSMENT

- Assess client for signs and symptoms of magnesium deficit or excess. Hypomagnesemia: tetany-like symptoms caused by hyperexcitability (tremors, twitching of the face) and ventricular tachycardia that leads to ventricular fibrillation and hypertension. Hypermagnesemia: lethargy, drowsiness, weakness, paralysis, loss of deep tendon reflexes, hypotension, and heart block.
- Check serum magnesium levels for magnesium imbalance. Symptoms of magnesium deficit may or may not be seen until serum level is below 1 mEq/L.
- Observe clients receiving digitalis preparations for digitalis toxicity. A magnesium deficit, as with a potassium deficit, enhances the action of digitalis, causing digitalis toxicity.

NURSING DIAGNOSES

- Imbalanced nutrition: less than body requirements related to insufficient intake of foods rich in magnesium
- Decreased cardiac output related to hypomagnesemia or hypermagnesemia
- Deficient knowledge related to signs and symptoms of magnesium imbalance

PLANNING

■ Client's serum magnesium level will be within normal range in 2 to 5 days.

NURSING INTERVENTIONS

■ Report to health care provider if client is NPO (nothing by mouth) and receiving IV fluids without magnesium salts for weeks. Slowly administer IV magnesium sulfate in solution to prevent a hot or flushed feeling. Monitor vital signs.

■ Monitor urinary output. Most of the body's magnesium is excreted by the kidneys. Report if urine output is <600 ml/day.

■ Moniter for digitalis toxicity (e.g., nausea, vomiting, bradycardia) in clients who have hypomagnesemia and

are taking digoxin. Magnesium deficit enhances the action of digitalis preparations.

■ Monitor vital signs. Report abnormal findings to health care provider.

■ Monitor serum electrolyte results. Report low serum potassium or serum calcium levels. Low serum magnesium levels may be attributed to hypokalemia or hypocalcemia. When correcting a potassium deficit, potassium is not replaced in cells until magnesium is replaced. A serum magnesium level of 1 mEq/L or less can cause cardiac arrest.

■ Check for Trousseau's and Chvostek's signs of severe hypomagnesemia. Tetany symptoms occur in both magnesium and calcium deficits.

■ Have IV calcium gluconate available for emergency reversal of hypermagnesemia from overcorrection of a magnesium deficit.

Client Teaching

• Advise client to eat foods rich in magnesium (green vegetables, fruits, fish and seafood, grains, nuts, and peanut butter).

• Instruct client with hypermagnesemia to avoid routine use of laxatives and antacids that contain magnesium. Suggest that client check drug labels.

Cultural Considerations ❖

• Use an interpreter as appropriate.

• Involve extended family in health teaching and support.

• Incorporate wise food choices that are culturally acceptable.

EVALUATION

■ Evaluate client's serum magnesium level. Report if magnesium imbalance continues.

■ Determine whether signs and symptoms caused by prior magnesium imbalance are absent.

Chloride

Chloride is the principal cation of the extracellular fluid (ECF). The chloride ion is a major contributor to acid-base balance, gastric juice acidity, and the osmolality of ECT. Normal serum chloride level is 95-108 mEq/L. **Hypochloremia** is a decreased serum chloride level and **hyperchloremia** is an elevated level. With increased serum osmolality, > 295mOsm/kg, there are more sodium and chloride ions proportional to the water. Sodium and chloride frequently work in combination. For example, during sodium retention chloride is also frequently retained, resulting in increased water retention. Clinical manifestations of hypochloremia include tremors, twitching, and slow/shallow breathing. With severe chloride loss, decreased blood pressure is seen. Clinical manifestations of hyperchloremia include weakness, lethargy, deep/rapid breathing, and unconsciousness (late).

Table 15–8

Drugs Affecting Magnesium Balance

Drugs	Rationale
Drugs Causing Hypomagnesemia (Serum Magnesium Deficit)	

Diuretics
    furosemide (Lasix)
    ethacrynic acid (Edecrin)
    mannitol
	Promote urinary loss of magnesium.

Antibiotics
    gentamicin
    tobramycin
    carbenicillin
    capreomycin
    neomycin
    polymyxin B
    amphotericin B
digitalis
calcium gluconate
insulin
	Can cause magnesium loss via kidney.

Laxatives cisplatin	Abuse can cause magnesium loss via gastrointestinal tract.

Corticosteroids
    cortisone
    prednisone
	Can decrease serum magnesium level.

Drugs Causing Hypermagnesemia (Serum Magnesium Excess)	

Magnesium salts
    Oral and enema
      magnesium hydroxide
      (MOM)
      magnesium sulfate
      (Epsom) salt
      magnesium citrate
	Excess use could increase serum magnesium level.

magnesium sulfate (maternity)	Use of excess magnesium sulfate in treatment of toxemia can cause hypermagnesemia.
lithium	Associated with hypermagnesemia.

Phosphorus

Phosphorus is a major anion with concentration in the intracellular fluid (ICF). Most phosphorus in the body is found in association with calcium. Serum phosphorus levels are decreased by parathyroid hormone (PTH) stimulation of the renal tubules to excrete phosphorus (and concomitantly increase serum calcium levels by causing calcium to leave bone). The normal serum phosphorus level is 1.7-2.6 mEq/L. Fifty five percent is ionized (free) and 45% is protein-bound. Phosphorus is essential in bone and teeth formation and for neuromuscular activity. Phosphorus is an important component of nucleic acids (DNA and RNA), assists in energy transfer in cells, helps maintain cellular osmotic pressure, and supports the acid-base balance of body fluids. Clinical manifestations of **hypophosphatemia** include muscle weakness, tremors, paresthesia, bone pain, hyporeflexia, seizures, hyperventilation, anorexia, and dysphagia. Symptoms of **hyperphosphatemia** include hyperreflexia, tetany (with decreased calcium), flaccid paralysis, muscular weakness, tachycardia, nausea, diarrhea, and abdominal cramps. Foods rich in phosphorus include whole grain cereals, nuts, milk, and meat.

Critical Thinking Case Study

JS, 72 years old, has had vomiting and diarrhea for 2 days. JS takes digoxin 0.25 mg/day and hydrochlorothiazide (HydroDIURIL) 50 mg/day. His serum potassium level is 3.2 mEq/L. He complains of being dizzy. His blood pressure is slightly lower than usual. The nurse assesses his physiologic status and notes that his muscles are weak and flabby, his abdomen is distended, and peristalsis is diminished.

1. What signs and symptoms indicate that JS is in potassium imbalance?
2. What contributing factors caused JS's potassium imbalance?
3. What interventions should be taken for alleviating this potassium imbalance?
4. How much potassium chloride would be needed to elevate JS's serum potassium by 1 mEq?

JS was ordered intravenous infusions of 1 L of 5% dextrose in water (D_5W) with 30 mEq of potassium chloride (KCl) and 1 L of 5% dextrose in 0.45% NaCl (½ normal saline). He was also prescribed oral KCl 15 mEq, three times a day for 2 days. Oral KCl is available in 15 mEq/10 ml.

5. Explain the method for diluting KCl in IV fluids. Can KCl be given intramuscularly, subcutaneously, or as an IV bolus (push)? Explain.
6. What instructions would you give JS for taking oral potassium supplements?
7. What happens if JS's urine output decreases while he is receiving IV and oral potassium? What would be your responsibility?
8. Because JS is taking a diuretic and digoxin, what should the nurse include with client teaching? Give examples.

NCLEX Study Questions

1. Your client has been vomiting and has weak, flabby muscles. The client's pulse is irregular. What type of imbalance would you suspect?
   a. hypokalemia
   b. hyperkalemia
   c. hypocalcemia
   d. hypercalcemia

2. Your client is receiving potassium supplements. An important nursing implication is:
   a. cannot be given as IV bolus
   b. must be diluted
   c. chill before administering
   d. give only at bedtime

3. Your client is due to receive Kayexalate. You are aware that this drug is used to treat:
   a. hypocalcemia
   b. severe hypercalcemia
   c. hypokalemia
   d. severe hyperkalemia

4. Drugs that may cause an elevated serum sodium level include:
   a. antifungals
   b. oral contraceptives
   c. cortisone preparations
   d. antiepileptics

5. Specific health teaching for clients with hypermagnesemia is:
   a. eat fruits, fish, and peanut butter
   b. avoid selected laxatives and antacids
   c. magnesium is very irritating to stomach
   d. measure weight daily

6. Your client is receiving fluid replacement. Your health teaching with this client includes all the following except:
   a. measure weight daily
   b. thirst means a mild fluid deficit
   c. monitor fluid intake
   d. avoid use of calcium supplements

7. Your client gained 10 pounds in 2 days. It is determined that the weight gain is caused by fluid retention. The weight gain may be equivalent to how many liters of fluid?
   a. 2
   b. 3
   c. 4
   d. 5

8. Your health teaching for a client with hypophosphatemia includes eating:
   a. meat, milk, whole grain cereals, nuts
   b. dairy products, vitamin D
   c. dairy products, protein rich foods
   d. dairy products, nuts, vitamin C

16
Nutritional Support

Outline

Objectives

Terms

Enteral Nutrition
Routes for Enteral Feedings
Enteral Solutions
Methods for Delivery
Complications

Enteral Medications
Nursing Process: Enteral Nutrition

Parenteral Nutrition
Total Parenteral Nutrition
Complications

Nursing Process: Total Parenteral
Nutrition

Transitional Feeding: Parenteral to Enteral

Key Websites

Critical Thinking Case Study

NCLEX Study Questions

Objectives

- Explain the differences between enteral nutrition and parenteral nutrition.
- Describe the routes for enteral feedings.
- Discuss examples of enteral solutions and explain the differences.
- Explain the advantages and differences of the methods used to deliver enteral nutrition.
- Describe the complications that may occur with use of enteral nutrition and parenteral nutrition.
- Discuss the nursing interventions for clients receiving enteral nutrition and parenteral nutrition

Terms

bolus, p. 257
continuous feedings, p. 257
cyclic method, p. 257
enteral nutrition, p. 255

hyperalimentation (HA), p. 255
intermittent enteral feedings, p. 257

intermittent infusion, p. 257
nasogastric tube, p. 255
nutritional support, p. 255

parenteral nutrition, p. 255
total parenteral nutrition (TPN), p. 255
Valsalva maneuver, p. 260

Nutrients are needed for cell growth, cellular function, enzyme activity, carbohydrate-fat-protein synthesis, muscular contraction, wound healing, immune competence, and gastrointestinal (GI) integrity. Inadequate nutrient intake can result from surgery, trauma, malignancy, and other catabolic illnesses. Without adequate nutritional support, protein catabolism (breakdown), malnutrition, and diminished organ functioning affect the GI, liver, renal, cardiac, and respiratory systems. The functioning of the immune system also is decreased.

Clients who are well nourished can usually tolerate a lack of nutrients for 14 days without major health problems. However, clients who are critically ill may only tolerate a lack of nutrient support for a short period (a few days to a week) before signs of impaired organ function, infection, or morbidity result. If nutritional support is started within hours of an injury, as in the cases of severe trauma or burns, recovery is more rapid. When injury is a result of minor surgery, no severe bodily harm results from lack of nutritional support for days, but for both the critically ill and for clients with minor injuries, early nutritional support improves intestinal and liver blood flow and function, enhances wound healing, decreases the occurrence of infection, and improves the general outcome of the health situation. "Early fed" injured clients have a positive nitrogen balance and less chance for bacterial infections; thus they also have a decrease in institutional length of stay.

Dextrose 5% in water (D₅W), normal saline, and lactated Ringer's solution are not forms of nutritional support, although these solutions do provide fluids and some electrolytes. A client requires 2000 calories per day; critically ill clients may require 3000 to 5000 calories per day. In cases of burns, the caloric need could be even greater. Clients who receive nothing by mouth (NPO) for an extended period become malnourished. Delayed nutritional support by as little as 5 days for a client experiencing trauma or neurologic damage (e.g., cervical fracture) could hamper wound healing and increase the risk of developing an infection.

There are two routes for administering **nutritional support**: enteral and parenteral. **Enteral nutrition**, which involves the GI tract, can be given orally or by feeding tubes (tube feeding). If the client can swallow, nutrient preparations can be taken by mouth; if the client is unable to swallow, a tube is inserted into the stomach or small intestine. **Parenteral nutrition** involves administering high-caloric nutrients through large veins, for example, the subclavian vein. This method is called **total parenteral nutrition (TPN)** or **hyperalimentation (HA)**. Parenteral nutrition is more costly (approximately three times more expensive) than enteral nutrition, and the benefits are not significant. In fact with TPN there is a higher infection rate. The use of TPN does not promote effective GI integrity, liver function, or body weight gain, as does enteral nutrition. But because enteral feedings require a functioning GI tract, TPN becomes necessary when the GI tract is incapacitated due to uncontrolled vomiting, malabsorption, or intestinal obstruction. TPN may also be necessary in cases where there is a high risk for aspiration or to supplement inadequate oral intake.

This chapter is divided into enteral nutrition and parenteral nutrition. Routes for nutritional administration, nutritional preparations, methods for delivery, complications, and the nursing process are discussed for each.

Enteral Nutrition

When enteral nutrition is prescribed there should be adequate small bowel function with digestion, absorption, and GI motility. To determine whether there is a lack of GI motility, the nurse assesses for abdominal distention and a decrease or absence of bowel sounds. In critically ill clients, frequently there is a decrease or absence in gastric emptying time; then TPN may be necessary. The preferred method for nutritional support is enteral feedings for clients with intact gastric emptying and with a decreased risk of aspiration.

Routes for Enteral Feedings

Oral, gastric by **nasogastric tube** or gastrostomy, and small intestinal by nasoduodenal/nasojejunal or jejunostomy tube are the routes used for enteral feedings. Use of nasogastric tube through oral (mouth) or nasal cavities is the most common route for short-term enteral feedings. The gastrostomy, nasoduodenal/nasojejunal, and jejunostomy tubes are used for long-term enteral feedings. Figure 16–1 displays the four types of GI tubes used for enteral feedings. If aspiration is a concern, the small intestinal route is suggested.

Enteral Solutions

Several types of liquid formulas are commercially available for enteral feedings. These solutions differ according to their various nutrients, caloric values, and osmolality. There are three groups of solutions for enteral nutrition: blenderized, polymeric (milk-based and lactose-free), and elemental or monomeric. Examples of commercial preparations are listed according to their groups in Table 16–1. Components of the enteral solutions include (1) carbohydrates in the form of dextrose, sucrose, lactose, starch or dextrin (the first three are simple sugars that can be absorbed quickly); (2) protein in the form of intact proteins, hydrolyzed proteins, or free amino acids; and (3) fat in the form of corn oil, soybean oil, or safflower oil (some have a higher oil content than others). With all enteral nutrition, sufficient water to maintain hydration is essential.

Blended formulas for enteral solutions are liquid in consistency so they are able to pass through the tube. These are individually prepared based on the client's nutritional need. Frequently baby food is used with liquid added. If food particles are too large, the tube can become clogged.

The two groups of polymeric solutions are milk-based and lactose-free. Most of the milk-based polymeric preparations come in powdered form to be mixed with milk or water. Many of these milk-based polymeric solutions do not provide complete nutritional requirements unless given in large amounts. Frequently they are used as a supplement to meet nutritional needs. The lactose-free polymeric solutions are commercially prepared in liquid form for replacement feedings. Many of these solutions are isotonic (300 to 340 mOsm/kg water), and the breakdown of nutrients includes 50% carbohydrates, 15% protein, 15% fat, and 20% other nutrients. Examples of polymeric solutions include Ensure, Isocal, and Osmolite (Figure 16–2). These solutions provide 1 calorie per milliliter of feeding.

Characteristics of the formula may be targeted to treat a specific group of disorders. For those with diabetes melli-

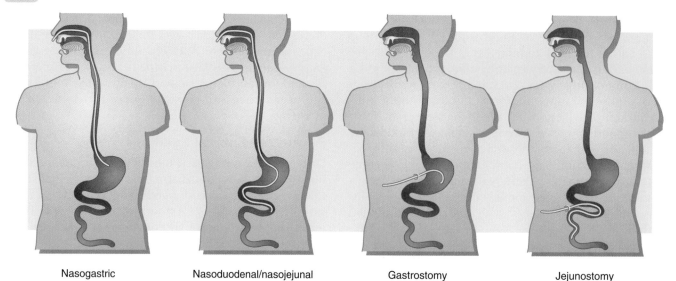

| Nasogastric | Nasoduodenal/nasojejunal | Gastrostomy | Jejunostomy |

FIGURE 16–1 Types of gastrointestinal tubes used for enteral feedings. A nasogastric tube is passed from the nose into the stomach. A weighted nasoduodenal/nasojejunal tube is passed through the nose into the duodenum/jejunum. A gastrostomy tube is introduced through a temporary or permanent opening on the abdominal wall (stoma) into the stomach. A jejunostomy tube is passed through a stoma directly into the jejunum.

Table 16–1

Commercial Preparations for Enteral Feeding

Type of Formula	Commercial Preparation	Description
Blenderized	Compleat	• Blended natural foods • Formulas come ready to use
Polymeric *Milk-based*	Meritene Instant Breakfast Sustacal	• Supplements prescribed for patients who have normal or near-normal gastrointestinal function • Usually taste good
Lactose-free	Boost Ensure Entrition Fibersource Isocal Osmolite Resource Ultracal	• Most commonly prescribed formula • May be used as tube feeding, meal replacement, or oral supplement • Contains protein, carbohydrates, and fat • Adequate quantities meet reference daily intakes for vitamins and minerals
Elemental (Mono- meric)	Criticare HN Peptamen Liquid Vital HN Vivonex TEN	• Partially digested nutrients for feeding • Contains nitrogen (free amino acids), carbohydrates (glucose polymers), and minimal fat (long-chain triglycerides) • Used for various gastrointestinal diseases.

tus, Glucerna and Diabetic Resource (low-carbohydrate, high-fat, lactose-free products), are most helpful. Nutri-Hep (low-fat, lactose-free product) is recommended to treat hepatic disorders. For individuals with pulmonary disorders, Pulmocare or Respalor (low-carbohydrate, high-fat products) are commonly prescribed. Nepro and Novasource Renal (low-fat amino acids, water-soluble vitamins) are used to treat those with renal disorders.

For partial GI tract dysfunction, the elemental or monomeric solutions are useful (i.e., Peptinex DT and Peptinex DT with probiotics). They are available in powdered and liquid forms. The nutrients from these solutions are

FIGURE 16–2 A typical selection of over-the-counter supplemental feeding products.

rapidly absorbed in the small intestine. They are more expensive than the other enteral solutions.

Methods for Delivery

Enteral feedings may be given by **bolus**, intermittent drip or infusion, continuous drip, or cyclic infusion. The bolus method was the first method used to deliver enteral feedings. With the bolus method, 250 to 400 ml of solution is rapidly administered through a syringe or funnel into the tube four to six times a day. This method takes about 10 minutes each feeding, and may not be tolerated well because a massive volume of solution is given in a short period. This method can cause nausea, vomiting, aspiration, abdominal cramping, and diarrhea, but a healthy client can normally tolerate the rapidly infused solution. This method is seldom used unless the client is ambulatory.

Intermittent enteral feedings are administered every 3 to 6 hours over 30 to 60 minutes by gravity drip or pump infusion. At each feeding, 300 to 400 ml of solution is usually given. A feeding bag is commonly used. **Intermittent infusion** is considered an inexpensive method for administering enteral nutrition.

Continuous feedings are prescribed for the critically ill or for those who receive feedings into the small intestine. The enteral feedings are given by an infusion pump such as the Kangaroo set at a slow rate over 24 hours. Approximately 50 to 125 ml of solution is infused per hour (Figure 16–3).

The **cyclic method** is another type of continuous feeding that is infused over 8 to 16 hours daily (day or night).

Administration during daytime hours is suggested for clients who are restless or for those who have a greater risk for aspiration. The nighttime schedule allows more freedom during the day for clients who are ambulatory.

Complications

Dehydration can occur if an insufficient amount of water is given with or between feedings. Some enteral solutions are hyperosmolar and can draw water out of the cells to maintain serum iso-osmolality.

Aspiration may occur if the client is fed while lying down or unconscious. The head of the bed should be elevated at least 30 degrees. The nurse should check for gastric residual by gently aspirating the stomach contents before administering the next enteral feeding.

One of the major problems of enteral feeding is diarrhea. This could be caused by rapid administration of feeding, high caloric solutions, malnutrition, GI bacteria (*Clostridium difficile*), and drugs. Antibacterials (antibiotics) and drugs that contain magnesium (e.g., antacids [Maalox] and sorbitol [used as a filler for certain drugs]), are associated with the occurrence of diarrhea. Many oral liquid drugs are hyperosmolar and tend to pull water into the GI tract and cause diarrhea.

Diarrhea can usually be managed or corrected by decreasing the rate of infusion of the enteral solution, diluting the solution, changing the solution, discontinuing the drug, or increasing the client's daily water intake.

Enteral Medications

Pancreatic enzymes such as precreatin (Creon) and pancrelipase (Viokase) are products used by individuals with pancreatic enzyme deficiency resulting from conditions such as pancreatectomy, pancreatic obstruction, and cystic fibrosis. Both these preparations promote digestion and absorption of foods normally accomplished by natural amylase, lipase, and protease. Best given before meals,

FIGURE 16–3 Examples of enteral infusion pumps for intermittent, continuous, and cyclic enteral feedings.

these artificial enzymes promote digestion and absorption of food.

Most drugs that can be administered orally can also be given via enteral tube. The drug must be in liquid form or dissolved into a liquid. Drugs that cannot be dissolved are time-release forms, enteric-coated forms, sublingual forms, and bulk-forming laxatives.

Liquid medication must be properly diluted when administered through the feeding tube. The drug dose is usually given as a bolus and then followed with water. Most liquid medications are hyperosmolar (>1000 mOsm/kg water) compared with the osmolality of the secretions of the GI tract (130 to 350 mOsm/kg water). Although the hyperosmolality of liquid medication was once thought to be well tolerated by the GI tract, abdominal distention and cramping, vomiting, and diarrhea can result from the administration of undiluted hyperosmolar liquid medications and electrolyte solutions. Liquid medication should be diluted with water to reduce the osmolality to 500 mOsm/kg H_2O (mildly hypertonic) to decrease GI intolerance. Table 16–2 lists the osmolalities of various commercial drug suspensions and solutions.

It is important to know about stopping the infusion when certain types of medications are administered. Some medications require the feeding be stopped for as long as thirty minutes to allow for adequate absorption. For example, absorption of phenytoin (Dilantin) is significantly reduced in the presence of protein, so it is important to stop the feeding for thirty minutes before administering this drug. The therapeutic effect of a drug may be affected as well. Sucralfate (Carafate), a treatment for gastric ulcers, may lose its effectiveness if the feeding is not held for thirty minutes after administering the medication.

Calculation for Dilution of Enteral Medications

The following three steps should be followed to determine the amount of water needed for diluting liquid medications:

Table 16–2
Osmolality of Selected Drugs

Drug	Average mOsm
acetaminophen elixir, 65 mg/ml	5400
amoxicillin suspension, 50 mg/ml	2250
cephalexin (Keflex) suspension, 50 mg/ml	1950
cimetidine (Tagamet) solution, 60 mg/ml	5500
digoxin elixir, 50 mcg/ml	1350
docusate sodium (Colace) syrup, 3.3 mg/ml	3900
furosemide (Lasix) solution, 10 mg/ml	2050
lithium citrate syrup, 1.6 mEq/ml	6850
milk of magnesia suspension	1250
potassium chloride liquid, 10%	3550
prochlorperazine syrup, 1 mg/ml	3250
theophylline solution, 5.33 mg/ml	800

Step 1. Calculate the drug order to find the volume of the drug:

$$D/H \times V \text{ or } H : V :: D : x$$

D: Desired dose: drug dose ordered by health care provider
H: On-hand dose: drug dose on label of container (e.g., bottle, vial, or ampule)
V: Vehicle: form and amount in which the drug is available (e.g., tablet, capsule, liquid)

Step 2. Find the osmolality of the drug (check drug literature or with pharmacist) and liquid dilution. Use 500 mOsm as a constant for the desired osmolality.

know mOsm/desired mOsm × volume of drug = total volume of liq

Step 3. Determine the volume of water for dilution:

total volume of liquid − volume of drug = volume of water for dilution

EXAMPLE

Order: acetaminophen 650 mg, q6h PRN for pain
Available: Acetaminophen elixir 65 mg/ml
Average mOsm/kg = 5400 (Table 16–2)

Step 1. Calculate the volume of drug:

$$D/H \times V = 650 \text{ mg}/65 \text{ mg} \times 1 \text{ ml} = 10 \text{ ml}$$

or

$$H : V \qquad D : x$$
$$65 \text{ mg} : 1 \text{ ml} :: 650 \text{ mg} : x \text{ ml}$$
$$65x = 650$$
$$x = 10 \text{ ml of drug}$$

Step 2. Find the osmolality of drug and total liquid dilution:

know mOsm (5400)/desired mOsm (500) × volume of drug (10) = 5400/500 × 10 = 108 ml of liquid

Step 3. Determine the volume of water for dilution:

total volume of liquid (108 ml) − volume of drug (10 ml) = 98 ml of water for dilution

Nursing Process

Enteral Nutrition

ASSESSMENT

■ Confirm that the tape around the tube is secured.
■ Assess client's tolerance to the enteral feeding, including possible GI disturbance (nausea, cramping, diarrhea—common complications of enteral feeding).

- Determine urine output. Record result for future comparison.
- Obtain client's weight to be used for future comparisons.
- Listen for bowel sounds. Diminished or absent bowel sounds should be reported immediately to health care provider.
- Assess baseline laboratory values. Compare with future laboratory results.

NURSING DIAGNOSES

- Risk for deficient fluid volume related to inadequate fluid intake or excess fluid loss
- Risk for diarrhea related to ingredients in enteral feedings
- Risk for aspiration related to enteral feedings via nasogastric tube

PLANNING

- Client will receive adequate nutritional support through enteral feedings.
- The complication of diarrhea related to enteral feedings will be managed.

NURSING INTERVENTIONS

- Check tube placement by aspirating gastric secretion or injecting air into tube to listen by stethoscope for air movement in the stomach. (However, injecting air to check for placement may be misleading, because the tube may be in the base of the lung and air flow there produces similar sounds as when the tube is placed in the stomach.) For placement of the tube for small intestine route, confirmation by radiograph may be needed.
- Determine gastric residual before enteral feeding. A residual of more than 50% of previous feeding indicates delayed gastric emptying. Notify health care provider. Usual residual is 0 to 100 ml.
- Check continuous route for gastric residual every 2 to 4 hours. If residual is more than 50 ml, stop infusion for 30 minutes to 1 hour then recheck.
- Before feeding, raise head of bed to a 30-degree angle. If elevating head of bed is not advisable, then position client on right side.
- Deliver enteral feeding according to method ordered: bolus, gastric, or small intestine.
- Flush feeding tube accordingly: intermittent feeding, 30 ml before and after; continuous feeding, every 4 hours; medications, 30 ml before and after. If tube obstruction occurs, flush with warm water or cola.
- Monitor adverse effects of enteral feedings such as diarrhea. To manage or correct diarrhea, decrease enteral feeding flow rate and as diarrhea lessens gradually increase feeding rate. Enteral solution may be diluted then gradually increased to full strength. However, diluted solution can decrease nutrient intake. Determine whether drugs could be causing the diarrhea.
- Dilute drug solution's osmolality to 500 mOsm when giving liquid medication through the tube. Use the formula in the text. Consult with health care provider.
- Monitor vital signs. Report abnormal findings.
- Give additional water during the day to prevent dehydration. Consult with health care provider.
- Weigh client to determine weight gain or loss. Compare with baseline weight. Client should be weighed at the same time each day with same scale and same amount of clothing.
- Change feeding bag daily. Do not add new solution to old solution in the feeding bag. The nutritional solution should not be ice cold but at room temperature.

Client Teaching

- Instruct client to report any problems related to enteral feedings such as diarrhea, sore throat, and abdominal cramping.

Cultural Considerations ❖

- Respect cultural beliefs concerning refusal to receive enteral or TPN. Explain the need for adequate nutrition, and find ways that nutritional needs can be met.
- Communicate, verbally or in writing, how enteral nutrition is used by various cultural groups such as those in third-world countries.
- Use an interpreter as appropriate.

EVALUATION

- Determine that client is receiving prescribed nutrients daily and is free of complications associated with enteral feedings.

Parenteral Nutrition

Total Parenteral Nutrition

Total parenteral nutrition (TPN), also called hyperalimentation (HA) or IV hyperalimentation (IVH), is the primary method for providing complete nutrients by the parenteral or IV route. TPN is an infusion of hyperosmolar glucose, amino acids, vitamins, electrolytes, minerals, and trace elements; it can meet a client's total nutritional needs. TPN is indicated for clients with severe burns who are in negative nitrogen balance; clients with GI disorders, when the GI tract needs a complete rest; and clients with debilitating diseases such as metastatic cancer or acquired immunodeficiency syndrome (AIDS).

The average percentage of dextrose in TPN is 25%. This high glucose concentration is mixed with commercially prepared protein and lipid sources. Fat emulsion supplement therapy provides an increased number of calories and is a carrier of fat-soluble vitamins. Vitamins and electrolytes are added before administration. Electrolytes are frequently added immediately before the infusion based on assessments of the client's serum electrolyte levels. High glucose concentrations are irritating to peripheral veins, so TPN is administered through central venous lines such as the subclavian or internal jugular.

Enteral feedings should be considered before TPN. Enteral feeding poses less risk of sepsis, maintains GI integrity, and is less costly. When enteral nutrition cannot be used because of severe GI disorders, TPN should be prescribed. TPN does enhance wound healing and provides the necessary nutrients to prevent cellular catabolism.

To avoid exogenous contamination during enteral feeding, the following guidelines are suggested: (1) Wash hands before handling the feeding system, (2) use a system with medication ports and wipe with alcohol before and after administering drugs, (3) wear nonsterile disposable gloves, (4) wear a mask if you have a cold, and (5) discard the feeding system every 24 hours (48 hours in a closed system). Do not touch any part of the system in contact with formula, and do not use any feeding system after the labeled expiration date.

It is important that the nurse be familiar with the specific equipment used in caring for the client on TPN. A variety of "set ups" are available for administration. Some tubings have antireflux valves, others have clamps. Each has implications for the administration of medications. Parenteral preparations must be administered by infusion pump. Policies and procedures for TPN therapy may vary by region and institution and must be researched and followed accordingly.

Complications

Complications associated with TPN can result from catheter insertion and TPN infusion. Table 16–3 lists the complications associated with TPN.

Complications include pneumothorax, hemothorax, hydrothorax, air embolism, infection, hyperglycemia, hypoglycemia, and fluid overload (hypervolemia). To prevent air embolism, the client should be taught the **Valsalva maneuver,** which is to take a breath, hold it, and bear down while the nurse is changing infusion bags or bottles and changing tubing. Strict asepsis is necessary when changing IV tubing and dressings at the insertion site. Gloves, masks, and antibacterial ointment are usually necessary. TPN solution is an excellent medium for organism growth. Hypertonic dextrose in a protein hydrolysate solution promotes yeast and bacterial growth. It has been reported that these organisms do not grow as rapidly in the preferred crystalline amino acid solution as they do in a protein hydrolysate solution. Most TPN solutions are prepared by the pharmacist with the use of a laminar airflow hood.

Hyperglycemia occurs primarily as a result of the hypertonic dextrose solution when TPN is initiated. This may be transient until the pancreas adjusts to the hyperglycemic load. Hyperglycemia also occurs when the infusion rate for TPN is too rapid. In some cases insulin is added to the TPN solution, which tends to be more effective than administering the insulin subcutaneously. Usually 1 L of solution is ordered for the first 24 hours when initiating TPN therapy. This allows the pancreas to accommodate to the increased glucose concentration of the solution. Additional

Table 16–3

Complications of Total Parenteral Nutrition

Complication	Causes	Symptoms
Catheter Insertion		
Pneumothorax	Accidental puncture of the pleural cavity	Sharp chest pain; decreased breath sounds
Hemothorax	Catheter damages the large vein	Same as pneumothorax
Hydrothorax	Catheter perforates the vein, releasing solution into the chest	Same as pneumothorax
Total Parenteral Nutrition Infusion		
Air embolism	Intravenous (IV) tubing disconnected. Catheter not clamped. Injection port fell off. Improper changing of IV tubing (no Valsalva maneuver).	Coughing, shortness of breath, chest pain, cyanosis
Infection	Poor aseptic technique when catheter inserted. Contamination when changing tubing, mixing solution, or changing dressing.	Temperature >100° F (37.7° C). Tachycardia; chills; sweating; redness; swelling; drainage at insertion site; pain in the neck, arm, or shoulder; lethargy
Hyperglycemia	Fluid infused too rapidly. Insufficient insulin coverage. Infection.	Nausea, headache, weakness, thirst, elevated blood glucose
Hypoglycemia	Fluids stopped abruptly. Too much insulin infused.	Pallor; cold, clammy skin. Increased pulse rate, "shaky feeling," headache, blurred vision
Fluid overload hypervolemia	Increased IV rate. Fluids shift from cellular to vascular spaces because of hypertonic solutions.	Cough, dyspnea, neck vein engorgement, chest rales, weight gain

daily increases of 500 to 1000 ml are ordered until the desired daily volume of 2.5 to 3 L is reached.

Sudden interruption of TPN therapy can cause hypoglycemia. After the glucose level is decreased the insulin level remains, causing a hypoglycemic state. It is suggested that an isotonic dextrose solution be administered for 12 to 24 hours after TPN therapy is discontinued. A gradual decrease in the hourly infusion rate of TPN may also be used to discontinue TPN therapy. This process decreases the possibility of a hypoglycemic reaction.

TPN solutions and tubing should be changed every 24 hours. Dressing changes are required every 48 to 72 hours, varying by health care facility policy. In some institutions, the dressing is changed every 24 hours for the first 7 to 10 days.

Nursing Process

Total Parenteral Nutrition

ASSESSMENT

- Obtain baseline vital signs for future comparison.
- Confirm baseline weight.
- Determine laboratory results. Electrolytes, glucose, and protein levels frequently change during TPN therapy. Early laboratory results are useful for future comparison.
- Check urine output. Report abnormal findings.
- Read the label on the TPN solution. Compare the solution with the order.

NURSING DIAGNOSES

- Risk for excess fluid volume related to excess fluid infusion or renal dysfunction
- Risk for deficient fluid volume related to osmotic diuresis resulting from hyperosmolar TPN solution
- Risk for infection related to TPN solution that has a high glucose concentration
- Ineffective breathing pattern related to complication from insertion of subclavian line

PLANNING

- Client's nutrient needs will be met via TPN.
- The common complication from TPN therapy—infection—will be avoided.

NURSING INTERVENTIONS

- Check vital signs. Report changes.
- Determine body weight and compare with baseline weight.
- Monitor laboratory results and report abnormal findings, especially electrolytes, protein, glucose. Compare laboratory changes with the baseline findings.

- Measure intake and output. Fluid volume deficit or excess could occur. Because the TPN solution is hyperosmolar, fluid shift occurs, which can cause osmotic diuresis.
- Monitor temperature changes for possible infection or febrile state. Use aseptic technique when changing dressings and solution bottles or bags.
- Check blood glucose level periodically. When TPN therapy is started, there may be a transient elevated glucose level until pancreatic beta cells adjust secretion of insulin. If this occurs, the flow rate for TPN should be started slowly and gradually increased as blood glucose level decreases. Regular insulin may be added to TPN fluids to correct elevated glucose levels.
- Refrigerate TPN solution that is not in use. High glucose concentration is an excellent medium for bacterial growth.
- Monitor flow rate of TPN. Start with 60 to 80 ml/hour and increase slowly to the ordered level to avoid hyperglycemia.
- Help clients avoid air embolism by instructing them how to perform the Valsalva maneuver: taking a breath, holding it, and bearing down. If parenteral line is opened to air when changing the solution bag or bottle and IV tubing, an air embolus could occur.
- Observe client's cardiac status during Valsalva maneuver; it can cause dysrhythmias.
- Check for signs and symptoms of overhydration: coughing, dyspnea, neck vein engorgement, or chest rales. Report findings.
- Follow the institution's procedure for changing dressing and tubing. Usually, tubing is changed daily and dressing is changed every 24 hours for the first 10 days then every 48 hours thereafter.
- Do not draw blood, give medications, or check central venous pressure via the TPN line. Results could be invalid.

Client Teaching

- Provide emotional support to client and family before and during TPN therapy.
- Be available to discuss client's concerns or refer client to appropriate health care provider.
- Instruct client to notify health care provider immediately if experiencing discomforts or reactions.
- Keep client informed of progress and effectiveness of TPN.

Cultural Considerations ❖

- Respect client's cultural beliefs about refusing TPN.
- Explain reasons for adequate nutrition and find ways to meet nutritional needs.
- Use an interpreter as appropriate.

EVALUATION

■ Evaluate client's positive and negative response to the TPN therapy.

■ Determine periodically whether client's serum electrolytes, protein, and glucose levels are within desired ranges.

■ Evaluate nutritional status by weight changes, energy level, feeling of well-being, symptom control, or healing.

Transitional Feeding: Parenteral to Enteral

The first stage of transitioning from parenteral to enteral feeding is determining a client's GI tolerance. This is usually accomplished by giving a small amount of enteral feeding at a slow rate of about 25 to 40 ml per hour. As the enteral rate is increased every 8 to 24 hours by increments of 25 to 40 ml, the parenteral preparation is reduced by the appropriate amount. Parenteral nutrition is typically discontinued when about 75% to 80% of a client's nutritional needs are being met through enteral feeding.

KEY WEBSITES

American Society for Parenteral and Enteral Nutrition (aspen)
www.nutritioncare.org

 Critical Thinking Case Study

MM had abdominal surgery and received D₅W and D₅ 0.45% NaCl for 4 days. A nasogastric tube was inserted for enteral nutrition. It was determined that the function of MM's GI tract was intact.

1. Why would MM receive enteral nutrition? Is it needed for short-term or long-term therapy?
2. Differentiate between the Ensure solution that MM is receiving and other forms of enteral solutions.
3. MM is at risk for complications related to enteral nutrition. Discuss potential complications and give specific nursing interventions for each.
4. Differentiate methods of delivery of enteral nutrition. Describe nursing interventions related to each method.
5. Give the rationale for changing MM's enteral nutrition from bolus method to intermittent method.

MM was ordered amoxicillin suspension 250 mg, q.i.d., and potassium chloride solution 10% (15 mEq/10 ml), every 12 hours. These medications are to be given through the enteral tubing.

6. How many milliliters of amoxicillin should MM receive per dose? How much water dilution is needed to reduce the drug osmolality to 500 mOsm?
7. How many milliliters of potassium chloride should MM receive per dose? How much water dilution is needed to reduce the drug osmolality to 500 mOsm?

 NCLEX Study Questions

1. You are about to determine your client's gastric residual before administering an enteral feeding; the last feeding was 240cc. A residual of more than what amount would indicate delayed gastric emptying?
   a. 100 cc
   b. 125 cc
   c. 150 cc
   d. 175 cc

2. The enteral feeding should be administered at what temperature?
   a. slightly warmed
   b. chilled
   c. ice cold
   d. room temperature

3. A frequent major complication of enteral feedings is:
   a. aspiration
   b. constipation
   c. diarrhea
   d. muscle weakness

4. Your client is receiving TPN. Health teaching includes the Valsalva maneuver to prevent:
   a. infection
   b. air embolism
   c. dehydration
   d. fat embolism

5. Sudden interruption of TPN therapy may cause:
   a. dehydration
   b. tremors
   c. hyperglycemia
   d. hypoglycemia

6. The average amount of dextrose in TPN solutions is:
   a. 15%
   b. 20%
   c. 25%
   d. 30%

7. Your client's care plan includes changing the TPN solution and tubing every how many hours?
   a. 24
   b. 36
   c. 48
   d. 72

Answers: 1. b; 2. d; 3. c; 4. b; 5. d; 6. c; 7. a.

FIVE

Autonomic Nervous System Agents

The *central nervous system* (CNS), the body's primary nervous system that consists of the brain and spinal cord, was previously discussed in the Unit IV introduction. The *peripheral nervous system (PNS)*, located outside the brain and spinal cord, is made up of two divisions: the autonomic and the somatic. After interpretation by the CNS, the PNS receives stimuli and initiates responses to those stimuli.

The *autonomic nervous system (ANS)*, also called the visceral system, innervates (acts on) smooth muscles and glands. Its functions include control and regulation of the heart, respiratory system, gastrointestinal (GI) tract, bladder, eyes, and glands. The ANS is an involuntary nervous system over which a person has little or no control. We breathe, our hearts beat, and peristalsis continues without our realizing it. However, unlike the ANS, the somatic nervous system is a voluntary system that innervates skeletal muscles over which there is control.

The two sets of neurons in the autonomic component of the PNS are the (1) afferent (sensory) neurons and the (2) efferent (motor) neurons. The *afferent neurons* send impulses to the CNS, where they are interpreted. The *efferent neurons* receive the impulses (information) from the brain and transmit those impulses through the spinal cord to the effector organ cells. The efferent pathways in the ANS are divided into two branches: the sympathetic and the parasympathetic nerves, collectively called the *sympathetic nervous system* and the *parasympathetic nervous system* (Figure V–1).

The sympathetic and parasympathetic nervous systems act on the same organs but produce opposite responses to provide homeostasis (balance) (Figure V–2). Drugs act on the sympathetic and parasympathetic nervous systems by either stimulating or depressing responses.

Sympathetic Nervous System

The *sympathetic nervous system* is also called the *adrenergic system*, because at one time it was believed that *adrenaline* was the *neurotransmitter* that innervated smooth muscle. The neurotransmitter is, however, *norepinephrine*.

The adrenergic receptor organ cells are of four types: alpha$_1$, alpha$_2$, beta$_1$, and beta$_2$ (Figure V–3). Norepinephrine is released from the terminal nerve ending and stimulates the cell receptors to produce a response.

Parasympathetic Nervous System

The **parasympathetic** nervous system is called the **cholinergic** system, because the neurotransmitter at the end of the neuron that innervates the muscle is **acetylcholine**.

263

FIGURE V–I Subdivisions of the peripheral nervous system.

FIGURE V–2 Sympathetic and parasympathetic effects on body tissues.

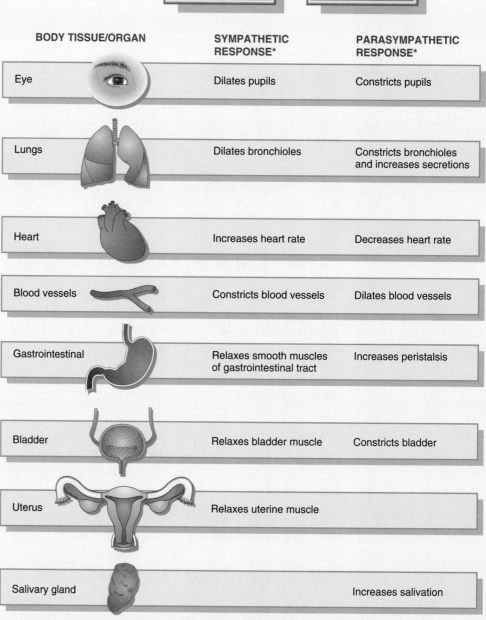

BODY TISSUE/ORGAN	SYMPATHETIC RESPONSE*	PARASYMPATHETIC RESPONSE*
Eye	Dilates pupils	Constricts pupils
Lungs	Dilates bronchioles	Constricts bronchioles and increases secretions
Heart	Increases heart rate	Decreases heart rate
Blood vessels	Constricts blood vessels	Dilates blood vessels
Gastrointestinal	Relaxes smooth muscles of gastrointestinal tract	Increases peristalsis
Bladder	Relaxes bladder muscle	Constricts bladder
Uterus	Relaxes uterine muscle	
Salivary gland		Increases salivation

*The sympathetic and parasympathetic nervous systems have opposite responses on body tissues and organs.

FIGURE V–3 Sympathetic and parasympathetic transmitters and receptors. *ACh*, Acetylcholine; *AChE*, acetylcholinesterase; *NE*, norepinephrine.

The cholinergic receptors at organ cells are either nicotinic or muscarinic, meaning that they are stimulated by the alkaloids nicotine and muscarine, respectively (see Figure V-3). Acetylcholine stimulates the receptor cells to produce a response, but the enzyme acetylcholinesterase may inactivate acetylcholine before it reaches the receptor cell.

Drugs that mimic the neurotransmitters norepinephrine and acetylcholine produce responses opposite to each other in the same organ. For example, an adrenergic drug (sympathomimetic) increases the heart rate, whereas a cholinergic drug (parasympathomimetic) decreases the heart rate (see Figure V–2). However, a drug that mimics the sympathetic nervous system and a drug that blocks the parasympathetic nervous system can cause similar responses in the organ. For instance, the sympathomimetic and the parasympatholytic drugs both increase the heart rate; the adrenergic blocker and the cholinergic drug both decrease heart rate.

Many name classifications are given to drugs that mimic or block both the sympathetic nervous system and the parasympathetic nervous system (Table V–1). The nurse needs to become familiar with these names. Drug names and specific actions are discussed in Chapters 17, Adrenergics and Adrenergic Blockers, and 18, Cholinergics and Anticholinergics.

Table V–I

Autonomic Nervous Systems: Sympathetic and Parasympathetic

Sympathetic Stimulants	Parasympathetic Stimulants
Sympathomimetics (adrenergics, adrenomimetics, or adrenergic agonists) Action: Increase blood pressure Increase pulse rate Relax bronchioles Dilate pupils of eyes Relax uterine muscles Increase blood sugar	**Direct-Acting** *Parasympathomimetics (cholinergics or cholinergic agonists)* Action: Decrease blood pressure Decrease pulse rate Constrict bronchioles Constrict pupils of eyes Increase urinary contraction Increase peristalsis **Indirect-Acting** *Cholinesterase inhibitors (anticholinesterase)* Action: Increase muscle tone
Sympathetic Depressants	**Parasympathetic Depressants**
Sympatholytics (adrenergic blockers, adrenolytics, or adrenergic antagonists) Action: Decrease pulse rate Decrease blood pressure Constrict bronchioles	*Parasympatholytics (anticholinergics, cholinergic antagonists, or antispasmodics)* Action: Increase pulse rate Decrease mucous secretions Decrease gastrointestinal motility Increase urinary retention Dilate pupils of eyes

Opposite responses on organ tissue are caused by sympathomimetics and parasympathomimetics and by sympatholytics and parasympatholytics. Sympathomimetics and parasympatholytics cause similar organ responses, as do sympatholytics and parasympathomimetics.

Summary

There are two subdivisions of the autonomic nervous system: the sympathetic and the parasympathetic nervous systems. These nervous systems have opposite effects on organ tissues. Drugs can either stimulate or block both of these nervous systems through their receptors. Table V–2 lists the organ responses from drugs that act on these systems.

Table V–2

Sympathetic and Parasympathetic Responses to Drugs

Sympathetic	Parasympathetic	Response
Sympathomimetic	Parasympathomimetic	Opposite response
Sympatholytic	Parasympatholytic	Opposite response
Sympathomimetic	Parasympatholytic	Similar response
Sympatholytic	Parasympathomimetic	Similar response

17

Adrenergics and Adrenergic Blockers

ELECTRONIC RESOURCES

evolve

Evolve website (http://evolve.elsevier.com/KeeHayes/pharmacology/):
- Case Studies
- Content Updates
- Frequently Asked Questions
- Student Review Activities
- WebLinks
- Additional Reference Material

Companion CD-ROM:
- NCLEX Examination Review Questions
- Pharmacology Animations
- IV Therapy Checklists
- Medication Error Checklists
- Drug Calculation Problems
- Electronic Calculators
- Top 200 Drugs with Pronunciations
- References from the Textbook

Outline

Objectives

- Explain the adrenergic receptors citing examples of their major responses.
- Differentiate between selective and nonselective adrenergic drugs.
- Discuss the major side effects of adrenergic drugs.
- Explain nursing interventions, including client teaching, associated with adrenergic drugs.
- Contrast the uses of alpha-blockers and beta-blockers.
- Explain the general side effects of adrenergic blockers.
- Describe nursing interventions, including client teaching, associated with adrenergic blockers.
- Apply the nursing process for the client taking beta-adrenergic blockers.

Terms

This chapter discusses two groups of drugs that affect the sympathetic nervous system: the adrenergics (**sympathomimetics** or adrenomimetics) and the adrenergic blockers (**sympatholytics** or adrenolytics). Adrenergic drugs and adrenergic blockers are listed here along with their dosages and uses.

Adrenergics

Drugs that stimulate the sympathetic nervous system are called adrenergics, adrenergic agonists, sympathomimetics, or adrenomimetics because they mimic the sympathetic neurotransmitters (i.e., norepinephrine, epinephrine). They act on one or more **adrenergic receptor** sites located in the cells of muscles, such as the heart, bronchiole walls, gastrointestinal (GI) tract, urinary bladder, and ciliary muscle of the eye. There are many adrenergic receptors; the four main receptors are alpha$_1$, alpha$_2$, beta$_1$, and beta$_2$, which mediate the major responses described in Table 17–1 and illustrated in Figure 17–1.

The alpha-adrenergic receptors are located in the vascular tissues (vessels) of muscles. When the alpha$_1$-receptor is stimulated, the arterioles and venules constrict, increasing peripheral resistance and blood return to the heart. Circulation is improved and blood pressure is increased. When there is too much stimulation, blood flow is decreased to the vital organs. The alpha$_2$-receptor is located in the postganglionic sympathetic nerve endings. When stimulated it inhibits the release of norepinephrine, leading to a decrease in vasoconstriction. This results in a decrease in blood pressure.

The beta$_1$-receptors are located primarily in the heart. Stimulation of the beta$_1$-receptor increases myocardial contractility and heart rate. The beta$_2$-receptors are found mostly in the smooth muscles of the lung, the arterioles of skeletal muscles, and the uterine muscle. Stimulation of the beta$_2$-receptor causes (1) relaxation of the smooth muscles of the lungs, resulting in bronchodilation; (2) an increase in blood flow to the skeletal muscles; and (3) relaxation of the uterine muscle, resulting in a decrease in uterine contraction (Table 17–1 and Figure 17–2).

Another adrenergic receptor is dopaminergic and is located in the renal, mesenteric, coronary, and cerebral arteries. When this receptor is stimulated, the vessels dilate and blood flow increases. Only dopamine can activate this receptor.

Inactivation of Neurotransmitters

After the transmitter (e.g., norepinephrine) has performed its function, the action must be stopped to prevent prolonging the effect. Transmitters are inactivated by (1) reuptake of the transmitter back into the neuron (nerve cell terminal), (2) enzymatic transformation or degradation, and (3) diffusion away from the receptor. The mechanism of norepinephrine reuptake plays a more important role in inactivation than the enzymatic action. Following the reuptake of the transmitter in the neuron, the transmitter may be degraded or reused. The two enzymes that inactivate the metabolism of norepinephrine are (1) monoamine oxidase (MAO), which is inside the neuron; and (2) catechol-O-methyltransferase (COMT), which is outside the neuron.

Drugs can stop the termination of the neurotransmitter (e.g., norepinephrine) by either (1) inhibiting the norepinephrine reuptake, which prolongs the action of the transmitter; or by (2) inhibiting the degradation of norepinephrine by enzyme action.

Classification of Sympathomimetics/ Adrenomimetics

The sympathomimetic drugs that stimulate adrenergic receptors are classified into three categories according to their effects on organ cells: (1) direct-acting sympathomimetics, which directly stimulate the adrenergic receptor (e.g., epinephrine or norepinephrine); (2) indirect-acting sympathomimetics, which stimulate the release of norepinephrine from the terminal nerve endings (e.g., amphetamine); and (3) mixed-acting sympathomimetics (both direct and indirect acting), which stimulate the adrenergic receptor sites and stimulate the release of norepinephrine from the terminal nerve endings (Figure 17–3).

Ephedrine is an example of a mixed-acting sympathomimetic. This drug acts indirectly by stimulating the release of norepinephrine from the nerve terminals and acts directly on the alpha$_1$-, beta$_1$-, and beta$_2$-receptors. Ephedrine-like epinephrine increases heart rate and blood pressure, but it is not as potent a vasoconstrictor as epinephrine. Ephedrine is helpful to treat idiopathic orthostatic hypotension and hypotension that results from spinal anesthesia. It also stimulates beta$_2$-receptors, which dilate bronchial tubes, and is useful to treat mild forms of bronchial asthma.

Catecholamines are the chemical structures of a substance (either endogenous or synthetic) that can produce a

Table 17–1

Effects of Adrenergics at Receptors

Receptor	Physiologic Responses
Alpha$_1$	Increases force of heart contraction; vasoconstriction increases blood pressure; mydriasis (dilation of pupils) occurs; salivary glands decrease secretion; increases urinary bladder relaxation and urinary sphincter contraction
Alpha$_2$	Inhibits release of norepinephrine; dilates blood vessels; produces hypotension; decreases gastrointestinal motility and tone
Beta$_1$	Increases heart rate and force of contraction; increases renin secretion, which increases blood pressure
Beta$_2$	Dilates bronchioles; promotes gastrointestinal and uterine relaxation; promotes increase in blood sugar through glycogenolysis in liver; increases blood flow in skeletal muscles

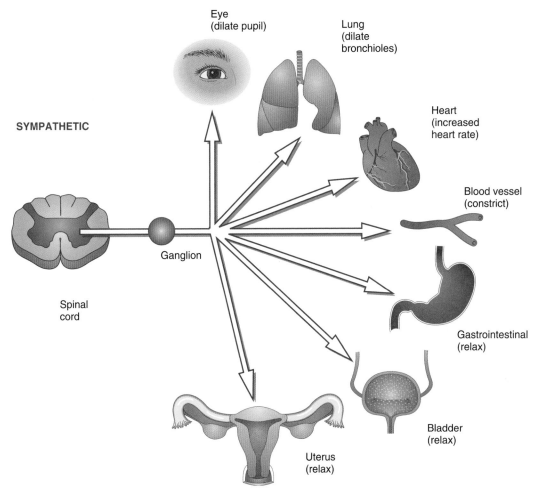

FIGURE 17–1 Sympathetic responses. Stimulation of the sympathetic nervous system or use of sympathomimetic (adrenergic) drugs can cause the pupils and bronchioles to dilate; the heart rate to increase; blood vessels to constrict; and the muscles of the gastrointestinal tract, bladder, and uterus to relax, thereby decreasing contractions.

sympathomimetic response. Examples of endogenous catecholamines are epinephrine, norepinephrine, and dopamine. The synthetic catecholamines are isoproterenol and dobutamine. Noncatecholamines (e.g., phenylephrine, metaproterenol, albuterol) stimulate the adrenergic receptors. Most noncatecholamines have a longer duration of action than the endogenous or synthetic catecholamines.

Many of the adrenergic drugs stimulate more than one of the adrenergic receptor sites. An example is epinephrine (Adrenalin), which acts on alpha$_1$-, beta$_1$-, and beta$_2$-adrenergic receptor sites. The responses from these receptor sites include an increase in blood pressure, pupil dilation, increase in heart rate (tachycardia), and bronchodilation. In certain types of shock (i.e., cardiogenic, anaphylactic), epinephrine is useful because it increases blood pressure, heart rate, and airflow through the lungs through bronchodilation. Because epinephrine affects three different adrenergic receptors, it is **nonselective** (excites all receptors approximately equally). Side effects result when more responses occur than are desired. Prototype Drug Chart 17–1 lists the pharmacologic behavior of epinephrine.

Epinephrine

Pharmacokinetics

Epinephrine can be administered subcutaneously, intravenously, topically, or by inhalation, intracardiac, and instillation methods. It should not be given orally, because it is rapidly metabolized in the GI tract and liver, which results in inadequate serum levels. The percentage by which the drug is protein-bound and its half-life are unknown. Epinephrine is metabolized by the liver and excreted in the urine.

Pharmacodynamics

Epinephrine is frequently used in emergencies to treat anaphylaxis, which is a life-threatening allergic response. Epinephrine is a potent inotropic (strengthens myocardial contraction) drug that increases cardiac output, promotes vasoconstriction and systolic blood pressure elevation, increases heart rate, and produces bronchodilation. High doses can result in cardiac dysrhythmias, therefore the electrocardiogram (ECG) should be monitored. Epinephrine can also cause renal vasoconstriction, thereby decreasing renal perfusion and urinary output.

The onset of action and peak concentration times are rapid. The use of decongestants with epinephrine has an additive effect. When epinephrine is administered with digoxin, cardiac dysrhythmias may occur. Beta-blockers, tricyclic antidepressants, and MAO inhibitors can cause a decrease in the action of epinephrine. Epinephrine is also discussed in Chapter 58 as one of the drugs used during emergencies.

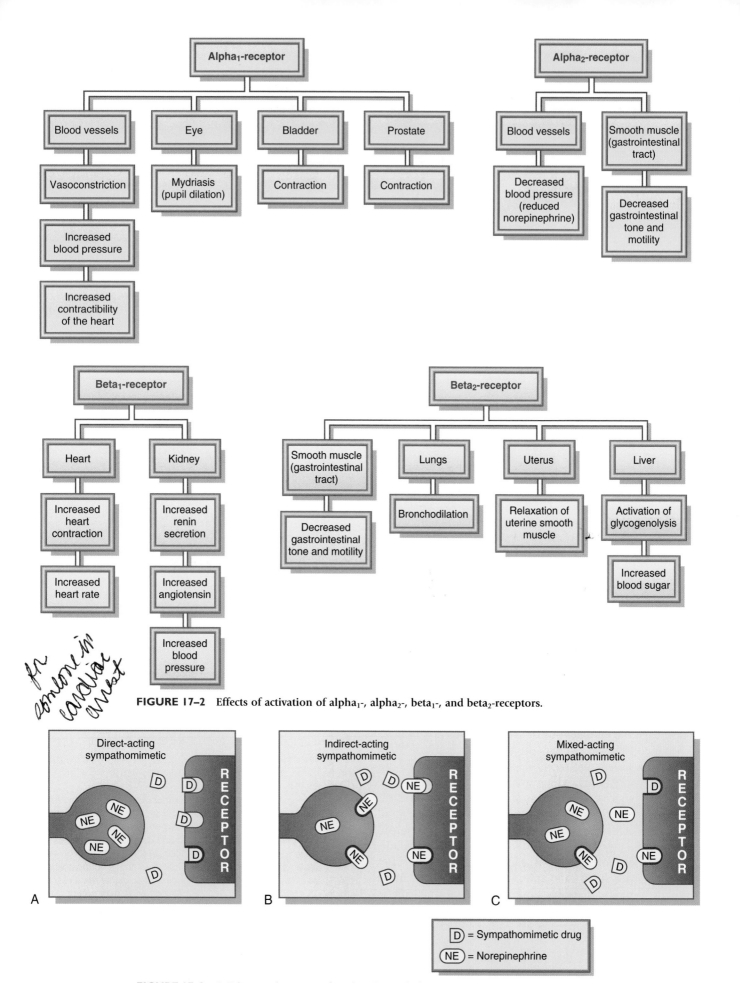

FIGURE 17–2 Effects of activation of alpha$_1$-, alpha$_2$-, beta$_1$-, and beta$_2$-receptors.

D = Sympathomimetic drug
NE = Norepinephrine

FIGURE 17–3 A, Direct-acting sympathomimetics; B, indirect-acting sympathomimetics; and C, mixed-acting sympathomimetics.

Prototype DRUG CHART 17-1

EPINEPHRINE

Drug Class

Sympathomimetic
Trade name: Adrenalin
Pregnancy Category: C

Dosage

Severe anaphylactic shock:
A: subQ: 0.1-0.5 ml of 1:1000 PRN
IV: 0.1-0.25 ml of 1:1000 with additional dilution
IV: 1-2.5 ml of 1:10,000 infused over 5-10 min
C: subQ: 0.01 ml/kg of 1:1000
V: 0.01 ml/kg of 1:1000 with additional dilution
IV: 0.1 mg or 10 ml of 1:100,000

Contraindications

Cardiac dysrhythmias, cerebral arteriosclerosis, pregnancy, narrow-angle glaucoma, cardiogenic shock
Caution: Hypertension, prostatic hypertrophy, hyperthyroidism, pregnancy, diabetes mellitus (hyperglycemia could result)

Drug-Lab-Food Interactions

Drug: Decrease epinephrine effect with methyldopa, beta blockers, and alpha-adrenergic blockers (e.g., phentolamine)
Lab: Increase blood glucose, serum lactic acid

Pharmacokinetics

Absorption: subQ/IM/IV: Rapidly
Distribution: PB: UK; in breast milk
Metabolism: t½: UK
Excretion: In urine unchanged

Pharmacodynamics

subQ/IM: Onset: 3-10 min
  Peak: 20 min
  Duration: 20-30 min
IV: Onset: Immediate
  Peak: 2-5 min
  Duration: 5-10 min
Inhal: Onset: 1 min
  Peak: 3-5 min
  Duration: 1-3

Therapeutic Effects/Uses

To treat allergic reaction, anaphylaxis, bronchospasm, cardiac arrest
Mode of Action: Action on one or more adrenergic sites; promotion of CNS and cardiac stimulation and bronchodilation

Side Effects

Anorexia, nausea, vomiting, nervousness, tremors, agitation, headache, pallor, insomnia, syncope, dizziness

Adverse Reactions

Palpitations, tachycardia, dyspnea
Life-threatening: Ventricular fibrillation, pulmonary edema

A, Adult; *C,* child; *CNS,* central nervous system; *IM,* intramuscular; *Inhal,* inhalation; *IV,* intravenous; *min,* minute; *PB,* protein-binding; *PRN,* as needed; *subQ,* subcutaneous; *t½,* half-life; *UK,* unknown.

Albuterol

Albuterol sulfate (Proventil) is **selective** for beta$_2$-adrenergic receptors, so the response is purely bronchodilation. An asthmatic client may respond better by taking albuterol than isoproterenol, because albuterol's primary action is on the beta$_2$-receptor. By using selective sympathomimetics, fewer undesired responses (i.e., side effects) will occur. However, high dosages of albuterol may affect the beta$_1$ receptors, causing an increase in heart rate. Prototype Drug Chart 17-2 lists the drug data related to albuterol.

Pharmacokinetics

Albuterol sulfate (Proventil, Ventolin) is well absorbed from the GI tract and is extensively metabolized by the liver. The half-life of the drug differs slightly according to the route of administration (oral route is 2.5 hours; inhalation route is 3.5 hours).

Pharmacodynamics

The primary use of albuterol is to prevent and treat bronchospasms. With inhalation, the onset of action of albuterol is faster than with oral administration, though the duration of action is the same for both oral and inhalation preparations.

Tremors, restlessness, and nervousness may occur when high doses of albuterol are taken. These side effects are most likely caused by the reflex effect of beta$_1$-receptors. If albuterol is taken with an MAO inhibitor, a hypertensive crisis can result. Beta-blockers may inhibit the action of albuterol. Albuterol and the beta$_2$ drugs are also discussed in Chapter 40.

Clonidine and Methyldopa

Clonidine (Catapres) and methyldopa (Aldomet) are selective alpha$_2$-adrenergic drugs used primarily to treat hypertension. The accepted theory for the action of alpha$_2$ drugs is that they regulate the release of norepinephrine by

Prototype DRUG CHART 17–2

ALBUTEROL

Drug Class	**Dosage**
Beta₂-adrenergic agonist Trade names: Proventil, Salbutamol, Ventolin, ✤Novo-Salmol *Pregnancy Category:* C	**A: PO:** 2-4 mg, t.i.d., q.i.d.; max: 32 mg/d in 4 divided doses **SR:** 4-8 mg, q12h **Inhal:** 1-2 puffs q4-6h PRN **Nebulizer:** 0.5 ml of 0.5% sol in 3 ml of 0.9% NaCl in 5-15 min **C 2-6 y:** PO: 0.1 mg/kg/t.i.d. **6-12 y:** PO: 2 mg, t.i.d., q.i.d. **6-12 y:** Inhal: Same as adult
Contraindications	**Drug-Lab-Food Interactions**
Caution: Severe cardiac disease, hypertension, hyperthyroidism, diabetes mellitus, pregnancy	*Drug: Increase* effect with other sympathomimetics; may *increase* effect with MAO inhibitors and tricyclic antidepressants *Antagonize* effect with beta-adrenergic blockers (beta-blockers) *Lab:* May *increase* glucose level slightly; may *decrease* serum potassium level
Pharmacokinetics	**Pharmacodynamics**

Absorption: Well absorbed from the GI tract
Distribution: PB: UK
Metabolism: t½: PO: 2.5–6 h; Inhal: 3.5–5 h
Excretion: 75% excreted in the urine
	PO: Onset: 30 min
	  Peak: 2-3 h
	  Duration: 4-6 h
	Inhal: Onset: 5-15 min
	  Peak: 0.5-2 h
	  Duration: 3-6 h

Therapeutic Effects/Uses

To treat bronchospasm, asthma, bronchitis, and other COPD
Mode of Action: Stimulates the beta₂-adrenergic receptors in the lungs, which relaxes the bronchial smooth muscles

Side Effects	**Adverse Reactions**
Tremor, dizziness, nervousness, restlessness	Palpitations, reflex tachycardia, hallucinations ***Life-threatening:*** Cardiac dysrhythmias

A, Adult; *C*, child; *COPD*, chronic obstructive pulmonary disease; *d*, day; *GI*, gastrointestinal; *h*, hour; *Inhal*, inhalation; *MAO*, monoamine oxidase; *min*, minute; *PB*, protein-binding; *PO*, by mouth; *PRN*, as needed; *q.i.d.*, four times a day; *SR*, sustained release; *t½*, half-life; *t.i.d.*, three times a day; *UK*, unknown; *y*, year; ✤, Canadian drug name.

inhibiting its release. Alpha₂ drugs are also believed to produce cardiovascular depression by stimulating alpha₂ receptors in the central nervous system (CNS), leading to a decrease in blood pressure (see Chapter 43).

Side Effects and Adverse Reactions

Side effects frequently result when the drug dosage is increased or the drug is nonselective (i.e., it acts on several receptors). Side effects commonly associated with adrenergic drugs include hypertension, tachycardia, palpitations, dysrhythmias, tremors, dizziness, urinary difficulty, nausea, and vomiting.

Names of adrenergic drugs, the receptors they activate, dosage information, and common uses are listed in Table 17–2.

Nursing Process

Adrenergic Agonist

ASSESSMENT

■ Record vital signs for future comparison. Epinephrine stimulates alpha₁ (increases blood pressure), beta₁ (increases heart rate), and beta₂ (dilates bronchial tubes) receptors. Albuterol (Proventil) stimulates the beta₂-receptor.

■ Assess the drugs client takes and report possible drug-drug interactions. Beta-blockers decrease the effect of epinephrine.

■ Determine client's health history. Most adrenergic drugs are contraindicated if client has cardiac dysrhythmias, narrow-angle glaucoma, or cardiogenic shock.
■ Compare results of laboratory tests with future laboratory findings.

Table 17–2

Adrenergic Drugs (Alpha₁, Beta₁, and Beta₂)

Generic (Brand)	Route and Dosage	Uses and Considerations
epinephrine (Adrenalin Chloride) Alpha₁, beta₁, and beta₂	See Prototype Drug Chart 17–1.	
ephedrine HCl, ephedrine sulfate (Ephedsol, Ectasule) Alpha₁, beta₁, and beta₂	A: PO: 25-50 mg t.i.d./q.i.d. subQ/IM: 12.5-50 mg; IV: 10-25 mg PRN; *max:* 150 mg/24 h C: >2 y: PO: 2-3 mg/kg/d in 4-6 divided doses; *max:* 75 mg/24 h	To treat hypotensive states, bronchospasm, nasal congestion, orthostatic hypotension. Effective for relief of symptoms of hay fever, sinusitis, allergic rhinitis. Also may be used to treat mild cases of asthma. Drug resistance may occur with prolonged use of ephedrine. If this occurs, stop drug for 3-5 d then resume. *Pregnancy category:* C; PB: UK; t½: 3-6 h
norepinephrine bitartrate (Levarterenol, Levophed) Alpha₁ and beta₁	A: IV: 4 mg in 250-500 ml of D₅W or NSS infused initially 8-12 mcg/min, then 4 mcg/min; monitor blood pressure	For shock. Potent vasoconstrictor. Increases blood pressure and cardiac output. Blood pressure should be closely monitored every 2-5 min during infusion. IV flow titrated according to blood pressure. *Pregnancy category:* D; PB: UK; t½: UK
dopamine HCl (Intropin) Alpha₁ and beta₁	A: IV/INF: 1-5 mcg/kg/min initially; gradually increase 5-10 mcg/kg/min; *max:* 50 mcg/kg/min C: IV: Usually the same	To correct hypotension. Does not decrease renal function in doses <5 mcg/kg/min. *Pregnancy category:* C; PB: UK; t½: 2 min
midodrine (ProAmatine) Alpha₁	A: PO: 10 mg t.i.d.	To treat symptomatic orthostatic hypotension. Blood pressure may increase by 15 to 30 mm Hg in 1 h with one 10-mg dose. *Pregnancy category:* C; PB: UK; t½: 3-4 h
phenylephrine HCl 12-hour spray/oxymetazoline HCl (Neo-Synephrine) Alpha	*Nasal decongestant:* A: Instill: 2-3 sprays or gtt of 0.25%-0.5% sol C: <6 y: Instill: 2-3 gtt of 0.125% sol C: 6-12 y: Instill: 2-3 gtt of 0.25% sol Also available IM, IV	To treat nasal congestion; acts as a decongestant. Used for clients with common cold, sinusitis, allergic rhinitis. Have client blow nose before drug is administered. *Pregnancy category:* C; PB: UK; t½: 2.5 h
pseudoephedrine HCl (Sudafed, Actifed, Co-Tylenol, PediaCare) Alpha and beta₁	*Nasal decongestant:* A: PO: 60 mg q.i.d./q6h PO/SR: 120 mg q12h; *max:* 240 mg/d C: 2-6 y: PO: 15 mg q6h; *max:* 60 mg/d C: 6-12 y: PO: 30 mg q6h; *max:* 120 mg/d	To treat nasal congestion. OTC drug. Check label for contraindications. Avoid taking with a history of hypertension, cardiac disease, diabetes mellitus. *Pregnancy category:* C; PB: UK; t½: 9-16 h
phenylpropanolamine HCl (Dimetapp, Dristan, Contac 12 Hour, Triaminicol, Triaminic)	Nasal decongestant: A: PO: 25 mg q4h PRN PO/SR: 75 mg q12h PRN C: 2-6 y: PO: 6.25 mg q4h PRN C: 6-12 y: 12.5 mg q4h PRN	To treat nasal congestion; acts as OTC drugs. FDA has required that phenylpropanolamine be withdrawn from OTC weight-control products and other OTC drugs. In some cases, pseudoephedrine has been used in place of phenylpropanolamine.
Dexatrim, Dietac, Control Alpha and beta₁	Appetite suppressant: A: PO/SR: 75 mg daily (before breakfast); PO: 25 mg t.i.d. a.c.	OTC drug used to control weight gain. Client should check with health care provider before taking an appetite suppressant. *Pregnancy category:* C; PB: UK; t½: 3-4 h
albuterol (Proventil, Ventolin) Beta₂	See Prototype Drug Chart 17–2.	To relieve bronchospasm caused by acute and chronic obstructive airway disease (e.g., asthma, bronchitis, emphysema). Stimulates beta₂-receptors of bronchi. Promotes bronchodilation. *Pregnancy category:* C; PB: UK; t½: 2.5-5 h

Continued

NURSING DIAGNOSES

- Risk for impaired tissue integrity related to severe hypotension
- Decreased cardiac output related to bradycardia

PLANNING

- Client's vital signs will be within normal or acceptable ranges.

NURSING INTERVENTIONS

- Record client's vital signs. Report signs of increasing blood pressure and increasing heart rate. If client receives an alpha-adrenergic drug intravenously for shock, blood pressure should be checked every 3 to 5 minutes or as indicated to avoid severe hypertension.
- Report side effects of adrenergic drugs: tachycardia, palpitations, tremors, dizziness, and increased blood pressure.

- Check client's urinary output and assess for bladder distention. Urinary retention can result from high drug dose or continuous use of adrenergic drugs.
- For cardiac resuscitation, administer epinephrine 1:1000 IV (1 mg/ml), which may be diluted in 10 ml of saline solution (as prescribed).
- Monitor IV site frequently when administering norepinephrine bitartrate (levarterenol) or dopamine (Intropin) because infiltration of these drugs causes tissue necrosis. These drugs should be diluted sufficiently in IV fluids. An antidote for norepinephrine (Levophed) and dopamine is phentolamine mesylate (Regitine) 5 to 10 mg, diluted in 10 to 15 ml of saline infiltrated into the area.
- To avoid nausea and vomiting, offer food to client when giving adrenergic drugs.
- Evaluate blood glucose levels because they may be increased.

Table 17–2

Adrenergic Drugs (Alpha₁, Beta₁, and Beta₂)—cont'd

Generic (Brand)	Route and Dosage	Uses and Considerations
metaproterenol sulfate (Alupent, Metaprel) Beta₁ (some) and beta₂	A & C: >9 y: PO: 10-20 mg t.i.d./q.i.d. C: <6 y: PO: 1-2.6 mg/kg/d in 3-4 divided doses C: 6-9 y: PO: 10 mg t.i.d./q.i.d. A & C: >12 yr: Inhal: 2-3 puffs q3-4h; max: 12 puffs/d	Treatment for bronchospasm, acute heart block (only used in atropine-refractory bradycardia). By stimulating beta₁-receptors, heart rate is increased but not as strongly as with isoproterenol HCl. Dilates bronchial tubes. *Pregnancy category:* C; PB: UK; t½: UK
dobutamine HCl (Dobutrex) Beta₁	A & C: IV: 2.5-10 mcg/kg/min initially; increase dose gradually; max: 40 mcg/kg/min	To treat cardiac decompensation by enhancing myocardial contractility, stroke volume, and cardiac output which may result from cardiogenic shock or cardiac surgery. *Pregnancy category:* C; PB: UK; t½: 2 min
isoetharine HCl (Bronkosol) Beta₂	A: IPPB: 0.5-1.0 ml of 0.5% sol OR 0.5 ml of 1% sol diluted in 3 ml of NSS A: Inhal: 1-2 puffs	To control asthma and chronic obstructive pulmonary disease by dilating bronchial tubes. *Pregnancy category:* C; PB: UK; t½: UK
terbutaline sulfate (Brethine, Brethaire, Bricanyl) Beta₂	*Bronchodilator:* A: PO: 2.5-5 mg t.i.d. OR q8h; SC: 0.25 mg initially; no more than 0.5 mg in 4 h Inhal: 2 puffs q4-6h C: >12 y: PO: 2.5 mg t.i.d. OR q8h *Premature labor:* A: PO: 2.5 mg q4-6h; IV: 10 mcg/min, gradually increase; *max:* 80 mcg/min	Primary use is to correct bronchospasm. Unofficial use during premature labor to prevent premature birth. *Pregnancy category:* B; PB: 25%; t½: 3-11 h
ritodrine HCl (Yutopar) Beta₂ and some beta₁	A: PO: Initially 10 mg q2h for first 24 h; maint: 10-20 mg q4-6h; *max:* 120 mg/d IV: 50-100 mcg/min; dose may gradually increase to 300 mcg/min	Used to decrease and/or stop uterine contraction. To be effective, heart rate must be more than 100 beats per minute. Because there are many side effects, drug is not used as frequently to control premature labor as it once was. *Pregnancy category:* C; PB: UK; t½: 1.6-2.6 h

A, Adult; *C*, child; *d*, day; *FDA*, Food and Drug Administration; *gtt*, drops; *h*, hour; *IM*, intramuscular; *inf*, infusion; *inhal*, inhalation; *IPPB*, intermittent positive pressure breathing; *IV*, intravenous; *min*, minute; *NSS*, normal saline solution; *OTC*, over-the-counter; *PB*, protein-binding; *PO*, by mouth; *PRN*, as needed; *q.i.d.*, four times a day; *SL*, sublingual; *SR*, sustained release; *subQ*, subcutaneous; *t½*, half-life; *t.i.d.*, three times a day; *UK*, unknown; *y*, year; *>*, greater than; *<*, less than.

Client Teaching

General

- Instruct client to read labels on all over-the-counter (OTC) drugs for cold symptoms and diet pills. Many of these have properties of sympathetic (adrenergic, sympathomimetics) drugs and should not be taken if client is hypertensive or has diabetes mellitus, cardiac dysrhythmias, or coronary artery disease.
- Advise mothers not to take drugs that contain sympathetic drugs while nursing infants. These drugs pass into breast milk.
- Explain to client that continuous use of nasal sprays or drops that contain adrenergics may result in nasal congestion rebound (inflamed and congested nasal tissue).

Self-Administration

- Inform client and family how to administer cold medications by spray or drops in the nostrils. Spray should be used with the head in an upright position. The use of nasal spray while lying down can cause systemic absorption. Coloration of nasal spray or drops might indicate deterioration.
- Direct client to use bronchodilator sprays conservatively. If client excessively uses a nonselective adrenergic drug that affects beta$_1$- and beta$_2$-receptors, tachycardia may occur.

Side Effects

- Encourage client to report side effects (e.g., rapid heart rate, palpitations, dizziness) to a health care provider.

Cultural Considerations ❖

- Decrease language barriers for clients with language difficulties and for those who do not work in the health care field by decoding the jargon of the health care environment.

EVALUATION

■ Evaluate client's response to the adrenergic drug. Continue monitoring client's vital signs and report abnormal findings.

Adrenergic Blockers (Antagonists)

Drugs that block the effects of the adrenergic neurotransmitter are called **adrenergic blockers,** adrenergic antagonists, or sympatholytics. They act as antagonists to adrenergic agonists by blocking the alpha- and beta-receptor sites. Most adrenergic blockers block either the alpha- or the beta-receptor. They block the effects of the neurotransmitter either directly by occupying the alpha- or the beta-receptors or indirectly by inhibiting the release of the neurotransmitters norepinephrine and epinephrine. The three sympatholytic receptors are alpha$_1$, beta$_1$, and beta$_2$. Table 17–3 lists the effects of alpha- and beta-blockers.

Table 17–3

Effects of Adrenergic Blockers at Receptors

Receptor	Responses
Alpha$_1$	Vasodilation: decreases blood pressure; reflex tachycardia might result; miosis (constriction of pupil) occurs; suppresses ejaculation; reduces contraction of smooth muscle in bladder neck and prostate gland
Beta$_1$	Decreases heart rate; reduces force of contractions
Beta$_2$	Constricts bronchioles; contracts uterus; inhibits glycogenolysis, which can decrease blood sugar

Alpha-Adrenergic Blockers

Drugs that block or inhibit a response at the alpha-adrenergic receptor site are called alpha-adrenergic blockers or **alpha-blockers.** Alpha-blocking agents are divided into two groups: selective alpha-blockers that block alpha$_1$ and nonselective alpha-blockers that block alpha$_1$ and alpha$_2$. Because alpha-adrenergic blockers can cause orthostatic hypotension and reflex tachycardia, many of these drugs are not as frequently prescribed as beta-blockers. Alpha-blockers are helpful in decreasing symptoms of benign prostatic hypertrophy (BPH).

Alpha-blockers promote vasodilation, causing a decrease in blood pressure. If vasodilation is longstanding, orthostatic hypotension can result. Dizziness may also be a symptom of a drop in blood pressure. As blood pressure decreases, pulse rate usually increases to compensate for the low blood pressure and inadequate blood flow. Alpha-blockers can be used to treat peripheral vascular disease (e.g., Raynaud's disease). Vasodilation occurs, permitting more blood flow to the extremities. Alpha blockers are also discussed in Chapter 43.

Beta-Adrenergic Blockers

Beta-adrenergic blockers, commonly called **beta-blockers,** decrease heart rate; a decrease in blood pressure usually follows. Some of the beta-blockers are nonselective, blocking both beta$_1$- and beta$_2$-receptors. Not only does the heart rate decrease because of beta$_1$-blocking, but bronchoconstriction also occurs. Nonselective beta-blockers (beta$_1$ and beta$_2$) should be used with extreme caution in any client who has chronic obstructive pulmonary disease (COPD) or asthma. A **selective** adrenergic blocker has a greater affinity for certain receptors. If the desired effect is to decrease pulse rate and blood pressure, then a selective beta$_1$-blocker such as metoprolol tartrate (Lopressor) may be ordered.

An intrinsic sympathomimetic activity (ISA) causes partial stimulation of beta receptors. Certain nonselective beta blockers (block both beta$_1$ and beta$_2$) that have ISA are carteolol, carvedilol, penbutolol, and pindolol. The selective blocker (blocks beta$_1$ only) that has ISA is acebutolol.

These agents reportedly cause fewer serious side effects and are helpful to clients experiencing severe bradycardia.

Propranolol hydrochloride (Inderal) was the first beta-blocker prescribed to treat angina, cardiac dysrhythmias, hypertension, and heart failure. This medication is given for the unlabeled use of migraine prophylaxis. Although it is still prescribed today, propranolol has many side effects, partly because of its nonselective response in blocking both beta$_1$- and beta$_2$-receptors. It is contraindicated for clients with asthma or second- or third-degree heart block. Propranolol is extensively metabolized by the liver (hepatic first-pass), so only a small amount of the drug reaches the systemic circulation. Prototype Drug Chart 17–3 describes the pharmacologic behavior of propranolol.

Pharmacokinetics

Propranolol is well absorbed from the GI tract. It crosses the blood-brain barrier and the placenta and is excreted in breast milk. It is metabolized by the liver and has a short half-life of 3 to 6 hours.

Pharmacodynamics

By blocking both types of beta-receptors, propranolol decreases the heart rate and, secondarily, the blood pressure. It also causes the bronchial tubes to constrict and the uterus to contract. It is available in tablets and sustained-release capsules and for intravenous administration. The onset of action of the sustained-release oral preparation is longer than that of the tablet; peak time and duration of action are also longer for the sustained-release formulation. This form is effective for dosing once a day, especially for clients who do not comply with drug doses of several times a day.

Prototype DRUG CHART 17–3

ATENOLOL

Drug Class
Beta$_1$-adrenergic blocker
Trade names: Tenormin, Apo-Atenolol
Pregnancy Category: C

Dosage
Hypertension:
A: PO: 50-100 mg/d
Elderly: PO: 25-50 mg/d
Myocardial infarction:
A: IV: 5 mg q5min × 2: then 10 min after second dose 50 mg PO, then 50 mg PO 12 h later, then 50 mg bid for 6-9 d

Contraindications
Sinus bradycardia, heart block > first degree, cardiogenic shock, overt cardiac failure
Caution: Renal dysfunction, peripheral arterial circulatory disorders, asthma, COPD, hyperthyroidism, concurrent use of diuretics and digitalis

Drug-Lab-Food Interactions
Drug: Increased absorption with atropine and other anticholinergics, *decreased* effects with NSAIDs, *increased* risk of hypoglycemia with insulin and sulfonylureas, *increased* hypotension with prazosin and terazosin, *increased* lidocaine and verapamil levels with toxicity

Pharmacokinetics
Absorption: Well-absorbed
Distribution: PB: 6-16%
Metabolism: t½: 6-7 h
Excretion: Urine

Pharmacodynamics
PO: Onset: 2.7-7.7 h
   Peak: 2-4 h
   Duration: 24 h
IV: Onset: UK
   Peak: 5 min
   Duration: 24 h

Therapeutic Effects/Uses
To treat hypertension, angina pectoris, and myocardial infarction
Mode of Action: Selectively blocks beta$_1$-adrenergic receptor sites, decreases sympathetic outflow to the periphery, suppresses renin-angiotensin-aldosterone system

Side Effects
Drowsiness, dizziness, fainting, depression, weakness, nausea, vomiting, diarrhea, cool extremities, leg pain

Adverse Reactions
Bradycardia, hypotension, heart failure, masking of hypoglycemia
Life-threatening: Agranulocytosis, pulmonary edema, dysrhythmias

rA, Adult; *COPD,* chronic obstructive pulmonary disease; *h,* hour; *IV,* intravenously; *min,* minute; *NSAID,* nonsteroidal antiinflammatory drug; *PB,* protein-binding; *PO,* by mouth; *t½,* half-life; *UK,* unknown.

Drug Interactions

Many drugs interact with propranolol. Phenytoin, isoproterenol, nonsteroidal antiinflammatory drugs (NSAIDs), barbiturates, and xanthines (caffeine, theophylline) decrease the drug effect of propranolol. When propranolol is taken with digoxin or a calcium blocker, atrioventricular (AV) heart block may occur. The blood pressure can be decreased if propranolol is taken with another antihypertensive, though this may be the desired result.

Beta-blockers are useful in treating cardiac dysrhythmias, mild hypertension, mild tachycardia, and angina pectoris. The use of beta-blockers as antihypertensives, antidysrhythmics, and drugs for angina is discussed in Chapters 41 and 43. Table 17–4 lists the alpha- and beta-blockers and their dosages, uses, and considerations.

Side Effects and Adverse Reactions

The side effects commonly associated with beta-blockers are bradycardia, palpitations, hypotension, headache, dizziness, hyperglycemia, hypoglycemia, bronchospasm, and agranulocytosis. General side effects of alpha-adrenergic blockers include cardiac dysrhythmias, flushing, hypotension, impotence or decreased libido, and depression. Usually the side effects are dose related.

Adrenergic Neuron Blockers

Drugs that block the release of norepinephrine from the sympathetic terminal neurons are called **adrenergic neuron blockers,** which are classified as a subdivision of the adrenergic blockers. The clinical use of neuron blockers is to decrease blood pressure. Guanadrel sulfate (Hylorel), an example of an adrenergic neuron blocker, is a potent antihypertensive agent.

Table 17–4
Adrenergic Blockers

Generic (Brand)	Route and Dosage	Uses and Considerations
tolazoline (Priscoline HCl) (alpha₁)	A: subQ/IM/IV: 10-50 mg q.i.d. *Pulmonary hypertension:* NB: IV: 1-2 mg/kg infused over 10 min, followed by 1-2 mg/kg/h for 24-48 h	For peripheral vascular disorder and persistent pulmonary hypertension in the newborn. Also for emergency hypertension. *Pregnancy category:* C; PB: UK; t½: 3-10 h
phentolamine mesylate (Regitine) (alpha₁)	A: IM/IV: 2.5-5 mg, repeat q5min until controlled, then q2-3h PRN C: IM/IV: 0.05-0.1 mg/kg, repeat PRN	Management of peripheral vascular disorder and hypertensive emergency. Antidote for dopamine infiltration. *Pregnancy category:* C; PB: UK; t½: 20 min
doxazosin mesylate (Cardura) (alpha₁)	A: PO: 1 mg/d, titrate dose up to *max:* 16 mg/d; maint: 4-8 mg/d Elderly: PO: 0.5 mg/d initially; may increase dose	For mild to moderate hypertension and BPH. Check for orthostatic hypotension. Dizziness, headache, syncope may occur. *Pregnancy category:* C; PB: 98%; t½: 9-12 h
prazosin HCl (Minipress) (alpha₁)	A: PO: 1 mg b.i.d./t.i.d.; maint: 3-15 mg/d; *max:* 20 mg/d in divided doses	Management of mild to moderate hypertension. May be used in combination with other antihypertensive drugs. *Pregnancy category:* C; PB: 95%; t½: 3 h
terazosin HCl (Hytrin) (alpha₁)	A: PO: 1 mg at bedtime, maint: 1-5 mg in 1-2 divided doses; *max:* 20 mg/d	For hypertension. May be used in combination with diuretic or other antihypertensive drugs. May also be used for BPH. May cause dizziness, headache, edema, orthostatic hypotension. *Pregnancy category:* C; PB: UK; t½: 9-12 h
carvedilol (Coreg) (alpha₁, beta₁, and beta₂)	A: PO: 6.25 mg b.i.d.; may increase to 12.5 mg b.i.d.; *max:* 50 mg/d	For treatment of hypertension. Can be used alone or with a thiazide diuretic. Used also for mild to moderate heart failure. *Pregnancy category:* C; PB: UK; t½: 7-10 h
labetalol (Normodyne, Trandate) (alpha₁, beta₁, and beta₂)	A: PO: 100 mg b.i.d.; dose may be increased; *max:* 2.4 g/d; IV: 20 mg OR 1-2 mg/kg; repeat 20-80 mg at 10-min interval; *max:* 300 mg/d	To treat mild to severe hypertension; angina pectoris; used during surgery to manage blood pressure. *Pregnancy category:* C; PB: 50%; t½: 6-8 h
carteolol HCl (Cartrol) (beta₁ and beta₂)	A: PO: 2.5-5.0 mg/d	For hypertension and glaucoma. Primarily blocks beta₁ adrenergic receptor; however, in large doses blocks beta₂. *Pregnancy category:* C; PB: 23%-30%; t½: 4-6 h
penbutolol (Levatol) (beta₁ and beta₂)	A: PO: 10-20 mg/d; *max:* 80 mg/d	To treat mild to moderate hypertension. Clients with asthma should avoid taking the drug. *Pregnancy category:* C; PB: 80%-98%; t½: 5 h
propranolol HCl (Inderal) (beta₁ and beta₂)	A: PO: Initially: 10-20 mg t.i.d.-q.i.d.; maint: 20-60 mg t.i.d.-q.i.d.; *max:* 320 mg/day; SR: 80-160 mg/day	Management of angina pectoris, myocardial infarction, hypertension, dysrhythmias, thyrotoxicosis. *Pregnancy category:* C; PB: 93%; t½: 2-4 h
nadolol (Corgard) (beta₁ and beta₂)	A: PO: 40-80 mg/d; *max:* 320 mg/d	Management of hypertension and angina pectoris. Contraindicated in bronchial asthma and severe COPD because it blocks beta₂. *Pregnancy category:* C; PB: 30%; t½: 10-24 h

Continued

Table 17-4

Adrenergic Blockers—cont'd

Generic (Brand)	Route and Dosage	Uses and Considerations
pindolol (Visken) (beta$_1$ and beta$_2$)	A: PO: 5 mg b.i.d./t.i.d.; maint: 10-30 mg in divided doses; *max:* 60 mg/d in divided doses	Management of hypertension and angina pectoris. Contraindicated in asthma, COPD, and second- and third-degree heart block. *Pregnancy category:* B; PB: 40%; t^1/$_2$: 3-4 h
sotalol (Betapace) (beta$_1$ and beta$_2$)	A: PO: 80 mg b.i.d.; may increase gradually. Average: 240-320 mg/d	To treat life-threatening ventricular arrhythmias and chronic angina pectoris. Pregnancy category: B; PB: 0; t^1/$_2$: 12 h
timolol maleate (Blocadren) (beta$_1$ and beta$_2$)	A: PO: Initially 10 mg b.i.d.; maint: 20-40 mg/d in 2 divided doses; *max:* 60 mg/d	Management of mild to moderate hypertension, dysrhythmias, and postmyocardial infarction. Also may be used as prophylaxis of migraine headache. For ophthalmic use to treat IOP. Use with caution for clients with asthma or COPD. *Pregnancy category:* C; PB: <10%; t^1/$_2$: 3-4 h

Selective Beta-Adrenergic Blockers

metoprolol tartrate (Lopressor) (beta$_1$)	Hypertension: A: PO: 50-100 mg/d in 1-2 divided doses; maint: 100-450 mg/d in divided doses; *max:* 450 mg/d in divided doses Myocardial infarction: A: IV: 5 mg q2min 3 doses, then PO: 100 mg b.i.d.	Management of hypertension, angina pectoris, postmyocardial infarction. Bradycardia, dizziness, and gastrointestinal distress may occur. *Pregnancy category:* C; PB: 12%; t^1/$_2$: 3-4 h
atenolol (Tenormin) (beta$_1$)	See Prototype Drug Chart 17-3.	
acebutolol HCl (Sectral) (beta$_1$)	A: PO: Initially: 200-400 mg/d A: PO: maint; 200-800 mg/d in 1-2 divided doses; *max:* 1200 mg/d	Treatment for mild to moderate hypertension, angina pectoris, and supraventricular dysrhythmias. Check apical pulse; do not give if <60 bpm. *Pregnancy category:* B; PB: 26%; t^1/$_2$: 3-13 h
betaxolol (Kerlone) (beta$_1$)	A: PO: 10-20 mg/d. Also for ophthalmic use: glaucoma	For hypertension and glaucoma. Ophthalmic preparation is used to decrease IOP. *Pregnancy category:* C; PB: UK; t^1/$_2$: 14-22 h
bisoprolol fumarate (Zebeta) (beta$_1$)	A: PO: Initially: 5 mg/d; maint: 2.5-20 mg/d	For hypertension and angina pectoris. Long-acting beta blocker. Heart rate and blood pressure may be decreased. *Pregnancy category:* C; PB: <30%; t^1/$_2$: 9-12 h
esmolol HCl (Brevibloc) (beta$_1$)	A: IV: Loading dose: 500 mcg/kg/min for 1 min; then 50 mcg/kg/min for 4 min	For treatment of supraventricular tachycardia, atrial fibrillation/flutter, and hypertension Contraindications: heart block, bradycardia, cardiogenic shock, uncompensated heart failure. *Pregnancy category:* C; PB: UK; t^1/$_2$: 9 min

A, Adult; *b.i.d.,* two times a day; *BPH,* benign prostatic hypertrophy; *bpm,* beats per minute; *C,* child; *COPD,* chronic obstructive pulmonary disease; *d,* day; *h,* hour; *IM,* intramuscular; *IOP,* intraocular pressure; *IV,* intravenous; *NB,* newborn; *PB,* protein-binding; *PO,* by mouth; *PRN,* as necessary; *q.i.d.,* four times a day; *subQ,* subcutaneous; *t^1/$_2$,* half-life; *t.i.d.,* three times a day; *UK,* unknown; *>,* greater than; *<,* less than.

Nursing Process

Adrenergic Neuron Blockers*

ASSESSMENT

■ Obtain baseline vital signs and electrocardiogram for future comparison. Bradycardia and decrease in blood pressure are common cardiac effects of beta-adrenergic blockers. Beta-adrenergic blockers are frequently called beta-blockers because they block beta$_1$ and beta$_2$ (nonselective) or beta$_1$ (cardiac selective) receptors.

■ Assess whether client has respiratory problems by listening for signs of wheezing or noting dyspnea (difficulty in breathing). If the beta-blocker is nonselective, not only does the pulse rate decrease but also bronchoconstriction can result. Clients with asthma should take a beta$_1$ blocker such as metoprolol (Lopressor) and avoid nonselective beta-blockers.

■ Determine the drugs that the client currently takes. Report if any are phenothiazines, digoxin, calcium channel blockers, or other antihypertensives.

■ Record client's urine output and use for future comparison.

NURSING DIAGNOSES

■ Ineffective breathing pattern related to dyspnea
■ Decreased cardiac output related to cardiac dysrhythmias
■ Risk for injury related to dizziness

PLANNING

■ Client will comply with the drug regimen.
■ Client's vital signs will be within the desired range.

NURSING INTERVENTIONS

■ Monitor client's vital signs. Report marked changes such as marked decrease in blood pressure and heart rate.
■ Administer IV propranolol undiluted or diluted in D_5W.
■ Note any complaints of excessive dizziness or light-headedness.
■ Report any complaint of stuffy nose. Vasodilation results from the use of alpha-adrenergic blockers, and nasal congestion can occur.
■ Determine whether client has diabetes and receives a beta-adrenergic blocker; insulin dose or oral hypoglycemic may need to be adjusted.
■ Have glucagon available. Clients who take beta-blockers do not have normal compensatory mechanisms while in shock states. To resuscitate such clients, glucagon must be given in high doses to counteract the sympatholytic effects of beta-blockers.

Client Teaching

General

● Advise client to avoid abruptly stopping a beta-blocker; rebound hypertension, rebound tachycardia, or angina attack could result.
● Instruct client to comply with the drug regimen.
● Educate clients about insulin therapy; early warning signs of hypoglycemia (e.g., tachycardia, nervousness) may be masked by the beta-blocker.
● Direct clients to monitor blood sugar carefully and follow diet orders when on insulin therapy.

Self-Administration

● Teach client and family how to take pulse and blood pressure.

Side Effects

● Encourage client to avoid orthostatic (postural) hypotension by slowly rising from supine or sitting positions to standing.
● Inform client and family of possible mood changes when taking beta blockers. Mood changes can include depression, nightmares, and suicidal tendencies.
● Warn clients that certain beta blockers (e.g., propranolol, metoprolol, pindolol) and alpha blockers (e.g.,

prazosin) may cause impotence or decreased libido, which is usually dose related.

Cultural Considerations ❖

● Obtain an interpreter when necessary; do not rely on family members, who may not fully disclose because of honor or shame.
● When translation is needed, discuss the ethnicity of the interpreter as well as the language desired. Provide an interpreter with the same ethnic background and gender if possible, especially when sensitive topics are being addressed.

EVALUATION

■ Evaluate the effectiveness of the adrenergic blocker. Vital signs must be stable within the desired range.

*Alpha- and beta-adrenergic blockers are also presented within the antidysrhythmic (see Chapter 41), antianginal (see Chapter 41), and antihypertensive (see Chapter 43) sections.

Critical Thinking Case Study

VT, age 79, has asthma. An adrenergic drug is selected.

1. What are the drug advantages and disadvantages associated with the use of ephedrine, isoproterenol, metaproterenol, albuterol, and terbutaline for VT? Explain.
2. Is age a factor in drug selection? Explain.

HP, age 69, has hypertension and asthma. An adrenergic blocker is selected.

1. What are the drug advantages and disadvantages associated with the use of doxazosin, prazosin, propranolol, metoprolol, atenolol, and acebutolol for HP? Explain.
2. What needs to be included when teaching HP about the use of an adrenergic blocker?

NCLEX Study Questions

1. For the client taking epinephrine, the nurse realizes there is a possible drug interaction with:
   a. albuterol (Proventil)
   b. metoprolol (Lopressor) — *both nonselective*
   c. bethanechol (Urecholine)
   d. tolterodine tartrate (Detrol)

2. The nurse will monitor the client taking albuterol (Proventil) for:
   a. palpitations — *from midose*
   b. hypoglycemia
   c. bronchospasm
   d. uterine contractions

3. A client is prescribed metoprolol (Lopressor) to treat hypertension. It is important for the nurse to monitor the client for:
   a. bradycardia
   b. hypertension
   c. ankle edema
   d. decreased respirations

4. Atenolol (Tenormin) is prescribed for a client. The nurse realizes that this drug is a beta-adrenergic blocker and this drug classification is contraindicated for clients with: — *relatively selective*
   a. hypothyroidism
   b. angina pectoris
   c. cardiogenic shock
   d. liver dysfunction

5. The nurse realizes that β1 receptor stimulation is differentiated from β2 stimulation in that stimulation of β1 receptors lead to:
   a. increased bronchodilation
   b. decreased uterine contractility
   c. increased myocardial contractility
   d. decreased blood flow to skeletal muscles

Answers: 1, b; 2, a; 3, a; 4, c; 5, c.

18

Cholinergics and Anticholinergics

ELECTRONIC RESOURCES

Evolve website (http://evolve.elsevier.com/KeeHayes/pharmacology/):
- *Case Studies*
- *Content Updates*
- *Frequently Asked Questions*
- *Student Review Activities*
- *WebLinks*
- *Additional Reference Material*

Companion CD-ROM:
- *NCLEX Examination Review Questions*
- *Pharmacology Animations*
- *IV Therapy Checklists*
- *Medication Error Checklists*
- *Drug Calculation Problems*
- *Electronic Calculators*
- *Top 200 Drugs with Pronunciations*
- *References from the Textbook*

Outline

Objectives

- Compare the two cholinergic receptors.
- Describe the responses of cholinergic drugs and anticholinergic drugs.
- Differentiate between direct-acting and indirect-acting cholinergic drugs.
- Contrast the major side effects of cholinergic and anticholinergic drugs.
- Differentiate the uses of cholinergics and anticholinergics.
- Explain the nursing process, including client teaching associated with cholinergics and anticholinergics.
- Apply the nursing process for the client taking neostigmine, a reversible cholinesterase inhibitor.

Terms

acetylcholine (ACh), p. 282
anticholinergics, p. 286
anticholinesterases, p. 282
cholinergic blocking agents, p. 286

cholinergics, p. 282
cholinesterase (ChE), p. 282
direct-acting cholinergics, p. 283

indirect-acting cholinergics, p. 285
miosis, p. 283
muscarinic receptors, p. 282

mydriasis, p. 286
nicotinic receptors, p. 282
parasympatholytics, p. 286
parasympathomimetics, p. 282

The two groups of drugs that affect the parasympathetic nervous system are the (1) *cholinergics* (parasympathomimetics) and the (2) *anticholinergics* (parasympatholytics). The Unit V opener offers a discussion and comparison of the parasympathetic nervous system (parasympathomimetics and parasympatholytics) and the sympathetic nervous system.

Cholinergics

Drugs that stimulate the parasympathetic nervous system are called **cholinergics,** or **parasympathomimetics,** because they mimic the parasympathetic neurotransmitter acetylcholine. Cholinergic drugs are also called *cholinomimetics, cholinergic stimulants,* or *cholinergic agonists.* **Acetylcholine (ACh)** is the neurotransmitter located at the ganglions and the parasympathetic terminal nerve endings. It innervates the receptors in organs, tissues, and glands. The two types of cholinergic receptors are (1) **muscarinic receptors,** which stimulate smooth muscle and slow the heart rate; and (2) **nicotinic receptors** (neuromuscular), which affect the skeletal muscles. Many cholinergic drugs are nonselective because they can affect both the muscarinic and nicotinic receptors. However, there are selective

cholinergic drugs for the muscarinic receptors that do *not* affect the nicotinic receptors. Figure 18–1 illustrates the effects of parasympathetic or cholinergic stimulation.

There are direct-acting cholinergic drugs and indirect-acting cholinergic drugs. *Direct-acting cholinergic drugs* act on the receptors to activate a tissue response (Figure 18–2, *A*). *Indirect-acting cholinergic drugs* inhibit the action of the enzyme **cholinesterase (ChE)** (acetylcholinesterase) by forming a chemical complex, thus permitting acetylcholine to persist and attach to the receptor (Figure 18–2, *B*). Drugs that inhibit cholinesterase are called *cholinesterase inhibitors, acetylcholinesterase (AChE) inhibitors,* or **anticholinesterases.** Cholinesterase may destroy acetylcholine before it reaches the receptor or after it has attached to the site. By inhibiting or destroying the enzyme cholinesterase, more acetylcholine is available to stimulate the receptor and remain in contact with it longer.

Cholinesterase inhibitors (anticholinesterases) can be separated into reversible inhibitors and irreversible inhibitors. The reversible inhibitors bind the enzyme cholinesterase for several minutes to hours, and the irreversible inhibitors bind the enzyme permanently. The resulting effects vary with how long the cholinesterase is bound.

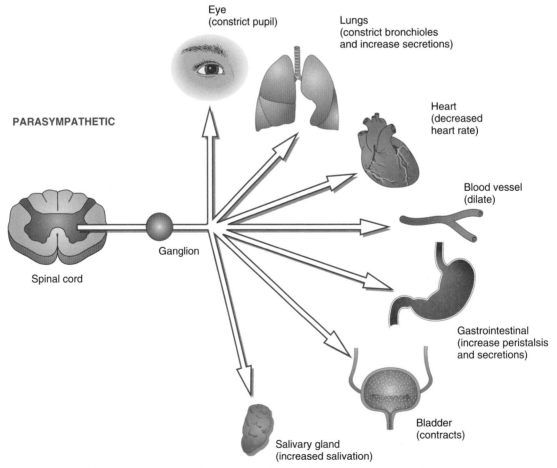

FIGURE 18–1   Parasympathetic responses. Stimulation of the parasympathetic nervous system or use of parasympathomimetic drugs will cause the pupils to constrict, bronchioles to constrict and bronchial secretions to increase, heart rate to decrease, blood vessels to dilate, peristalsis and gastric secretions to increase, the bladder muscle to contract, and salivary glands to increase salivation.

FIGURE 18–2 A, Direct-acting parasympathomimetic (cholinergic drugs). Cholinergic drugs resemble acetylcholine and act directly on the receptor. B, Indirect-acting parasympathomimetic (cholinesterase inhibitors). Cholinesterase inhibitors inactivate the enzyme acetylcholinesterase (cholinesterase) thus permitting acetylcholine to react to the receptor. *ACh,* Acetylcholine; *AChE,* acetylcholinesterase or cholinesterase; *D,* cholinergic drug; *DD,* cholinesterase inhibitor (anticholinesterase).

The major responses of cholinergic drugs are to stimulate bladder and gastrointestinal (GI) tone, constrict the pupils of the eyes **(miosis),** and increase neuromuscular transmission. Other effects of cholinergic drugs include decreased heart rate and blood pressure and increased salivary, GI, and bronchial glandular secretions. Table 18–1 lists the functions of direct- and indirect-acting cholinergic drugs.

Direct-Acting Cholinergics

Many drugs classified as **direct-acting cholinergics** are primarily selective to the muscarinic receptors but are nonspecific because the muscarinic receptors are located in the smooth muscles of the GI and genitourinary tracts, glands, and heart. Bethanechol chloride (Urecholine), a direct-acting cholinergic drug, acts on the muscarinic (cholinergic) receptor and is used primarily to increase urination. Metoclopramide HCl (Reglan) is a direct-acting cholinergic drug that is usually prescribed to treat gastroesophageal reflux disease (GERD). Metoclopramide increases gastric emptying time. Prototype Drug Chart 18–1 details the pharmacologic behavior of bethanechol.

Direct-Acting Cholinergics: Eye

Pilocarpine is a direct-acting cholinergic drug that constricts the pupils of the eyes thus opening the canal of Schlemm to promote drainage of aqueous humor (fluid). This drug is used to treat glaucoma by relieving fluid (intraocular) pressure in the eye. Pilocarpine also acts on the nicotinic receptor, as does carbachol. Both agents are discussed in more detail in Chapter 48.

Pharmacokinetics

Bethanechol chloride (Urecholine) is poorly absorbed from the GI tract. The percentage of protein-binding and the half-life are unknown. The drug is most likely excreted in the urine.

Pharmacodynamics

The principal use of bethanechol is to promote micturition (urination) by stimulating the muscarinic cholinergic receptors to increase urine output. The client voids approximately 30 minutes to 1.5 hours after taking

Table 18–1	
Effects of Cholinergic Drugs	
Body Tissue	**Response**
Cardiovascular*	Decreases heart rate, lowers blood pressure because of vasodilation, and slows conduction of atrioventricular node.
Gastrointestinal†	Increases tone and motility of smooth muscles of stomach and intestine. Peristalsis is increased and sphincter muscles are relaxed.
Genitourinary	Contracts muscles of the urinary bladder, increases tone of ureters, and relaxes bladder's sphincter muscles. Stimulates urination.
Ocular†	Increases pupillary constriction, or miosis (pupil becomes smaller), and increases accommodation (flattening or thickening of eye lens for distant or near vision).
Glandular*	Increases salivation, perspiration, and tears.
Bronchial (lung)*	Stimulates bronchial smooth muscle contraction and increases bronchial secretions.
Striated muscle†	Increases neuromuscular transmission and maintains muscle strength and tone.

*Tissue responses to large doses of cholinergic drugs.
†Major tissue responses to normal doses of cholinergic drugs.

an oral dose of bethanechol because of the increased tone of the detrusor urinae muscle. Bethanechol also increases peristalsis in the GI tract. The drug should be taken on an empty stomach. It should not be administered intramuscularly (IM) or intravenously (IV), but it can be given subcutaneously (subQ). Micturition usually occurs within 15 minutes via the subQ route. The duration of action is 4 to 6 hours for oral administration and 2 hours for the subQ route.

Prototype **DRUG CHART 18–1**

BETHANECHOL CHLORIDE

Drug Class	Dosage
Cholinergic/parasympathomimetic Trade names: Urecholine, ✽Duvoid *Pregnancy Category:* C	**A: PO:** 10-50 mg b.i.d./ t.i.d./q.i.d.; *max:* 120 mg/d **subQ:** 2.5-5 mg, repeat at 15-30 min intervals; PRN Do *NOT* give IM or IV. **C: PO:** 0.5 mg/kg/d in 3-4 divided doses
Contraindications	**Drug-Lab-Food Interactions**

Severe bradycardia or hypotension, chronic
    obstructive pulmonary disease, asthma, peptic
    ulcer, parkinsonism, hyperthyroidism
	Drug: Decrease bethanechol effect with
	    antidysrhythmics
	Lab: Increase AST, bilirubin, amylase, lipase

Pharmacokinetics	**Pharmacodynamics**

Absorption: PO: Poorly absorbed
Distribution: PB: UK
Metabolism: t½: UK
Excretion: In urine
	PO: Onset: 0.5-1.5 h
	    Peak: 1-2 h
	    Duration: 4-6 h
	subQ: Onset: 5-15 min
	    Peak: 0.5 h
	    Duration: 2 h

Therapeutic Effects/Uses

To treat urinary retention, abdominal distention
Mode of Action: Stimulate the cholinergic (muscarinic) receptor; promote contraction of the bladder; increase GI
    peristalsis, GI secretion, pupillary constriction, and bronchoconstriction

Side Effects	Adverse Reactions

Nausea, vomiting, diarrhea, salivation, sweating,
    flushing, frequent urination, rash, miosis,
    blurred vision, abdominal discomfort
	Orthostatic hypotension, bradycardia, muscle weakness
	Life-threatening: Acute asthmatic attack, heart block,
	    circulatory collapse, cardiac arrest

A, Adult; *AST*, aspartate aminotransferase; *b.i.d.*, two times a day; *d*, day; *GI*, gastrointestinal; *h*, hour; *IM*, intramuscular; *IV*, intravenous; *min*, minute; *PB*, protein-binding; *PO*, by mouth; *PRN*, as needed; *q.i.d.*, four times a day; *subQ*, subcutaneous; *t½*, half-
life; *t.i.d.*, three times a day; *UK*, unknown; ✽,Canadian drug name.

Side Effects and Adverse Reactions

Mild to severe side effects of most muscarinic agonists
such as bethanechol include hypotension, bradycardia,
excessive salivation, increased gastric acid secretion, abdominal cramps, diarrhea, bronchoconstriction, and, in
some cases, cardiac dysrhythmias. This group of agents
should be prescribed cautiously for clients with low blood
pressure and heart rates. Muscarinic agonists are contraindicated for clients with intestinal or urinary tract obstruction and for those with active asthma.

Nursing Process

**Cholinergic, Direct Acting:
Bethanechol (Urecholine)**

ASSESSMENT

■ Note baseline vital signs for future comparison.
■ Assess urine output (should be >600 ml/d). Report
decrease in urine output.

■ Obtain history from client of health problems such
as peptic ulcer, urinary obstruction, or asthma. Cholinergics can aggravate symptoms of these conditions.

NURSING DIAGNOSES

■ Impaired urinary elimination related to urinary re-
tention
■ Anxiety related to wheezing
■ Risk for impaired skin integrity related to rash

PLANNING

■ Client will have increased bladder and GI tone after
taking cholinergics.
■ Client will have increased neuromuscular strength.

NURSING INTERVENTIONS

Direct Acting
• Monitor client's vital signs. Heart rate and blood pressure decrease when large doses of cholinergics are

taken. Orthostatic hypotension is a side effect of a cholinergic such as bethanechol.

- Record fluid intake and output. Decreased urinary output should be reported because it may be related to urinary obstruction.
- Give cholinergics 1 hour before or 2 hours after meals. If client complains of gastric pain, the drug may be given with meals.
- Check serum amylase, lipase, aspartate aminotransferase, and bilirubin levels. These laboratory values may increase slightly when taking cholinergics.
- Observe client for side effects such as gastric pain or cramping, diarrhea, increased salivary or bronchial secretions, bradycardia, and orthostatic hypotension.
- Auscultate for bowel sounds. Report decreased or hyperactive bowel sounds.
- Auscultate breath sounds for rales (cracking sounds from fluid congestion in lung tissue) or rhonchi (rough sounds resulting from mucous secretions in lung tissue). Cholinergic drugs can increase bronchial secretions.
- Have IV atropine sulfate (0.6 mg) available as an antidote for cholinergic overdose. Early signs of overdosing include salivation, sweating, abdominal cramps, and flushing.
- Note that diaphoresis (excessive perspiration) may occur; linens should be changed as needed.

Indirect Acting

- Beware of the possibility of cholinergic crisis (overdose); symptoms include muscular weakness and increased salivation.

Client Teaching

Direct Acting

General

- Instruct client to take the cholinergic as prescribed. Compliance with the drug regimen is essential.

Side Effects

- Direct client to report severe side effects such as profound dizziness or a decrease in heart rate below 60 beats/min.
- Teach client to arise from a lying position slowly to avoid dizziness; this is most likely a result of orthostatic hypotension.
- Encourage client to maintain effective oral hygiene if excess salivation occurs.
- Advise client to report any difficulty in breathing as a result of respiratory distress.

Indirect Acting (see drugs for myasthenia gravis)

- Direct client to take the drug on time to avoid respiratory muscle weakness.
- Instruct client to assess changes in muscle strength. Cholinesterase inhibitors (anticholinesterases) increase muscle strength.

Cultural Considerations ❖

- When offering a prescription, instructions, or pamphlets to Asians and Pacific Islanders, use both hands to show respect.
- The extended family structure is important for teaching health strategies and providing support. Recognize the importance of including women in decision making and disseminating health information.

EVALUATION

- Determine the effectiveness of the cholinergic or anticholinesterase drug.
- Evaluate the stability of client's vital signs and note the presence of side effects or adverse reactions.

Indirect-Acting Cholinergics

The **indirect-acting cholinergics** do not act on receptors; instead they inhibit or inactivate the enzyme cholinesterase, permitting acetylcholine to accumulate at the receptor sites (Figure 18–2, *B*). This action gives them the name *cholinesterase (ChE) inhibitors, acetylcholinesterase (AChE) inhibitors,* or *anticholinesterases,* of which there are two types: reversible and irreversible.

The function of the enzyme cholinesterase is to break down into choline and acetic acid. A small amount of cholinesterase can break down a large amount of acetylcholine in a short period. A cholinesterase inhibitor drug binds with cholinesterase, allowing acetylcholine to activate the muscarinic and nicotinic cholinergic receptors. This action permits skeletal muscle stimulation, which increases the force of muscular contraction. Because of this action, cholinesterase inhibitors are useful to increase muscle tone for clients with myasthenia gravis (a neuromuscular disorder). By increasing acetylcholine, additional effects occur such as increase in GI motility, bradycardia, miosis, bronchial constriction, and increased micturition.

The primary use of cholinesterase inhibitors is to treat myasthenia gravis. Other uses are to treat glaucoma, Alzheimer's disease, and muscarinic antagonist poisoning.

Reversible Cholinesterase Inhibitors

Reversible cholinesterase inhibitors are used (1) to produce pupillary constriction in the treatment of glaucoma and (2) to increase muscle strength in clients with myasthenia gravis. Drug effects persist for several hours. Drugs used to increase muscular strength in myasthenia gravis include neostigmine (Prostigmin [short-acting]), pyridostigmine bromide (Mestinon [moderate-acting]), ambenonium chloride (Mytelase [long-acting]), and edrophonium chloride (Tensilon [short-acting for diagnostic purposes]). These drugs are discussed in more detail in Chapter 23. A reversible ophthalmic anticholinesterase drug is physostigmine (Antilirium). Ophthalmic agents are further discussed in Chapter 48.

Side Effects

Caution in taking reversible cholinesterase inhibitors is required for clients who have bradycardia, asthma, peptic ulcers, or hyperthyroidism. Cholinesterase inhibitors are contraindicated for clients with intestinal or urinary obstruction.

Irreversible Cholinesterase Inhibitors

Irreversible cholinesterase inhibitors are potent agents because of their long-lasting effect. The enzyme cholinesterase must be regenerated before the drug effect diminishes, a process that may take days or weeks. These drugs are used to produce pupillary constriction and to manufacture organophosphate insecticides.

With irreversible cholinesterase inhibitors, the bond between the irreversible cholinesterase inhibitor and cholinesterase is considered permanent; however, this bond can be broken with the use of the drug pralidoxime (Protopam). Pralidoxime is an antidote to reverse the irreversible organophosphate. It has its effect at the neuromuscular junction. Table 18–2 lists examples of cholinergic drugs and their standard dosages and common uses.

Anticholinergics

Drugs that inhibit the actions of acetylcholine by occupying the acetylcholine receptors are called **anticholinergics** or **parasympatholytics**. Other names for anticholinergics are **cholinergic blocking agents,** *cholinergic* or *muscarinic antagonists, antiparasympathetic agents, antimuscarinic agents,* and *antispasmodics*. The major body tissues and organs affected by the anticholinergic group of drugs are the heart, respiratory tract, GI tract, urinary bladder, eyes, and exocrine glands. By blocking the parasympathetic nerves, the sympathetic (adrenergic) nervous system dominates. Anticholinergic and adrenergic drugs produce many of the same responses.

Anticholinergic and cholinergic drugs have opposite effects. The major responses to anticholinergics are a decrease in GI motility, a decrease in salivation, dilation of pupils **(mydriasis)**, and an increase in pulse rate. Other effects of anticholinergics include decreased bladder contraction, which can result in urinary retention, and decreased rigidity and tremors related to neuromuscular excitement. An anticholinergic can act as an antidote to the toxicity caused by cholinesterase inhibitors and organophosphate ingestion. The various effects of anticholinergics are described in Table 18–3.

Muscarinic receptors, also called *cholinergic receptors*, are involved in tissue and organ responses to anticholinergics, because anticholinergics inhibit the actions of acetylcholine by occupying these receptor sites. Figure 18–3 illustrates this action of anticholinergic drugs. Anticholinergic drugs may block the effect of direct-acting parasympathomimetics such as bethanechol and pilocarpine and of indirect-acting parasympathomimetics such as physostigmine and neostigmine.

Atropine

Atropine sulfate, first derived from the belladonna plant *(Atropa belladonna)* and purified in 1831, is a classic anticholinergic, or muscarinic antagonist drug. Scopolamine was the second belladonna alkaloid produced. Atropine and scopolamine act on the muscarinic receptor, but they have little effect on the nicotinic receptor. Atropine is useful (1) as a preoperative medication to decrease salivary secretions; (2) as an antispasmodic drug to treat peptic ulcers, because it relaxes the smooth muscles of the GI tract and decreases peristalsis; and (3) as an agent to increase the heart rate when bradycardia is present. Atropine can also be used as an antidote for muscarinic agonist poisoning caused by an overdose of a cholinesterase inhibitor or a muscarinic drug such as bethanechol. However, if a client takes atropine or an atropine-like drug (antihistamine) for a long period, side effects can occur. Prototype Drug Chart 18–2 details the pharmacologic behavior of atropine.

Synthetic anticholinergic drugs are also used as antispasmodics to treat peptic ulcers and intestinal spasticity. One example is propantheline bromide (Pro-Banthine), which has been available for several decades. It decreases gastric secretions and GI spasms. Since the introduction of the histamine (H_2) blockers, anticholinergic agents such as propantheline are not used as frequently to decrease gastric secretions.

Pharmacokinetics

Atropine sulfate is well absorbed orally and parenterally. It crosses the blood-brain barrier and exerts its effect on the central nervous system (CNS). The protein binding is unknown. It crosses the placenta. Atropine has a short half-life, so there is little cumulative effect. Most of the absorbed atropine is excreted in the urine (75% to 95%).

Pharmacodynamics

Atropine sulfate blocks acetylcholine by occupying the muscarinic receptor. It increases the heart rate by blocking vagus stimulation and promotes dilation of the pupils by paralyzing the iris sphincter. The two most frequent uses of atropine are to decrease salivation and respiratory secretions preoperatively and to treat sinus bradycardia by increasing the heart rate. Atropine also is used ophthalmically for mydriasis and cycloplegia before eye refraction and to treat inflammation of the iris (iritis) and uveal tract.

Its onset of action orally is between 0.5 to 1 hour and peaks at 2 to 4 hours. For the IM route, the onset of action is 10 to 30 minutes and peaks at 30 minutes. The duration for oral and IM routes is 4 hours; via the IV route, the onset of action is immediate and peak action is at 5 minutes.

Side Effects and Adverse Reactions

The common side effects of atropine and atropine-like drugs include dry mouth, decreased perspiration, blurred vision, tachycardia, constipation, and urinary retention. Other side effects and adverse reactions are nausea, headache, dry skin, abdominal distention, hypotension or hypertension, impotence, photophobia, and coma.

Table 18–2

Cholinergics

Generic (Brand)	Route and Dosage	Uses and Considerations
Direct-Acting Cholinergics		
bethanechol Cl (Urecholine)	See Prototype Drug Chart 18–1.	
metoclopramide HCl (Reglan, Maxolon)	A: PO: 10-15 mg t.i.d. a.c. C: PO/IM/IV: 0.4-0.8 mg/kg/d in 4 divided doses	For GERD and gastroparesis. Central dopamine receptor antagonist. Increases gastric emptying time. *Pregnancy category:* B; PB: UK; t^1/$_2$: 2.5-6 h
carbachol (Miostat)	Ophthalmic: 0.75%-3%, 1-2 gtt, 3 daily	To reduce IOP, miosis. See Chapter 48.
pilocarpine HCl (Pilocar)	Ophthalmic: 0.5%-4%, 1 gt	To reduce IOP, miosis. See Chapter 48.
Cholinesterase Inhibitor		
tacrine HCl (Cognex)	*Alzheimer's disease:* A: PO: 10 mg, q.i.d., increase dose at 6 wk intervals A: PO: 40-160 mg/d p.c.; *max:* 160 mg/d	To improve memory in mild to moderate Alzheimer's dementia. Drug enhances cholinergic function. *Pregnancy category:* C; PB: 55%; t^1/$_2$: 1.5-3.5 h
donepezil HCl (Aricept); rivastigmine (Exelon)	See Chapter 22, Table 22–8.	
Indirect-Acting Cholinergics or Cholinesterase Inhibitors for the Eye		
demecarium bromide (Humorsol)	0.125%-0.25%, 1 gt q12-48 h	To reduce IOP in glaucoma; long-acting miotic. See Chapter 48.
echothiophate iodide (Phospholine Iodide)	0.03%-0.25%, 1 gt daily or b.i.d.	To reduce IOP; long-acting miotic. See Chapter 48.
isoflurophate (Floropryl)	0.25%, ointment q8-72 h	To treat glaucoma. Apply to the conjunctival sac. See Chapter 48.
Reversible Cholinesterase Inhibitors: Myasthenia Gravis		
ambenonium Cl (Mytelase)	A: PO: 2.5-5.0 mg t.i.d./q.i.d.; dose may be increased; maint: 5-25 mg t.i.d./q.i.d.	To increase muscle strength in myasthenia gravis; long acting. May be used with glucocorticoids. *Pregnancy category:* C; PB: UK; t^1/$_2$: UK
edrophonium Cl (Tensilon)	A: IV: 2 mg; then 8 mg if no response IM: 10 mg; may repeat with 2 mg in 30 min C: 34 kg: IV: 1 mg; repeat in 30-45 sec if no response; *max:* 5 mg C: 34 kg: IV: 2 mg; repeat with 1 mg if no response; *max:* 10 mg	To diagnose myasthenia gravis; very short-acting. *Pregnancy category:* C; PB: UK; t^1/$_2$: 1.2-2 h
neostigmine (Prostigmin); neostigmine methylsulfate (injectable form)	A: PO: Initially 15 mg t.i.d.; maint: 150 mg/d in divided doses; range: 15-375 mg/d IM/IV: 0.5-2.5 mg PRN C: PO: 2 mg/kg/d in 6 divided doses	To increase muscle strength in myasthenia gravis; short acting. Used also to prevent or treat postoperative urinary retention. *Pregnancy category:* C; PB: 15%-25%; t^1/$_2$: 1-1.5 h
physostigmine salicylate (Eserine Salicylate)	0.25%-0.5%, 1 gt daily or q.i.d.	To reduce IOP, miosis; short-acting
pyridostigmine bromide (Mestinon)	A: PO: 60-120 mg t.i.d./q.i.d.; maint: 600 mg/d in 3-4 divided doses; *max:* 1.5 g/d SR: 180-540 mg daily or b.i.d. IM/IV: 2 mg q2-3h C: PO: 7 mg/kg/d in 5-6 divided doses	To increase muscle strength in myasthenia gravis; moderate-acting. Prevents destruction of the neurotransmitter acetylcholine. *Pregnancy category:* C; PB: 10%; t^1/$_2$: 3-4 h
Antidote for Irreversible and Reversible Cholinesterase Inhibitors		
pralidoxime Cl (Protopam)	A: IM: 1-2 g, repeat in 1-2 h, then 10 to 12 h intervals A: IV: 1-2 g in 100 ml of saline solution infused over 15-30 min A: PO: 1-3 g, repeat in 5 h PRN C: IV: 20-40 mg/kg/dose; repeat in 1-2 h; 10- to 12-h intervals PRN	To treat overdose of organophosphate pesticides that cause muscle paralysis and to treat overdose of a cholinesterase inhibitor for myasthenia gravis. *Pregnancy category:* C; PB: UK; t^1/$_2$: 1-2.7 h

A, Adult; *a.c.,* before meals; *b.i.d.,* two times a day; *C,* child; *d,* day; *GERD,* gastroesophageal reflux disease; *GI,* gastrointestinal; *gt,* drop; *gtt,* drops; *h,* hour; *IM,* intramuscular; *IOP,* intraocular pressure; *IV,* intravenous; *maint,* maintenance; *PB,* protein-binding; *p.c.,* after meals; *PO,* by mouth; *PRN,* as needed; *q.i.d.,* four times a day; *sec,* second; *SR,* sustained-release; *t^1/$_2$,* half-life; *t.i.d.,* three times a day; *UK,* unknown; *>,* greater than; *<,* less than.

Table 18–3

Effects of Anticholinergic Drugs

Body Tissues	Responses
Cardiovascular	Increases heart rate with large doses. Small doses can decrease heart rate.
Gastrointestinal (GI)	Relaxes smooth muscle tone of GI tract, decreasing GI motility and peristalsis. Decreases gastric and intestinal secretions.
Urinary tract	Relaxes the bladder detrusor muscle and increases constriction of the internal sphincter. Urinary retention can result.
Ocular	Dilates pupils (mydriasis) and paralyzes ciliary muscle (cycloplegia), causing a decrease in accommodation.
Glandular	Decreases salivation, perspiration, and bronchial secretions.
Bronchial	Dilates the bronchi and decreases bronchial secretions.
Central nervous system	Decreases tremors and rigidity of muscles. Drowsiness, disorientation, and hallucination can result from large doses.

FIGURE 18–3 Anticholinergic response. The anticholinergic drug occupies the receptor sites, blocking acetylcholine. *ACh*, Acetylcholine; *D*, anticholinergic drug.

Anticholinergic Drugs: Atropine

ASSESSMENT

■ Obtain baseline vital signs for future comparison. Tachycardia is a side effect that occurs with large doses of anticholinergics such as atropine sulfate.
■ Assess urine output. Urinary retention may occur.
■ Check client's medical history. Atropine and atropine-like drugs are contraindicated if client has narrow-angle glaucoma, obstructive gastrointestinal (GI) disorder, paralytic ileus, ulcerative colitis, benign prostatic hypertrophy, or myasthenia gravis.
■ Determine a history of the drugs client takes. Phenothiazines and antidepressants increase the effect of anticholinergics.

NURSING DIAGNOSES

■ Impaired urinary elimination related to urinary retention
■ Impaired oral mucous membrane related to decreased oral secretions
■ Risk for injury related to acute confusion

PLANNING

■ Client's secretions will be decreased before surgery.
■ Client will not have side effects that may become a health problem.

NURSING INTERVENTIONS

■ Monitor client's vital signs. Report if tachycardia occurs.
■ Determine fluid intake and output. Encourage client to void before taking the medication. Report decreased urine output. Anticholinergics can cause urinary retention. Maintain adequate fluid intake.
■ Record bowel sounds. Absence of bowel sounds may indicate paralytic ileus resulting from a decrease in GI motility (peristalsis).
■ Check for constipation caused by decrease in GI motility. Encourage client to ingest foods that are high in fiber, to drink adequate amounts of fluids, and to exercise if able.
■ Raise bedside rails for clients who are confused and debilitated. Atropine could cause central nervous system stimulation (excitement, confusion) or drowsiness.
■ Provide mouth care. Atropine decreases oral secretions and can cause dryness.
■ Administer IV atropine undiluted or diluted in 10 ml of sterile water. Rate of administration is 0.6 mg/min.

Client Teaching

General
• Direct client to avoid hot environments and excess physical exertion. Elevations in body temperature can result from diminished sweat gland activity.
• Teach client with glaucoma to avoid atropine-like drugs. Anticholinergics cause mydriasis and increase the intraocular pressure. Clients should be alerted to check labels on over-the-counter drugs to determine whether they are contraindicated for glaucoma.
• Instruct client not to drive a motor vehicle or participate in activities that require alertness. Drowsiness is common.
• Advise client to avoid alcohol, cigarettes, caffeine, and aspirin at bedtime to decrease gastric acidity.

- Tell client with mydriasis following an eye examination to use sunglasses in bright light because of photophobia (intolerance of bright light).

Side Effects

- Advise client of common side effects such as dry mouth, decrease in urination, and constipation that occur as a result of long-term use of anticholinergics.
- Direct client to increase fluid intake to prevent constipation when taking anticholinergics for a prolonged period.
- Instruct client to urinate before taking the anticholinergic. Urinary retention can be a problem. Client should report a marked decrease in urine output.

- Suggest that client use hard candy, ice chips, or chewing gum. Maintain effective oral hygiene if client's mouth is dry. Anticholinergics decrease salivation.
- Encourage client to use eye drops to moisten dry eyes that result from decreased lacrimation (tearing).

Diet

- Suggest that client's diet include foods high in fiber and increased water intake to prevent constipation.

Cultural Considerations ❖

- Obtain an interpreter when necessary; do not rely on family members, who may not fully disclose because of honor and shame.

Prototype DRUG CHART 18–2

ATROPINE

Drug Class

Anticholinergic/parasympatholytic
Trade names: Atropine, Atropisol (Optic), ✽Atropair
Pregnancy Category: C

Dosage

A: PO/IM/IV: 0.4-0.6 mg q4-6h PRN
C: PO/IM/IV: 0.01 mg/kg/dose; *max:* 0.4 mg/dose, q4-6h, PRN

Contraindications

Narrow-angle glaucoma, obstructive GI disorders, paralytic ileus, ulcerative colitis, tachycardia, benign prostatic hypertrophy, myasthenia gravis, myocardial ischemia
Caution: Renal or hepatic disorders, COPD, heart failure

Drug-Lab-Food Interactions

Drug: Increase anticholinergic effect with phenothiazines, antihistamines, tricyclic antidepressants, amantadine, quinidine may *increase* effects of atenolol

Pharmacokinetics

Absorption: PO/IM: Well absorbed
Distribution: PB: UK; crosses the placenta
Metabolism: t½: 2-3 h
Excretion: 75% excreted in urine

Pharmacodynamics

PO: Onset: 0.5-1 h
  Peak: 1-2 h
  Duration: 4h
IM: Onset: 10-30 min
  Peak: 0.5 h
  Duration: 4 h
IV: Onset: Immediate
  Peak: 5 min
  Duration: UK
Instill: Onset: 20-30 min
  Peak: 30-40 min
  Duration: days

Therapeutic Effects/Uses

Preoperative medication to reduce salivation, increase heart rate, dilate pupils
Mode of Action: Inhibition of acetylcholine by occupying the receptors; increase heart rate by blocking vagus stimulation; promote dilation of the pupils by blocking iris sphincter muscle

Side Effects

Dry mouth, nausea, headache, constipation, rash, dry skin, flush, blurred vision, photophobia, urinary retention

Adverse Reactions

Tachycardia, hypotension, pupillary dilation, abdominal distension, palpitations, nasal congestion
Life-threatening: Paralytic ileus, coma

A, Adult; *C,* child; *COPD,* chronic obstructive pulmonary disease; *GI,* gastrointestinal; *h,* hour; *IM,* intramuscular; *instill,* instillation; *IV,* intravenous; *MAOI,* monoamine oxidase inhibitor; *min,* minute; *PB,* protein-binding; *PO,* by mouth; *PRN,* as needed; *t½,* half-life; *UK,* unknown; >, greater than; ✽,Canadian drug name.

- Ask open-ended questions and have clients demonstrate rather than verbalize their understanding of treatments. Because politeness and "saving face" prevail, do not assume that a positive response means a definite yes.

EVALUATION

- ■ Evaluate client's response to the anticholinergic.
- ■ Determine whether constipation, urine retention, or increased pulse rate is or remains a problem.

Antiparkinson–Anticholinergic Drugs

At one time atropine was given to clients with Parkinson's disease to decrease salivation and drooling. It was also found to have some effect on the motor manifestation of this disease by decreasing tremors and rigidity. Additional studies indicate that anticholinergic (antimuscarinic) agents affect the CNS as well as the parasympathetic nervous system. These anticholinergic drugs affect the CNS by suppressing the tremors and muscular rigidity of parkinsonism, but they have little effect on mobility and muscle weakness. As a result of these findings, several anticholinergic drugs were developed (e.g., trihexyphenidyl hydrochloride [Artane], procyclidine [Kemadrin], biperiden [Akineton], and benztropine [Cogentin]), for the treatment of Parkinson's disease. These drugs can be used alone in early stages of parkinsonism. They may be used in combination with levodopa to control parkinsonism or used alone to treat pseudoparkinsonism, which results from the side effects of the phenothiazines in antipsychotic drugs. Drugs used to treat parkinsonism are described in more detail in Chapter 22. Prototype Drug Chart 18–3 lists the drug data related to trihexyphenidyl, which is used for pseudoparkinsonism.

Pharmacokinetics

Trihexyphenidyl is well absorbed from the GI tract. Its protein-binding percentage and half-life are unknown. It is excreted in the urine.

Prototype DRUG CHART 18-3

TRIHEXYPHENIDYL HCL

Drug Class Antiparkinson: anticholinergic agent Trade names: Artane, Trihexane, Trihexy, ✣Aparkane, Apo-Trihex, Novohexidyl *Pregnancy Category:* C	**Dosage** *Parkinsonism:* A: PO: Initially 1-2 mg/d; increase to 6-10 mg/d in 3 divided doses; *max:* 15 mg/dl *Extrapyramidal symptoms (drug induced):* A: PO: 1 mg/d; increase to 5-15 mg/d in divided doses
Contraindications Narrow-angle glaucoma, GI obstruction, urinary retention, severe angina pectoris, myasthenia gravis *Caution:* Tachycardia, benign prostatic hypertrophy, children, elderly, nursing mothers	**Drug-Lab-Food Interactions** **Drug:** *Increase* anticholinergic effect with phenothiazines, antihistamines, tricyclic antidepressants, amantadine, quinidine *Decrease* trihexyphenidyl absorption with antacids
Pharmacokinetics **Absorption:** PO: Well absorbed **Distribution:** PB: UK **Metabolism:** t½: 5-10 h **Excretion:** In urine	**Pharmacodynamics** **PO:** Onset: 1 h Peak: 2-3 h Duration: 6-12 h **SR/PO:** Onset: UK Peak: UK Duration: 12-24 h

Therapeutic Effects/Uses
To decrease involuntary symptoms of parkinsonism or drug-induced parkinsonism by inhibiting acetylcholine
Mode of Action: Blocks cholinergic (muscarinic) receptors to decrease involuntary movements.

Side Effects Nausea, vomiting, dry mouth, constipation, anxiety, restlessness, headache, flushing, dizziness, blurred vision, photophobia, pupil dilation, dysphagia	**Adverse Reactions** Tachycardia, palpitations, urticaria, postural hypotension, urinary retention *Life-threatening:* Paralytic ileus

A, Adult; *d*, day; *GI*, gastrointestinal; *h*, hour; *IV*, intravenous; *PB*, protein-binding; *PO*, by mouth; *SR*, sustained-release; *t½*, half-life; *UK*, unknown; ✣, Canadian drug name.

Pharmacodynamics

Trihexyphenidyl decreases involuntary movement and diminishes the signs and symptoms of tremors and muscle rigidity that occur with Parkinson's disease and pseudoparkinsonism. It is available as a tablet, elixir, and sustained-release capsule. The duration of action of the sustained-release preparation is twice as long as that for the oral and elixir forms. Alcohol, narcotics, amantadine, phenothiazines, and antihistamines may increase the effect of trihexyphenidyl. The side effects are similar to other anticholinergic drugs.

Antihistamines for Treating Motion Sickness

The effects of anticholinergics on the CNS benefit clients prone to motion sickness. An example of such an anticholinergic, classified as an antihistamine for motion sickness, is scopolamine. It is available topically as a skin patch (Transderm Scōp) that is placed behind the ear. Prevention of motion sickness is also provided via wrist bands and ginger gum. Transdermal scopolamine is delivered over 3 days and is frequently prescribed for activities such as flying, cruising on the water, and bus or automobile trips. Other drugs classified as antihistamines for motion sickness are dimenhydrinate (Dramamine), cyclizine (Marezine), and meclizine hydrochloride (Bonine). Most of these drugs can be purchased over-the-counter (OTC), with the exception of Transderm Scōp.

Examples of anticholinergic drugs and their dosages and common uses are found in Table 18–4. Dosages may vary according to age, sex, and weight. Because anticholinergic drugs can increase intraocular pressure, they should not be administered to clients diagnosed with glaucoma.

Table 18–4

Anticholinergics

Generic (Brand)	Route and Dosage	Uses and Considerations
Anticholinergics: Gastrointestinal or Cholinergic Blockers		
atropine sulfate	See Prototype Drug Chart 18–2.	
dicyclomine HCl (Bentyl, Antispas, Di-Spaz)	A: PO: 10-20 mg t.i.d./q.i.d. IM: 20 mg q6h C: >2 y: PO: 10 mg t.i.d./q.i.d.	For IBS. Avoid use in clients with narrow-angle glaucoma, severe ulcerative colitis, paralytic ileus. *Pregnancy category:* B; PB: UK; t$^{1/2}$: 9-10 h
Glycopyrrolate (Robinul)	*GI disorders:* A: PO: 1-2 mg b.i.d./t.i.d. IM/IV: 0.1-0.2 mg t.i.d./q.i.d. *Preoperative:* A: IM: 4.4 mcg/kg 30 min-1 h before surgery	Presurgery to reduce secretions and for peptic ulcer. Contraindicated in clients with narrow-angle glaucoma, obstructive GI tract, ulcerative colitis. *Pregnancy category:* B; PB: UK; t$^{1/2}$: 1-4.5 h
hyoscyamine SO$_4$ (Cystospaz, Anaspaz, Levsin)	A: PO/SL: 0.125-0.25 mg t.i.d./q.i.d. a.c. and at bedtime SR: 0.375-0.75 mg/q12h subQ/IM/IV: 0.25-0.5 mg b.i.d./q.i.d., PRN C: 2-10 y: half adult dose or individualized	Treatment of peptic ulcer and IBS. Controls gastric secretion and spastic bladder. Contraindicated in clients with narrow-angle glaucoma and severe ulcerative colitis. *Pregnancy category:* C; PB: 50%-60%; t$^{1/2}$: 3.5 h
isopropamide iodide (Darbid)	A: PO: 5 mg b.i.d. or q12h; may increase to 10 mg b.i.d.	To treat peptic ulcer and IBS. Not for use in children under 12 y. *Pregnancy category:* C; PB: UK; t$^{1/2}$: UK
methscopolamine bromide (Pamine)	A: PO: 2.5 mg a.c. and 2.5-5.0 mg at bedtime	Treatment of peptic ulcer, IBS. Avoid use in clients with prostatic hypertrophy and intestinal atony. *Pregnancy category:* C; PB: UK; t$^{1/2}$: UK
oxyphencyclimine HCl (Daricon)	A: PO: 5-10 mg b.i.d., t.i.d.	For peptic ulcer, IBS. Not for use in children under 12 y. *Pregnancy category:* C; PB: UK; t$^{1/2}$: UK
propantheline bromide (Pro Banthine)	A: PO: 15 mg a.c. t.i.d.; 30 mg at bedtime; *max:* 120 mg/d Elderly: 7.5 mg a.c. t.i.d.; *max:* 90 mg/d	Antispasmodic for peptic ulcer, IBS. Also used for pancreatitis and urinary bladder spasm. Pregnancy category: C; PB: UK; t$^{1/2}$: 9 h
scopolamine hydrobromide (also hyoscine hydrobromide)	*Preoperative:* A: PO: 0.5-1 mg subQ/IM/IV: 0.3-0.6 mg C: subQ: 0.006 mg/kg or 0.2 mg/m^2; *max:* 0.3 mg *Motion sickness:* A: PO: 0.3-0.6 mg; transderm patch: 1 patch behind ear q72h	For preanesthetic drug, IBS, motion sickness, and delirium. Contraindicated in clients with narrow-angle glaucoma, obstructive GI disease, severe ulcerative colitis, and paralytic ileus. *Pregnancy category:* C; PB: 30%; t$^{1/2}$ 8 h

A, Adult; *a.c.*, before meals; *b.i.d.*, two times a day; *C*, child; *d*, day; *EPR*, extrapyramidal reaction; *GI*, gastrointestinal; *gtt*, drops; *h*, hour; *IBS*, irritable bowel syndrome; *IM*, intramuscular; *inhal*, inhalation; *IV*, intravenous; *maint*, maintenance; *min*, minute; *PB*, protein-binding; *p.c.*, after meals; *PO*, by mouth; *PRN*, as needed; *q.i.d.*, four times a day; *subQ*, subcutaneous; *SL*, sublingual; *sol*, solution; *SR*, sustained-release; *t$^{1/2}$*, half life; *t.i.d.*, three times a day; *UK*, unknown; *>*, greater than; *<*, less than.

Continued

Table 18-4

Anticholinergics—cont'd

Generic (Brand)	Route and Dosage	Uses and Considerations
Cholinergic Antagonists: Eye		
cyclopentolate HCl (Cyclogyl)	0.5%-2%, sol, 1-2 gtt	For mydriasis and cycloplegia for eye examination. See Chapter 48.
homatropine (Isopto Homatropine)	2%-5% sol, 1-2 gtt	For mydriasis and cycloplegia (paralysis of ciliary muscle resulting in loss of accommodation) for eye examination. See Chapter 48.
tropicamide (Mydriacyl Ophthalmic)	0.5%-1% sol, 1-2 gtt	For mydriasis and cycloplegia for eye examination. See Chapter 48.
Anticholinergic–Antiparkinson Drugs		
benztropine mesylate (Cogentin)	*Parkinsonism:* A: PO: IV: Initially 0.5-1.0 mg/d in 1-2 divided doses (larger dose at bedtime); maint: 0.5-6 mg/d in 1-2 divided doses EPR: A: PO: 1-2 mg, b.i.d.	Treatment of parkinsonism and drug-induced extrapyramidal syndrome. See Chapter 22.
biperiden lactate (Akineton)	*Parkinsonism:* A: PO: 2 mg t.i.d./q.i.d. IM/IV: 2 mg q30min for 4 doses Elderly: PO: 2 mg in 1 or 2 divided doses	Same as benztropine mesylate. See Chapter 22.
procyclidine HCl (Kemadrin)	Parkinsonism: A: PO: 2.5-5 mg p.c. t.i.d.; maint: 10-20 mg/d	Same as benztropine mesylate. See Chapter 22.
trihexyphenidyl HCl (Artane, Trihexy)	See Prototype Drug Chart 18-3.	
Anticholinergic–Antimuscarinic Drugs		
tolterodine tartrate (Detrol, Detrol LA)	See Prototype Drug Chart 18-4.	
Others		
ipratropium bromide (Atrovent)	A: Inhal: 2 inhal q.i.d. C: >3 y: Inhal: 1 or 2 inhal t.i.d.	Anticholinergic bronchodilator to treat chronic obstructive pulmonary disease by blocking action of acetylcholine at bronchial smooth muscle sites, promoting bronchodilation. *Pregnancy category:* B; PB: UK; t½: UK. See Chapter 40.

Side Effects and Adverse Reactions

Side effects of antihistamines used as anticholinergics include dry mouth, visual disturbances (especially blurred vision resulting from pupillary dilation), constipation secondary to decreased GI peristalsis, urinary retention related to decreased bladder tone, tachycardia (when taken in large doses), hypotension, skin rash, muscle weakness, and flushing.

Critical Thinking Case Study

JS, age 56, is scheduled for surgery to remove gallstones. He has been in good health, and his only other clinical problem is glaucoma. Preoperative medications, meperidine 75 mg and atropine sulfate 0.4 mg, were given intramuscularly 1 hour before surgery.

1. What are the advantages of giving atropine sulfate before surgery?
2. If JS received an atropine-like drug for several months, what assessments should be made related to its effects?
3. How does atropine sulfate differ from bethanechol chloride?

JS receives ophthalmic pilocarpine drops to control glaucoma.

4. How does pilocarpine differ from physostigmine? Explain.
5. What client teaching should the nurse include related to the use of pilocarpine?

Prototype DRUG CHART 18–4

TOLTERODINE TARTRATE

Drug Class

Antimuscarinic agent: Anticholinergic
Trade names: Detrol, Detrol LA
Pregnancy Category: C

Dosage

A: PO: 2 mg b.i.d. or 4 mg SR daily

Contraindications

Hypersensitivity, urinary retention, gastric
retention, uncontrolled narrow-angle glaucoma
Caution: Controlled narrow-angle glaucoma,
cardiovascular disease, urinary bladder outflow
obstruction, pyloric stenosis or other GI obstructive
disorders, paralytic ileus, ulcerative colitis, renal or
hepatic dysfunction, lactation

Drug-Lab-Food Interactions

Drug: *Increased* effects with amantadine, amoxapine,
bupropion, clozapine, cyclobenzaprine, disopyramide,
maprotiline, olanzapine, orphenadrine, H_1 blockers,
phenothiazines, and tricyclic antidepressants;
decreased effects with azole antifungals (e.g., ketoconazole) or macrolide antibiotics (e.g., erythromycin), cyclosporine, and fluoxetine

Pharmacokinetics

Absorption: GI absorption decreased with food
Distribution: PB: 96%
Metabolism: t½: 2-4 h
Excretion: urine and feces

Pharmacodynamics

PO: Onset: UK
     Peak: 1-2 h
     Duration: UK

Therapeutic Effects/Uses

To decrease urinary frequency, urgency, and incontinence.
Mode of Action: Blocks cholinergic (muscarinic) receptors selectively in urinary bladder

Side Effects

Dry mouth and eyes, headache, dizziness, fainting,
nervousness, nausea, vomiting, diarrhea, abdominal
pain, dyspepsia, flatulence, dysuria, weight gain,
arthralgia, urinary retention, UTI, URI, rash, pruritus,
dry skin

Adverse Reactions

Bronchitis, visual abnormalities, chest pain,
hypertension

A, Adult; *b.i.d.,* two times a day; *GI,* gastrointestinal; *H1,* histamine 1; *h,* hour; *PB,* protein-binding; *PO,* by mouth; *SR,* sustained-
release; *t½,* half-life; *UK,* unknown; *URI,* upper respiratory tract infection; *UTI,* urinary tract infection.

NCLEX Study Questions

1. A client is receiving bethanechol (Urecholine). The
   nurse realizes that the action of this drug is to treat:
   a. glaucoma
   b. urinary retention
   c. delayed gastric emptying
   d. gastroesophageal reflux disease

2. The nurse teaches the client receiving atropine to expect
   which of the following side effects?
   a. diarrhea
   b. bradycardia
   c. blurred vision
   d. frequent urination

3. When benztropine (Cogentin) is ordered for a client,
   the nurse acknowledges that this drug is an effective
   treatment for:
   a. paralytic ileus
   b. motion sickness
   c. urinary retention
   d. Parkinson's disease

4. Isopropamide (Darbid) is an anticholinergic, which the
   nurse realizes is given to treat:
   a. mydriasis
   b. constipation
   c. urinary retention
   d. irritable bowel syndrome

5. The nurse realizes that cholinergic drugs mimic the
   parasympathetic neurotransmitter:
   a. dopamine
   b. acetylcholine
   c. cholinesterase
   d. monoamine oxidase

SIX

Neurologic and Neuromuscular Agents

The nervous system is composed of all nerve tissues: brain, spinal cord, nerves, and ganglia. The purpose of the nervous system is to receive stimuli and transmit information to nerve centers for an appropriate response. There are two types of nervous systems: the central nervous system and the peripheral nervous system.

The *central nervous system (CNS)*, composed of the brain and spinal cord, regulates body functions (Figure VI–1). The CNS interprets information sent by impulses from the *peripheral nervous system (PNS)* and returns the instruction through the PNS for appropriate cellular actions. Stimulation of the CNS may either increase nerve cell (*neuron*) activity or block nerve cell activity.

The PNS consists of two divisions: the *somatic nervous system (SNS)* and the *autonomic nervous system (ANS)*. The SNS is voluntary and acts on skeletal muscles to produce locomotion and respiration. The ANS, also called the *visceral system*, is involuntary and controls and regulates the functioning of the heart, respiratory system, gastrointestinal system, and glands. The ANS, a large nervous system that functions without our conscious control, has two subdivisions: the sympathetic and the parasympathetic nervous systems.

The sympathetic nervous system of the ANS is called the *adrenergic system*, because its neurotransmitter is norepinephrine. The parasympathetic nervous system is called the *cholinergic system*, because its neurotransmitter is acetylcholine. Because organs are innervated by both the sympathetic and the parasympathetic systems, they can produce opposite responses. The sympathetic response is excitability, and the parasympathetic response is inhibition.

The sympathetic and the parasympathetic nerve pathways originate from different locations in the spinal cord. These nervous systems send information by two types of nerve fibers, the preganglionic and the postganglionic, and by the ganglion between these fibers (Figure VI–2). The preganglionic nerve fiber carries messages from the CNS to the ganglion, and the postganglionic fiber transmits impulses from the ganglion to body tissues and organs.

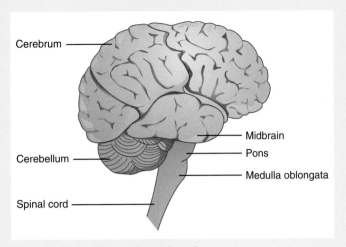

FIGURE VI–I   Brain and spinal cord.

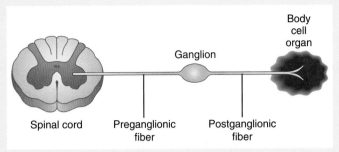

FIGURE VI–2   Preganglionic and postganglionic nerve fibers.

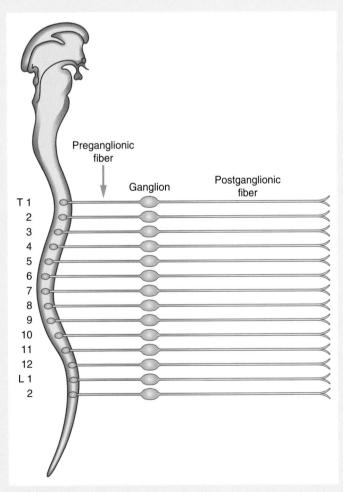

FIGURE VI–3   Sympathetic nerve fibers.

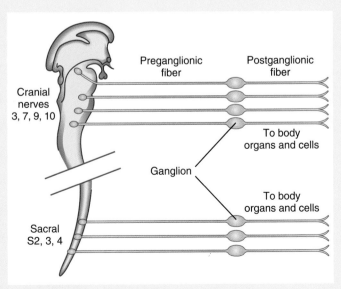

FIGURE VI–4   Parasympathetic nerve fibers.

The sympathetic nervous system is also called the *thoracolumbar division* of the ANS, because the preganglionic fibers originate from the thoracic (T1 to T12) and the upper lumbar (L1 and L2) segments of the spinal cord. The sympathetic preganglionic fibers are short from the spinal cord to the ganglion, and the sympathetic postganglionic fibers are long from the ganglion to the body cells. Figure VI–3 illustrates the sympathetic preganglionic fibers from the spinal cord.

The parasympathetic nervous system is called the *craniosacral division* of the ANS, because the preganglionic fibers originate with the cranial nerves III, VII, IX, and X from the brainstem and the sacral segments (S2, S3, and S4) of the spinal cord. The parasympathetic preganglionic fibers are long from the spinal cord to the ganglion, and the parasympathetic postganglionic fibers are short from the ganglion to the body cells. Figure VI–4 illustrates the parasympathetic preganglionic fibers from the spinal cord.

Drugs that stimulate and depress the CNS are discussed in Chapters 19, Central Nervous System Stimulants; 20, Central Nervous System Depressants; and 25, Drugs for Pain Management: Nonopioid and Opioid Analgesics. Amphetamines, amphetamine-like drugs, anorexiants, an-aleptics, and xanthines (caffeine) stimulate the CNS. Some of these drugs are used therapeutically for attention deficit/hyperactivity disorder (ADHD) and narcolepsy. The groups of drugs that depress the CNS are sedative-hypnotics, anesthetics, narcotics, and nonnarcotic agents. Drugs used to control convulsions (Chapter 21, Anticonvulsants) are considered CNS depressants. The drug groups used to control psychiatric and depressive disorders (Chapters 26, Antipsychotics and Anxiolytics, and 27, Antidepressants and Mood Stabilizers) also affect CNS response. Drugs that affect the sympathetic and the parasympathetic nervous systems are discussed in Chapters 17, Adrenergics and Adrenergic Blockers, and 18, Cholinergics and Anticholinergics. The drugs used to treat neuromuscular disorders, such as parkinsonism, myasthenia gravis, multiple sclerosis, and Alzheimer's disease, have varying effects on the nervous system and muscles (Chapters 22, Drugs for Neurologic Disorders: Parkinsonism and Alzheimer's Disease, and 23, Drugs for Neuromuscular Disorders: Myasthenia Gravis, Multiple Sclerosis, and Muscle Spasms).

Figure VI–5 is a schematic breakdown of the nervous systems in the body.

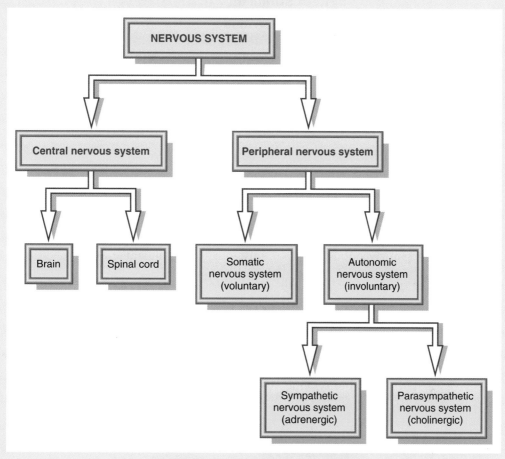

FIGURE VI–5 The body's nervous system.

19

Central Nervous System Stimulants

ELECTRONIC RESOURCES

Evolve website (http://evolve.elsevier.com/KeeHayes/pharmacology/):
- *Case Studies*
- *Content Updates*
- *Frequently Asked Questions*
- *Student Review Activities*
- *WebLinks*
- *Additional Reference Material*

Companion CD-ROM:
- *NCLEX Examination Review Questions*
- *Pharmacology Animations*
- *IV Therapy Checklists*
- *Medication Error Checklists*
- *Drug Calculation Problems*
- *Electronic Calculators*
- *Top 200 Drugs with Pronunciations*
- *References from the Textbook*

Outline

Objectives

- Explain the effects of stimulants on the central nervous system (CNS).
- Discuss attention deficit/hyperactivity disorder and narcolepsy.
- Explain the action of drugs used for attention deficit/hyperactivity disorder and narcolepsy.
- Contrast the common side effects of amphetamines, anorexiants, analeptics, doxapram, and caffeine.
- Discuss the drugs used in the treatment of migraine headaches.
- Describe at least four nursing interventions when administering CNS stimulants.
- Apply the nursing process for the client taking doxapram (Dopram).

Terms

Numerous drugs can stimulate the **central nervous system (CNS),** which involves the brain and spinal cord that regulates body functions. Medically approved use of these drugs is limited to the treatment of attention deficit/hyperactivity disorder (ADHD) in children, narcolepsy, obesity, and the reversal of respiratory distress. The major group of CNS stimulants includes amphetamines and caffeine, which stimulate the cerebral cortex of the brain; analeptics and caffeine, which act on the brainstem and medulla to stimulate respiration; and anorexiants, which act to some degree on the cerebral cortex and on the hypothalamus to suppress appetite. Amphetamines and related anorexiants are greatly abused. Long-term use of amphetamines can produce psychologic **dependence** or **tolerance,** a condition in which larger and larger doses of a drug are needed to reproduce the initial response. Gradually increasing a drug dose and then abruptly stopping the drug may result in depression and withdrawal symptoms.

Drugs used to treat migraine and cluster headaches include analgesics, ergot alkaloids, and selective serotonin₁ receptor agonists (triptans). The frequently prescribed triptan group causes vasoconstriction of blood vessels in the cortex.

Pathophysiology

Attention deficit/hyperactivity disorder (ADHD), formerly called *attention deficit disorder (ADD),* might be caused by a dysregulation of the transmitters serotonin, norepinephrine, and dopamine. ADHD occurs primarily in children, usually before the age of 7, and may continue through the teenage years. In some cases it may not be identified until early adulthood. The incidence of ADHD is three to seven times more common in boys than in girls. Characteristic behaviors include inattentiveness, inability to concentrate, restlessness (fidgety), hyperactivity (excessive and purposeless activity), inability to complete tasks, and impulsivity.

The child with ADHD may display poor coordination, and there may be abnormal electroencephalographic (EEG) findings. Intelligence is usually not affected. This disorder has also been called *minimal brain dysfunction, hyperactivity* in children, **hyperkinesis,** and *hyperkinetic syndrome with learning disorder.* Some professionals state that ADHD is often incorrectly diagnosed, resulting in many children receiving unnecessary treatment for months or years.

Narcolepsy is characterized by falling asleep during normal waking activities such as driving a car or talking with someone. Sleep paralysis, the condition of muscle paralysis that is normal during sleep, usually accompanies narcolepsy and affects the voluntary muscles. The narcoleptic is unable to move and may collapse.

Amphetamines

Amphetamines stimulate the release of **neurotransmitters**—norepinephrine and dopamine—from the brain and sympathetic nervous system (peripheral nerve terminals).

Amphetamines ordinarily cause euphoria and alertness, but they can also cause sleeplessness, restlessness, tremors, and irritability. Cardiovascular problems such as increased heart rate, palpitations, cardiac dysrhythmias, and increased blood pressure can result from continuous use of amphetamines.

The half-life of amphetamines varies from 4 to 30 hours. Acidic urine excretes amphetamines faster than alkaline urine. When CNS toxicity or cardiac toxicity is suspected, decreasing the urine pH (acidity) aids in the excretion of the drug. Acidic urine decreases the half-life of amphetamines. Amphetamines are prescribed for narcolepsy and in some cases for ADHD, when amphetamine-like drugs are ineffective. Amphetamine (Adderall) has been effective for controlling ADHD. Dextroamphetamine (Dexedrine) and methamphetamine (Desoxyn) may also be prescribed for some ADHD clients.

Side Effects and Adverse Reactions

Amphetamines can cause adverse effects in the central nervous system and the cardiovascular, gastrointestinal (GI), and endocrine systems. The side effects and adverse reactions include restlessness, insomnia, tachycardia, hypertension, heart palpitations, dry mouth, anorexia, weight loss, diarrhea, constipation, and impotence.

Amphetamine-Like Drugs for ADHD and Narcolepsy

Methylphenidate (Ritalin) and dexmethylphenidate (Focalin), classed as amphetamine-like drugs, are given to increase a child's attention span and cognitive performance (e.g., memory, reading) and to decrease impulsiveness, hyperactivity, and restlessness. Methylphenidate is also used to treat narcolepsy. There may be potential abuse of methylphenidate; thus it is classified as a controlled-substance schedule (CSS) II drug. Prototype Drug Chart 19–1 illustrates the pharmacokinetics, pharmacodynamics, and therapeutic effects of methylphenidate in the treatment of ADHD and narcolepsy. Amphetamine and amphetamine-like drugs should not be taken in the evening or before bedtime, because insomnia may result.

Modafinil (Provigil) is another drug prescribed for narcolepsy. It increases the amount of time clients with narcolepsy feel awake. Its mechanism of action is not fully known.

Methylphenidate is the most frequently prescribed drug to treat ADHD. Table 19–1 lists the amphetamines and amphetamine-like drugs and their dosages, uses, and considerations.

Pharmacokinetics

Methylphenidate is well absorbed from the GI mucosa. Methylphenidate is usually administered to children twice a day before breakfast and lunch. Because food affects its absorption rate, this drug should be given 30 to 45 minutes before meals. Methylphenidate should be given 6 hours or less before sleep, because it may cause insomnia. Transder-

Prototype DRUG CHART 19–1

METHYLPHENIDATE

Drug Class

Amphetamine-like drug (CNS stimulant)
Trade names: Ritalin, Ritalin SR, Metadate CD, Concerta SR, Daytrana transdermal patch
CSS II
Pregnancy Category: C

Dosage

Attention deficit/hyperactivity disorder (ADHD):
C>6 y: PO: 5 mg before breakfast and lunch; if necessary increase dosage weekly by 5-10 mg; *max:* 60 mg/d
SR: Not recommended for initial treatment
Narcolepsy:
A: PO: 10 mg, 2-3 times/day 30 min before meals

Contraindications

Hypersensitivity, hyperthyroidism, anxiety, history of seizures, motor tics, Tourette syndrome, glaucoma
Caution: Not to be used for children <6 y
Hypertension, depression, alcoholism, pregnancy

Drug-Lab-Food Interactions

Drug: May decrease effects of decongestants, antihypertensives, barbiturates; may alter effects of insulin therapy
Increases hypertensive crisis with MAOIs; *increases* effects of oral anticoagulants, anticonvulsants, tricyclic antidepressants
Food: Caffeine (coffee, tea, colas, chocolate) may *increase* effects

Pharmacokinetics

Absorption: Well absorbed from GI tract
Distribution: *PB: UK*
Metabolism: t½: 1-3 h
Excretion: 40% excreted unchanged in urine

Pharmacodynamics

PO: Onset: 0.5-1 h
Peak: 1-3 h
Duration: 4-6 h
SR: 4-8 h

Therapeutic Effects/Uses

To correct hyperactivity caused by ADHD, increase attention span, treat fatigue, and control narcolepsy
Mode of action: Acts primarily on the reticular activating system and cerebral cortex.

Side Effects

Anorexia, vomiting, diarrhea, insomnia, dizziness, nervousness, restlessness, irritability, tremors hypervitaminosis A, bulging fontanelles in infants

Adverse Reactions

Tachycardia, hypertension, growth suppression
Palpitations, transient loss of weight in children, increased hyperactivity
Life-threatening: Exfoliative dermatitis, uremia, thrombocytopenia

A, Adult; *ADHD,* attention deficit/hyperactivity disorder; *C,* child; *CD,* controlled dose; *CNS,* central nervous system; *CSS,* Controlled Substances Schedule; *d,* day; *GI,* gastrointestinal; *h,* hour; *MAOI,* monoamine oxidase inhibitor; *min,* minute; *PB,* protein-binding; *PO,* by mouth; *SR,* sustained release; *t½,* half life; *UK,* unknown; *y,* year.

---

mal patches may be worn for 9 hours. This drug is excreted in the urine; 40% of methylphenidate is excreted unchanged.

Pharmacodynamics

Methylphenidate helps to correct ADHD by decreasing hyperactivity and improving attention span. This drug may also be prescribed for treating narcolepsy. Amphetamine-like drugs are considered more effective in treating ADHD than amphetamines, except for Adderall. Amphetamines are generally avoided because they have a higher potential for abuse, habituation, and tolerance. Sympathomimetic drugs such as decongestants enhance the actions of methylphenidate. Antihypertensives and barbiturates can decrease the action of these drugs. Foods that contain caffeine should be avoided, because they increase drug action.

Nursing Process

Central Nervous System Stimulant: Methylphenidate HCl (Ritalin)

ASSESSMENT

■ Determine whether there is a history of heart disease, hypertension, hyperthyroidism, parkinsonism, or glaucoma; in such cases, drug is usually contraindicated.
■ Record vital signs to be used for future comparisons. Pay close attention to clients with cardiac disease, because drug may reverse effects of antihypertensives.

- Ascertain client's mental status (e.g., mood, affect, aggressiveness).
- Evaluate height, growth, weight of children.
- Assess complete blood count (CBC), differential white blood cells (WBCs), and platelets before and during therapy.

NURSING DIAGNOSES

- Disorganized behavior (e.g., impulsiveness, short attention span, distractibility) that interferes with peer relationships, learning, and discipline
- Interrupted family processes related to dysfunctional behavior
- Risk for delayed development related to treatment regimen

PLANNING

- Client will be free of hyperactivity.

- Client will increase attention span.
- Client's blood pressure and heart rate will be within normal limits.
- Client will behave in a calm manner.

NURSING INTERVENTIONS

- Monitor vital signs. Report irregularities.
- Record height, weight, and growth of children.
- Observe client for withdrawal symptoms (e.g., nausea, vomiting, weakness, headache).
- Monitor client for side effects (e.g., insomnia, restlessness, nervousness, tremors, irritability, tachycardia, elevated blood pressure). Report findings.

Client Teaching

General
- Instruct client to take drug before meals.
- Direct client to avoid alcohol consumption.

Table 19-1

Amphetamines and Amphetamine-Like Drugs

Generic (Brand Name)	Route and Dosage	Uses and Considerations
Amphetamines		
Amphetamine sulfate (Adderall) CSS II	Narcolepsy: A: PO: 5-20 mg, daily-t.i.d.; *max*: 60 mg/d C: >6-12 y: PO: 5 mg/d ADHD: C: 3-5 y: PO: 2.5 mg/d C: 6-12 y: PO: 5 mg/d, *max*: 40 mg/d	For narcolepsy, ADHD. Dosage should be minimal to control symptoms in ADHD. CNS and cardiac toxicity could occur. *Pregnancy category*: C; PB: UK; t½: 10-30 h
Dextroamphetamine sulfate (Dexedrine) CSS II	ADHD: C: 3-5 y: PO: 2.5 mg/d C: 6-12 y: PO: 5 mg/d, *max*: 40 mg/d	Uses similar to those of amphetamines. Drug has been used for obesity and narcolepsy. *Pregnancy category*: C; PB: UK; t½: UK
Methamphetamine HCl (Desoxyn) CSS II	C: PO: 2.5-5 mg daily; increase to 20 mg as needed in two divided doses	For ADHD. Could cause CNS and cardiac toxicity. *Pregnancy category*: C; PB: UK; t½: UK
Lisdexamfetamine dimesylate (Vyvanse) CSS II	ADHD: C: 6-12 y: PO: 30 mg/d in morning, may increase 20 mg/d weekly, *max*: 70 mg/d	For ADHD. *Pregnancy category*: C; PB: UK; t½: < 1 h
Amphetamine-Like Drugs		
Methylphenidate HCl (Ritalin) CSS II	See Prototype Drug Chart 19–1.	
Modafinil (Provigil) CSS IV	A: PO: 200 mg/d. With hepatic dysfunction: 100 mg/d Elderly: Reduce dose	For narcolepsy. It does not disrupt nighttime sleep. Common side effects include headaches, nausea, diarrhea, and nervousness. *Pregnancy category*: C; PB: UK; t½: 15 h.
Dexmethylphenidate (Focalin)	A & C: PO: >6 y 2.5 mg twice daily; may increase 2.5 mg/d at weekly intervals; *max*: 20 mg/d	For ADHD. *Pregnancy category*: C; PB: UK; t½: 2.2 h
Atomoxetine (Strattera)	A: PO: 40 mg/d; may increase after 3 d; max: 100 mg/d; C: PO: 0.5 mg/kg/d; may increase after 3 d; *max*: 1.4 mg/kg/d or 100 mg, whichever is less	For ADHD. *Pregnancy category*: C; PB: 98%; t½: 2.2 h
Armodafinil (Nuvigil)	A & C: PO: >16 y 150-250 mg qd in morning	For narcolepsy. *Pregnancy category*: C; PB: 60%; t½: 15 h.

A, Adult; *ADHD*, attention deficit/hyperactivity disorder; *C*, child; *CNS*, central nervous system; *CSS*, controlled substance schedule; *d*, day; *h*, hour; *PB*, protein binding; *PO*, by mouth; *t½*, half life; *UK*, unknown; *y*, year; *>*, greater than.

- Encourage use of sugarless gum to relieve dry mouth.
- Teach client to monitor weight twice a week and report weight loss.
- Advise client to avoid driving and using hazardous equipment when experiencing tremors, nervousness, or increased heart rate.
- Instruct client not to abruptly discontinue the drug; dose must be tapered off to avoid withdrawal symptoms. Consult health care provider before modifying dose.
- Encourage client to read labels on OTC products, because many contain caffeine. A high plasma caffeine level could be fatal.
- Teach nursing mothers to avoid taking all CNS stimulants. These drugs are excreted in breast milk and can cause hyperactivity or restlessness in infants.
- Direct family to seek counseling for children with attention deficit/hyperactivity disorder. Drug therapy alone is not an appropriate therapy program. Notify school nurse of drug therapy regimen.
- Explain to client or family that long-term use may lead to drug abuse.

Diet
- Advise client to avoid foods that contain caffeine.
- Instruct parents to provide children with a nutritional breakfast; drug may have anorexic effects.

Side Effects
- Teach client about drug side effects and the need to report tachycardia and palpitations. Monitor children for onset of Tourette syndrome.

Cultural Considerations ❖
- Decrease language barriers by decoding the jargon of the health care environment for those with language difficulties and for those who are not in the health care field.

EVALUATION

- Evaluate effectiveness of drug therapy, level of hyperactivity, and presence of adverse effects.
- Monitor weight, sleep patterns, and mental status.

Anorexiants

Obesity has been treated with prescribed amphetamines or over-the-counter (OTC) amphetamine-like drugs for decades. Amphetamines were once freely prescribed as **anorexiants** (appetite suppressants) for short-term use (4 to 12 weeks), but because of tolerance, psychologic dependence, and abuse, they are not currently recommended for use as appetite suppressants. The Food and Drug Administration (FDA) has ordered the removal of phenylpropanolamine from OTC weight loss drugs and cold remedies. A study has shown an increased risk of hemorrhagic stroke in young women who take drugs containing phenylpropanolamine and a 16 times greater risk in women who take the

drugs as appetite suppressants. However, this drug was not associated with an increased risk of stroke in men. It has been suggested that phenylpropanolamine might also cause renal failure, psychosis, hypertension, and cardiac dysrhythmias. Topical use of the drug has not been associated with systemic effects. Most of the anorexiants used to suppress appetite (Table 19–2) do not have the serious side effects associated with amphetamines. To lose weight, emphasis should be placed on proper diet, exercise, and behavioral modifications. Reliance on appetite suppressants should be discouraged. Individuals who take anorexiants should be under the care of a health care provider.

Side Effects and Adverse Reactions

Children younger than 12 years should not be given anorexiants, and self-medication with anorexiants should be discouraged. Long-term use of these drugs frequently results in such severe side effects as nervousness, restlessness, irritability, insomnia, heart palpitations, and hypertension.

Analeptics

Analeptics, which are CNS stimulants, mostly affect the brainstem and spinal cord but also affect the cerebral cortex. The primary use of an analeptic is to stimulate respiration. One subgroup of analeptics is the xanthines (methylxanthines), of which caffeine and theophylline are the main drugs. Depending on the dose, caffeine stimulates the CNS, and large doses stimulate respiration. The concentration of caffeine in various beverages is listed on the *Evolve* website (*www.evolve.elsevier.com*). Newborns with respiratory distress might be given caffeine to increase respiration. Theophylline is used mostly to relax the bronchioles; however, it has also been used to increase respiration in newborns. See Chapter 40 for further explanation of theophylline. Table 19–2 lists the analeptics and their dosages, uses, and considerations.

Side Effects and Adverse Reactions

Side effects from caffeine are similar to those from anorexiants: nervousness, restlessness, tremors, twitching, palpitations, and insomnia. Other side effects include diuresis (increased urination), GI irritation (e.g., nausea, diarrhea), and, rarely, tinnitus (ringing in the ear). More than 500 mg of caffeine affects the CNS and heart. High doses of caffeine in coffee, chocolate, and cold-relief medications can cause psychologic dependence. The half-life of caffeine is 3.5 hours; however, in clients with liver disease and who are pregnant, metabolism is slowed and the half-life prolonged. Caffeine is contraindicated during pregnancy, because its effect on the fetus is unknown.

Respiratory Central Nervous System Stimulant

Doxapram (Dopram), a CNS and respiratory stimulant, is used to treat respiratory depression caused by drug overdose, pre- and postanesthetic respiratory depression,

Table 19–2

Anorexiants and Analeptics

Drug	Route and Dosage	Uses and Considerations
Anorexiants		
benzphetamine HCl (Didrex) CSS III	A: PO: 25-50 mg daily-t.i.d.	Similar to amphetamines. Potential for abuse. Avoid taking drug during pregnancy. *Pregnancy category:* X; PB: UK, $t^{1/2}$: 6-12 h
dextroamphetamine sulfate (Dexedrine) CSS II	A: PO: 5-10 mg 1 to 3 × 3 d 30-60 min a.c.	To treat obesity. Can cause restlessness and insomnia. For short-term use. *Pregnancy category:* C; PB: UK; $t^{1/2}$: 30-35 h
diethylpropion HCl (Dospan, Tenuate, Tepanil, ♣Nobesine) CSS IV	A: PO: 25 mg t.i.d.; SR: 75 mg daily	For appetite suppression by stimulating the appetite control center in the hypothalamus. Take 1 h before meals. For short-term use. *Pregnancy category:* B; PB: UK; $t^{1/2}$: 2-3 h
sibutramine (Meridia) CSS IV	A: PO: 10 mg qd; may increase to 15 mg if < 4 lb weight loss in 4 weeks	For long-term appetite suppression to promote weight loss in clients with a BMI of 30 or greater. Should be taken in the morning. *Pregnancy category:* C; PB: UK; $t^{1/2}$: 14-16 h
mazindol (Mazanor, Sanorex) CSS IV	A: PO: 1 mg t.i.d. a.c. or 2 mg qd 60 min before lunch	To treat obesity. May give with meals to avoid GI discomfort. *Pregnancy category:* C; PB: UK; $t^{1/2}$: 2.5-9 h
phentermine HCl (Fastin, Ionamin, Zantryl, Adipex-P, Obe-Nix 30) CSS IV	A: PO: 8 mg 3 × daily or 15-37.5 mg daily	For appetite suppression *Pregnancy category:* C; PB: UK; $t^{1/2}$: 19-24 h
Without phenylpropanolamine HCl: Acutrim, Control, Dexatrim, Dexatrim Natural, Prolamine	A: PO: 1 tablet in morning	To control weight gain. FDA has ordered removal of drugs containing phenylpropanolamine HCl because it may cause stroke, hypertension, or cardiac dysrhythmias.
Orlistat (Xenical)	A: PO: greater than 16 years, 60-120 mg t.i.d. with each main meal containing fat	For long-term weight loss and weight maintenance by reducing fat absorption in GI tract. Pregnancy category: B; PB: UK; $t^{1/2}$: 1-2 h
Analeptics *Methylxanthines*		
caffeine	*Neonatal apnea:* Infant and C: PO IM IV: 5 10 mg/kg on day 1; then 2.5-5 mg/d *Therapeutic range:* 5 20 mg/ml	Used for newborns with apnea to stimulate respiration; increases heart rate and blood pressure. Given through an NGT, IM, or IV. *Pregnancy category:* C; PB: 25% 35%; $t^{1/2}$: A: 3-5 h, neonate: 40-144 h
OTC drugs (NōDōz, Tirend), coffee	A: 100-200 mg q3-4h as needed	Restores mental alertness. Contains citrated caffeine. Brewed coffee contains 60-180 mg of caffeine per cup.
theophylline	Infants: NGT: 5 mg/kg on day 1; then 2 mg in divided doses	Used for newborns with apnea to stimulate respiration. Given through an NGT.
Respiratory Stimulants		
doxapram HCl (Dopram)	A: IV: 0.5-1 mg/kg; infusion: 1-2 mg/ min; *max:* 3 g/d *Neonatal apnea:* Initially: 0.5 mg/kg/h; maint: 0.5-2.5 mg/kg/h titrated to lowest effective rate	Used for respiratory depression. It can increase blood pressure. *Pregnancy category:* B; PB: UK; $t^{1/2}$: A: 2.5-4 h, neonate: 7-10 h

A, Adult; *a.c.*, before meals; *C*, child; *CSS*, Controlled Substances Schedule; *d*, day; *FDA*, Food and Drug Administration; *h*, hour; *IM*, intramuscular; *IV*, intravenous; *MAOI*, monoamine oxidase inhibitor; *max*, maximum; *min*, minute; *NGT*, nasogastric tube; *OTC*, over the counter; *PB*, protein binding; *PO*, by mouth; *subQ*, subcutaneous; *SR*, sustained release; $t^{1/2}$, half life; *t.i.d.*, three times a day; *UK*, unknown; ♣ Canadian drug name.

and chronic obstructive pulmonary disease (COPD). It should be used with caution for the treatment of neonatal apnea. It is administered intravenously, and its onset of action is within 20 to 40 seconds with a peak action within 2 minutes. Side effects are infrequent; however, with an overdose, hypertension, tachycardia, trembling, and convulsions may occur. Mechanical ventilation is more effective than doxapram for treating clients who experience respiratory distress as a result of using certain drugs.

Headaches: Migraine and Cluster

Migraine headaches are characterized by a unilateral throbbing head pain accompanied by nausea, vomiting, and photophobia. These symptoms frequently persist for 4 to 24 hours and for several days in some cases. Two thirds of migraine headaches are experienced by women in their 20s and 30s. Symptoms usually decrease or are absent during pregnancy and menopause. The intensity of migraine pain can disrupt daily activities.

Pathophysiology

Migraine headaches are caused by inflammation and dilation of the blood vessels in the cranium. The etiology is unknown, but some theories suggest an imbalance in the neurotransmitter serotonin (5-hydroxytryptamine [5-HT]) that causes vasoconstriction and suppresses migraine headaches. The tendency of calcitonin gene-related peptide (CGRP) is to promote a migraine attack. Serum CGRP levels are elevated during a migraine attack. Foods such as cheese, chocolate, and red wine can trigger an attack.

The two types of migraine are (1) classic migraines, which are associated with an aura that occurs minutes to 1 hour before onset, and (2) common migraines, which are not associated with an aura.

Cluster headaches are characterized by a severe unilateral nonthrobbing pain usually located around the eye. They occur in a series of cluster attacks—one or more attacks every day for several weeks. They are not associated with an aura and do not cause nausea and vomiting. Men are more commonly affected by cluster headaches than women.

Table 19–3

Drugs to Treat Severe Migraine Headaches

Drug	Route and Dosage	Uses and Considerations
Ergot Alkaloids		
ergotamine tartrate	A: SL: 2 mg, may repeat in 30 min; *max:* 6 mg/24 h A: Inhal: 1 inhal; may repeat in 5 min A: Intranasal: 1 spray (0.5 mg) in each nostril; repeat in 15 min A: IM/IV: 1 mg at start of headache; repeat 1 h later	An antimigraine drug. To prevent or abort migraine attack. Not for prolonged use. *Pregnancy category:* D; PB: UK; $t^{1/2}$: varies
dihydroergotamine mesylate (Migranal)	A: Intranasal: 1 spray in each nostril; may repeat in 15 min A: IM/IV: 1 mg; may repeat in 1 h; *max:* 3 mg IM and 2 mg IV	To prevent or abort migraine attack. *Pregnancy category:* X; PB: UK; $t^{1/2}$: 21-32 h
Selective Serotinin₁ Receptor Agonists (Triptans)		
sumatriptan succinate (Imitrex)	A: PO: 25 mg; may repeat in 2 h; max: 100 mg A: subQ: 6 mg, may repeat in 1 h A: Intranasal: 5-10-20 mg in nostril; repeat once in 2 h	To treat acute migraine attacks and cluster headaches. Promotes vasoconstriction *Pregnancy category:* C; PB: 10%-20%; $t^{1/2}$: 2 h
naratriptan (Amerge)	A: PO: 1-2.5 mg; may repeat in 4 h; *max:* 5 mg/24 h	For acute migraines. Has a longer half-life, thus duration of action is longer. Causes vasoconstriction of cranial carotid arteries. Avoid if client has severe hypertension, IHD, MI. *Pregnancy category:* C; PB: 28%-31%; $t^{1/2}$: 6 h
rizatriptan benzoate (Maxalt, Maxalt MLT)	A: PO: 5-10 mg; may repeat in 2 h; *max:* 30 mg/24 h	For acute migraines. Two types of tablets: regular and melt-in-mouth. Second tablet does not need to be taken by water. Avoid if client has uncontrolled hypertension, IHD, previous MI. *Pregnancy category:* C; PB: UK; $t^{1/2}$: 2-3 h
zolmitriptan (Zomig)	A: PO: 2.5-5 mg; may repeat in 2 h; *max:* 10 mg/24 h	For acute migraines. 65% of clients respond in 2 h. Avoid if client has uncontrolled hypertension, IHD, previous MI. *Pregnancy category:* C; PB: 25%; $t^{1/2}$: 3 h
almotriptan (Axert)	A: PO: 6.25-12.5 mg; may repeat in 2 h; *max:* 25 mg/24 h	To treat acute migraines. *Pregnancy category:* C; PB: 35%; $t^{1/2}$: 3-4 h
frovatriptan (Frova)	A: PO: 2.5 mg; may repeat in 2 h; *max:* 7.5 mg/24 h	To treat acute migraines. *Pregnancy category:* C; PB: 15%; $t^{1/2}$: 26 h
eletriptan (Relpax)	A: PO: 20-40 mg; may repeat in 2 h; *max:* 80 mg/24 h	To treat acute migraines. *Pregnancy category:* C; PB: 85%; $t^{1/2}$: 4 h

A, Adult; *h,* hour; *IHD,* ischemic heart disease; *IM,* intramuscular; *IV,* intravenous; *max,* maximum; *MI,* myocardial infarction; *min,* minute; *PB,* protein-binding; *PO,* by mouth; *SL,* sublingual; *subQ,* subcutaneous; $t^{1/2}$, half-life; *UK,* unknown.

Treatment of Migraine Headaches

Preventive treatment for migraines includes (1) beta-adrenergic blockers such as propranolol (Inderal) and atenolol (Tenormin); (2) anticonvulsants such as valproic acid (Depakote) and gabapentin (Neurontin); and (3) tricyclic antidepressants such as amitriptyline (Elavil) and imipramine (Tofranil).

Treatment or cessation of a migraine attack depends on the intensity of pain. Drugs used to treat migraines include analgesics, opioid analgesics, ergot alkaloids, and selective serotonin$_1$ (5-HT) receptor agonists, also known as *triptans*. For mild migraine attacks, aspirin, acetaminophen, or nonsteroidal antiinflammatory drugs (NSAIDs), such as ibuprofen or naproxen (Aleve), may be prescribed. Aspirin may be used in combination with caffeine. Meperidine (Demerol) and butorphanol nasal spray (Stadol NS) are opioid analgesics that are occasionally used.

Ergotamine tartrate, a nonspecific serotonin agonist and vasoconstrictor, has been prescribed for years to treat moderate to severe migraine headaches. It should be taken early during a migraine attack. Nausea and vomiting might occur; antiemetics decrease these symptoms. Ergotamine is available in sublingual tablets or with caffeine in oral tablets and suppositories. Dihydroergotamine, an ergot alkaloid, can be administered subcutaneously, intramuscularly, intravenously, and by means of a nasal spray.

The triptans (5-HT$_1$ receptor agonists) are the most recently developed group of drugs for the treatment of migraine headaches. Sumatriptan (Imitrex), a selective serotonin receptor agonist with a short duration of action, was the first triptan drug. It is considered more effective than ergotamine in treating acute migraine attacks. Table 19–3 lists the ergot alkaloids and the selective serotonin$_1$ (5-HT) receptor agonists and their dosages, uses, and considerations. Do not confuse sumatriptan with zolmitriptan. Both drugs are triptans but have different dosages. Also, do not confuse Amerge (triptan used for migraines) with Amaryl (sulfonylurea used for diabetes mellitus) or Altace (angiotensin-converting enzyme inhibitor) used for hypertension and heart failure. Prototype Drug Chart 19–2 provides further pharmacology of sumatriptan.

Prototype DRUG CHART 19–2

SUMATRIPTAN

Drug Class

5-HT$_1$ receptor agonist (antimigraine)
Trade name: Imitrex
Pregnancy Category: C

Dosage

A: PO: 25-50 mg for 1 dose, may repeat once after 2 h, *max*: 200 mg/24 h
A: subQ: 6 mg, may repeat with 6 mg at least 1 h after first injection, *max*: 12 mg/24 h
A: Intranasal: 5-20 mg in one nostril, may repeat after 2 h, *max*: 40 mg/24 h

Contraindications

Hypersensitivity, coronary artery disease, hypertension, obesity, diabetes mellitus, smoking
Caution: Liver or renal dysfunction

Drug-Lab-Food Interactions

Drug: Risk of vasospasm and blood pressure elevation with dihydroergotamine and other ergo alkaloids; Increased levels and toxicity within 2 wks of MAO inhibitors

Pharmacokinetics

Absorption: Rapidly absorbed following subQ injection
Distribution: PB: 10%-20%
Metabolism: t½: 2 h
Excretion: Urine and feces

Pharmacodynamics

PO: Onset: 1-1½ h
Peak: 2-4 h
Duration: UK
subQ: Onset: 10 min
Peak: 2 h
Duration: UK

Therapeutic Effects/Uses

To treat migraine and cluster headaches
Mode of action: Causes vasoconstriction of cranial carotid arteries to relieve migraine attacks

Side Effects

Dizziness, fainting, tingling, numbness, warm sensation, drowsiness, muscle cramps, nausea, vomiting, diarrhea, abdominal cramping

Adverse Reactions

Hypotension, hypertension, heart block, angina, dysrhythmias, thromboembolism, seizures, central nervous system hemorrhage, stroke
Life-threatening: Coronary artery vasospasm, myocardial infarction, cardiac arrest

A, Adult; *h*, hour; *MAO*, monoamine oxidase inhibitor; *max*, maximum; *min*, minute; *PB*, protein-binding; *PO*, by mouth; *subQ*, subcutaneous; *t½*, half life; *UK*, unknown; *wk*, week.

KEY WEBSITES

NIDA InfoFacts: Methylphenidate (Ritalin): http://www.nida.nih.gov/Infofacts/Ritalin.html

National Attention Deficit Disorder Association: http://www.add.org/

Information on zolmitriptan (Zomig): http://www.zomig.com/index.aspx?ce=set

Critical Thinking Case Study

MP, 67 years old, wants to lose 30 pounds. She wants to take an OTC diet pill but does not want to exercise or be on a diet.

1. Would you suggest a diet pill? Why or why not?
2. What does the nurse need to assess concerning this client's physical status before suggesting a diet pill or weight loss program?
3. What behavior modification might you suggest related to losing weight?
4. In what ways could diet control and exercise help this client? Explain.
5. Would you suggest a weight-loss program such as Weight Watchers or Jenny Craig? How do these programs differ? Would one program benefit MP more than the other? Explain.

NCLEX Study Questions

1. The nurse should know that _____ are used to treat migraine attacks.
   a. triptans
   b. anticonvulsants
   c. tricyclic antidepressants
   d. beta-adrenergic blockers

2. When a 12-year-old child is prescribed methylphenidate, it is most important for the nurse to monitor the child's:
   a. temperature
   b. respirations
   c. intake and output
   d. height and weight

3. Which individual is most likely to be demonstrating attention deficit/hyperactivity disorder?
   a. a girl who is fidgety
   b. a girl who lacks impulsivity
   c. a boy with smooth coordination
   d. a boy with an inability to complete tasks

4. Which statement is true regarding benzphetamine?
   a. has a potential for abuse
   b. is similar to amphetamines
   c. should be avoided during pregnancy
   d. may have a side effect of hypotension

5. The nurse should know that a common side effect of analeptics is:
   a. twitching
   b. bradycardia
   c. constipation
   d. urinary retention

Answers: 1, a; 2, d; 3, d; 4, d; 5, a.

20

Central Nervous System Depressants

Outline

Objectives

- Explain the types and stages of sleep.
- Discuss several nonpharmacologic ways to induce sleep.
- Differentiate these adverse effects: *hangover, dependence, tolerance, withdrawal symptoms,* and *rapid eye movement (REM) rebound.*
- Contrast short-acting and intermediate-acting barbiturates used as sedative hypnotics. Discuss the uses of benzodiazepines.
- Apply the nursing process for the client taking benzodiazepines for hypnotic use.
- Differentiate nursing interventions related to barbiturates and benzodiazepine hypnotics.
- Describe the stages of anesthesia.
- Explain the uses for topical anesthetics.
- Differentiate general and local anesthetics and their major side effects.

Terms

Drugs that are central nervous system (CNS) depressants cause varying degrees of depression (reduction in functional activity) within the CNS. The degree of depression depends primarily on the drug and the amount of drug taken. The broad classification of CNS depressants includes sedative-hypnotics, general and local anesthetics, analgesics, narcotic and nonnarcotic analgesics, anticonvulsants, antipsychotics, and antidepressants. The last five groups of depressant drugs are presented in separate chapters. Sedative-hypnotics and general and local anesthetics are discussed in this chapter.

Types and Stages of Sleep

Sleep disorders such as **insomnia** (inability to fall asleep) occur in 5% to 10% of healthy adults, 20% to 25% of hospitalized clients, and approximately 75% of psychiatric clients. Insomnia occurs more frequently in women and increases with age. Sedative-hypnotics are commonly ordered for treatment of sleep disorders.

People spend approximately one third of their lives, or as much as 25 years, sleeping. Normal sleep is composed of two definite phases: **rapid eye movement (REM) sleep** and **nonrapid eye movement (NREM) sleep.** Both REM and NREM occur cyclically during sleep at about 90-minute intervals (Figure 20–1). The four succeedingly deeper stages of NREM sleep end with an episode of REM sleep, and the cycle begins again. If sleep is interrupted the cycle begins again with stage 1 of NREM sleep.

It is during the REM sleep phase that individuals experience most of their recallable dreams. Individuals perform better during their waking hours if they experience all types and stages of sleep. Children have few REM sleep periods and have longer periods of stage 3 and 4 NREM sleep. Older adults experience a decrease in stages 3 and 4 of NREM sleep and have frequent waking periods.

It is difficult to rouse a person during REM sleep. The period of REM sleep episodes becomes longer during the sleep process. Frequently if a person is roused from REM sleep, a vivid, bizarre dream may be recalled. If these dreams are unpleasant, they may be called *nightmares.* Sleep-walking or nightmares that occur in children take place during NREM sleep.

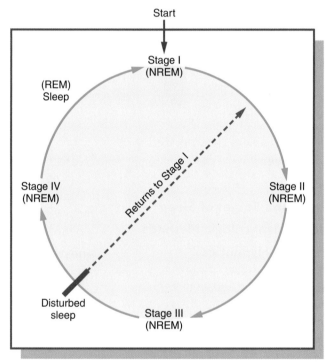

FIGURE 20–1 Types and stages of sleep. NREM, Nonrapid eye movement (four stages); REM, rapid eye movement (dreaming).

Nonpharmacologic Methods

Before using sedative-hypnotics or over-the-counter (OTC) sleep aids, various nonpharmacologic methods should be used to promote sleep. Once the nurse discovers why the client cannot sleep, the following ways to promote sleep may be suggested:

1. Arise at a specific hour in the morning.
2. Take few or no daytime naps.
3. Avoid drinks that contain caffeine 6 hours before bedtime.
4. Avoid heavy meals or strenuous exercise before bedtime.
5. Take a warm bath, read, or listen to music before bedtime.
6. Decrease exposure to loud noises.
7. Avoid drinking copious amounts of fluids before sleep.
8. Drink warm milk before bedtime.

Sedative-Hypnotics

The mildest form of CNS depression is **sedation,** which diminishes physical and mental responses at lower dosages of certain CNS depressants but does not affect consciousness. Sedatives are used mostly during the daytime. Increasing the drug dose can produce a **hypnotic effect**—not hypnosis but a form of "natural" sleep. Sedative-hypnotic drugs are sometimes the same drug; however, certain drugs are used more often for their hypnotic effect. With very high doses of sedative-hypnotic drugs, anesthesia may be achieved. An example of an ultrashort-acting barbiturate used to produce anesthesia is thiopental sodium (Pentothal).

Sedatives were first prescribed to reduce tension and anxiety. Barbiturates were initially used for their antianxiety effect until the early 1960s, when benzodiazepines were introduced. Because of the many side effects of barbiturates and their potential for physical and mental dependency, they are now less frequently prescribed. The chronic use of any sedative-hypnotic should be avoided.

Because of the high incidence of sleep disorders, hypnotics are one of the most frequently prescribed drugs. More than $35 million is spent each year on OTC sleep aids such as Nytol, Sominex, Sleep-Eze, and Tylenol PM. The primary ingredient in OTC sleep aids is an antihistamine like diphenhydramine and not barbiturates or benzodiazepines.

There are short-acting hypnotics and intermediate-acting hypnotics. Short-acting hypnotics are useful in achieving sleep, because they allow the client to awaken early in the morning without experiencing lingering side effects. Intermediate-acting hypnotics are useful for sus-taining sleep; however, after using one the client may experience residual drowsiness, or **hangover,** in the morning. This may be undesirable if the client is active and requires mental alertness. The ideal hypnotic promotes natural sleep without disrupting normal patterns of sleep and produces no hangover or undesirable effect. Table 20–1 lists the common side effects and adverse reactions associated with sedative-hypnotic use and abuse.

Hypnotic drug therapy should be short-term to prevent drug **dependence** and drug **tolerance.** Interrupting hypnotic therapy can decrease drug tolerance, but abruptly discontinuing a high dose of hypnotic taken over a long period can cause **withdrawal symptoms.** In such cases the dose should be tapered to avoid withdrawal symptoms. As a general rule the lowest dose should be taken to obtain sleep. Clients with severe respiratory disorders should avoid hypnotics, which could cause an increase in respiratory distress. Normally hypnotics are contraindicated during pregnancy.

The category of sedative-hypnotics includes barbiturates, benzodiazepines, and nonbenzodiazepines, among others. Each category is discussed separately. Prototype drug charts are included for barbiturates and benzodiazepines.

Barbiturates

Barbiturates were introduced as a sedative in the early 1900s. More than 2000 barbiturates have been developed, but only 12 are currently marketed. Barbiturates are classified as long-acting, intermediate-acting, short-acting, and ultrashort-acting.

- The *long-acting* group includes phenobarbital and mephobarbital and is used to control seizures in epilepsy. Phenobarbital, introduced in 1912, is still in use.

Table 20–1

Common Side Effects and Adverse Reactions of Sedative-Hypnotics

Side Effects and Adverse Reactions	Explanation of the Effects
Hangover	A hangover is residual drowsiness resulting in impaired reaction time. The intermediate- and long-acting hypnotics are frequently the cause of drug hangover. The liver biotransforms these drugs into active metabolites that persist in the body, causing drowsiness.
REM rebound	REM rebound, which results in vivid dreams and nightmares, frequently occurs after taking a hypnotic for a prolonged period then abruptly stopping. However, it may occur after taking only one hypnotic dose.
Dependence	Dependence is the result of chronic hypnotic use. Physical and psychologic dependence can result. Physical dependence results in the appearance of specific withdrawal symptoms when a drug is discontinued after prolonged use. The severity of withdrawal symptoms depends on the drug and dosage. Symptoms may include muscular twitching and tremors, dizziness, orthostatic hypotension, delusions, hallucinations, delirium, and seizures. Withdrawal symptoms start within 24 hours and can last for several days.
Tolerance	Tolerance results when there is a need to increase the dosage over time to obtain the desired effect. It is mostly caused by an increase in drug metabolism by liver enzymes. The barbiturate drug category can cause tolerance after prolonged use. Tolerance is reversible when the drug is discontinued.
Excessive depression	Long-term use of a hypnotic may result in depression, which is characterized by lethargy, sleepiness, lack of concentration, confusion, and psychologic depression.
Respiratory depression	High doses of sedative-hypnotics can suppress the respiratory center in the medulla.
Hypersensitivity	Skin rashes and urticaria can result when taking barbiturates. Such reactions are rare.

REM, Rapid eye movement.

- The *intermediate-acting* barbiturates, such as butabarbital (Butisol), are useful as sleep sustainers for maintaining long periods of sleep. Because these drugs take approximately 1 hour for the onset of sleep, they are not prescribed for those who have trouble getting to sleep. Vital signs should be closely monitored in persons who take intermediate-acting barbiturates.

- The *short-acting* barbiturates secobarbital (Seconal) and pentobarbital (Nembutal) are used to induce sleep for those who have difficulty falling asleep. These drugs may

Table 20–2

Sedative-Hypnotics: Barbiturates and Others

Generic (Brand)	Route and Dosage	Uses and Considerations
Barbiturates: Short-Acting		
pentobarbital sodium (Nembutal Sodium) CSS II	*Sedative:* A: PO: 20-30 mg t.i.d. C: PO: 2-6 mg/kg/d in 3 divided doses. *max:* 100 mg/d *Hypnotic:* A: PO: 100-200 mg at bedtime; IM: 150-200 mg C: PO: 30-100 mg at bedtime; IM 2-6 mg/kg; *max:* 100 mg/d *Preoperative:* A: PO/IM/IV: 100-200 mg in 2 divided doses	For sedation, sleep, or preanesthetic. *Pregnancy category:* D; PB: 35%-45%; $t^{1/2}$: 4-50 h
secobarbital sodium (Seconal Sodium) CSS II	See Prototype Drug Chart 20–1.	
Barbiturates: Intermediate-Acting		
butabarbital sodium (Butisol Sodium) CSS III	*Sedative:* A: PO: 15-30 mg t.i.d., q.i.d. *Hypnotic:* A: PO: 50-100 mg at bedtime *Preoperative sedative:* A: PO: 50-100 mg, 1-1.5 h before surgery	To relieve anxiety and as short-term hypnotic for insomnia. Avoid alcohol with all barbiturates. *Pregnancy category:* D; PB: 50%; $t^{1/2}$: 60-120 h
Barbiturates: Long-Acting		
mephobarbital (Mebaral) CSS IV	*Sedative:* A: PO: 32-100 mg t.i.d., q.i.d. C: PO: < 5 y 16-32 mg t.i.d., q.i.d. > 5 y 32-64 mg t.i.d., q.i.d.	To control convulsive episodes, agitation, anxiety, and delirium tremens. *Pregnancy category:* D; PB: UK; $t^{1/2}$: 34 h
Other Sedative-Hypnotics		
chloral hydrate CSS IV	*Sedative:* A: PO: 250 mg t.i.d. p.c. C: PO: 8.3 mg/kg t.i.d. p.c.; *max:* 1000 mg/d or 500 mg/dose *Hypnotic:* A: PO: 500 mg-1g at bedtime C: PO: 50 mg/kg at bedtime; *max:* 1000 mg	For sedative or sleep. Used since mid-1800s. No hangover and less respiratory depression. Give with meals or fluids to prevent gastric irritation. Give 15-30 min before sleep. *Pregnancy category:* C; PB: 70%-80%; $t^{1/2}$: 8-10 h
ethchlorvynol (Placidyl) CSS IV	*Sedative:* A: PO: 100-200 mg, b.i.d., t.i.d. *Hypnotic:* A: PO: 0.5-1 g, at bedtime for 1 wk only	Barbiturate-like drug. For sedation and sleep. Use no longer than 1 wk. *Caution:* renal or liver disease and drug abuse. Give with food or fluid to decrease nausea and vomiting. Has a short duration of action. *Pregnancy category:* C; PB: UK; $t^{1/2}$: 20-100 h
paraldehyde (Paral) CSS IV	*Sedative:* A: PO: 5-0 ml q4-6h PRN in water or juice; *max:* 30 ml C: PO: 0.3 ml/kg *Hypnotic:* A: PO: 10-30 ml at bedtime	Exhaled via the lungs. Strong odor and disagreeable taste. Seldom used today; has been used to control delirium tremens (DTs) in alcoholics. Can be used for drug poisoning and to control convulsions, such as status epilepticus. *Pregnancy category:* C; PB: UK; $t^{1/2}$: 7.5 h
ramelteon (Rozerem)	A: PO: 8 mg within 30 minutes of bedtime	For treatment of insomnia. *Pregnancy category:* C; PB: 82%; $t^{1/2}$: 1-2.5 h

A, Adult; *b.i.d.,* two times a day; *C*, child; *CSS*, Controlled Substances Schedule; *d*, day; *h*, hour; *IM*, intramuscular; *IV*, intravenous; *max*, maximum; *PB*, protein-binding; *p.c.,* after meals; *PO*, by mouth; *PRN*, as needed; *q.i.d.,* four times a day; $t^{1/2}$, half-life; *t.i.d.,* three times a day; *UK*, unknown; *wk*, week; <, less than; >, greater than.

cause the person to awaken early in the morning. Vital signs should be closely monitored in persons who take short-acting barbiturates.

• The *ultrashort-acting* barbiturate, thiopental sodium (Pentothal), is used as a general anesthetic.

Barbiturates should be restricted to short-term use (2 weeks or less) because of their numerous side effects, including tolerance to the drug. In the United States barbiturates are classified as class II in the schedule of the Controlled Substances Act. In Canada, barbiturates are classified as schedule G. Barbiturates are listed in Table 20–2 and described in more detail in Prototype Drug Chart 20–1, with a focus on the short-acting barbiturate secobarbital (Seconal). The nursing process is based on the drug data.

Pharmacokinetics

Pentobarbital (Nembutal) has been available for nearly half a century and was the hypnotic of choice until the introduction of benzodiazepines in the 1960s. It has a slow absorption rate and is moderately protein-bound. The long half-life is mainly because of the formation of active metabolites resulting from liver metabolism.

Pharmacodynamics

Pentobarbital and secobarbital are used primarily for sleep induction and for sedation needs. They have a rapid onset with a short duration of action and are considered short-acting barbiturates. The onset of action of pentobarbital is slower when administered intramuscularly (IM) than when administered orally (PO). Do not confuse pentobarbital with phenobarbital (Herbal Alert 20–1).

Many drug interactions are associated with barbiturates. Alcohol, narcotics, and other sedative-hypnotics used in combination with barbiturates may further depress the CNS. Pentobarbital increases hepatic enzyme action, causing an increased metabolism and decreased effect of drugs such as oral anticoagulants, glucocorticoids, tricyclic antidepressants, and quinidine. Pentobarbital may cause hepatotoxicity if taken with large doses of acetaminophen.

Herbal ALERT 20–1

Sedatives

Kava kava should not be taken in combination with CNS depressants such as barbiturates and opioids. This herb may increase the sedative effect.

Valerian, when taken with alcohol and other CNS depressants such as barbiturates, may increase the sedative effects of the prescribed drug.

Prototype DRUG CHART 20–1

SECOBARBITAL SODIUM

Drug Class	**Dosage**
Sedative-hypnotic: Barbiturate	*Sedative:*
Trade name: Seconal Sodium	A: PO: 100-300 mg/d
CSS II	C: PO: 4-6 mg/kg/d in 3 divided doses
Pregnancy Category: D	*Hypnotic:*
	A: PO: 100-200 mg at bedtime
	Preoperative:
	A: PO: 100-300 mg 1-2 h before surgery
Contraindications	**Drug-Lab-Food Interactions**
Respiratory depression, severe hepatic disease, pregnancy (fetal immaturity), nephrosis, hypersensitivity	*Drug: Decrease* respiration with alcohol, CNS depressants, and MAOIs
Caution: liver or kidney dysfunction; elderly, children, and debilitated individuals	
Pharmacokinetics	**Pharmacodynamics**
Absorption: PO: 90% absorbed from GI tract	PO: Onset: 15-30 min
Distribution: PB: UK	Peak: 0.5-1 h
Metabolism: t½: 15-40 h	Duration: 3-4 h
Excretion: In urine as metabolites	

Therapeutic Effects/Uses

To treat insomnia; used for sedation, preoperative medication
Mode of Action: Depression of the CNS, including the motor and sensory activities

Side Effects	**Adverse Reactions**
Lethargy, drowsiness, hangover, dizziness, paradoxical excitement in the elderly	Drug dependence or tolerance
	Life threatening: Respiratory distress, laryngospasm

A, Adult; *C,* child; *CNS,* central nervous system; *CSS,* Controlled Substances Schedule; *d,* day; *GI,* gastrointestinal; *h,* hour; *MAOIs,* monoamine oxidase inhibitors; *min,* minute; *PB,* protein-binding; *PO,* by mouth; *t½,* half-life; *UK,* unknown.

Nursing Process

Sedative-Hypnotic: Barbiturate

ASSESSMENT

■ Obtain a drug history of current drugs and herbs client is taking.

■ Record baseline vital signs for future comparison.

■ Determine whether there is a history of insomnia or sleep disorder.

■ Assess renal function. Urine output should be 600 ml/day. Renal impairment could prolong drug action by increasing half-life of the drug.

■ Assess potential for fluid volume deficit, which would potentiate hypotensive effects.

NURSING DIAGNOSES

■ Sleep deprivation related to anxiety and stress

■ Risk for injury related to dizziness

PLANNING

■ Client will receive adequate sleep without hangover when taking hypnotic.

NURSING INTERVENTIONS

■ Recognize that continuous use of a barbiturate might result in drug abuse.

■ Monitor vital signs, especially respirations and blood pressure.

■ Raise bedside rails of older adults and clients receiving a hypnotic for the first time. Confusion may occur, and injury may result.

■ Observe client, especially an older adult or a debilitated client, for adverse reactions to secobarbital (Prototype Drug Chart 20-1).

■ Check client's skin for rashes. Skin eruptions may occur in clients taking barbiturates.

■ Assess client for withdrawal symptoms when barbiturates have been taken over a prolonged period of time and abruptly discontinued.

■ Administer IV pentobarbital at a rate of less than 50 mg/min. *Do not* mix pentobarbital with other medications. IM injection should be given deep in a large muscle such as the gluteus medius.

Client Teaching

General

• Teach client to use nonpharmacologic ways to induce sleep (enjoying a warm bath, listening to music, drinking warm fluids, and avoiding drinks with caffeine for 6 hours before bedtime).

• Instruct client to avoid alcohol and antidepressant, antipsychotic, and narcotic drugs while taking the barbiturate. Respiratory distress may occur when these drugs are combined.

• Inform client that certain herbs (Herbal Alert 20–1) may interact with CNS depressants such as barbiturates. Herbal supplement may need to be discontinued or prescription drug dose may need to be modified.

• Advise client not to drive a motor vehicle or operate machinery. Caution is always encouraged.

• Instruct client to take hypnotic 30 minutes before bedtime. Short-acting hypnotics take effect within 15 to 30 minutes.

• Encourage client to check with health care provider about OTC sleeping aids. Drowsiness may result from taking these drugs; therefore caution while driving is advised.

Side Effects

• Advise client to report adverse reactions such as hangover to health care provider. Drug selection or dosage might need to be changed.

• Instruct client that hypnotics such as secobarbital should be gradually withdrawn, especially if it has been taken for several weeks. Abrupt cessation of the hypnotic may result in withdrawal symptoms (e.g., tremors, muscle twitching).

Cultural Considerations ❖

• Use an interpreter as appropriate and involve extended family in health teaching and support.

• Provide written instruction (or videos) in client's preferred language.

EVALUATION

■ Assess the effectiveness of barbiturates.

■ Evaluate respiratory status to ensure that respiratory distress has not occurred.

Benzodiazepines

Selected benzodiazepines (minor tranquilizer or anxiolytic), introduced with chlordiazepoxide (Librium) in the 1960s as antianxiety agents, are ordered as sedative-hypnotics for inducing sleep. Several benzodiazepines marketed as hypnotics include flurazepam (Dalmane), temazepam (Restoril), triazolam (Halcion), estazolam (ProSom), and quazepam (Doral) (Table 20–2). Increased anxiety might be the cause of insomnia for some clients, so lorazepam (Ativan) and diazepam (Valium) can be used to alleviate the anxiety. These drugs are classified as schedule IV according to the Controlled Substances Act. The benzodiazepines increase the action of the inhibitory neurotransmitter gamma-aminobutyric acid (GABA) to the GABA receptors. Neuron excitability is reduced. Do not confuse lorazepam with alprazolam.

Benzodiazepines (except for temazepam) can suppress stage 4 of NREM sleep, which may result in vivid dreams or nightmares and can delay REM sleep. Benzodiazepines are effective for sleep disorders for several weeks longer than other sedative-hypnotics; to prevent *REM rebound*, however, they should not be used for longer than 3 to 4 weeks.

Flurazepam (Dalmane) was the first benzodiazepine hypnotic introduced. Triazolam (Halcion) is a short-acting hypnotic with a half-life of 2 to 5 hours. It does not produce any active metabolites. Complaints of adverse reactions to prolonged use of triazolam (e.g., loss of memory) led to its removal from the market in Great Britain, but a British advisory group is recommending that the legislative body reinstate triazolam. Its use is under review by the U.S. Food and Drug Administration (FDA). Currently it is seldom prescribed.

Small doses of benzodiazepine are recommended for clients with renal or hepatic dysfunction. For benzodiazepine overdose, the benzodiazepine antagonist flumazenil may be prescribed. Benzodiazepines prescribed as antianxiety drugs are discussed in Chapter 26.

Pharmacokinetics

Benzodiazepines are well absorbed through the gastrointestinal (GI) mucosa. Flurazepam is rapidly metabolized in the liver to active metabolites, and it has a long half-life of 45 to 100 hours. Flurazepam is highly protein-bound, and if taken with other highly protein-bound drugs, more free drug is available, increasing the risk of adverse effects.

Pharmacodynamics

Benzodiazepines are used to treat insomnia by inducing and sustaining sleep. They have a rapid onset of action and intermediate- to long-acting effects. The normal recommended dose of a benzodiazepine may be too much for the older adult, so half the dose is recommended initially to prevent overdosing.

Alcohol or narcotics taken with a benzodiazepine may cause an additive depressive CNS response. Triazolam (Halcion) may cause rebound insomnia and temazepam (Restoril) may cause euphoria and palpitations.

Nonbenzodiazepines

Zolpidem (Ambien) is a nonbenzodiazepine that differs in chemical structure from benzodiazepines. It is used for short-term treatment (<10 days) of insomnia. Its duration of action is 6 to 8 hours with a short half-life of 2 to 2.5 hours. Zolpidem is metabolized in the liver to three inactive metabolites and excreted in bile, urine, and feces. When zolpidem is prescribed for older adults, the dose should be decreased. Table 20–3 lists the benzodiazepines and nonbenzodiazepines used as sedative-hypnotics and their dosages, uses, and considerations. Zolpidem is described in Prototype Drug Chart 20–2.

Chloral Hydrate

Chloral hydrate was first introduced in the 1860s. It is used to induce sleep and decrease nocturnal awakenings; it does not suppress REM sleep. There is less occurrence of hangover, respiratory depression, and tolerance with chloral hydrate than with other sedative-hypnotics. Its use is effective in older adults. Chloral hydrate can be given to clients with mild liver dysfunction, but it should be avoided if severe liver or renal disorder is present. Gastric irritation may occur, so the drug should be taken with sufficient water. Drugs that interact with chloral hydrate include other CNS depressants, furosemide, and oral anticoagulants.

Sedatives and Hypnotics for Older Adults

Identifying the cause of insomnia in an older adult should be the first diagnostic consideration, and nonpharmacologic methods should be used before sleep medications are prescribed. Because of physiologic changes in older adults, the use of hypnotics can cause a variety of side effects.

Barbiturates increase CNS depression and confusion in older adults and should not be taken for sleep. The short- to intermediate-acting benzodiazepines such as estazolam (ProSom), temazepam (Restoril), and triazolam (Halcion) are considered safer than barbiturates. Long-acting hypnotic benzodiazepines such as flurazepam (Dalmane), quazepam (Doral), and diazepam (Valium) should be avoided. In many cases, older adults should be instructed to take the prescribed benzodiazepine no more than four times a week to avoid side effects and drug dependency. They can choose selected nights to take the hypnotic.

The main sleep problem experienced by older adults is frequent nighttime awakening. Reports have shown that older women experience more troublesome sleep patterns than men. Sleep disturbance may be caused by discomfort or pain. To alleviate pain and aid sleep the OTC drug Tylenol PM, which contains acetaminophen and diphenhydramine (an antihistamine), may be taken. Occasionally a non-steroidal antiinflammatory drug (NSAID) such as ibuprofen may alleviate the discomfort that prevents sleep.

Nursing Process

Sedative-Hypnotic: Benzodiazepine

ASSESSMENT

- Record baseline vital signs and laboratory tests (e.g., AST, ALT, bilirubin) for future comparisons.
- Obtain drug history. Taking CNS depressants with benzodiazepine hypnotics can depress respirations.
- Ascertain client's problem with sleep disturbance.

NURSING DIAGNOSES

- Sleep deprivation related to anxiety

PLANNING

- Client will remain asleep for 6 to 8 hours.

NURSING INTERVENTIONS

■ Monitor vital signs. Check for signs of respiratory depression (slow, irregular breathing patterns).

■ Raise bedside rails of older adults or clients receiving sedative-hypnotics for the first time. Confusion may occur, and injury may result.

■ Observe client for side effects of sedative-hypnotics (hangover [residual sedation], light-headedness, dizziness, confusion).

Client Teaching

General

• Teach client to use nonpharmacologic ways to induce sleep (enjoying a warm bath, listening to music, drinking warm fluids such as milk, avoiding drinks with caffeine after dinner).

• Instruct client to avoid alcohol, antidepressant, antipsychotic, and narcotic drugs while taking sedative-hypnotics. Severe respiratory distress may occur when these drugs are combined.

• Advise client to take sedative-hypnotic before bedtime. Flurazepam takes effect within 15 to 45 minutes.

• Suggest that client urinate before taking sedative-hypnotic to prevent sleep disruption.

• Encourage client to check with health care provider about OTC sleeping aids. Drowsiness may result from taking these drugs, so caution while driving is advised.

Table 20–3

Sedative-Hypnotics: Benzodiazepines and Nonbenzodiazepines

Generic (Brand)	Route and Dosage	Uses and Considerations
Benzodiazepines		
alprazolam (Xanax) CSS IV	A: PO: 0.25-0.5 mg at bedtime	For alleviating anxiety that may cause sleeplessness. *Pregnancy category:* D; PB: UK; t½: 12-15 h
estazolam (ProSom) CSS IV	A: PO: 1-2 mg at bedtime Elderly: PO: 0.5 mg at bedtime	New benzodiazepine hypnotic for treatment of insomnia. Should not be used for longer than 6 wk. Decreases frequency of nocturnal awakening. *Pregnancy category:* X; PB: 93%; t½: 10-24 h
flurazepam HCl (Dalmane) CSS IV	A: PO: 15-30 mg at bedtime Elderly: PO: 15 mg at bedtime	For insomnia. *Pregnancy category:* X; PB: 97%; t½: 2-3 h
lorazepam (Ativan) CSS IV	*Insomnia:* A: PO: 2-4 mg at bedtime	Used as a preoperative sedative and to reduce anxiety. *Pregnancy category:* D; PB: 85%; t½: 12-14 h
quazepam (Doral) CSS IV	A: PO: 7.5-15 mg at bedtime	To treat insomnia and decrease nocturnal awakenings. Avoid alcohol with this drug and all benzodiazepines. *Pregnancy category:* X; PB: 95%; t½: 39 h
temazepam (Restoril) CSS IV	*Hypnotic:* A: PO: 15-30 mg at bedtime	To treat insomnia and decrease nocturnal awakenings. Also has sedative effects. *Pregnancy category:* X; PB: 96%; t½: 10-20 h
triazolam (Halcion) CSS IV	Hypnotic: A: PO: 0.125-0.5 mg at bedtime (0.5 mg with caution) Elderly: PO: 0.125-0.25 mg at bedtime	For management of insomnia. Should not be used longer than 7-10 d at a time to avoid tolerance. Avoid alcohol and smoking when taking triazolam. *Pregnancy Category:* X; PB: 89%; t½: 2-4 h
Benzodiazepine Antagonists		
flumazenil (Romazicon)	A: IV: 0.2 mg over 30 sec; may repeat with 0.3 mg in 30 sec; *max:* 3 mg total dose	Management of benzodiazepine overdose or reversal of sedative effects of benzodiazepine with general anesthesia. *Pregnancy category:* UK; PB: UK; t½: UK.
Nonbenzodiazepines		
zolpidem tartrate (Ambien) CSS IV	See Prototype Drug Chart 20–2.	
eszopiclone (Lunesta) CSS IV	*Insomnia:* A: PO: 2 mg at bedtime; may increase to 3 mg	To treat insomnia. *Pregnancy category:* C; PB: UK; t½: 6 h
zaleplon (Sonata) CSS IV	*Insomnia:* A: PO: 10 mg at bedtime; *max:* 20 mg at bedtime Elderly: PO: 5 mg at bedtime; *max:* 10 mg at bedtime	For ultrashort-term treatment of insomnia. *Pregnancy category:* C; PB: 60%; t½: 1 h

A, Adult; *CSS,* Controlled Substances Schedule; *d,* day; *h,* hour; *IV,* intravenous; *max,* maximum; *PB,* protein-binding; *PO,* by mouth; *sec,* second; *t½,* half-life; *UK,* unknown; *wk,* week.

Side Effects

- Instruct client to report adverse reactions such as hangover to health care provider. Drug selection or dosage may need to be changed if hangover occurs.

Cultural Considerations ❖

- Ask the transcultural person about methods family members have used to promote sleep.
- Suggest nonpharmacologic alternatives that may be effective in inducing sleep.

EVALUATION

- ■ Evaluate the effectiveness of sedative-hypnotic in promoting sleep.
- ■ Determine whether side effects such as hangover occur after several days of taking sedative-hypnotic. Another hypnotic may be prescribed if side effects persist.

Anesthetics

Anesthetics are classified as *general* and *local*. General anesthetics depress the CNS, alleviate pain, and cause a loss of consciousness. The first anesthetic, nitrous oxide ("laugh-ing gas"), was used for surgery in the early 1800s. It is still an effective anesthetic and is frequently used in dental surgery. In the mid-1800s, ether and chloroform were introduced. Ether, a highly flammable volatile liquid, has a pungent odor and can cause nausea and vomiting after it has been administered. Ether is seldom used now, probably because of the hazard of possible explosion and its noxious odor. Chloroform is toxic to liver cells and is no longer used.

Pathophysiology

Several theories exist regarding how inhalation anesthetics cause CNS depression and a loss of consciousness. The differing theories suggest the following about inhalation anesthetics:

1. The lipid structure of cell membranes is altered, resulting in impaired physiologic functions.
2. The inhibitory neurotransmitter gamma-aminobutyric acid (GABA) is activated to the GABA receptor that pushes chloride ions into the neurons. This greatly decreases the fire action potentials of the neurons.
3. The ascending reticular activating system is altered, and the neurons cease to transmit information (stimuli) to the brain.

Prototype DRUG CHART 20–2

ZOLPIDEM TARTRATE

Drug Class Sedative-Hypnotic: Non-benzodiazepine Trade name: Ambien CSS IV *Pregnancy Category:* B	**Dosage** A: PO: 5-10 mg at bedtime; *max:* 7-10 mg/d Elderly: PO: 5 mg at bedtime; *max:* 7-10 mg/d
Contraindications Hypersensitivity to benzodiazepine, lactation *Caution:* Renal or liver dysfunction; pregnancy; children, elderly, and debilitated individuals	**Drug-Lab-Food Interactions** *Drug: Decrease* CNS function with alcohol, CNS depressants, anticonvulsants, and phenothiazines *Food: Decreases* absorption
Pharmacokinetics **Absorption:** PO: well absorbed **Distribution:** PB: 79%-96% **Metabolism:** t½: 2-2.5 h **Excretion:** In bile, urine, and feces	**Pharmacodynamics** PO: Onset: 7-27 min Peak: 0.5-2.3 h Duration: 6-8 h

Therapeutic Effects/Uses

To treat insomnia
Mode of Action: Depression of CNS, neurotransmitter inhibition

Side Effects Drowsiness, lethargy, hangover (residual sedation), irritability, dizziness, anxiety, nausea, vomiting, hypervitaminosis A, bulging fontanelles in infants	**Adverse Reactions** Tolerance, psychologic or physical dependence

A, Adult; *CNS,* central nervous system; *CSS,* Controlled Substances Schedule; *d,* day; *h,* hour; *min,* minute; *PB,* protein-binding; *PO,* by mouth; *t½,* half-life.

Balanced Anesthesia

Balanced anesthesia, a combination of drugs, is frequently used in general anesthesia. Balanced anesthesia generally includes the following:

1. A hypnotic given the night before
2. Premedication with a narcotic analgesic or benzodiazepine (e.g., midazolam [Versed]) plus an anticholinergic (e.g., atropine) given about 1 hour before surgery to decrease secretions
3. A short-acting barbiturate such as thiopental sodium (Pentothal)
4. An inhaled gas—often a combination of nitrous oxide and oxygen
5. A muscle relaxant given as needed

Balanced anesthesia minimizes cardiovascular problems, decreases the amount of general anesthetic needed, reduces possible postanesthetic nausea and vomiting, minimizes the disturbance of organ function, and decreases pain. Because the client does not receive large doses of general anesthetics, fewer adverse reactions occur. Recovery is enhanced by allowing quicker mobility.

Stages of General Anesthesia

General anesthesia proceeds through four stages (Table 20–4). The surgical procedure is usually performed during the third stage. If an anesthetic agent is given immediately before inhalation anesthesia, the third stage can occur without the early stages of anesthesia being observed. However, if the drug is given slowly, all stages of anesthesia are usually observed.

Assessment before Surgery

The client's response to anesthesia may differ according to variables related to the health status of the individual. These variables include age (young and elderly), a current health disorder (e.g., renal or liver), pregnancy, history of heavy smoking, obesity, and frequent use of alcohol and drugs. These problems must be identified *before* surgery because the type and amount of anesthetic required might need adjustment.

Inhalation Anesthetics

During the third stage of anesthesia, inhalation anesthetics (i.e., gas or volatile liquids administered as gas) are used to deliver general anesthesia. Certain gases, notably nitrous oxide and cyclopropane, are absorbed quickly, have a rapid action, and are eliminated rapidly. Cyclopropane was a popular inhalation anesthetic from 1930 to 1960, but because of its highly flammable state as ether, it is no longer used. In the late 1950s, halothane was introduced as a nonflammable alternative. Other inhalation drugs introduced as anesthetics include methoxyflurane in the 1960s, enflurane in the 1970s, isoflurane in the 1980s, desflurane in 1992, and the newest, seroflurane, in 1995.

Inhalation anesthetics typically provide smooth induction. Upon discontinuing administration of halothane (Fluothane), isoflurane (Forane), and enflurane (Ethrane), recovery of consciousness usually occurs in approximately 1 hour. Recovery from desflurane (Suprane) and sevoflurane (Ultane) is within minutes. Inhalation anesthetics are usually combined with a barbiturate (e.g., thiopental), a strong analgesic (e.g., morphine), and a muscle relaxant (e.g., pancuronium) for surgical procedures.

Adverse effects from inhalation anesthetics include respiratory depression, hypotension, dysrhythmias, and hepatic dysfunction. In clients at risk, these drugs may trigger malignant hyperthermia. The newer drugs primarily cause less nausea and vomiting than the older anesthetics.

Intravenous Anesthetics

Intravenous (IV) anesthetics may be used for general anesthesia or for the induction stage of anesthesia. For outpatient surgery of short duration, an intravenous anesthetic might be the preferred form of anesthesia. Previously thiopental sodium (Pentothal), an ultrashort-acting barbiturate, was the general anesthetic used for short-term surgery. It is still used for the rapid induction stage of anesthesia and in dental procedures. Presently droperidol (Innovar), etomidate (Amidate), and ketamine hydrochloride (Ketalar) are also used intravenously as general anesthetics. IV anesthetics have rapid onsets and short durations of ac-

Table 20–4		
Stages of Anesthesia		
Stage	**Name**	**Description**
1	Analgesia	Begins with consciousness and ends with loss of consciousness. Speech is difficult; sensations of smell and pain are lost. Dreams and auditory and visual hallucinations may occur. This stage may be called the *induction stage*.
2	Excitement or delirium	Produces a loss of consciousness caused by depression of the cerebral cortex. Confusion, excitement, or delirium occur. Short induction time.
3	Surgical	Surgical procedure is performed during this stage. There are four phases. The surgery is usually performed in phase 2 and upper phase 3. As anesthesia deepens, respirations become more shallow and respiratory rate is increased.
4	Medullary paralysis	Toxic stage of anesthesia. Respirations are lost and circulatory collapse occurs. Ventilatory assistance is necessary.

tion. Table 20–5 describes the inhalation and intravenous anesthetics used for general anesthesia.

Midazolam (Versed) and propofol (Diprivan) are commonly administered for the induction and maintenance of anesthesia or conscious sedation for minor surgery or pro-

cedures like mechanical ventilation or intubation. Clients are sedated and relaxed but responsive to commands.

Adverse effects from IV anesthetics include respiratory and cardiovascular depression. Propofol supports microbial growth and may increase the risk of bacterial infec-

Table 20–5

Inhalation and Intravenous Anesthetics

Drug	Induction Time	Considerations
Inhalation: Volatile Liquids		
ether	Slow	Highly flammable. Has no severe effect on the cardiovascular system or liver.
halothane (Fluothane)	Rapid	Introduced in the 1950s. Highly potent anesthetic. Rapid recovery. Could decrease blood pressure. Has a bronchodilator effect. Contraindicated in obstetrics.
methoxyflurane (Penthrane)	Slow	Introduced in the 1960s. Used during labor. Drug dose is usually less than other anesthetics and does not suppress uterine contraction. Could cause hypotension. Contraindicated in renal disorders.
enflurane (Ethrane)	Rapid	Introduced in the 1970s. Similar to halothane. Can depress respiratory function; ventilatory support may be necessary. Not to be used during labor, because uterine contractions could be suppressed. Avoid with clients with seizure disorders.
isoflurane (Forane)	Rapid	Introduced in the 1980s. Frequently used in inhalation therapy. Has a smooth and rapid induction of anesthesia and rapid recovery. Could cause hypotension and respiratory depression. Not to be used during labor, because it suppresses uterine contractions. Has minimal cardiovascular effect.
desflurane (Suprane)	Rapid	Introduced in 1992 as a volatile liquid anesthetic. Similar to isoflurane. Rapid recovery after anesthetic administration has ceased. Could cause hypotension and respiratory depression.
sevoflurane (Ultane)	Rapid	For induction and maintenance during surgery. May be given alone or combined with nitrous oxide. Rate of elimination similar to desflurane.
Inhalation: Gas		
nitrous oxide (laughing gas)	Very rapid	Rapid recovery. Has minimal cardiovascular effect. Should be given with oxygen. Low potency.
cyclopropane	Very rapid	Highly flammable and explosive. Seldom used.
Intravenous (Ultra-Short Barbiturates)		
thiopental sodium (Pentothal)	Rapid	Has short duration of action. Used for rapid induction of general surgery. Keep client warm; shivering and tremors may occur. Can depress respiratory center; ventilatory assistance might be necessary.
methohexital sodium (Brevital sodium)	Rapid	Has short duration. Frequently used for induction and with other drugs as part of balanced anesthesia. An inhalation anesthesia usually follows.
thiamylal sodium (Surital)	Rapid	Used for induction of anesthesia and as anesthesia for electroshock therapy.
Benzodiazepines		
diazepam (Valium)	Moderate to rapid	For induction of anesthesia. No analgesic effect.
midazolam (Versed)	Rapid	For induction of anesthesia and for endoscopic procedures. IV drug can cause conscious sedation. Avoid if cardiopulmonary disorder is present.
Others		
droperidol and fentanyl (Innovar)	Moderate to rapid	A neuroleptic analgesic when combined with fentanyl (potent opiate narcotic). Frequently used with a general anesthetic. Can also be used as a preanesthetic drug. Also used for diagnostic procedures. May cause hypotension and respiratory depression.
etomidate (Amidate)	Rapid	Used for short-term surgery, for induction of anesthesia, or with a general anesthetic to maintain the anesthetic state.
ketamine hydrochloride (Ketalar)	Rapid	Used for short-term surgery or induction of anesthesia. Increases salivation, blood pressure, and heart rate. May be used for diagnostic procedures. Avoid with history of psychiatric disorders.
propofol (Diprivan)	Rapid	For induction of anesthesia; may be used with general anesthesia. Short duration of action. May cause hypotension and respiratory depression. Pain can occur at injection site, so may be mixed with a local anesthetic (lidocaine) to decrease pain.

h, Hour; *IV*, intravenous; *min*, minute.

tion. Discarding opened vials within 6 hours is a necessary precaution in the prevention of sepsis.

Topical Anesthetics

Use of topical anesthetic agents is limited to mucous membranes, broken or unbroken skin surfaces, and burns. Topical anesthetics come in different forms: solution, liquid spray, ointment, cream, gel, and powder. Topical anesthetics decrease the sensitive nerve endings of the affected area.

Local Anesthetics

Local anesthetics block pain at the site where the drug is administered, allowing consciousness to be maintained. Local anesthetics are useful in dental procedures, suturing skin lacerations, short-term (minor) surgery at a localized area, blocking nerve impulses (nerve block) below the insertion of a spinal anesthetic, and diagnostic procedures such as lumbar puncture and thoracentesis.

Most local anesthetics are divided into two groups, the esters and the amides, according to their basic structures. The amides have a very low incidence of allergic reaction.

The first local anesthetic used was cocaine hydrochloride in the late 1800s. Procaine hydrochloride (Novocain), a synthetic of cocaine, was discovered in the early 1900s. Lidocaine hydrochloride (Xylocaine) was developed in the mid-1950s to replace procaine, except in dental procedures. Lidocaine has a rapid onset and a long duration of action, is more stable in solution, and causes fewer hypersensitivity reactions than procaine. Since the introduction of lidocaine, many local anesthetics have been marketed. Table 20–6 describes the various types of local anesthetics according to short-, moderate-, and long-acting effects.

The PainFree pump system, developed by Sgarlato Labs, controls discomfort in the first 24 to 96 hours postoperatively. This spring-loaded pump administers a local anesthetic by continuous infusion to surgical wound sites. The pump is portable and can be worn in its accompanying carrying case.

Benefits of the pump include increased mobility and reduced narcotic use, drowsiness, nausea, and hospital stay. The PainFree pump method complies with The Joint Commission (TJC) recommendations for pain management. Orthopedic joint surgeries, mastectomy, cesarean section, hysterectomy, hernia repair, and cholecystectomy frequently use the postoperative pain control provided by the pump method. For example, the client who has a bilateral hernia repair has a catheter inserted into deep fascia of the lower abdominal area. A continuous flow of bupivacaine (Marcaine), a local anesthetic, is delivered via a Y-connector to both sides at a flow rate of approximately 2 ml per hour.

Spinal Anesthesia

Spinal anesthesia requires that a local anesthetic be injected in the subarachnoid space at the third or fourth lumbar space. If the local anesthetic is given too high in the spinal column, the respiratory muscles could be affected, and respiratory distress or failure could result. Headaches might result following spinal anesthesia (a "spinal"), possibly because of a decrease in cerebrospinal fluid pressure caused by a leak of fluid at the needle insertion point. Encouraging the client to remain flat following surgery with spinal anesthesia and to take increased fluids usually decreases the likelihood of leaking spinal fluid. Hypotension also can result following spinal anesthesia.

Table 20–6

Local Anesthetics

Anesthetics	Type	Uses and Considerations
Short Acting (½-1 h)		
chloroprocaine (Nesacaine)	Ester	For infiltration, caudal, and epidural anesthesia. Onset of action 6-12 min.
procaine HCl (Novocain)	Ester	Introduced in 1905. For nerve block, infiltration, epidural, and spinal anesthesias. Useful in dentistry. Caution in use for clients allergic to ester-type anesthetics
Moderate Acting (1-3 h)		
lidocaine (Xylocaine)	Amide	Introduced in 1948. For nerve block, infiltration, epidural, and spinal anesthesias. Allergic reaction is rare. Used to treat cardiac dysrhythmias (see Chapter 40).
mepivacaine HCl (Carbocaine HCl; Isocaine; Polocaine)	Amide	For nerve block, infiltration, caudal, and epidural anesthesias. May be used in dentistry.
prilocaine HCl (Citanest)	Amide	For peripheral nerve block, infiltration, caudal, and epidural anesthesias. May be used in dentistry.
Long Acting (3-10 h)		
bupivacaine (Marcaine, Sensorcaine)	Amide	For peripheral nerve block, infiltration, caudal, and epidural anesthesias.
dibucaine HCl (Nupercainal)	Amide	For topical use (creams and ointment) to affected areas.
etidocaine (Duranest)	Amide	For peripheral nerve block, infiltration, caudal, and epidural anesthesias.
tetracaine HCl (Pontocaine)	Ester	For spinal anesthesia (high and low saddle block). Also for topical use to affected areas such as to the eye to anesthetize cornea, to nose and throat for bronchoscopy, to skin for relief of pain and pruritus (itching).

Various sites of the spinal column can be used for a **nerve block** with a local anesthetic (Figure 20–2). A **spinal block** is the penetration of the anesthetic into the subarachnoid membrane, the second layer of the spinal cord. An **epidural block** is the placement of the local anesthetic in the outer covering of the spinal cord, or the dura mater. A **caudal block** is placed near the sacrum. A **saddle block** is given at the lower end of the spinal column to block the perineal area. Blood pressure should be monitored during administration of these types of anesthesia, because a decrease in blood pressure resulting from the drug and procedure might occur. A saddle block is frequently used for women in labor during childbirth. Further discussion of labor and delivery drugs may be found in Chapter 53.

Nurses play an important role in client assessment before and after general and local anesthesia is administered. Preparing the client for surgery by explaining the preparations and completing the preoperative orders, including premedications, are necessary to enhance the safety and effectiveness of anesthesia and surgery.

FIGURE 20–2 Positioning a client for spinal anesthetic.

Nursing Process

Anesthetics

ASSESSMENT

- Record baseline vital signs.
- Obtain a drug history, noting drugs that affect the cardiopulmonary systems.

NURSING DIAGNOSES

- Pain related to injury
- Ineffective breathing pattern related to central nervous system depression

PLANNING

- Client will participate in preoperative preparation and understand postoperative care.
- Client's vital signs will remain stable following surgery.

NURSING INTERVENTIONS

- Monitor client's postoperative state of sensorium. Report if client remains nonresponsive or confused for a time.
- Check preoperative and postoperative urine output. Report deficit of hourly or 8-hour urine output.
- Record vital signs following general and local anesthesia; hypotension and respiratory distress may result.
- Administer an analgesic or a narcotic-analgesic with caution until client fully recovers from anesthetic. To prevent adverse reactions, dosage might need to be adjusted if client is under the influence of anesthetic.

Client Teaching

- Explain to client the preoperative preparation and postoperative nursing assessment and interventions.

Cultural Considerations ❖

- Failing to allow adequate time for information processing may result in an inaccurate response or no response. Allow time for people to respond to questions, especially for those who have language barriers. Speak clearly and slowly, giving time for translation. Obtain an interpreter if necessary.

EVALUATION

- Evaluate client's response to the anesthetics. Continue to monitor client for adverse reactions.

KEY WEBSITES

Anesthetic Risk and the Elderly: http://www.asahq.org/clinical/geriatrics/anesth.htm

Information on Zolpidem: http://www.nlm.nih.gov/medlineplus/druginfo/medmaster/a693025.html

Preanesthetic Evaluation for the Elderly Patient: http://www.asahq.org/clinical/geriatrics/prean_eval.htm

Critical Thinking Case Study

JZ, a 72-year-old woman, has difficulty staying asleep. She asks the nurse whether she should take Nytol or Sominex before bedtime.

1. Before JZ takes any sleep aid or hypnotic, what nursing assessments should be made?
2. Describe a nursing plan that may help alleviate JZ's sleep disturbance.
3. Would JZ be a candidate for taking a barbiturate or a benzodiazepine? Explain.
4. What follow-up plan should the nurse have related to JZ's sleep problem?

NCLEX Study Questions

1. Secobarbital (Seconal) has been ordered for a client to prevent insomnia. The nurse knows that secobarbital is:
   a. a short-acting drug that may cause one to awaken early in the morning
   b. an intermediate-acting drug that frequently causes REM rebound
   c. an intermediate-acting drug that frequently causes a hangover effect
   d. a long-term acting drug that is frequently associated with dependence

2. Lorazepam (Ativan) is a benzodiazepine that acts by:
   a. depressing the central nervous system (CNS), leading to a loss of consciousness
   b. depressing the CNS, including the motor and sensory activities
   c. increasing the action of the inhibitory neurotransmitter gamma-aminobutyric acid (GABA) to GABA receptors
   d. creating an epidural block by placement of the local anesthetic in the outer covering of the spinal cord

3. A client is taking zolpidem (Ambien) for insomnia. The nurse knows that this drug is classified as a:
   a. barbiturate
   b. benzodiazepine
   c. piperidinedione
   d. nonbenzodiazepine

4. A client received spinal anesthesia. Which of the following is most important for the nurse to monitor?
   a. loss of consciousness
   b. hangover effects and dependence
   c. hypotension and headaches
   d. excitement or delirium

5. Which of the following is true regarding zolpidem?
   a. maximum dose is 20 mg/day
   b. may lead to psychologic dependence
   c. for the elderly, dose is 15 mg at bedtime
   d. should only be used for 21 days or less

Answers: 1, a; 2, c; 3, d; 4, c; 5, b.

21
Anticonvulsants

Outline

Objectives

- Contrast the two international classifications of seizures with characteristics of each type.
- Differentiate between the types of seizures.
- Summarize the pharmacokinetics, side effects and adverse reactions, therapeutic plasma phenytoin level, contraindications for use, and drug interactions of phenytoin (Dilantin).
- Describe the uses for hydantoins, long-acting barbiturates, succinimides, oxazolidones, benzodiazepines, iminostilbenes, and valproate.
- Apply the nursing process to anticonvulsants.

Terms

anoxia, p. 322
anticonvulsants, p. 322
atonic seizure, p. 322
clonic seizure, p. 322

electroencephalogram (EEG), p. 321
gingival hyperplasia, p. 323
grand mal, p. 322

hydantoins, p. 323
idiopathic, p. 322
nystagmus, p. 323
petit mal, p. 322

psychomotor, p. 322
status epilepticus, p. 324
teratogenic, p. 323
tonic seizure, p. 322

It is estimated that approximately 2.7 million people in the United States have active epilepsy, a seizure disorder. The seizure associated with epilepsy results from abnormal electric discharges from the cerebral neurons and is characterized by a loss or disturbance of consciousness and usu-ally by a convulsion (abnormal motor reaction). The **electroencephalogram (EEG)**, computerized tomography (CT), and magnetic resonance imaging (MRI) are useful in diagnosing epilepsy. The EEG records abnormal electric discharges of the cerebral cortex. Of all epilepsy cases, 50%

are considered to be primary, or **idiopathic** (of unknown cause), and 50% are considered to be secondary to trauma, brain **anoxia** (absence of oxygen), infection, or cerebrovascular disorders (e.g., cerebrovascular accidents or stroke).

Epilepsy is a chronic, usually lifelong, disorder. The majority of persons with seizures had their first seizure before 20 years of age. Isolated seizures could result from fever, hypoglycemic reaction, electrolyte imbalance (hyponatremia), acid-base imbalance (acidosis or alkalosis), and alcohol or drug withdrawal. When these conditions are corrected, the seizures cease. Recurrent seizures may result from birth and perinatal injuries, head trauma, congenital malformations, neoplasms (tumors), and idiopathic or unknown causes.

International Classification of Seizures

There are various types and names of seizures, such as **grand mal** (tonic-clonic), **petit mal** (absence), and **psychomotor**. The international classification of seizures (Table 21–1) describes two categories of seizure: generalized and partial. A person may have more than one type of seizure.

Anticonvulsants

Drugs used for epileptic seizures are called **anticonvulsants** or antiepileptic drugs (AEDs). Anticonvulsant drugs suppress the abnormal electric impulses from the seizure focus to other cortical areas, thus preventing the seizure but not eliminating the cause of the seizure. Anticonvulsants are classified as central nervous system (CNS) depressants.

With the use of anticonvulsants, approximately 70% of persons with epilepsy are free of seizures. Anticonvulsants are usually taken throughout the person's lifetime. In some cases, the health care provider might discontinue the anticonvulsant if there has not been a seizure in the past 3 to 5 years.

Before 1850 there were various remedies for control of seizures. In 1857 potassium bromide was the first treatment to successfully control seizures. Bromide was the primary anticonvulsant used for years, although the drug was habit forming and caused side effects. Phenobarbital was introduced in 1918 and phenytoin (Dilantin) in 1938. Both are still used for seizure disorders.

There are many types of anticonvulsants used to treat epilepsy, including the hydantoins (phenytoin, mephenytoin, ethotoin), long-acting barbiturates (phenobarbital, me-

Table 21–1

International Classification of Seizures

Category	Characteristics
Generalized Seizures	Convulsive and nonconvulsive; involve both cerebral hemispheres of the brain
Tonic-clonic seizure	Also called *grand mal seizure*; most common form of seizure. In the tonic phase, skeletal muscles contract or tighten in a spasm lasting 3 to 5 seconds. In the clonic phase, there is a dysrhythmic muscular contraction, or jerkiness, of legs and arms lasting 2 to 4 minutes
Tonic seizure	Sustained muscle contraction
Clonic seizure	Dysrhythmic muscle contraction
Absence seizure	Also called *petit mal seizure*; brief loss of consciousness lasting less than 10 seconds; fewer than three spike waves on the electroencephalogram (EEG) printout; usually occurs in children
Myoclonic seizure	Isolated clonic contraction or jerks lasting 3 to 10 seconds; may be limited to one limb (focal myoclonic) or involve the entire body (massive myoclonic); may be secondary to a neurologic disorder such as encephalitis or Tay-Sachs disease
Atonic seizure	Head drop; loss of posture; sudden loss of muscle tone. If lower limbs are involved, client could collapse
Infantile spasms	Muscle spasm
Partial Seizures	Involve one hemisphere of the brain. No loss of consciousness in simple partial seizures, but there is a loss of consciousness in complex partial seizures
Simple seizure	Occurs in motor, sensory, autonomic, and psychic forms; no loss of consciousness
Motor	Formerly called the *jacksonian seizure*; involves spontaneous movement that spreads; can develop into a generalized seizure
Sensory	Visual, auditory, or taste hallucinations
Autonomic response	Paleness, flushing, sweating, or vomiting
Psychologic	Personality changes
Complex seizure	There is a loss of consciousness. Client does not recall behavior immediately before, during, and immediately after seizure
Psychomotor	Complex symptoms: automatisms (repetitive behavior such as chewing or swallowing motions), behavioral changes, and motor seizures
Cognitive	Confusion or memory impairment
Affective	Bizarre behavior
Compound	May lead to generalized seizures such as tonic-clonic, tonic

phobarbital, primidone), succinimides (ethosuximide), oxazolidones (trimethadione), benzodiazepines (diazepam, clonazepam), carbamazepine, and valproate (valproic acid). Anticonvulsants are not used for all types of seizures. For example, the hydantoin phenytoin is effective in treating grand mal (tonic-clonic) seizures and psychomotor seizures but is not effective in treating petit mal (absence) seizures.

Pharmacophysiology: Action of Anticonvulsants

The anticonvulsant drugs work in one of three ways: (1) by suppressing sodium influx through the drug binding to the sodium channel when it is inactivated, prolonging the channel inactivation and thereby preventing neuron firing; (2) by suppressing the calcium influx, preventing the electric current generated by the calcium ions to the T-type calcium channel; and (3) by increasing the action of gamma-aminobutyric acid (GABA), which inhibits neurotransmitter throughout the brain. The drugs that suppress sodium influx are phenytoin, fosphenytoin, carbamazepine, oxcarbazepine, valproic acid, topiramate, zonisamide, and lamotrigine. Valproic acid and ethosuximide are examples of drugs that suppress calcium influx. Examples of drug groups that enhance the action of GABA are barbiturates, benzodiazepines, and tiagabine. Gabapentin promotes GABA release. A new anticonvulsant, vigabatrin, inhibits the degradation of GABA from enzyme action.

Hydantoins

The first anticonvulsant used to treat seizures was phenytoin, a hydantoin discovered in 1938 that is still the most commonly used drug for controlling seizures. **Hydantoins** act by inhibiting sodium influx, stabilizing cell membranes, reducing repetitive neuronal firing, and limiting seizures. By increasing the electrical stimulation threshold in cardiac tissue, it also acts as an antidysrhythmic. It has a small effect on general sedation, and is nonaddicting. However, this drug should not be used during pregnancy, because it can have a **teratogenic** effect on the fetus.

Drug dosage for phenytoin, as well as for other anticonvulsants, varies according to the age of the client. Newborns, persons with liver disease, and older adults require a lower dosage because of a decrease in metabolism resulting in more available drug. Children and young and middle-aged adults have an increased metabolic rate. The drug dosage is adjusted according to the therapeutic plasma or serum level. Phenytoin has a narrow therapeutic range of 10-20 mcg/ml. The benefits of an anticonvulsant become apparent when the serum drug level is within the therapeutic range; if, however, the drug level is below the desired range, the client is not receiving the required drug dosage to prevent seizures. If the drug level is above the desired range, drug toxicity may result. Monitoring the therapeutic serum drug range is of utmost importance to ensure drug effectiveness. Prototype Drug Chart 21–1 lists the pharmacologic data associated with phenytoin.

Pharmacokinetics

Phenytoin is slowly absorbed from the small intestine. It is a highly protein-bound (85% to 95%) drug; a decrease in serum protein or albumin can increase the free phenytoin serum level. With a small to average drug dose, the half-life of phenytoin is approximately 22 hours, but the range can be from 6 to 45 hours. Phenytoin is metabolized to inactive metabolites, and that portion is excreted in the urine.

Pharmacodynamics

The pharmacodynamics of orally administered phenytoin include onset of action within 30 minutes to 2 hours, peak serum concentration in 1.5 to 3 hours, steady state of serum concentration in 7 to 10 days, and a duration of action dependent on the half-life. Oral phenytoin is most commonly ordered as a sustained-release (SR) capsule. The peak SR concentration time is 4 to 12 hours.

Intravenous (IV) infusion of phenytoin should be administered by direct injection into a large vein. The drug may be diluted in saline solution; however, dextrose solution should be avoided because of drug precipitation. Continuous IV infusion of phenytoin should not be used. IV phenytoin, 50 mg or fraction thereof, should be administered over a period of 1 minute for adults and, when the client is elderly, at a rate of 25 mg per minute. Infusion rates of more than 50 mg per minute may cause hypotension or cardiac dysrhythmias, especially with older and debilitated clients. Local irritation at the injection site may be noted, and sloughing may occur. Intramuscular (IM) injection of phenytoin irritates tissues and may cause damage. For this reason and because of its erratic absorption rate, IM administration of phenytoin is discouraged.

Mephenytoin is a potent hydantoin and much more toxic than phenytoin. It is used for severe grand mal or psychomotor seizures that do not respond to phenytoin or other anticonvulsant therapy. The newest hydantoin, ethotoin, produces similar responses as phenytoin and has a shorter half-life of 3 to 6 hours; therefore the chance of cumulative drug effects decreases.

Side Effects and Adverse Reactions

The severe side effects of hydantoins include **gingival hyperplasia,** or overgrowth of the gum tissues (reddened gums that bleed easily); neurologic and psychiatric effects, such as slurred speech, confusion, depression, and thrombocytopenia (low platelet count); and leukopenia (low white blood cell count). Clients on hydantoins for long periods might have an elevated blood sugar (hyperglycemia), which results from the drug inhibiting the release of insulin. Less severe side effects include nausea, vomiting, constipation, drowsiness, headaches, alopecia, hirsutism, and **nystagmus** (constant, involuntary, cyclical movement of the eyeball).

Drug-Drug Interactions

Drug-drug interaction is common with hydantoins, because they are highly protein-bound. Hydantoins compete with other drugs (e.g., anticoagulants and aspirin) for plasma protein-binding sites. The hydantoins displace anticoagulants and aspirin, causing more free drug and increasing their activity. Barbiturates, rifampin, and a chronic ingestion of ethanol increase hydantoin metabolism. Drugs like sulfonamides and cimetidine (Tagamet) can increase the action of hydantoins by inhibiting liver metabolism, which is necessary for drug excretion. Absorption of hydantoins can be decreased by antacids, calcium preparations, sucralfate (Carafate) and antineoplastic

Prototype **DRUG CHART 21–1**

PHENYTOIN

Drug Class

Anticonvulsant, hydantoin
Trade name: Dilantin
Pregnancy Category: D

Dosage

A: PO: 100 mg, t.i.d., q.i.d.
IV: LD: 10-15 mg/kg/d; infusion ,<50 mg/min; *max:* 300 mg/d in divided doses
C: Initially 5 mg/kg/d in 2-3 divided doses; 4-8 mg/kg/d in divided doses
Therapeutic serum range: 10-20 mcg/ml
Toxic level: 30-50 mcg/ml

Contraindications

Hypersensitivity, heart block, psychiatric disorders, pregnancy

Drug-Lab-Food Interactions

Drug: Increase effects with cimetidine, isoniazid, chloramphenicol; *decrease* effects with folic acid, calcium, antacids, sucralfate, vinblastine, cisplatin
Decrease effects of anticoagulants, oral contraceptives, antihistamines, corticosteroids, theophylline, cyclosporin, quinidine, dopamine, rifampin
Food: Decreased effects of folic acid, calcium, and vitamin D absorption by phenytoin

Pharmacokinetics

Absorption: PO: Slowly absorbed; IM: Erratic rate of absorption
Distribution: PB: 85%-95%
Metabolism: t½: 6-45 h; average: 22 h
Excretion: In urine, small amount; in bile and feces, moderate amount

Pharmacodynamics

PO: Onset: 0.5-2 h
      Peak: 1.5-3 h
      Duration: 6-12 h
IV: Onset: within min-1 h
      Peak: 2 h
      Duration: >12 h

Therapeutic Effects/Uses

To prevent tonic-clonic (grand mal) and complex partial seizures
Mode of Action: Reduces motor cortex activity by altering transport of ions

Side Effects

Headache, diplopia, confusion, dizziness, sluggishness, decreased coordination, ataxia, slurred speech, rash, anorexia, nausea, vomiting, hypotension (IV), pink-red/brown discoloration of urine

Adverse Reactions

Leukopenia, hepatitis, depression, gingival hyperplasia, gingivitis, nystagmus, hirsutism, osteoporosis
Life-threatening: Aplastic anemia, thrombocytopenia, agranulocytosis, Stevens-Johnson syndrome, hypotension, ventricular fibrillation, encephalopathy

A, Adult; *C*, child; *d*, day; *h*, hour; *IM*, intramuscular; *IV*, intravenous; *LD*, loading dose; *max*, maximum; *min*, minute; *PB*, protein-binding; *PO*, by mouth; *q.i.d.*, four times a day; *t½*, half-life; *t.i.d.*, three times a day; >, greater than; <, less than.

---

drugs. Antipsychotics and certain herbs can lower the seizure threshold and increase seizure activity (Herbal Alert 21–1). The client should be closely monitored for seizure occurrence.

Barbiturates

Phenobarbital, a long-acting barbiturate, is still prescribed to treat partial seizures, grand mal seizures and acute episodes of **status epilepticus** seizures (rapid succession of epileptic seizures), meningitis, toxic reactions, and eclampsia. Barbiturates reduce seizures by enhancing the activity of GABA, which is an inhibitory neurotransmitter. Possible teratogenic effects and other side effects related to phenytoin are less pronounced with phenobarbital. The

Herbal **ALERT 21–1**

Anticonvulsants

Evening primrose and borage may lower seizure threshold when these herbs are taken with anticonvulsants. The anticonvulsant dose may need modification.
• Ginkgo may decrease phenytoin effectiveness.

therapeutic serum range of phenobarbital is 15-40 mcg/ml. Problems associated with phenobarbital include sedation and client tolerance to the drug. Discontinuance of phenobarbital should be gradual to avoid recurrence of seizures.

Succinimides

The succinimide drug group is used to treat absence or petit mal seizures, and it may be used in combination with other anticonvulsants to treat such seizures. Ethosuximide (Zarontin) is the succinimide of choice. Succinimides act by decreasing calcium influx through the T-type calcium channels. The therapeutic serum range of ethosuximide is 40-100 mcg/ml. Adverse affects include blood dyscrasias, renal and liver impairment, and systemic lupus erythematosus.

Oxazolidones/Oxazolidinedione

The oxazolidones, trimethadione and paramethadione, are also prescribed to treat petit mal seizures. Trimethadione was the first drug developed for petit mal. There are many severe side effects associated with this group of anticonvulsants. Trimethadione may be used in combination with other drugs or singly to treat refractory petit mal seizures.

Benzodiazepines

The three benzodiazepines that have anticonvulsant effects are clonazepam, clorazepate dipotassium, and diazepam. Clonazepam is effective in controlling petit mal (absence) seizures, but tolerance may occur 6 months after drug therapy starts, and consequently clonazepam dosage has to be adjusted. The therapeutic serum range of clonazepam is 20-80 ng/ml. Clorazepate dipotassium is frequently administered in adjunctive therapy for treating partial seizures.

Diazepam is primarily prescribed for treating acute status epilepticus and must be administered IV to achieve the desired response. The drug has a short-term effect; thus other anticonvulsants such as phenytoin or phenobarbital need to be given during or immediately after administration of diazepam.

Iminostilbenes

Carbamazepine, an iminostilbene, is effective in treating refractory seizure disorders that have not responded to other anticonvulsant therapies. It is used to control grand mal and partial seizures and a combination of these seizures.

Carbamazepine is also used for psychiatric disorders (e.g., bipolar disease), trigeminal neuralgia (as an analgesic), and alcohol withdrawal. The therapeutic serum range of carbamazepine is 5-12 mcg/ml.

An interaction may occur when grapefruit juice is taken with carbamazepine (Tegretol), causing possible toxicity. Therefore drug concentrations must be monitored carefully.

Valproate

Valproic acid has been prescribed for petit mal, grand mal, and mixed types of seizures. Care should be taken when giving this drug to very young children and clients with liver disorders, because hepatotoxicity is one of the possible adverse reactions. Liver enzymes should be monitored. The therapeutic serum range is 40-100 mcg/ml. The FDA has approved divalproex sodium (Depakote) for treatment of manic episodes associated with bipolar disorder.

Table 21–2 lists the various anticonvulsants and their dosages, uses, and considerations. Table 21–3 lists selected

---

Table 21–2

Anticonvulsants

Generic (Brand)	Route and Dosage	Uses and Considerations
Barbiturates		
mephobarbital (Mebaral) CSS II	A: PO: 400-600 mg/d in divided doses C: PO: 6-12 mg/kg/d in divided doses or C: 5 y: 32-64 mg t.i.d./q.i.d. C: <5 y: 16-32 mg t.i.d./q.i.d.	For grand mal and petit mal (absence) seizures. May be used in combination with other anticonvulsants. Also used to manage delirium tremens. May cause drowsiness and dizziness. *Pregnancy category:* D; PB: UK; t½: 34 h
phenobarbital (generic) CSS IV	Status epilepticus: Neonate: IV: LD: 15-20 mg/kg single or divided dose A & C: IV: 15-18 mg/kg; *max:* 30 mg/kg Maintenance: Neonate: PO/IV: 3-4 mg/kg/d in 1-2 divided doses Infant: 5-6 mg/kg/d in 1-2 divided doses C: 1-5 y: PO: 6-8 mg/kg/d in 1-2 divided doses C: 6-12 y: PO: 4-6 mg/kg/d in 1-2 divided doses A: PO: 1-3 mg/kg/d; 100-300 mg/d in divided doses Therapeutic serum range: 15-40 mcg/ml	Long-acting barbiturate. Used for grand mal (tonic-clonic), partial seizures, and to control status epilepticus. May be used in combination with phenytoin. High doses given to older adults or children may cause confusion, depression, irritability. Long-term use with high doses could cause physical dependence. *Pregnancy category:* D; PB: 20%-40%; t½: A: 50-140 h; C: 35-75 h
primidone (Mysoline)	A: PO: 125-250 mg b.i.d./q.i.d.; *max:* 2 g/d C: <8 y: PO: half of adult dose Therapeutic serum range: 5-10 mcg/ml	Barbiturate-like drug. Used to manage grand mal and psychomotor seizures. Take with food if drug causes GI distress. *Pregnancy category:* D; PB: 99%; t½: 10-24 h

A, Adult; *b.i.d.*, twice a day; *C*, child; *CSS*, Controlled Substances Schedule; *GI*, gastrointestinal; *d*, day; *h*, hour; *IV*, intravenous; *LD*, loading dose; *max*, maximum; *min*, minute; *PB*, protein-binding; *PE*, phenytoin equivalents; *PO*, by mouth; *PRN*, as needed; *q.i.d.*, four times a day; *t½*, half-life; *UK*, unknown; *y*, year; *>*, greater than; *<*, less than.

Continued

Table 21–2

Anticonvulsants—cont'd

Generic (Brand)	Route and Dosage	Uses and Considerations
Benzodiazepines (Anxiolytics)		
clonazepam (Klonopin) CSS IV	A: PO: 0.5-1 mg t.i.d.; gradually increase dose q3d until seizures are controlled C: PO: 0.01-0.03 mg/kg/d; gradually increase Therapeutic serum range: 20-80 ng/ml	For petit mal, myoclonus, and status epilepticus. May be used when petit mal (absence) seizures are refractory to succinimides or valproic acid. *Pregnancy category:* C; PB: 85%; t^{1}/$_{2}$: A: 20-50 h; C: 24-36 h
clorazepate (Tranxene) CSS IV	A: PO: 7.5 mg t.i.d. C: >9 y: PO: 7.5 mg b.i.d.	May be used for partial seizures and as adjunctive therapy for seizures. Also treats anxiety and acute alcohol withdrawal. *Pregnancy category:* D; PB: 97%; t^{1}/$_{2}$: 48 h
diazepam (Valium) CSS IV	Status epilepticus: A: IV: 5-10 mg; repeat if needed at 10- to 15-min intervals; *max:* 30 mg C <5 y: IV: 0.2-0.5 mg over 2-5 min; *max:* 5 mg C >5 y: IV 1 mg slowly; repeat if needed	For status epilepticus (drug of choice). Administer IV and repeat q10-15min up to 30 mg PRN; then q2-4h PRN. Also treats anxiety and acute alcohol withdrawal. *Pregnancy category:* D; PB: 98%; t^{1}/$_{2}$: 20-50 h
lorazepam (Ativan) CSS IV	Status epilepticus: Neonate: IV: 0.05 mg/kg over 2-5 min; may repeat in 10-15 min Infants & C: 0.1 mg/kg over 2-5 min; *max:* 4 mg/single dose A: IV: 4 mg over 2-5 min; *max:* 8 mg; may repeat in 10-15 min for all ages Therapeutic serum range: 50-240 ng/ml	To control status epilepticus. Infusion rate should not exceed 2 mg/min. Also treats anxiety and acute alcohol withdrawal. *Pregnancy category:* D; PB: 85%; t^{1}/$_{2}$: 10-16 h
Hydantoins		
fosphenytoin (Cerebyx)	A: IV: LD: 10-20 mg PE/kg Maintenance: 4-6 mg PE/kg/d Status epilepticus: IV: LD: 15-20 mg PE/kg infused at 100-150 mg PE/min	To treat grand mal seizures, complex partial seizures, and status epilepticus. Decreases sodium and calcium ion influx in the neurons. Converts to phenytoin. Dilute in D$_{5}$W or 0.9% NaCl. *Pregnancy category:* D; PB: 95-99%; t^{1}/$_{2}$: 8-15 min
mephenytoin (Mesantoin)	A: PO: Initially: 50-100 mg; 100-200 mg t.i.d. C: PO: Initially: 50-100 mg; 100-400 mg/d in 3 divided doses or 3-15 mg/kg/d in Therapeutic serum range: 25-40 mcg/ml	For grand mal, psychomotor, focal (simple) seizures. Severe adverse reaction may include blood dyscrasias. *Pregnancy category:* C; PB: UK; t^{1}/$_{2}$: 7 h; metabolite: 100-144 h
phenytoin (Dilantin)	See Prototype Drug Chart 21–1.	
Iminostilbene		
carbamazepine (Tegretol)	A: PO: 200 mg b.i.d.; increasing doses as needed C: PO: 10-20 mg/kg/d in divided doses or 100 mg b.i.d. Therapeutic serum range: 5-12 mcg/ml	For grand mal, psychomotor, mixed seizures. Used in treating seizures that do not respond to other anticonvulsants. *Pregnancy category:* C; PB: 75%-90%; t^{1}/$_{2}$: 15-30 h
oxcarbazepine (Trileptal)	A: PO: 300 mg b.i.d.; increase to 1200-2400 mg/d C: PO: 8-10 mg/kg; *max:* 600 mg/d	To control refractory partial seizures as monotherapy. Can be used for generalized tonic-clonic seizures. Blocks the sodium channel. Less severe side effects than carbamazepine. *Pregnancy category:* D; PB: UK; t^{1}/$_{2}$: 8-10 h
Oxazolidones		
paramethadione (Paradione)	A: PO: 300-600 mg t.i.d./q.i.d. C: PO: 13 mg/kg t.i.d. or 335 mg/m^{2} t.i.d. or 300-900 mg/d in divided doses	For petit mal (absence) seizures. May be used when refractory to other anticonvulsants. *Pregnancy category:* D; PB: UK; t^{1}/$_{2}$: 1-4 h
trimethadione (Tridione)	Same as paramethadione	For petit mal seizures. May be used when refractory to other anticonvulsants. Has many side effects. After prolonged use, drug should be withdrawn gradually. *Pregnancy category:* D; PB: ,10%; t^{1}/$_{2}$: 6-12 d
Succinimides		
ethosuximide (Zarontin)	A: PO: 250 mg b.i.d.; increase dose gradually C: 3-6 y: PO: 250 mg/d Therapeutic serum range: 40-100 mcg/ml	For petit mal and myoclonic seizures. Gastric irritation is common; may take with food. *Pregnancy category:* C; PB: UK; t^{1}/$_{2}$: A: 50-60 h, C: 25-30 h

GABA, Gamma aminobutyric acid; *SR,* sustained release.

Table 21-2

Anticonvulsants—cont'd

Generic (Brand)	Route and Dosage	Uses and Considerations
Valproate valproic acid (Depakene) Divalproex Na (Depakote)	A & C: PO: 15 mg/kg; *max:* 60 mg/kg/d in divided doses Therapeutic serum range: 40-100 mcg/ml	For grand mal, petit mal, psychomotor, and myoclonic seizures. Doses may be increased weekly by 5-10 mg/kg/d until seizures are controlled. Avoid during pregnancy. *Pregnancy category:* D; PB: 90%; t$\frac{1}{2}$: 6-16 h
Miscellaneous acetazolamide (Diamox)	Commonly used with other anticonvulsants: A: PO/IM/IV: 375 mg/d; *max:* 250 mg q.i.d. or PO SR: 250-500 mg daily or b.i.d. C: PO: 8-30 mg/kg in divided doses; *max:* 1.5 g/d	For grand mal, petit mal (absence), and focal seizures. Adequate fluid intake should be maintained to prevent kidney stones. *Pregnancy category:* D; PB: 90%; t$\frac{1}{2}$: 2.5-6 h
gabapentin (Neurontin)	Adjunctive therapy for partial seizures: A: PO: 900-1800 mg/d in 3 divided doses; *max time between doses:* 12 h; *max:* 2400 mg/d in divided doses	Used as adjunctive therapy for partial seizures. Promotes GABA release. To avoid GI upset, give drug with food. If drug is discontinued, dose should be gradually reduced to avoid occurrence of seizures. *Pregnancy category:* C; PB: 3%; t$\frac{1}{2}$: 5-7 h
felbamate (Felbatol)	A: PO: 1200 mg/d in divided doses C: >2 y: PO: 45 mg/kg/d in divided doses	To treat partial and secondary generalized seizures. Also used in adjunctive therapy for treatment of Lennox-Gastaut syndrome in children. Weak inhibitory effect on GABA-receptor binding. CONTRAINDICATIONS: Client with a blood disorder (reported incidences of aplastic anemia from use of the drug). *Pregnancy category:* C; PB: UK; t$\frac{1}{2}$: UK
Miscellaneous lamotrigine (Lamictal)	A: PO: Initially: 25-50 mg/d for 2 wk; then 50 mg b.i.d. for 2 wk *Maintenance:* 300-500 mg/d in 2 divided doses; if used with valproic acid, daily doses need to be reduced	Used for partial seizures and in adjunctive anticonvulsant therapy. Also to treat tonic-clonic, absence, atypical absence, and myoclonic seizures, and for treatment of Lennox-Gastaut syndrome in infants and children. Blocks the sodium influx. May be given with other anticonvulsants. *Pregnancy category:* C; PB: UK; t$\frac{1}{2}$: 12.5-25 h (half-life is increased when given with other anticonvulsants)
levetiracetam (Keppra)	A: PO: 500 mg b.i.d.; may increase dose by 1000 mg/d; *max:* 3000 mg/d	To treat complex partial seizures. For adjunctive and monotherapy. Unlikely to cause drug interactions. *Pregnancy category:* UK; PB: 0%; t$\frac{1}{2}$: 6-8 h
tiagabine (Gabitril)	A: PO: 4 mg/d; may increase by 4-8 mg/d; *max:* 56 mg/d C: 12-18 y: PO: 4 m/g/d; may increase by 4-8 mg; *max:* 32 mg/d	For partial seizures as adjunctive therapy. Increases GABA levels. *Pregnancy category:* UK; PB: UK; t$\frac{1}{2}$: UK
topiramate (Topamax)	A: PO: 25-50 mg/d; *max:* 400 mg/d; may be increased by weekly increment C: 2-16 y: PO: Initially 25 mg/d; increase 1-3 mg/kg/d to 5-9 mg/kg/d in divided doses	For partial seizures and generalized tonic-clonic seizures. Inhibits calcium channels and increases action of GABA. Older adults can take adult dose. *Pregnancy category:* UK; PB: UK; t$\frac{1}{2}$: UK.
zonisamide (Zonegran)	A & C >16 y: PO: 100 mg/d for 2 wk; may increase 100 mg/d at intervals of 2 wk; *max:* 400 mg/d	For adjunctive treatment of partial seizures. Blocks sodium and calcium channels. Does not affect serum levels of phenytoin or valproic acid. Contraindicated if sensitive to sulfonamides. *Pregnancy category:* X; PB: UK; t$\frac{1}{2}$: 60 h
magnesium sulfate	Preeclampsia or eclampsia: A: IV: Initially: 4 g in 250 ml D$_5$W; then 4 g IM: follow with 4 g IM q4h PRN or Inf: 1-4 g/h Hypomagnesemic seizures: A: IV: 1-2 g (19% sol) over 20 min; follow with 1 g IM q4-6h based on blood levels	To control seizures in toxemia of pregnancy caused by eclampsia or preeclampsia. *Pregnancy category:* B; PB: UK; t$\frac{1}{2}$: UK
pregabalin (Lyrica)	Adjunctive therapy for partial seizures: A: PO: 50-600 mg/d bid; *max:* 600 mg/d	For partial seizures and neuralgia. Binds alpha2-delta receptor sites affecting calcium channels in CNS tissues. *Pregnancy category:* C; PB: 0%; t$\frac{1}{2}$: 6 h

CNS, Central nervous system; *IM*, intramuscular; *sol*, solution.

anticonvulsants that are frequently prescribed to treat seizure disorders.

Anticonvulsant dosages usually start low and gradually increase over a period of weeks until the serum drug level is within therapeutic range or the seizures stop. Serum anticonvulsant drug levels should be closely monitored to prevent toxicity.

Anticonvulsants and Pregnancy

During pregnancy, seizure episodes increase 25% in women with epilepsy. Hypoxia that may occur during seizures places both the pregnant woman and her fetus at risk.

Many anticonvulsant drugs have teratogenic properties that increase the risk for fetal malformations, but many women with epilepsy give birth to normal infants. Phenytoin and carbamazepine have been linked to fetal anomalies such as cardiac defects and cleft lip and palate. Trimethadione should not be given to women of childbearing age because of its strong teratogenic effect. It has been reported that valproic acid is known to cause major congenital malformation in infants in 4% to 8% of pregnant women who take the drug. As expected, the highest incidence of birth defects occurs when the woman takes combinations of anticonvulsant drugs.

Anticonvulsant drugs increase the loss of folate (folic acid) in pregnant women, so daily folate supplements should be taken. Anticonvulsants tend to act as inhibitors of vitamin K, contributing to hemorrhaging in infants shortly after birth. Frequently pregnant women taking anticonvulsants are given an oral vitamin K supplement during the last week or 10 days of the pregnancy, or vitamin K is administered to the infant soon after birth.

Anticonvulsants and Febrile Seizures

Seizures associated with fever usually occur in children between the ages of 3 months and 5 years. Epilepsy develops in approximately 2.5% of children who have had one or more febrile seizures. Prophylactic anticonvulsant treatment such as phenobarbital or diazepam may be indicated for high-risk clients. Valproic acid should not be given to children because of its possible hepatotoxic effect.

Table 21–3

Selected Anticonvulsants for Seizure Disorders

Seizure Disorder	Drug Therapy
Tonic-clonic (grand mal)	phenytoin carbamazepine fosphenytoin valproic acid lamotrigine primidone phenobarbital
Partial (complex-secondarily generalized)	phenytoin carbamazepine oxcarbazepine levetiracetam primidone phenobarbital tiagabine topiramate zonisamide
Absence (petit mal)	ethosuximide valproic acid lamotrigine clonazepam
Myoclonic, atonic, atypical absence	valproic acid lamotrigine clonazepam
Status epilepticus	diazepam fosphenytoin lorazepam phenytoin

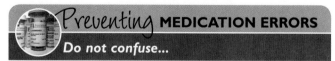

Preventing MEDICATION ERRORS

Do not confuse...

Cerebyx (hydantoin anticonvulsant) with **Celebrex** (nonsteroid antiinflammatory drug). The names of these drugs look and sound alike but are different in their pharmacology.

Nursing Process

Anticonvulsants: Phenytoin

ASSESSMENT

■ Obtain a drug history of current drugs and herbs client is taking. Report if a drug-drug or herb-drug interaction is probable.

■ Check urinary output to determine if adequate (>600 ml/d).

■ Determine laboratory values related to renal and liver function. If both BUN and creatinine levels are elevated, a renal disorder should be suspected. Elevated serum liver enzymes (alkaline phosphatase, alanine aminotransferase, gamma-glutamyl transferase, 59-nucleotidase) indicate a hepatic disorder.

NURSING DIAGNOSES

■ Risk for injury related to decreased coordination
■ Impaired oral mucous membranes related to blood dyscrasias
■ Imbalanced nutrition: less than body requirements related to anorexia

PLANNING

■ Client will be free of seizures and will adhere to anticonvulsant therapy.

■ Client's side effects from phenytoin will be minimal.

NURSING INTERVENTIONS

■ Monitor serum drug levels of anticonvulsant to determine overdosing or underdosing of drug.

■ Promote client's compliance to medication regimen.

■ Monitor client's CBC levels for early detection of blood dyscrasias.

■ Protect client from hazards in the environment such as sharp objects and table corners during a seizure.

■ Determine whether client is receiving adequate nutrients; phenytoin may cause anorexia, nausea, and vomiting.

■ Advise women taking oral contraceptives and anticonvulsants to use an additional contraceptive method.

Client Teaching

General

• Instruct client to shake the suspension form thoroughly to assure accurate dosage.

• Advise client not to drive or perform other hazardous activities when beginning anticonvulsant therapy. Until client adapts to drug dosage, drowsiness is likely to occur.

• Instruct female clients contemplating pregnancy to consult with health care provider, because phenytoin and valproic acid may have a teratogenic effect.

• Monitor serum phenytoin levels closely during pregnancy, because seizures tend to become more frequent due to increased metabolic rates. Most anticonvulsants are classified as pregnancy category D.

• Inform client that alcohol and other CNS depressants can cause an added depressive effect on the body and should be avoided.

• Explain to client that certain herbs can interact with an anticonvulsant drug (Herbal Alert 21–1). Anticonvulsant dose may need to be adjusted.

• Encourage client to obtain a medical alert identification card, medical alert bracelet, or tag that indicates the health problem and drug taken.

• Teach client not to abruptly stop drug therapy, but rather to withdraw the prescribed drug gradually under medical supervision to prevent seizure rebound (recurrence of seizures) and status epilepticus.

• Counsel client of the need for preventive dental check-ups.

• Warn client to take the prescribed anticonvulsant, get laboratory tests as ordered, and keep follow-up visits with health care provider.

• Teach client not to self-medicate with OTC drugs without first consulting health care provider.

• Instruct client with diabetes to monitor serum glucose levels more closely than usual because phenytoin may inhibit insulin release, causing an increase in glucose level.

• Inform client of the existence of national, state, and local associations that provide resources, current information, and support for persons with epilepsy.

Diet

• Educate client to take anticonvulsant at the same time every day with food or milk.

Side Effects

• Tell client that urine may be a harmless pinkish red or reddish brown.

• Instruct client to maintain good oral hygiene and to use a soft toothbrush to prevent gum irritation and bleeding.

• Teach client to report symptoms of sore throat, bruising, and nosebleeds, which may indicate a blood dyscrasia.

• Encourage client to inform health care provider of adverse reactions such as gingivitis, nystagmus (involuntary movement of the eyeball), slurred speech, rash, and dizziness.

Cultural Considerations ❖

• Communicate respect for cultural beliefs concerning refusal or reluctance to take anticonvulsant medications daily for life; use an interpreter and the extended family as needed to help client understand importance of keeping to prescribed drug regimen.

• Use a written drug schedule in client's preferred language to support adherence to prescribed drug regimen.

• Encourage client's compliance with follow up by a community nurse.

• When language barriers exist, videos and pictures showing client's own cultural group may help strengthen compliance with health interventions.

EVALUATION

■ Evaluate the effectiveness of the drug in controlling seizures.

■ Continue to monitor serum phenytoin levels to determine whether they are within the desired range. High serum levels of phenytoin are frequently indicators of phenytoin toxicity.

■ Monitor client for hydantoin overdose. Symptoms are nystagmus and ataxia (impaired coordination) initially, later hypotension, unresponsive pupils, and coma. Respiratory and circulatory support, as well as hemodialysis are usually used in the treatment of phenytoin overdose.

Anticonvulsants and Status Epilepticus

Status epilepticus, a continuous seizure state, is considered a medical emergency. If treatment is not begun immediately, death could result. The choices of pharmacologic agents are diazepam (Valium) administered IV or lorazepam (Ativan) followed by IV administration of phenytoin

Table 21–4

Selected Anticonvulsants: Pharmacokinetics, Pharmacodynamics, and Therapeutic Ranges

	Pharmacokinetics			Pharmacodynamics			
Drug	Protein-Binding (%)	t½	Excretion	PO Onset	Peak Time (h)	Duration of Action (h)	Therapeutic Serum Range
phenytoin (Dilantin)	85-95	6-45 h (average 22 h)	Kidneys, bile, and GI	30 min-2 h	1.5-3	6-12	10-20 mcg/ml
phenobarbital	20-45	2-6 d	50%-75% in urine	30-60 min	8-12	6-24	15-40 mcg/ml
ethosuximide (Zarontin)	UK	30 h (child)	25% in urine unchanged	UK	>4	12-60	40-100 mcg/ml
clonazepam (Klonopin)	UK	20-50 h	Kidneys and feces	20-60 min	1-2	6-12	20-80 ng/ml
carbamazepine (Tegretol)	75	25-65 h	75% in urine, 25% in feces	Varies	4-7	6-12	5-12 mcg/ml
valproic acid (Depakene)	90	6-16 h	Kidneys	20-30 min	1-4	24	40-100 mcg/ml

d, Day; *GI*, gastrointestinal; *h*, hour; *min*, minute; *PO*, by mouth; *t*½, half-life; *UK*, unknown; *>*, greater than.

(Dilantin). For continued seizures, midazolam (Versed) or propofol (Diprivan), then high-dose barbiturates are used. These drugs should be administered slowly to avoid respiratory depression.

Summary

The pharmacologic behavior of specific anticonvulsants is summarized in Table 21–4.

KEY WEBSITES

Management of Status Epilepticus: http://www.aafp.org/afp/20030801/469.html

Phenytoin (Dilantin): http://www.mentalhealth.com/drug/p30-d05.html

Seizure Disorders in the Elderly: http://www.aafp.org/afp/20030115/325.html

Critical Thinking Case Study

SS, 26 years old, takes phenytoin (Dilantin) 100 mg, t.i.d., to control grand mal seizures. SS and her husband are contemplating starting a family.

1. What action should the nurse take in regard to client family planning?

SS complains of frequent "upset stomach" and "bleeding gums" when brushing her teeth.

2. To decrease GI distress, what can be suggested?
3. To alleviate bleeding gums, what client teaching for SS may be included?
4. The nurse checks SS's serum phenytoin level. What are the indications of an abnormal serum level? What appropriate actions should be taken?

NCLEX Study Questions

1. The nurse witnesses a client's seizure involving generalized contraction of the body followed by jerkiness of arms and legs. The nurse realizes this is a _____ seizure.
   a. myoclonic
   b. petit mal
   c. tonic clonic
   d. psychomotor

2. Phenytoin (Dilantin) has been prescribed for a client with seizures. Which is an appropriate nursing intervention?
   a. monitoring CBC levels
   b. reporting a phenytoin level of 18 mcg/ml
   c. encouraging the client to brush teeth vigorously to prevent plaque buildup
   d. teaching the client to stop the drug immediately when passing pinkish-red or reddish-brown urine

3. When administering phenytoin (Dilantin), the nurse realizes more teaching is needed if the client states:
   a. "I must shake the oral suspension very well prior to pouring in the dose cup."
   b. "I cannot drink alcoholic beverages when taking phenytoin."
   c. "I should take phenytoin one hour before meals."
   d. "I will need to get periodic dental checkups."

4. A client is taking clonazepam for absence (petit mal) seizures. Which value does the nurse know is the therapeutic serum range for clonazepam?
   a. 5-12 mcg/ml
   b. 10-20 mcg/ml
   c. 15-40 mcg/ml
   d. 20-80 ng/ml

5. Which of the following drugs would most likely be used for status epilepticus?
   a. carbamazepine (Tegretol)
   b. fosphenytoin (Cerebyx)
   c. gabapentin (Neurontin)
   d. levetiracetam (Keppra)

22

Drugs for Neurologic Disorders: Parkinsonism and Alzheimer's Disease

Outline

Objectives

- Summarize the pathophysiology of parkinsonism and Alzheimer's disease.
- Contrast the actions of anticholinergics, dopaminergics, dopamine receptors, MAO-B inhibitors, and COMT inhibitors in the treatment of parkinsonism.
- Describe the side effects of antiparkinson drugs.
- Apply the nursing process to anticholinergics, dopaminergics, and acetylcholinesterase inhibitors.
- Differentiate the phases of Alzheimer's disease with corresponding symptoms.
- Discuss the drug group used to treat Alzheimer's disease.

Terms

Parkinsonism (Parkinson's disease), a chronic neurologic disorder that affects the extrapyramidal motor tract (which controls posture, balance, and locomotion), is considered a syndrome (combination of symptoms) because of its three major features: rigidity, **bradykinesia** (slow movement), and tremors. Rigidity (abnormally increased muscle tone) increases with movement. Postural changes caused by rigidity and bradykinesia include the chest and head thrust forward with the knees and hips flexed, a shuffling gait, and the absence of arm swing. Other characteristic symptoms are masked facies (no facial expression), involuntary tremors of the head and neck, and pill-rolling motions of the hands. The tremors may be more prevalent at rest.

Alzheimer's disease is a chronic, progressive, neurodegenerative condition with marked cognitive dysfunction. Various theories exist as to the cause of Alzheimer's disease: neuritic plaques, degeneration of the cholinergic neurons, and deficiency in acetylcholine.

Parkinsonism

In 1817 Dr. James Parkinson described six clients as having "shaking palsy." Three symptoms were described by Parkinson: (1) involuntary tremors of the limbs, (2) rigidity of muscles, and (3) slowness of movement. In the United States there are approximately one million persons with parkinsonism, and 50,000 new cases are diagnosed each year. Because parkinsonism generally affects clients between the ages of 50 and 70 years and older, many consider the health problem to be part of the aging process caused by loss of neurons. The three cardinal symptoms are rigidity, tremors, and bradykinesia. Normally the symptoms have a gradual onset and are usually mild and unilateral in the beginning.

There are different types of parkinsonism. **Pseudoparkinsonism** frequently occurs as an adverse reaction to antipsychotic drugs, especially the phenothiazines. In addition, parkinsonism symptoms could result from poisons (e.g., carbon monoxide, manganese), arteriosclerosis, and Wilson's disease (hepatolenticular degeneration).

Nonpharmacologic Measures

Symptoms of parkinsonism can be lessened through the use of nonpharmacologic measures such as client teaching, exercise, nutrition, and group support. Exercise can improve mobility and flexibility; the client with Parkinson's disease should enroll in a therapeutic exercise program tailored to this disorder. A balanced diet with fiber and fluids helps prevent constipation and weight loss. Clients with Parkinson's disease and their family members should be encouraged to attend a support group to help cope with and understand parkinsonism.

Pathophysiology

Parkinsonism is caused by an imbalance of the neurotransmitters dopamine (DA) and acetylcholine (ACh). It is marked by degeneration of neurons that originate in the substantia nigra of the midbrain and terminate at the basal ganglia of the extrapyramidal motor tract. The reason for the degeneration of neurons is unknown.

There are two neurotransmitters within neurons of the striatum of the brain: dopamine, an inhibitory neurotransmitter, and acetylcholine, an excitatory neurotransmitter. Dopamine is released from the dopaminergic neurons; acetylcholine is released from the cholinergic neurons. Dopamine normally maintains control of acetylcholine and inhibits its excitatory response. In Parkinson's disease there is an unexplained degeneration of the dopaminergic neurons, and an imbalance between dopamine and acetylcholine occurs. With less dopamine production, acetylcholine is unopposed, thereby causing the excitation and stimulation of neurons that release gamma-aminobutyric acid (GABA). With increased stimulation of GABA, the symptomatic movement disorders of parkinsonism occur.

By the time early symptoms of Parkinson's disease appear, 80% of the striatal dopamine has already been depleted. The remaining striatal neurons synthesize dopamine from levodopa and release dopamine as needed. Before the next dose of levodopa, symptoms (e.g., slow walking, loss of dexterity) return or worsen, but within 30 to 60 minutes of receiving a dose, the client's functioning is much improved.

Drugs used to treat parkinsonism reduce the symptoms or replace the dopamine deficit. These drugs fall into five categories: (1) anticholinergics, which block the cholinergic receptors; (2) dopaminergics, which convert to dopamine; (3) dopamine agonists, which stimulate the dopamine receptors; (4) MAO-B inhibitor, which inhibits the monoamine oxidase-B (MAO-B) enzyme that interferes with dopamine; and (5) COMT inhibitors, which inhibit the catechol-O-methyltransferase enzyme that inactivates dopamine. Table 22–1 compares the various parkinsonism drugs.

$\mathcal{Herbal}$ **ALERT 22–1**

Orphenadrine Citrate
🍃 Valerian and kava kava potentiate sedation.

$\mathcal{Preventing}$ **MEDICATION ERRORS**
Do not confuse...

- Symmetrel with Synthroid.

- Parlodel with pindolol.

- Mirapex with MiraLax. These drug names look alike, but the pharmacology is different.

Anticholinergics

Anticholinergic drugs reduce the rigidity and some of the tremors characteristic of parkinsonism but have minimal effect on bradykinesia. The anticholinergics are parasympatholytics that inhibit the release of acetylcholine. Anticholinergics are still used to treat drug-induced parkinsonism, or pseudoparkinsonism, a side effect of the antipsychotic drug group phenothiazines. Examples of anticholinergics used for parkinsonism include trihexyphenidyl (Artane), benztropine (Cogentin), biperiden (Akineton), procyclidine (Kemadrin), ethopropazine (Parsidol), and orphenadrine (Norflex). The latter two drugs are the newest anticholinergics. *Do not confuse Artane with Altace.*

Diphenhydramine (Benadryl), an antihistamine, has similar anticholinergic properties. It is sometimes used to treat mild parkinsonism and for older adults who may not be able to tolerate the dopamine agonist group of drugs.

Table 22–2 lists the anticholinergics and their dosages, uses, and considerations. Anticholinergics used to treat parkinsonism are also discussed in Chapter 18.

Nursing Process

Antiparkinson: Anticholinergic Agent

ASSESSMENT

■ Obtain client's health history. Report if client has a history of glaucoma, GI dysfunction, urinary retention, angina pectoris, or myasthenia gravis. All anticholinergics are contraindicated if client has glaucoma.
■ Obtain a drug history. Report if a drug-drug interaction is probable. Phenothiazines, tricyclic antidepressants, and antihistamines increase the effect of trihexyphenidyl.

Table 22–1

Comparison of Drugs Used to Treat Parkinson's Disease

Drug	Purpose
Dopaminergics	
carbidopa-levodopa	Decrease symptoms of parkinsonism. Carbidopa, a decarboxylase inhibitor, permits more levodopa to reach the striatum nerve terminals (where levodopa is converted to dopamine). With the use of carbidopa, less levodopa is needed.
Dopamine Agonists	
amantadine	Amantadine was first used as an antiviral drug for influenza A. It decreases symptoms of parkinsonism. It can be given as an early treatment for Parkinson's disease, which could delay the necessity of levodopa. Amantadine is effective in treating drug-induced parkinsonism and has fewer side effects than anticholinergics.
bromocriptine	A D_2-dopamine receptor agonist. Bromocriptine may be used for early treatment of Parkinson's disease. With increasing motor symptoms, bromocriptine can be given with levodopa therapy.
pramipexole (Mirapex) ropinirole HCl (Requip)	D_2- and D_3-dopamine receptor agonists. These drugs can be used in combination with levodopa. They have fewer side effects than older dopamine agonists.
MAO-B Inhibitor	
selegiline HCl (Eldepryl)	Inhibits the catabolic enzymes of dopamine. MAO-B inhibitor extends the action of dopamine. It can be given in the early phase of Parkinson's disease. If the drug is given with levodopa, the dosage of levodopa is usually decreased.
rasagiline (Azilect)	Interferes with dopamine reuptake at synapses in the brain. Prevents the enzyme monoamine oxidase B from breaking down in brain.
COMT Inhibitors	
entacapone (Comtan), tolcapone (Tasmar)	Inhibits the COMT enzyme, increasing concentration of levodopa. These drugs are used in combination with levodopa-carbidopa (Sinemet). With COMT inhibitors, a smaller dose of levodopa is needed.
Anticholinergics; Antiparkinson	
	Anticholinergics were the first group of drugs used to treat Parkinson's disease before levodopa and dopamine agonists were introduced. Anticholinergics are useful in decreasing tremors related to Parkinson's disease. The major use of these agents currently is to treat drug-induced parkinsonism. Treatment should start with low dosages, then the dose should gradually be increased. Older adults are more susceptible to the many side effects of anticholinergics. Clients with memory loss or dementia should not be on anticholinergic therapy.

COMT, Catechol-O-methyltransferase; MAO-B, monoamine oxidase-B.

■ Assess baseline vital signs for future comparison. Pulse rate may increase.

■ Determine usual urinary output as a baseline for comparison. Urinary retention may occur with continuous use of anticholinergics.

NURSING DIAGNOSES

■ Impaired physical mobility related to muscle rigidity, tremors, and bradykinesia

■ Impaired urinary elimination related to urinary retention

PLANNING

■ Client will have decreased involuntary symptoms caused by parkinsonism or drug-induced parkinsonism.

NURSING INTERVENTIONS

■ Monitor vital signs, urine output, and bowel sounds. Increased pulse rate, urinary retention, and constipation are side effects of anticholinergics.

■ Observe for involuntary movements.

Client Teaching

General

• Advise client to avoid alcohol, cigarettes, caffeine, and aspirin to decrease gastric acidity.

Side Effects

• Encourage client to relieve dry mouth with hard candy, ice chips, or sugarless chewing gum. Anticholinergics decrease salivation.

• Suggest that client use sunglasses in direct sunlight because of possible photophobia.

Table 22-2

Antiparkinson Drugs: Anticholinergics

Generic (Brand)	Route and Dosage	Uses and Considerations
benztropine mesylate (Cogentin)	*Parkinsonism:* A: PO: Initially 0.5-1.0 mg/d in 1-2 divided doses (larger dose at bedtime); maint: 0.5-6 mg/d in 1-2 divided doses *Extrapyramidal syndrome:* A: PO: 1-4 mg/d in 1-2 divided doses IM/IV: 1-2 mg/d	For parkinsonism and drug-induced parkinsonism to reduce dystonia. May be taken with other antiparkinson drugs. Contraindicated in glaucoma, GI obstruction, severe ulcerative colitis, prostatic hypertrophy, myasthenia gravis. *Pregnancy category:* C; PB: UK; t$\frac{1}{2}$: UK
biperiden HCl (Akineton)	*Parkinsonism:* A: PO: 2 mg in 1-4 divided doses IM/IV: 2 mg every 30 min to 4 doses; *max:* 8 mg/d C: IM/IV: 0.04 mg/kg or 1.2 mg/m^2, repeat PRN	For parkinsonism and drug-induced parkinsonism (EPS). With prolonged use, drug tolerance may occur. Similar contraindications as benztropine. Avoid taking drug with alcohol or CNS depressants. Dry mouth, blurred vision, drowsiness, muscle weakness, and constipation may occur. *Pregnancy category:* C; PB: UK; t$\frac{1}{2}$: UK
ethopropazine HCl (Parsidol)	*Parkinsonism:* A: PO: Initially 50 mg daily/b.i.d.; maint: 100-400 mg/d in divided doses; *max:* 600 mg/d in divided doses	For all types of parkinsonism. A phenothiazine derivative with anticholinergic and antihistamine effects. Common side effects include dry mouth, drowsiness, dizziness, confusion, urinary retention, constipation. Contraindications: glaucoma, GU obstruction, prostatic hypertrophy. *Pregnancy category:* C; PB: UK; t$\frac{1}{2}$: UK
orphenadrine HCl or citrate (Norflex)	A: PO: 50 mg t.i.d. or 100 mg b.i.d.	For parkinsonism. Antihistamine with some anticholinergic effects. Has slight CNS stimulation and can cause euphoria. *Pregnancy category:* C; PB: UK; t$\frac{1}{2}$: 14 h
procyclidine HCl (Kemadrin)	*Parkinsonism:* A: PO: 2.5 mg p.c. t.i.d. *Extrapyramidal syndrome:* A: PO: Initially 2.5 mg p.c. t.i.d.; maint: 2.5-5 mg p.c. t.i.d.	For parkinsonism and drug-induced parkinsonism. Relieves rigidity more than tremors. May be taken with other antiparkinson drugs. Contraindicated in glaucoma. *Pregnancy category:* C; PB: UK; t$\frac{1}{2}$: UK
trihexyphenidyl HCl (Artane)	(Prototype Drug Chart 18-4)	
Rotigotine (Neupro)	A: Transdermal patch: 1 patch qd	For parkinsonism and restless leg syndrome *Pregnancy category:* C; PB: 92%; t$\frac{1}{2}$: 3 h

A, Adult; *b.i.d.*, two times a day; *C*, child; *CNS*, central nervous system; *d*, day; *EPS*, extrapyramidal symptoms; *GI*, gastrointestinal; *GU*, genitourinary; *h*, hour; *IM*, intramuscular; *IV*, intravenous; *min*, minute; *PB*, protein-binding; *p.c.*, after meals; *PO*, by mouth; *PRN*, as needed; *t$\frac{1}{2}$*, half-life; *t.i.d.*, three times a day; *UK*, unknown.

- Advise client to void before taking the drug to minimize urinary retention.
- Advise client who takes an anticholinergic for control of symptoms of parkinsonism to have routine eye examinations; because clients who have glaucoma should not take anticholinergics.

Diet

- Encourage client to ingest foods high in fiber and increase fluid intake to prevent constipation.

Cultural Considerations ❖

- Assess personal beliefs of client or family and modify communications to meet cultural needs; use an interpreter and community nurse follow-up as needed.

EVALUATION

■ Evaluate client's response to trihexyphenidyl or benztropine mesylate to determine whether parkinsonism symptoms are controlled.

Dopaminergics

Carbidopa and Levodopa

The first dopaminergic drug was levodopa (L-dopa), which was introduced in 1961 but is no longer available in the United States. When introduced, levodopa was effective in diminishing symptoms of Parkinson's disease and increasing mobility, because the blood-brain barrier admits levodopa but not dopamine. The enzyme dopa decarboxylase converts levodopa to dopamine in the brain, but this enzyme is also found in the peripheral nervous system and allows 99% of levodopa to be converted to dopamine *before* it reaches the brain. Therefore only about 1% of levodopa taken is available to be converted to dopamine once it reaches the brain, and large doses are needed to achieve a pharmacologic response. These high doses could cause many side effects, including nausea, vomiting, dyskinesia, orthostatic hypotension, cardiac dysrhythmias, and psychosis.

Because of the side effects of levodopa and the fact that so much levodopa is metabolized before reaching the brain, an alternative drug, carbidopa, was developed to inhibit the enzyme dopa decarboxylase. By inhibiting the enzyme in the peripheral nervous system, more levodopa reaches the brain. The carbidopa is combined with levodopa in a ratio of 1 part carbidopa to 10 parts levodopa. Figure 22–1 illustrates the comparative action of levodopa and carbidopa-levodopa.

The advantages of combining levodopa with carbidopa are the following:

- More dopamine reaches the basal ganglia.
- Smaller doses of levodopa are required to achieve the desired effect.

The disadvantage of the carbidopa-levodopa combination is that with more available levodopa, more side effects

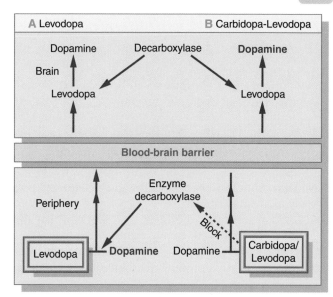

FIGURE 22–1 A, When levodopa is used alone only 1% reaches the brain because 99% converts to dopamine while in the peripheral nervous system. B, By combining carbidopa with levodopa, carbidopa can inhibit the enzyme decarboxylase in the periphery, thereby allowing more levodopa to reach the brain.

may be noted. Side effects may include nausea, vomiting, **dystonic movement** (involuntary abnormal movement), and psychotic behavior. The peripheral side effects of levodopa are not as prevalent; however, cardiac dysrhythmia, palpitations, and orthostatic hypotension may occur. The carbidopa-levodopa combination is usually not used to treat drug-related parkinsonism. Prototype Drug Chart 22–1 lists the pharmacologic behavior of carbidopa-levodopa.

Nursing Process

Antiparkinson: Dopaminergic Agent: Carbidopa-Levodopa

ASSESSMENT

■ Obtain client's vital signs to use for future comparison.

■ Assess client for signs and symptoms of parkinsonism, including stooped forward posture, shuffling gait, masked facies, and resting tremors.

■ Obtain a history from client of glaucoma, heart disease, peptic ulcers, kidney or liver disease, and psychosis.

■ Report if drug-drug interaction is probable. Drugs that should be avoided or closely monitored are levodopa, bromocriptine, and anticholinergics.

■ Obtain a drug history.

NURSING DIAGNOSES

■ Impaired physical mobility related to dizziness

■ Risk for activity intolerance related to fatigue

PLANNING

■ Symptoms of parkinsonism will be decreased or absent after 1 to 4 weeks of drug therapy.

NURSING INTERVENTIONS

■ Monitor client's vital signs and electrocardiogram. Orthostatic hypotension may occur during early use of levodopa and bromocriptine. Instruct client to rise slowly to avoid faintness.

■ Check for weakness, dizziness, or syncope, which are symptoms of orthostatic hypotension.

■ Administer carbidopa-levodopa (Sinemet) with low-protein foods. High-protein diets interfere with drug transport to the CNS.

■ Observe for symptoms of parkinsonism.

Client Teaching

General

• Advise client not to abruptly discontinue the medication. Rebound parkinsonism (increased symptoms of parkinsonism) can occur.

• Inform client that urine may be discolored and will darken with exposure to air. Perspiration also may be dark. Explain that both are harmless but clothes may be stained.

• Advise client to avoid chewing or crushing extended-release tablets.

Side Effects

• Instruct client to report side effects and symptoms of dyskinesia. Explain to client that it may take weeks or months before symptoms are controlled.

Diet

• Suggest to client that taking levodopa with food may decrease GI upset, but food will slow the drug absorption rate.

Prototype DRUG CHART 22–1

CARBIDOPA-LEVODOPA

Drug Class Antiparkinson: Dopaminergic Trade name: Sinemet *Pregnancy Category:* C	**Dosage** **A: PO:** 1:10 ratio; initially 10 carbidopa/100 levodopa t.i.d.; maint: 25/250 mg t.i.d. **Extended-release:** 5 mg carbidopa/200 mg levodopa b.i.d. to 10/100 t.i.d. or q.i.d.; may increase to 1 tablet daily or every other day (maximum 8 tablets)
Contraindications Narrow-angle glaucoma; severe cardiac, renal, or hepatic disease *Caution:* Peptic ulcer, psychiatric disorders	**Drug-Lab-Food Interactions** *Drug: Increase* hypertensive crisis with MAOIs *Decrease* levodopa effect with anticholinergics, **Lab:** *May increase* BUN, AST, ALT, ALP, LDH **Food:** Avoid foods containing vitamin B$_6$ (pyridoxine)
Pharmacokinetics **Absorption:** PO: Well absorbed **Distribution:** PB: Carbidopa: 36%; levodopa: UK **Metabolism:** t½: 1-2 h **Excretion:** In urine as metabolites	**Pharmacodynamics** **PO: Onset:** 15 min Peak: 1-3 h Duration: 5-12 h

Therapeutic Effects/Uses

To treat parkinsonism; to relieve tremors and rigidity

Mode of Action: Transmission of levodopa to brain cells for conversion to dopamine; carbidopa blocks the conversion of levodopa to dopamine in the peripheral nervous system

Side Effects	**Adverse Reactions**
Anorexia, nausea, vomiting, dysphagia, fatigue, dizziness, headache, dry mouth, bitter taste, twitching, blurred vision, insomnia	Involuntary choreiform movements, palpitations, orthostatic hypotension, urinary retention, psychosis, severe depression, hallucinations *Life-threatening:* Agranulocytosis, hemolytic anemia, cardiac dysrhythmias, leukopenia

A, Adult; *ALP*, alkaline phosphatase; *ALT*, alanine aminotransferase; *AST*, aspartate aminotransferase; *b.i.d.*, two times a day; *BUN*, blood urea nitrogen; *h*, hour; *LDH*, lactic dehydrogenase; *maint*, maintenance; *MAOIs*, monoamine oxidase inhibitors; *min*, minute; *PB*, protein-binding; *PO*, by mouth; *q.i.d.*, four times a day; *t½*, half-life; *t.i.d.*, three times a day; *UK*, unknown.

- Advise client to avoid vitamins that contain vitamin B$_6$ (pyridoxine) and an excess of foods high in vitamin B$_6$ such as beans (lima, navy, kidney) and cereals. Vitamin B$_6$ inhibits conversion of levodopa to dopamine, but vitamin B$_6$ deficiency can produce peripheral neuritis and muscle weakness, so a conservative amount is needed.
- Encourage client who takes high doses of selegiline to avoid foods high in tyramine (i.e., aged cheese, red wine, cream, yogurt, chocolate, bananas, and raisins). Encourage client to check with a dietitian regarding these foods.

Amantadine and Bromocriptine
- Suggest that client taking amantadine report any signs of skin lesions, seizures, or depression. A history of these health problems should have been previously reported to health care provider.
- Advise client taking bromocriptine to report symptoms of light-headedness when changing positions (a symptom of orthostatic hypotension).
- Instruct client to avoid alcohol when taking bromocriptine.
- Teach client to check heart rate and report changes in rate or irregularity.
- Warn client not to abruptly stop the drug without first notifying health care provider.

Cultural Considerations ❖
- Recognize that various cultural groups will need guidance in understanding the disease process of parkinsonism. Support client and family member who may be dismayed about the symptoms of parkinsonism and lack knowledge of the disease process.
- For clients who speak little or no English an interpreter may be needed to support understanding of drug doses and schedules and recognition of severe side effects that need to be reported to health care provider.

EVALUATION
- Evaluate the effectiveness of the drug therapy in controlling the symptoms of parkinsonism.
- Determine whether there is an absence of side effects.

Dopamine Agonists

Other dopaminergics called **dopamine agonists** stimulate the dopamine receptors. For example, amantadine hydrochloride (Symmetrel) is an antiviral drug that acts on the dopamine receptors. It may be taken alone or in combination with levodopa or an anticholinergic drug. Initially, amantadine produces improvement in symptoms of parkinsonism in approximately two thirds of clients, but this improvement is usually not sustained, because drug tolerance develops. Amantadine can also be used to treat drug-induced parkinsonism.

Bromocriptine mesylate (Parlodel) acts directly on dopamine receptors in the central nervous system (CNS), cardiovascular system, and gastrointestinal (GI) tract. Bromocriptine is more effective than amantadine and the anticholinergics; however, it is not as effective as carbidopa-levodopa in alleviating parkinsonian symptoms. Clients who do not tolerate carbidopa-levodopa are frequently given bromocriptine.

MAO-B Inhibitor

The enzyme monoamine oxidase-B (MAO-B) causes catabolism (breakdown) of dopamine. Selegiline inhibits MAO-B, thus prolonging the action of levodopa. It may be ordered for newly diagnosed clients with Parkinson's disease. The use of selegiline could delay levodopa therapy by a year. It decreases "on-off" fluctuations. Rasagiline (Azilect) is an MAO-B inhibitor used for the treatment of Parkinson's disease.

Large doses of selegiline may inhibit MAO-A, an enzyme that promotes metabolism of tyramine in the GI tract. If they are not metabolized by MAO-A, ingestion of foods high in tyramine (aged cheese, red wine, and bananas) can cause a hypertensive crisis. Severe adverse drug interactions can occur between selegiline and various tricyclic antidepressants (TCA) or selective serotonin reuptake inhibitors (SSRIs).

COMT Inhibitors

The enzyme catechol-O-methyltransferase (COMT) inactivates dopamine. When taken with a levodopa preparation, COMT inhibitors increase the amount of levodopa concentration in the brain. Tolcapone (Tasmar) was the first COMT inhibitor taken with levodopa for advanced Parkinson's disease. This drug can affect liver cell function; therefore serum liver enzymes should be closely monitored. Entacapone (Comtan) does not affect liver function.

Table 22–3 lists dopaminergics, dopamine agonists, MAO-B inhibitor, and COMT inhibitors with their dosages, uses, and considerations.

Precautions for Drugs Used to Treat Parkinson's Disease
Side Effects and Adverse Reactions

The common side effects of anticholinergics include dry mouth and dry secretions, urinary retention, constipation, blurred vision, and an increase in heart rate. Mental effects such as restlessness and confusion may occur in the older adult.

The side effects of carbidopa-levodopa are numerous. GI disturbances are common because dopamine stimulates the chemoreceptor trigger zone (CTZ) in the medulla, which stimulates the vomiting center. Taking the drug with food can decrease nausea and vomiting, but food slows the absorption rate. **Dyskinesia** (impaired voluntary movement) may occur with high levodopa dosages. Cardiovascular side effects include orthostatic hypotension and increased heart rate during early use of levodopa. Cardiac dysrhythmias may occur as

Table 22–3

Antiparkinson: Dopaminergics

Generic (Brand)	Route and Dosage	Uses and Considerations
Dopaminergics		
carbidopa-levodopa (Sinemet)	(Prototype Drug Chart 22–1) A: PO: 0.5-1.0 g/d in 2-4 divided doses; increase dose gradually; average maint: 3-6 g/d with food, in divided doses; *max:* 8 mg/d	For parkinsonism. Not for drug-induced parkinsonism. Can cause GI upset; drug should be taken with food. Many side effects: nausea, vomiting, orthostatic hypotension, cardiac dysrhythmias, psychosis. *Pregnancy category:* C; PB: UK; t½: 1-3 h
Dopamine Agonists		
amantadine HCl; (Symmetrel)	Parkinsonism: A: PO: 100 mg b.i.d.; may increase dose; *max:* 400 mg/d	For early-onset parkinsonism, drug-induced parkinsonism, and influenza A respiratory virus. Effective for rigidity and bradykinesia; less effective for decreasing tremors. May be used alone or in combination. Has fewer side effects than anticholinergic drugs. *Pregnancy category:* C; PB: 60%-70%; t½: 12-24 h
bromocriptine mesylate (Parlodel)	A: PO: Initially 1.25-2.5 mg/d; may gradually increase dose; maint: 30-60 mg/d in 3 divided doses; *max:* 100 mg/d	For parkinsonism. Response is better than with amantadine. Can be taken in adjunct with levodopa or carbidopa-levodopa. Hypotension, lightheadedness, and syncope are major side effects. Initially, small doses are given then gradually increased over several weeks. *Pregnancy category:* C; PB: 90%-96%; t½: 6-8 h; terminal phase: 50 h
pramipexole dihydrochloride (Mirapex)	A: PO: Initially: 0.375 mg/d in 3 divided doses; maint: 1.5-4.5 mg/d in 3 divided doses	Stimulates dopamine receptors in striatum. *Pregnancy category:* C; PB: 15%; t½: 8-12 h
ropinirole HCl (Requip)	A: PO: Initially: 0.25 mg t.i.d.; *max:* 24 mg/d	Stimulates dopamine receptors in striatum. *Pregnancy category:* C; PB: 30%-40%; t½: 6 h
MAO-B Inhibitor		
selegiline HCl (Eldepryl)	A: PO: 10 mg/d in 2 divided doses	For early onset parkinsonism. May delay use of levodopa therapy by 1 y. Can be given with levodopa preparations; dose of levodopa would need to be decreased. *Pregnancy category:* C; PB: >90%; t½: 2-20 h
rasagiline (Azilect)	A: PO: 1 mg/d for monotherapy; 0.5-1 mg/d when adjunctive	For treatment of Parkinson's disease. *Pregnancy category:* C; PB: 88-94%; t½: 3 h
COMT Inhibitors		
tolcapone (Tasmar)	A: PO: 50-200 mg t.i.d. Elderly: 50-100 mg t.i.d.	To potentiate dopamine activity by inhibiting the enzyme COMT. Used in conjunction with levodopa-carbidopa (Sinemet); prolongs action of levodopa. *Pregnancy category:* UK; PB: 99%; t½: 2-3 h
entacapone (Comtan)	A: PO: 200 mg with each dose of levodopa-carbidopa; *max:* 2 g/d Elderly: same as adult	Used in combination with levodopa-carbidopa. Prevents peripheral COMT; thus more levodopa reaches the brain. Prolongs half-life of levodopa and decreases "on-off" fluctuations. Levodopa dose should be decreased when it is taken with a COMT inhibitor. *Pregnancy category:* UK; PB: UK; t½: 1.5-3 h

A, Adult; *COMT,* catechol-O-methyltransferase; *d,* day; *GI,* gastrointestinal; *h,* hour; *max,* maximum; *PB,* protein-binding; *PO,* by mouth; *t½,* half-life; *t.i.d.,* three times a day; *UK,* unknown; >, greater than.

carbidopa-levodopa dosages are increased. Nightmares, mental disturbances, and suicidal tendencies may occur.

Amantadine has few side effects, but they can intensify when the drug is combined with other antiparkinson drugs. Orthostatic hypotension, confusion, urinary retention, and constipation are common side effects of amantadine.

Side effects from bromocriptine are more common than from amantadine. These include GI disturbances (nausea), orthostatic hypotension, palpitations, chest pain, edema in the lower extremities, nightmares, delusions, and confusion. If bromocriptine is taken with carbidopa-levodopa,

usually the drug dosages are reduced and side effects and drug intolerance decrease.

Pramipexole (Mirapex) and ropinirole (Requip) can cause nausea, dizziness, somnolence, weakness, and constipation. These drugs intensify the dyskinesia and hallucination caused by levodopa. *(Do not confuse Mirapex with MiraLax.)*

Large doses of selegiline (Eldepryl, Carbex) may inhibit MAO-A. Hypertensive crisis might occur if foods high in tyramine such as aged cheese, red wine, and bananas are ingested.

Tolcapone (Tasmar) may cause severe liver damage. Clients with liver dysfunction should not take this drug. Entacapone (Comtan) is not known to affect liver function. With entacapone, the urine can be dark yellow to orange; with tolcapone, the urine can be bright yellow. Both tolcapone and entacapone can intensify the adverse reactions of levodopa (e.g., hallucinations, orthostatic hypotension, constipation, dizziness), because these drugs prolong the effect of levodopa.

Contraindications

Anticholinergics or any drugs that have anticholinergic effects are contraindicated for persons with glaucoma. Persons with severe cardiac, renal, or psychiatric health problems should avoid levodopa drugs because of adverse reactions. Clients with chronic obstructive lung diseases such as emphysema can have dry, thick mucous secretions caused by large doses of anticholinergic drugs.

Drug-Drug Interactions

Pyridoxine (vitamin B_6) increases dopa decarboxylase action, which metabolizes levodopa in the peripheral nervous system to dopamine. Foods rich in pyridoxine such as beans (lima, navy, kidney) and certain cereals therefore should be avoided. Antipsychotic drugs block the receptors for dopamine. Carbidopa-levodopa taken with a monoamine oxidase (MAO) inhibitor antidepressant can cause a hypertensive crisis.

Alzheimer's Disease

Alzheimer's disease is an incurable dementia illness characterized by chronic, progressive neurodegenerative conditions with marked cognitive dysfunction. The onset occurs between ages 45 and 65 (Table 22–4). It affects about four million Americans, and about 250,000 new cases are diagnosed annually. Approximately 50% of clients in nursing homes are admitted with Alzheimer's disease. This health problem is the fourth leading cause of death in adults.

Pathophysiology

Many physiologic changes contribute to Alzheimer's disease. Currently theories related to the changes that cause Alzheimer's disease include the following:

- Degeneration of the cholinergic neuron and deficiency in acetylcholine

- Neuritic plaques that form mainly outside the neurons and in the cerebral cortex
- Apolipoprotein E_4 (apo E_4) that promotes formation of neuritic plaques, which binds beta-amyloid in the plaques
- Beta-amyloid protein accumulation in high levels that may contribute to neuronal injury
- Presence of neurofibrillary tangles with twists inside the neurons

Figure 22–2 illustrates the normal neuron and the neuron affected by Alzheimer's disease. Other factors thought to influence the occurrence of Alzheimer's are genetic predisposition and a slow virus or infection that attacks brain cells.

Symptoms of Alzheimer's disease progress from confusion to memory loss to dementia (Table 22–5). With loss of memory, loss of logical thinking and judgment and time disorientation occur. As the disease progresses, memory loss becomes more severe; personality changes occur; and hyperactivity, hostility, paranoia, tendency to wander, and the inability to speak or express oneself result. Custodial care becomes necessary.

Acetylcholinesterase Inhibitors/ Cholinesterase Inhibitors

There is no known cure for Alzheimer's disease. FDA approved medications to treat Alzheimer's disease symptoms include ergoloid mesylate (Hydergine), which has not been very successful for treating memory loss, and

FIGURE 22–2 Histologic changes in Alzheimer's disease. A, Healthy neuron. B, Neuron affected by Alzheimer's disease showing characteristic neuritic plaques and cellular neurofibrillary tangles. (Modified from Lehne RA: *Pharmacology for nursing care*, ed 6, Philadelphia, 2007, Saunders.)

Table 22-4	
Prevalence of Alzheimer's Disease in the United States	
Age (Years)	**Percentage**
45-64	2
65-74	3-5
75-84	19
85 or older	47

Table 22–5

Stages of Cognitive Decline Due to Alzheimer's Disease

Stage	Clinical Phase	Symptoms
1	Normal	No change in cognition
2	Very mild	Forgets object location; some deficit in word-finding
3	Mild (early confusion)	Early cognitive decline in one or more areas, memory loss, decreased ability to function in work situation, name-finding deficit, some decrease in social functioning, recall difficulties, anxiety
4	Moderate	Unable to perform complex tasks such as managing personal finances, planning a dinner party, concentrating, and knowing current events
5	Moderately severe (early dementia)	Usually needs assistance for survival, reminders to bathe, help in selecting clothes and other daily functions; may be disoriented as to time and recent events although this can fluctuate; may become tearful
6	Severe (dementia)	Needs assistance with dressing, bathing, and toilet functions (e.g., flushing); may forget names of spouse/family/caregivers and details of their personal lives; generally unaware of their surroundings; incontinence of urine and feces may occur; CNS disturbances such as agitation, delusions, paranoia, obsessive anxiety, and potential for violent behavior may increase
7	Very severe (late dementia)	Unable to speak (speech limited to five words or less), may scream or make other sounds; unable to ambulate, sit up, smile, or feed self; unable to hold head erect, ultimately slips into stupor or coma

From McKenry LM, Tessier E, Hogan MA: *Pharmacology in nursing*, ed 22, St Louis, 2006, Mosby, p. 483. Data from Alzheimer's Association: Stages of Alzheimer's. Retrieved June 29, 2007, from *http://www.alz.org/alzheimers_disease_stages_of_alzheimers.asp*.

acetylcholinesterase (AChE) inhibitors. (AChE is an enzyme responsible for breaking down ACh and is also known as *cholinesterase*.) The AChE inhibitors are tacrine (Cognex); donepezil (Aricept); and rivastigmine (Exelon), a drug that permits more acetylcholine in the neuron receptors. Rivastigmine has effective penetration into the CNS; thus cholinergic transmission is increased. These AChE inhibitors increase cognitive function for clients with mild to moderate Alzheimer's disease. A reversible AChE inhibitor used to treat mild to moderate Alzheimer's disease is galantamine (Razadyne).

Several drugs for treating Alzheimer's disease are under investigation. Some of these are certain nonsteroidal anti-inflammatory drugs (piroxicam, indomethacin), calcium channel blockers, MAO-B inhibitor (selegiline), serotonin antagonists, CNS stimulants (methylphenidate [Ritalin]), angiotensin-converting enzyme (ACE) inhibitors, and Vitamin E.

Tacrine

Tacrine (Cognex), an AChE inhibitor, is prescribed to improve cognitive function for clients with mild to moderate Alzheimer's disease (Prototype Drug Chart 22–2). This drug increases the amount of ACh at the cholinergic synapses. Tacrine tends to slow the disease process, but only 30% of clients have an effective response to tacrine, and even for those it has a short-lasting effect. Table 22–6 lists the drugs used to treat Alzheimer's disease. *Do not confuse Cognex with Corgard.*

Pharmacokinetics

Tacrine is absorbed faster through the GI tract without food. Because it has a relatively short half-life, tacrine is given four times a day, and the dose is gradually increased. The protein-binding power is average.

Pharmacodynamics

Tacrine has been somewhat successful in improving memory in the early phase of Alzheimer's disease. The onset of action is 0.5 to 1.5 hours; peak action is 2 hours. However, the duration of action is prolonged to 24 to 36 hours; side effects should be closely monitored. This drug is contraindicated for clients with liver disease because hepatotoxicity may occur. Cumulative drug effect is likely to occur in older adults and in clients with liver and renal dysfunction.

Drug Treatment for Alzheimer's Disease: Tacrine

ASSESSMENT

■ Record client's mental and physical abilities. Note limitation of cognitive function and self-care.

■ Obtain a history of liver or renal disease or dysfunction.

■ Assess for memory and judgment losses. Elicit from family members a history of behavioral changes (e.g., memory loss, declining interest in people or home, difficulty in following through with simple activities, and tendency to wander from home).

■ Observe for signs of behavioral disturbances such as hyperactivity, hostility, and wandering.

■ Check for signs of aphasia or difficulty in speech.

■ Note client's motor function.

■ Determine family members' ability to cope with client's mental and physical changes.

Prototype DRUG CHART 22–2

TACRINE

Drug Class Acetylcholinesterase inhibitor Trade name: Cognex *Pregnancy Category:* C	**Dosage** **A: PO:** Initially: 10 mg q.i.d.; after 6 wk: 20 mg q.i.d.; after 12 wk: 30 mg q.i.d.; after 16 wk: 40 mg q.i.d.; *max:* 160 mg/d
Contraindications Liver and renal diseases	**Drug-Lab-Food Interactions** *Drug: Increase* effect of theophylline *Increase* effect with cimetidine *Lab:* Increase ALT, AST
Pharmacokinetics **Absorption:** PO: Food decreases absorption rate **Distribution:** PB: 50% **Metabolism:** t½: 3 h **Excretion:** In urine	**Pharmacodynamics** **PO:** Onset: 0.5 h Peak: 2 h Duration: 24-36 h
Therapeutic Effects/Uses Improves memory loss **Mode of Action:** Elevates acetylcholine concentration	
Side Effects Anorexia, nausea, vomiting, diarrhea, dizziness, headache, constipation, rhinitis, depression	**Adverse Reactions** *Life threatening:* Hepatotoxicity

A, Adult; *ALT,* alanine aminotransferase; *AST,* aspartate aminotransferase; *d,* day; *h,* hour; *max,* maximum; *PB,* protein-binding; *PO,* by mouth; *q.i.d.,* four times a day; *t½,* half-life.

Table 22–6

Acetylcholinesterase (AChE) Inhibitors for Alzheimer's Disease

Generic (Brand)	Route and Dosage	Uses and Considerations
donepezil (Aricept)	A: PO: 5-10 mg/d	AChE inhibitor. To treat mild to moderate phase of Alzheimer's disease. *Pregnancy category:* C; PB: 90%; t½: 70 h
ergoloid mesylates (Hydergine)	A: PO: Initially, 1 mg	To increase cognitive function. Actual improvement is uncertain. *Pregnancy category:* C; PB: UK; t½: 3.5 h
rivastigmine (Exelon)	A: PO: Initial dose: 1.5 mg, b.i.d.; increase every 2 wk PRN; *max:* 6 mg b.i.d.	AChE inhibitor. To treat mild to moderate Alzheimer's disease. GI upset is common adverse effect. Weight loss may be a problem. This drug is not considered to cause hepatotoxicity. *Pregnancy category:* B; PB: UK; t½: 1.5 h
tacrine HCl (Cognex)	(See Prototype Drug Chart 22–3)	
memantine (Namenda)	A: PO: 5 mg/d, may increase dose in 5 mg increments every week to 20 mg/d	Neurotransmitter inhibitor. To treat mild to severe Alzheimer's disease. *Pregnancy category:* B; PB: 45%; t½: 60-80 h
galantamine (Razadyne, formerly called *Reminyl*)	A: PO: Initially 4 mg bid, may increase 4 mg every 4 wk if well tolerated Maintenance dose: 16-24 mg qd in 2 divided doses	Reversible AChE inhibitor. To treat mild to moderate Alzheimer's disease. *Pregnancy category:* B; PB: 18%; t½: 7 h

A, Adult; *AChE,* acetylcholinesterase; *b.i.d.,* twice a day; *d,* day; *GI,* gastrointestinal; *h,* hour; *max,* maximum; *PB,* protein-binding; *PO,* by mouth; *t½,* half-life; *UK,* unknown; *wk,* week.

NURSING DIAGNOSES

- Disturbed thought processes related to confusion
- Self-care deficit: dressing, feeding, toileting related to memory loss
- Chronic confusion related to memory loss
- Interrupted family processes related to decreased cognition
- Compromised family coping related to overwhelming disruption of lifestyle
- Risk for injury related to hyperactivity and dizziness
- Imbalanced nutrition: less than body requirement related to anorexia, nausea, and vomiting

PLANNING

- Client's loss of memory will proceed slower with the medication AChE inhibitor than without medication.
- Client can maintain self-care of body functions with assistance.

NURSING INTERVENTIONS

- Maintain consistency in care.
- Assist client in ambulation and activity.
- Check for side effects related to continuous use of AChE inhibitors.
- Record vital signs periodically. Note signs of bradycardia and hypotension.
- Monitor client's behavioral changes and record improvement or decline.

Client Teaching

General

- Explain to client and family members the purpose for prescribed drug therapy.
- Teach the time for drug dosing and the schedule for increasing drug dosing to the family member responsible for client's medications.
- Instruct family member in safety techniques (e.g., removing obstacles from client's foot path so that client can avoid injury when wandering).
- Inform family member of support groups that are available, for instance, Alzheimer's Disease and Related Disorders Association.

Side Effects

- Inform client and family member that client should rise slowly to avoid dizziness and loss of balance.

Diet

- Instruct family member about foods that may be prepared for client's consumption and tolerance.

Cultural Considerations ❖

- Recognize that various cultural groups may need guidance in understanding the disease process of Alzheimer's disease.

- Communicate respect for variant cultural beliefs and practices; help family members understand that their family member has a neurologic problem that may be part of the aging process. Explain how symptoms may become more progressive.

EVALUATION

- Evaluate the effectiveness of drug regimen by determining whether client's mental and physical status shows improvement from drug therapy

KEY WEBSITES

Tacrine: http://www.nlm.nih.gov/medlineplus/druginfo/medmaster/a693039.html

Update on Parkinson's Disease: http://www.aafp.org/afp/990415ap/2155.html

National Institute of Neurological Disorders and Stroke: http://www.ninds.nih.gov/

 Critical Thinking Case Study

TR, age 79, was diagnosed with Parkinson's disease 10 years ago. During his early treatment, he took selegiline. The drug dosage was increased to alleviate symptoms.

1. How does selegiline alleviate symptoms of parkinsonism?
2. What assessments should be made before and during the time TR takes selegiline?

Because TR developed numerous side effects and adverse reactions to selegiline, the health care provider changed the drug to carbidopa-levodopa (Sinemet). TR asks the nurse why the drug was changed.

3. What are the similarities and differences between selegiline and Sinemet??
4. What are the advantages of carbidopa-levodopa?

TR's family says they know a person with Parkinson's disease who takes the antiviral drug amantadine (Symmetrel). The family asks whether Symmetrel is the same as Sinemet and, if so, should TR take that drug instead of a drug containing carbidopa-levodopa.

5. What is the effect of amantadine on symptoms of parkinsonism?
6. What would be an appropriate response to the family's question concerning the use of Symmetrel for TR?
7. What are the uses for dopamine agonists and COMT inhibitors?
8. Certain anticholinergic drugs may be used to control parkinsonism symptoms. What is the action of these drugs and what are their side effects? These anticholinergic drugs are usually prescribed for parkinsonism symptoms resulting from what?

NCLEX Study Questions

1. A client with parkinsonism asks the nurse to explain what causes this condition. The most accurate response by the nurse is that the cause of parkinsonism is the degeneration of:
   a. cholinergic neurons
   b. dopaminergic neurons
   c. acetylcholine neurotransmitters
   d. monamine oxidase-B neurotransmitters

2. A client is receiving carbidopa-levodopa for parkinsonism. Which of the following statements is true regarding medication therapy for parkinsonism?
   a. carbidopa-levodopa may lead to hypertension
   b. carbidopa-levodopa may lead to excessive saliva
   c. dopaminergic and anticholinergic therapy may lead to drowsiness and sedation
   d. dopaminergics and anticholinergics are contraindicated in clients with glaucoma

3. A family member of a client with Alzheimer's disease asks the nurse what causes this disorder. The nurse realizes that in Alzheimer's disease there is:
   a. an excess of acetylcholine
   b. neurofibrillary tangles inside neurons
   c. degeneration of dopaminergic neurons
   d. neuritic plaques form inside neurons in the cerebellum

4. A client is taking rivastigmine (Exelon). Which of the following is true regarding rivastigmine?
   a. hepatotoxicity may occur
   b. the initial dose is 6 mg t.i.d.
   c. GI distress is a common side effect
   d. weight gain may be an adverse effect

5. Nursing interventions for the client taking carbidopa-levodopa for parkinsonism include:
   a. encouraging client to adhere to a high-protein diet
   b. informing client that perspiration may be dark and stain clothing
   c. advising client that glucose levels should be checked through urine testing
   d. warning client that it may take 4 to 5 days before symptoms are controlled

Answers: 1, b; 2, d; 3, b; 4, c; 5, b.

23

Drugs for Neuromuscular Disorders: Myasthenia Gravis, Multiple Sclerosis, and Muscle Spasms

ELECTRONIC RESOURCES

Evolve website (http://evolve.elsevier.com/KeeHayes/pharmacology/):
- *Case Studies*
- *Content Updates*
- *Frequently Asked Questions*
- *Student Review Activities*
- *WebLinks*
- *Additional Reference Material*

Companion CD-ROM:
- *NCLEX Examination Review Questions*
- *Pharmacology Animations*
- *IV Therapy Checklists*
- *Medication Error Checklists*
- *Drug Calculation Problems*
- *Electronic Calculators*
- *Top 200 Drugs with Pronunciations*
- *References from the Textbook*

Outline

Objectives

- Contrast the pathophysiology of myasthenia gravis and multiple sclerosis.
- Discuss the drug group used to treat myasthenia gravis.
- Explain the treatment strategies for the three phases of multiple sclerosis.
- Differentiate between the muscle relaxants used for spasticity and those used for muscle spasms.
- Apply the nursing process to drugs used to treat myasthenia gravis and muscle spasms.

Terms

Myasthenia gravis (MG), a lack of nerve impulses and muscle responses at the myoneural (nerves in muscle endings) junction, causes fatigue and muscular weakness of the respiratory system, facial muscles, and extremities. Because of cranial nerve involvement, ptosis (drooping eyelid) and difficulty in chewing and swallowing occur. Respiratory arrest may result from respiratory muscle paralysis. The symptoms of MG are caused by inadequate secretion of acetylcholine (ACh) or a loss of ACh because of an increase in the enzyme acetylcholinesterase, which destroys ACh at the myoneural junction.

The neuromuscular disorder **multiple sclerosis (MS)** attacks the myelin sheath of nerve fibers, causing lesions known as *plaques*. While there are no definitive diagnostic tests, the sclerotic plaques are usually detected and measured by magnetic resonance imaging (MRI). Pharmacologic treatment is necessary to control the symptoms of this disorder.

Muscle spasms have various causes, including injury or motor neuron disorders that lead to conditions such as cerebral palsy, MS, spinal cord injuries (paraplegia [paralysis of the legs]), cerebral vascular accident (stroke), or hemiplegia (paralysis of one side of the body). Spasticity of muscles can be reduced with the use of skeletal **muscle relaxants**.

Myasthenia Gravis

Myasthenia gravis (MG) is a chronic autoimmune neuromuscular disease that affects approximately 14 in 100,000 persons. It can occur at any age; however, MG occurs more commonly in women younger than 30 years and men older than 50. It is not a genetic disorder, but there can be a familial tendency.

Pathophysiology

Myasthenia gravis results from a lack of acetylcholine (ACh) receptor sites. This autoimmune disorder involves an antibody response against an alpha subunit of the acetylcholine receptor (AChR) site at the neuromuscular junction. Antibodies attack AChR sites, obstructing the binding of ACh and eventually destroying receptor sites. When AChR sites are reduced, ACh molecules are prevented from binding to receptors and stimulating normal neuromuscular transmission. The result is ineffective muscle contraction and muscle weakness. About 90% of clients with MG have anti-acetylcholine antibodies that can be detected through serum testing.

The thymus gland is involved in systemic immunity that is active during infancy and early childhood, but the gland normally shrinks during adulthood. Approximately 60% of MG clients have thymic hyperplasia. It has been suggested in some cases that if the thymus gland is removed during the early onset of MG, clinical symptoms are greatly decreased. Thymectomy has been an option for clients younger than 50 years of age.

Myasthenia gravis is characterized primarily by weakness and fatigue of the skeletal (voluntary) muscles. Other characteristics of MG include dysphagia (difficulty chewing and swallowing), dysarthria (slurred speech), and respiratory muscle weakness. Early symptoms of MG are ptosis (drooping eyelids) and diplopia (double vision).

The group of drugs used to control MG is the AChE inhibitors, also called *cholinesterase inhibitors* and *anticholinesterase*, which inhibit the action of the enzyme. As a result of this action, more acetylcholine is available to activate the cholinergic receptors and promote muscle contraction. The AChE inhibitors are classified as parasympathomimetics.

When muscular weakness of the client with MG becomes generalized, **myasthenic crisis** may occur. This complication is a severe generalized muscle weakness and may involve the muscles of respiration, such as the diaphragm and intercostal muscles. Triggers of myasthenic crisis include inadequate dosing of AChE inhibitors, infection, emotional stress, menses, pregnancy, surgery, trauma, hypokalemia, temperature extremes, and alcohol intake. Myasthenic crisis can also occur three to four hours after taking certain medications (e.g., aminoglycoside antibiotics, calcium channel blockers, phenytoin, psychotropics). If muscle weakness remains untreated, death could result from paralysis of the respiratory muscles. Neostigmine, a fast-acting AChE inhibitor, can relieve myasthenia crisis.

Overdosing with AChE inhibitors may cause another complication of MG called **cholinergic crisis,** which is an acute exacerbation of symptoms. A cholinergic crisis usually occurs within 30 to 60 minutes after taking anticholinergic medications. This complication is due to continuous depolarization of postsynaptic membranes that create neuromuscular blockade. The client with cholinergic crisis often has severe muscle weakness that can lead to respiratory paralysis and arrest. Accompanying symptoms include **miosis** (abnormal pupil constriction), pallor, sweating, vertigo, excess salivation, nausea, vomiting, abdominal cramping, diarrhea, bradycardia, and **fasciculations** (involuntary muscle twitching).

Acetylcholinesterase Inhibitors/ Cholinesterase Inhibitors

The first drug used to manage MG was neostigmine (Prostigmin). It is a short-acting **acetylcholinesterase (AChE)** inhibitor with a half-life of 0.5 to 1 hour. The drug is given every 2 to 4 hours and must be given on time to prevent muscle weakness. The AChE inhibitor pyridostigmine bromide (Mestinon) has an intermediate action and is given every 3 to 6 hours. Ambenonium chloride (Mytelase) is a long-acting AChE inhibitor and is usually prescribed when the client does not respond to neostigmine or pyridostigmine. Prototype Drug Chart 23–1 presents drug data related to pyridostigmine. Table 23–1 lists the AChE inhibitors. The cholinesterase (AChE) inhibitors are discussed in Chapter 22.

Prototype **DRUG CHART 23–1**

PYRIDOSTIGMINE BROMIDE

Drug Class	**Dosage**
Cholinesterase inhibitor Trade name: Mestinon *Pregnancy Category:* C	**A: PO:** 60-120 mg t.i.d./q.i.d.; *max:* 1.5 g/d **SR:** 180-540 mg q.d. or b.i.d. **IM/IV:** 2 mg q2-3h **C: PO:** 7 mg/kg/d in 5-6 divided doses

Contraindications	**Drug-Lab-Food Interactions**
GI and GU obstruction, severe renal disease *Caution:* Asthma, bradycardia, peptic ulcer, cardiac dysrhythmias, pregnancy	*Drug: Decrease* pyridostigmine effect with atropine, muscle relaxants, antidysrhythmics, magnesium

Pharmacokinetics	**Pharmacodynamics**

Absorption: PO: Poorly absorbed; SR: 50% absorbed
Distribution: PB: UK
Metabolism: t½: PO: 3.5-4 h; IV: 2 h
Excretion: In urine and by liver
	PO: Onset: 30-45 min
	  Peak: UK
	  Duration: 3-6 h
	PO SR: Onset: 0.5-1 h
	  Peak: UK
	  Duration: 6-12 h
	IM: Onset: 15 min
	  Peak: UK
	  Duration: 2-4 h
	IV: Onset: 2-5 min
	  Peak: UK
	  Duration: 2-3 h

Therapeutic Effects/Uses

To control and treat myasthenia gravis
Mode of Action: Transmission of neuromuscular impulses by preventing destruction of acetylcholine

Side Effects	**Adverse Reactions**
Nausea, vomiting, diarrhea, headache, dizziness, abdominal cramps, excess saliva, sweating, rash, miosis	Hypotension, bradycardia, urticaria *Life-threatening:* Respiratory depression, bronchospasm, cardiac dysrhythmias, seizures

A, Adult; *ALP*, alkaline phosphatase; *ALT*, alanine aminotransferase; *AST*, aspartate aminotransferase; *b.i.d.*, twice a day; *BUN*, blood urea nitrogen; *C*, child; *d*, day; *GI*, gastrointestinal; *GU*, genitourinary; *h*, hour; *IM*, intramuscular; *IV*, intravenous; *LDH*, lactic dehydrogenase; *MAOIs*, monoamine oxidase inhibitors; *max*, maximum; *min*, minute; *PB*, protein-binding; *PO*, by mouth; *q.i.d.*, four times a day; *SR*, sustained-release; *t½*, half-life; *t.i.d.*, three times a day; *UK*, unknown.

Pharmacokinetics

Pyridostigmine is poorly absorbed from the GI tract. Half of the sustained-release capsule is absorbed readily, but the balance is poorly absorbed. The half-life of oral pyridostigmine is 3.5 to 4 hours; when given intravenously (IV), it is 2 hours. Because of its short half-life, pyridostigmine must be administered several times a day. The drug is metabolized by the liver and excreted in the urine.

Pharmacodynamics

Pyridostigmine increases muscle strength of clients with muscular weakness resulting from MG. The onset of action of oral preparations is 0.5 to 1 hour. The duration of action is longer with the sustained-release drug capsule. One thirtieth of the oral dose of pyridostigmine can be administered IV. Overdosing of pyridostigmine can result in signs and symptoms of cholinergic crisis (extreme muscle weakness; increased salivation, tears, sweating; miosis); the antidote atropine sulfate should be available. This crisis requires emergency medical intervention because of respiratory muscle weakness.

Clients who do not respond to AChE inhibitors may require prednisone or immunosuppressive drugs. Prednisone decreases MG symptoms and promotes remission, but long-term use can cause adverse dermatologic effects (see Chapter 49).

The immunosuppressive agent azathioprine (Imuran) can be used in conjunction with a lower dose of prednisone. With azathioprine the white blood cell (WBC) count and liver enzymes should be closely monitored to avoid leukopenia and hepatotoxicity.

Overdosing and underdosing of AChE inhibitors have similar symptoms: muscle weakness, dyspnea (difficulty breathing), and dysphagia (difficulty swallowing). Additional symptoms that may be present with overdosing are increased salivation (drooling), bradycardia, abdominal cramping, and increased tearing and sweating. All doses of

Table 23–1

Acetylcholinesterase (AChE) Inhibitors: Myasthenia Gravis

Generic (Brand)	Route and Dosage	Uses and Considerations
ambenonium (Mytelase)	A: PO: 2.5-5.0 mg t.i.d./q.i.d.; dose may be increased; *maint:* 5-40 mg t.i.d./q.i.d.	For myasthenia gravis. A long-acting AChE inhibitor. It is 6 times more potent than neostigmine. Frequently used when client cannot take neostigmine or pyridostigmine because of the bromide component. It can be taken in adjunct with glucocorticoid drug. *Pregnancy category:* C; PB: UK; t½: UK
edrophonium Cl (Tensilon)	A: IV 2 mg; then 8 mg if no response IM: 10 mg; may repeat with 2 mg in 30 min C: <34 kg: IV: 1 mg, repeat in 30-45 sec if no response; *max:* 5 mg C: >34 kg: IV: 2 mg, repeat with 1 mg if no response; *max:* 10 mg	For diagnosing myasthenia gravis. Ptosis should be absent in 1-5 min. Very short-acting drug. *Pregnancy category:* C; PB: UK; t½: 1.2-2 h
neostigmine bromide (Prostigmin)	A: PO: 15-30 mg in 3-4 divided doses; *maint:* 150 mg/d in divided doses; *range:* 15-375 mg/d IM/IV: 0.5-2 mg PRN C: PO: 2 mg/kg/d in divided doses or 10 mg/m² q4h	For controlling myasthenia gravis. Must be given on time to prevent myasthenia crisis. Parenteral route is used if chewing, swallowing, and breathing are affected. Because of its short half-life, dose is usually given in 3 to 6 divided doses. Overdose can cause cholinergic reaction, nausea, abdominal cramps, excessive salivation, and sweating. *Pregnancy category:* C; PB: 15%-25%; t½: 1-1.5 h
pyridostigmine bromide (Mestinon)	(Prototype Drug Chart 23–2)	

A, Adult; *C,* child; *d,* day; *h,* hour; *IM,* intramuscular; *IV,* intravenous; *PB,* protein-binding; *PO,* by mouth; *PRN,* as needed; *q.i.d.,* four times a day; *t½,* half-life; *t.i.d.,* three times a day; *UK,* unknown; <, less than; >, greater than.

AChE inhibitors should be administered *on time,* because late administration of the drug could result in muscle weakness.

Underdosing can result in myasthenia crisis, and overdosing can result in cholinergic crisis. Edrophonium chloride (Tensilon) is a very short-acting AChE inhibitor that may be used to distinguish between myasthenia crisis and cholinergic crisis. These two different crises have a similar major symptom: severe muscle weakness. After edrophonium is administered, if the symptoms are alleviated because of an increase in ACh, the cause is myasthenia crisis. However, if the muscle weakness becomes more severe, the cause is cholinergic crisis due to drug overdosing.

Edrophonium may also be used to diagnose MG. Its ultra-short duration of 5 to 20 minutes increases muscle strength immediately. If ptosis is immediately corrected after administration of this drug, the diagnosis is most likely MG. Table 23–1 lists the AChE inhibitors.

Side Effects and Adverse Reactions

Side effects and adverse reactions of AChE inhibitors include GI disturbances (nausea, vomiting, diarrhea, abdominal cramps), increased salivation and tearing. Other side effects include miosis (constricted pupil of the eye), blurred vision, bradycardia, and hypotension.

 Nursing Process

Drug Treatment for Myasthenia Gravis: Pyridostigmine (Mestinon)

ASSESSMENT

■ Obtain a drug history of drugs client currently takes. Report if a drug-drug interaction is likely. Client should avoid atropine, atropine-like drugs, and muscle relaxants.
■ Record baseline vital signs for future comparison.
■ Assess client for signs and symptoms of myasthenia crisis such as muscle weakness with difficulty breathing and swallowing.

NURSING DIAGNOSES

■ Ineffective breathing pattern related to weak respiratory muscles
■ Risk for activity intolerance related to fatigue
■ Anxiety related to possible recurrence of myasthenia crisis and dyspnea

PLANNING

■ Client's symptoms of muscle weakness and difficulty breathing and swallowing caused by myasthenia gravis will be eliminated or reduced in 2 to 3 days.

NURSING INTERVENTIONS

■ Monitor effectiveness of drug therapy (acetylcholinesterase [AChE] inhibitors). Muscle strength should be increased. Both depth and rate of respirations should be assessed and maintained within normal range.
■ Administer pyridostigmine IV undiluted at rate of 0.5 mg/min. Do *not* add the drug to IV fluids.
■ Observe client for signs and symptoms of cholinergic crisis caused by overdosing: muscle weakness; increased salivation, sweating, tearing; miosis.
■ Have readily available an antidote for cholinergic crisis (atropine sulfate).

Client Teaching

General
• Instruct client to take drugs as prescribed to avoid recurrence of symptoms.
• Encourage client to wear a medical identification bracelet or necklace (e.g., MedicAlert) that indicates health problem and drugs taken.

Side Effects
• Advise client to report to health care provider recurrence of symptoms of myasthenia gravis. Drug therapy may need to be modified.

Diet
• Inform client to take drug before meals for best drug absorption. If gastric irritation occurs, take drug with food.

Cultural Considerations ❖

• Use simple and clear instructions. Involve family members in teaching about prescriptive therapies and disease process. Communicate respect for client/family culture and beliefs.
• Accommodate cultural values and assess whether client/family is accustomed to not taking all of medication as ordered or using medicines prescribed for other people. Stress that medications need to be taken as prescribed; medications are ordered specifically for each ailment; unused drugs should be discarded; and use of medications by individuals other than the intended may have serious consequences.

EVALUATION

■ Evaluate effectiveness of the drug therapy to maintain muscle strength.
■ Determine the absence of respiratory distress.

Multiple Sclerosis

Multiple sclerosis (MS) is an autoimmune disorder that attacks the myelin sheath of nerve fibers in the brain and spinal cord, causing lesions that are called *plaques.* In the United States, MS affects approximately 300,000 persons (ages 20 to 40), mostly white women. It is uncommon in African and Asian populations. Onset of MS is usually slow. It is a condition in which there are remissions and exacerbations of multiple symptoms (sensory and cerebellar) such as diplopia, weakness in the extremities, or spasticity. MS is difficult to diagnose, because there is no specific diagnostic test. Available laboratory tests that may suggest MS include elevated immunoglobulin G (IgG) in the cerebrospinal fluid, increased IgG/albumin ratio, and multiple lesions observable through MRI. A study cited by Noronha and Arnason states that monthly MRI scans of clients with MS can readily identify new lesions before clients have clinical symptoms; however, this can be costly. Scheduling regular treatment protocols to avoid clinical MS attacks is not recommended, because of the side effects of the drugs (e.g., glucocorticoids) used.

There are treatment strategies for three types or phases of MS: the acute attack, remission-exacerbation, and chronic progressive MS. Table 23–2 describes these three phases. Goals for treatment strategies are to decrease the inflammatory process of nerve fibers and improve conduction of demyelinating axons.

Various drug regimens for treating MS are currently in research and development. It is known, however, that clients with MS should avoid the following drugs: (1) histamine (H_2) blockers such as cimetidine and ranitidine, (2) indomethacin (a nonsteroidal antiinflammatory drug [NSAID]), and (3) beta-blockers like propranolol.

Skeletal Muscle Relaxants

Muscle relaxants relieve muscular spasms and pain associated with traumatic injuries and spasticity from chronic debilitating disorders (e.g., MS, stroke [cerebrovascular accident], cerebral palsy, head and spinal cord injuries). Spasticity results from increased muscle tone from hyperexcitable neurons caused by increased stimulation from the cerebral neurons or lack of inhibition in the spinal cord or at the skeletal muscles. The centrally acting muscle relaxants depress neuron activity in the spinal cord or brain and act directly on the skeletal muscles.

Centrally Acting Muscle Relaxants

The mechanism of action of centrally acting muscle relaxants is not fully known. Centrally acting muscle relaxants are used in cases of spasticity to suppress hyperactive reflex and for muscle spasms that do not respond to antiinflammatory agents, physical therapy, or other forms of therapy. The centrally acting muscle relaxants are described in Table 23–3. Prototype Drug Chart 23–2 gives the drug data for the centrally acting muscle relaxant carisoprodol (Soma).

Table 23–2

Treatment Strategies for the Three Phases of Multiple Sclerosis

Phases of Multiple Sclerosis	Characteristics	Treatment Strategies
Acute attack	Fatigue; motor weakness; optic neuritis	Tapering course of glucocorticoids (prednisone) Adrenocorticotropic hormone (ACTH) stimulates the adrenal cortex to secrete cortisol ACTH can be given IM or IV: Aqueous ACTH, 80 units in 500 ml of D_5W for 1-5 d Tapering doses of ACTH gel, IM for 25-30 d, starting with 40 units, b.i.d. 6-alpha methylprednisolone sodium succinate (MP): MP 1 g/d, IV, for 5-7 d Tapering doses of oral glucocorticoid
Remission-exacerbation	Recurrence of clinical MS symptoms; spasticity	Biologic (immune) response modifiers (BRMs); see Chapter 38. Betaseron, an interferon-β (IFN-β): 0.25 mg (8 million international units) every other day. Reduces spasticity and improves muscle movement. Also, interferon β-1a includes Rebif (given subQ in doses of 44 mcg 3 times per week) and Avonex (given IM in doses of 30 mcg every week), used in relapsing forms of MS. Immunosuppressant drug azathioprine (Imuran). Reduces exacerbation (relapses). Used for MS to decrease steroid use.
Chronic progressive	Progressive MS symptoms (wheelchair bound)	Immunosuppressant cyclophosphamide (Cytoxan) *Possible treatment protocol:* Cytoxan 600 mg/m² in 250 ml of D_5W every other day × 5 doses. Monitor WBC values. ACTH, tapering doses for 14 d. Starting with 40 units, IM, b.i.d.

b.i.d., Twice a day; *d*, day; *IM*, intramuscular; *IV*, intravenous; *WBC*, white blood cell count.

Spasticity

Skeletal muscle spasticity is muscular hyperactivity that causes contraction of the muscles, resulting in pain and limited mobility. Centrally acting muscle relaxants act on the spinal cord. Examples of centrally acting muscle relaxants used to treat spasticity are baclofen (Lioresal), dantrolene (Dantrium), and tizanidine (Zanaflex). Diazepam (Valium), a benzodiazepine, has also been effective for treating spasticity.

Muscle Spasms

Various centrally acting muscle relaxants are used for muscle spasm to decrease pain and increase range of motion. They have a sedative effect and should not be taken concurrently with CNS depressants such as barbiturates, narcotics, and alcohol. These agents, with the exception of cyclobenzaprine, can cause drug dependence. In addition, dizziness and drowsiness are common side effects. Exam-

Preventing MEDICATION ERRORS

Do not confuse...

- **baclofen** (skeletal muscle relaxant) with **Bactroban** (topical antibacterial) or **Beclovent** (corticosteroid inhalant). These drug names look alike, but the actions and pharmacology are very different.

Herbal ALERT 23–1

Diazepam

Kava kava and valerian may potentiate central nervous system depression.

ples of this group of centrally acting muscle relaxants are carisoprodol (Soma), chlorzoxazone (Paraflex), cyclobenzaprine (Flexeril), metaxalone (Skelaxin), methocarbamol (Robaxin), and orphenadrine citrate (Norflex).

Pharmacokinetics

Carisoprodol is well absorbed from the GI tract, and its half-life is moderate. The protein-binding percentage for carisoprodol is unknown. Carisoprodol is metabolized in the liver and excreted in urine.

Pharmacodynamics

Carisoprodol alleviates muscle spasm associated with acute painful musculoskeletal conditions. When carisoprodol is taken with alcohol, sedative-hypnotics, barbiturates, or tricyclic antidepressants (TCAs), increased central nervous system (CNS) depression occurs. The onset of action, peak concentration time, and duration of action for carisoprodol is short.

Side Effects and Adverse Reactions

The side effects from centrally acting muscle relaxants include drowsiness, dizziness, light-headedness, headaches, and occasional GI sensitivity (nausea, vomiting, diarrhea, abdominal distress). Cyclobenzaprine and orphenadrine have anticholinergic effects.

Table 23–3

Muscle Relaxants

Generic (Brand)	Route and Dosage	Uses and Considerations
Anxiolytics		
diazepam (Valium) CSS IV	A: PO: 2-10 mg b.i.d./q.i.d. IM/IV: 5-10 mg; may repeat	Diazepam has many uses, one of which is to relieve muscle spasms associated with paraplegia and cerebral palsy. Contraindicated in narrow-angle glaucoma. *Pregnancy category:* D; PB: 98%; $t^{1/2}$: 20-50 h
meprobamate (Miltown) CSS IV	A: PO: 400 mg-1.2 g/d in divided doses	This anxiolytic has a muscle relaxant effect. *Pregnancy category:* D; PB: UK; $t^{1/2}$: 10-12 h
Muscle Relaxants		
Spasticity (Centrally Acting)		
baclofen (Lioresal)	A: PO: Initially 5 mg t.i.d.; may increase dose; *maint:* 10-20 mg t.i.d./q.i.d.; *max:* 80 mg/d	For muscle spasms caused by MS and spinal cord injury. Overdose may cause CNS depression. Drowsiness, dizziness, nausea, hypotension may occur. *Pregnancy category:* C; PB: 30%; $t^{1/2}$: 3-4 h
tizanidine (Zanaflex)	A: PO: 4 mg q6-8h; adjust dose by 2 mg PRN; *max:* single dose of 12 mg	To manage spasticity, especially for spinal cord injury and multiple sclerosis. *Pregnancy category:* C; PB: UK; $t^{1/2}$: 2.5 h (half-life is longer for metabolites)
Spasticity (Direct Acting)		
dantrolene sodium (Dantrium)	A: PO: Initially 25 mg/d; increase gradually; *maint:* 100 mg b.i.d.-q.i.d. C: PO: Initially 0.5 mg/kg b.i.d.; increase dose gradually by 0.5 mg/kg t.i.d./q.i.d.; *max:* 100 mg q.i.d	For chronic neurologic disorders causing spasms: spinal cord injuries, stroke, MS. Start with low doses and increase every 4 to 7 d. Avoid taking with alcohol and CNS depressants. *Pregnancy category:* C; PB: 95%; $t^{1/2}$: 8 h
Centrally Acting Muscle Relaxants		
carisoprodol (Soma)	(Prototype Drug Chart 23–4)	
chlorzoxazone (Parafon forte)	A: PO: 250-500 mg t.i.d./q.i.d.; *max:* 3 g/d C: PO: 20 mg/kg/d or 600 mg m²/d in 3-4 divided doses	For acute or severe muscle spasms. Not effective for cerebral palsy. Take with food to decrease GI upset. *Pregnancy category:* C; PB: UK; $t^{1/2}$: 1 h
cyclobenzaprine HCl (Flexeril, Cycoflex)	A: PO: 10 mg t.i.d.; may increase dose; *maint:* 20-40 mg/d in 2-4 divided doses; *max:* 60 mg/d	For short-term treatment of muscle spasms. Not effective for relieving cerebral or spinal cord disease. Take with food or milk to decrease GI upset. *Pregnancy category:* B; PB: 93%; $t^{1/2}$: 1-3 d
methocarbamol (Robaxin, Marbaxin)	A: PO: Initially 1.5 g q.i.d.; *maint:* 1 g q.i.d. IM/IV: 0.5-1 g q8h; *max:* 3 g/d	For acute muscle spasms; drug used for treatment of tetanus. Has CNS depressant effects (sedation). Avoid taking alcohol or CNS depressants. Urine may be green, brown, or black. Drowsiness that may occur usually decreases with continued drug use. *Pregnancy category:* C; PB: UK; $t^{1/2}$: 1-2 h
metaxalone (Skelaxin)	A: PO: 800 mg t.i.d.- q.i.d.	For acute painful muscle spasticity *Pregnancy category:* UK; PB: UK; $t^{1/2}$: 2-3 hr
orphenadrine citrate (Norflex, Flexon)	A: PO: 100 mg b.i.d. IM/IV: 60 mg; may repeat in 12 h	For acute muscle spasm. Can be toxic with a mild overdose. Used in combination with aspirin and caffeine (Norgesic). *Pregnancy category:* C; PB: <20%; $t^{1/2}$: 14 h
Depolarizing Muscle Relaxants (Adjunct to Anesthesia)		
pancuronium bromide (Pavulon)	A: IV: 0.04-0.1 mg/kg; then 0.01 mg/kg every 30-60 min PRN C: >10 y: same as for adult	Used in surgery for relaxation of skeletal muscle (e.g., abdominal wall). Considered to be five times as potent as tubocurarine chloride. Does not cause hypotension or bronchospasm. *Pregnancy category:* C; PB: <10%; $t^{1/2}$: 2 h
succinylcholine Cl (Anectine Cl, Quelicin, Sucostrin)	A: IM: 2.5-4 mg/kg; *max:* 150 mg; IV: 0.3-1.1 mg/kg; *max:* 150 mg C: IM/IV: 1-2 mg/kg; *max:* IM: 150 mg	Used in surgery with anesthesia for skeletal muscle relaxation. Also used in endoscopy and intubation. *Pregnancy category:* C; PB: UK; $t^{1/2}$: UK
vecuronium bromide (Norcuron)	A & C: >9 y: IV: Initially 0.04-0.1 mg/kg/dose, then 0.05-0.1 mg/kg/h PRN	Use is similar as succinylcholine chloride. Can be used for clients with asthma, renal disease, or limited cardiac reserve. Given after general anesthesia has been started. *Pregnancy category:* C; PB: 60%-80%; $t^{1/2}$: 0.5-1.5 h
tubocurarine Cl	Anesthesia intubation: A: IV: Initially: 6-9 mg, followed by 3-4.5 mg in 3-5 min if needed C: IV: 0.2-0.5 mg/kg	Adjunct to general anesthesia. To induce skeletal muscle relaxation. *Pregnancy category:* C; PB: UK; $t^{1/2}$: 1-3 h

A, Adult; *b.i.d.,* twice a day; *C,* child; *CNS,* central nervous system; *CSS,* Controlled Substances Schedule; *d,* day; *GI,* gastrointestinal; *h,* hour; *IM,* intramuscular; *IV,* intravenous; *MS,* multiple sclerosis; *PB,* protein-binding; *PO,* by mouth; *PRN,* as needed; *q.i.d.,* four times a day; $t^{1/2},$ half-life; *t.i.d.,* three times a day; *UK,* unknown; *y,* year; >, greater than; <, less than.

Prototype DRUG CHART 23–2

CARISOPRODOL

Drug Class	**Dosage**
Centrally acting muscle relaxants Trade names: Soma, Soprodol *Pregnancy Category:* C	**A:** PO: 350 mg t.i.d. at bedtime **C: >5y: PO:** 25 mg/kg/d in 4 divided doses
Contraindications	**Drug-Lab-Food Interactions**
Severe liver or renal disease	*Drug: Increase* CNS depression with alcohol, narcotics, sedative-hypnotics, antihistamines, tricyclic anti-depressants May *increase* risk of ventricular fibrillation with calcium channel blockers
Pharmacokinetics	**Pharmacodynamics**
Absorption: PO: Well absorbed **Distribution:** PB: UK **Metabolism:** t½: 8 h **Excretion:** In urine	**PO:** Onset: 30 min Peak: 3-4 h Duration: 4-6 h

Therapeutic Effects/Uses

To relax skeletal muscles. Baclofen, dantrolene, and tizanidine are used to treat spasticity associated with stroke, spinal cord injury, multiple sclerosis, cerebral palsy
Mode of Action: Blocks interneuronal activity.

Side Effects	**Adverse Reactions**
Nausea, vomiting, dizziness, weakness, insomnia	Asthmatic attack, tachycardia, hypotension, diplopia

A, Adult; *C*, child; *CNS*, central nervous system; *d*, day; *h*, hour; *min*, minute; *PB*, protein-binding; *PO*, by mouth; *t½*, half-life; *t.i.d.*, three times a day; *UK*, unknown; >, greater than.

Nursing Process

Muscle Relaxant: Carisoprodol

ASSESSMENT

- Collect medical history. Carisoprodol is contraindicated if client has severe renal or liver disease.
- Obtain baseline vital signs for future comparison.
- Secure client's health history to identify the cause of muscle spasm and determine whether it is acute or chronic.
- Gather a drug history. Report if a drug-drug interaction is probable.
- Note if there is a history of narrow-angle glaucoma or myasthenia gravis. Cyclobenzaprine and orphenadrine are contraindicated with these health problems.

NURSING DIAGNOSES

- Impaired physical mobility related to dizziness and hyperactive reflexes
- Activity intolerance related to drowsiness and hyperactive reflexes

PLANNING

- Client will be free of muscular pain within 1 week.

NURSING INTERVENTIONS

- Monitor serum liver enzyme levels of clients taking dantrolene and carisoprodol. Report elevated levels of liver enzymes such as alkaline phosphatase (ALP), alanine aminotransferase (ALT), and gamma-glutamyl transferase (GGT).
- Record vital signs. Report abnormal results.
- Observe for CNS side effects (e.g., dizziness).

Client Teaching

General

- Instruct client that the muscle relaxant should not be abruptly stopped. Drug should be tapered over 1 week to avoid rebound spasms.
- Advise client not to drive or operate dangerous machinery when taking muscle relaxants. These drugs have a sedative effect and can cause drowsiness.
- Inform client that most of the centrally acting muscle relaxants for acute spasms are usually taken for no longer than 3 weeks.

- Teach client to avoid alcohol and CNS depressants. If muscle relaxants are taken with these drugs, CNS depression may be intensified.
- Warn client that these drugs are contraindicated for pregnant women or nursing mothers. Check with health care provider.

Side Effects
- Tell client to report side effects of the muscle relaxant: nausea, vomiting, dizziness, faintness, headache, and diplopia. Dizziness and faintness are most likely caused by orthostatic (postural) hypotension.

Diet
- Educate client to take muscle relaxants with food to decrease gastrointestinal upset.

Cultural Considerations ❖

- When offering a prescription, instructions, or pamphlets to Asian and Pacific Islanders use both hands, which show respect. Health care practitioners are held in high regard.
- Demonstrate respect by addressing client formally until told otherwise, and do not ask private questions in public.

EVALUATION

- Evaluate effectiveness of the muscle relaxant to determine whether client's muscular pain has decreased or disappeared.

KEY WEBSITES

Facts About Myasthenia Gravis (MG): www.myasthenia.org

How to handle myasthenic crisis: Essential steps in patient care: http://www.postgradmed.com/issues/2000/04_00/bedlack.htm

Pyridostigmine: http://www.nlm.nih.gov/medlineplus/druginfo/medmaster/a682229.html

 Critical Thinking Case Study

FR, age 29, was diagnosed with myasthenia gravis 2 years ago. She is receiving pyridostigmine 120 mg t.i.d. Last evening FR was involved in an automobile accident. She was taken to the emergency room unconscious and missed two evening does of pyridostigmine.

1. How does pyridostigmine alleviate the symptoms of myasthenia gravis?
2. What are the potential side effects and adverse effects of pyridostigmine?
3. What problems are likely to develop following delayed pyridostigmine dosing?

FR is scheduled for surgery to repair a fractured femur suffered in the accident. During surgery FR develops bradycardia.

4. What medications may lead to drug interactions with pyridostigmine?
5. What problems may develop from pyridostigmine overdosing?
6. What are the similarities between myasthenia crisis and cholinergic crisis?

 NCLEX Study Questions

1. Which of the following best explains the pathophysiology of myasthenia gravis?
   a. degeneration of cholinergic neurons and a deficit in acetylcholine leads to neuritic plaques and neurofibrillary tangles
   b. decreased amount of acetylcholine to cholinergic receptors produces weak muscles and reduced nerve impulses
   c. myelin sheaths of nerve fibers in brain and spinal cord develop lesions or plaques
   d. imbalance of dopamine and acetylcholine leads to degeneration of neurons in midbrain and extrapyramidal motor tracts.

2. The nurse realizes that pyridostigmine administration may lead to which adverse reaction?
   a. hypertension
   b. bronchospasm
   c. thrombocytopenia
   d. Stevens-Johnson syndrome

3. A client has spasticity following a spinal cord injury. Which of the following drugs might be prescribed to treat this client's spasticity?
   a. tacrine
   b. ropinirole
   c. carisoprodol
   d. pyridostigmine

4. A client with multiple sclerosis is in the chronic progressive phase. Which drug would be most helpful at this time?
   a. interferon β-1a (Avonex, Rebif)
   b. glucocorticoids
   c. azathioprine (Imuran)
   d. cyclophosphamide (Cytoxan)

5. Which of the following statements is true regarding carisoprodol (Soma)?
   a. may cause hypertension
   b. may lead to bradycardia
   c. blocks interneuronal activity
   d. its action is decreased by antihistamines

Answers: 1. b; 2, b; 3, c; 4, d; 5, c.

SEVEN

Antiinflammatory and Pain Management Agents

Introduction

Unit VII discusses agents prescribed to alleviate an inflammatory process. Included in this unit are antiinflammatory drugs.

Inflammation

Inflammation is a reaction to tissue injury caused by the release of chemical mediators that trigger both a vascular response and the migration of fluid and cells (leukocytes, or white blood cells) to the injured site. The chemical mediators are (1) histamines, (2) kinins, and (3) prostaglandins. *Histamine*, the first mediator in the inflammatory process, causes dilation of the arterioles and increases capillary permeability, allowing fluid to leave the capillaries and flow into the injured area. *Kinins*, such as bradykinin, also increase capillary permeability and the sensation of pain. *Prostaglandins* are released, causing an increase in vasodilation, capillary permeability, pain, and fever. The antiinflammatory drugs, such as nonsteroidal antiinflammatory drugs (NSAIDs) and steroids (cortisone preparations), inhibit chemical mediators, thus decreasing the inflammatory process. Figure VII–1 illustrates the process of chemical mediators acting on injured tissues. The five responses to tissue injury are called the *cardinal signs of inflammation:* redness, swelling, pain, heat, and loss of function.

Inflammation may or may not be the result of an infection. (Only a small percentage of inflammations are caused by infections.) Other causes of inflammation include trauma, surgical interventions, extreme heat or cold, and caustic chemical agents. Antiinflammatory drugs reduce fluid migration and pain, lessening loss of function and increasing the client's mobility and comfort.

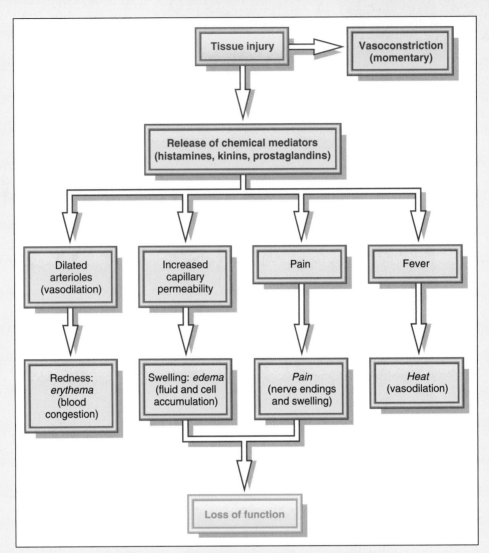

FIGURE VII–I   Chemical mediator response to tissue injury.

24

Antiinflammatory Drugs

> **ELECTRONIC RESOURCES**
>
> **Evolve website (http://evolve.elsevier.com/KeeHayes/pharmacology/):**
> - *Case Studies*
> - *Content Updates*
> - *Frequently Asked Questions*
> - *Student Review Activities*
> - *WebLinks*
> - *Additional Reference Material*
>
> **Companion CD-ROM:**
> - *NCLEX Examination Review Questions*
> - *Pharmacology Animations*
> - *IV Therapy Checklists*
> - *Medication Error Checklists*
> - *Drug Calculation Problems*
> - *Electronic Calculators*
> - *Top 200 Drugs with Pronunciations*
> - *References from the Textbook*

Outline

Objectives

- Explain the pathophysiologic basis of five cardinal signs of inflammation.
- Describe the action of nonsteroidal antiinflammatory drugs (NSAIDs).
- Explain the use of disease-modifying antirheumatic drugs (DMARDs).
- Differentiate between the side effects and adverse reactions of NSAIDs and DMARDs.
- Correlate the nursing processes associated with NSAIDs and corticosteroids, including client teaching.
- Apply the nursing process to the client taking DMARDs.
- Explain the action of antigout medications.

Terms

Inflammation is a response to tissue injury and infection. When the inflammatory process occurs, a vascular reaction takes place in which fluid, elements of blood, leukocytes (white blood cells [WBCs]), and chemical mediators accumulate at the injured tissue or infection site. The process of inflammation is a protective mechanism in which the body attempts to neutralize and destroy harmful agents at the site of injury and to establish conditions for tissue repair.

Although there is a relationship between inflammation and infection, these terms should *not* be used interchangeably. **Infection** is caused by microorganisms and results in inflammation, but *not* all inflammations are caused by infections.

Pathophysiology

The five characteristics of inflammation, called *the cardinal signs of inflammation,* are redness, swelling (edema), heat, pain, and loss of function. Table 24–1 gives the description and explanation of the cardinal signs of inflammation. The two phases of inflammation are the *vascular phase,* which occurs 10 to 15 minutes after an injury, and the *delayed phase.* The vascular phase is associated with vasodilation and increased capillary permeability, during which blood substances and fluid leave the plasma and go to the injured site. The delayed phase occurs when leukocytes infiltrate the inflamed tissue.

Various chemical mediators are released during the inflammation process. Prostaglandins that have been isolated from the exudate at inflammatory sites are among them. **Prostaglandins** (chemical mediators) have many effects: vasodilation, relaxation of smooth muscle, increased capillary permeability, and sensitization of nerve cells to pain.

Cyclooxygenase (COX) is the enzyme responsible for converting arachidonic acid into prostaglandins and their products. This synthesis of prostaglandins causes inflammation and pain at a tissue injury site. There are two enzyme forms of cyclooxygenase: COX-1 and COX-2. COX-1 protects the stomach lining and regulates blood platelets, and COX-2 triggers inflammation and pain.

Antiinflammatory Agents

Drugs such as aspirin inhibit the biosynthesis of prostaglandin and are therefore called *prostaglandin inhibitors.* Because prostaglandin inhibitors affect the inflammatory process, they are more commonly called *antiinflammatory agents.*

Antiinflammatory agents also relieve pain (analgesic), reduce elevated body temperature (antipyretic), and inhibit platelet aggregation (anticoagulant). Aspirin is the oldest antiinflammatory drug, but it was first used for its analgesic and antipyretic properties. As a result of searching for a more effective drug with fewer side effects, many other antiinflammatory agents, or prostaglandin inhibitors, have been discovered. Although these drugs have potent antiinflammatory effects that mimic the effects of corticosteroids (cortisone), they are *not* chemically related to corticosteroids and therefore are called **nonsteroidal antiinflammatory drugs (NSAIDs).** Most NSAIDs are used to decrease inflammation and pain for clients who have some type of arthritic condition.

Nonsteroidal Antiinflammatory Drugs

NSAIDs are aspirin and aspirin-like drugs that inhibit the enzyme COX, which is needed for the biosynthesis of prostaglandins. Chapters 25 and 44 present expanded discussions of NSAIDs in their roles as analgesics and anticoagulants. These drugs may be called *prostaglandin inhibitors* with varying degrees of analgesic and antipyretic effects, but they are used primarily as antiinflammatory agents to relieve inflammation and pain. Their antipyretic effect is less than their antiinflammatory effect. With several exceptions, NSAID preparations are not suggested for use in alleviating mild headaches and mildly elevated temperature.

Table 24–1

Cardinal Signs of Inflammation

Signs	Description and Explanation
Erythema (redness)	Redness occurs in the first phase of inflammation. Blood accumulates in the area of tissue injury because of the release of the body's chemical mediators (kinins, prostaglandins, and histamine). Histamine dilates the arterioles.
Edema (swelling)	Swelling is the second phase of inflammation. Plasma leaks into the interstitial tissue at the injury site. Kinins dilate the arterioles, increasing capillary permeability.
Heat	Heat at the inflammatory site can be caused by increased blood accumulation and may result from pyrogens (substances that produce fever) that interfere with the temperature-regulating center in the hypothalamus.
Pain	Pain is caused by tissue swelling and the release of chemical mediators.
Loss of function	Function is lost because of the accumulation of fluid at the tissue injury site and because of pain, which decreases mobility at the affected area.

Preferred drugs for headaches and fever are aspirin, acetaminophen, and ibuprofen (given to children and adults with high fever). NSAIDs are more appropriate for reducing swelling, pain, and stiffness in joints.

NSAIDs cost more than aspirin. Other than aspirin, the only NSAIDs that can be purchased over-the-counter (OTC) are ibuprofen (Motrin, Nuprin, Advil, Medipren) and naproxen (Aleve). Ibuprofen is also available in generic form in 200 mg tablets or capsules. All other NSAIDs require a prescription. Examples of prescription products on the market that contain NSAID contents alone or in combination include Anaprox, Celebrex, Clinoril, Daypro, Equagesic, Naprosyn, Percodan, Relafen, Soma Compound, Talwin, and Toradol. If a client can take aspirin for the inflammatory process without gastrointestinal (GI) upset, salicylate products are usually recommended.

There are seven groups of NSAIDs:
1. Salicylates
2. *Para*-Chlorobenzoic acid derivatives, or indoles
3. Phenylacetic acids
4. Propionic acid derivatives
5. Fenamates
6. Oxicams
7. Selective COX-2 inhibitors

The first six NSAID groups on the list are now known as *first-generation NSAIDs,* and the COX-2 inhibitors are called *second-generation NSAIDs.*

Table 24–2 provides dosage information and considerations for use for the most commonly used NSAIDs. The half-lives of NSAIDs differ greatly—some have a short half-life, others have a moderate to long half-life with a general range of 8 to 24 hours. Aspirin should not be taken with an NSAID because of the side effects. In addition, combined therapy does not increase effectiveness.

Salicylates

Aspirin comes from the family of salicylates derived from salicylic acid. Aspirin is also called *acetylsalicylic acid (ASA)* after the acetyl group used in the composition of aspirin. The abbreviation frequently used for aspirin is ASA.

Aspirin was developed in 1899 by Adolph Bayer, making it the oldest antiinflammatory agent. It was the most frequently used antiinflammatory agent before the introduction of ibuprofen. Aspirin is a prostaglandin inhibitor that decreases the inflammatory process. It is also considered an antiplatelet drug for clients with cardiac or cerebrovascular disorders; aspirin decreases platelet aggregation, and thus blood clotting is decreased. Because high doses of aspirin are usually needed to relieve inflammation, gastric distress is a common problem. In such cases, enteric-coated (EC) tablets may be used. Aspirin should *not* be taken with other NSAIDs because it decreases the blood level and effectiveness of NSAIDs.

Aspirin and other NSAIDs relieve pain by inhibiting the enzyme COX, which is needed for the biosynthesis of prostaglandins. There are two enzyme forms of cyclooxygenase, symbolized as COX-1 and COX-2. (Figure 24–1)

COX-1 protects the stomach lining and regulates blood platelets, promoting blood clotting. COX-2 triggers pain and inflammation at the injured site. Usually NSAIDs inhibit or block both COX-1 and COX-2. Inhibition of COX-1 produces the desirable effect of decreasing platelet aggregation, but the undesirable effect of decreasing protection to the stomach lining. Stomach bleeding and ulcers may occur with aspirin and NSAID agents. When COX-2 is inhibited, pain and fever are reduced and inflammation is suppressed, but COX-2 inhibitors do not cause gastric ulceration and have no effect on platelet function.

Newer NSAIDs block only COX-2 and not COX-1. These drugs leave protection for the stomach lining intact (no gastric bleeding and ulcers), but still deliver relief for pain and inflammation.

A COX-2 inhibitor approved by the Food and Drug Administration (FDA) is celecoxib (Celebrex, manufactured by Pfizer). Drugs similar to COX-2 inhibitors include meloxicam (Mobic) and nabumetone (Relafen, manufactured by SmithKline Beecham), which allow some stomach protection. Clients at risk for stroke or heart attack who take aspirin to prevent blood clotting (decreases platelet aggregation) would not benefit from COX-2 inhibitors. If COX-1 enzyme were not blocked, increased blood clotting would remain even though the stomach lining is protected.

Many researchers believe that COX-2 inhibitors may prevent some types of cancer (e.g., colon cancer). Fruits and vegetables block COX-2 enzyme naturally, protecting the colon from malignant growths.

Pharmacokinetics

Aspirin is well absorbed from the GI tract (Prototype Drug Chart 24–1). It can cause GI upset, so it should be taken with water, milk, or food. The EC or buffered form can decrease gastric distress. Enteric coated tablets should not be crushed or broken.

Aspirin has a short half-life. It should not be taken during the last trimester of pregnancy, because it could cause premature closure of the ductus arteriosus in the fetus. Aspirin should not be taken by children with flu symptoms, because it may cause the potentially fatal Reye syndrome.

Pharmacodynamics

Aspirin, like other NSAIDs, inhibits prostaglandin synthesis by inhibiting COX-1 and COX-2; thus it decreases inflammation and pain. The onset of action for aspirin is within 30 minutes. It peaks in 1 to 2 hours, and the duration of action is an average of 4 to 6 hours. The action for the rectal preparation of aspirin can be erratic because of blood supply and fecal material in the rectum; it may take a week or longer for a therapeutic antiinflammatory effect.

Hypersensitivity to Salicylate Products

Clients may be hypersensitive to aspirin. Tinnitus (ringing in the ears), vertigo (dizziness), and bronchospasm—especially in asthmatic clients—are symptoms of aspirin overdose or hypersensitivity to aspirin. Clients should not take diflunisal if they are hypersensitive to aspirin. Diflunisal is a derivative of salicylic acid, although it is not converted to salicylic acid in the body.

Salicylates are present in numerous foods (e.g., prunes, raisins, licorice) and in spices (e.g., curry powder, paprika).

Table 24–2

Antiinflammatory: Nonsteroidal Antiinflammatory

Generic (Brand)	Route and Dosage	Uses and Considerations
First-Generation NSAIDs		
Salicylates		
aspirin (ASA, Bayer, Ecotrin)	(Prototype Drug Chart 24–1)	
diflunisal (Dolobid)	A: PO: Initially: 1 g (1000 mg); *maint:* 500 mg q8-12h	Relief of mild to moderate pain; used to treat osteoarthritis and rheumatoid arthritis. Acts by inhibiting prostaglandin synthesis. Avoid if hypersensitive to aspirin. Do not use during third trimester of pregnancy. *Pregnancy category:* C; PB: 80%-90%; t½: 8-12 h
Salicylate Derivatives		
olsalazine sodium (Dipentum)	A: PO: 500 mg q12h; may increase dose every 2 to 4 wk; *max:* 3 g/d in divided doses	To treat inflammatory bowel disease, especially ulcerative colitis. Excretion is mainly in feces as 5-ASA. *Pregnancy category:* C; PB: UK; t½: 6 h
sulfasalazine (Azulfidine)	A: PO: 0.5 g daily initially then 2 g daily in divided doses; *max:* 75 mg/kg/d C: PO: 40-50 mg/kg/d in 4 divided doses	For treatment of ulcerative colitis and rheumatoid arthritis. Avoid if allergic to sulfonamides or aspirin. *Pregnancy category:* B (D if near term); PB: UK; t½: 5-10 h
Para-Chlorobenzoic Acid (Indoles)		
indomethacin (Indocin)	A: PO: 25-50 mg b.i.d./t.i.d. with food; SR: 75 mg daily/b.i.d.; *max:* 200 mg/d C: PO: 1-2 mg/kg/d in 2-4 divided doses; may increase to 4 mg/kg/d; *max:* 150-200 mg/d	For moderate to severe arthritic conditions. Potent drug. GI upset and ulceration are common. Take drug with food. Avoid indomethacin if allergic to aspirin. *Pregnancy category:* B (D near term); PB: 90%-99%; t½: 3-120 h
sulindac (Clinoril)	A: PO: 150-200 mg b.i.d.	For acute and chronic arthritis, bursitis, and tendinitis. Not as potent as indomethacin. Give with food. *Pregnancy category:* C; PB: 93%; t½: 7-18 h
tolmetin (Tolectin)	A: PO: Initially: 400 mg t.i.d.; *maint:* 600-1800 mg/d in divided doses; *max:* 2 g/d C: >2 y: PO: 20 mg/kg/d in divided doses; *max:* 30 mg/kg/d	For acute and chronic arthritis, including juvenile rheumatoid arthritis. Less potent than indomethacin; more effective than aspirin. Take drug with food. *Pregnancy category:* B (D near term); PB: 90%-99%; t½: 1-1.5 h
Phenylacetic Acid		
diclofenac sodium (Voltaren)	A: PO: 25-50 mg t.i.d./q.i.d. or 75 mg b.i.d.	For rheumatoid arthritis, osteoarthritis, and spondylitis. Also for acute gout, juvenile rheumatoid arthritis, bursitis, and tendinitis. If GI distress occurs, take with food. *Pregnancy category:* B; PB: 90%-99%; t½: 2 h
etodolac (Lodine)	A: PO: 600-1200 mg/d in 2-4 divided doses PRN; *max:* 1200 mg/d *Rheumatoid arthritis:* A: PO: 500 mg b.i.d.	Used for acute pain, rheumatoid arthritis, and osteoarthritis. Take with food or antacid to avoid GI distress. *Pregnancy category:* C; PR: 99%; t½: 6-7 h
ketorolac tromethamine (Toradol)	A: PO: 10 mg q6h PRN; *max:* 40 mg/day IM/IV: 30 mg q6h PRN; *max:* 120 mg/day Elderly: PO: 5-10 mg q6h PRN; *max:* 40 mg/day IM/IV: 15 mg q6h PRN; *max:* 60 mg/day	First injectable NSAID. For short-term pain management of 5 days or less. Also available for ophthalmic use to relieve itching caused by allergic conjunctivitis. *Pregnancy category:* B; PB: 99%; t½: 3-8 h; increase in elderly
Propionic Acid		
fenoprofen calcium (Nalfon)	A: PO: 300-600 mg t.i.d./q.i.d.; *max:* 3.2 g/d C: PO: 900 mg/m² in divided doses	Treatment of mild to moderate pain. Also for arthritic conditions. Most effective after 2-3 wk of therapy. Take with food. *Pregnancy category:* B (D at term); PB: 90%-99%; t½: 3 h
flurbiprofen sodium (Ansaid, Ocufen)	A: PO: 50-300 mg/d in 2-4 divided doses; *max:* 300 mg/d *Ophthalmic use:* 0.03% sol	Treatment of acute and chronic arthritis. Take drug with food. *Pregnancy category:* C; PB: UK; t½: 5 h

A, Adult; *b.i.d.*, twice a day; *C*, child; *d*, day; *GI*, gastrointestinal; *h*, hour; *IM*, intramuscular; *maint*, maintenance; *max*, maximum; *NSAID*, nonsteroidal antiinflammatory drug; *PB*, protein-binding; *PO*, by mouth; *PRN*, as needed; *q.i.d.*, four times a day; *sol*, solution; *SR*, sustained-release; *t½*, half-life; *t.i.d.*, three times a day; *UK*, unknown; *wk*, week; *y*, year; *>*, greater than; *<*, less than.

Table 24–2

Antiinflammatory: Nonsteroidal Antiinflammatory—cont'd

Generic (Brand)	Route and Dosage	Uses and Considerations
ibuprofen (Motrin, Advil, Nuprin, Medipren)	(Prototype Drug Chart 24–2)	
ketoprofen (Orudis, Actron)	*Inflammatory:* A: PO: *maint:* 150-300 mg/d in 3-4 divided doses; *max:* 300 mg/d *Mild to moderate pain:* A: PO: 25-50 mg q6-8h PRN; *max:* 300 mg/d	Relief of mild to moderate pain and acute and chronic arthritis. Take with food or 8 ounces of water to avoid GI upset. *Pregnancy category:* B (D at term); PB: 99%; t½: 3-4 h
naproxen (Naprosyn)	A: PO: 250-500 mg b.i.d. C: PO: 5-10 mg/kg/d in 2 divided doses	Relief of mild to moderate pain. Also for arthritic, gout, bursitis conditions and dysmenorrhea. Similar OTC drug: Aleve. Take with food or with a full glass of water. *Pregnancy category:* B; PB: 99%; t½: 8-20 h
oxaprozin (Daypro)	A: PO: Initially: 1200 mg/d; *maint:* 600 mg/d; *max:* 1800 mg/d in divided doses	Treatment of acute and chronic arthritis. Take with food for GI discomfort. *Pregnancy category:* C; PB: 99%; t½: 40 h
Anthranilic Acids (Fenamates)		
meclofenamate (Meclomen)	A: PO: 200-400 mg in 3-4 divided doses	For acute and chronic arthritis. GI symptoms can be severe. Used when other NSAIDs are not effective. Take with food to avoid GI upset. *Pregnancy category:* B (D at term); PB: 99%; t½: 3 h
mefenamic acid (Ponstel)	A: PO: Initially: 500 mg; then 250 mg q6h PRN; *max:* 1 g/d	For acute and chronic arthritis. Diarrhea is a common problem. Usually discontinued after 7 days. *Pregnancy category:* C; PB: 90%; t½: 2-4 h
Oxicams		
piroxicam (Feldene)	A: PO: 10 mg b.i.d. or 20 mg daily	For arthritic conditions. Long half-life; effective at 2 weeks. GI upset may occur. *Pregnancy category:* C; PB: 99%; t½: 30-86 h
meloxicam (Mobic)	A: PO: 7.5-15 mg daily	For treatment of osteoarthritis. Some COX-2 selectivity. *Pregnancy category:* C (first and second trimester), D (third trimester); PB: 99%; t½: 15-20 h
Naphthylalkanones		
nabumetone (Relafen)	A: PO: 500-1000 mg/d or in 2 divided doses	To treat chronic inflammation and pain, especially for arthritic conditions such as rheumatoid arthritis. Inhibits cyclooxygenase, particularly COX-2 more than COX-1; fewer GI problems. *Pregnancy category:* C; PB: 99%; t½: 22-30 h
COX-2 Inhibitors (Second-Generation NSAIDs)		
celecoxib (Celebrex)	A: PO: 100-200 mg/d Elderly: Same dose	To treat arthritic-type pain. Relieves inflammation and pain without causing GI distress. Should not be used like aspirin for cardiac precautions. Avoid during third trimester of pregnancy. *Pregnancy category:* C (D at late pregnancy); PB: 97%; t½: 11 h

OTC, Over-the-counter.

Nursing Process

Salicylate: Aspirin

ASSESSMENT

■ Determine a medical history. Determine whether there is any history of gastric upset, gastric bleeding, or liver disease. Aspirin can cause gastric irritation. It prolongs bleeding time by inhibiting platelet aggregation.

■ Obtain a drug history. Report if a drug-drug interaction is probable.

NURSING DIAGNOSES

■ Risk for injury related to vertigo
■ Chronic pain related to tissue swelling of rheumatoid arthritis

PLANNING

■ Client will be free of mild pain in 12 to 24 hours and mild inflammation within 1 week. Aspirin may be ordered for mild to severe arthritic condition, pain relief, antiinflammatory effects, fever reduction, and inhibition of platelet aggregation.

NURSING INTERVENTIONS

■ Monitor serum salicylate (aspirin) level when client takes high doses of aspirin for chronic conditions such as arthritis. The normal therapeutic range is 15 to 30 mg/dl. Mild toxicity occurs at serum level of >30 mg/dl, and severe toxicity occurs at >50 mg/dl.
■ Observe client for signs of bleeding such as dark (tarry) stools, bleeding gums, petechiae (round red spots), ecchymosis (excessive bruising), and purpura (large red spots) when client takes high doses of aspirin.

Client Teaching

General

• Advise client not to take aspirin with alcohol or drugs such as the anticoagulant warfarin (Coumadin) that are highly protein-bound. Aspirin displaces drugs like warfarin from the protein-binding site, causing increased anticoagulant levels.
• Suggest that client inform the dentist before a dental visit if taking high doses of aspirin.
• With the health care provider's approval, instruct client to discontinue aspirin 3 to 7 days before surgery to reduce risk of bleeding.
• Keep aspirin bottle out of reach of small children.
• Educate parent to call the poison control center immediately if a child has taken a large or unknown amount of aspirin (also acetaminophen).
• Warn client not to administer aspirin for virus or flu symptoms in children. Reye syndrome (vomiting, lethargy, delirium, and coma) has been linked with aspirin and viral infections. Acetaminophen is usually prescribed for cold and flu symptoms.
• Inform client that aspirin tablets can cause GI distress.
• Inform client with dysmenorrhea to take acetaminophen instead of aspirin 2 days before and during the first 2 days of the menstrual period.

Side Effects

• Direct client to report side effects such as drowsiness, tinnitus (ringing in the ears), headaches, flushing, dizziness, GI symptoms (bleeding, heartburn), visual changes, and seizures.

Diet

• Instruct client to take aspirin (also ibuprofen) with food, at mealtime, or with plenty of fluids. Enteric-coated aspirin helps prevent GI disturbance.

Cultural Considerations ❖

• Do not misunderstand loud voice volume as necessarily reflecting anger among some African Americans and Arabs, who may be merely expressing their thoughts in a dynamic manner.

EVALUATION

■ Evaluate the effectiveness of aspirin in relieving pain. If pain persists, another analgesic such as ibuprofen may be prescribed.
■ Determine whether client has any side effects to aspirin.

*Aspirin is only one of the NSAIDs.

FIGURE 24–1 Uses of COX-1 and COX-2 inhibitors.

Para-Chlorobenzoic Acid

One of the first NSAIDs introduced was indomethacin (Indocin), a *para*-chlorobenzoic acid. It is used for rheumatoid arthritis, gouty arthritis, and osteoarthritis and is a potent prostaglandin inhibitor. It is highly protein bound (90%) and displaces other protein-bound drugs, resulting in potential toxicity. It has a moderate half-life (4 to 11 hours). Indomethacin is very irritating to the stomach and should be taken with food.

Prototype DRUG CHART 24–1

ASPIRIN

Drug Class

Analgesic, antiinflammatory drug
Trade names: ASA, Bayer, Ecotrin, Alka Seltzer,
  Empirin, ✣Astrin, Entrophen, Novasen
Pregnancy Category: D

Dosage

Analgesic:
A: PO: 325-650 mg q4h prn; *max:* 4 g/d
C: PO: 40-65 mg/d or 10-15 mg/kg in 4-6 divided doses;
  max: 3.5 g/d
TIA and thromboembolic condition:
A: PO: 325-650 mg/d or b.i.d.
Arthritis:
A: PO: 3.6-5.4 g/d in divided doses
TDM: 15-30 mg/dl; 150-300 mcg/ml

Contraindications

Hypersensitivity to salicylates or NSAIDs, flu or virus
  symptoms in children, third trimester of pregnancy
Caution: Renal or hepatic disorders

Drug-Lab-Food Interactions

Drug: increase risk of bleeding with anticoagulants;
  increase risk of hypoglycemia with oral hypoglycemic
  drugs; *increase* ulcerogenic effect with glucocorticoids
Lab: Decrease cholesterol and potassium, T_3, T_4 levels;
  increase PT, bleeding time, uric acid

Pharmacokinetics

Absorption: PO: 80%-100%
Distribution: PB: 80%-90%, crosses placenta
Metabolism: t½: 2-3 h (low dose); 2-20 h (high dose)
Excretion: 50% in urine

Pharmacodynamics

PO: Onset: 15-30 min
  Peak: 1-2 h
  Duration: 4-6 h
PR: Onset: 1-2 h
  Peak: 3-5 h
  Duration: 4-7 h

Therapeutic Effects/Uses

To reduce pain and inflammatory symptoms; to decrease body temperature; to inhibit platelet aggregation
Mode of Action: Inhibition of prostaglandin synthesis, inhibition of hypothalamic heat-regulator center

Side Effects

Anorexia, nausea, vomiting, diarrhea, dizziness,
  confusion, hearing loss, heartburn, rash, stomach
  pains, drowsiness

Adverse Reactions

Tinnitus, urticaria, ulceration
Life-threatening: agranulocytosis, hemolytic anemia,
  bronchospasm, anaphylaxis, thrombocytopenia,
  hepatotoxicity, leukopenia

A, Adult; *ASA*, acetylsalicylic acid; *b.i.d.*, two times a day; *C*, child; *d*, day; *h*, hour; *max*, maximum; *min*, minute; *NSAIDs*, nonsteroidal antiinflammatory drugs; *PB*, protein-binding; *PO*, by mouth; *PR*, per rectum; *PRN*, as necessary; *PT*, prothrombin time; *t½*, half-life; *TDM*, therapeutic drug monitoring; *TIA*, transient ischemic attack; ✣, Canadian drug name.

Two other *para*-chlorobenzoic acid derivatives—sulindac (Clinoril) and tolmetin (Tolectin)—produce less severe adverse reactions than indomethacin. Tolmetin is not as highly protein-bound as indomethacin, and sulindac and has a short half-life. This group of NSAIDs may cause sodium and water retention and increased blood pressure.

Phenylacetic Acid Derivatives

Diclofenac sodium (Voltaren), a phenylacetic acid derivative, has a plasma half-life of 8 to 12 hours. Its analgesic and antiinflammatory effects are similar to those of aspirin, but it has minimal to no antipyretic effects. It is indicated for rheumatoid arthritis, osteoarthritis, and ankylosing spondylitis. Adverse reactions are similar to those of other NSAIDs.

Ketorolac (Toradol), another phenylacetic acid derivative, is the first injectable NSAID. Like other NSAIDs, it inhibits prostaglandin synthesis, but it has greater analgesic properties than other antiinflammatory agents. Ketorolac is recommended for short-term management of pain. For postsurgical pain it has shown analgesic efficacy equal or superior to that of opioid analgesics. It is administered intramuscularly in doses of 30 to 60 mg every 6 hours for adults.

Propionic Acid Derivatives

The propionic acid group is a relatively new group of NSAIDs. These drugs are aspirin-like but have stronger effects and create less GI irritation. Drugs in this group are highly protein-bound, so drug interactions might occur, especially when given with another highly protein-bound drug. Propionic acid derivatives are better tolerated than other NSAIDs. Gastric upset occurs, but it is not as severe as with aspirin and indomethacin. Severe adverse reactions such as blood dyscrasias are not frequently seen. Ibuprofen (Motrin) is the most widely used propionic acid NSAID, and it may be purchased OTC in lower doses (200 mg). Prototype Drug Chart 24–2 details the pharmacologic behavior of ibuprofens. Six other propionic acid agents are fenoprofen calcium (Nalfon), naproxen (Naprosyn), suprofen (Profenal), ketoprofen (Orudis), flurbiprofen (Ansaid), and oxaprozin (Daypro).

Pharmacokinetics

Ibuprofens are well absorbed from the GI tract. These drugs have a short half-life but are highly protein-bound. If ibuprofen is taken with another highly protein-bound drug, severe side effects may occur. The drug is metabolized in the liver to inactivate metabolites and is excreted as inactive metabolites in the urine.

Pharmacodynamics

Ibuprofens inhibit prostaglandin synthesis and are therefore effective in alleviating inflammation and pain. They have a short onset of action, peak concentration time, and duration of action. It may take several days for the antiinflammatory effect to be evident.

There are many drug interactions associated with ibuprofen. It can increase the effects of warfarin (Coumadin), sulfonamides, many of the cephalosporins, and phenytoin. When taken with aspirin, its effect can be decreased. Hypoglycemia may result when ibuprofen is taken with insulin or an oral hypoglycemic drug. There is a high risk of toxicity when ibuprofen is taken concurrently with calcium blockers.

Fenamates

The fenamate group includes potent NSAIDs used for acute and chronic arthritic conditions. Like most NSAIDs, gastric irritation is a common side effect of fenamates, and clients with a history of peptic ulcer should avoid taking this group of drugs. Other side effects include edema, dizziness, tinnitus, and pruritus. Two fenamates are meclofenamate sodium monohydrate (Meclomen) and mefenamic acid (Ponstel).

Oxicams

Piroxicam (Feldene), an oxicam, is indicated for long-term arthritic conditions such as rheumatoid arthritis and osteoarthritis. It too can cause gastric problems like ulceration and epigastric distress, but the incidence is lower than for some other NSAIDs. It is well tolerated, and its

---

Prototype DRUG CHART 24–2

IBUPROFEN

Drug Class

Nonsteroidal antiinflammatory drug, propionic acid derivative
Trade names: Motrin, Advil, Nuprin, Medipren, Rufen, ✽Amersol
Pregnancy Category: B

Dosage

A: PO: 200-800 mg t.i.d./q.i.d.; *max:* <3.2 g/d (<3200 mg/d)
C: PO: Average: 5-10 mg/kg/d; *max:* 40 mg/kg/d
1-4 y or <20 kg: 400 mg/d in divided doses
5-7 y or 20-30 kg: 600 mg/d in divided doses
>8 y or 30-40 kg: 800 mg/d in divided doses

Contraindications

Severe renal or hepatic disease, asthma, peptic ulcer
Caution: Bleeding disorders, pregnancy, lactation, systemic lupus erythematosus

Drug-Lab-Food Interactions

Drug: Increase bleeding time with oral anticoagulants; *increase* effects of phenytoin, sulfonamides, warfarin; *decrease* effect with aspirin; may *increase* severe side effects of lithium

Pharmacokinetics

Absorption: PO: Well absorbed
Distribution: PB: 98%
Metabolism: t½: 2-4 h
Excretion: In urine, mostly as inactive metabolites; some in bile

Pharmacodynamics

PO: Onset: 0.5 h
Peak: 1-2 h
Duration: 4-6 h

Therapeutic Effects/Uses

To reduce inflammatory process; to relieve pain; antiinflammatory effect for arthritic conditions; to reduce fever
Mode of Action: Inhibition of prostaglandin synthesis, thus relieving pain and inflammations

Side Effects

Anorexia, nausea, vomiting, diarrhea, edema, rash, purpura, tinnitus, fatigue, dizziness, lightheadedness, anxiety, confusion, fluid retention with edema

Adverse Reactions

GI bleeding
Life-threatening: Blood dyscrasias, cardiac dysrhythmias, nephrotoxicity, anaphylaxis

A, Adult; *C,* child; *d,* day; *GI,* gastrointestinal; *h,* hour; *max,* maximum; *PB,* protein-binding; *PO,* by mouth; *q.i.d.,* four times a day; *t½,* half-life; *t.i.d.,* three times a day; *y,* year; *<,* less than; *>,* greater than; ✽, Canadian drug name.

major advantage over other NSAIDs is its long half-life, which allows it to be taken only once daily.

Full clinical response to piroxicam may take 1 to 2 weeks. This drug is also highly protein-bound and may interact with another highly protein-bound drug if taken together. Piroxicam should not be taken with aspirin or other NSAIDs.

General Side Effects and Adverse Reactions for First-Generation NSAIDs

Most NSAIDs tend to have fewer side effects than aspirin when taken at antiinflammatory doses, but gastric irritation is still a common problem when NSAIDs are taken without food. In addition, sodium and water retention may occur. Alcoholic beverages consumed with NSAIDs may increase gastric irritation and should be avoided.

Nonsteroidal Antiinflammatory Drug: Ibuprofen

ASSESSMENT

■ Check client's history of allergy to NSAIDs such as ibuprofen. If an allergy is present, notify health care provider.
■ Obtain a drug and herbal history and report any possible drug-drug or herb-drug interactions. NSAIDs can increase the effects of phenytoin (Dilantin), sulfonamides, and warfarin. Most NSAIDs are highly protein-bound and can displace other highly protein-bound drugs like warfarin (Coumadin).
■ Determine a medical history. NSAIDs are contraindicated if client has a severe renal or liver disease, peptic ulcer, or bleeding disorder.
■ Assess client for GI upset and peripheral edema, which are common side effects of NSAIDs.

NURSING DIAGNOSES

■ Risk for injury related to dizziness
■ Risk for activity intolerance related to fatigue

PLANNING

■ The inflammatory process will subside in 1 to 3 weeks.

NURSING INTERVENTIONS

■ Observe client for bleeding gums, petechiae, ecchymoses, or black (tarry) stools. Bleeding time can be prolonged when NSAIDs are taken, especially with a highly protein-bound drug such as warfarin (anticoagulant).

■ Report if client has GI discomfort. Administer the NSAIDs at mealtime or with food to prevent GI upset.
■ Monitor vital signs and check for peripheral edema, especially in the morning.
■ Do not give directions such as take one "blue" pill at a specified time. Instead, provide the name and dosage of the medication.

Client Teaching

General
• Inform client not to take aspirin and acetaminophen with NSAIDs. Taking an NSAID with aspirin could cause GI upset and possible GI bleeding.
• Inform client to avoid alcohol when taking NSAIDs. GI upset or gastric ulcer may result.
• Alert client that many herbal products may interact with NSAIDs and could cause bleeding. Doses of NSAIDs and/or herbs may need to be modified to avoid possible bleeding occurrence. (Herbal Alert 24–1)
• Direct client to inform the dentist or surgeon before a procedure when taking ibuprofen or other NSAIDs for a continuous period.
• Warn women not to take NSAIDs 1 to 2 days before menstruation to avoid heavy menstrual flow. If discomfort occurs, acetaminophen is usually prescribed.
• Advise pregnant women to avoid NSAIDs. Congenital abnormalities may occur when NSAIDS are taken during early pregnancy, and excess bleeding might occur during delivery.
• Tell client that it may take several weeks to experience the desired drug effect of some NSAIDs and disease-modifying antirheumatic drugs (DMARDs).

Side Effects
• Educate client of the common side effects of NSAIDs. Nausea, vomiting, peripheral edema, GI upset, purpura or petechiae, or dizziness might occur. Report occurrences of side effects.

Diet
• Advise client to take NSAIDs with meals or food to reduce GI upset.

Cultural Considerations ❖

• Recognize that clients from various cultural backgrounds respond to pain and inflammation in various ways. In some cultures, the use of drugs to alleviate pain and inflammation is not acceptable. Herbal

Herbal ALERT 24–1

NSAIDs

🌿 Dong quai, feverfew, garlic, ginger, and ginkgo, when taken with nonsteroidal antiinflammatory drugs (NSAIDs), may cause bleeding.

medicine and acupuncture may be used to alleviate pain.

- Be supportive of client's methods for pain control. Explain the purpose of medications and their action and side effects.

EVALUATION

■ Evaluate the effectiveness of the drug therapy, such as a decrease in pain and in swollen joints and an increase in mobility.

Selective COX-2 Inhibitors (Second-Generation NSAIDs)

COX-2 inhibitors became available in the last several years to decrease inflammation and pain. Most NSAIDs are non-selective inhibitors that inhibit COX-1 and COX-2. By in-

hibiting COX-1, protection of the stomach lining is decreased and the clotting time is also decreased, which may benefit the client with cardiovascular or coronary artery disease (CAD). Selective COX-2 inhibitors are drugs of choice for clients with severe arthritic conditions who need high doses of an antiinflammatory drug, because large doses of NSAIDs may cause peptic ulcer and gastric bleeding.

Currently there is one drug, celecoxib (Celebrex), classified as a COX-2 inhibitor. Nabumetone (Relafen) is a similar drug that can be used; however it is not considered a "true" COX-2 inhibitor. Nabumetone inhibits COX-2 more than COX-1 (Prototype Drug Chart 24–3).

Use of NSAIDs in Older Adults

Older adults frequently use NSAIDs to treat pain associated with inflammation caused by osteoarthritis, rheumatoid arthritis, and neuromuscular-skeletal disorders. As older adults age, the number of drugs taken daily increases; therefore drug interactions are more common, especially

---

Prototype DRUG CHART 24–3

CELECOXIB

Drug Class

Nonsteroidal antiinflammatory: COX-2 inhibitor
Trade name: Celebrex
Pregnancy Category: C (first and second trimester), D (third trimester)

Dosage

Arthritis:
A: PO: 100-200 mg daily or b.i.d.
Dysmenorrhea:
A: PO: 400 mg first dose, follow with 200 mg same day if needed, then 200 mg twice daily PRN

Contraindications

Hypersensitivity, advanced renal disease, severe hepatic failure, anemia, concurrent use of diuretics and ACE inhibitors
Caution: Renal or hepatic dysfunction, hypertension, fluid retention, heart failure, infection, history of GI bleeding or ulceration, concurrent anticoagulant therapy, steroids, or alcohol use

Drug-Lab-Food Interactions

Drug: Decrease effect of ACE inhibitors, increased INR and GI bleeding with warfarin, may increase toxicity with lithium, fluconazole increases celecoxib levels

Pharmacokinetics

Absorption: Well absorbed in GI tract
Distribution: PB: 97%
Metabolism: t½: 11.2 h
Excretion: Primarily in feces

Pharmacodynamics

PO: Onset: UK
     Peak: 3 h
     Duration: UK

Therapeutic Effects/Uses

To treat osteoarthritis and rheumatoid arthritis, to relieve dysmenorrhea
Mode of Action: Inhibits COX-2 (which normally promotes prostaglandin synthesis and inflammatory response) but does not inhibit COX-1

Side Effects

Headache, dizziness, sinusitis, nausea, flatulence, diarrhea, rash

Adverse Reactions

Peripheral edema

A, Adult; *ACE,* angiotensin-converting enzyme; *b.i.d.,* twice a day; *COX,* cyclooxygenase; *GI,* gastrointestinal; *h,* hour; *INR,* international normalized ratio; *PB,* protein-binding; *PO,* by mouth; *PRN,* as needed; *t½,* half-life; *UK,* unknown.

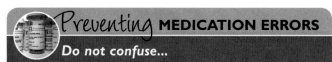

when numerous drugs are taken with NSAIDs. With the use of NSAIDs, GI distress (including ulceration) is four times more common in older adults; hospitalization is often necessary.

The introduction of COX-2 inhibitors (second-generation NSAIDs) has decreased the incidence of GI problems associated with their use; however, edema is likely to occur. Renal function should be evaluated, and older adults should increase their fluid intake for adequate hydration. To decrease possible complications, the NSAID dose should be lowered.

Corticosteroids

Corticosteroids such as prednisone, prednisolone, and dexamethasone are frequently used as antiinflammatory agents. This group of drugs controls inflammation by suppressing or preventing many of the components of the inflammatory process at the injured site. Corticosteroids have been widely prescribed for arthritic conditions, and although they are not the drug of choice for arthritis because of their numerous side effects, they are frequently used to control arthritic flare-ups.

The half-life of a corticosteroid is long (greater than 24 hours), and it is administered once a day in a large prescribed dose. When discontinuing steroid therapy, the dosage should be tapered over a period of 5 to 10 days. Steroids are discussed in more detail in Chapter 50.

Disease-Modifying Antirheumatic Drugs

When NSAIDs do not control immune-mediated arthritic disease sufficiently, other drugs, although more toxic, can be prescribed to alter the disease process. The **disease-modifying antirheumatic drugs (DMARDs)** include gold drug therapy, immunosuppressive agents, immunomodulators, and antimalarials. DMARDs help alleviate the symptoms of rheumatoid arthritis for the 2 million persons in the United States affected by the disorder.

Gold

Gold drug therapy, called **chrysotherapy** or heavy metal therapy, is the most frequently used DMARD. It is used to arrest progression of rheumatoid arthritis and prevent de-

formities caused by the disease. It depresses migration of leukocytes and suppresses prostaglandin activity. Gold preparations are thought to inhibit destructive lysosomal enzymes contained in leukocytes which are released in the joints. The effect of gold on the immune mechanism is limited.

Gold is not used in the early stages of arthritis unless the illness is progressing rapidly and is unresponsive to other therapy, nor is it used in far-advanced arthritis. It is used for palliative (relief of symptoms), not curative, effects. Response in alleviating symptoms is slow. With injectable gold, results may take up to 2 months; oral dosages could take 3 to 6 months for clinical response. The half-life of gold is 7 to 25 days, and gold drugs are highly protein-bound. Blood should be monitored for blood dyscrasia before and during parenteral or oral gold therapy.

The gold salt auranofin (Ridaura) is the only gold preparation that can be administered orally. The two parenteral gold salts are aurothioglucose (Solganal) and gold sodium thiomalate (Myochrysine). Oral gold may be absorbed erratically, so parenteral gold may be advisable. Switching from parenteral to oral gold preparations may be necessary for long-term use. Prototype Drug Chart 24–4 presents drug data for the gold preparation auranofin (Ridaura).

Pharmacokinetics

The GI tract absorbs 25% of auranofin. It is moderately highly protein-bound. Its half-life is long, both in the blood (26 days) and in the body tissues (40 to 120 days). Although 60% of auranofin is excreted in the urine, the drug may be present in the urine for up to 15 months after chrysotherapy has been discontinued.

Pharmacodynamics

Auranofin is prescribed to relieve inflammation and pain from rheumatoid arthritis when NSAIDs and other measures are ineffective. The therapeutic effect may take 3 to 6 months; steady state (the average therapeutic effect that is maintained) of the drug is achieved after 2 to 4 months. Side effects and adverse reactions need to be closely monitored.

Table 24–3 details the dosages and considerations for the three gold drugs used as antiinflammatory agents for rheumatoid arthritis.

Side Effects and Adverse Reactions

Approximately 25% to 45% of clients receiving gold therapy experience side effects. The side effects may occur anytime during and up to several months after therapy. The numerous possible side effects include dermatitis, urticaria (hives), erythema, alopecia (loss of hair), stomatitis (mouth ulcers), pharyngitis, gastritis, colitis, hepatitis, severe blood dyscrasias (agranulocytosis, aplastic anemia), and even anaphylactic shock.

Contraindications

Gold therapy is contraindicated for clients with eczema, urticaria, colitis, hemorrhagic conditions, and systemic lupus erythematosus.

Prototype **DRUG CHART 24–4**

GOLD

Drug Class

Disease-modifying antirheumatic drug
Trade name: Ridaura
Pregnancy Category: C

Dosage

A: PO: 6 mg/d in single or divided doses; may increase
  dose to 9 mg/d
C: Initial: 0.1 mg/kg/d in 1-2 divided doses; *maint:*
  0.15 mg/kg/d in 1-2 divided doses; *max:* 0.2 mg/kg/d
  in 1-2 divided doses

Contraindications

Severe renal or hepatic disease, colitis, systemic
  lupus erythematosus, pregnancy, blood dyscrasias
Caution: Diabetes mellitus, heart failure

Drug-Lab-Food Interactions

Drug: With anticancer drugs, may cause bone marrow
  depression
Lab: Slightly *increase* liver enzyme tests

Pharmacokinetics

Absorption: PO: 25% absorbed
Distribution: PB: 60%
Metabolism: t½: 26 d in blood; 40-120 d in tissue
Excretion: >60% in urine (may appear for 15 mo);
  in feces

Pharmacodynamics

PO: Onset: UK
  Peak: 1-2 h
  Duration: Months

Therapeutic Effects/Uses

To alleviate inflammation and pain of rheumatoid arthritis
Mode of Action: Inhibition of prostaglandin synthesis and decreased phagocytosis

Side Effects

Anorexia, nausea, vomiting, diarrhea, stomatitis,
  abdominal cramps, pruritus, dizziness, headache,
  metallic taste, rash, dermatitis, photosensitivity

Adverse Reactions

Corneal gold deposits, urticaria, hematuria, proteinuria,
  bradycardia
Life-threatening: Nephrotoxicity, agranulocytosis,
  thrombocytopenia, interstitial pneumonitis

A, Adult; *C,* child; *d,* day; *h,* hour; *maint,* maintenance; *max,* maximum; *mo,* month; *PB,* protein-binding; *PO,* by mouth; *t½,* half-
life; *UK,* unknown; >, greater than.

Nursing Process

Disease-Modifying Antirheumatic Drug: Gold

ASSESSMENT

■ Determine client's health history. Usually, gold drugs
such as auranofin are contraindicated if there is renal or
hepatic dysfunction, marked hypertension, heart failure, systemic lupus erythematosus, or uncontrolled diabetes mellitus.

■ Check for proteinuria and hematuria before giving
initial gold dose and during gold therapy.

■ Observe client for 30 minutes after gold injection for
possible allergic reaction after the first and second injections. It takes approximately 10 to 15 minutes for a serious allergic reaction (anaphylaxis) to occur.

■ Obtain baseline vital signs and hematology laboratory findings for future comparison.

NURSING DIAGNOSES

■ Impaired physical mobility related to severe pain
■ Chronic pain related to swelling of tissues
■ Risk for impaired skin integrity related to effects of
imposed immobility

PLANNING

■ Client will have reduced inflammation and pain
while taking the gold treatment without adverse drug
reaction.

NURSING INTERVENTIONS

■ Record client's vital signs. Report abnormal findings.
■ Monitor laboratory tests (e.g., complete blood count).
Report abnormal findings.
■ Check periodically for signs of side effects and ad-
verse reactions to gold therapy. Side effects may include
anorexia, nausea, vomiting, diarrhea, gingivitis, stoma-

Antiinflammatory Drugs: DMARDs

Generic (Brand)	Route and Dosage	Uses and Considerations
auranofin (Ridaura) aurothioglucose (Solganal)	(Prototype Drug Chart 24–3) Increase dose weekly: A: IM: 10, 25, 50 mg (sol in oil) C: IM: 6-12 y: 0.25 mg-1 mg	For rheumatoid arthritis when unresponsive to NSAIDs. Start with low dose. Check laboratory values, especially white blood cell count, hemoglobin, and hematocrit. Check renal and liver function. *Pregnancy category:* C; PB: 95%; $t^{1/2}$: 3-27 d
gold sodium thiomalate (Myochrysine)	Increase dose weekly: A: IM: 10, 25, 50 mg (aqueous sol) until 1 g cumulative dose; *maint:* 25-50 mg q2-3 wk; *max:* 1 g/wk C: TD: 10 mg, followed by 1 mg/kg/wk 3 20 wk; *maint:* 1 mg/kg/dose every 2-4 wk; *max:* 50/kg/dose	Same considerations as aurothioglucose. Contains 50% gold. *Pregnancy category:* C; PB: 95%; $t^{1/2}$: 3-27 d
anakinra (Kineret)	A: subQ: 100 mg daily	For treatment of rheumatoid arthritis unresponsive to other DMARDs. *Pregnancy category:* B; PB: UK; $t^{1/2}$: 4-6 h
etanercept (Enbrel)	A: subQ: 25 mg 2 times/wk C: >4 y: subQ: 0.4 mg/kg 2 times/wk; *max:* 25 mg/dose	For treatment of rheumatoid arthritis unresponsive to other DMARDs. *Pregnancy category:* B; PB: UK; $t^{1/2}$: 115 h
infliximab (Remicade)	*Rheumatoid arthritis* A: IV: 3 mg/kg over 2 h, then 2 mg/kg on wk 2 and 6 *Crohn's disease* A: IV: 5 mg/kg over 2 h, then 2 mg/kg on wk 2 and 6	For treatment of moderate to severe rheumatoid arthritis and Crohn's disease. *Pregnancy category:* C; PB: UK; $t^{1/2}$: 9.5 d
adalimumab (Humira)	A: subQ: 40 mg every 2 wk	For treatment of rheumatoid arthritis unresponsive to other DMARDs. *Pregnancy category:* X; PB: UK; $t^{1/2}$: 16.5 d
leflunomide (Arava)	A: PO: 100 mg/d for 3 d initially, then 20 mg daily	For treatment of rheumatoid arthritis unresponsive to other DMARDs. *Pregnancy category:* X; PB: 99%; $t^{1/2}$: 19 d
abatacept (Orencia)	A: IV: 500 mg for < 60 kg; 750 mg for 60-100 kg; 1 gram for >100 kg; initial dose followed by additional doses at 2- and 4-week intervals, then q4wk	For treatment of moderate to severe rheumatoid arthritis. *Pregnancy category:* C; PB: UK; $t^{1/2}$: UK

A, Adult; *C,* child; *d,* day; *DMARDs,* disease-modifying antirheumatic drugs; *h,* hour; *IM,* intramuscular; *IV,* intravenous; *maint,* maintenance; *NSAIDs,* nonsteroidal antiinflammatory drugs; *PB,* protein-binding; *sol,* solution; *subQ,* subcutaneous; $t^{1/2}$, half-life; *TD,* test dose; *UK,* unknown; *wk,* week; *y,* year; *>,* greater than; *<,* less than.

titis, rash, itching, and decreased urine output. Most gold drugs have a long half-life; a cumulative effect can result. Auranofin causes less severe adverse reactions than other gold preparations.

Client Teaching

General

- Instruct client to perform frequent dental hygiene, including brushing the teeth with a soft toothbrush and flossing to prevent or control gingivitis and stomatitis. Use of diluted hydrogen peroxide can be helpful in mild stomatitis.
- Advise client to adhere to scheduled laboratory blood tests and appointments with the health care provider so any adverse reactions can be monitored.
- Inform client that the desired therapeutic effect may take as long as 3 to 4 months.

Side Effects

- Direct client to report early symptoms of possible gold toxicity such as a metallic taste or pruritus. A rash may occur. These symptoms should be reported to health care provider.
- Teach client the side effects and to report them immediately. (Prototype Drug Chart 24–4 has a list of side effects and adverse reactions.)
- Warn client to avoid direct sunlight, because the gold drug may cause photosensitivity. Use of sun block is necessary.
- Alert client to report skin conditions such as dermatitis, bruising, and petechiae. Bleeding gums and blood in the stools should be reported to the health care provider.

Diet

- Suggest high-fiber diet or antidiarrheal drugs to control diarrhea. If diarrhea is continuous or severe for a prolonged time, the gold drug is usually discontinued.

Cultural Considerations ❖

- Develop a sound, trusting relationship and listen attentively.
- Use simple, clear instructions and an interpreter as needed.
- Include family members in the plan of care.

EVALUATION

■ Determine the effectiveness of gold therapy by determining whether client has less pain and inflammation.

■ Evaluate client for present or repeated side effects. The gold therapy regimen may need to be changed or discontinued.

Immunosuppressive Agents

Immunosuppressives are used to treat refractory rheumatoid arthritis (arthritis that does not respond to antiinflammatory drugs). In low doses, selected immunosuppressive agents have been effective in the treatment of rheumatoid arthritis. Drugs such as azathioprine (Imuran), cyclophosphamide (Cytoxan), and methotrexate (Mexate), primarily used to suppress cancer growth and proliferation, might be used to suppress the inflammatory process of rheumatoid arthritis when other treatments fail. In one study of clients receiving cyclophosphamide, few new erosions of joint cartilage were present, suggesting that the disease process was not active. These agents are not the first or second choice for treatment of rheumatoid arthritis.

Immunomodulators

Immunomodulators treat moderate to severe rheumatoid arthritis by disrupting the inflammatory process and delaying the disease progression. Interleukin (IL-1) receptor antagonists and tumor necrosis factor (TNF) blockers are two groups of drugs classified as immunomodulators.

Anakinra (Kineret), an IL-1 receptor antagonist, blocks activity of IL-1 by inhibiting IL-1 from binding to interleukin receptors located in cartilage and bone. IL-1 is a proinflammatory cytokine that contributes to synovial inflammation and joint destruction. Anakinra is administered subcutaneously. The peak is 3 to 7 hours, and the half-life is 6 hours.

The TNF blockers bind to the TNF and block it from attaching to TNF receptors on the synovial cell surfaces. By neutralizing TNF, a contributor to synovitis, inflammatory disease process is delayed. Etanercept (Enbrel) was the first TNF blocker developed and is administered subcutane-

---

Prototype **DRUG CHART 24–5**

INFLIXIMAB

Drug Class	**Dosage**
Immunomodulator: Tumor necrosis factor blocker Trade name: Remicade *Pregnancy Category:* C	*Rheumatoid arthritis:* A: IV: 3 mg/kg wk 1 then 2 mg/kg wk 2 and 6 then 2 mg/kg q8wk *Crohn's disease:* A: IV: 5 mg/kg wk 1 may repeat wk 2 and 6

Contraindications	**Drug-Lab-Food Interactions**
Hypersensitivity, heart failure *Caution:* Renal or hepatic dysfunction, immunosuppression, multiple sclerosis, elderly	*Drug:* May decrease effectiveness of vaccines

Pharmacokinetics	**Pharmacodynamics**

Absorption: UK
Distribution: UK
Metabolism: t½: 9.5 d
Excretion: UK
	IV: Onset: UK
	  Peak: UK
	  Duration: UK

Therapeutic Effects/Uses

To treat moderate to severe rheumatoid arthritis and Crohn's disease

Side Effects	**Adverse Reactions**
Headache, dizziness, coughing, fatigue, chills, hot flashes, anxiety, insomnia, depression, nausea, vomiting, diarrhea, constipation, flatulence, rash, alopecia, dry skin, urinary frequency	Severe infections, chest pain, hypotension, hypertension, increased hepatic enzymes

A, Adult; *d,* day; *IV,* intravenous; *t½,* half-life; *UK,* unknown; *wk,* week.

ously. The peak half-life is 115 hours. Signs and symptoms of rheumatoid arthritis are suppressed rapidly with etanercept therapy but reappear if the drug is discontinued. Other TNF blockers include infliximab (Remicade), adalimumab (Humira), and leflunomide (Arava). Infliximab is administered intravenously (IV) over at least 2 hours, adalimumab is administered subcutaneously, and leflunomide is administered orally (Prototype Drug Chart 24–5).

Both IL-1 receptor antagonists and TNF blockers predispose the client to severe infections; they are contraindicated in active infection and should be discontinued when an infection occurs. Immunomodulators are usually very expensive: approximately $14,000 to $37,000 per year.

Antimalarials

Antimalarial drugs may be used to treat rheumatoid arthritis when other methods of treatment fail. The mechanism of action of antimalarials in suppressing rheumatoid arthritis is unclear. The effect may take 4 to 12 weeks to become apparent, and antimalarials are usually used in combination with NSAIDs in clients whose arthritis is not under control.

Antigout Drugs

Gout has been called the "disease of kings," because in the past royalty ate rich foods, drank wine and alcohol, and suffered from gout. It was also called the "unwalkable disease." Hippocrates (460-357 BC) referred to gout as *podagra* (foot seizure). He recognized gout as affecting other joints of the large toe, hand, elbow, knee, and shoulder. Hippocrates' recommendation of treatment included purgatives (strong laxatives). Galen (131-200 AD) attributed gout to "intemperance" and heredity.

Gout is an inflammatory condition that attacks joints, tendons, and other tissues. It may be called *gouty arthritis*. The most common site of acute gouty inflammation is at the joint of the big toe. Gout is characterized by a uric acid metabolism disorder and a defect in purine (products of certain proteins) metabolism, resulting in an increase in urates (uric acid salts) and an accumulation of uric acid (hyperuricemia) or an ineffective clearance of uric acid by the kidneys. Uric acid solubility is poor in acid urine and urate crystals may form, causing urate calculi. Gout may appear as bumps, or *tophi*, in the subcutaneous tissue of earlobes, elbows, hands, and the base of the large toe. In addition to tophi, the complications of untreated or prolonged periods of gout include gouty arthritis, urinary calculi, and gouty nephropathy.

Fluid intake should be increased while taking antigout drugs to promote uric acid excretion and prevent renal calculi. Foods rich in purine (e.g., organ meats, sardines, salmon, gravy, herring, liver, meat soups) and alcohol (especially beer) should be avoided. Alcohol causes both an overproduction and underexcretion of uric acid. Acetaminophen should be taken for discomfort instead of aspirin (salicylic acid) to reduce acidity.

Antiinflammatory Gout Drug: Colchicine

The first drug used to treat gout was colchicine, introduced in 1936. This antiinflammatory gout drug inhibits the migration of leukocytes to the inflamed site. It is effective in alleviating acute symptoms of gout, but it is not effective in decreasing inflammation occurring in other inflammatory disorders. Colchicine does not inhibit uric acid synthesis and does not promote uric acid excretion. It should not be used if the client has a severe renal, cardiac, or GI problem. Gastric irritation is a common problem, so colchicine should be taken with food. With high doses, nausea, vomiting, diarrhea, or abdominal pain occurs in approximately 75% of clients taking the drug.

Colchicine is well absorbed in the GI tract, and its peak concentration time is within 2 hours. Most of the drug is excreted in the feces, but 10% to 20% is excreted in the urine.

Uric Acid Inhibitor

Allopurinol (Zyloprim), first marketed in 1963, is not an antiinflammatory drug; instead, it inhibits the final steps of uric acid biosynthesis and therefore lowers serum uric acid levels, preventing the precipitation of an attack. This drug is frequently used as a prophylactic to prevent gout. It is a drug of choice for clients with chronic tophaceous gout. Allopurinol is also indicated for gout clients with renal impairment. It is useful for clients who have renal obstructions caused by uric acid stones and for clients with blood disorders such as leukemia and polycythemia vera. It is also given to clients who do not respond well to uricosuric drugs such as probenecid. Increased fluid intake is recommended to promote diuresis and alkalinization of the urine. Prototype Drug Chart 24–6 presents the pharmacologic behavior of allopurinol.

Pharmacokinetics

Eighty percent of allopurinol is absorbed from the GI tract. Biosynthesis of uric acid occurs in the liver in pure form and active metabolites. The half-life of the drug itself is 2 to 3 hours and 20 to 24 hours for its active metabolites. The protein-binding percentage is unknown. Most of the drug and its metabolites are excreted in feces and some in urine.

Pharmacodynamics

Allopurinol inhibits the production of uric acid by inhibiting the enzyme xanthine oxidase, which is needed in the synthesis of uric acid. Allopurinol also improves the solubility of uric acid. Its onset of action occurs within 30 to 60 minutes; its peak time averages 2 to 4 hours. Allopurinol has a long duration of action.

Alcohol, caffeine, and thiazide diuretics increase the uric acid level. Use of ampicillin or amoxicillin with allopurinol increases the risk of rash formation. Allopurinol can increase the effect of warfarin (Coumadin) and oral hypoglycemic drugs.

Uricosurics

Uricosurics increase the rate of uric acid excretion by inhibiting its reabsorption. These drugs are effective in alleviating chronic gout, but they should not be used during

Prototype **DRUG CHART 24–6**

ALLOPURINOL

Drug Class

Antigout: Uric acid biosynthesis inhibitor
Trade names: Zyloprim, ✳Alloprin, Apo-Allopurinol, Novopurinol
Pregnancy Category: C

Dosage

A: **PO:** Initially: 100 mg/dl, may increase; 200-300 mg/d (for mild gout); 400-600 mg/d (for severe gout); *max:* 800 mg/d
C: ≤**10 y: PO:** 10 mg/kg/d in 2-3 divided doses

Contraindications

Hypersensitivity, severe renal disease
Caution: Hepatic disorder

Drug-Lab-Food Interactions

Drug: Increase effect of warfarin, phenytoin, theophylline, anticancer drugs, ACE inhibitors; *increase* rash with ampicillin, amoxicillin; *increase* toxicity with thiazide diuretics; *decrease* allopurinol effect with antacids
Lab: Increase AST, ALT, BUN

Pharmacokinetics

Absorption: PO: 80% absorbed
Distribution: PB: UK
Metabolism: t½: 2-3 h
Metabolite: 20-24 h
Excretion: 10%-20% in urine; 80%-90% in feces

Pharmacodynamics

PO: Onset: 0.5-1 h
Peak: 2-4 h
Duration: 18-30 h

Therapeutic Effects/Uses

To treat gout and hyperuricemia; prevent urate calculi
Mode of Action: Reduction of uric acid synthesis

Side Effects

Anorexia, nausea, vomiting, diarrhea, stomatitis, dizziness, headache, rash, pruritus, malaise, metallic taste

Adverse Reactions

Cataracts, retinopathy
Life-threatening: Bone marrow depression, aplastic anemia, thrombocytopenia, agranulocytosis, leukopenia

A, Adult; *ACE,* angiotensin-converting enzyme; *ALT,* alanine aminotransferase; *AST,* aspartate aminotransferase; *BUN,* blood urea nitrogen; *C,* child; *d,* day; *h,* hour; *max,* maximum; *PB,* protein-binding; *PO,* by mouth; *t½,* half-life; *UK,* unknown; *y,* year; ≤, equal to or less than; ✳, Canadian drug name.

---

acute attacks. Probenecid (Benemid) is a uricosuric that has been available since 1945. It blocks the reabsorption of uric acid and promotes its excretion. Probenecid can be taken with colchicine. To begin initial therapy for relieving symptoms of gout and inhibiting uric acid reabsorption, small doses of colchicine should be given before adding probenecid. If gastric irritation occurs, probenecid should be taken with meals. It has an average half-life of 8 to 10 hours and is 85% to 95% protein-bound. Use caution when administering this drug with other highly protein-bound drugs.

Another uricosuric is sulfinpyrazone (Anturane). This drug is a metabolite of phenylbutazone and is more potent than probenecid. Sulfinpyrazone should be taken with meals or with antacids to prevent gastric irritation. Severe blood dyscrasias might occur, especially in clients with a history of blood dyscrasia. Table 24–4 gives dosages and considerations for the commonly used antigout drugs.

Side Effects and Adverse Reactions

Side effects may include flushed skin, sore gums, and headache. Kidney stones resulting from the uric acid could be prevented by increasing water intake and maintaining a urine pH above 6. Blood dyscrasias occur rarely. Aspirin use should be avoided, because it causes uric acid retention.

Nursing Process

Antigout: Allopurinol

ASSESSMENT

■ Determine a medical history from client of any gastric, renal, cardiac, or liver disorders. Antigout drugs are excreted via kidneys, so sufficient renal function is

Table 24-4

Antigout Drugs

Generic (Brand)	Route and Dosage	Uses and Considerations
Antiinflammatory Gout Drug		
colchicine (✤Novocolchine)	A: PO: Initially: 0.5-1.2 mg; then 0.5-0.6 mg q1-2h for pain relief; *max:* 4 mg/d; IV: Initially: 2 mg, then 0.5 mg q6h PRN; *max:* 4 mg/d	Treatment of acute gout and prophylaxis of recurrent gouty arthritis. Not for clients with renal or gastric disorders. Take with food. *Pregnancy category:* C; PB: 10%-30%; t½: 20-30 min
Uric Acid Biosynthesis Inhibitor		
allopurinol (Zyloprim)	(Prototype Drug Chart 24-4)	
Uricosurics		
probenecid (Benemid)	A: PO: First week: 250 mg b.i.d.; *maint:* 500 mg b.i.d.; *max:* 2 g/d C: <50 kg: PO: 25-40 mg/kg/d in 4 divided doses	Treatment for hyperuricemia; promotes urinary excretion of uric acid. For gout and gouty arthritis. Alkaline urine helps prevent renal stones. Increase fluid intake. *Pregnancy category:* B; PB: 90%; t½: 4-10 h
sulfinpyrazone (Anturane)	A: PO: First week: 100-200 mg b.i.d.; maint: 200-400 mg b.i.d.; may reduce to 200 mg/d; *max:* 800 mg/d	Used in the management of hyperuricemia; decreases gouty attacks. Can cause GI distress. Take with food. *Pregnancy category:* C; PB: 90%; t½: 3 h

A, Adult; *b.i.d.*, twice a day; *C*, child; *d*, day; *GI*, gastrointestinal; *h*, hour; *IV*, intravenous; *maint*, maintenance; *max*, maximum; *min*, minute; *PB*, protein-binding; *PO*, by mouth; *PRN*, as needed; *t½*, half-life; <, less than; ✤, Canadian drug.

needed. Drug dosage and drug selection might need to be changed.
- Obtain a drug history. Report possible drug-drug interactions (Prototype Drug Chart 24-2).
- Assess serum uric acid value for future comparison.
- Record urine output. Use initial urine output for future comparison.
- Check laboratory tests (e.g., blood urea nitrogen [BUN], serum creatinine, alkaline phosphatase [ALP], aspartate aminotransferase [AST], alanine aminotransferase [ALT], lactate dehydrogenase [LDH]) and compare with future laboratory test results.

NURSING DIAGNOSES

- Impaired tissue integrity related to inflammation of great toe
- Acute pain related to tissue swelling

PLANNING

- Client's "gouty pain" is absent or controlled without side effects.

NURSING INTERVENTIONS

- Report GI symptoms, gastric pain, nausea, vomiting, or diarrhea when taking antigout drugs. Take these drugs with food to alleviate gastric distress.
- Record client's urine output. Because the drugs and uric acid are excreted through the urine, kidney stones

might occur, so both water intake and urine output should be increased.
- Monitor laboratory tests for renal and liver function (BUN, serum creatinine, ALP, AST, ALT).

Client Teaching
General
- Encourage client to keep medical appointments and have regular scheduled laboratory tests for renal, liver, and complete blood count functions. Some antigout drugs may cause blood dyscrasias; blood tests should be monitored.
- Instruct client to increase fluid intake; it will increase drug and uric acid excretion.

Side Effects
- Inform client to report to health care provider side effects of antigout drugs: anorexia, nausea, vomiting, diarrhea, stomatitis, dizziness, rash, pruritus, and metallic taste.
- Advise client to have a yearly eye examination, because visual changes can result from prolonged use of allopurinol.

Diet
- Warn client to avoid alcohol and caffeine, because they can increase uric acid levels.
- Suggest to client not to take large doses of vitamin C while taking allopurinol; kidney stones may occur.
- Tell client not to ingest foods high in purine content (e.g., organ meats, salmon, sardines, gravy, and legumes). Purine foods increase uric acid levels.

- Direct client to report any gastric distress. Encourage client to take antigout drugs with food or at mealtime.

Cultural Considerations ❖

- Provide additional explanation as needed related to the disease process and the purpose of the drug and its side effects.
- Identify conflicts in values and beliefs.
- Suggest follow-up by a community health nurse to determine client's compliance to the drug regimen and the effectiveness of the prescribed drug therapy.

EVALUATION

■ Evaluate client's response to the antigout drug. If pain persists, drug regimen may need modification.
■ Determine the presence of adverse reactions. Drug therapy for gout pain may need to be changed.

KEY WEBSITES

Aspirin: http://www.nlm.nih.gov/medlineplus/druginfo/medmaster/a682878.html

Celecoxib: www.nlm.nih.gov/medlineplus/druginfo/medmaster/a699022.html

Colchicine: www.rxlist.com/cgi/generic2/colch.htm

Critical Thinking Case Study

PQ, age 72, had taken 650 mg of aspirin four times a day for 8 months to alleviate her chronic symptoms of pain and inflammation associated with arthritis. Four weeks ago, a peptic ulcer developed.

1. Explain the process in which PQ could have a peptic ulcer. How could this have been prevented?
2. Compare the similarities and differences in the side effects of salicylates with those of acetic acid agents, propionic acid agents, COX-2 inhibitors, and phenylacetic acid.
3. What client teaching points should PQ receive before and during the time she takes aspirin?
4. How would COX-2 inhibitors prevent the development of a peptic ulcer?
5. Would the DMARD group be more helpful to alleviate PQ's symptoms? Explain your rationale.
6. Compare the differences in the various types of DMARDs.

NCLEX Study Questions

1. The nurse understands the differences between COX-1 and COX-2 inhibitors, in that ibuprofen is more likely to lead to _____ than celecoxib.
   a. fever
   b. constipation
   c. peptic ulcers
   d. metallic taste

2. A nurse is administering gold, a disease-modifying antirheumatic drug to a client. Which needs to be monitored carefully in this client?
   a. hypertension
   b. blood in urine
   c. peripheral edema
   d. respiratory depression

3. When teaching the client who is receiving allopurinol, the nurse should encourage the client to:
   a. eat more meat.
   b. increase vitamin C intake.
   c. have annual eye examinations.
   d. take medication 2 hours before meals.

4. A client is admitted to the hospital with an acute gout attack. The nurse realizes that which of the following medications is best to treat acute gout?
   a. colchicine
   b. allopurinol
   c. probenecid
   d. sulfinpyrazone

5. A client is taking aspirin for arthritis. Which adverse reaction should the nurse teach the client to report to the health care provider?
   a. tinnitus
   b. seizures
   c. sinusitis
   d. palpitations

Answers: 1, c; 2, b; 3, c; 4, a; 5, a.

25

Nonopioid and Opioid Analgesics

Outline

Objectives

- Differentiate between acute and chronic pain.
- Compare indications for nonopioid and opioid analgesics.
- Describe the serum therapeutic ranges of acetaminophen and aspirin.
- Contrast the side effects of aspirin and opioids.
- Explain the methadone treatment program.
- Discuss nursing interventions and client teaching related to nonopioid and opioid analgesics.
- Apply the nursing process to the client with patient-controlled analgesia (PCA).

Terms

Pain is defined by the International Association for the Study of Pain (IASP) as *an unpleasant sensory and emotional experience related to tissue injury*. Due to the subjective nature of pain, the nurse must be knowledgeable and skillful in the assessment and measurement of pain to achieve optimal pain management.

Pain management is regarded as such a significant component of nursing care that pain has become known as the "fifth vital sign." The Joint Commission (TJC), formerly the Joint Commission on the Accreditation of Healthcare Organizations (JCAHO), has incorporated the assessment, documentation, and management of pain into its standards (JCAHO 2003), which reflects the importance of this vital sign. The nurse's role is to assess the client's pain level, alleviate the client's pain through nonpharmacologic and pharmacologic treatments, thoroughly document the client's response to treatment, and teach clients and their significant others to manage pain control themselves when appropriate.

An individual's **pain threshold** reflects the level of stimulus needed to create a painful sensation. Individual genetic makeup contributes to the variations in pain threshold from person to person. The mu (μ) opioid receptor gene controls the number of μ receptors present. When an individual has a large amount of μ receptors, the pain threshold is high and pain sensitivity is reduced.

The amount of pain a person can endure without having it interfere with normal functioning is called **pain tolerance.** This psychological aspect of pain varies greatly in individuals, because it is very subjective. Pain tolerance is influenced by factors such as age, gender, culture, ethnicity, previous experience, anxiety level, and specific circumstances.

Analgesics, both nonopioid and opioid, are prescribed for the relief of pain. The choice of analgesic depends upon the severity of the pain. Mild to moderate pain is frequently relieved with the use of nonopioid (also known as *nonnarcotic*) analgesics. Moderate to severe pain usually requires an opioid (also known as *narcotic*) analgesic.

Drugs used for pain relief are presented in this chapter. Many of the same nonopioid analgesics that are taken for pain, such as the **nonsteroidal antiinflammatory drugs (NSAIDs),** are also taken for antiinflammatory purposes. This application for these drugs is covered in Chapter 24.

The most common classification of pain is by duration. *Acute pain* can be mild, moderate, or severe and is usually associated with a specific tissue injury. The onset of acute pain is usually sudden and of short duration. *Chronic pain* usually has a vague origin and onset with a prolonged duration.

Pain may also be classified by its origin. **Nociceptors** (sensory pain receptors) are activated by noxious stimuli (mechanical, thermal, and chemical) in peripheral tissues. When tissue damage occurs, injured cells release chemical mediators that affect the exposed nerve endings of the nociceptors. Pain that originates from tissue injury is nociceptor pain, which includes somatic (structural tissues: bones, muscles) and visceral (organ) pain. **Neuropathic pain** is an unusual sensory disturbance often involving neural supersensitivity. This pain is due to injury or disease of the peripheral or central nervous system (CNS). The client with neuropathic pain usually complains of burning, tingling, or electrical shocks in the affected area, often triggered by light touch. Diabetic neuropathy associated with diabetes mellitus is an example of peripheral neuropathic pain. Severe, intractable pain from a herniated disk or spinal cord injury is evidence of neuropathic pain in the CNS.

Pathophysiology

The most common pain theory is called the *gate theory*, proposed by Melzack and Wall in 1965. According to this theory, tissue injury activates nociceptors and causes the release of chemical mediators such as substance P, prostaglandins, bradykinin, histamine, serotonin, acetylcholine, glutamate, adenosine triphosphate, leukotrienes, and potassium. These substances initiate an action potential along a sensory nerve fiber and sensitize pain receptors. Nociceptive action potentials are transmitted via afferent nerve fibers. One type of pain fiber that primarily transmits impulses from the periphery is the A delta (δ) fiber. Because A δ pain fibers are wrapped in a myelin sheath, they transmit impulses rapidly in acute pain. The C fiber is a type of pain fiber that is small and unmyelinated, and because C fibers are unmyelinated, they transmit impulses slowly. C fibers are more often associated with chronic, dull pain.

A pain signal begins at the nociceptors in the periphery and proceeds throughout the CNS. Knowing how and where pharmacologic agents work is essential to controlling pain. The body produces neurohormones called **endorphins** (peptides) that naturally suppress pain conduction, although the method is not completely understood. Opioids such as morphine activate the same receptors as endorphins to reduce pain. Nonsteroidal antiinflammatory drugs (NSAIDs) control pain at the peripheral level by blocking the action of cyclooxygenase (pain-sensitizing chemical) and interfering with the production of prostaglandins. Cortisone decreases pain by blocking the action of phospholipase, reducing the production of both prostaglandins and leukotrienes. In neuropathic pain, anticonvulsant drugs prevent the production of nerve impulses by stabilizing the neuronal membrane and inactivating peripheral sodium channels.

To ascertain severity of pain, the health care provider should ask the client to rate the degree of pain on a scale of 1 to 10, with 10 being the worst or most severe pain. The client's comfort level should also be determined. A client who indicates a pain level of 9 may verbalize a decrease in pain to a level of 3 within 30 to 45 minutes after receiving pain medication. Table 25–1 lists the types of pain and the drug groups that may be effective in relieving each type of pain.

Undertreatment of Pain

Undertreatment of pain is a major issue in health care today. The National Pharmaceutical Council and The Joint Commission state that up to 75% of clients have unrelieved pain. Some reasons for undertreatment are sociocultural variables that mediate a client's willingness to acknowledge being in pain, the client's inability to describe pain, the nurse's inability to measure pain, lack of regular pain assessment rounds, attitudes of the health care team, an unwillingness to believe the client's report of pain, inaccurate knowledge of the health care provider concerning addiction and tolerance, and prescription of an inadequate analgesic dose. Many scales and instruments are available to the nurse for assessment and measurement of the client's pain level.

Unrelieved pain leads to a multitude of harmful effects involving almost all organs of the body. As a result of unrelieved pain, the client may develop increased respiratory rate and heart rate, hypertension, increased stress response, urinary retention, fluid overload, electrolyte imbalance, glucose intolerance, hyperglycemia, pneumonia, atelectasis, anorexia, paralytic ileus, constipation, weakness, confusion, and infection.

In addition to psychological and physical suffering, inadequate pain management leads to high health care costs. It is estimated the cost of extended hospital stays, readmissions to the hospital, and outpatient visits due to inadequate pain management is $100 billion per year.

Nonopioid Analgesics

Nonopioid analgesics (aspirin, acetaminophen, ibuprofen, naproxen) are less potent than opioid analgesics. They are used to treat mild to moderate pain. Nonopioids are usually purchased over-the-counter (OTC), but (COX-2 inhibitors) require a prescription. Nonopioids are effective for the dull, throbbing pain of headaches, dysmenorrhea (menstrual pain), inflammation, minor abrasions, muscular aches and pain, and mild to moderate arthritis. Most analgesics also have an antipyretic effect and will lower an elevated body temperature. Some, such as aspirin, have antiinflammatory and antiplatelet effects as well.

Table 25–I

Types of Pain

Type of Pain	Definition	Drug Treatment
Acute	Pain occurs suddenly and responds to treatment; can result from trauma, tissue injury, inflammation, or surgery	Mild pain: Scheduled nonopioid (acetaminophen, NSAIDs [aspirin, Motrin, Advil] q6h) Moderate pain: Scheduled combination of nonopioid and opioid (oxycodone 5 mg and acetaminophen 325 mg q4h) Severe pain: Scheduled potent opioid (morphine 15 mg q4h)
Chronic	Pain persists for greater than 6 mo *and* is difficult to treat or control	Nonopioid drugs are suggested. Opioids, if used, should meet these criteria: Oral or transdermal Long duration of action Include adjunct therapy Cause minimal respiratory depression
Cancer	Pain from pressure on nerves and organs, blockage to blood supply or metastasis to bone	NSAIDs and opioid drugs administered PO, transdermal, IM, IV, or PCA
Somatic	Pain of skeletal muscle, ligaments, and joints	Nonopioids: NSAIDs (aspirin, Motrin, Advil); also act as antiinflammatories and muscle relaxants
Superficial	Pain from surface areas such as skin and mucous membranes	Mild pain: Nonopioid Moderate pain: Combination of opioid and nonopioid analgesic drug
Vascular	Pain from vascular or perivascular tissues contributing to headaches or migraines	Nonopioid drugs
Visceral	Pain from smooth muscle and organs	Opioid drugs

IM, Intramuscular; *IV,* intravenous; *NSAIDs,* nonsteroidal antiinflammatory drugs; *PCA,* patient-controlled analgesia; *PO,* by mouth.

Nonsteroidal Antiinflammatory Drugs

All nonsteroidal antiinflammatory drugs (NSAIDs) have an analgesic effect as well as an antipyretic and antiinflammatory action. NSAIDs such as aspirin (ASA), ibuprofen (Motrin IB, Nuprin, Advil, Medipren), and naproxen (Aleve) can be purchased as OTC drugs. Aspirin, a salicylate NSAID, is the oldest nonopioid analgesic drug still in use. Adolf Bayer marketed the original formulation in 1899, and currently aspirin can be purchased under many names and with added ingredients. Examples are Bufferin, Ecotrin (enteric-coated tablet), Anacin (containing caffeine), and Alka-Seltzer.

In children younger than 12 years of age, aspirin should not be used and is contraindicated for any elevated temperature, regardless of the cause, because of the danger of Reye syndrome (neurologic problems associated with viral infection treated with salicylates). In these circumstances, acetaminophen (Tylenol) is recommended instead of aspirin.

In addition to its analgesic, antipyretic, and antiinflammatory properties, aspirin decreases platelet aggregation (clotting). Some health care providers may therefore prescribe one 81-mg, 162-mg, or 325-mg aspirin tablet every day or one 325-mg tablet every other day as a preventive measure against transient ischemic attacks (TIAs, or "small strokes"), heart attacks, or any thromboembolic episode. Aspirin is discussed in depth in Chapter 24 along with other NSAIDs.

Aspirin and other NSAIDs relieve pain by inhibiting biosynthesis of prostaglandin by different forms of the enzyme cyclooxygenase (COX). Inhibition of COX-2 decreases inflammation and pain, but inhibition of COX-1 decreases protection of the stomach lining. As a result of an NSAID's inhibition of COX-1, stomach ulcers and bleeding may occur. Aspirin is the drug of choice for alleviating pain and inflammation in arthritic conditions, but when given in high doses, severe GI problems develop in approximately 20% of clients. Some pharmaceutical companies have developed antiinflammatory and analgesic drugs that inhibit only COX-2. The COX-2 inhibitors were developed to eliminate the GI side effects associated with aspirin and other NSAIDs. COX-2 inhibitors are discussed in depth in Chapter 24.

Side Effects and Adverse Reactions

A common side effect of NSAIDs is gastric irritation. These drugs should be taken with food, at mealtime, or with a full glass of fluid to help reduce this problem.

If an NSAID is taken for dysmenorrhea during the first two days of menstruation, excess bleeding might occur (more so with aspirin than with ibuprofen).

Some clients are hypersensitive to aspirin. Tinnitus, vertigo, bronchospasm, and urticaria are some of the symptoms that indicate hypersensitivity or overdose of the salicylate product. Certain foods also contain salicylates: prunes, raisins, paprika, and licorice. Those who have a hypersensitivity to aspirin and salicylate products may be sensitive to other NSAIDs. This hypersensitivity may be related to inhibition of the enzyme cyclooxygenase by the salicylate product.

Acetaminophen

The analgesic acetaminophen (paraaminophenol derivative) is a popular nonprescription drug for the relief of pain, discomfort, and fever in infants, children, adults, and older adults (Figure 25–1). Acetaminophen is a nonopioid drug, but it is not an NSAID. Acetaminophen does not have the antiinflammatory properties of aspirin, so it is not the drug of choice for any inflammatory process. It constitutes 25% of all OTC drugs sold. Examples of OTC products that contain acetaminophen include Actifed: Cold & Allergy, Sinus; Anacin; Excedrin; Goody's Powders; Midol: Maximum Strength Menstrual Formula; Percogesic; and Vicks: Cold & Flu Relief. Examples of prescription products on the market that contain acetaminophen include Darvocet-N 100, Lortab, Percocet, and Vicodin. Acetaminophen (Tylenol, Panadol, Tempra), first marketed in the mid-1950s, is a safe, effective analgesic and antipyretic drug used for muscular aches and pains and for fever caused by viral infections. It causes little to no gastric distress and does not interfere with platelet aggregation. There is no link between acetaminophen and Reye syndrome, and it does not increase the potential for excessive bleeding if taken for dysmenorrhea, as do aspirin and NSAIDs (Prototype Drug Chart 25–1).

Pharmacokinetics

Acetaminophen is well absorbed from the gastrointestinal (GI) tract. Rectal absorption may be erratic because of the presence of fecal material or a decrease in blood flow to the colon. Because of acetaminophen's short half-life, it can be administered every 4 hours as needed with a maximum dose of 4 g/day. However, it is suggested that a client who frequently takes acetaminophen limit the dose to 2000 mg/day (2 g/d) to avoid the possibility of hepatic or renal dysfunction. More than 85% of acetaminophen is metabolized to drug metabolites by the liver.

FIGURE 25–1   This 12-year-old girl injured her foot playing soccer. Which of these analgesics—acetaminophen (Tylenol) or ibuprofen (Motrin)—should she choose to relieve her pain and inflammation?

Prototype DRUG CHART 25–1

ACETAMINOPHEN

Drug Class

Analgesic
Trade names: Tylenol, Tempra, Panadol, ✽Robigesic, Atasol
Pregnancy Category: B

Dosage

A: PO: 325-650 mg q4-6h PRN; *max:* 4000 mg/d;
   rectal supp: 650 mg q.i.d.
C: 0-3 mo: PO: 40 mg 4-53/d
4 mo-1 y: PO: 80 mg 4-53/d
1-2 y: PO: 120 mg 4-53/d
2-3 y: PO: 160 mg 4-53/d
4-5 y: PO: 240 mg 4-53/d
6-8 y: PO: 320 mg 4-53/d
9-10 y: PO: 400 mg 4-53/d
>11 y: PO: 480 mg 4-53/d
C: 2-5 y: Rectal: 120 mg 4-53/d
6-12 y: Rectal: 325 mg 4-53/d

Contraindications

Severe hepatic or renal disease, alcoholism;
   hypersensitivity

Drug-Lab-Food Interactions

Increase effect with caffeine, diflunisal
Decrease effect with oral contraceptives, anticholinergics, cholestyramine, charcoal

Pharmacokinetics

Absorption: PO: rapidly absorbed; rectal: erratic
Distribution: PB: 20%-50%; crosses the placenta,
   excreted in breast milk
Metabolism: t½: 1-3.5 h
Excretion: In urine as metabolites

Pharmacodynamics

PO: Onset: 10-30 min
   Peak: 1-2 h
   Duration: 3-5 h
Rectal: Onset: UK
   Peak: UK
   Duration: 4-6 h

Therapeutic Effects/Uses

To decrease pain and fever
Mode of Action: Inhibition (weak) or prostaglandin synthesis, inhibition of hypothalamic heat-regulator center

Side Effects

Anorexia, nausea, vomiting, rash

Adverse Reactions

Severe hypoglycemia, oliguria, urticaria
Life-threatening: Hemorrhage, hepatotoxicity,
   hemolytic anemia, leukopenia, thrombocytopenia

A, Adult; *C*, child; *d*, day; *h*, hour; *min*, minute; *PB*, protein-binding; *PO*, by mouth; *q.i.d.*, four times a day; *t½*, half-life; *UK*, unknown; *y*, year; *>*, greater than; ✽, Canadian drug name.

Large doses or overdoses can be toxic to the hepatic cells, so when large doses are administered over a long period, the serum level of acetaminophen should be monitored. The therapeutic serum range is 5 to 20 mcg/ml. Liver enzyme levels (aspartate aminotransferase [AST], alanine aminotransferase [ALT], alkaline phosphatase [ALP]), and serum bilirubin should also be monitored.

Pharmacodynamics

Acetaminophen weakly inhibits prostaglandin synthesis, which decreases pain sensation. It is effective in eliminating mild to moderate pain and headaches and is useful for its antipyretic effect. Acetaminophen does not possess antiinflammatory action. Its onset of action is rapid, and the duration of action is 5 hours or less. Severe adverse reactions may occur with an overdose, so acetaminophen in liquid or chewable form should be kept out of a child's reach.

Side Effects and Adverse Reactions

An overdose of acetaminophen can be extremely toxic to liver cells, causing hepatotoxicity. Death could occur in 1 to 4 days from hepatic necrosis. If a child or adult ingests excessive amounts of acetaminophen tablets or liquid, a poison control center should be contacted *immediately* and the child or adult should be taken to the emergency department. Early symptoms of hepatic damage include nausea, vomiting, diarrhea, and abdominal pain.

Table 25–2 lists the commonly used nonopioid analgesics, their dosage, uses, and considerations.

Nursing Process

Analgesic: Acetaminophen

ASSESSMENT

■ Obtain a medical history of liver dysfunction. Overdosing or extremely high doses of acetaminophen can cause hepatotoxicity.

Table 25–2

Analgesics

Generic (Brand)	Route and Dosage	Uses and Considerations
Paraaminophenol		
acetaminophen (Tylenol, Panadol, Tempra)	(Prototype Drug Chart 25-1)	
NSAIDs		
aspirin (Bayer, Ecotrin, Astrin)	Analgesic: A: PO: 325-650 mg, q4h, *max:* 4 g/d C: PO: 40-65 mg/kg/d in 4-6 divided doses; *max:* 3.6 g/d	Effective in relieving headaches, muscle pain, inflammation and pain from arthritis; mild anticoagulant. Serum therapeutic range: *headache:* 5 mg/ dl; *inflammation:* 15-30 mg/dl. Can displace other highly protein-bound drugs. If taken with acetaminophen, GI bleeding could result. Side effects: gastric discomfort, tinnitus, vertigo, deafness (reversible), increased bleeding. Should be taken with foods or at mealtime. Should *not* be taken with alcohol. *Pregnancy category:* D; PB: 55%-90%; t½: 2-20 h (high doses)
diflunisal (Dolobid)	A: PO: Initially 1000 mg; *maint:* 500 mg q8-12h	Used for mild to moderate pain. Considered to be less toxic than aspirin. *Pregnancy category:* C; PB: 99%, t½: 8-12 h
Propionic Acid		
ibuprofen (Motrin, Advil, Nuprin, Medipren)	Pain: A: PO 200-800 mg q4-6h; *max:* 3200 mg/d	For mild to moderate muscle aches and pains. Causes some gastric distress but less than aspirin. Should be taken with food, at mealtime, or with plenty of fluids. *Pregnancy category:* B; PB: 98%; t½: 2-4 h
naproxen (Naprosyn, Naprelan, EC-Naprosyn, Aleve, Anaprox, Anaprox-DS)	Mild to moderate pain: A: PO: initially 500 mg, then 200-250 mg q6-8h; *max:* 1250 mg/d C: PO: >2 y: 5-7 mg/kg q8-12h Inflammatory disease: A: PO: 250-500 mg b.i.d.; *max:* 1000 mg/d; C: PO: >2 y: 10-15 mg/kg q8-12h; *max:* 1000 mg/d	Treatment of inflammation and pain from osteoarthritis, rheumatoid arthritis, ankylosing spondylitis, gout, and dysmenorrhea. *Pregnancy category:* B; PB: UK; t½: 12-15 h
ketorolac (Toradol, Acular)	A: PO: 10 mg q6h PRN; *max:* 40 mg/day IM/IV: 30 mg q6h PRN; *max:* 120 mg/day Elderly: PO: 5-10 mg q6h PRN; *max:* 40 mg/day IM/IV: 15 mg q6h PRN; *max:* 60 mg/day	For short-term pain management (5 days or less). *Pregnancy category:* B; PB: UK; t½: 4-6 h
Oxicams meloxicam (Mobic)	A: PO: Initially 7.5 mg/d; *max:* 15 mg/d	Treatment of pain from osteoarthritis. *Pregnancy category:* C (first and second trimester), D (third trimester); PB: 99%; t½: 15-20 h
Naphthylalkanones nabumetone (Relafen)	A: PO: 1000 mg/d; *max:* 2000 mg/d	Treatment of pain from osteoarthritis, rheumatoid arthritis. *Pregnancy category:* C; PB: 99%; t½: 24 h
COX-2 Inhibitors celecoxib (Celebrex)	A: PO: 200 mg/d or 100 mg b.i.d. Elderly: Same as adult dose	Treatment of osteoarthritis and rheumatoid arthritis. Not indicated for clients <18 y. Use caution for clients with severe renal or liver disorders and for those allergic to sulfonamides. *Pregnancy category:* C; PB: UK; t½: 11.2 h
Miscellaneous tramadol (Ultram)	*Postanalgesia:* A & C: >12 y: IM: 2.5-7.5 mg q4-6h PRN A: PO: 50-100 mg q4-6h PRN; *max:* 400 mg/d Elderly: >75 y: *max:* 300 mg/d *Hepatic dysfunction:* 50 mg q12h *Renal disorder:* CL$_{cr}$ (CrCl) <30 ml/min: 50-100 mg q12h	Used for moderate to severe pain. Contraindicated in severe alcoholism or with use of opioids. Nausea, vomiting, dizziness, constipation, headache, anxiety, and seizures may occur. *Pregnancy category:* C; PB: UK; t½: UK

A, Adult; *b.i.d.,* twice a day; *C,* child; *d,* day; *GI,* gastrointestinal; *h,* hour; *IM,* intramuscular; *IV,* intravenous; *maint,* maintenance; *max,* maximum; *min,* minute; *NSAIDs,* nonsteroidal antiinflammatory drugs; *PB,* protein-binding; *PO,* by mouth; *PRN,* as needed; *t½,* half-life; *UK,* unknown; *y,* year.

Table 25–2

Analgesics—cont'd

Generic (Brand)	Route and Dosage	Uses and Considerations
Methotrimeprazine HCl (Levoprome)	*Sedative-analgesic:* A & C: >12 y: PO: 6-25 mg/d in divided doses with meals IM: 10-12 mg q4-6h PRN (deep IM) Elderly: IM: 5-10 mg q4-6h	Treatment of moderate to severe pain. May be used before and after surgery for pain and sedation. Has properties of phenothiazines, analgesia, and sedative-hypnotics. *Pregnancy category:* C; PB: UK; t½: 20 hr

>, Greater than; <, less than.

■ Ascertain the severity of pain. Nonopioid NSAIDs such as ibuprofen or an opioid may be necessary to relieve pain.

NURSING DIAGNOSES

■ Risk for injury related to analgesic effect on sensorium
■ Acute pain related to edema from surgical incision

PLANNING

■ Client's pain will be relieved or diminished.

NURSING INTERVENTIONS

■ Check liver enzyme tests such as alanine aminotransferase, alkaline phosphatase, gamma-glutamyl transferase, 5′ nucleotidase, and bilirubin for elevations in clients taking high doses or overdoses of acetaminophen.

Client Teaching

General

• Instruct client to keep acetaminophen out of children's reach. Acetaminophen for children is available in flavored tablets and liquid. High doses can cause hepatotoxicity.
• Teach client not to self-medicate with acetaminophen longer than 10 days. Teach adult caregiver not to medicate child longer than 5 days without health care provider's approval.
• Direct parent to call the poison control center immediately if a child has taken a large or unknown amount of acetaminophen.
• Check acetaminophen dosage on package level of OTC drugs. Do *not* exceed the recommended dosage. Suggested safe adult acetaminophen dose is 2000 mg/d (2 g/day), not to exceed 4 g/day to avoid liver damage (Prototype Drug Chart 25–1).

Side Effects

• Teach client to report side effects. Overdosing can cause severe liver damage and death.
• Inform parent that liver damage may occur with excess use of acetaminophen.

• Check serum acetaminophen level if toxicity is suspected. Normal serum level is 5 to 20 mcg/ml; toxic level is >50 mcg/ml. Levels of >200 mcg/ml could indicate hepatotoxicity. The antidote for acetaminophen is acetylcysteine (Mucomyst). Dosage is based on serum acetaminophen level.

Cultural Considerations ❖

• The extended family structure is important for teaching health strategies and providing support. Recognize the importance of including women in decision making and disseminating health information.

EVALUATION

■ Evaluate the effectiveness of acetaminophen in relieving pain. If pain persists, another analgesic may be needed.
■ Determine whether client is taking the dose as recommended. Observe and report any side effects.

Herbal ALERT 25–1

🍃 Kava kava helps relieve pain by relaxing the body.
• Capsaicin, which is found naturally in cayenne pepper, is selective for C fiber nociceptors and relieves some arthritis pain in topical cream or gel form.

Opioid Analgesics

Opioid analgesics, called **opioid agonists**, are prescribed for moderate and severe pain. In the United States the Harrison Opioid Act of 1914 required that all forms of opium be sold with a prescription and that it no longer be used as a nonprescription drug. The Controlled Substances Act of 1970 classified addicting drugs, opioids among them, in five schedule categories according to their potential for drug abuse (see Chapter 8). **Addiction** is defined as a psychologic and physical dependence upon a substance beyond normal voluntary control, usually after prolonged use of a substance.

Herbal ALERT 25-2

Opioids taken with kava kava, valerian, and St. John's wort may increase sedation.

Opium was used as early as 350 BC to relieve pain. In 1803 a German pharmacist isolated morphine from opium. Morphine, a prototype opioid, is obtained from the sap of seed pods of the opium poppy plant. Codeine is another drug obtained from opium. In the past 40 years, many synthetic and semisynthetic opioids have been developed.

While nonopioid analgesics act on the peripheral nervous system at the pain receptor sites, opioid analgesics act mostly on the CNS. Opioids act primarily by activating the μ receptors, while also exerting a weak activation of the kappa (k) receptors. Analgesia, respiratory depression, euphoria, and sedation are effects of μ activation. Activation of k receptors leads to analgesia and sedation, having no effect on respiratory depression and euphoria.

Opioids not only suppress pain impulses but also respiration and coughing by acting on the respiratory and cough centers in the medulla of the brainstem. One example of such an opioid is morphine, a potent analgesic that can readily depress respirations. Codeine is not as potent as morphine ($^{1}/_{15}$ to $^{1}/_{20}$ as potent), but it also relieves mild to moderate pain and suppresses cough, which allows it also to be classified as an antitussive. Most opioids, with the exception of meperidine (Demerol), have an antitussive (cough suppression) effect. The opioids have two isomers, *levo* and *dextro*. The levo-isomers of opioids produce an analgesic effect only; however, both levo- and dextro-isomers possess an antitussive response. The dextro-isomers do not cause physical dependence, but the levo-isomers do. Synthetic cough suppressants are discussed in Chapter 39.

In addition to pain relief and antitussive effects, many opioids possess antidiarrheal effects. Common side effects with high doses of most opioids include nausea and vomiting (particularly in ambulatory clients), constipation, a moderate decrease in blood pressure, and orthostatic hypotension. High doses of opioids may also cause respiratory depression, urinary retention (usually in older adults), and antitussive effects.

Morphine

Morphine, an extraction from opium, is a potent opioid analgesic (Prototype Drug Chart 25–2). Morphine is effective against acute pain resulting from acute myocardial infarction (AMI), cancer, and dyspnea resulting from pulmonary edema. It may be used as a preoperative medication. Although it is effective in relieving severe pain, it can cause respiratory depression, orthostatic hypotension, miosis, urinary retention, constipation resulting from reduced bowel motility, and cough suppression. An antidote for morphine excess or overdose is the opioid antagonist naloxone (Narcan).

Pharmacokinetics

Morphine may be taken orally, although GI absorption can be somewhat erratic. For severe pain, such as with AMI, it is given intravenously (IV). Morphine is 30% protein-bound and may also be administered rectally and epidurally. Oral morphine undergoes first hepatic pass, meaning the liver metabolizes the drug before bioavailability to the rest of the body occurs. Only a small amount of morphine crosses the blood-brain barrier to produce an analgesic effect. It has a short half-life, and 90% is excreted in the urine. Morphine crosses the placenta and is excreted in breast milk.

Pharmacodynamics

Morphine binds with the opiate receptor in the CNS. Parenterally the onset of action is rapid, especially IV. Onset of action is slower for subcutaneous (subQ) and intramuscular (IM) injections. Duration of action with most types of drug administration is 3 to 5 hours; with controlled-release morphine sulfate tablets (MS Contin) duration is 8 to 12 hours.

 Nursing Process

Opioid Analgesic: Morphine Sulfate

ASSESSMENT

■ Obtain a medical history. Contraindications for morphine include severe respiratory disorders, increased intracranial pressure, and severe renal disease. Morphine may cause seizures.
■ Determine a drug history. Report if a drug-drug interaction is probable. Morphine increases the effects of alcohol, sedatives or hypnotics, antipsychotic drugs, and muscle relaxants and might cause respiratory depression.
■ Assess vital signs, noting rate and depth of respirations for future comparisons; opioids commonly decrease respirations and systolic blood pressure.
■ Monitor urinary output; morphine can cause urinary retention.
■ Assess type of pain, location, and duration before giving opioids.

NURSING DIAGNOSES

■ Acute pain related to surgical tissue injury
■ Ineffective breathing patterns related to excess morphine dosage

PLANNING

■ Client's pain will be diminished or alleviated.

NURSING INTERVENTIONS

■ Administer morphine before pain reaches its peak to maximize effectiveness of the drug.
■ Monitor vital signs at frequent intervals to detect respiratory changes. Respirations of <10/min can indicate respiratory distress.

Prototype **DRUG CHART 25–2**

MORPHINE SULFATE

Drug Class

Opioid
Trade names: Duramorph, MS Contin, Roxanol SR,
♣Epimorph, Statex
CSS II
Pregnancy Category: B

Dosage

A: PO: 10-30 mg q4h PRN
SR: 15-30 mg, q8-12h PRN
IM/subQ: 5-15 mg PRN
IV: 4-10 mg q4h PRN: diluted; inject over 5 min Epidural:
    2-10 mg over 24h
C: IM/subQ: 0.1-0.2 mg/kg PRN; *max:* <15 mg/dose
Neonate: subQ/IM/IV: 0.05 mg/kg q4-8h; *max:* 0.1 mg/kg

Contraindications

Asthma with respiratory depression, increased
    intracranial pressure, shock
Caution: Respiratory, renal, or hepatic diseases;
    myocardial infarction; older adults; very young

Drug-Lab-Food Interactions

Drug: Increase effects of alcohol, sedatives-hypnotics,
    antipsychotic drugs, muscle relaxants
Lab: Increase AST, ALT

Pharmacokinetics

Absorption: PO: varies; **IV:** rapid
Distribution: PB: UK; crosses placenta, excreted
    in breast milk
Metabolism: t½: 2.5-3 h
Excretion: 90% in urine

Pharmacodynamics

PO: Onset: Variable
    Peak: 1-2 h
    Duration: 4-5 h; SR: 8-12 h
subQ/IM: Onset: 15-30 min
    Peak: SC: 50-90 min
    IM: 0.5-1 h
    Duration: 3-5 h
IV: Onset: rapid
    Peak: 20 min
    Duration: 3-5 h

Therapeutic Effects/Uses

To relieve severe pain
Mode of Action: Depression of the CNS; depression of pain impulses by binding with the opiate receptor in the CNS

Side Effects

Anorexia, nausea, vomiting, constipation, drowsiness,
    dizziness, sedation, confusion, urinary retention,
    rash, blurred vision, bradycardia, flushing, euphoria,
    pruritus

Adverse Reactions

Hypotension, urticaria, seizures
Life-threatening: Respiratory depression, increased
    intracranial pressure

A, Adult; *ALT*, alanine aminotransferase; *AST*, aspartate aminotransferase; *C*, child; *CNS*, central nervous system; *CSS*, Controlled Substances Schedule; *h*, hour; *IM*, intramuscular; *IV*, intravenous; *min*, minute; *PB*, protein binding; *PO*, by mouth; *PRN*, as necessary; *subQ*, subcutaneous; *SR*, sustained-release; *t½*, half-life; *UK*, unknown; <, less than; ♣, Canadian drug name.

■ Record client's urine output because urinary retention is a side effect of morphine. Urine output should be at least 600 ml/day.

■ Check bowel sounds for decreased peristalsis; constipation is a side effect of morphine. Dietary change or mild laxative might be needed.

■ Check for pupil changes and reaction. Pinpoint pupils can indicate morphine overdose.

■ Have naloxone (Narcan) available as an antidote to reverse respiratory depression if morphine overdose occurs.

■ Validate child's dose of morphine before its administration. Recommended dose is 0.1 to 0.2 mg/kg/q4h, intramuscularly or subcutaneously; maximum dose is 15 mg/dose.

■ Check older adults for alertness and orientation, because confusion is a side effect of morphine. Side rails and other safety precautions should be taken as well as administration of decreased dosages.

Client Teaching

General

• Encourage client not to use alcohol or CNS depressants with any opioid analgesics such as morphine. Respiratory depression can result.

• Suggest nonpharmacologic measures to relieve pain as client recuperates from surgery. As recovery progresses, a nonopioid analgesic may be prescribed.

Side Effects

- Alert client that with continuous use, opioids such as morphine can become addicting. If addiction occurs, inform client about methadone treatment programs and other resources in the area.
- Instruct client to report dizziness while taking morphine. Dizziness could be due to orthostatic hypotension. Advise client to ambulate with caution or only with assistance.
- Teach client to report difficulty in breathing, blurred vision, and headaches.

Cultural Considerations ❖

- Identify conflicts in values and beliefs about pain and its management.
- Respect cultural and religious differences concerning refusal of opioid analgesics.
- Incorporate traditional practices into Western medicine when possible.

EVALUATION

- Evaluate the effectiveness of morphine in lessening or alleviating pain. If pain persists after several days, dose should be increased or opioid changed.
- Determine stability of vital signs. Any decrease in respiration and blood pressure should be reported.

Meperidine

One of the first synthetic opioids, meperidine (Demerol), became available in the mid-1950s. It is classified as a schedule II drug according to the Controlled Substances Act. Meperidine has a shorter duration of action than morphine, and its potency varies according to the dosage. Meperidine, which can be given orally, IM, and IV, is primarily effective in GI procedures. It does not have the antitussive property of opium preparations.

During pregnancy meperidine is preferred to morphine, because it does not diminish uterine contractions and causes less neonatal respiratory depression. Meperidine causes less constipation and urinary retention than morphine. Meperidine is not indicated for clients with chronic pain, severe liver dysfunction, sickle cell disease, a history of seizures, severe coronary artery disease (CAD), and cardiac dysrhythmias. When older adults and clients with advanced cancer receive large doses of meperidine, neurotoxicity (e.g., nervousness, tremors, agitation, irritability, seizures) have been reported. Meperidine should not be prescribed for long-term use; the dose is frequently limited to 600 mg in a 24-hour period for no longer than 48 to 72 hours.

Meperidine is metabolized in the liver to an active metabolite; therefore the dose should be decreased for clients with hepatic or renal insufficiency. It is excreted in the urine in a metabolite form called *normeperidine*. Meperidine should not be taken with alcohol or sedative-hypnotics, because the combination of these drugs causes an additive CNS depression. A major side effect of meperidine is a decrease in blood pressure, which should be monitored, especially if the client is an older adult.

Table 25–3 lists opioids and their dosages, uses, and considerations.

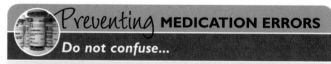

Preventing MEDICATION ERRORS

Do not confuse...

- **meperidine** with **morphine**, **meprobamate**, or **hydromorphone**.
- **Demerol** with **Desyrel**, **Dilaudid**, or **Temaril**. These drug names look alike, but the drugs are different.

Table 25–3

Opioids: Opium and Synthetics

Generic (Brand)	Route and Dosage	Uses and Considerations
codeine (sulfate, phosphate) CSS II	A: PO/subQ/IM: 15-60 mg q4-6h PRN C: PO/subQ/IM: 0.5-1 mg/kg q4-6h	Effective for mild to moderate pain. Can be used with a nonopioid (acetaminophen) for pain relief. Has antitussive properties. Can decrease respiration and cause physical dependence and constipation. *Pregnancy category:* C; PB: 70%, $t^{1/2}$: 2.5 h
hydrocodone bitartrate (Hycodan, Vicodin with acetaminophen) CSS II	*Analgesic:* A: C >12 y: PO: 5-10 mg q4-6h C: 2-12 y: PO: 1.25-5 mg q4-6h Elderly: PO: 2.5-5 mg q4-6h *Extended-release:* A: PO: 10 mg q12h C: 6-12 y: PO: 5 mg q12h	Treatment of moderate to moderately-severe pain. Combination with acetaminophen (Lortab, Vicodin), aspirin (Lortab ASA), ibuprofen (Vicoprofin), and chlorpheniramine (Tussionex). Can be prescribed for analgesic and antitussive purposes. *Pregnancy category:* C; PB: UK; $t^{1/2}$: 4 h (longer $t^{1/2}$ in older adults)

A, Adult; *C,* child; *CSS,* Controlled Substances Schedule; *h,* hour; *IM,* intramuscular; *PB,* protein-binding; *PO,* by mouth; *PRN,* as necessary; *subQ,* subcutaneous; $t^{1/2}$, half-life; *UK,* unknown; *y,* year.

Table 25-3

Opioids: Opium and Synthetics—cont'd

Generic (Brand)	Route and Dosage	Uses and Considerations
hydromorphone HCl (Dilaudid) CSS II	A: PO/subQ/IM/IV: 1-4 mg q4-6 h PRN *Extended-release:* A: 12-32 mg q24h Rectal: 3 mg q4-6h C: PO 0.03-0.08 mg/kg q4-6h (max: 5 mg/dose) IV 0.015 mg/kg q4-6h	Treatment of moderate to severe pain. Can be prescribed for analgesic and antitussive purposes. *Pregnancy category:* C; PB: UK; t$^{1}/_{2}$: UK
levorphanol tartrate (Levo-Dromoran) CSS II	A: PO/subQ: Initially: 2 mg PO/subQ: 2-3 mg q6-8h PRN	For moderate to severe pain. Has side effects similar to morphine. *Pregnancy category:* B; PB: 50%-60%; t$^{1}/_{2}$: 11-16 h
meperidine (Demerol) CSS II	A: PO/subQ/IM/IV: 50-150 mg q3-4h PRN C: PO/subQ/IM/IV: 1-1.5 mg/kg q3-4h PRN; *max:* 100 mg q4h for children	For relief of moderate to severe pain, GI procedures, and preoperative sedation. *Pregnancy category:* B; PB: 60%-80%; t$^{1}/_{2}$: 3-8 h
morphine sulfate CSS II	(Prototype Drug Chart 25–2)	For relief of moderate to moderately severe pain, including postoperative and postpartum pain. Avoid taking drug over an extended period of time. As potent as morphine. Take with food to avoid GI distress. *Pregnancy category:* B to D; PB: UK; t$^{1}/_{2}$: 2-3 h
oxycodone HCl (OxyContin) CSS II	A: PO: 5-10 mg q6h PRN C: >12 y: PO: 2.5 mg q6h PRN C: 6-12 y: PO: 1.25 mg q6h PRN	
oxycodone HCl with acetaminophen (Percocet) and oxycodone terephthalate with aspirin (Percodan) CSS II	A: PO: 5 mg q4-6h PRN or 5-10 mg q6h PRN C: 6-12 y: 1.25 mg q6h PRN C: 12-17 y: 2.5 mg q6h PRN	For moderate to severe pain. *Percocet* contains acetaminophen. *Percodan* contains aspirin and can cause gastric irritation, so it should be taken with food or plenty of liquid. *Pregnancy category:* B; PB: UK; t$^{1}/_{2}$: 2-3 h
propoxyphene HCl (Darvon) CSS IV propoxyphene napsylate (Darvon-N) CSS IV	A: PO: HCl: 65 mg q4h PRN; *max:* 390 mg/d A: PO: napsylate: 100 mg q4h PRN; *max:* 600 mg/d	For mild pain. Weak analgesic. *Darvocet-N* contains acetaminophen and *Darvon-compound* contains aspirin, so should be taken with food or plenty of liquid. Not a constipating drug; has little physical dependence. *Pregnancy category:* C; PB: .90%; t$^{1}/_{2}$: 12 h
alfentanil (Alfenta) CSS II	A: IV: 8-40 mcg/kg for surgery Continuous infusion: 0.5-1 mcg/kg/min Total dose: 8-40 mcg/kg	Opioid analgesic with rapid onset of action. May be given to induce anesthesia or administered by continuous infusion with nitrous oxide and oxygen. *Pregnancy category:* C; PB: UK; t$^{1}/_{2}$: UK
fentanyl (Duragesic, Sublimaze) CSS II	A: IM: 50-100 mcg q1-2h PRN C: 2-12 y: IM: 1.7-3.3 mcg q1-2h PRN *Lozenge:* A: Suck on 400-mcg lozenge until sedated C: 35-40 kg: Suck on 400-mcg lozenge until sedated C: 25-35 kg: Suck on 400-mcg lozenge until sedated *Transdermal patch:* A: Initially 25 mcg/h patch q3d	Short-acting potent opioid analgesic. May be used with short-term surgery. Dose varies according to age. Drug available as a transdermal patch for controlling chronic pain. *Pregnancy category:* C; PB: 80%-89%; t$^{1}/_{2}$: 7 h IV; 17 h transdermal
sufentanil citrate (Sufenta) CSS II	*Primary anesthetic:* A: IV: 8-30 mcg/kg with 100% oxygen and muscle relaxant C: IV: 10-25 mcg/kg with 100% oxygen and muscle relaxant *Adjunct to anesthesia:* IV: 1-8 mcg/kg	Potent synthetic opioid; used as part of the balanced anesthesia group. May be used as a primary anesthetic. *Pregnancy category:* C; PB: 93%; t$^{1}/_{2}$: 1-3 h
remifentanil (Ultiva) CSS II	A: IV: Infusion rate: 0.05-2 mcg/min IV: Post-op: 0.025-0.2 mcg/min	Newest opioid analgesic. Rapid onset of action, short-acting duration (5-10 min). Can cause respiratory depression, hypotension, and bradycardia. *Pregnancy category:* UK; PB: UK; t$^{1}/_{2}$: UK
methadone (Dolophine) CSS II	*Moderate to severe acute pain:* A: PO/subQ/IM: 2.5-10 mg q3-4h PRN C: PO/IV: 0.1 mg/kg q4h for 2-3 doses, then q6-12h PRN; *max:* 10 mg/dose *Detoxification:* A: PO/subQ/IM: 15-40 mg/d; *max:* 120 mg/d Neonate: PO/IV: 0.05-0.2 mg/dk q12-24h; taper dose by 10%-20%/wk over 1-1$^{1}/_{2}$ mo	Similar to morphine but longer duration of action. Used in drug abuse programs. Helps alleviate craving for opioids. Peak action 30-60 min. *Pregnancy category:* C; PB: UK; t$^{1}/_{2}$: 15-25 h

GI, Gastrointestinal; *IV,* intravenous; *maint;* maintenance; *max,* maximum; *min,* minute.

Hydromorphone

Hydromorphone (Dilaudid) is a semisynthetic opioid similar to morphine. The analgesic effect is approximately six times more potent than morphine with fewer hypnotic effects and less GI distress. This opioid has a faster onset and shorter duration of action than morphine. Hydromorphone is classified as a schedule II drug according to the Controlled Substances Act. Tolerance to hydromorphone increases gradually.

This drug is given orally, rectally, subQ, IM, and IV for the relief of moderate to severe pain. When given IV, dilution of each dose with 5 ml of sterile water or normal saline is preferred. Direct IV administration of 2 mg or less should be given over 2 to 5 minutes. Hydromorphone is readily absorbed in the body and excreted in the urine. Respirations should be monitored closely, and adequate hydration should be provided.

Side Effects and Adverse Reactions

Many side effects are known to accompany the use of opioids. Of particular importance are signs of respiratory depression (respiration <10/min). Other side effects include **orthostatic hypotension** (decrease in blood pressure when rising from sitting or lying position), tachycardia, drowsiness and mental clouding, constipation, and urinary retention. In addition, pupillary constriction (a sign of toxicity), tolerance, and psychological and physical dependence may occur with prolonged use.

Increased metabolism of opioids contributes to tolerance, which causes an increased need for higher doses of the opioid. If chronic use of the opioid is discontinued, withdrawal (cessation of drug administration) symptoms usually occur within 24 to 48 hours after the last opioid dose. **Withdrawal syndrome** is caused by physical dependence. Symptoms of withdrawal syndrome include irritability, diaphoresis (sweating), restlessness, muscle twitching, and an increase in pulse rate and blood pressure. Withdrawal symptoms from opioids are unpleasant but not as severe or life-threatening as those that accompany withdrawal from sedative-hypnotics—a process that may lead to convulsions.

Contraindications

Use of opioid analgesics is contraindicated for clients with head injuries. Opioids decrease respiration, thus causing an accumulation of carbon dioxide (CO_2). With an increase in carbon dioxide retention, blood vessels dilate (vasodilation), especially cerebral vessels, which causes increased intracranial pressure.

Opioid analgesics given to a client with a respiratory disorder only intensify the respiratory distress. In the client with asthma, opiates decrease respiratory drive while simultaneously increasing airway resistance.

Opioids may cause hypotension and are not indicated for clients in shock or for those who have very low blood pressure. If an opioid is necessary, the dosage needs to be adjusted accordingly; otherwise, the hypotensive state may

worsen. For an older adult or a person who is debilitated, the opioid dose usually needs to be decreased.

Morphine is the opioid analgesic prototype, and all other opioids are measured in comparison to morphine. The following Equianalgesic Opioid Dose Table illustrates the comparison of various opioid dosages to a standard dose of Morphine 10 mg IM.

Combination Drugs

To treat moderate to severe pain, combination drugs of an NSAID and an opioid analgesic may be used. Examples are hydrocodone and ibuprofen (Vicoprofin), which is a combination of an NSAID and an opioid. Another combination for the treatment of mild to moderate pain is acetaminophen and codeine. Using a combination of drugs for pain helps to decrease drug dependency that may result from possible long-term use of an opioid agent.

Patient-Controlled Analgesia (PCA)

Patient-controlled analgesia is an alternative route for opioid administration for self-administered pain relief as needed. Usually a loading dose (e.g., 2-10 mg of morphine) is given initially to achieve pain relief. Then within predetermined safety limits, the client controls administration of the opioid analgesic, depending on the amount of pain. To receive the opioid, the client pushes a button on the PCA device, releasing a specific dose of analgesic (e.g., 1 mg morphine) into the IV line. The nurse titrates the opioid analgesic dose by regulating the time intervals (every several minutes) at which the drug can be received. A lockout mechanism on the electronically controlled infusion pump prevents the client from constantly pushing the button and causing a drug overdose. The PCA device maintains a near-constant analgesic level, avoiding episodes of severe pain and oversedation. Morphine is used most often for PCA, but fentanyl (Sublimaze) and hydromorphone (Dilaudid) may also be given.

Transdermal Opioid Analgesics

Transdermal opioid analgesics provide a continuous "around-the-clock" pain control that is helpful to clients who suffer from chronic pain. The transdermal method is

Equianalgesic Opioid Dose Table

Opioid Analgesic	Oral	Intra-muscular	Intravenous
morphine	30 mg	10 mg	10 mg
fentanyl	—	0.1 mg	—
codeine	200 mg	130 mg	—
hydromorphone	7.5 mg	1.5 mg	1.5 mg
meperidine	300 mg	75 mg	75 mg
oxycodone	20 mg	—	—
hydrocodone	30 mg	—	—
oxymorphone	10 mg rectal	1 mg	1 mg
methadone	20 mg	10 mg	10 mg

Adapted from Lehne RA: *Pharmacology for nursing care*, ed 7, St. Louis, 2007, Saunders, p. 266.

not useful for acute or postoperative pain. An example of a transdermal opioid analgesic is fentanyl (Duragesic), which is administered via a transdermal patch. This patch comes in various strengths—25, 50, 75, and 100 mcg/hour. Maximum serum fentanyl levels occur within 24 hours of when the patch is first applied. Fentanyl is also available for IM and IV use. Fentanyl is more potent than morphine. For older adults, the use of a lower fentanyl transdermal dose is usually suggested. The health care provider must exercise caution when prescribing fentanyl for clients who weigh less than 110 pounds.

Analgesic Titration

Analgesics may be titrated to increase or decrease the dosage. Usually postoperative pain will decrease over time, and analgesics will be titrated downward. However, the client with cancer-related pain usually has a continual increase in pain and will require an upward titration. Titration can be accomplished by changing the dose, the interval between doses, the route of administration, or the drug. When titrating analgesics, the dosage is decided after assessing the client's respiratory rate and pain level.

Opioid Use in Special Populations
Children

Pain management in children is complex, because it is more difficult to assess their pain. Some children will not verbalize discomfort when they are in severe pain, and some are fearful of treatments like injections that relieve pain. Nurses should use age-appropriate communication skills to ascertain a child's need for pain relief. The "ouch scale" illustrated in Figure 25–2 can be helpful in determining a child's level of pain. Also, the parent may help identify the presence and degree of the child's pain. Crying and whining may be indicators of a need for pain relief or may represent other needs.

A child, like an adult, should be given medication before the pain becomes severe. The use of oral liquid medication for pain relief, if appropriate, is generally more acceptable to the child. The nurse, using drawings and pictures related to areas of pain in the body and pain relief with smiling faces, may alleviate the child's fear and help with drug compliance.

Older Adults

Usually, adults who are 65 years of age or older require adjustment to drug doses to avoid severe side effects. Merely decreasing the usual adult dosage of opioid analgesic is not always the answer for older adults. Many take an array of medications for their health problems, increasing the possibility of drug interactions and drug side effects. In older adults, side effects from the use of opioids become more pronounced. The nurse needs to closely monitor for adverse reactions in older adults who take opioid analgesics. As a person ages, liver and renal functions decrease, causing the rate of metabolism and excretion of the drug to decrease. As a result, drug accumulation may occur.

Older adults tend to have different beliefs and fears than younger generations regarding opioids. They may believe that pain is inevitable due to aging or fear addiction. Older adults may not want to report pain, because they do not want to be a burden. The nurse must perform pain assessment with a supportive approach in an unhurried manner and teach the client accurate drug information.

Pain assessment may be more difficult with older adults due to the decrease in cognitive and sensory-perceptual abilities. Dementia or hearing and visual deficits may interfere with communication. The nurse may need to

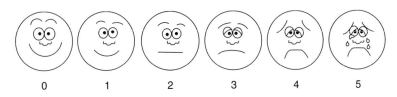

0	1	2	3	4	5

1. Explain to the child that each face is for a person who feels happy because he has no pain (hurt, or whatever word the child uses) or feels sad because he has some or a lot of pain.

2. Point to the appropriate face and state, "This face is . . ."
   0-"very happy because he doesn't hurt at all."
   1-"hurts just a little bit."
   2-"hurts a little more."
   3-"hurts even more."
   4-"hurts a whole lot."
   5-"hurts as much as you can imagine, although you don't have to be crying to feel this bad."

3. Ask the child to choose the face that best describes how he feels. Be specific about which pain (e.g., "shot" or incision) and what time (e.g., now? earlier? before lunch?).

FIGURE 25–2 A scale used to rate the intensity of pain in children. (From Hockenberry M: *Wong's essentials of pediatric nursing,* ed 8, St. Louis, 2009, Mosby.)

rely on a more thorough physical assessment to discover the presence of pain, because self-reporting may not be reliable.

In the presence of decreased renal and hepatic function, drugs that tend to be more toxic in older adults include meperidine (Demerol), pentazocine (Talwin), and propoxyphene (Darvon). Analgesics are usually metabolized in the liver and excreted in the urine. Usual doses of analgesics in older adults may result in excessive sedation and prolonged duration of action. Chronological age is one of several factors that influence medication use and dosage. Comorbidity must also be considered.

Cognitively Impaired Individuals

Any cognitively impaired individual may be unable to report pain adequately. The nurse should use a measurement scale that is appropriate for the client. Some physical signs of pain include moans, grimacing, clenched teeth, noisy respirations, and restlessness.

Oncology Clients

Cancer pain is managed according to three levels of analgesia based upon the World Health Organization (WHO) Ladder as followed:

  Step 1—Mild Pain: Nonopioids with or without an adjuvant medication

  Step 2—Moderate Pain: Nonopioids and mild opioid with or without an adjuvant medication

  Step 3—Severe Pain: Stronger opioid at higher dosage levels with or without an adjuvant medication

Opioids are titrated for oncology clients until pain relief is achieved or the side effects become intolerable. For effective pain management in clients with cancer, extremely high doses may be required. There are no set dosage limits for oncology clients.

Individuals with a History of Substance Abuse

Often clients with a history of substance abuse require pain medication. A thorough pain assessment is necessary to find out the cause of pain. The nurse needs to know that opioids are effective and safe in this population, even though larger doses in greater frequency may be required. Studies have shown that withholding opioids in this population has not increased recovery from addiction. However, opioid agonist-antagonists such as pentazocine (Talwin) should be avoided in chemically dependent clients, because these drugs may precipitate withdrawal syndrome.

Adjuvant Therapy

Medications used as **adjuvant analgesics** have been developed for other purposes and later found to be effective for pain relief in neuropathy. Adjuvant therapy is usually used along with a nonopioid and opioid. Examples of adjuvant analgesics include anticonvulsants, antidepressants, corticosteroids, antidysrhythmics, and local anesthetics.

Anticonvulsant medications (gabapentin [Neurontin]) act on the peripheral nerves and CNS by inhibiting spontaneous neuronal firing. They are used for neuropathic pain and the prevention of migraine headaches. Tricyclic antidepressants (amitriptyline [Elavil]) prevent the reuptake of serotonin and norepinephrine in the cells. Lower doses of tricyclic antidepressants than those usually prescribed for depression are effective in treating peripheral neuropathy. Corticosteroids serve as effective analgesics by reducing nociceptive stimuli. Antidysrhythmics (mexiletine [Mexitil]) block sodium channels to reduce pain. Local anesthetics (lidocaine patch) can be effective analgesics by interrupting the transmission of pain signals to the brain.

Adjuvant medications potentiate opioid analgesia for severe persistent pain in diabetic neuropathy, cancer, migraine headaches, and rheumatoid arthritis. When any of the adjuvant medications are used in conjunction with an NSAID and opioid, dosages may be kept lower to reduce adverse effects.

Treatment for Opioid-Addicted Individuals

Throughout the country there are many treatment programs that help the opioid-addicted individual withdraw from heroin or similar opioids without experiencing withdrawal symptoms. When opioids are discontinued suddenly, withdrawal symptoms and rebound pain (temporary increase in pain) usually occur. Withdrawal symptoms include diarrhea, abdominal cramps, restlessness, watery eyes, runny nose, and nausea.

One type of program is the **methadone treatment program.** This program works by replacing opioids with methadone, also an opioid but one that causes less dependency than the opioids it replaces. Oral methadone does not lead to the euphoria ("high") achieved with injectable opioids. The half-life of methadone is longer than most opioids, so it needs to be given only once a day. The dosage range is 15 to 40 mg daily; the maximum dosage is 120 mg daily.

Other types of methadone treatment programs include weaning programs and maintenance programs. In a weaning program, the recovering addict receives a dose of methadone for the first 2 days that approximates the same dose as the "street" drug used. After 2 days, the methadone dose may be decreased by 5 to 10 mg daily or as indicated until the client is completely weaned off methadone. In a maintenance program, a client is given the same methadone dose every day. The dose may be less than that of the street drug, but it remains consistent throughout the course of treatment.

Opioid Agonist-Antagonists

In the past 20 years **opioid agonist-antagonists,** medications in which an opioid antagonist (e.g., naloxone [Narcan]) is added to an opioid agonist, were developed in hopes of decreasing opioid abuse. Pentazocine (Talwin), the first opioid analgesic, can be given orally (tablet) and by injection (subQ, IM, and IV). Pentazocine is classified as a schedule IV drug. Butorphanol tartrate (Stadol), buprenorphine (Buprenex), and nalbuphine hydrochloride (Nubain) are examples of other opioid agonist-antagonist analgesics. Reports say that pentazocine and butorphanol can cause dependence. Opioid agonist-antagonist drugs are not given for cancer pain, because of the risk of potential CNS toxicity from the high doses required. These analgesics are considered safe for use during labor, but their safety during early pregnancy has not been established.

Prototype Drug Chart 25–3 details the pharmacologic behavior of nalbuphine, and Table 25–4 lists the various opioid agonist-antagonists.

Pharmacokinetics

Nalbuphine can be administered orally, IM, subQ, or IV. It is rapidly absorbed parenterally. Nalbuphine has a short half-life. It is metabolized in the liver and excreted in the urine.

Pharmacodynamics

Nalbuphine is effective in alleviating moderate to severe pain. Onset of action is rapid, and peak time occurs within 30 minutes with IV administration. Duration of action is the same for all routes of administration: approximately 5 hours.

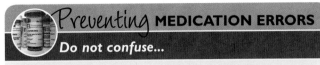

Preventing MEDICATION ERRORS

Do not confuse...

- **Nubain** (narcotic agonist-antagonist analgesic for moderate to severe pain) with **Nebcin** (aminoglycoside antibiotic) or **Nuprin** (OTC analgesic, antipyretic, NSAID). Their names may look alike, but their drug classes and actions are very different.

Prototype DRUG CHART 25–3

NALBUPHINE

Drug Class
Opioid, agonist-antagonist
Trade name: Nubain
Pregnancy Category: B

Dosage
A: IV/IM/subQ: 10-20 mg q3-6h; *max:* 160 mg/d
C: IV/IM/subQ: 0.1-0.15 mg/kg q3-6h

Contraindications
Hypersensitivity
Caution: History of drug abuse or emotional instability, impaired respirations, head injury, increased intracranial pressure, MI, biliary tract surgery, renal or hepatic dysfunction

Drug-Lab-Food Interactions
Drug: CNS depression is potentiated with alcohol or other CNS depressants

Pharmacokinetics
Absorption: readily occurs parenterally
Distribution: PB: <30%; crosses placenta, excreted in breast milk
Metabolism: t½: 5 h
Excretion: In urine

Pharmacodynamics
PO: Onset: 2-3 min IV; 15 minutes IM
  Peak: 30 min IV
  Duration: 3-6 h

Therapeutic Effects/Uses
To relieve moderate to severe pain
Mode of Action: Inhibition of pain impulses transmitted in the CNS by binding with opiate receptor and increasing pain threshold

Side Effects
Dizziness, confusion, hallucinations, blurred vision, headache, flushing, sedation, nervousness, restlessness, euphoria, depression, crying, dysphoria, unusual dreams, dry mouth, bitter taste, nausea, vomiting, abdominal cramps, clammy skin, urinary urgency

Adverse Reactions
Bradycardia, tachycardia, hypotension, hypertension, dyspnea
Life-threatening: Respiratory depression

CNS, Central nervous system; *d,* day; *h,* hour; *IM,* intramuscular; *IV,* intravenous; *max,* maximum; *MI,* myocardial infarction; *min,* minute; *PB,* protein-binding; *subQ,* subcutaneous; *t½,* half-life.

Table 25–4

Opioids: Agonist-Antagonists

Generic (Brand)	Route and Dosage	Uses and Considerations
buprenorphine HCl (Buprenex) CSS V	Pain: A: IM/IV: Initially: 0.3 mg q6h; may increase to 0.6 mg q6h PRN; IV infusion: 25-50 mcg/h Opioid dependence/cocaine withdrawal: A: SL 8 mg qd within 4 h of last opioid dose on day 1; 16 mg on day 2, then switch to maintenance dose of 4-24 mg qd	For moderate to severe pain associated with surgery, cancer, urinary calculi, myocardial infarction, and trauma. Avoid alcohol and CNS depressants. *Pregnancy category:* C; PB: 96%; t½: 2-3 h
butorphanol tartrate (Stadol) CSS IV	A: IM: 1-4 mg q3-4h PRN IV: 0.5-2 mg q3-4h PRN Nasal spray: 1 mg (1 spray) q3-4h	Management of moderate to severe pain for cancer, urinary calculi, labor, musculoskeletal, and burns. *Pregnancy category:* C; PB: >90%; t½: 2.5-4 h
dezocine (Dalgan) CSS IV	A: IM: 5-20 mg q3-6h PRN; *max:* 120 mg/d IV: 2.5-10 mg q3-6h PRN	To control moderate to severe pain. *Pregnancy category:* C; PB: UK; t½: 2.2-2.6 h
nalbuphine HCl (Nubain) CSS IV	(Prototype Drug Chart 25–3)	
pentazocine lactate (Talwin) CSS IV	A: PO: 50-100 mg q3-4h PRN; *max:* 360 mg/d A: subQ/IM/IV: 30 mg q3-4 h PRN; *max:* 360 mg/d Elderly: PO: 50 mg q4h Elderly: IM: 30 mg q4h	To control moderate to severe pain. *Pregnancy category:* C; PB: 60%; t½: 2-3 h

A, Adult; *CNS,* central nervous system; *CSS,* Controlled Substances Schedule; *d,* day; *h,* hour; *IM,* intramuscular; *IV,* intravenous; *max,* maximum; *PB,* protein-binding; *PO,* by mouth; *PRN,* as needed; *subQ,* subcutaneous; *t½,* half-life; *UK,* unknown; *>,* greater than.

Nursing Process

Opioid Agonist-Antagonist Analgesic: Nalbuphine (Nubain)

ASSESSMENT

■ Obtain a drug history from client. Report if a drug-drug interaction is probable. When taken with nalbuphine, CNS depressants can cause respiratory depression.
■ Note baseline vital signs for future comparison.
■ Assess the type of pain, duration, and location before giving the drug.

NURSING DIAGNOSIS

■ Acute pain related to trauma

PLANNING

■ Client's intensity of pain will be lessened.

NURSING INTERVENTIONS

■ Monitor vital signs. Note any changes in respirations.
■ Check bowel sounds and date of last bowel movement to identify constipation. Decreased peristalsis may result in constipation. A mild laxative may be necessary.

■ Determine urine output. Report if urine output is <30 ml/hour or <600 ml/day.
■ Administer IV nalbuphine undiluted. Do not mix with barbiturates.

Client Teaching

General
• Instruct client not to use alcohol or CNS depressants while taking nalbuphine. Respiratory depression can occur.
• Suggest nonpharmacologic methods for lessening pain like changing position or ambulation.

Side Effects
• Instruct client to report side effects of nalbuphine: dizziness, headaches, constipation, dysuria, rash, or blurred vision. Hallucinations, tachycardia, and respiratory depression are adverse reactions that might occur.

Cultural Considerations ❖
• Accept various cultural groups' use of alternative methods in relief of pain.

EVALUATION

■ Evaluate effectiveness of nalbuphine in relieving pain. If ineffective, another opioid analgesic may need to be ordered.
■ Determine stability of vital signs. Note whether there is a change in respirations, pulse rate, or blood pressure. Report abnormal findings.

Opioid Antagonists

Opioid antagonists are antidotes for overdoses of natural and synthetic opioid analgesics. The opioid antagonists have a higher affinity to the opiate receptor site than the opioid being taken. An opioid antagonist blocks the receptor and displaces any opioid that would normally be at the receptor, inhibiting the opioid action. Indications for opioid antagonists include reversal of postoperative opioid depression and opioid overdose.

Naloxone (Narcan), administered IM or IV; naltrexone hydrochloride (ReVia), administered orally by tablet or liquid; and nalmefene (Revex) are opioid antagonists. These drugs are perfect examples of pharmacologic antagonists because they reverse the respiratory and CNS depression (sedation and hypotension) caused by opioids. Table 25–5 lists the opioid antagonists.

When receiving opioid antagonists, the client should be monitored continuously. The opioid action may exceed that of opioid antagonists and further analgesia may be needed. For example, fentanyl and a combination of drugs given during surgery may lead to excessive respiratory depression. Naloxone may be given as an opioid antidote. The client's respiratory and CNS status should be monitored closely for indications of analgesic reversal (tachycardia, nausea, vomiting, and sweating) and possible need of further analgesia. The client receiving naloxone should also be observed for bleeding, because this drug may cause an elevated partial thromboplastin time.

Table 25–5

Opioid Antagonists

Generic (Brand)	Route and Dosage	Uses and Considerations
nalmefene (Revex)	A: IM/IV: 0.25 mcg/kg initially; repeat 0.25 mcg/kg at 2- to 5-min intervals PRN	Reverses opioid overdose and respiratory depression. Long half-life. *Pregnancy category:* B; PB: UK; $t^{1/2}$: 8.5-10.8 h
naloxone HCl (Narcan)	*Opiate overdose;* Opioid-induced respiratory distress: A: IV: 0.4-2 mg; may repeat q 2-3 min; *max:* 10 mg C: IV: 0.01-0.1 mg/kg; may repeat q 2-3 min; *max:* 10 mg *Postoperative respiratory depression:* A: IV: 0.1-0.2 mg; may repeat q 2-3 min PRN C: IV/IM: 0.005-0.01 mg/kg; may repeat q 2-3 min PRN	To treat opioid overdose. Approved for use in neonates to reverse respiratory depression induced by maternal opioid use. *Pregnancy category:* B; PB: UK; $t^{1/2}$: 1-1.5 h
naltrexone HCl (Trexan, ReVia)	A: PO: 25 mg/d; repeat 25 mg in 1 h if no withdrawal response	Treatment of opioid abuse and alcohol abuse. Three to five times more potent than naloxone. Decreases but does not prevent craving for opioids. Use after client is off opioids for 7 or more days. Do not give if client is in opiate withdrawal; can precipitate a withdrawal reaction. High doses can cause hepatotoxicity. *Pregnancy category:* C; PB: 21% ; $t^{1/2}$: 4-13 h

A, Adult; *C,* child; *h,* hour; *IM,* intramuscular; *IV,* intravenous; *max,* maximum; *min,* minute; *PB,* protein-binding; *PO,* by mouth; *PRN,* as needed; $t^{1/2}$, half-life; *UK,* unknown.

KEY WEBSITES

Duragesic (fentanyl transdermal patch): http://www.rxlist.com/cgi/generic/fentanyl.htm

acetaminophen: http://www.nlm.nih.gov/medlineplus/druginfo/medmaster/a681004.html

Use of opioids for treatment of chronic pain: http://www.painmed.org/productpub/statements/opioidstmt.html

Critical Thinking Case Study

RJ, a 79-year-old man, underwent abdominal surgery for resection of his colon. His physician prescribed morphine 10 mg every 3 to 4 hours PRN after the surgery. RJ did not ask for "pain medication," because he worried he might become addicted. A day after the surgery his nurse noted he was restless and grimaced whenever he moved in bed. He refused to breathe deeply or cough when instructed to do so. The nurse compared RJ's vital signs to his baseline findings and noted an increased pulse rate and a drop in systolic blood pressure of 6 mm Hg.

1. Should the nurse give morphine? Explain.
2. What would your reaction be to RJ in regard to his restlessness, grimacing, and refusal to deep breathe and cough?

3. What is the significance of the change in vital signs?
4. What classic side effects of opioid analgesics should the nurse assess?
5. What are some possible nonpharmacologic measures that might be helpful in alleviating RJ's pain?

The second postoperative day RJ began asking for morphine every 3 hours. On the fifth day the physician discontinued RJ's morphine and prescribed acetaminophen with codeine.

6. Why was the opioid analgesic order changed?
7. RJ does not want to ambulate. What is an appropriate nursing response?

NCLEX Study Questions

1. Of the following medications, the nurse knows that _____ will cause the least gastrointestinal distress.
   a. aspirin
   b. ketorolac
   c. celecoxib
   d. ibuprofen

2. A client states during a medical history that he takes several acetaminophen throughout the day. The nurse teaches the client that he should not exceed:
   a. 1 gram/day
   b. 2 grams/day
   c. 4 grams/day
   d. 6 grams/day

3. For the client receiving periodic morphine IV push, which is most critical for the nurse to monitor?
   a. fever
   b. diarrhea
   c. respirations
   d. white blood cell count

4. A client is admitted to the emergency room in respiratory depression following self-injection with hydromorphone. The admitting nurse knows that _____ will reverse respiratory depression caused by opioid overdose.
   a. fentanyl
   b. naloxone
   c. butorphanol
   d. Sufenta

5. Assessing a client following IV morphine administration, the nurse notes cold clammy skin, a pulse of 40 beats/min, respirations of 10/min, and constricted pupils. Which of the following medications will the client likely need next?
   a. naloxone (Narcan)
   b. meloxicam (Mobic)
   c. pentazocine (Talwin)
   d. propoxyphene (Darvon)

Answers: 1, c; 2, c; 3, c; 4, b; 5, a.

Eight

Psychiatric Agents

People normally experience moods and emotions such as excitement, anxiety, and depression. However, *pathology* may develop when moods and emotions become extreme. This imbalance may affect the performance of daily activities, perception of reality, ability to carry out responsibilities, fulfillment of work requirements, and establishment of interpersonal relationships.

From moods and emotions flow the various thoughts, feelings, and actions of individuals, which are communicated throughout the central nervous system (CNS) by chemical neurotransmitters. An impulse is communicated by traveling through the presynaptic neuron across the synaptic cleft and binding to a receptor on the postsynaptic neuron, as illustrated in the figure.

Neurotransmitters (chemicals in the body) are synthesized in the cytoplasm in the presynaptic neuron and stored in vesicles. The vesicle safeguards neurotransmitters from being destroyed by enzymes. When an impulse arrives by way of an action potential at a presynaptic neuron, vesicles are triggered to move to the cell membrane wall and release the transmitter into the synaptic cleft.

Neurotransmitters function with the help of receptors, which are embedded in the membrane of the postsynaptic neuron. Receptors are configured in size and shape to interlock with specific transmitters. Immediately upon connection of neurotransmitters to receptors, an action is exerted and the transmitter is removed. Once released, transmitters can be broken down into inactive substances by enzymes, diffused away from the synapse into intracellular fluid, or returned to the presynaptic neuron in a process called *reuptake*.

The major neurotransmitters affecting psychopathology include gamma-aminobutyric acid (GABA), serotonin, dopamine, norepinephrine, and acetylcholine. The GABA neurotransmitter is associated with the regulation of anxiety. When the level of GABA neurotransmitters is reduced, anxiety disorders may result. Benzodiazepines (antianxiety drugs) act by binding to a GABA receptor site, making the postsynaptic receptor more sensitive to GABA and its neurotransmission. This connection decreases signs and symptoms of anxiety.

Action potential

Vesicle

Presynaptic cell

Neurotransmitters

Synaptic cleft

Postsynaptic neuron

Stimulus (gated Na$^+$ channel)

Serotonin neurotransmission is associated with arousal and general activity levels of the CNS. Serotonin functions to regulate sleep, wakefulness, and mood, as well as the delusions, hallucinations, and withdrawal of schizophrenia. Antidepressants block the reuptake of serotonin into the presynaptic neuron. A structurally specific drug is more likely to affect only the specific receptors for which it is intended and not the receptors specific for other neurochemicals, which would produce unintended effects or side effects. Selective serotonin reuptake inhibitor (SSRI) drugs are specific and generally produce fewer side effects in the treatment of depression than older antidepressants such as monamine oxidase inhibitors (MAOIs).

Dopamine-containing neurons are thought to be involved in regulation of cognition, emotional responses, and motivation, and dopamine neurotransmitters are associated with schizophrenia and other psychoses. Antipsychotic drugs block dopamine receptors in the postsynaptic neuron.

Norepinephrine is associated with control of arousal, attention, vigilance, mood, affect, and anxiety. This transmitter is involved with thinking, planning, and interpreting. Tricyclic antidepressants block the reuptake of norepinephrine into the presynaptic neuron and effectively treat depressive disorders. MAOIs inactivate norepinephrine, dopamine, and serotonin by inhibiting the monoamine oxidase enzyme to relieve signs and symptoms of depression.

Acetylcholine plays a role in sleep and wakefulness. Alzheimer's disease is associated with a reduction of acetylcholine.

Faulty release, reuptake, or elimination of neurotransmitters may lead to an imbalance of neurotransmission and pathology. Mental disorders can then develop and affect an individual's thoughts, feelings, and behaviors.

Knowledge of psychopharmacology is essential to psychiatric mental health nursing. A basic understanding of the actions of psychotropic drugs will help nurses rapidly comprehend and apply information and enhance the effectiveness of pharmacologic treatment. Essential responsibilities of the psychiatric mental health nurse in administering psychotropic medications are to assess behavior, monitor for side effects, and educate the client and family. These actions are crucial to successful psychopharmacologic therapy.

This unit discusses drugs used to treat psychoses and anxiety in Chapter 26, Antipsychotics and Anxiolytics. Antidepressants and mood stabilizers are discussed in Chapter 27.

26
Antipsychotics and Anxiolytics

ELECTRONIC RESOURCES

evolve

Evolve website (http://evolve.elsevier.com/KeeHayes/pharmacology/):
- *Case Studies*
- *Content Updates*
- *Frequently Asked Questions*

- *Student Review Activities*
- *WebLinks*
- *Additional Reference Material*

Companion CD-ROM:
- *NCLEX Examination Review Questions*
- *Pharmacology Animations*
- *IV Therapy Checklists*
- *Medication Error Checklists*

- *Drug Calculation Problems*
- *Electronic Calculators*
- *Top 200 Drugs with Pronunciations*
- *References from the Textbook*

Outline

Objectives

- Differentiate between the two groups of drugs: antipsychotics and anxiolytics.
- Contrast the action, uses, side effects, and adverse effects of traditional/typical and atypical antipsychotics.
- Plan nursing interventions, including client teaching, for the client taking anxiolytics.
- Apply the nursing process to the client taking an atypical antipsychotic.

Terms

acute dystonia, p. 395
akathisia, p. 395
antiemetic, p. 394
antipsychotics, p. 393
anxiolytics, p. 403
atypical antipsychotics,
 p. 394

blood dyscrasias, p. 399
dopamine, p. 394
dystonia, p. 399
extrapyramidal symptoms
 (EPS)/extrapyramidal
 reactions, p. 394

neuroleptic, p. 393
neuroleptic malignant syndrome, p. 395
orthostatic hypotension,
 p. 396
parkinsonism, p. 394

phenothiazines, p. 395
psychosis, p. 394
schizophrenia, p. 394
tardive dyskinesia, p. 395
typical antipsychotics,
 p. 394

This chapter discusses the CNS depressants antipsychotics and anxiolytics, which are used to manage symptoms of psychosis and anxiety disorders. **Antipsychotics** are also known as *neuroleptics* or *psychotropics*, but the preferred name for this group is either *antipsychotics* or *neuroleptics*. **Neuroleptic** refers to any drug that modifies

psychotic behavior and exerts an antipsychotic effect. Anxiolytics are also called *antianxiety drugs* or *sedative-hypnotics*. Certain anxiolytics are used to treat sleep disorders, seizures, and withdrawal symptoms from alcohol intoxication. Some of these drugs are also used for conscious sedation and anesthesia supplementation. However, the anxiolytics described in this chapter are used specifically to treat anxiety.

Psychosis

Psychosis, or losing contact with reality, is manifested in a variety of mental or psychiatric disorders. Psychosis is usually characterized by more than one symptom, but these may include difficulty in processing information and coming to a conclusion, delusions, hallucinations, incoherence, catatonia, and aggressive or violent behavior. **Schizophrenia,** a chronic psychotic disorder, is the major category of psychosis in which many of these symptoms are manifested.

The symptoms of schizophrenia usually develop in adolescence or early adulthood. The symptoms of this psychotic disorder are divided into two groups: "positive" symptoms and "negative" symptoms. Positive symptoms may be characterized by exaggeration of normal function (e.g., agitation), incoherent speech, hallucination, delusion, and paranoia. Negative symptoms are characterized by a decrease or loss in function and motivation. There is a poverty of speech content, poor self-care, and social withdrawal. The negative symptoms tend to be more chronic and persistent. The typical or traditional group of antipsychotics is more helpful for managing positive symptoms than negative symptoms. Since 1984 a new group of antipsychotics called *atypical* have been found to be more useful in treating both the positive and negative symptoms of schizophrenia. Antipsychotics comprise the largest group of drugs used to treat mental illness. Specifically these drugs improve the thought processes and behavior of clients with psychotic symptoms, especially those with schizophrenia and other psychotic disorders. They are not used to treat anxiety or depression. The theory is that psychotic symptoms result from an imbalance in the neurotransmitter **dopamine** in the brain. Sometimes these antipsychotics are called *dopamine antagonists.* Antipsychotics block D_2 dopamine receptors in the brain, reducing psychotic symptoms. Many antipsychotics block the chemoreceptor trigger zone and vomiting (emetic) center in the brain, producing an **antiemetic** (an agent that prevents or relieves nausea and vomiting) effect. When dopamine is blocked, however, **extrapyramidal symptoms (EPS)** or **extrapyramidal reactions** of **parkinsonism** (Parkinson's disease, a chronic neurologic disorder that affects the extrapyramidal motor tract) such as tremors, masklike facies, rigidity, and shuffling gait may develop. Many clients who take high-potency antipsychotic drugs may require long-term medication for parkinsonian symptoms.

Antipsychotic Agents

Antipsychotics are divided into two major categories: *typical* (or *traditional*) and *atypical.* The **typical antipsychotics,** introduced in 1952, are subdivided into phenothiazines and nonphenothiazines. Nonphenothiazines include bu-

tyrophenones, dibenzoxazepines, dihydroindolones, and thioxanthenes. The phenothiazines and thioxanthenes block norepinephrine, causing sedative and hypotensive effects early in treatment. The butyrophenones block only the neurotransmitter dopamine.

Atypical antipsychotics make up the second category of antipsychotics. Clozapine, discovered in the 1960s and made available in Europe in 1971, was the first atypical antipsychotic agent. It was not marketed in the United States until 1990 because of adverse hematologic reactions. Atypical antipsychotics are effective for treating schizophrenia and other psychotic disorders in clients who do not respond to or are intolerant of typical antipsychotics. Because of their decreased side effects, atypical antipsychotics may be used instead of traditional typical antipsychotics as first-line therapy.

Pharmacophysiologic Mechanisms of Action

Antipsychotics block the actions of dopamine and thus may be classified as dopaminergic antagonists. There are five subtypes of dopamine receptors: D_1 through D_5. All antipsychotics block the D_2 (dopaminergic) receptor, which in turn promotes the presence of EPS, resulting in pseudoparkinsonism. Atypical antipsychotics have a weak affinity to D_2 receptors, a stronger affinity to D_4 receptors, and they block the serotonin receptor. These agents cause fewer EPS than the typical (phenothiazines) antipsychotic agents, which have a strong affinity to D_2 receptors.

Adverse Reactions
Extrapyramidal Syndrome

Pseudoparkinsonism, which resembles symptoms of Parkinson's disease, is a major side effect of typical antipsychotic drugs. Symptoms of pseudoparkinsonism, or EPS, include stooped posture, masklike facies, rigidity, tremors at rest, shuffling gait, pill-rolling motion of the hand, and bradykinesia. When clients take high-potency typical antipsychotic drugs, these symptoms are more pronounced. Clients who take low-strength antipsychotics such as chlorpromazine (Thorazine) are not as likely to have symptoms of pseudoparkinsonism as those who take fluphenazine (Prolixin).

During early treatment with typical antipsychotic agents for schizophrenia and other psychotic disorders, two adverse extrapyramidal reactions that may occur are acute dystonia and akathisia. Tardive dyskinesia is a later phase of extrapyramidal reaction to antipsychotics. Use of anti-

Herbal ALERT 26–1

Antipsychotic Agents

- Kava kava may increase the risk and severity of dystonic reactions when taken with phenothiazines.
- Kava kava may increase the risk and severity of dystonia when taken concurrently with fluphenazine.

cholinergic drugs helps decrease pseudoparkinsonism symptoms, acute dystonia, and akathisia, but has little effect on alleviating tardive dyskinesia.

The symptoms of **acute dystonia** usually occur in 5% of clients within days of taking typical antipsychotics. Characteristics of the reaction include muscle spasms of face, tongue, neck, and back; facial grimacing; abnormal or involuntary upward eye movement; and laryngeal spasms that can impair respiration. This condition is treated with anticholinergic/antiparkinsonism drugs such as benztropine (Cogentin). The benzodiazepine lorazepam (Ativan) may also be prescribed.

Incidence of **akathisia** occurs in approximately 20% of clients who take a typical antipsychotic drug. With this reaction, the client has trouble standing still, is restless, paces the floor, and is in constant motion (e.g., rocks back and forth). Akathisia is best treated with a benzodiazepine (e.g., lorazepam) or a beta-blocker (e.g., propranolol).

Tardive dyskinesia is a serious adverse reaction occurring in clients who have taken a typical antipsychotic drug for more than a year. The likelihood of developing tardive dyskinesia depends on the dose and duration of the antipsychotic factor. Characteristics of tardive dyskinesia include protrusion and rolling of the tongue, sucking and smacking movements of the lips, chewing motion, and involuntary movement of the body and extremities. In older adults, these reactions are more frequent and severe. The antipsychotic drug should be stopped in all who experience tardive dyskinesia. Other benzodiazepines, calcium channel blockers, or beta-blockers are helpful in some cases in decreasing tardive dyskinesia. No one agent is effective for all clients. High doses of vitamin E may be helpful, and its use to treat tardive dyskinesia is currently under investigation. Clozapine has also been effective for treating tardive dyskinesia. Figure 26–1 shows the characteristics of pseudoparkinsonism, acute dystonia, akathisia, and tardive dyskinesia.

Neuroleptic Malignant Syndrome

Neuroleptic malignant syndrome (NMS) is a rare but potentially fatal condition associated with antipsychotic drugs. NMS symptoms involve muscle rigidity, sudden high fever, altered mental status, blood pressure fluctuations, tachycardia, dysrhythmias, seizures, rhabdomyolysis, acute renal failure, respiratory failure, and coma. Treatment of NMS involves immediate withdrawal of antipsychotics, adequate hydration, hypothermic blankets, and administration of antipyretics, benzodiazepines, and muscle relaxants such as dantrolene (Dantrium).

Phenothiazines

In 1952 chlorpromazine hydrochloride (Thorazine) was the first phenothiazine introduced for treating psychotic behavior in clients in psychiatric hospitals. The **phenothiazines** are subdivided into three groups: aliphatic, piperazine, and piperidine, which differ mostly in their side effects.

The *aliphatic phenothiazines* produce a strong sedative effect, decreased blood pressure, and may cause moderate EPS (pseudoparkinsonism). Chlorpromazine (Thorazine)

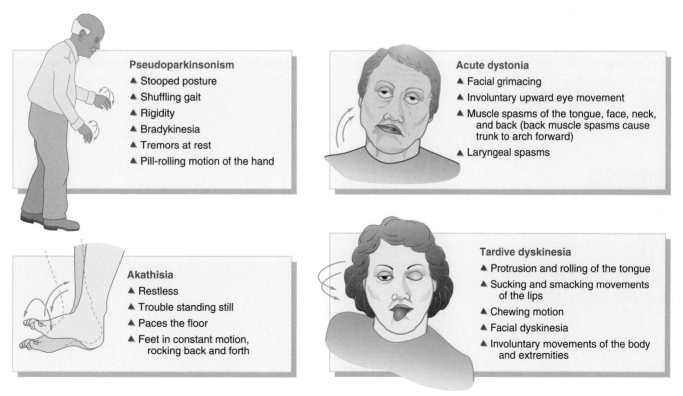

FIGURE 26–1 Characteristics of pseudoparkinsonism, acute dystonia, akathisia, and tardive dyskinesia.

is in the aliphatic group and may produce pronounced **orthostatic hypotension** (low blood pressure that occurs when an individual assumes an upright position from a supine position).

The *piperazine phenothiazines* produce a low sedative and strong antiemetic effect but have little effect on blood pressure. They cause more EPS than other phenothiazines. Examples of piperazine phenothiazines are fluphenazine (Prolixin) and perphenazine (Trilafon).

The *piperidine phenothiazines* have a strong sedative effect, cause few EPS, have a low to moderate effect on blood pressure, and have no antiemetic effect. Thioridazine (Mellaril) is an example of piperidine phenothiazines. Table 26–1 summarizes the effects of the phenothiazines.

Most antipsychotics can be given orally (tablet or liquid), intramuscularly (IM), or intravenously (IV). For oral use, the liquid form might be preferred, because some clients hide tablets to avoid taking them. In addition the absorption rate is faster with the liquid form. Peak serum drug level occurs in 2 to 3 hours. The antipsychotics are highly protein-bound (>90%), and excretion of the drugs and their metabolites is slow. Phenothiazines are metabolized by liver enzymes into phenothiazine metabolites. Metabolites can be detected in the urine several months after the medication has been discontinued. Phenothiazine metabolites may cause a harmless pinkish to red-brown urine color. The *full* therapeutic effects of antipsychotics may not be evident for 3 to 6 weeks following initiation of therapy, but an observable therapeutic response may be apparent after 7 to 10 days.

Noncompliance with antipsychotics is common. Many ethnocultural groups from countries outside the United States, and some people from within the United States as well, may be accustomed to not taking all of their medications as ordered or use medicines prescribed for other people. Encourage the client to take the medication as prescribed. Also, explain and reexplain essential information to compensate for client's knowledge deficit or language limitations.

Prototype Drug Chart 26–1 illustrates the drug characteristics of fluphenazine (Prolixin), a phenothiazine antipsychotic used to manage psychosis.

Pharmacokinetics

Oral absorption of fluphenazine is rapid and not affected by food. This drug is strongly protein-bound and has a long half-life; therefore, the drug may accumulate. Fluphenazine is metabolized by the liver, crosses the blood-brain barrier and placenta, and is excreted as metabolites primarily in the urine. With hepatic dysfunction, the phenothiazine dose may need to be decreased. Lack of drug metabolism in the liver will cause an elevation in serum drug level.

Pharmacodynamics

Fluphenazine is prescribed primarily for psychotic disorders. This drug has anticholinergic properties and should be cautiously administered to clients with glaucoma, especially narrow-angle glaucoma. Because hypotension is a side effect of these phenothiazines, any antihypertensives simultaneously administered can cause an additive hypotensive effect. Narcotics and sedative-hypnotics administered simultaneously with these phenothiazines can cause an additive CNS depression. Antacids decrease the absorption rate of both drugs and all phenothiazines, so they should be given 1 hour before or 2 hours after an oral phenothiazine.

The onset of action for fluphenazine hydrochloride is 1 hour, with a duration rate of 6 to 8 hours. Fluphenazine decanoate has delayed absorption, with the onset of action 24 to 72 hours and duration of 1 to 6 weeks.

Nonphenothiazines

The many groups of nonphenothiazine antipsychotics include butyrophenone, dibenzoxazepines, dihydroindolone, and thioxanthene.

In the *butyrophenone* group, a frequently prescribed nonphenothiazine is haloperidol (Haldol). Haloperidol's pharmacologic behavior is similar to that of the phenothiazines. It is a potent antipsychotic drug in which the equivalent prescribed dose is smaller than drugs of lower

Table 26–1				
Effects of Phenothiazines (Varies Within Class)				
Group	**Sedation**	**Hypotension**	**EPS**	**Antiemetic**
Aliphatic	+++	+++	++	++
chlorpromazine and triflupromazine				+++
Piperazine	++	+	+++	+++
Piperidine	+++	+++	+	—
Nonphenothiazines				
haloperidol	+	+	+++	++
loxapine	++	++	+++	—
molindone	+/++	+	+++	—
thiothixene	+	+	+++	—
Atypical antipsychotics				
risperidone	+	+	+/0	—

—, No effect; +, mild effect; ++, moderate effect; +++, severe effect; *EPS,* extrapyramidal symptoms.

Prototype DRUG CHART 26–1

FLUPHENAZINE

Drug Class	**Dosage**
Antipsychotic: Neuroleptic, piperazine phenothiazine Trade names: Prolixin, Permitil, ✸Moditen HCl *Pregnancy Category:* C	*Psychoses:* **A: PO:** 0.5-10 mg/d; *max:* 20 mg/d **IM/subQ:** HCl 2.5-10 mg/d q6-8h; *max:* 10 mg/d **Elderly:** 1-2.5 mg/d **Decanoate:** 12.5-25 mg q1-4wk
Contraindications	**Drug-Lab-Food Interactions**
Hypersensitivity, subcortical brain damage, blood dyscrasias, renal or liver damage, coma	*Drug: Increase* depressive effects when taken with alcohol or other CNS depressants *Food:* Kava kava may increase dystonia
Pharmacokinetics	**Pharmacodynamics**
Absorption: Rapidly absorbed **Distribution:** PB 90% **Metabolism:** t½: 5-15 h **Excretion:** In urine	**PO: HCl:** Onset: 1 h Peak: 0.5 h Duration: 6-8 h **IM: Peak:** 1.5-2 h **IM: Decanoate:** Onset: 24-72 h Duration:1-6 wk

Therapeutic Effects/Uses

To manage symptoms of psychosis including schizophrenia
Mode of Action: Blocks dopamine receptors in the brain and controls psychotic symptoms

Side Effects	**Adverse Reactions**
Sedation, dizziness, headache, dry mouth, nasal congestion, blurred vision, photosensitivity, nausea, constipation, urinary retention, polyuria, peripheral edema	Hypertension, hypotension, tachycardia, tardive dyskinesia, impaired thermoregulation, extra- pyramidal symptoms, convulsions *Life-threatening:* granulocytosis

A, Adult; *CNS,* central nervous system; *d,* day; *h,* hour; *IM,* intramuscular; *max,* maximum; *PB,* protein-binding; *PO,* by mouth; *t½,*
half-life; *wk,* week; ✸, Canadian drug name.

potency (e.g., chlorpromazine). The drug dose for haloperidol is 0.5 to 5 mg, whereas the drug dose for chlorpromazine is 10 to 25 mg. Long-acting preparations (haloperidol decanoate [Haldol] and fluphenazine decanoate
[Prolixin]) are given for slow release via injection every 2
to 4 weeks. Administration precautions should be taken to
prevent soreness and inflammation at the injection site.
Because the medication is a viscous liquid, a large-gauge
needle (e.g., 21-gauge) should be used with the Z-track
method for administration in a deep muscle. See Chapter
3 for further explanation of the Z-track method of injection. The injection site should not be massaged, and sites
should be rotated. These medications should not remain
in a plastic syringe longer than 15 minutes. Prototype Drug
Chart 26–2 provides the drug data related to haloperidol.

Pharmacokinetics

Haloperidol is absorbed well through the gastrointestinal (GI) mucosa. It
has a long half-life and is highly protein-bound, so the drug may accumulate. Haloperidol is metabolized in the liver and excreted in urine and
feces.

Pharmacodynamics

Haloperidol alters the effects of dopamine by blocking dopamine receptors; thus sedation and EPS may occur. The drug is used to control
psychoses and decrease agitation in adults and children. Dosages need
to be decreased in older adults because of decreased liver function and
potential side effects. It may be prescribed for children with hyperactive
behavior. Haloperidol has anticholinergic activity, so care should be
taken when administering it to clients with a history of glaucoma.

Haloperidol has a similar onset of action, peak time of concentration,
and duration of action as phenothiazines. It has strong EPS effects. Skin
protection is necessary for prolonged use because of the possible side
effect of photosensitivity.

From the *dibenzoxazepine* group, loxapine (Loxitane) is a
moderately potent agent. It has moderate sedative and orthostatic hypotensive effects and a strong EPS effect.

The typical antipsychotic molindone hydrochloric acid
(Moban) from the *dihydroindolone* group is a moderately
potent agent. It has low sedative and orthostatic hypotensive effects and a strong EPS effect.

In the nonphenothiazine group known as *thioxanthenes*
is thiothixene (Navane), a highly potent typical antipsy-

Prototype **DRUG CHART 26–2**

HALOPERIDOL AND HALOPERIDOL DECANOATE

Drug Class

Antipsychotic, neuroleptic (nonphenothiazine)
Trade names: Haldol, ✜Peridol
Pregnancy Category: C

Dosage

A: PO: 0.5-5 mg b.i.d.- t.i.d.
IM: 2-5 mg q4h PRN
C: PO: 0.05-0.15 mg/kg/d in divided doses; 0.5 mg/d in 2-3 divided doses (not for child <3 y)
Elderly: Decreased doses PO: 0.5-2 mg b.i.d.- t.i.d.

Contraindications

Narrow-angle glaucoma; severe hepatic, renal, and cardiovascular diseases; bone marrow depression; Parkinson's disease; blood dyscrasias; CNS depression; subcortical brain damage

Drug-Lab-Food Interactions

Drug: Increase sedation with alcohol, CNS depressants; *increase* toxicity with anticholinergics, CNS depressants, lithium; *decrease* effects with phenobarbital, carbamazepine; *decrease* effects with caffeine

Pharmacokinetics

Absorption: PO: 60% absorbed
Distribution: PB: 80%-90%
Metabolism: t½: 15-35 h
Excretion: In urine and feces

Pharmacodynamics

PO: Onset: erratic
Peak: 2-6 h
Duration: 24-72 h
IM: Onset: 15-30 min
Peak: 30-45 min
Duration: 4-8 h
IM: Decanoate: Onset: UK
Peak: 6-7 d
Duration: 3-4 wk

Therapeutic Effects/Uses

To treat acute and chronic psychoses, to treat children with severe behavior problems who are combative, to suppress narcotic withdrawal symptoms, to treat schizophrenia resistant to other drugs, to treat Tourette syndrome, to treat symptoms of dementia in older adults
Mode of Action: Alteration of the effect of dopamine on CNS; mechanism for antipsychotic effects are unknown

Side Effects

Sedation, extrapyramidal symptoms, orthostatic hypotension, headache, photosensitivity, dry mouth and eyes, blurred vision

Adverse Reactions

Tachycardia, seizures, urinary retention, tardive dyskinesia
Life-threatening: Laryngospasm, respiratory depression, cardiac dysrhythmias, neuromalignant syndrome

A, Adult; *b.i.d.,* twice a day; *C,* child; *CNS,* central nervous system; *d,* day; *h,* hour; *IM,* intramuscular; *min,* minute; *PB,* protein-binding; *PO,* by mouth; *PRN,* as needed; *t½,* half-life; *t.i.d.,* three times a day; *UK,* unknown; *wk,* week; *y,* year; <, less than; ✜, Canadian drug name.

Symptoms and Suggested Treatment for Overdose of Phenothiazines

Symptoms

- Unable to arouse, blood pressure fluctuations, tachycardia, agitation, delirium, convulsions, dysrhythmias, neuroleptic malignant syndrome, extrapyramidal symptoms, and renal, cardiac, and respiratory failure.

Treatment

- Maintain airway, gastric lavage, activated charcoal administration, adequate hydration, anticholinergics, and norepinephrine.

chotic drug. It has side effects similar to those of molindone with low sedative and orthostatic hypotensive effects and a strong EPS effect.

Side Effects and Adverse Reactions

There are several common side effects associated with antipsychotics. The most common side effect for all antipsychotics is drowsiness. Many of the antipsychotics have some anticholinergic effects: dry mouth, increased heart rate, urinary retention, and constipation. Blood pressure decreases with the use of antipsychotics; aliphatics and piperidines cause a greater decrease in blood pressure than the others.

Extrapyramidal symptoms can begin 5 to 30 days after initiation of antipsychotic therapy and are most prevalent with the phenothiazines, butyrophenones, and thioxanthenes. These symptoms include pseudoparkinsonism, akathisia, **dystonia** (prolonged muscle contractions with twisting, repetitive movements), and tardive dyskinesia. Tardive dyskinesia may develop in 20% of clients taking antipsychotics for long-term therapy. Antiparkinsonian anticholinergic drugs may be given to control EPS, but they are not always effective in treating tardive dyskinesia.

High dosing or long-term use of some antipsychotics can cause **blood dyscrasias** (blood cell disorders) such as agranulocytosis. White blood cell (WBC) count should be closely monitored and reported to the health care provider if there is an extreme decrease in leukocytes.

Dermatologic side effects seen early in drug therapy are pruritus and marked photosensitivity. Clients are urged to use sunscreen, hats, and protective clothing and to stay out of the sun.

Drug Interactions

Because phenothiazine lowers the seizure threshold, dosage adjustment of an anticonvulsant may be necessary. If either aliphatic phenothiazine or the thioxanthene group is administered, a higher dose of anticonvulsant might be necessary to prevent seizures.

Antipsychotics interact with alcohol, hypnotics, sedatives, narcotics, and benzodiazepines to potentiate the sedative effects of antipsychotics. Atropine counteracts EPS and potentiates antipsychotic effects. Use of antihypertensives can cause an additive hypotensive effect.

Antipsychotics should *not* be given with other antipsychotic or antidepressant drugs except to control psychotic behavior for selected individuals who are refractory to drug therapy. Under ordinary circumstances if one antipsychotic drug is ineffective, a different one is prescribed. Individuals should *not* take alcohol or other CNS depressants (e.g., narcotic analgesics, barbiturates) with antipsychotics, because additive depression is likely to occur.

When discontinuing antipsychotics, the drug dosage should be reduced gradually to avoid sudden recurrence of psychotic symptoms. Table 26–2 lists common antipsychotic drugs (phenothiazines and nonphenothiazines) and their dosages, uses, and considerations.

Antipsychotic Dosage for Older Adults

Older adults usually require smaller doses of antipsychotics—from 25% to 50% less than young and middle-aged adults. Regular to high doses of antipsychotics increase the risk of severe side effects. Dosage amounts need to be individualized according to the client's age and physical status. In addition, dosage changes may be necessary during antipsychotic therapy.

Table 26–2

Phenothiazines and Nonphenothiazines

Generic (Brand)	Drug Potency	Route and Dosage	Uses and Considerations
Phenothiazines			
Aliphatics			
chlorpromazine HCl (thorazine)	Low	A: PO: 25-100 mg t.i.d. or q.i.d. A: IM/IV: 25-50 mg q4-6h A: PR: 50-100 mg q6-8h C: PO: >6 mo: 0.55 mg/kg q4-6h C: IM/IV: >6 mo: 0.55 mg/kg q6-8h C: PR: >6 mo: 1 mg/kg q6-8h	For psychosis, schizophrenia, intractable hiccups, preoperative sedation, behavioral problems in children, nausea, and vomiting. *Pregnancy category:* C; PB: 95%; t½: 8-30 h
Piperazines			
fluphenazine HCl (Prolixin)	High	(Prototype Drug Chart 26–1)	
perphenazine (Trilafon)	Moderate	A: PO: 4-16 mg b.i.d., t.i.d., or q.i.d.	For psychotic disorders; to control severe nausea and vomiting; to treat intractable hiccups. Used also before chemotherapy to prevent nausea. *Pregnancy category:* C; PB: 90%; t½: 9.5 h
Piperidines			
thioridazine HCl (Mellaril)*	Low	A: PO: 50-100 mg t.i.d.; *max:* 800 mg/d Elderly: ⅓ to ½ adult dose	For psychosis only when unresponsive to other medications. Higher doses for severe psychosis. Lower doses (10-50 mg t.i.d.) for marked depression, alcohol withdrawal, intractable pain. Few EPS. Little antiemetic effect. Can cause life-theatening dysrhythmias. *Pregnancy category:* C; PB: 90%; t½: 24-34 h

A, Adult; *b.i.d.*, twice a day; C, child; *d*, day; *EPS*, extrapyramidal symptoms; *h*, hour; *IM*, intramuscular; *IV*, intravenous; *max*, maximum; *mo*, month; *PB*, protein-binding; *PO*, by mouth; *PR*, rectally; *q.i.d.*, four times a day; *t½*, half-life; *t.i.d.*, three times a day; *UK*, unknown; >, greater than.
*Avoid spilling liquid on skin. Contact dermatitis could result.

Continued

Table 26–2

Phenothiazines and Nonphenothiazines—cont'd

Generic (Brand)	Drug Potency	Route and Dosage	Uses and Considerations
Nonphenothiazines			
Butyrophenone			
haloperidol (Haldol)	High	(Prototype Drug Chart 26–2)	
Dibenzoxazepine			
loxapine (Loxitane)	Moderate	A: PO: Initially: 10 mg b.i.d.; then may increase to 50-100 mg/d in 2-4 divided doses Elderly: ⅓ to ½ adult dose A: IM: 12.5-50 mg q4-6h	For acute psychosis and schizophrenia. Likely to cause EPS. Overdose can cause cardiac toxicity or neurotoxicity. *Pregnancy category:* C; PB: 95%; t½: 5 h
Dihydroindolone			
molindone HCl (Moban)	Moderate	A: PO: Initial: 50-75 mg in 3-4 divided doses A: PO: 5-50 mg t.i.d.-q.i.d.; *max:* 225 mg/d Elderly: ⅓ to ½ adult dose	Management of schizophrenia. Can cause EPS. Has less sedative effect. *Pregnancy category:* C; PB: UK; t½: 1.5 h
Thioxanthenes			
thiothixene hcl (navane)	high	A: PO: 2 mg t.i.d.; *max:* 60 mg/d; im: 4 mg b.i.d.-q.i.d.; *max:* 30 mg/d	Management of psychotic disorders, especially acute and chronic schizophrenia. Can cause EPS. *Pregnancy category:* C; PB: 90%; t½: 24-34 h
Atypical Antipsychotics			
clozapine (Clozaril)	Low	A: PO: Initially: 25-50 mg/d; if tolerated, gradually increase to 300-450 mg/d in divided doses; *max:* 900 mg/d	For severely ill schizophrenic clients, especially those who do not respond to other antipsychotics. With long-term use, monitor white blood cell count. *Pregnancy category:* B; PB: 95%; t½: 8-12 h
olanzapine (Zyprexa)	UK	A: PO: 5 mg/d initially, 5-10 mg/d thereafter	Treatment of schizophrenia. Does not cause EPS symptoms. May cause headaches, dizziness, agitation, insomnia, and somnolence. *Pregnancy category:* C; PB: UK; t½: 27-30 h
quetiapine (Seroquel)	UK	A: PO: 25 mg/d initially, 25-50 mg b.i.d. first week; *max:* 400 mg/d	Treatment of schizophrenia. Not likely to cause EPS. May cause dizziness, headache, sedation. *Pregnancy category:* UK; PB: UK; t½: UK
risperidone (Risperdal)	Low	(Prototype Drug Chart 26–3)	
ziprasidone (Geodon)	UK	A: PO: 20 mg b.i.d. may increase q2d; *max:* 80 mg b.i.d. A: IM: 10 mg q2h or 20 mg q4h; *max:* 40 mg/day	For management of schizophrenia. *Pregnancy category:* C; PB: 99%; t½: 7 h
aripiprazole (Abilify)	UK	A: PO: 10-15 mg/day may increase q2wk; *max:* 30 mg q day	For management of schizophrenia. *Pregnancy category:* C; PB: 99%; t½: 75 h
paliperidone (Invega)	UK	A: PO: 6-12 mg qd in the morning; *max:* 12 mg/d	Treatment of schizophrenia. *Pregnancy category:* C; PB: 74%; t½: 23 h

Atypical (Serotonin/Dopamine Antagonists) Antipsychotics

A new category of antipsychotics was marketed in the United States in the early 1990s. This group, atypical antipsychotics, differs from the typical/traditional antipsychotics, because the atypical agents are effective in treating both positive and negative symptoms of schizophrenia. The typical antipsychotics have not been effective in the treatment of negative symptoms. Two advantages of the atypical agents are that (1) they are effective in treating negative symptoms, and (2) they are not likely to cause EPS or tardive dyskinesia. The atypical drugs available include clozapine (Clozaril), risperidone (Risperdal), olanzapine (Zyprexa), quetiapine (Seroquel), and paliperidone (Invega). These agents have a greater affinity for blocking serotonin and dopaminergic D_4 receptors than primarily blocking the dopaminergic D_2 receptor responsible for mild and severe EPS. Weight gain is a common side effect of atypical antipsychotics.

Clozapine (Clozaril) was the first atypical antipsychotic agent used to treat schizophrenia and other psychoses. It does not cause acute EPS, although tremors and occasional rigidity have been reported. Serious adverse reactions of clozapine are seizures and agranulocytosis, a decrease in the production of granulocytes which involves the body's immune defenses. Currently clozapine is only indicated for the treatment of severely ill schizophrenic clients who have not responded to traditional antipsychotic drugs. The WBC count needs to be closely monitored for leukopenia; if the WBC (leukocytes) level falls below 3000 mm³, clozapine should be discontinued. Seizures have been reported in 3% of clients taking the drug. Dizziness, sedation, tachycardia, orthostatic hypotension, and constipation are common side effects.

Another atypical agent used to treat positive and negative symptoms of schizophrenia is risperidone (Risperdal). Its action is similar to that of clozapine, and the occurrence of EPS and tardive dyskinesia is low. It does not cause agranulocytosis. Paliperidone (Invega), approved by the FDA in December 2006, is the major active metabolite of risperidone and is an extended-release tablet with once-a-day dosing. Paliperidone should be swallowed whole and not chewed, divided, or crushed. The most common adverse effects include EPS, insomnia, headache, and akathisia.

The atypical antipsychotic olanzapine (Zyprexa), like clozapine and risperidone, is effective for treating positive and negative symptoms of schizophrenia. It does not cause agranulocytosis.

Quetiapine (Seroquel), like all the other atypical antipsychotics, is less likely to cause EPS. Tardive dyskinesia for long-term use has not been determined.

Ziprasidone (Geodon) was approved by the Food and Drug Administration (FDA) in 2001, and aripiprazole (Abilify) was FDA approved in 2002. For individuals with cardiac dysrhythmias, Ziprasidone must be prescribed with caution, because its use may lead to prolonged Q-T interval; ECGs should be monitored. Ziprasidone is contraindicated in clients with a history of prolonged Q-T interval or with other concurrent drugs known to prolong Q-T interval. Clients taking quetiapine, clozapine, risperidone, olanzapine, ziprasidone, and aripiprazole should be monitored for hyperglycemia and other symptoms of diabetes mellitus.

Prototype Drug Chart 26–3 illustrates drug characteristics of risperidone (Risperdal), an atypical antipsychotic.

Prototype DRUG CHART 26–3

RISPERIDONE

Drug Class	**Dosage**
Nonphenothiazine, atypical antipsychotic Trade name: Risperdal *Pregnancy Category:* C	*Psychosis:* **A: PO:** 1 mg b.i.d.; increase by 1 mg b.i.d. daily to initial target of 3 mg b.i.d.; *max:* 8 mg/d **Elderly: PO:** 0.5 mg b.i.d.; increase by 0.5 mg b.i.d. daily to initial target of 1.5 mg/d; *max:* 4 mg/d
Contraindications	**Drug-Lab-Food Interactions**
Hypersensitivity, lactation, dysrhythmias, blood dyscrasias, liver damage	*Drug:* Increased effects of antihypertensives; decreased risperidone levels with concurrent use of carbamazepine; concurrent use of cisapride may cause dysrhythmias *Lab:* Increased AST, ALT, ALP, and blood glucose
Pharmacokinetics	**Pharmacodynamics**
Absorption: Rapidly absorbed **Distribution:** PB: 90% **Metabolism:** t½: 24 h **Excretion:** In urine 70% and feces 14%	**PO:** Onset: UK Peak: 1-2 h Duration: UK

Therapeutic Effects/Uses

To manage symptoms of psychosis, including schizophrenia
Mode of Action: Interferes with the binding of dopamine to dopamine (D_2) and serotonin 5-hydroxytryptamine ($5\text{-}HT_2$) receptors

Side Effects	**Adverse Reactions**
Sedation, weight gain, headaches, dry mouth, photosensitivity, urinary retention, sexual dysfunction, hyperglycemia	Orthostatic hypotension, tachycardia, EPS, ECG changes, convulsions *Life-threatening:* Neuroleptic malignant syndrome

A, Adult; *ALP,* alkaline phosphatase; *ALT,* alanine aminotransferase; *AST,* aspartate aminotransferase; *b.i.d.,* twice a day; *d,* day; *ECG,* electrocardiogram; *EPS,* extrapyramidal symptom; *h,* hour; *max,* maximum; *PB,* protein-binding; *PO,* by mouth; *t½,* half-life; *UK,* unknown.

When anxiety, hallucination, agitation, mania, confusion, or depression and other symptoms are noted, the health care provider should check the medications that the client is taking.

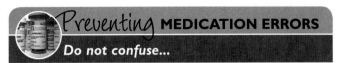

Preventing MEDICATION ERRORS

Do not confuse...

- **Seroquel** with **Serzone** (an antidepressant). Seroquel may also be confused with **sertindole (Serlect)** because the words look alike.

Nursing Process

Phenothiazine and Nonphenothiazine

ASSESSMENT

- Record baseline vital signs for use in future comparison.
- Obtain a health history from client of present drug therapy. If client is taking an anticonvulsant, drug dose might need to be increased, because antipsychotics tend to lower seizure threshold.
- Assess mental status and cardiac, eye, and respiratory disorders before start of drug therapy and continue daily assessment.

NURSING DIAGNOSES

- Disturbed thought processes related to delusions
- Activity intolerance related to sedation
- Disturbed sensory-perceptual responses related to hallucinations
- Self-care deficit related to loss of motivation
- Noncompliance related to loss of motivation

PLANNING

- Client's psychotic behavior will improve with drug(s) and psychotherapy.

NURSING INTERVENTIONS

- Monitor vital signs. Orthostatic hypotension is likely to occur.
- Remain with client while medication is taken and swallowed; some clients hide antipsychotics in the mouth to avoid taking them.
- Avoid skin contact with liquid concentrates to prevent contact dermatitis. Liquid must be protected from light and should be diluted with fruit juice.
- Administer oral doses with food or milk to decrease gastric irritation.
- Administer by IM route deep into muscle, because drug irritates fatty tissue. Do *not* inject into subQ tissue.

Check blood pressure for marked decrease 30 minutes after drug is injected.
- Do *not* mix in same syringe with heparin, pentobarbital, cimetidine, or dimenhydrinate.
- Chill suppository in refrigerator for 30 minutes before removing foil wrapper.
- Observe for EPS: *acute dystonia* (spasms of tongue, face, neck, and back), *akathisia* (restlessness, inability to sit still, foot-tapping), *pseudoparkinsonism* (muscle tremors, rigidity, shuffling gait), and *tardive dyskinesia* (lip smacking, protruding and darting tongue, and constant chewing movement). Report these promptly to the health care provider.
- Assess for symptoms of neuroleptic malignant syndrome (NMS): increased fever, pulse, and blood pressure; muscle rigidity; increased creatine phosphokinase and WBC count; altered mental status; acute renal failure; varying levels of consciousness; pallor; diaphoresis; tachycardia; and dysrhythmias.
- Record urine output. Urinary retention may result.
- Monitor serum glucose level.

Client Teaching

General

- Instruct client to take the drug exactly as ordered. In schizophrenia and other psychotic disorders, antipsychotics do not cure the mental illness but do alleviate symptoms. Many clients on medication can function outside the institution setting. Compliance with drug regimen is extremely important.
- Inform client that medication may take 6 weeks or longer to achieve full clinical effect.
- Caution client not to consume alcohol or other CNS depressants such as narcotics; these drugs intensify the depressant effect on the body.
- Recommend client not to abruptly discontinue the drug. Seek advice from health care provider before making any changes in dosage.
- Encourage client to read labels on OTC preparations. Some are contraindicated when taking antipsychotics.
- Teach smoking cessation, because smoking increases metabolism of some antipsychotics.
- Guide client to maintain good oral hygiene by frequently brushing and flossing teeth.
- Encourage client to talk with health care provider regarding family planning. The effect of antipsychotics on the fetus is not fully known; however, there may be teratogenic effects on the fetus.
- Explain to client that phenothiazine passes into breast milk. This could cause drowsiness and unusual muscle movement in the baby.
- Instruct client on the importance of routine follow-up examinations.
- Encourage client to obtain laboratory tests on schedule. WBCs are monitored for 3 months, especially

during the start of drug therapy. Leukopenia, or decreased WBCs, may occur. Be alert to symptoms of malaise, fever, and sore throat, which may be an indication of agranulocytosis, a serious blood dyscrasia. Report this promptly to the health care provider, especially when client is taking clozapine.

- Advise client to wear an identification bracelet indicating the medication taken.
- Inform client that tolerance to sedative effect develops over a period of days or weeks.

Side Effects

- Direct client to avoid potentially dangerous situations, such as driving, until drug dosing has been stabilized.
- Inform client about EPS; instruct client to promptly report symptoms to health care provider.
- Instruct client to wear sunglasses for photosensitivity, to limit exposure to direct sunlight, and to use sunscreen and protective clothing to prevent a skin rash.
- Advise client of orthostatic hypotension and possible dizziness.
- Teach client who is taking aliphatic phenothiazines like chlorpromazine that the urine might be pink or red-brown; this discoloration is harmless.
- Inform client that changes may occur related to sexual functioning and menstruating. Women could have irregular menstrual periods or amenorrhea, and men might experience impotence and gynecomastia (enlargement of breast tissue).
- Suggest lozenges or hard candy if mouth dryness occurs. Advise client to consult health care provider if dry mouth persists for more than 2 weeks.
- Encourage client to avoid extremes in environmental temperatures and exercise.
- Advise client to rise slowly from sitting or lying to standing to prevent a sudden decrease in blood pressure.

Cultural Considerations ❖

- Recognize that various cultural groups may have difficulty in accepting the client's mental disorder.

EVALUATION

- Evaluate the effectiveness of the drug and whether the client has acceptably reduced psychotic symptoms at the *lowest* dose possible.
- Ascertain whether client can cope with everyday living situations and attend to activities of daily living.
- Determine if any side effects of or adverse reactions to the drug have occurred.

Anxiolytics

Anxiolytics, or *antianxiety drugs,* are primarily used to treat anxiety and insomnia. The major anxiolytic group is benzodiazepines (a minor tranquilizer group). Long before benzodiazepines were prescribed for anxiety and insomnia, barbiturates were used. Benzodiazepines are considered more effective than barbiturates, because they enhance the action of gamma-aminobutyric acid (GABA), an inhibitory neurotransmitter within the CNS. Benzodiazepines have fewer side effects and may be less dangerous in overdosing. Long-term use of barbiturates causes drug tolerance and dependence and may cause respiratory distress. Currently barbiturates are not drugs of choice for treating anxiety.

Table 26–3 lists the approved uses for benzodiazepines. Drugs used to treat insomnia, which include the benzodiazepines, are discussed in Chapter 20.

A certain amount of anxiety may make one more alert and energetic, but when anxiety is excessive, it can be disabling, and anxiolytics may be prescribed. The action of anxiolytics resembles that of the sedative-hypnotics but *not* that of the antipsychotics.

There are two types of anxiety—primary and secondary. *Primary anxiety* is not caused by a medical condition or by drug use; *secondary anxiety* is related to selected drug use or medical or psychiatric disorders. Anxiolytics are not usually given for secondary anxiety unless the medical prob-

Table 26–3

Approved Uses for Benzodiazepines

Prescribed Uses	Drugs
Anxiety	alprazolam (Xanax) chlordiazepoxide (Librium) chlorazepate (Tranxene) diazepam (Valium) ketazolam (Loftan) lorazepam (Ativan) prazepam (Centrax)
Anxiety Associated with Depression	alprazolam (Xanax) clonazepam (Klonopin) lorazepam (Ativan)
Insomnia: Short-Term Use	estazolam (Prosom) flurazepam (Dalmane) quazepam (Doral) temazepam (Restoril) triazolam (Halcion)
Seizures and Status Epilepticus	clonazepam (Klonopin) clorazepate (Tranxene) diazepam (Valium)—status epilepticus lorazepam (Ativan)—status epilepticus
Alcohol Withdrawal	clorazepate (Tranxene) chlordiazepoxide (Librium) diazepam (Valium)
Skeletal Muscle Spasms	diazepam (Valium)
Preoperative Medications	chlordiazepoxide (Librium) diazepam (Valium) lorazepam (Ativan) midazolam (Versed)

lem is untreatable, severe, and causes disability. In this case, an anxiolytic could be given for a short period to alleviate any acute anxiety attacks. These agents treat the symptoms but do not cure them. Long-term use of anxiolytics is discouraged, because tolerance develops within weeks or months, depending on the agent. Drug tolerance can occur in less than 2 to 3 months in clients who take meprobamate or phenobarbital.

Nonpharmacologic Measures

Some of the symptoms of a severe or *panic attack* of anxiety include dyspnea (difficulty in breathing), choking sensation, chest pain, heart palpitations, dizziness, faintness, sweating, trembling and shaking, and fear of losing control. Before giving anxiolytics, nonpharmacologic measures should be used for decreasing anxiety. These measures might include using a relaxation technique, psychotherapy, or support groups.

Benzodiazepines

Benzodiazepines have multiple uses as anticonvulsants, sedative-hypnotics, preoperative drugs, and anxiolytics. Most of the benzodiazepines are used mainly for severe or prolonged anxiety. Examples include chlordiazepoxide (Librium), diazepam (Valium), clorazepate dipotassium (Tranxene), lorazepam (Ativan), alprazolam (Xanax), and prazepam (Centrax). The most frequently prescribed benzodiazepine is lorazepam (Ativan). Table 26–4 describes the various uses for benzodiazepines. Many of the benzodiazepines are used for more than one purpose.

Benzodiazepines are lipid-soluble and are absorbed readily from the GI tract. They are highly protein-bound (80% to 98%). Benzodiazepines are primarily metabolized by the liver and excreted in urine, so the drug dosage for clients with liver or renal disease should be lowered accordingly to avoid possible cumulative effects. Traces of benzodiazepine metabolites could be present in the urine for weeks or months after the person has stopped taking the drug. These are controlled substance schedule IV (CSS IV) drugs.

In 1962 the first benzodiazepine, chlordiazepoxide (Librium), became widely used for its sedative effect. Diazepam (Valium) was the most frequently prescribed drug in the early 1970s and was called a miracle drug by many. Lorazepam (Ativan) is the prototype drug of benzodiazepine and is described in Prototype Drug Chart 26–4.

Pharmacokinetics

Lorazepam is highly lipid-soluble, and the drug is rapidly absorbed from the GI tract. The drug is highly protein-bound, and the half-life is 10 to 20 hours. Lorazepam is excreted primarily in the urine.

Herbal ALERT 26-2

Benzodiazepines

Kava kava should not be combined with benzodiazepines, because it increases the sedative effect.

Pharmacodynamics

Lorazepam acts on the limbic, thalamic, and hypothalamic levels of the CNS. The onset of action is 15 to 30 minutes by mouth and 1 to 5 minutes by IV. The serum levels of most oral doses of benzodiazepines peak in 2 hours. Oxazepam levels peak in 3 hours, and prazepam levels peak in 6 hours. Duration of action varies. The average is 2 to 3 hours when given orally; when given IV, the longest duration of action is 1 hour.

It is recommended that benzodiazepines be prescribed for no longer than 3 to 4 months. Beyond 4 months, the effectiveness of the drug lessens. Table 26–4 lists the anxiolytics and their dosages, uses, and considerations.

Miscellaneous Anxiolytics

The anxiolytic buspirone hydrochloride (BuSpar) might not become effective until 1 to 2 weeks after continuous use. It has fewer side effects of sedation and physical and psychologic dependency associated with many benzodiazepines. NOTE: Buspirone has an interaction with grapefruit juice that can lead to toxicity. To avoid this interaction, buspirone users should be advised to limit intake of grapefruit juice to 8 ounces daily or half a fresh grapefruit.

Side Effects and Adverse Reactions

The side effects associated with benzodiazepines are sedation, dizziness, headaches, dry mouth, blurred vision, rare urinary incontinence, and constipation. Adverse reactions include leukopenia (decreased WBC count) with symptoms of fever, malaise, and sore throat; tolerance to the drug dosage with continuous use; and physical dependency. Box 26–1 lists guidelines for treating benzodiazepine overdose.

Benzodiazepines should not be abruptly discontinued, because withdrawal symptoms are likely to occur. Withdrawal symptoms caused by short-term benzodiazepine use are similar to those from the sedative-hypnotics (agitation, nervousness, insomnia, tremor, anorexia, muscular cramps, sweating). However, they are slow to develop, taking 2 to 10 days, and can last several weeks, depending on the benzodiazepine's half-life. When discontinuing a benzodiazepine, the drug dosage should be gradually de-

Box 26-1

Suggested Treatment for Overdose of Benzodiazepines

1. Administer an emetic and follow with activated charcoal if the client is conscious; use gastric lavage if the client is unconscious.
2. Administer the benzodiazepine antagonist flumazenil (Romazicon) IV if required.
3. Maintain an airway, give oxygen as needed for decreased respirations, and monitor vital signs.
4. Give IV vasopressors for severe hypotension.
5. Request a mental health consultation for the client.

NOTE: Dialysis has little value in removing benzodiazepine from the bloodstream.

Table 26–4

Anxiolytics

Generic (Brand)	Route and Dosage	Uses and Considerations
Benzodiazepines		
alprazolam (Xanax) CSS IV	A: PO: 0.25-0.5 mg t.i.d. Elderly: 0.125-0.25 mg b.i.d.; *max:* 4 mg/d	Management of anxiety and panic disorders and anxiety associated with depression. Side effects include drowsiness, dry mouth, and light-headedness. *Pregnancy category:* D; PB: 80%; t$^{1/2}$: 12-15 h
chlordiazepoxide HCl (Librium) CSS IV	*Anxiety disorders:* A: PO: 5-25 mg t.i.d.-q.i.d. C: PO: 5 mg b.i.d.-q.i.d. *Acute alcohol withdrawal:* A: PO/IM/IV: 50-100 mg; *max:* 300 mg/d Elderly: $^{1/2}$ adult dose	Effective for alcohol withdrawal syndrome (DTs), anxiety, and tension. Dose should be less for the older adult. *Pregnancy category:* D; PB: 90%-98%; t$^{1/2}$: 6-30 h
clorazepate dipotassium (Tranxene) CSS IV	A: PO: 15-60 mg/d in divided doses (daily dose range) Elderly: 7.5 mg b.i.d. or at bedtime	For anxiety, alcohol withdrawal syndrome, and partial seizures. Avoid taking alcohol or CNS depressants with clorazepate. Drowsiness and dizziness may occur. *Pregnancy category:* C; PB: 80%-90%; t$^{1/2}$: 0.5-1 h
diazepam (Valium) CSS IV	*Anxiety, muscle spasm, and alcohol withdrawal:* A: PO/IM/IV: 2-10 mg b.i.d.-q.i.d. Elderly: PO: 1-2 mg qd-b.i.d.; *max:* 10 mg/d C: <6 mo: PO: 1-2.5 mg b.i.d.- t.i.d. *Preoperative sedation:* A: IV: 5-15 mg 15 min prior to surgery/procedure *Status epilepticus:* A: IV: 5-10 mg q10-20min, *max:* 30 mg C: <6 yr: IV: 0.2-0.5 mg/kg q15-30min; *max:* 5 mg C: >6 yr: IV: 0.2-0.5 mg/kg q15-30min; *max:* 10 mg	Management of anxiety, muscle spasms, alcohol withdrawal, status epilepticus, and preoperative sedation. *Pregnancy category:* D; PB: 98%; t$^{1/2}$: 25-50 h
lorazepam (Ativan) CSS IV	(Prototype Drug Chart 26–4)	For mild to moderate anxiety. To control alcohol syndrome. Drowsiness, dizziness may occur. *Pregnancy category:* C; PB: 85%-95%; t$^{1/2}$: 3.5-21 h
Azapirones		
buspirone HCl (BuSpar)	A: PO: Initial: 5 mg b.i.d.-t.i.d. A: PO: 15-30 mg/d in divided doses; *max:* 60 mg/d Elderly: *max:* 30 mg/d	For anxiety and anxiety-related depression. Takes several weeks before anxiolytic effects occur. Common side effects include drowsiness, dizziness, headache, and nausea. *Pregnancy category:* B; PB: 95%; t$^{1/2}$: 2-3 h
Benzodiazepine Antagonists		
flumazenil (Romazicon)	A: IV: 0.2 mg over 15-30 sec; repeat 0.2 mg at 1-min intervals; *max:* 1 mg	Used to partially or completely reverse benzodiazepine dose from sedation, anesthesia, and overdose. Should not be used with antipsychotics or antidepressants. *Pregnancy category:* C; PB: UK; t$^{1/2}$: UK

A, Adult; *b.i.d.*, twice a day; *C*, child; *CNS*, central nervous system; *CSS*, Controlled Substances Schedule; *d*, day; *h*, hour; *IM*, intramuscular; *IV*, intravenous; *max*, maximum; *min*, minute; *PB*, protein-binding; *PO*, by mouth; *q.i.d.*, four times a day; *t$^{1/2}$*, half-life; *t.i.d.*, three times a day; *UK*, unknown.

creased over a period of days, depending on dose or length of time on the drug. Withdrawal symptoms from long-term, high-dose benzodiazepine therapy include paranoia, delirium, panic, hypertension, and status epilepticus. Convulsions during withdrawal may be prevented with simultaneous substitution of an anticonvulsant. Alcohol and other CNS depressants should *not* be taken with benzodiazepines, because respiratory depression could result. Tobacco, caffeine, and sympathomimetics decrease the effectiveness of benzodiazepines. Benzodiazepines are contraindicated during pregnancy because of possible teratogenic effects on the fetus.

Prototype **DRUG CHART 26–4**

LORAZEPAM

Drug Class	**Dosage**
Anxiolytic, benzodiazepine Trade name: Ativan *Pregnancy Category:* D	*Anxiety:* **A: PO:** 2-6 mg/d; *max:* 10 mg/d **C: PO/IV:** 0.05 mg/kg q4-8 h; *max:* 2 mg per dose **Elderly: PO:** 0.5-1 mg/d; *max:* 2 mg/d
Contraindications	**Drug-Lab-Food Interactions**
Hypersensitivity, CNS depression, shock, coma, narrow-angle glaucoma, pregnancy, lactation *Caution:* Hepatic or renal dysfunction, suicidal	*Drug:* Increases CNS depression when taken with alcohol, CNS depressants, and anticonvulsants, cimetidine increases lorazepam plasma levels, increases phenytoin levels, decreases levodopa effects, smoking decreases antianxiety effects *Food:* Kava kava may potentiate sedation
Pharmacokinetics	**Pharmacodynamics**
Absorption: Rapid from GI tract **Distribution:** PB: 90% **Metabolism:** t½: 10-20 h **Excretion:** In urine	**PO: Onset:** UK Peak: 2 h Duration: 12-24 h **IM: Onset:** 15-30 min Peak: 60-90 min Duration: UK **IV: Onset:** 1-5 min Peak: UK Duration: UK

Therapeutic Effects/Uses

To control anxiety and to treat status epilepticus; preoperative sedation
Mode of Action: Potentiate gamma-aminobutyrate (GABA) effects by binding to specific benzodiazepine receptors
and inhibiting GABA neurotransmission

Side Effects	**Adverse Reactions**
Drowsiness, dizziness, weakness, confusion, blurred vision, nausea, vomiting, anorexia, sleep disturbance, restlessness, hallucinations	Hypertension, hypotension

A, Adult; *C,* child; *CNS,* central nervous system; *d,* day; *GI,* gastrointestinal; *h,* hour; *IM,* intramuscular; *IV,* intravenous; *max,* maximum; *min,* minute; *PB,* protein-binding; *PO,* by mouth; *t½,* half-life; *UK,* unknown.

 Nursing Process

Benzodiazepines

ASSESSMENT

- Assess for suicidal ideation.
- Obtain a history of client's anxiety reaction.
- Determine client's support system (family, friends, groups), if any.
- Obtain client's drug history. Report possible drug-drug interaction.

NURSING DIAGNOSES

- Anxiety related to panic
- Impaired physical mobility related to drowsiness and weakness

PLANNING

- Client's anxiety and stress will be reduced through non-pharmacologic methods, anxiolytic drugs, or support/group therapy.

NURSING INTERVENTIONS

■ Observe client for side effects of anxiolytics. Recognize that drug tolerance and physical and psychologic dependency can occur with most anxiolytics.

■ Recognize that anxiolytic dosages should be lower for older adults, children, and debilitated persons than for middle-aged adults.

■ Monitor vital signs, especially blood pressure and pulse; orthostatic hypotension may occur.

■ Encourage the family to be supportive of client.

Client Teaching

General

• Advise client not to drive a motor vehicle or operate dangerous equipment when taking anxiolytics, because sedation is a common side effect.

• Instruct client not to consume alcohol or CNS depressants such as narcotics while taking an anxiolytic.

• Teach client ways to control excess stress and anxiety (relaxation techniques, long walks).

• Inform client that effective response may take 1 to 2 weeks.

• Encourage client to follow drug regimen and not to abruptly stop taking the drug after prolonged use because withdrawal symptoms can occur. Drug dose is usually tapered when the drug is discontinued.

Side Effects

• Instruct client to rise slowly from the sitting to standing position to avoid dizziness from orthostatic hypotension.

Cultural Considerations ❖

• Use simple and clear instructions, modifying methods and materials to meet client/family cultural needs. Ask family members to assist with translation only if an interpreter is not available, and do not ask private questions in public.

EVALUATION

■ Evaluate the effectiveness of drug therapy by determining if client is less anxious and more able to cope with stresses and anxieties.

■ Determine if client is taking the anxiolytic drug as prescribed and adhering to client teaching instructions.

KEY WEBSITES

Antipsychotic Medications and the Elderly: http://www.psychweekly. com/aspx/article/ArticleDetail.aspx?articleid=57

Risperidone (Risperdal): http://psyweb.com/Drughtm/jsp/risper.jsp

SSRI Meds: http://www.drugawareness.org/Ribbon/ SSRIMeds.html

Critical Thinking Case Study

FS, 35 years old, is receiving risperidone, 3 mg b.i.d., to control a psychotic disorder. She has taken the drug for 6 months, but has recently become agitated and is complaining of insomnia.

1. What is the relation between FS's drug dose and her complaints? Explain.
2. What further assessment should be made concerning FS and the drug regimen?
3. How does risperidone compare with other antipsychotics such as chlorpromazine and haloperidol regarding actions and adverse effects?

NCLEX Study Questions

1. Facial grimacing, involuntary upward eye movement, and muscle spasms of the tongue and face are indicative of:
   a. akathisia
   b. acute dystonia
   c. tardive dyskinesia
   d. pseudoparkinsonism

2. The nurse understands that antipsychotics act by:
   a. blocking actions of dopamine
   b. blocking actions of epinephrine
   c. promoting prostaglandin synthesis
   d. enhancing the action of gamma-aminobutyric acid

3. An antipsychotic agent, fluphenazine (Prolixin), is ordered for a client with psychosis. The nurse knows that this agent can lead to extrapyramidal symptoms (EPS) that may be treated with:
   a. quetiapine (Seroquel)
   b. aripiprazole (Abilify)
   c. benztropine (Cogentin)
   d. chlorpromazine (Thorazine)

4. An atypical antipsychotic is prescribed for a client with psychosis. The nurse understands that this category of medications includes:
   a. clozapine (Clozaril)
   b. loxapine (Loxitane)
   c. haloperidol (Haldol)
   d. thiothixene (Navane)

5. Which of the following statements is true concerning lorazepam (Ativan)?
   a. May cause confusion and blurred vision
   b. Maximum adult dose is 25 mg per day
   c. Cimetidine decreases lorazepam plasma levels
   d. Interferes with the binding of dopamine receptors

Answers: 1, b; 2, a; 3, c; 4, a; 5, a.

27

Antidepressants and Mood Stabilizers

ELECTRONIC RESOURCES

Evolve website (http://evolve.elsevier.com/KeeHayes/pharmacology/):
- Case Studies
- Content Updates
- Frequently Asked Questions
- Student Review Activities
- WebLinks
- Additional Reference Material

Companion CD-ROM:
- NCLEX Examination Review Questions
- Pharmacology Animations
- IV Therapy Checklists
- Medication Error Checklists
- Drug Calculation Problems
- Electronic Calculators
- Top 200 Drugs with Pronunciations
- References from the Textbook

Outline

Objectives

- Contrast the various categories of antidepressants, giving an example of one drug for each category.
- Describe the side effects and adverse reactions of antidepressants.
- Plan nursing interventions, including client teaching, for antidepressants (tricyclics, monoamine oxidase inhibitors [MAOIs] and selective serotonin reuptake inhibitors [SSRIs]).
- Explain the uses of lithium and its serum/plasma therapeutic ranges, side effects and adverse reactions, and nursing interventions.
- Apply the nursing process to the client taking Lithium.

Terms

antidepressants, p. 409
atypical (heterocyclic) antidepressants, p. 411
bipolar affective disorder, p. 409
depression, p. 409

dysphoria, p. 409
electroconvulsive therapy (ECT), p. 409
manic-depressive illness, p. 409

monoamine oxidase inhibitors (MAOIs), p. 412
reactive depression, p. 409

selective serotonin reuptake inhibitors (SSRIs), p. 411
tricyclic antidepressants (TCAs), p. 409

Antidepressants have been called *mood elevators*. They are used for depressive episodes that are accompanied by feelings of hopelessness and helplessness. There are various drug categories of antidepressants that can be prescribed for more than 1 month to 12 months and perhaps longer.

Mood-stabilizer agents such as lithium are effective for bipolar affective disorder (manic-depressive illness). Drug therapy for treating reactive, unipolar, and bipolar disorders is discussed in this chapter.

Depression

Depression is the most common psychiatric problem, affecting approximately 10% to 20% of the population. Only one third of depressed persons receive medical or psychiatric help. Women between the ages of 25 and 45 are two to three times more likely to experience major depression than men. Depression is characterized primarily by mood changes and loss of interest in normal activities. It is second only to hypertension as the most common chronic clinical condition.

Contributing causes of depression include genetic predisposition, social and environmental factors, and biologic conditions. Some signs of major depression include loss of interest in most activities, depressed mood, weight loss or gain, insomnia or hypersomnia, loss of energy, fatigue, feelings of despair, decreased ability to think or concentrate, and suicidal thoughts. Approximately two thirds of all suicides are related to depression. Depressed men, especially older white men, are more likely to commit suicide than depressed women. Antidepressants can mask suicidal tendencies.

The three types of depression are (1) *reactive*, (2) *major*, and (3) *bipolar affective disorder* (previously referred to as manic-depression). **Reactive depression** usually has a sudden onset after a precipitating event (e.g., depression resulting from a loss, such as death of a loved one). The client knows why he or she is depressed and may call this the "blues." Usually this type of depression lasts for months. A benzodiazepine agent may be prescribed. *Major depression* is characterized by loss of interest in work and home, inability to complete tasks, and deep depression (**dysphoria**). Major depression can be either primary (i.e., not related to other health problems) or secondary to a health problem (e.g., physical or psychiatric disorder or drug use). Antidepressants have been effective in treating major depression. **Bipolar affective disorder (manic-depressive illness)** involves swings between two moods, the manic (euphoric) and the depressive (dysphoria). Lithium was originally the drug of choice for treating this type of disorder. However, divalproex sodium (Depakote) is currently the drug of choice for bipolar disorder.

Electroconvulsive therapy (ECT) was used to treat psychosis and depression before the introduction of antipsychotics and antidepressants. Although not used as frequently as in the past, ECT may still be prescribed for clients who are extremely depressed, suicidal, or do not respond to antidepressant therapy. The use of thiopental (short-acting anesthetic) and succinylcholine (short-acting neuromuscular blocking agent which reduces the severe convulsive movements) has made ECT not as traumatic as it once was, and therefore a safer method for treating depression. The use of ECT does not affect the person's intellectual function, but may temporarily affect short-term memory.

Pathophysiology

There are many theories about the cause of major depression. A common one suggests an insufficient amount of brain monoamine neurotransmitters (norepinephrine, serotonin, perhaps dopamine). It is thought that decreased levels of serotonin permit depression to occur, and decreased levels of norepinephrine cause depression. However, there can be other physiologic causes of depression as well as social and environmental factors.

Herbal Supplements for Depression

St. John's wort and gingko biloba have been suggested for the management of mild depression. St. John's wort can decrease reuptake of the neurotransmitters serotonin, norepinephrine, and dopamine. The use of these and many herbal products should be discontinued 1 to 2 weeks before surgery. The client should check with the health care provider regarding herbal treatments (Herbal Alert 27–1).

Antidepressant Agents

Antidepressants are divided into four groups: (1) tricyclic antidepressants (TCAs), or tricyclics; (2) selective serotonin reuptake inhibitors (SSRIs); (3) atypical antidepressants that affect various neurotransmitters; and (4) monoamine oxidase inhibitors (MAOIs). The tricyclics and MAOIs were marketed in the late 1950s, and many of the SSRIs and atypical antidepressants were available in the 1980s. The SSRI agents are popular antidepressants, because they do not cause sedation, hypotension, anticholinergic effects, or cardiotoxicity as do many of the TCAs. Users of SSRIs can experience sexual dysfunction, which can be managed.

Tricyclic Antidepressants

The **tricyclic antidepressants (TCAs)** are used to treat major depression, because they are effective and less expensive than SSRIs and other drugs. Imipramine was the first TCA marketed in the 1950s.

Herbal **ALERT 27–1**

Selective Serotonin Reuptake Inhibitors (SSRIs)

🍃 Feverfew may interfere with SSRI antidepressants such as fluoxetine (Prozac).

• St. John's wort interacts with SSRIs, which may cause serotonin syndrome (dizziness, headache, sweating, and agitation).

The action of TCAs is to block the uptake of the neurotransmitters norepinephrine and serotonin in the brain. The clinical response of TCAs occurs after 2 to 4 weeks of drug therapy. If there is no improvement after 2 to 4 weeks, the antidepressant is slowly withdrawn and another antidepressant is prescribed. *Polydrug therapy,* the practice of giving several antidepressants or antipsychotics together, should be avoided because of possible serious side effects.

The effectiveness of TCAs in treating major depression is well documented. This group of drugs elevates mood, increases interest in daily living and activity, and decreases insomnia. For agitated depressed persons, amitriptyline (Elavil), doxepin (Sinequan), or trimipramine (Surmontil) may be prescribed, because of their highly sedative effect. Frequently TCAs are given at night to minimize problems caused by their sedative action. When discontinuing TCAs, the drugs should be gradually decreased to avoid withdrawal symptoms such as nausea, vomiting, anxiety, and akathisia. Imipramine hydrochloride (Tofranil) is used for the treatment of enuresis (involuntary discharge of urine during sleep in children).

The TCA drugs include amitriptyline, imipramine, trimipramine, doxepin, desipramine, nortriptyline, and protriptyline. The TCA drugs desipramine and nortriptyline are major metabolites of imipramine and amitriptyline. Prototype Drug Chart 27–1 describes the drug characteristics of amitriptyline.

Pharmacokinetics

Amitriptyline is strongly protein-bound. The half-life is 10 to 50 hours, and a cumulative drug effect may result. Amitriptyline is primarily excreted in urine.

Prototype DRUG CHART 27–1

AMITRIPTYLINE HCl

Drug Class

Antidepressant, tricyclic antidepressant
Trade names: Elavil, ✦Apo-Amitriptyline, Novotriptyn
Pregnancy Category: D

Dosage

A: PO: 25 mg b.i.d.- q.i.d.; increase to 150-200 mg/d; dose may be given as a single bedtime dose
IM: 20-30 mg q.i.d.
C: >13 y: PO: 10 mg t.i.d. and 20 mg at bedtime
Elderly: PO: 10 mg t.i.d., 10-25 mg at bedtime
Therapeutic serum range: 100-200 ng/ml

Contraindications

Acute myocardial infarction (AMI), taking MAOIs
Caution: Severe depression with suicidal tendency, severe liver or kidney disease
Narrow-angle glaucoma, seizures, prostatic disease

Drug-Lab-Food Interactions

Drug: Increase effects of CNS, respiratory depression, and hypotensive effect with alcohol and CNS depressants
Increase sedation, anticholinergic effects with phenothiazines, and haloperidol; *increase* toxicity with cimetidine; *decrease* effect of clonidine, guanethidine
Hypertensive crisis and death may occur with MAOIs.
Lab: Altered ECG readings

Pharmacokinetics

Absorption: PO: well absorbed
Distribution: PB: 95%
Metabolism: t½: 10-50 h
Excretion: Excreted primarily in urine

Pharmacodynamics

PO: Onset: 1-3 wk
Peak: 2-6 wk
Duration: UK

Therapeutic Effects/Uses

To treat depression with or without melancholia, manic and depressive phases of bipolar disorder, depression associated with organic disease, alcoholism, migraine headaches, mixed symptoms of anxiety and depression, or urinary incontinence
Mode of Action: Serotonin and norepinephrine are increased in nerve cells because of blockage from nerve fibers.

Side Effects

Sedation, drowsiness, blurred vision, dry mouth and eyes, urinary retention, constipation, weight gain, dizziness, nervousness, nausea, anorexia, sexual dysfunction

Adverse Reactions

Orthostatic hypotension, cardiac dysrhythmias, extrapyramidal syndrome (EPS)
Life threatening: Agranulocytosis, thrombocytopenia, leukopenia, seizures

A, Adult; *b.i.d.,* twice a day; *C,* child; *CNS,* central nervous system; *d,* day; *ECG,* electrocardiogram; *h,* hour; *IM,* intramuscular; *MAOI,* monoamine oxidase inhibitor; *PB,* protein-binding; *PO,* by mouth; *q.i.d.,* four times a day; *t½,* half-life; *t.i.d.,* three times a day; *UK,* unknown; *wk,* week; *>,* greater than; ✦, Canadian drug name.

Pharmacodynamics

Amitriptyline is well absorbed, but antidepressant effects develop slowly over several weeks. The onset of the antidepressant effect of amitriptyline is 1 to 4 weeks, and the peak concentration is 2 to 12 hours. Drug doses are decreased for elderly clients to reduce side effects.

Side Effects and Adverse Reactions

The TCAs have many side effects: orthostatic hypotension, sedation, anticholinergic effects, cardiac toxicity, and seizures. Rising from a sitting position too rapidly can cause dizziness and light-headedness, so the client should be instructed to rise slowly to an upright position to avoid *orthostatic hypotension*. This group of antidepressants blocks the histamine receptors; thus sedation is likely to occur initially but decreases with continuous use of the drug. Because TCAs block the cholinergic receptors, they can cause anticholinergic effects such as tachycardia, urinary retention, constipation, dry mouth, and blurred vision. Other side effects of TCAs include allergic reactions (skin rash, pruritus, and petechiae) and sexual dysfunction (impotence and amenorrhea). Most TCAs can cause blood dyscrasias (leukopenia, thrombocytopenia, and agranulocytosis) requiring close monitoring of blood cell counts. Amitriptyline may lead to extrapyramidal symptoms (EPS). Clomipramine may cause neuroleptic malignant syndrome (NMS). Seizure threshold is decreased by TCAs; therefore clients with seizure disorders may need to have the TCA dose adjusted. The most serious adverse reaction to TCAs is cardiac toxicity, such as dysrhythmias that may result from high doses of the drug.

Drug Interactions

Alcohol, hypnotics, sedatives, and barbiturates potentiate central nervous system (CNS) depression when taken with TCAs. Concurrent use of MAOIs with amitriptyline may lead to cardiovascular instability and toxic psychosis. Antithyroid medications taken with amitriptyline may increase the risk of dysrhythmias.

Selective Serotonin Reuptake Inhibitors

In the late 1980s a group of antidepressants that did not have TCA chemical structure were identified. This group was first classified as second-generation antidepressants. Today they have been reclassified as **selective serotonin reuptake inhibitors (SSRIs)**. The SSRIs block the reuptake of serotonin into the nerve terminal of the CNS, thereby enhancing its transmission at the serotonergic synapse. These drugs do not block the uptake of dopamine or norepinephrine, nor do they block cholinergic and alpha$_1$-adrenergic receptors. Selective serotonin reuptake inhibitors are more commonly used to treat depression than are the TCAs. They are more costly but have fewer side effects than TCAs.

The primary use of SSRIs is for major depressive disorders. They are also effective for treating anxiety disorders such as obsessive-compulsiveness, panic, phobias, posttraumatic stress disorders, and other forms of anxiety.

Fluvoxamine (Luvox) is useful for treating obsessive-compulsive disorders in children and adults. SSRIs have also been used to treat eating disorders and selected drug abuses. Miscellaneous uses for SSRIs include decreasing premenstrual tension syndrome, preventing migraine headaches, and preventing or minimizing aggressive behavior in clients with borderline personality disorder.

The SSRIs include fluoxetine (Prozac), fluvoxamine (Luvox), sertraline (Zoloft), paroxetine (Paxil), citalopram (Celexa), and escitalopram (Lexapro). Fluoxetine (Prozac) has been effective in 50% to 60% of clients who fail to respond to TCA therapy (TCA-refractory depression). Of all the SSRIs, sertraline (Zoloft) is the most commonly prescribed antidepressant. The Food and Drug Administration (FDA) approved of a weekly fluoxetine dose of 90 mg. However, before taking the weekly dose, the client should respond to a daily maintenance dose of 20 mg per day without serious effects. It has been reported that there are some side effects to the weekly 90 mg fluoxetine dose. NOTE: Many SSRIs have an interaction with grapefruit juice that can lead to possible toxicity. It is recommended that daily intake be limited to 8 ounces of grapefruit juice or one half a grapefruit. Do not confuse **Celexa** with **Celebrex** (anti-inflammatory), because the names look similar. Prototype Drug Chart 27–2 describes drug characteristics of the SSRI fluoxetine (Prozac). Table 27–1 lists the side effects of the various antidepressants.

Pharmacokinetics

Fluoxetine is strongly protein-bound. The half-life is 2 to 3 days; therefore a cumulative drug effect may result from long-term use. Fluoxetine is metabolized and excreted by the kidneys.

Pharmacodynamics

Fluoxetine is well absorbed; however, its antidepressant effect develops slowly over several weeks. The onset of fluoxetine's antidepressant effect is between 1 and 4 weeks, and peak concentration is at 4 to 8 hours after ingestion. The drug dose for older adults should be decreased to reduce side effects.

Side Effects and Adverse Reactions

Fluoxetine produces common side effects such as dry mouth, blurred vision, insomnia, headache, nervousness, anorexia, nausea, diarrhea, and suicidal ideation. Fluoxetine has fewer side effects than amitriptyline (Table 27–1).

Some clients may experience sexual dysfunction when taking SSRIs. Men have discontinued taking fluoxetine (Prozac) after experiencing a decrease in sexual arousal. Some women have become anorgasmic when taking paroxetine HCl (Paxil). The side effects often decrease or cease over the 2- to 4-week period of waiting for the therapeutic effect to emerge.

Atypical Antidepressants

Atypical (heterocyclic) antidepressants, or *second-generation antidepressants*, became available in the 1980s and have been used for major depression, reactive depression, and anxiety. They affect one or two of the three

Prototype **DRUG CHART 27–2**

FLUOXETINE

Drug Class

Antidepressant, selective serotonin reuptake inhibitor
Trade name: Prozac
Pregnancy Category: B

Dosage

A: PO: 20 mg in AM *max:* 80 mg/d in divided doses
Elderly: 10 mg/d initially; may increase by 10-20 mg q2wk
Therapeutic range: 90-300 ng/ml

Contraindications

Acute myocardial infarction (AMI), taking MAOIs
Caution: Severe depression with suicidal tendency, severe liver or kidney disease

Drug-Lab-Food Interactions

Drug: Increase effects of CNS, respiratory depression, and hypotensive effect with alcohol and CNS depressants
Lab: Altered ECG readings

Pharmacokinetics

Absorption: PO: well absorbed
Distribution: PB: 95%
Metabolism: *fluoxetine:* t½: 2-3 d
Excretion: Excreted primarily in urine

Pharmacodynamics

PO: Onset: 2-4 wk
Peak: 2-4 wk
Duration: weeks

Therapeutic Effects/Uses

To treat depression with or without melancholia, manic and depressive phases of bipolar disorder, depression associated with organic disease, alcoholism, migraine headaches, mixed symptoms of anxiety and depression, or urinary incontinence
Mode of Action: Serotonin is increased in nerve cells because of blockage from nerve fibers.

Side Effects

Headache, nervousness, restlessness, insomnia, tremors, GI distress, sexual dysfunction

Adverse Reactions

Seizures

A, Adult; *CNS*, central nervous system; *d*, day; *ECG*, electrocardiogram; *GI*, gastrointestinal; *MAOI*, monoamine oxidase inhibitor; *max*, maximum; *PB*, protein-binding; *PO*, by mouth; *t½*, half-life; *wk*, week.

neurotransmitters: serotonin, norepinephrine, and dopamine. One of the first atypical antidepressants marketed was amoxapine (Asendin), and others include bupropion (Wellbutrin), maprotiline (Ludiomil), nefazodone (Serzone), trazodone (Desyrel), mirtazapine (Remeron), and venlafaxine (Effexor). Amoxapine and maprotiline are sometimes considered to be TCAs because of their pharmacologic similarities. Atypical antidepressant agents should not be taken with MAOIs and should not be used within 14 days after discontinuing MAOIs. Trazodone may have a potential drug interaction with ketoconazole, ritonavir, and indinavir that may lead to increased trazodone levels and adverse effects. Table 27–2 lists the drugs and how each affects the various neurotransmitters.

Monoamine Oxidase Inhibitors

The fourth group of antidepressants is the **monoamine oxidase inhibitors (MAOIs).** The enzyme monoamine oxidase inactivates norepinephrine, dopamine, epinephrine, and serotonin. By inhibiting monoamine oxidase, the levels of these neurotransmitters rise. In the body there are two forms of monoamine oxidase (MAO) enzyme: MAO-A and MAO-B. These enzymes are found primarily in the liver and brain. MAO-A inactivates dopamine in the brain, whereas MAO-B inactivates norepinephrine and serotonin. The MAOIs are nonselective, inhibiting both MAO-A and MAO-B. Inhibition of MAO by MAOIs is thought to relieve the symptoms of depression. Three MAOIs are currently prescribed: tranylcypromine sulfate (Parnate), isocarboxazid (Marplan), and phenelzine sulfate (Nardil). These MAOIs are detailed in Table 27–2.

For the treatment of depression, MAOIs are as effective as TCAs, but because of adverse reactions such as the risk of hypertensive crisis resulting from food and drug interactions, only 1% of clients taking antidepressants take an MAOI. Currently MAOIs are not the antidepressants of choice and are usually prescribed when the client does not respond to TCAs or second-generation antidepressants. However, MAOIs are still used for mild, reactive, and atypical depression (chronic anxiety, hypersomnia, fear). MAOIs and TCAs should *not* be taken together when treating depression.

Table 27-1

Side Effects of Antidepressants

Antidepressant Category	Anticholinergic Effect	Sedation	Hypotension	GI Distress	Cardiotoxicity	Seizures	Insomnia/ Agitation
Tricyclic Antidepressants							
amitriptyline (Elavil)	++++	++++	+++	−	++++	+++	−
clomipramine (Anafranil)	++++	++++	++	−	++++	++	−
desipramine (Norpramin)	+	++	++	−	++	++	+
doxepin (Sinequan)	+++	++++	++	−	++	++	−
imipramine (Tofranil)	+++	+++	+++	+	++++	++	+
nortriptyline (Aventyl)	+	+++	+	−	+++	++	−
protriptyline (Vivactil)	+++	+	++	−	+++	++	+
trimipramine (Surmontil)	+++	++++	+++	−	++++	++	−
Selective Serotonin Reuptake Inhibitors							
citalopram (Celexa)	+	0	0	++	−	−	+
fluoxetine (Prozac)	−	+	−	+++	−	0/+	++
fluvoxamine (Luvox)	−	++	−	+++	−	−	++
paroxetine (Paxil)	−	+	−	+++	−	−	++
sertraline (Zoloft)	−	+	−	+++	−	−	++
Atypical (Heterocyclic) Antidepressants							
amoxapine (Asendin)	+++	++	+	−	+	+++	++
bupropion (Wellbutrin)	++	−	0/+	+	+	++++	++
trazodone (Desyrel)	−	+++	++	+	+	+	−
maprotiline (Ludiomil)	+++	+++	+	−	++	+++	−
venlafaxine (Effexor)	0	0	0	0	0/+	+	−
Monoamine oxidase Inhibitors (MAOIs)	−	+	++	+	−	−	++

−, No effect; +, mild effect; ++, moderate effect; +++, strong effect; ++++, severe effect; 0, no data available.

Table 27-2

Antidepressants

Generic (Brand)	Route and Dosage	Uses and Considerations
Tricyclic Antidepressants		
amitriptyline HCl (Elavil, Endep, Enovil)	(Prototype Drug Chart 27–1) *Therapeutic serum range:* 100-200 ng/ml	
clomipramine HCl (Anafranil)	A: PO: 25-100 mg/d in divided doses; *max:* 250 mg/d; after titration, entire dose may be given at bedtime Elderly: 20-30 mg/d C: >10 y: PO: 25-100 mg/d in divided doses or 3 mg/kg/d	To treat obsessive-compulsive disorder. May be used to alleviate anxiety or panic disorder. Tremor, dizziness, weight gain, and dry mouth are common side effects. *Pregnancy category:* C; PB: 97%; t$^{1/2}$: 20-30 h

Continued

Table 27–2

Antidepressants—cont'd

Generic (Brand)	Route and Dosage	Uses and Considerations
desipramine HCl (Norpramin, Pertofrane)	A: PO: 25 mg t.i.d. or 75 mg at bedtime; increase to 200 mg/d; *max:* 300 mg/d Elderly: 25-50 mg/d in divided doses; *max:* 150 mg/d *Therapeutic serum range:* 150-250 ng/ml	For depression. Has been used for attention deficit/hyperactivity disorder (ADHD). Take with food if GI distress occurs. Common side effects include drowsiness, dry mouth, increased appetite, urinary retention, and postural hypotension. *Pregnancy category:* D; PB: 90%-95%; t$^{1}/_{2}$: 12-60 h
doxepin HCl (Sinequan, Zonalon)	A: PO: 75-100 mg/d at bedtime or in divided doses; *max:* 300 mg/d Elderly: 25-50 mg/d *Therapeutic serum range:* 30-50 ng/ml	For depression and anxiety related to involutional depression or manic-depressive disorder. Has less effect on cardiac status than other drugs in this group. *Pregnancy category:* C; PB: 80%-85%; t$^{1}/_{2}$: 6-8 h
imipramine HCl (Tofranil)	A: PO: 75 mg/d (at bedtime or 25 mg t.i.d.); *max:* 300 mg/d IM: Initially: *max:* 100 mg/d in divided doses Elderly: 25-100 mg in divided doses C: <12 y: PO: 25-50 mg at bedtime C: >12 y: PO: 75 mg at bedtime *Therapeutic serum range:* 150-250 ng/ml	For depression. Can be taken at bedtime to lessen dangers from sedative effect. Take with food if GI distress occurs. Avoid taking with alcohol or CNS depressants. Common side effects include drowsiness, dry mouth, hypotension, delayed micturition. *Pregnancy category:* D; PB: 90%-95%; t$^{1}/_{2}$: 8-15 h
nortriptyline HCl (Aventyl)	A: PO: 25 mg t.i.d.- q.i.d.; *max:* 150 mg/d Elderly: 30-50 mg/d in divided doses or 10-25 mg at bedtime *Therapeutic serum range:* 50-150 ng/ml	For depression. Similar to imipramine HCl. *Pregnancy category:* D; PB: 90%-95%; t$^{1}/_{2}$: 18-28 h
protriptyline HCl (Vivactil)	A: PO: 15-40 mg/d in divided doses; increase gradually; *max:* 60 mg/d Elderly: 5 mg t.i.d.; *max:* 20 mg/d *Therapeutic serum range:* 70-250 ng/ml	For depression. Has little sedative effect. Effects are similar to imipramine HCl. *Pregnancy category:* C; PB: 92%; t$^{1}/_{2}$: 60-98 h
trimipramine maleate (Surmontil)	A: 75-150 mg/d in divided doses or at bedtime; *max:* 200 mg/d Elderly: *max:* 100 mg/d	For depression. Similar to imipramine HCl. *Pregnancy category:* C; PB: 95%; t$^{1}/_{2}$: 20-26 h
Selective Serotonin Reuptake Inhibitors (SSRIs)		
citalopram (Celexa)	A: PO: 20-40 mg/d; *max:* 80 mg/d Elderly: 10-20 mg/d	For depression, panic disorder, obsessive-compulsive disorder. Wait 14 days after stopping MAOIs. May cause sexual dysfunction, insomnia, nausea, and dry mouth. *Pregnancy category:* C; PB: UK; t$^{1}/_{2}$: 35 h
fluoxetine HCl (Prozac)	(Prototype Drug Chart 27–2)	
paroxetine HCl (Paxil)	*Depression:* A: PO: 10-50 mg/d; *max:* 80 mg/d Elderly: PO: Initially: 10 mg/d; *max:* 40 mg/d *Obsessive-compulsive disorder:* A: PO: 20-60 mg/d *Panic attack:* A: PO: 40 mg/d	For depression and obsessive-compulsive disorders. Lower dose for older adults and those with renal and hepatic disorders. Side effects include dizziness, insomnia, headache, nausea, dry mouth, tremors, postural hypotension. *Pregnancy category:* B; PB: 90%-95%; t$^{1}/_{2}$: 21 h, elderly: 68 h
sertraline HCl (Zoloft)	A: PO: 50 mg/d; *max:* 200 mg/d Elderly: 25 mg/d; dose may be increased	Management of major depressive disorders. Do not take with MAOIs or TCAs. Take with food if GI distress occurs. Urine may be pink-red-brown color. *Pregnancy category:* B; PB: 98%; t$^{1}/_{2}$: 26 h
fluvoxamine (Luvox)	A: PO: 50 mg at bedtime, increase by 50 mg in 5 to 7 d; *max:* 300 mg/d C: 8-18 y: PO: 25 mg at bedtime, increase by 25 mg; *max:* 200 mg/d Elderly: decrease dose	To treat obsessive-compulsive disorder and depression. *Caution:* Do not use in renal or hepatic disorder. *Pregnancy category:* C; PB: UK; t$^{1}/_{2}$: 13-15 h
escitalopram (Lexapro)	A: PO: 10 mg/d, may increase to 20 mg/d after 1 wk Elderly: 10 mg/d	For management of depression. *Pregnancy category:* C; PB: 89%; t$^{1}/_{2}$: 25 h

A, Adult; *b.i.d.,* twice a day; *C,* child; *CNS,* central nervous system; *d,* day; *EPS,* extrapyramidal symptoms; *GI,* gastrointestinal; *h,* hour; *IM,* intramuscular; *maint,* maintenance; *MAOIs,* monoamine oxidase inhibitors; *max,* maximum; *PB,* protein-binding; *PO,* by mouth; *q.i.d.,* four times a day; *t$^{1}/_{2}$,* half-life; *t.i.d.,* three times a day; *TCAs,* tricyclic antidepressants; *UK,* unknown; *y,* year; <, less than; >, greater than; *b.i.d.,* twice a day; *EPS,* extrapyramidal symptoms; *maint,* maintenance.

Table 27–2

Antidepressants—cont'd

Generic (Brand)	Route and Dosage	Uses and Considerations
duloxetine (Cymbalta)	A: PO: 40-60 mg/d in single or divided doses	For treatment of major depression. *Pregnancy category:* C; PB: UK; t^1/$_2$: 8-17 h
Atypical (Heterocyclic or Second Generation) Antidepressants		
amoxapine (Asendin)	A: PO: 25 mg b.i.d.-q.i.d.; increase 150-200 mg/d; dose may be given as a single one	For depression with anxiety and reactive depression. Do not take with MAOIs. Side effects include drowsiness, dizziness, EPS, postural hypotension, increased appetite, urinary retention. *Pregnancy category:* C; PB: >90%; t^1/$_2$: 8 h
maprotiline HCl (Ludiomil)	A: PO: 75 mg at bedtime or in divided doses; *max:* 150 mg/d in single or divided doses Elderly: 25 mg at bedtime; *max:* 75 mg/d	Same as amoxapine. Can be taken at bedtime. *Pregnancy category:* B; PB: 88%; t^1/$_2$: 21-25 h
trazodone HCl (Desyrel)	A: PO: 75 mg at bedtime or 50 mg t.i.d.- q.i.d.; *max:* 600 mg/d	For depression. Can be taken at bedtime to lessen dangers from sedative effect. Drowsiness, light-headedness, orthostatic hypotension, and dry mouth might occur. Take with food to decrease GI distress. *Pregnancy category:* C; PB: 85%-95%; t^1/$_2$: 5-10 h
Norepinephrine and Dopamine Reuptake Inhibitors (NDRIs)		
bupropion HCl (Wellbutrin)	A: PO: Initially: 200 mg/d as b.i.d.; increase gradually to 300 mg/d in divided doses; *max:* 450 mg/d	For depression. May cause increased risk of seizures. Avoid with a history of seizures. Many side effects. *Pregnancy category:* B; PB: >80%; t^1/$_2$: 50 h
Serotonin Antagonists		
mirtazapine (Remeron)	A: PO: 15-30 mg at bedtime; *maint:* 15-45 mg at bedtime; *max:* 60 mg/d	For depression, anxiety, and insomnia. Increases both norepinephrine and serotonin neurotransmitters. Has low anticholinergic activity. *Pregnancy category:* C/D; PB: UK; t^1/$_2$: 20-40 h
Serotonin and Norepinephrine Reuptake Inhibitors		
venlafaxine (Effexor)	A: PO: 75-150 mg/d in 2-3 divided doses; *max:* 375 mg/d in 3 divided doses	For depression, feelings of guilt, worthlessness, and anxiety. Dose decreased with renal and hepatic disorders and for anxiety. Does not cause cardiovascular problems or sedation. *Pregnancy category:* C; PB: UK; t^1/$_2$: 3-7 h, metabolites 9-13 h.
Monoamine Oxidase Inhibitors (MAOIs)		
isocarboxazid (Marplan)	A: PO: 10-20 mg/d; *max:* 60 mg/d	For depression that is refractory to TCAs. Avoid certain foods such as cheese, beer, figs, shrimp, bananas, and chocolate and avoid drugs (e.g., TCAs). *Pregnancy category:* C; PB: UK; t^1/$_2$: UK
phenelzine sulfate (Nardil)	A: PO: 15 mg t.i.d.; 1 mg/kg in divided doses; *max:* 90 mg/d Elderly: *max:* 45-60 mg/d	For depression. Avoid certain foods and drugs (see isocarboxazid). *Pregnancy category:* C; PB: UK; t^1/$_2$: UK
tranylcypromine sulfate (Parnate)	A: PO: 30 mg/d in 2 divided doses (20 mg in AM and 10 mg in PM); *max:* 60 mg/d Elderly: *max:* 45 mg/d	Same as isocarboxazid and phenelzine sulfate.
Selegiline HCl (Emsam, Eldepryl, Zelapar)	A: Transdermal: 6 mg/d; may increase 3 mg/d q2wk to 12 mg/d	For treatment of major depression. Avoid certain foods and drugs (see isocarboxazid). *Pregnancy category:* C; PB: 90%; t^1/$_2$: 2-20 h
Mood Stabilizers		
lithium citrate (Eskalith, Lithibid)	(Prototype Drug Chart 27–3)	
carbamazepine (Equetro, Carbatrol, Tegretol)	A: PO: 200 mg b.i.d.; increase dose 200 mg/d as needed; *max:* 1600 mg/d	For treatment of acute manic and mixed episodes associated with bipolar disorder. Contraindicated in bone marrow depression. *Pregnancy category:* C; PB: 76%; t^1/$_2$: 35-40 h

Drug and Food Interactions

Certain drug and food interactions with MAOIs can be fatal. Any drugs that are CNS stimulants or sympathomimetics, vasoconstrictors and cold medications containing phenylephrine and pseudoephedrine, for example, can cause a hypertensive crisis when taken with an MAOI. In addition, foods that contain tyramine (cheese [cheddar, Swiss, bleu], cream, yogurt, coffee, chocolate, bananas, raisins, Italian green beans, liver, pickled herring, sausage, soy sauce, yeast, beer, and red wines) have sympathomimetic-like effects and can cause a hypertensive crisis (Table 27–3). These types of food and drugs *must be avoided* by MAOI users. Frequent blood pressure monitoring is essential, and client teaching regarding foods and over-the-counter (OTC) drugs to avoid is an important nursing responsibility. Because of the danger associated with a hypertensive crisis, many psychiatrists will not prescribe MAOIs for depression unless they sense the client's ability to comply with the drug and food regimen. However, if properly taken this group of drugs is effective for treating depression.

In teaching clients about the foods and drugs to avoid when taking MAOIs, some individuals respond better to verbal instructions and education with reinforcement from videos than to printed communications. Herbal Alert Box 27–2 details herb interactions with MAOIs.

Table 27–3

Foods that Can Cause a Hypertensive Crisis When Taken with Monoamine Oxidase Inhibitors

Foods	Effects
Cheese (cheddar, Swiss, bleu)	Sweating, tremors
Bananas, raisins	Bounding heart rate
Pickled foods	Increased blood pressure
Red wine, beer	Increased temperature
Cream, yogurt	
Chocolate, coffee	
Italian green beans	
Liver	
Yeast	
Soy sauce	

Avoid taking barbiturates, tricyclic antidepressants, antihistamines, central nervous system depressants, and over-the-counter cold medications with monoamine oxidase inhibitors.

Herbal ALERT 27–2

Monoamine Oxidase Inhibitors (MAOIs)

🌿 Ginseng, ephedra, ma-huang, and St. John's wort may lead to palpitations, heart attack, and hypertensive crisis when taken with antidepressant MAOIs.

- Ginseng may lead to manic episodes when given in combination with MAOIs such as tranylcypromine sulfate.
- Excessive dose of anise may interfere with MAOIs.
- An increased use of brewer's yeast with MAOIs can increase blood pressure.

Side Effects and Adverse Reactions

Side effects of MAOIs include CNS stimulation (agitation, restlessness, insomnia), orthostatic hypotension, and anticholinergic effects.

Nursing Process

Antidepressants

ASSESSMENT

- Record client's baseline vital signs and weight for future comparison.
- Check client's liver and renal function by assessing urine output (>600 ml/d), blood urea nitrogen (BUN), and serum creatinine and liver enzyme levels.
- Obtain a health history of episodes of depression; assess mental status and assess for suicidal tendencies.
- Secure a drug history of the current drugs, alcohol, and herbs client is taking. CNS depressants can cause an additive effect. Antidepressants that cause anticholinergic-like symptoms are contraindicated if client has glaucoma.
- Assess for tardive dyskinesia and neuroleptic malignant syndrome (NMS), including hyperpyrexia, muscle rigidity, tachycardia, and cardiac dysrhythmias.

NURSING DIAGNOSES

- Risk for self-directed violence and injury related to feelings of despair
- Anxiety related to situational crises
- Social isolation related to feelings of sadness
- Ineffective coping related to negative thought patterns
- Hopelessness related to feelings of despair
- Deficient knowledge related to inexperience with escitalopram (Lexapro)
- Ineffective health maintenance related to lack of interest

PLANNING

- Client's depression or manic-depressive behavior will be decreased.

NURSING INTERVENTIONS

- Observe client for signs and symptoms of depression: mood changes, insomnia, apathy, or lack of interest in activities.
- Check client's vital signs. Orthostatic hypotension is common. Check for anticholinergic-like symptoms: dry mouth, increased heart rate, urinary retention, or constipation. Check weight two or three times per week.
- Monitor client for suicidal tendencies when marked depression is present.

■ Observe client for seizures when client is taking an anticonvulsant; antidepressants lower the seizure threshold. The anticonvulsant dose might need to be increased.

■ Monitor for drug-drug and food-drug interactions. Provide client with a list of foods to avoid when taking monoamine oxidase inhibitors (MAOIs). These include cheese, red wine, beer, liver, bananas, yogurt, and sausage.

■ Check client for extremely high blood pressure when taking MAOIs. Sympathomimetic-like drugs and foods containing tyramine may cause a hypertensive crisis if taken with MAOIs.

Client Teaching

General

- Teach client to take the medication as prescribed. Compliance is important.
- Inform client that full effectiveness of drug may not be evident until 1 to 2 weeks after start of therapy.
- Encourage client to keep medical appointments.
- Instruct client not to consume alcohol or any CNS depressants because of their addictive effect.
- Inform client that many herbal products interact with antidepressants, especially MAOIs and selective serotonin reuptake inhibitors (SSRIs). Herbs may need to be discontinued or the antidepressant drug dosage may need modification (Herbal Alerts 27–1 and 27-2).
- Teach client not to drive or be involved in potentially dangerous mechanical activity until stabilization of drug dose has been established.
- Instruct client not to abruptly stop taking the drug. Drug dose should be gradually decreased.
- Encourage client who is planning pregnancy to consult with health care provider about possible teratogenic effects of the drug on the fetus.
- Take with food if GI distress occurs.

Side Effects

- Advise client that antidepressants may be taken at bedtime to decrease dangers from the sedative effect. Have client check with health care provider. Transient side effects include nausea, drowsiness, headaches, and nervousness.

Cultural Considerations ❖

- If Asian client is taking an antipsychotic such as a tricyclic antidepressant (TCA) or lithium, the drug dose may need to be decreased. Explain this to client.
- Explain to Hispanic client that the dose for the antidepressant drug may be lower than is required for other cultural groups.

EVALUATION

■ Evaluate the effectiveness of the drug therapy regarding whether client's depression is controlled or has ceased.

Mood Stabilizers

Mood stabilizers are used to treat bipolar affective disorder. Lithium was the first drug used to manage this disorder. Lithium was first used as a salt substitute in the 1940s, but because of lithium poisoning, it was banned from the market. Some refer to lithium as an *antimania drug* that is effective in controlling manic behavior that arises from underlying bipolar disorder. Lithium has a calming effect without impairing intellectual activity. It controls any evidence of flight of ideas and hyperactivity. If the person stops taking lithium, manic behavior may return.

Lithium is an inexpensive drug that must be closely monitored. Lithium has a narrow therapeutic serum range: 0.5 to 1.5 mEq/L. Serum lithium levels greater than 1.5 to 2 mEq/L are toxic. The serum lithium level should be monitored biweekly until the therapeutic level has been obtained and then monitored monthly on the maintenance dose. Serum sodium levels also need to be monitored because lithium tends to deplete sodium. Lithium must be used with caution, if at all, by clients taking diuretics. Prototype Drug Chart 27–3 lists the pharmacologic behavior of lithium.

Pharmacokinetics

More than 95% of lithium is absorbed through the gastrointestinal (GI) tract. The average half-life of lithium is 24 hours; however, in older adults the half-life can be up to 36 hours. Because of its long half-life, cumulative drug action may result. Lithium is metabolized by the liver, and most of the drug is excreted unchanged in the urine.

Pharmacodynamics

Lithium is prescribed mostly for the stabilization of bipolar affective disorder. The onset of action is fast, but the client may not achieve the desired effect for 5 to 6 days. Increased sodium intake increases renal excretion, so the sodium intake needs to be closely monitored. Increased urine output can result in body fluid loss and dehydration. Adequate fluid intake of 1 to 2 L should be maintained daily.

Anticonvulsants, such as carbamazepine (Tegretol), lamotrigine (Lamictal), and divalproex/valproic acid (Depakote) have been used in place of lithium for some clients. These agents are further discussed in Chapter 21. The antipsychotic drugs olanzapine (Zyprexa), ziprasidone (Geodon), and aripiprazole (Abilify) are approved to treat acute mania and mixed episodes of bipolar disorder. Antipsychotic drugs are discussed further in Chapter 26.

Side Effects and Adverse Reactions

The many side effects of lithium—dry mouth, thirst, increased urination (loss of water and sodium), weight gain, bloated feeling, metallic taste, and edema of the hands and ankles—can be annoying to the client. If taken during pregnancy, lithium may have teratogenic effects on the fetus.

Lithium and nonsteroidal antiinflammatory drugs (NSAIDs) should *not* be given together on a continuous basis and should not be prescribed for clients who have a cardiac "sick sinus syndrome." If the client has taken lithium for a long period, laboratory tests to determine thyroid function should be closely monitored.

Prototype **DRUG CHART 27–3**

LITHIUM

Drug Class

Mood stabilizer
Trade names: Eskalith, Lithane, Lithonate, Lithobid,
✦Carbolith, Lithizine
Pregnancy Category: D

Contraindications

Liver and renal disease, pregnancy, lactation,
severe cardiovascular disease, severe dehydration,
brain tumor or damage, sodium depletion,
children <12 y of age
Caution: Thyroid disease

Dosage

A: PO: 300-600 mg t.i.d.; *maint:* 300 mg t.i.d.-q.i.d.;
max: 2.4 g/d
Elderly: Lower dosage
Therapeutic drug range: 0.5-1.5 mEq/L

Drug-Lab-Food Interactions

Drug: May *increase* lithium level with thiazide diuretics,
methyldopa, haloperidol, NSAIDs, antidepressants,
carbamazepine, theophylline, aminophylline, sodium
bicarbonate, phenothiazines
Lab: Increase urine and blood glucose, protein; decrease
serum sodium level
Food: Increase sodium intake; lithium may cause sodium
depletion

Pharmacokinetics

Absorption: PO: well absorbed
Distribution: PB: UK
Metabolism: t½: 21-30 h; >36 h with renal
impairment or in elderly
Excretion: 98% in urine, mostly unchanged

Pharmacodynamics

PO: Onset: UK
Peak: 2-4 h
Duration: 24 h

Therapeutic Effects/Uses

To treat bipolar manic-depressive psychosis, manic episodes
Mode of Action: Alteration of ion transport in muscle and nerve cells; increased receptor sensitivity to serotonin

Side Effects

Headache, lethargy, drowsiness, dizziness, tremors,
slurred speech, dry mouth, anorexia, vomiting,
diarrhea, polyuria, hypotension, abdominal pain,
muscle weakness, restlessness

Adverse Reactions

Urinary incontinence, clonic movements, stupor,
azotemia, leukocytosis, nephrotoxicity
Life-threatening: Cardiac dysrhythmias, circulatory
collapse

A, Adult; *C,* child; *d,* day; *h,* hour; *max,* maximum; *NSAIDs,* nonsteroidal antiinflammatory drugs; *PB,* protein-binding; *PO,* by
mouth; *q.i.d.,* four times a day; *SR,* sustained release; *t.i.d.,* three times a day; *t½,* half-life; *UK,* unknown; <, less than; >, greater
than; ✦, Canadian drug name.

Nursing Process

Mood Stabilizer: Lithium

ASSESSMENT

- Assess for suicidal ideation.
- Record client's baseline vital signs for future comparison.
- Evaluate client's neurologic status, including gait, level of consciousness, reflexes, and tremors.
- Check client's hepatic and renal function by assessing urine output (>600 ml/d) and whether blood urea nitrogen (BUN) and serum creatinine and liver enzyme levels are within normal range. Assess for toxicity. Draw weekly blood levels initially and then every 1 to 2 months. Therapeutic serum levels for acute mania are 1 to 1.5 mEq/L; for maintenance, levels are 0.5 to 1.5 mEq/L. Signs and symptoms of toxicity at serum levels of 1.5 to 2 mEq/L are persistent nausea and vomiting, severe diarrhea, ataxia, blurred vision, and tinnitus. At 2 to 3.5 mEq/L, signs and symptoms of toxicity are excessive output of dilute urine, increasing tremors, muscular irritability, psychomotor retardation, mental confusion, and giddiness. At 3.5 mEq/L or higher, levels are life threatening and may result in impaired consciousness, nystagmus, seizures, coma, oliguria/anuria, cardiac dysrhythmias, myocardial infarction, and cardiovascular collapse. Withhold medication and notify health care provider immediately if any of these occur.

- Obtain a health history of episodes of depression or manic-depressive behavior.
- Obtain client's drug history. Diuretics, nonsteroidal antiinflammatory drugs (NSAIDs) (e.g., ibuprofen), tet-

racyclines, methyldopa, and probenecid decrease renal clearance of lithium, causing drug accumulation.

NURSING DIAGNOSES

- Risk for injury or violence related to impulsiveness
- Ineffective coping related to manic behavior
- Noncompliance related to lack of adequate education regarding lithium

PLANNING

- Client's manic-depressive behavior will be decreased.

NURSING INTERVENTIONS

- Observe client for signs and symptoms of depression: mood changes, insomnia, apathy, or lack of interest in activities.
- Record client's vital signs. Orthostatic hypotension is common.
- When drawing blood to check for lithium levels, draw samples immediately before the next dose (8 to 12 hours after the previous dose). Monitor for signs of lithium toxicity. Report high (greater than 1.5 mEq/L) or toxic (greater than 2.0 mEq/L) serum lithium levels immediately to health care provider.
- Monitor client for suicidal tendencies when marked depression is present.
- Evaluate client's urine output and body weight. Fluid volume deficit may occur as a result of polyuria.
- Observe client for fine and gross motor tremors and presence of slurred speech, which are signs of adverse reaction.
- Check client's cardiac status. Loss of fluids and electrolytes may cause cardiac dysrhythmias.
- Monitor client's serum electrolytes. Report abnormal findings.

Client Teaching

General

- Teach client to take lithium as prescribed. Emphasize importance of adherence to the therapy, laboratory tests, and follow-up visits with health care provider. If lithium is stopped, manic symptoms will reappear.
- Encourage client to keep medical appointments. Have client check with health care provider before taking OTC preparations.
- Instruct client not to drive a motor vehicle or be involved in potentially dangerous mechanical activity until stable lithium level is established.
- Advise client to maintain adequate fluid intake: 2 to 3 L/d initially and 1 to 2 L/d maintenance. Fluid intake should increase in hot weather.
- Teach client to take lithium with meals to decrease gastric irritation.

- Inform client that effectiveness of drug may not be evident until 1 to 2 weeks after the start of therapy. Compliance in taking the prescribed lithium doses on a daily basis is a major problem with bipolar clients. When client has a period of emotional stability, he or she does not believe that the drug is needed; thus, client stops taking the lithium.
- Advise client who is planning pregnancy to consult with health care provider about possible teratogenic effects of the drug on the fetus, especially during the first 3 months.
- Encourage client to wear or carry an identification tag or bracelet indicating the drug taken.

Diet

- Inform client to avoid caffeine products (coffee, tea, cola), because they can aggravate the manic phase of bipolar disorder.
- Instruct client to maintain adequate sodium intake and to avoid crash diets that affect physical and mental health.

Side Effects

- Advise client to contact health care provider if experiencing symptoms of toxicity. Early symptoms: diarrhea, drowsiness, loss of appetite, muscle weakness, nausea, vomiting, slurred speech, trembling. Late symptoms: blurred vision, confusion, increased urination, convulsions, severe trembling, unsteadiness.

Cultural Considerations ❖

- Obtain an interpreter when necessary; do not rely on family members, who may not fully disclose because of honor and shame.

EVALUATION

- Evaluate the effectiveness of the drug therapy. Client is free of bipolar behavior.
- Allow client to verbalize understanding of symptoms of toxicity.
- Determine whether client demonstrates a subsiding or resolution of the symptoms.

KEY WEBSITES

Information on Antidepressants: http://www.nlm.nih.gov/medlineplus/antidepressants.html

Depression: http://www.nlm.nih.gov/medlineplus/depression.html

Use of Psychoactive Medication During Pregnancy and Possible Effects on the Fetus and Newborn: http://aappolicy.aappublications.org/cgi/content/full/pediatrics;105/4/880

St. John's Wort and the Treatment of Depression: http://nccam.nih.gov/health/stjohnswort/index.htm

Critical Thinking Case Study

ST, 37 years old, is receiving fluoxetine (Prozac) 20 mg in the evening for depression. ST complains of insomnia and GI upset.

1. What could you suggest to ST to help her avoid insomnia? Explain.
2. How might ST avoid GI upset when taking fluoxetine?

ST states that she does not think the fluoxetine is helping. She has heard that there are herbal supplements that may be taken for depression. She has also heard that fluoxetine can be taken weekly.

3. Is ST's fluoxetine dose within normal dosage range? Explain.
4. How would you respond to ST about the use of certain herbal supplements for depression?
5. What would your response be concerning the use of fluoxetine in a weekly dose?

NCLEX Study Questions

1. A client is admitted with bipolar affective disorder. The nurse acknowledges that _____ is a drug used to treat this disorder for some clients in place of lithium.
   a. thiopental
   b. gingko biloba
   c. fluvoxamine (Luvox)
   d. divalproex (Depakote)

2. The nurse realizes that some herbs interact with selective serotonin reuptake inhibitors (SSRIs). Which herb interaction may cause serotonin syndrome?
   a. feverfew
   b. ma-huang
   c. St. John's wort
   d. gingko biloba

3. An SSRI is prescribed for a client. The nurse realizes that which of the following is an SSRI?
   a. paroxetine (Paxil)
   b. amitriptyline (Elavil)
   c. divalproex sodium (Depakote)
   d. bupropion HCl (Wellbutrin)

4. A client is taking tranylcypromine sulfate (Parnate) for depression. Which of the following should the nurse include in the teaching plan of this medication?
   a. warn of severe hypotension
   b. avoid beer and cheddar cheese
   c. encourage ginseng and ephedra
   d. encourage fruit such as bananas

5. Which of the following statements is true concerning lithium?
   a. The maximum dose is 3.4 g/day.
   b. The therapeutic drug range is 2.5 to 3.5 mEq/L.
   c. Lithium increases receptor sensitivity to GABA.
   d. Concurrent NSAIDs may increase lithium levels.

Answers: 1. d; 2. c; 3. a; 4. b; 5. d.

Nine

Antibacterial Agents

Introduction

Unit IX discusses agents prescribed to combat disease-producing microorganisms (pathogens). Included in this unit are antibacterials-antibiotics (penicillins, cephalosporins, macrolides, tetracyclines, aminoglycosides, and fluoroquinolones) and sulfonamides.

Infection

Disease-producing microorganisms may be gram-positive or gram-negative bacteria, viruses, or fungi. The degree to which they are pathogenic depends on the microorganism and its virulence. The cell walls of bacteria differ in their structure: bacilli are elongated, cocci are spherical, and spirilla are helical.

Bioterrorism

Bioterrorism is a current threat to humanity. In recent years anthrax has been developed as a biological weapon, usually in a powder form for inhalation. While there are three types of anthrax affecting the skin, gastrointestinal systems, and lungs, inhalation is the most lethal form. An aerosol cloud of anthrax spores is colorless, odorless, and invisible, creating the same exposure for individuals indoors as those outside. The World Health Organization analyzed the release of aerosolized anthrax in 1970 and concluded that in appropriate weather and wind conditions, upwind, in a population of 5 million, approximately 250,000 individuals would be affected, and the expected mortality rate would be 100,000.

Often the first sign of anthrax use as a biological weapon is the recognition of symptoms. Infectious symptoms of anthrax are fever, chills, headache, nausea, vomiting, nasal congestion, shortness of breath, cough, malaise, joint pain and stiffness, and chest pain. Onset of symptoms of anthrax may appear from 7 days to 8 weeks after exposure.

Anthrax may be prevented by a vaccination. The Centers for Disease Control and Prevention (CDC) is working with state and local officials to prepare for an anthrax attack. When appropriate antibiotics are not initiated before the development of symptoms, the mortality rate is approximately 90%. Anthrax is caused by the spore-forming *Bacillus anthracis*. This acute infectious disease can be treated with fluoroquinolones, such as ciprofloxacin (Cipro); tetracyclines, such as doxycycline (Vibramycin); or penicillins, such as Penicillin V.

28
Penicillins and Cephalosporins

> **ELECTRONIC RESOURCES**
>
> **Evolve website (http://evolve.elsevier.com/KeeHayes/pharmacology/):**
> - Case Studies
> - Content Updates
> - Frequently Asked Questions
> - Student Review Activities
> - WebLinks
> - Additional Reference Material
>
> **Companion CD-ROM:**
> - NCLEX Examination Review Questions
> - Pharmacology Animations
> - IV Therapy Checklists
> - Medication Error Checklists
> - Drug Calculation Problems
> - Electronic Calculators
> - Top 200 Drugs with Pronunciations
> - References from the Textbook

Objectives

- Explain the mechanisms of action of antibacterial drugs.
- Differentiate between bacteria that are naturally resistant and those that have acquired resistance to an antibiotic.
- Summarize the three general adverse effects associated with antibacterial drugs.
- Differentiate between narrow-spectrum and broad-spectrum antibiotics.
- Describe the effects of the natural, broad-spectrum (extended), penicillinase-resistant, and antipseudomonal penicillins.
- Contrast the effects of first-, second-, third-, and fourth-generation cephalosporins.
- Apply the nursing process for clients receiving penicillins and cephalosporins.

Terms

This chapter discusses the antibacterials and their effects, which include mechanisms of antibacterial action, body defenses, resistance to antibacterials, use of antibacterial combinations, general adverse reactions to antibacterials, and narrow- and broad-spectrum antibiotics. This chapter also discusses two antibacterials in detail: penicillin and cephalosporin.

Pathophysiology

Bacteria, known as *prokaryotes*, are single-celled organisms lacking a true nucleus and nuclear membrane. Most bacteria have a rigid cell wall, and the structure of the cell wall determines the shape of the bacteria. One classification of bacteria involves the appearance or shape under a microscope. A *bacillus* is a rod-shaped organism. *Cocci* are spherical. When cocci appear in clusters, they are called *staphylococci*; when cocci are arranged in chains, they are called *streptococci*. Bacteria reproduce by cell division about every 20 minutes.

Another classification of bacteria involves staining properties of the cell. The Gram staining method was devised in 1882 by Hans Christian Gram, a Danish bacteriologist. Gram staining is determined by the ability of the bacterial cell wall to retain a purple stain by a basic dye. Crystal violet is normally used in the staining process but may be substituted with methylene blue. If bacteria retain a purple stain, they are classified as *gram-positive* microorganisms. Those bacteria not stained are known as *gram-negative* microorganisms. Examples of *gram-positive* bacteria include *Staphylococcus aureus*, *Streptococcus pneumoniae*, *Group B streptococcus*, and *Clostridium perfringens*. Examples of *gram-negative* bacteria include *Neisseria meningitides*, *Escherichia coli*, and *Haemophilus influenzae*.

Bacteria produce toxins that cause cell lysis (cell death). Many bacteria produce the enzyme beta-lactamase, which destroys beta-lactam antibiotics such as penicillins and cephalosporins.

Antibacterial Drugs

Antibacterials/Antibiotics

Although the terms *antibacterial*, *antimicrobial*, and *antibiotic* are frequently used interchangeably, there are some subtle differences in meaning. **Antibacterials** and **antimicrobials** are substances that inhibit bacterial growth or kill bacteria and other **microorganisms** (microscopic organisms including viruses, fungi, protozoa, and rickettsiae). Technically the term *antibiotic* refers to chemicals produced by one kind of microorganism that inhibits the growth of or kills another. For practical purposes, however, these terms may be used interchangeably. Several drugs, including antiinfective and chemotherapeutic agents, have actions similar to those of antibacterial and antimicrobial agents. Antibacterial drugs do not act alone in destroying bacteria. Natural body defenses, surgical procedures to excise infected tissues, and dressing changes may be needed along with antibacterial drugs to eliminate the infecting bacteria.

Antibacterial drugs are either obtained from natural sources or manufactured. The use of moldy bread on wounds to fight infection dates back 3500 years. In 1928 Alexander Fleming, a British bacteriologist, noted that "mold" was contaminating his bacterial cultures and inhibiting bacterial growth. The mold was called *Penicillium notatum*; thus Fleming called the substance *penicillin*. In 1939 Howard Florey expanded on Fleming's findings and purified the penicillin so it could be used commercially. Penicillin was used during World War II and marketed in 1945. Sulfonamide, a synthetic antibacterial, was introduced in 1935. Sulfonamides are discussed in greater detail in Chapter 30.

Bacteriostatic drugs inhibit the growth of bacteria, whereas **bactericidal** drugs kill bacteria. Some antibacterial drugs (tetracycline and sulfonamides) have a bacteriostatic effect, whereas other antibacterials (penicillins and cephalosporins) have a bactericidal effect. Depending on the drug dose and serum level, certain drugs can have both bacteriostatic and bactericidal effects.

For drugs with a narrow therapeutic index—aminoglycosides, for example—peaks and troughs of serum antibiotic levels are monitored to determine whether the drug is within the therapeutic range for its desired effect. If the serum *peak* level is too high, drug toxicity could occur. If the serum *trough* level (drawn minutes before administration of the next drug dose) is below the therapeutic range, the client is not receiving an adequate antibiotic dose to kill the targeted microorganism.

Mechanisms of Antibacterial Action

Five mechanisms of antibacterial action are responsible for the inhibition of growth or destruction of microorganisms: (1) inhibition of bacterial cell-wall synthesis, (2) alteration of membrane permeability, (3) inhibition of protein synthesis, (4) inhibition of the synthesis of bacterial ribonucleic acid (RNA) and deoxyribonucleic acid (DNA), and (5) interference with metabolism within the cell (Table 28–1).

Pharmacokinetics

Antibacterial drugs must not only penetrate the bacterial cell wall in sufficient concentration, but also must have an affinity (attraction) to the binding sites on the bacterial cell. The time the drug remains at the binding sites increases the effect of the antibacterial action. This time factor is controlled by the pharmacokinetics (distribution, half-life, and elimination) of the drug. Antibacterials that have a longer half-life usually maintain a greater concentration at the binding site; therefore frequent dosing is not required. Most antibacterials are not highly protein-bound, with a few exceptions (e.g., oxacillin, ceftriaxone, cefoperazone, cefonicid, cefprozil, cloxacillin, nafcillin, clindamycin). Protein-binding does not have a major influence on the effectiveness of most antibacterial drugs. The steady state of the antibacterial drug occurs after the fourth to fifth half-lives, and the drug is eliminated from the body, mainly through urine, after the seventh half-life.

Pharmacodynamics

The drug concentration at the site or the exposure time for the drug plays an important role in bacterial eradication. Antibacterial drugs are used to achieve the minimum effective concentration (MEC) necessary to halt the growth of a microorganism. Many antibacterials have a bactericidal effect against the pathogen when the drug concentration remains constantly above the MEC during the dosing interval. Duration of time for use of the antibacterial varies according to the type of pathogen, site of infection, and immunocompetence of the host. With some severe infections, a continuous infusion regimen is more effective than intermittent dosing because of constant drug concentration and time exposure. Once-daily antibacterial dosing (e.g., aminoglycosides, macrolides, fluoroquinolones) has been effective in eradicating pathogens and, in most of those cases, has not caused severe adverse reactions (ototoxicity, nephrotoxicity). The ease of compliance with once- or twice-daily drug dosing also increases the client's adherence to the drug regimen.

Figure 28–1 illustrates the effect of three methods of drug dosing. The drug dose is effective when it remains above the MEC.

Table 28–1

Mechanisms of Actions of Antibacterial Drugs

Action	Effect	Drugs
Inhibitions of cell wall synthesis	Bactericidal effect. Enzyme breakdown of cell wall. Inhibition of enzyme in synthesis of cell wall.	penicillin cephalosporins bacitracin vancomycin
Alteration in membrane permeability	Bacteriostatic or bactericidal effect. Membrane permeability increased. Loss of cellular substances causes lysis of the cell.	amphotericin B nystatin polymyxin colistin
Inhibition of protein synthesis	Bacteriostatic or bactericidal effect. Interferes with protein synthesis without affecting normal cell. Inhibits the steps of protein synthesis.	aminoglycosides tetracyclines erythromycin lincomycin
Inhibition of synthesis of bacterial RNA and DNA	Inhibits synthesis of RNA and DNA in bacteria. Binds to nucleic acid and enzymes needed for nucleic acid synthesis.	fluoroquinolones
Interference with cellular metabolism	Bacteriostatic effect. Interferes with steps of metabolism within cells.	sulfonamides trimethoprim isoniazid (INH) nalidixic acid rifampin

DNA, Deoxyribonucleic acid; *RNA*, ribonucleic acid.

FIGURE 28–1   Effects of concentrated drug dosing.

Body Defenses

Body defenses and antibacterial drugs work together to stop the infectious process. The effect that antibacterial drugs have on an infection depends not only on the drug but also on the host's defense mechanisms. Factors such as age, nutrition, immunoglobulins, white blood cells (WBCs), organ function, and circulation influence the body's ability to fight infection. Elderly and undernourished individuals have less resistance to infection than younger, well nourished populations. If the host's natural body defense mechanisms are inadequate, drug therapy might not be as effective. As a result, drug therapy may need to be closely monitored or revised. When circulation is impeded, an antibacterial drug may not be distributed properly to the infected area. In addition, **immunoglobu-** lins (antibody proteins such as IgG and IgM) and other elements of the immune response system (WBCs) needed to combat infections may be depleted in individuals with poor nutritional status.

Resistance to Antibacterials

Bacteria may be sensitive or resistant to certain antibacterials. When bacteria are sensitive to a drug, the pathogen is inhibited or destroyed. If bacteria are resistant to an antibacterial, the pathogen continues to grow, despite administration of that antibacterial drug.

Bacterial resistance may result naturally **(inherent resistance)** or it may be acquired. A natural, or inherent, resistance occurs without previous exposure to the antibacterial drug. For example, the gram-negative (non-gram-staining) bacterium *Pseudomonas aeruginosa* is inherently resistant to penicillin G. An **acquired resistance** is caused by prior exposure to the antibacterial. Although *Staphylococcus aureus* was once sensitive to penicillin G, repeated exposures have caused this organism to evolve and become resistant to it. Penicillinase, an enzyme produced by the microorganism, is responsible for causing its penicillin resistance. Penicillinase metabolizes penicillin G, causing the drug to be ineffective. Penicillinase-resistant penicillins that are effective against *S. aureus* are currently available.

Antibiotic resistance is a major problem. In the early 1980s pharmaceutical companies thought that enough antibiotics were on the market, so these companies concentrated on developing antiviral and antifungal drugs. As a result fewer new antibiotics were developed during the 1980s. Now pharmaceutical companies have developed many new antibiotics, but antibiotic resistance continues to develop, especially when antibiotics are used frequently. As bacteria reproduce, some mutation occurs, and eventually the mutant bacteria survive the effects of the drug. One explanation is that the mutant bacteria strain may have grown a thicker cell wall.

In large health care institutions, there is a tendency toward drug resistance in bacteria. Mutant strains of organisms have developed, thus increasing their resistance to antibiotics that were once effective against them. Infections acquired while clients are hospitalized are called **nosocomial infections.** Many of these infections are caused by drug-resistant bacteria and can prolong hospitalization, which is costly to both the client and third-party health care insurers.

Another problem related to antibiotic resistance is that bacteria can transfer their genetic instruction to another bacterial species, and the other bacterial species becomes resistant to that antibiotic as well. Bacteria can pass along high resistance to a more virulent and aggressive bacterium (e.g., *S. aureus,* enterococci). Many enterococcal strains are resistant to penicillin, ampicillin, gentamicin, streptomycin, and vancomycin. One of the biggest resistance problems is vancomycin-resistant enterococci (VRE), which can cause death in many persons with weakened immune systems. The incidence of VRE in hospitals has increased. Staphylococcal bacteria tend to be resistant to every drug except vancomycin. If VRE transfers to *Staphylococcus* its resistance to vancomycin, a major medical problem could result.

One antibiotic after another is ineffective against new resistant strains of bacteria. As new drugs are developed, drug resistance will probably develop as well. Pharmaceutical companies and biotechnical firms are working on new classes of drugs to "beat" the problem of bacterial resistance to antibiotics. Ziracin has been approved in the classification of antibiotic called *everninomicin.* Another class of antibiotics, oxazolidinones, was discovered by a pharmaceutical company in 1988, but the company could not overcome toxicity problems in this class of drug. Another pharmaceutical company has taken the compound and made it less toxic. This antibiotic, linezolid, is effective against methicillin-resistant staphylococci, VRE, and penicillin-resistant streptococci. Quinupristin/dalfopristin (Synercid), two streptogramin antibacterials, is marketed in a combination of 30:70 for intravenous (IV) use against life-threatening infection caused by VRE and for treatment of bacteremia, *S. aureus,* and *Streptococcus pyogenes.*

Another way to attack antimicrobial resistance is to develop drugs that disable the antibiotic-resistant mechanism in the bacteria. Clients would take the antibiotic-resistance disabler along with the antibiotic already on the market, making the drug effective again. Developing bacterial vaccine is another way to combat bacteria and lessen the need for antibiotics. The bacterial vaccine against pneumococcus has been effective in decreasing the occurrence of pneumonia and meningitis among various age groups.

Antibiotic misuse, a major problem today, may decrease antibiotic resistance. Studies reveal that 23% to 37.8% of clients in hospitals receive antibiotics and 50% of this population is receiving antibiotics inappropriately. When antibiotics are taken unnecessarily (i.e., for viral infections or when no infection is present) or incorrectly (i.e., skipping doses, not taking the full antibiotic regimen), one may develop resistance to antibacterials. Consumer education is important because many clients "demand" antibiotics for viral conditions. Antibiotics are ineffective against viruses. However, viral infections that persist could decrease the body's immune system thus promoting a bacterial infection. The nurse should teach clients proper use of antibiotics to prevent situations that promote drug-resistance to bacteria.

Cross-resistance can also occur between antibacterial drugs that have similar actions, such as the penicillins and cephalosporins. To ascertain the effect antibacterial drugs have on a specific microorganism, culture and sensitivity or antibiotic susceptibility testing is performed. A *culture and sensitivity* laboratory test (C & S) can detect the infective microorganism present in a sample (blood, sputum, swab, etc.) and what drug can kill it. The organism causing the infection is determined by culture, and the antibiotics the organism is sensitive to are determined by sensitivity. The susceptibility or resistance of one microorganism to several antibacterials can be determined by this method. Multiantibiotic therapy (daily use of several antibacterials) delays the development of microorganism resistance.

Use of Antibiotic Combinations

Combination antibiotics should not be routinely prescribed or administered except for specific uncontrollable infections. Usually a single antibiotic will successfully treat a bacterial infection. When there is a severe infection that persists and is of unknown origin or has been unsuccessfully treated with several single antibiotics, a combination of two or three antibiotics may be suggested. Before antibiotic therapy, a culture or cultures should be taken to identify the bacteria.

When two antibiotics are combined, the result is additive, potentiative, or antagonistic. The *additive* effect is equal to the sum of the effects of two antibiotics. The *potentiative* effect occurs when one antibiotic potentiates the effect of the second antibiotic, increasing their effectiveness. The *antagonistic* result is a combination of a drug that is bactericidal, such as penicillin, and a drug that is bacteriostatic, such as tetracycline. When these two drugs are used together, the desired effect may be greatly reduced.

General Adverse Reactions to Antibacterials

Three major adverse reactions associated with the administration of antibacterial drugs are allergic (hypersensitivity) reactions, superinfection, and organ toxicity. Table 28–2 describes these adverse reactions, all of which require close monitoring of the client.

Table 28–2

General Adverse Reactions to Antibacterial Drugs

Type	Considerations
Allergy or hypersensitivity	Allergic reactions to drugs may be mild or severe. Examples of mild reactions are rash, pruritus, and hives. An example of a severe response is anaphylactic shock. Anaphylaxis results in vascular collapse, laryngeal edema, bronchospasm, and cardiac arrest. Shortness of breath is frequently the first symptom of anaphylaxis. Severe allergic reaction generally occurs within 20 minutes. Mild allergic reaction is treated with an antihistamine; anaphylaxis requires treatment with epinephrine, bronchodilators, and antihistamines.
Superinfection	Superinfection is a secondary infection that occurs when the normal microbial flora of the body are disturbed during antibiotic therapy. Superinfections can occur in the mouth, respiratory tract, intestine, genitourinary tract, or skin. Fungal infections frequently result in superinfections, although bacterial organisms (e.g., *Proteus, Pseudomonas,* staphylococci) may be the offending microorganisms. Superinfections rarely develop when the drug is administered for less than a week. They occur more commonly with the use of broad-spectrum antibiotics. For fungal infection of the mouth, nystatin is frequently used.
Organ toxicity	The liver and kidneys are involved in drug metabolism and excretion. Antibacterials may result in damage to these organs. For example, aminoglycosides can be *nephrotoxic* (as well as ototoxic [ears]).

Narrow-Spectrum and Broad-Spectrum Antibiotics

Antibacterial drugs are either narrow spectrum or broad spectrum. The **narrow-spectrum antibiotics** are primarily effective against one type of organism. For example, penicillin and erythromycin are used to treat infections caused by gram-positive bacteria. Certain **broad-spectrum antibiotics** (tetracycline and cephalosporins) can be effective against both gram-positive and gram-negative organisms. Because narrow-spectrum antibiotics are selective, they are more active against those single organisms than the broad-spectrum antibiotics. Broad-spectrum antibiotics are frequently used to treat infections when the offending microorganism has not been identified by C & S.

Penicillins and Cephalosporins

Penicillins

Penicillin, a natural antibacterial agent obtained from the mold genus *Penicillium,* was introduced to the military during World War II and is considered to have saved many soldiers' lives. It became widely used in 1945 and was labeled a "miracle" drug. With the advent of penicillin, many clients survived who would have normally died from wound and severe respiratory infections.

Penicillin's beta-lactam structure (beta-lactam ring) interferes with bacterial cell-wall synthesis by inhibiting the bacterial enzyme that is necessary for cell division and cellular synthesis. The bacteria die of cell lysis (cell breakdown). The penicillins can be both bacteriostatic and bactericidal, depending on the drug and dosage. Penicillin G is primarily bactericidal.

Penicillins are mainly referred to as *beta-lactam antibiotics.* Bacteria can produce a variety of enzymes, beta-lactamases, that can inactivate penicillin and other beta-lactam antibiotics such as the cephalosporins. The beta-lactamases, which attack penicillins, are called *penicillinases.*

Penicillin G was the first penicillin administered orally and by injection. With oral administration, only about one third of the dose is absorbed. Because of its poor absorption, penicillin G given by injection (intramuscular [IM] and intravenous [IV]) is more effective in achieving a therapeutic serum penicillin level. Aqueous penicillin G has a short duration of action, and the IM injection is very painful, because it is an aqueous drug solution. As a result, a longer-acting form of penicillin, procaine penicillin (milky color), was produced to extend the activity of the drug. Procaine in the penicillin decreases the pain related to injection.

Penicillin V was the next type of penicillin produced. Although two thirds of the oral dose is absorbed by the gastrointestinal (GI) tract, it is a less potent antibacterial drug than penicillin G. Penicillin V is effective against mild to moderate infections, including anthrax as a biological weapon of bioterrorism.

Initially penicillin was overused. It was first introduced for the treatment of staphylococcal infections, but after a few years mutant strains of *Staphylococcus* developed that were resistant to penicillins G and V because of the bacterial enzyme penicillinase, which destroys penicillin. This led to the development of new broad-spectrum antibiotics with structures similar to penicillin to combat infections resistant to penicillins G and V.

Food may decrease the absorption of many oral penicillins, so those penicillins should be taken with a full glass of water 1 hour before food intake or 2 hours after. Amoxicillins and bacampicillin are penicillins that are unaffected by food.

Broad-Spectrum Penicillins (Aminopenicillins)

Broad-spectrum penicillins are used to treat both gram-positive and gram-negative bacteria. They are not, however, as "broadly" effective against all microorganisms as they were once considered to be. This group of drugs is costlier than penicillin and therefore should not be used when ordinary penicillins, such as penicillin G, are effective. The broad-spectrum penicillins are effective against some gram-negative organisms: *Escherichia coli, Haemophilus influenzae, Shigella dysenteriae, Proteus mirabilis,* and *Salmonella.* However, these drugs are not penicillinase resistant. They are readily inactivated by beta-lactamases, thus ineffective against *S. aureus.* Examples of this group are ampicillin (Omnipen), amoxicillin (Amoxil), and bacampicillin (Spectrobid) (Table 28–3). Amoxicillin is the most prescribed penicillin derivative for adults and children.

Penicillinase-Resistant Penicillins (Antistaphylococcal Penicillins)

Penicillinase-resistant penicillins (antistaphylococcal penicillins) are used to treat penicillinase-producing *S. aureus.* Cloxacillin (Cloxapen) and dicloxacillin (Dynapen) are oral preparations of these antibiotics; nafcillin (Unipen) and oxacillin (Prostaphin) are IM and IV preparations. This group of drugs is not effective against gram-negative organisms and is less effective than penicillin G against gram-positive organisms. Prototype Drug Chart 28–1 compares the similarities and differences in the broad-spectrum penicillin amoxicillin and the penicillinase-resistant penicillin dicloxacillin.

Extended-Spectrum Penicillins (Antipseudomonal Penicillins)

The antipseudomonal penicillins are a group of broad-spectrum penicillins. This group of drugs is effective against *Pseudomonas aeruginosa,* a gram-negative bacillus that is difficult to eradicate. These drugs are also useful against many gram-negative organisms such as *Proteus* spp., *Serratia* spp., *Klebsiella pneumoniae, Enterobacter* spp., and *Acinetobacter* spp. The antipseudomonal penicillins are not penicillinase-resistant. Their pharmacologic action is similar to that of aminoglycosides, but they are less toxic.

Table 28–3 lists the drugs in the four categories of penicillin-type antibacterials. The administration route of various types of penicillins (oral, IM, IV), along with the cephalosporins, are available on the Evolve website.

Beta-Lactamase Inhibitors

When a broad-spectrum antibiotic (e.g., amoxicillin) is combined with a beta-lactamase (enzyme) inhibitor (e.g., clavulanic acid), the resulting antibiotic (e.g., amoxicillin-clavulanic acid [Augmentin]) inhibits the bacterial beta-

Table 28–3

Antibacterials: Penicillins

Generic (Brand)	Route and Dosage	Uses and Considerations
Basic Penicillins		
penicillin G procaine (Crysticillin, Wycillin)	A: IM: 600,000-1.2 million units/d in 1-2 divided doses C: IM: 300,000-600,000 units/d in 1-2 divided doses NB: IM: 50,000 units/kg/d	For moderately serious infections. Slow IM absorption with prolonged action. The solution is milky. *Pregnancy category:* B; PB: 65%; t½: 0.5 h
penicillin G benzathine (Bicillin)	A: IM: 1.2 million units as a single dose C: IM: >27 kg: 900,000 units/dose IM: <27 kg: 50,000 units/kg/dose or 300,000-600,000 units/dose	Long-acting penicillin when given by injection. Used as a prophylaxis for rheumatic fever. *Pregnancy category:* B; PB: 65%; t½: 1 h
penicillin G sodium/potassium (Pentids, Pfizerpen)	A: PO: 200,000-500,000 units q6h IM: 500,000-5 million units/d in divided doses IV: 4-20 million units/d in divided doses, diluted in IV fluids C: PO: 25,000-90,000 units/d in divided doses IV: 50,000-100,000 units/kg/d in divided doses	Poorly absorbed orally because of gastric acidity and food. Take 1 h before or 2 h after meals. Penicillin G is available in salts (potassium [K] and sodium [Na]). With high doses, electrolyte levels should be monitored. Injectable solution is clear. *Pregnancy category:* B; PB: 60%; t½: 0.5-1 h
penicillin V potassium (V-Cillin K, Veetids, Betapen VK)	A: PO: 125-500 mg q6h C: PO: 15-50 mg/kg/d in 3-4 divided doses	Acid-stable and less active than penicillin G against some bacteria. Not recommended in renal failure. Take drug after meals. *Pregnancy category:* B; PB: 80%; t½: 0.5 h
Broad-Spectrum Penicillins		
amoxicillin (Amoxil) amoxicillin-clavulanate (Augmentin)	(Prototype Drug Chart 28–1) A: PO: 250-500 mg q8-12h C: PO: <40 kg: 20-40 mg/kg/d	Treatment of lower respiratory infections, otitis media, sinusitis, skin infections, and UTIs. *Pregnancy category:* B; PB: UK; t½: 1-3 h

A, Adult; *C,* child; *d,* day; *h,* hour; *IM,* intramuscular; *IV,* intravenous; *NB,* newborn; *PB,* protein-binding; *PO,* by mouth; *t*½, half-life; *UK,* unknown; *UTI,* urinary tract infection; >, greater than; <, less than.

Continued

Table 28–3

Antibacterials: Penicillins—cont'd

Generic (Brand)	Route and Dosage	Uses and Considerations
ampicillin (Polycillin, Omnipen)	A: PO: 250-500 mg q6h IM/IV: 2-8 g/d in divided doses (250 mg-2 g q6h) C: PO: 25-50 mg/kg/d in 4 divided doses IM/IV: 25-100 mg/kg/d in 4 divided doses	First broad-spectrum penicillin. 50% of drug is absorbed by GI tract. Effective against gram-negative and gram-positive bacteria. Individuals with penicillin allergies may also be allergic to ampicillin. *Pregnancy category*: B; PB: 15%-28%; $t^{1/2}$: 1-2 h
ampicillin-sulbactam (Unasyn)	A: IV: 1.5-3.0 g q6h C: IV: 100-300 mg/kg/d, divided q6h	Same as ampicillin. Sulbactam inhibits beta lactamase thus extending the spectrum. *Pregnancy category*: B; PB: 28%-38%; $t^{1/2}$: 1-2 h
bacampicillin HCl (Spectrobid)	A: PO: 400-800 mg q12h C: PO: 12.5-25 mg/kg/d in 2 divided doses	Same as ampicillin. 90% absorbed. Hydrolyzed to ampicillin during absorption from GI tract. *Pregnancy category*: B; PB: 17%-20%; $t^{1/2}$: 1 h
Penicillinase-Resistant Penicillins		
cloxacillin (Tegopen)	A: PO: 250-500 mg q6h C: PO: <20 kg: 12.5-25 mg/kg q6h; *max*: 4 g/d	For most gram-positive bacterial infections. *Pregnancy category*: B; PB: 90%-95%; $t^{1/2}$: 30-60 min
dicloxacillin sodium (Dynapen) methicillin (Staphcillin)	(Prototype Drug Chart 28–1) A: IM: 1 g q6h IV: 1-2 g q6h diluted in NSS C: IM/IV: 100-200 mg/kg/d in 4-6 divided doses	First penicillinase-resistant penicillin. Used to treat staphylococcal infection. *Pregnancy category*: B; PB: 25%-40%; $t^{1/2}$: 0.5-1 h
nafcillin (Nafcin, Unipen)	A: PO: 250 mg-1 g q4-6h IM: 250-500 mg q6h IV: 500 mg-2 g q4-6h C: PO: 25-100 mg/kg/d in 4 divided doses IM: 25 mg/kg b.i.d. IV: 50-300 mg/kg/d in 4-6 divided doses	Highly effective against penicillin G-resistant *Staphylococcus aureus*. Not recommended for oral use because of its instability in gastric juices. *Pregnancy category*: B; PB: 90%; $t^{1/2}$: 0.5-1.5 h
oxacillin sodium (Prostaphlin, Bactocill)	A: PO: 250-1 g q4-6h IM/IV: 500 mg-2 g q4h; *max*: IM/IV: 12 g C: PO/IM/IV: 50-100 mg/kg/d in divided doses IM/IV: 50-150 mg/kg/d in divided doses	For penicillin-resistant staphylococci. As effective as methicillin. *Pregnancy category*: B; PB: 95%; $t^{1/2}$: 0.5-1 h
Extended-Spectrum Penicillins		
carbenicillin indanyl (Geocillin, Geopen)	A: PO: 382-764 mg q6h	The first penicillin-like drug developed to treat infections caused by *Pseudomonas aeruginosa* and *Proteus* spp. Contains large amounts of sodium. Use with caution when administering to clients with hypertension or heart failure. *Pregnancy category*: B; PB: 50%; $t^{1/2}$: 1-1.5 h
mezlocillin sodium (Mezlin)	A: IM/IV: 3-4 g q6h or 100-300 mg/kg/d in 4 divided doses; *max*: 24 g/d C: IM/IV: 50 mg/kg q4h	For serious infections, especially because of *Pseudomonas aeruginosa*. Can be given in combination with aminoglycosides and cephalosporins to obtain synergistic effect. *Pregnancy category*: B; PB: 30%-40%; $t^{1/2}$: 1 h
piperacillin-tazobactam (Zosyn)	A: IV: 3.375 g, q6h over 30 min, 7-10 d Reduce for renal insufficiency	To treat severe appendicitis, skin infections, pneumonia, beta-lactamase-producing bacteria. Tazobactam is a beta-lactamase inhibitor. *Pregnancy category*: B; PB: UK; $t^{1/2}$: 0.7-1.2 h
ticarcillin-clavulanate (Timentin)	A: IV: 3.1 g q6h C: >12 y: IV: 200-300 mg/kg/d in 4-6 divided doses	Clavulanic acid protects ticarcillin from degradation by beta-lactamase enzymes. Effective for treating septicemia and lower respiratory tract, urinary tract, skin, bone, and joint infections. *Pregnancy category*: B; PB: 45%-65%; $t^{1/2}$: 1.1-1.5 h

GI, Gastrointestinal; *max*, maximum; *NSS*, normal saline solution; *y*, year.

Prototype DRUG CHART 28-1

AMOXICILLIN AND DICLOXACILLIN

Drug Class

amoxicillin: Broad-spectrum penicillin
dicloxacillin: Penicillinase-resistant penicillin
Trade names:
amoxicillin: Amoxil, ✦Apo-Amoxi
dicloxacillin: Dynapen, Dycill, Pathocil
Pregnancy Category: B

Dosage

amoxicillin:
A: PO: 250-500 mg q8h
C: PO: 20-40 mg/kg/d in 3 divided doses
dicloxacillin:
A: PO: 125-500 mg q6h
C: PO: 12.5-25 mg/kg/d q6h

Contraindications

amoxicillin/dicloxacillin: Allergic to penicillin
amoxicillin: Severe renal disorder
Caution: amoxicillin/dicloxacillin: Hypersensitivity
   to cephalosporins

Drug-Lab-Food Interactions

Drug: amoxicillin/dicloxacillin: Increase effect with
   aspirin, probenecid; *decrease* effect with tetracycline,
   erythromycin
Lab: Increase serum AST, ALT, BUN, and creatinine
Food: Decrease affect with acidic fruits or juices

Pharmacokinetics

Absorption: PO:
amoxicillin: >80% in intestine
dicloxacillin: 35%-76% in GI tract
Distribution: PB:
amoxicillin: 20%
dicloxacillin: 95%
Metabolism: t½:
amoxicillin: 1-1.5 h
dicloxacillin: 0.5-1 h
Excretion:
amoxicillin: 70% in urine; clavulanate: 30%-40%
   in urine *dicloxacillin:* Excreted in bile and urine

Pharmacodynamics

amoxicillin:
PO: Onset: 0.5 h
   Peak: 1-2 h
   Duration: 6-8 h
dicloxacillin:
PO: Onset: 0.5 h
   Peak: 1 h
   Duration: 4-6 h

Therapeutic Effects/Uses

amoxicillin: To treat respiratory tract infection, urinary tract infection, otitis media, sinusitis
dicloxacillin: To treat *Staphylococcus aureus* infection
Mode of Action: *amoxicillin/dicloxacillin:* Inhibition of the enzyme in cell wall synthesis; bactericidal effect

Side Effects

amoxicillin/dicloxacillin: Nausea, vomiting, diarrhea, rash
amoxicillin: Edema, stomatitis
dicloxacillin: Abdominal pain, flatulence

Adverse Reactions

amoxicillin/dicloxacillin: Superinfections (vaginitis)
Life-threatening: amoxicillin/dicloxacillin: Blood
   dyscrasias, hemolytic anemia, bone marrow
   depression
amoxicillin: Respiratory distress
dicloxacillin: Eosinophilia, liver toxicity

A, Adult; *ALT,* alanine aminotransferase; *AST,* aspartate aminotransferase; *BUN,* blood urea nitrogen; *C,* child; *d,* day; *GI,* gastrointestinal; *h,* hour; *PB,* protein-binding; *PO,* by mouth; *t½,* half-life; *>*greater than; ✦, Canadian drug name.

lactamases, making the antibiotic effective and extending its antimicrobial effect. There are three beta-lactamase inhibitors: clavulanic acid, sulbactam, and tazobactam. These inhibitors are not given alone but combined with a penicillinase-sensitive penicillin such as amoxicillin, ampicillin, piperacillin, or ticarcillin. The combined drugs currently marketed include the following:

• *Oral use:* amoxicillin-clavulanic acid (Augmentin)

• *Parenteral use:* ampicillin-sulbactam (Unasyn), piperacillin-tazobactam (Zosyn), and ticarcillin-clavulanic acid (Timentin)

Pharmacokinetics

Amoxicillin is well absorbed from the GI tract, whereas cloxacillin is only partially absorbed. Protein-binding power differs between the two drugs—amoxicillin is 25% protein-bound and cloxacillin is highly protein-bound (>90%). Drug toxicity may result when other highly protein-bound drugs are used with cloxacillin. Both drugs have short half-lives. Seventy percent of amoxicillin is excreted in the urine; cloxacillin is excreted in bile and urine.

Pharmacodynamics

Both amoxicillin and cloxacillin are penicillin derivatives and are bactericidal. These drugs interfere with bacterial cell-wall synthesis, causing cell lysis. Amoxicillin may be produced with or without clavulanic acid, an agent that prevents the breakdown of amoxicillin by decreasing resistance to the antibacterial drug. The addition of clavulanic acid intensifies the effect of amoxicillin. The amoxicillin-clavulanic acid preparation (Augmentin) and amoxicillin trihydrate (Amoxil) have similar pharmacokinetics and pharmacodynamics, as well as similar side effects and adverse reactions. When aspirin and probenecid are taken with amoxicillin or cloxacillin, the serum antibacterial levels may be increased. The effects of amoxicillin and cloxacillin are decreased when taken with erythromycin and tetracycline. The onset of action, serum peak concentration time, and duration of action for amoxicillin and cloxacillin are very similar.

Geriatrics

Most beta-lactam antibiotics are excreted via the kidneys. With older adults, assessment of renal function is most important. Serum blood urea nitrogen (BUN) and serum creatinine should be monitored. With a decrease in renal function, the antibiotic dose should be decreased.

Side Effects and Adverse Reactions

Common adverse reactions to penicillin administration are hypersensitivity and **superinfection** (occurrence of a secondary infection when the flora of the body is disturbed) (Table 28–2). Nausea, vomiting, and diarrhea are common GI disturbances. Rash is an indicator of a mild to moderate allergic reaction. Severe allergic reaction leads to anaphylactic shock. Clinical manifestations of a severe allergic reaction include laryngeal edema, severe bronchoconstriction with stridor, and hypotension. Allergic effects occur in 5% to 10% of persons receiving penicillin compounds; therefore close monitoring during the first dose and subsequent doses of penicillin is essential.

Drug Interactions

The broad-spectrum penicillins—amoxicillin and ampicillin—may decrease the effectiveness of oral contraceptives. Potassium supplements can increase serum potassium levels when taken with potassium penicillin G or V. When penicillin is mixed with an aminoglycoside in IV solution, the actions of both drugs are inactivated.

Nursing Process

Antibacterials: Penicillins

ASSESSMENT

■ Assess for allergy to penicillin or cephalosporins. Client who is hypersensitive to amoxicillin should not take any type of penicillin products. Severe allergic reaction could occur. A small percentage of clients who are allergic to penicillin could also be allergic to a cephalosporin product.

■ Check laboratory results, especially liver enzymes. Report elevated alkaline phosphatase, alanine aminotransferase, aspartate aminotransferase.

■ Record urine output. If amount is inadequate (<30 ml/h or <600 ml/d), drug or drug dosage may need to be changed.

NURSING DIAGNOSES

■ Risk for infection related to invasion of bacteria through the surgical incision
■ Risk for impaired tissue integrity related to rash
■ Noncompliance with drug regimen related to decreased finances

PLANNING

■ Client's infection will be controlled and later eliminated.

NURSING INTERVENTIONS

■ Send sample (swab, blood, sputum, etc.) to laboratory for culture and antibiotic sensitivity testing of infective organism (also known as *C & S*) before antibiotic therapy is started.
■ Check for signs and symptoms of superinfection, especially in clients taking high doses of the antibiotic for a prolonged time. Signs and symptoms include stomatitis (mouth ulcers), genital discharge (vaginitis), and anal or genital itching.
■ Examine client for allergic reaction to the penicillin product, especially after the first and second doses. This may be a mild reaction, such as a rash, or a severe reaction, such as respiratory distress or anaphylaxis.
■ Have epinephrine available to counteract a severe allergic reaction.
■ Do not mix aminoglycosides with a high-dose or extended-spectrum penicillin G, because this combination may inactivate the aminoglycoside.
■ Check client for bleeding if high doses of penicillin are being given; a decrease in platelet aggregation (clotting) may result.
■ Monitor body temperature and infected area.
■ Dilute the antibiotic for IV use in an appropriate amount of solution as indicated in the drug pamphlet.

Client Teaching

General

• Instruct client to take the *entire* prescribed penicillin product, such as amoxicillin, until the bottle is empty. If only a portion of the penicillin is taken, drug resistance to that antibacterial agent may develop in the future.

- Advise client who is allergic to penicillin to wear a medical alert (MedicAlert) bracelet or necklace and carry a card that indicates the allergy. Client should notify health care provider of any allergy to penicillin when reporting health history.
- Keep drugs out of the reach of small children. Request childproof containers.
- Inform client to report any side effects or adverse reaction that may occur while taking the drug.
- Encourage client to increase fluid intake; fluids aid in decreasing the body temperature and in excreting the drug.
- Instruct client or child's parent that chewable tablets must be chewed or crushed before swallowing.

Diet
- Advise client to take medication with food to avoid gastric irritation.

Cultural Considerations ❖

- Recognize that clients and family members from various cultural backgrounds may have alternative practices for alleviating infections. Accept adjunctive alternative methods if they are not harmful to client. Explain the purpose of the antibiotic.
- If client does not speak English, request a translator to obtain a history of symptoms related to the infection and any allergies to antibiotics.

EVALUATION

- Evaluate the effectiveness of the antibacterial agent by determining whether the infection has ceased and whether any side effects, including superinfection, have occurred.

Cephalosporins

In 1948 a fungus called *Cephalosporium acremonium* was discovered in seawater at a sewer outlet off the coast of Sardinia. This fungus was found to be active against gram-positive and gram-negative bacteria and resistant to beta-lactamase (an enzyme that acts against the beta-lactam structure of penicillin). In the early 1960s cephalosporins were used with clinical effectiveness. For cephalosporins to be effective against numerous organisms, their molecules were chemically altered, and semisynthetic cephalosporins were produced. Like penicillin the cephalosporins have a beta-lactam structure and act by inhibiting the bacterial enzyme necessary for cell wall synthesis. Lysis to the cell occurs, and the bacterial cell dies.

First-, Second-, Third-, and Fourth-Generation Cephalosporins

Cephalosporins are a major antibiotic group used in hospitals and in health care offices. These drugs are bactericidal with actions similar to penicillin. For antibacterial activity, the beta-lactam ring of cephalosporins is necessary.

Four groups of cephalosporins have been developed, identified as *generations*. Each generation is effective against a broader spectrum of bacteria (Table 28–4).

Not all cephalosporins are affected by the beta-lactamases. The first-generation cephalosporins are destroyed by beta-lactamases, but not all of the second generation is affected by beta-lactamases. Third-generation cephalosporins are resistant to beta-lactamases. Most of the third- and fourth-generation cephalosporins (e.g., aztreonam, imipenem-cilastatin) are effective in treating sepsis and many strains of gram-negative bacilli. The cephalosporins ceftazidime and cefepime, along with aztreonam and imipenem-cilastatin, are effective against most strains of *Pseudomonas aeruginosa*. Table 28–5 lists the other unclassified beta-lactam antibiotics.

Approximately 10% of persons allergic to penicillin are also allergic to cephalosporins, because both groups of antibacterials have similar molecular structures. If a client is allergic to penicillin and taking a cephalosporin, the nurse should watch for a possible allergic reaction to the cephalosporin, although the likelihood of a reaction is small.

Only a few cephalosporins are administered orally. These include cephalexin (Keflex), cefadroxil (Duricef), cephradine (Velosef), cefaclor (Ceclor), cefuroxime axetil (Ceftin), cefuroxime sodium (Zinacef), cefdinir (Omnicef), and ceftibuten (Cedax). The rest of the cephalosporins are administered IM and IV. Prototype Drug Chart 28–2 compares the

Table 28–4	
Activity of the Four Generations of Cephalosporins	
Generation	Activity
First	Effective against gram-positive bacteria (streptococci and most staphylococci). Effective against most gram-negative bacteria (*Escherichia coli* and species of *Klebsiella, Proteus, Salmonella,* and *Shigella*).
Second	Same effectiveness as first generation. These antibiotics possess a broader spectrum against other gram-negative bacteria (*Haemophilus influenzae, Neisseria gonorrhoeae, Neisseria meningitidis, Enterobacter* spp., and several anaerobic organisms).
Third	Same effectiveness as first and second generations. Also effective against gram-negative bacteria (*Pseudomonas aeruginosa, Serratia* spp., and *Acinetobacter* spp). Less effective against gram-positive bacteria.
Fourth	Similar to third generation. Resistant to most beta-lactamase bacteria. Broader gram-positive coverage than the third generations. Effective against *E. coli, Klebsiella, Proteus,* streptococci, certain staphylococci, and *P. aeruginosa.*

Table 28–5

Other Beta-Lactam Antibiotics

Generic (Brand)	Route and Dosage	Uses and Considerations
aztreonam (Azactam)	*Severe infections:* A: IM/IV: 1.0-2.0 g q6-8h; *max*: 8 g/d	For treatment of gram-negative infections of the lower respiratory tract, urinary tract, skin, and vagina. Not effective against gram-positive organisms. May be used in combination with other antibiotics. *Pregnancy category*: B; PB: 56%; t½: 1.7-2.1 h
imipenem-cilastatin (Primaxin)	A: IM: 500-750 mg q12h IV: 250 mg-1 g q6-8h C: IV: 15-25 mg/kg q6h	For treatment of septicemia and severe infections of the lower respiratory tract, urinary tract, skin, bones, and joints. Effective against most gram-negative organisms including *Pseudomonas aeruginosa*. *Pregnancy category*: C; PB: 20%; t½: 1 h
meropenem (Merrem)	A: IV: 1-2 g q8h C: >3 mo: 20-40 mg/kg q8h	A carbapenem antibiotic, similar to cephalosporins. Effective against most strains of gram-negative organisms, including *Pseudomonas aeruginosa*, and effective for complicated appendicitis, peritonitis, meningitis, and soft tissue infections. *Pregnancy category*: B; PB: UK; t½: 1 h

A, Adult; *C*, child; *d*, day; *h*, hour; *IM*, intramuscular; *IV*, intravenous; *max*, maximum; *min*, minute; *PB*, protein-binding; *PO*, by mouth; *t½*, half-life; *UK*, unknown; *y*, year; >, greater than.

similarities and differences in a first-generation cephalosporin, cefazolin sodium (Ancef, Kefzol), and a second-generation cephalosporin, cefaclor (Ceclor).

Pharmacokinetics

Cefazolin is administered IM and IV, and cefaclor is given orally. The protein-binding power of cefazolin is greater than that of cefaclor. The half-life of each drug is short, and the drugs are excreted 60% to 80% unchanged in the urine.

Pharmacodynamics

Cefazolin and cefaclor inhibit bacterial cell-wall synthesis and produce a bactericidal action. For IM and IV use of cefazolin, the onset of action is almost immediate, and peak concentration time is 5 to 15 minutes for IV use. The peak concentration time for an oral dose of cefaclor is 30 to 60 minutes.

When probenecid is administered with either of these drugs, urine excretion of cefazolin or cefaclor is decreased, which increases the action of the drug. The effects of cefazolin and cefaclor can be decreased if the drug is given with tetracyclines or erythromycin. These drugs can cause false-positive laboratory results for proteinuria and glucosuria, especially when they are taken in large doses.

Table 28–6 lists the cephalosporins in their designated generation, dosages, and considerations.

Side Effects and Adverse Reactions

The side effects and adverse reactions to cephalosporins include GI disturbances (nausea, vomiting, diarrhea), alteration in blood clotting time (increased bleeding) with administration of large doses, and **nephrotoxicity** (toxicity to the kidney) in individuals with a preexisting renal disorder.

Drug Interactions

Drug interactions can occur with certain cephalosporins and alcohol. For example, alcohol consumption may cause flushing, dizziness, headache, nausea, vomiting, and muscular cramps while taking cefamandole, cefoperazone, or moxalactam. Taking uricosuric drugs concurrently can decrease the excretion of cephalosporins, thereby greatly increasing serum levels. Uricosurics increase the excretion rate of uric acid by inhibiting its reabsorption.

Antibacterials: Cephalosporins

ASSESSMENT

■ Assess for allergy to cephalosporins. If allergic to one type or class of cephalosporin, client should not receive any other type of cephalosporin.

■ Record vital signs and urine output. Report abnormal findings, which may include elevated temperature or decreased urine output.

■ Check laboratory results, especially those that indicate renal and liver function (blood urea nitrogen, serum creatinine, aspartate aminotransferase, alanine aminotransferase, alkaline phosphatase, bilirubin). Report abnormal findings. Use these laboratory results for baseline values.

NURSING DIAGNOSES

■ Risk for impaired tissue integrity related to rash
■ Risk for infection related to invasive procedure
■ Ineffective tissue perfusion: renal related to adverse effects of cefdinir
■ Noncompliance with drug regimen related to lack of knowledge relevant to regimen behavior

PLANNING

■ Client's infection will be controlled and later eliminated.

NURSING INTERVENTIONS

■ Culture the infected area before cephalosporin therapy is started. The organism causing the infection can be determined by culture, and the antibiotics the organism

Prototype DRUG CHART 28–2

CEFAZOLIN AND CEFACLOR

Drug Class

cefazolin: first-generation cephalosporin
cefaclor: second-generation cephalosporin
Trade names:
cefazolin: Ancef, Kefzol
cefaclor: Ceclor
Pregnancy Category: B

Dosage

cefazolin:
A: IM/IV: 250 mg-2 g q6-8h; *max:* 12 g/d
C: IM/IV: 25-100 mg/kg/d in 3 divided doses; *max:* 4 g/d
cefaclor:
A: PO: 250-500 mg q8h; *max:* 4 g/d
C: PO: 20-40 mg/kg/d in 3 divided doses; *max:* 1 g/d

Contraindications

cefazolin/cefaclor: Hypersensitivity to cephalosporins
Caution: cefazolin/cefaclor: Hypersensitivity to
   penicillins; renal disease, lactation

Drug-Lab-Food Interactions

Drug: cefazolin/cefaclor: Increase effect with probenecid; increase toxicity with loop diuretics, aminoglycosides, colistin, vancomycin; *decrease* effect with
   tetracyclines, erythromycin
Lab: May *increase* BUN, serum creatinine, AST, ALT, ALP,
   LDH, bilirubin

Pharmacokinetics

Absorption:
cefazolin: IM, IV
cefaclor: PO: Well absorbed
Distribution: PB:
cefazolin: 75%-85%
cefaclor: 25%
Metabolism: t½:
cefazolin: 1.5-2.5 h
cefaclor: 0.5-1 h
Excretion:
cefazolin: 70% excreted unchanged in urine
cefaclor: 60%-80% excreted unchanged in urine

Pharmacodynamics

cefazolin:
IM: Onset: rapid
   Peak: 0.5-2 h
   Duration: UK
IV: Onset: immediate
   Peak: 5-15 min
   Duration: UK
cefaclor:
PO: Onset: rapid
   Peak: 0.5-1 h
   Duration: UK

Therapeutic Effects/Uses

cefazolin/cefaclor: To treat respiratory, urinary, and skin infections
cefazolin: To treat bone and joint infection, genital infections, and endocarditis
cefaclor: To treat ear infection, ampicillin-resistant strains, and certain gram-negative organisms; *E. coli, Proteus,*
   H. influenzae, and gram-positive strains; *Streptococcus pneumoniae, S. pyogenes,* and *S. aureus*
Mode of Action: Inhibition of cell wall synthesis, causing cell death; bactericidal effect

Side Effects

cefazolin/cefaclor: Anorexia, nausea, vomiting,
   diarrhea, rash
cefazolin: Abdominal cramps, fever
cefaclor: Pruritus, headaches, vertigo, weakness

Adverse Reactions

cefazolin/cefaclor: Superinfections, urticaria
Life-threatening:
cefazolin: Seizures (high doses), anaphylaxis
cefaclor: Renal failure

A, Adult; *ALP,* alkaline phosphatase; *ALT,* alanine aminotransferase; *AST,* aspartate aminotransferase; *BUN,* blood urea nitrogen;
C, child; *d,* day; *h,* hour; *IM,* intramuscular; *IV,* intravenous; *LDH,* lactic dehydrogenase; *max,* maximum; *min,* minute; *PB,* protein-
binding; *PO,* by mouth; *t½,* half-life; *UK,* unknown.

is sensitive to are determined by sensitivity (C & S).
(Antibiotic therapy may be started before culture result
is reported. The antibiotic may need to be changed after
C & S test results are received.)

■ Check for signs and symptoms of a superinfection,
especially if client takes high doses of a cephalosporin
product for a prolonged period. Superinfection is usually caused by the fungal organism *Candida* in the

mouth (mouth ulcers) or in the genital area (vaginitis in
females).

■ Refrigerate oral suspensions. For IV cephalosporins,
dilute in an appropriate amount of IV fluids (50-100
ml) according to the drug pamphlet.

■ Administer IV cephalosporins over 30 to 45 minutes
2 to 4 times a day.

■ Monitor vital signs, urine output, and laboratory results. Report abnormal findings.

Table 28–6

Antibacterials: Cephalosporins

Generic (Brand)	Route and Dosage	Uses and Considerations
First Generation		
cefadroxil (Duricef)	A: PO: 500 mg-2 g/d in 1-2 divided doses C: PO: 30 mg/kg/d in 2 divided doses	To treat urinary tract infections, beta-hemolytic streptococcal infections, and staphylococcal skin infection. Well absorbed by GI tract and not affected by food. *Pregnancy category:* B; PB: 20%; $t^{1}/_{2}$: 1-2 h
cefazolin sodium (Ancef, Kefzol)	A: IM/IV: 250 mg-1 g q6-8h; *max:* 12 g/d C: IM/IV: 25-100 mg/kg/d in 3 divided doses; *max:* 6 g/d	Similar to cephalothin but more effective against *Escherichia coli* and *Klebsiella. Pregnancy category:* B; PB: 75%-85%; $t^{1}/_{2}$: 1.5-2.5 h
cephalexin (Keflex)	*Infection:* A: PO: 250-500 mg q6h C: PO: 25-50 mg/kg/d in 3-4 divided doses *Otitis media:* C: PO: 25-100 mg/kg/d in 4 divided doses	First acid-stable cephalosporin sufficiently absorbed from the GI tract. Useful for treating urinary tract infections. *Pregnancy category:* B; PB: 10%-15%; $t^{1}/_{2}$: 0.5-1.2 h
cephapirin sodium (Cefadyl)	A: IM/IV: 500 mg-1 g q4-6h; *max:* 12 g/d C: IM/IV: 40-80 mg/kg/d in 4 divided doses	Treatment is the same as for cephalothin. *Pregnancy category:* B; PB: 40%-50%; $t^{1}/_{2}$: 0.5-1 h
cephradine (Velosef)	A: PO: 250-500 mg q6h or 500 mg-1 g q12h IM/IV: 500 mg-1 g q6-12h C: PO: 25-50 mg/kg/d in 4 divided doses IM/IV: 50-100 mg/kg/d in 4 divided doses	Treatment is the same as for cephalothin. Oral drug is similar to cephalexin. Well absorbed from GI tract. *Pregnancy category:* B; PB: 20%; $t^{1}/_{2}$: 1-2 h
Second Generation		
cefaclor (Ceclor)	(Prototype Drug Chart 28–2)	
cefmetazole sodium (Zefazone)	A: IV: 1-2 g q6-12h	For treatment of lower respiratory and urinary tract infections. Also used for preoperative prophylaxis for surgery. *Pregnancy category:* B; PB: 68%; $t^{1}/_{2}$: 1.5-3 h
cefonicid sodium (Monocid)	A: IM/IV: 500 mg-2 g/d single dose or b.i.d.	Similar to cefamandole. Also used for surgical prophylaxis. *Pregnancy category:* B; PB: 98%; $t^{1}/_{2}$: 4.5 h
cefotetan (Cefotan)	A: IM/IV: 500 mg-2g q12h C: IM/IV: 40-80 mg/kg/d in 2 divided doses; *max:* 6 g/d	Effective against some gram-negative organisms, except *Pseudomonas aeruginosa. Pregnancy category:* B; PB: 85%; $t^{1}/_{2}$: 3-5 h
cefoxitin sodium (Mefoxin)	A: IM/IV: 1-2 g q6-8h; *max:* 12 g/d C: IM/IV: 80-160 mg/kg/d in divided doses	Used to treat severe infections and septicemia. *Pregnancy category:* B; PB: 70%; $t^{1}/_{2}$: 45 min-1 h
cefprozil monohydrate (Cefzil)	A: PO: 250-500 mg daily or q12h C: PO: 15 mg/kg q12h × 10 d	Effective against gram-positive bacilli including *Staphylococcus aureus.* With impaired renal function, dose is usually decreased by 50%. *Pregnancy category:* B; PB: 99%; $t^{1}/_{2}$: 1-2 h
cefuroxime (Ceftin, Zinacef)	A: PO: 250-500 mg q12h IM/IV: 750 mg-1.5 g q8h C: PO: 125-250 mg q12h IM/IV: 50-100 mg/kg/d in divided doses	Similar to cefamandole. Effective in treating meningitis and septicemia and for cardiothoracic procedures and surgical prophylaxis. *Pregnancy category:* B; PB: 50%; $t^{1}/_{2}$: 1.5-2 h
Third Generation		
cefdinir (Omnicef)	A: PO: 300 mg q12h or 600 mg/d C: PO: 7 mg/kg q12h or 14 mg/kg/d Preferred: q12h dosing because of short $t^{1}/_{2}$	New third-generation cephalosporin. To treat otitis media, acute sinusitis, chronic bronchitis, pharyngitis/tonsillitis, pneumonia, and skin infections. Active for *Haemophilus influenzae, Streptococcus pyogenes, Neisseria gonorrhoeae,* and many strains of enteric gram-negative bacilli. Not active for *P. aeruginosa, Enterococcus, Legionella, Chlamydia. Pregnancy category:* B; PB: 60%-70%; $t^{1}/_{2}$: 1.7 h
cefoperazone (Cefobid)	A: IM/IV: 2-4 g/d in 2 divided doses C: IV: 25-100 mg/kg q12h	To treat respiratory, urinary tract, and female genital tract infections. Most effective against *Pseudomonas. Pregnancy category:* B; PB: 70%-80%; $t^{1}/_{2}$: 2.5 h

A, Adult; *b.i.d.,* two times a day; *C,* child; *d,* day; *GI,* gastrointestinal; *h,* hour; *IM,* intramuscularly; *IV,* intravenously; *PB,* protein-binding; *PO,* by mouth; $t^{1}/_{2}$, half-life.

Table 28–6

Antibacterials: Cephalosporins—cont'd

Generic (Brand)	Route and Dosage	Uses and Considerations
cefotaxime (Claforan)	A: IM/IV: 1-2 g q8-12h C: IM/IV: 50-200 mg/kg/d in 4-6 divided doses *Life-threatening infection:* 2 g q4	First of the third generation. Effective against *P. aeruginosa*. Also used in treating gram-negative meningitis. *Pregnancy category:* B; PB: 30%-40%; t$^{1}/_{2}$: 1-1.5 h
cefpodoxime (Vantin)	A: PO: 200 mg q12h × 1-2 wk C: 6 mo-12 y: PO: 10 mg/kg/d in 2 divided doses	To treat otitis media and respiratory and urinary tract infection. Food enhances drug absorption. *Pregnancy category:* B; PB: 20%-40%; t$^{1}/_{2}$: 2-3 h
ceftazidime (Fortaz, Tazicef)	A: IM/IV: 500 mg-2 g q8-12h C: IV: 30-50 mg/kg q8h; *max:* 6 g/d	Most effective against *Pseudomonas* spp. *Pregnancy category:* B; PB: 10%-17%; t$^{1}/_{2}$: 1-2 h
ceftriaxone (Rocephin)	A: IM/IV: 500 mg-2 g in single dose or q12h; *max:* 4 g/d C: IM/IV: 50-75 mg/kg/d in 2 divided doses	Similar to ceftizoxime and cefotaxime. Has a very long half-life, so is given once or twice a day. Used against Neisseria and gonococcal infections and in the treatment of Lyme disease. *Pregnancy category:* B; PB: 85%-95%; t$^{1}/_{2}$: 8 h
ceftizoxime sodium (Cefizox)	A: IM/IV: 500 mg-2 g q8-12h C: IV: 50 mg/kg q6-8h; *max:* 200 mg/kg/d	For treatment of respiratory, urinary tract, skin, bone, and joint infections. For surgical prophylaxis. *Pregnancy category:* B; PB: 30%-60%; t$^{1}/_{2}$: 2 h
ceftibuten (Cedax)	A: PO: 400 mg/d × 10 d (for renal insufficiency, reduced dose) C: (6 mo-12 yr): PO: 9 mg/kg/d × 10d; *max:* 400 mg/d	Treatment for chronic bronchitis, pharyngitis, and tonsillitis. Active against gram-positive and gram-negative bacteria, *H. influenzae, Streptococcus pneumoniae,* and *Streptococcus pyogenes.* Poor activity against staphylococci and pneumococci. *Pregnancy category:* B; PB: UK; t$^{1}/_{2}$: 1.5-3 h
moxalactam disodium (Moxam)	A: IM/IV: 2-6 g/d in 2-3 divided doses; *max:* 4 g q8h C: IM/IV: 50 mg/kg q6-8h	For lower respiratory, urinary tract, bone, and joint infection. Also for septicemia and meningitis. Less active against gram-positive cocci, *S. aureus,* and streptococci. Active against *E. coli, Klebsiella pneumoniae,* and *Serratia.* Variable activity for *P. aeruginosa.* Can be used with an aminoglycoside. *Pregnancy category:* C; PB: UK; t$^{1}/_{2}$: 2-3.5 h
cefditoren pivoxil (Spectracef)	A: PO: 200-400 mg b.i.d. for 10 d	For chronic bronchitis, pharyngitis, tonsillitis, skin infections and other mild to moderate bacterial infections. *Pregnancy category:* B; PB: 88%; t$^{1}/_{2}$: 1.6 h
Fourth Generation		
cefepime (Maxipime)	A: IM/IV: 0.5-1g q12h *Severe infection:* A: IV: 2 g q12h × 10 d	Similar to third-generation cephalosporins. Resistant to most beta-lactamase bacteria. Effective against pneumonia, *E. coli, Klebsiella, Proteus,* streptococci, certain staphylococci, and *P. aeruginosa.* Has a broader gram-positive coverage than the third-generation cephalosporins. *Pregnancy category:* B; PB: UK; t$^{1}/_{2}$: 2 h

UK, Unknown.

Client Teaching

General

- Keep drugs out of reach of small children. Request childproof containers.
- Instruct client to report signs of superinfection, such as mouth ulcers or discharge from the anal or genital area.
- Advise client to ingest buttermilk or yogurt to prevent superinfection of the intestinal flora with long-term use of a cephalosporin.
- Instruct client to take the complete course of medication, even when symptoms of infection have ceased.
- Infuse all IV cephalosporins over 30 minutes or as ordered to prevent pain and irritation.
- Observe for hypersensitivity reactions.

Side Effects

- Instruct client to report any side effects from use of oral cephalosporin drugs; these may include anorexia, nausea, vomiting, headache, dizziness, itching, and rash.

Diet
- Advise client to take medication with food if gastric irritation occurs.

Cultural Considerations ❖

- Failing to allow adequate time for information processing may result in an inaccurate response or no response. Allow time for people to respond to questions, especially for those who have language barriers. Speak clearly and slowly, giving time for translation. Obtain an interpreter if necessary.

EVALUATION

- Evaluate the effectiveness of the cephalosporin by determining if the infection has ceased and no side effects, including superinfection, have occurred.

KEY WEBSITES

Oral Ampicillin: http://www.nlm.nih.gov/medlineplus/druginfo/medmaster/a685002.html

Management of Patients Who Have a History of Penicillin Allergy: http://www.cdc.gov/std/treatment/2006/penicillin-allergy.htm

Site of b-lactamase attack in penicillins and cephalosporins: http://www.ncbi.nlm.nih.gov/books/bv.fcgi?call=bv.View..ShowTOC&rid=mmed.TOC&depth=1

Critical Thinking Case Study

SA, age 6, has otitis media. The health care provider ordered amoxicillin 250 mg every 8 hours. The nurse asks SA's mother if SA is allergic to any drugs, and her mother says she is allergic to penicillin.

1. What are the similarities and differences in penicillin and amoxicillin? Explain.
2. What nursing action should the nurse take? Why?

The health care provider changed the amoxicillin order to cefaclor (Ceclor) 250 mg every 8 hours. The therapeutic dosage for children is 20 to 40 mg/kg/d in three divided doses. SA weighs 40 pounds.

3. What are the similarities and differences in amoxicillin and cefaclor? Explain.
4. Is the prescribed cefaclor dosage for SA within safe parameters? Explain.
5. Explain the significance of the nurse asking about allergies to antibiotics such as penicillin. What is the relationship of penicillin and cefaclor in regard to allergies?
6. What should the nurse include in client teaching for SA and her mother?

NCLEX Study Questions

1. A client is receiving amoxicillin (Amoxil). The nurse knows that the action of this drug is by:
   a. inhibition of protein synthesis
   b. alteration of membrane permeability
   c. inhibition of bacterial cell-wall synthesis
   d. alteration of synthesis of bacterial ribonucleic acid

2. The nurse knows that amoxicillin (Amoxil) is a penicillin. Knowledgeable about the different groups of penicillins, the nurse realizes that amoxicillin is in the _____ group.
   a. beta-lactamase inhibitor
   b. broad-spectrum penicillin
   c. extended-spectrum penicillin
   d. penicillinase-resistant penicillin

3. Side effects/adverse reactions of penicillins include:
   a. seizures
   b. renal failure
   c. hypertension
   d. hemolytic anemia

4. A client is taking cefoperazone (Cefobid), which is a:
   a. first-generation cephalosporin
   b. second-generation cephalosporin
   c. third-generation cephalosporin
   d. fourth-generation cephalosporin

5. Which of the following is true regarding cefaclor (Ceclor)?
   a. Normal adult dose is 2 grams q6h
   b. A common side effect is hypotension
   c. Used to treat respiratory infection.
   d. Route of administration is intramuscularly

Answers: 1, c; 2, b; 3, d; 4, c; 5, c.

29

Macrolides, Tetracyclines, Aminoglycosides, and Fluoroquinolones

ELECTRONIC RESOURCES

Evolve website (http://evolve.elsevier.com/KeeHayes/pharmacology/):
- *Case Studies*
- *Content Updates*
- *Frequently Asked Questions*
- *Student Review Activities*
- *WebLinks*
- *Additional Reference Material*

Companion CD-ROM:
- *NCLEX Examination Review Questions*
- *Pharmacology Animations*
- *IV Therapy Checklists*
- *Medication Error Checklists*
- *Drug Calculation Problems*
- *Electronic Calculators*
- *Top 200 Drugs with Pronunciations*
- *References from the Textbook*

Objectives

- Describe the pharmacokinetics and pharmacodynamics of erythromycin.
- Apply the nursing process for tetracyclines, including client teaching.
- Summarize the nurse's role in detecting ototoxicity and nephrotoxicity associated with the administration of aminoglycosides.
- Discuss the reasons for ordering serum aminoglycosides for peak and trough concentration levels.
- Write a teaching plan to include the mechanism for action of fluoroquinolones (quinolones).
- Contrast the nursing interventions for each of the drug categories: macrolides, tetracyclines, aminoglycosides, and fluoroquinolones.

Terms

bactericidal, p. 438
bacteriostatic, p. 438
hepatotoxicity, p. 438
nephrotoxicity, p. 443
ototoxicity, p. 442
pathogen, p. 438
photosensitivity, p. 443
superinfection, p. 443

The groups of antibacterials discussed in this chapter include macrolides (erythromycin, clarithromycin, azithromycin, dirithromycin), lincosamides, vancomycin, ketolides, tetracyclines, glycylcyclines, aminoglycosides, fluoroquinolones (quinolones), and lipopeptides. The macrolides, lincosamides, and tetracyclines are primarily **bacteriostatic** (inhibit bacterial growth) drugs and may be **bactericidal** (kill bacteria), depending on the drug dose or **pathogen** (microorganism capable of producing disease). Vancomycin, aminoglycosides, and fluoroquinolones are bactericidal drugs.

Macrolides, Lincosamides, Vancomycin, and Ketolides

These four groups of drugs are discussed together, because they have spectrums of antibiotic effectiveness similar to penicillin, although they differ in structure. Drugs from these groups are used as penicillin substitutes, especially in individuals who are allergic to penicillin. Erythromycin is the drug frequently prescribed if the client has a hypersensitivity to penicillin.

Macrolides

Macrolides, including azithromycin (Zithromax), clarithromycin (Biaxin), and erythromycin (E-Mycin), are called *broad-spectrum antibiotics*, reflecting their large size. Erythromycin, the first macrolide, was derived from the funguslike bacteria *Streptomyces erythreus* and was first introduced in the early 1950s. Macrolides bind to the 50S ribosomal subunits and inhibit protein synthesis. At low to moderate drug doses, macrolides have a bacteriostatic effect, and with high drug doses, their effect is bactericidal. Macrolides can be administered orally or intravenously (IV) but not intramuscularly (IM), because it is too painful. Administration of IV macrolides should be infused slowly to avoid unnecessary pain (phlebitis).

Gastric acid destroys erythromycin in the stomach; therefore acid-resistant salts are added to erythromycin (e.g., ethylsuccinate, stearate, estolate) to decrease dissolution (breakdown in small particles) in the stomach. This allows the drug to be absorbed in the intestine. Normally food does not hamper the absorption of acid-resistant macrolides. Table 29–1 lists the dosages, uses, and considerations of macrolides.

Macrolides are active against most gram-positive bacteria and moderately active against some gram-negative bacteria. Resistant organisms may emerge during treatment. Macrolides are used to treat mild to moderate infections of the respiratory tract, sinuses, gastrointestinal tract (GI), skin and soft tissue, and diphtheria, impetigo contagiosa, and sexually transmitted diseases (STDs).

Erythromycin is the drug of choice for the treatment of mycoplasmal pneumonia and Legionnaire's disease. The first macrolide developed after the introduction of erythromycin was clarithromycin (Biaxin), which has been effec-

tive against many bacterial infections. Biaxin XL is clarithromycin in a once-a-day extended-release tablet to be taken for 7 days. Azithromycin is frequently prescribed for upper and lower respiratory infections, STDs, and uncomplicated skin infections (Figure 29–1). Table 29–1 lists the drugs developed from the derivatives of erythromycin. Prototype Drug Chart 29–1 details the pharmacologic behavior of azithromycin.

Pharmacokinetics

Clarithromycin and erythromycin are readily absorbed from the GI tract, mainly by the duodenum. Azithromycin is incompletely absorbed from the GI tract, and only 37% reaches systemic circulation. Azithromycin and erythromycin are available IV, but intermittent infusions should be diluted in normal saline (NS) or in dextrose 5% in water (D_5W) to prevent phlebitis or burning sensations at the injection site. Azithromycin 500 mg should be diluted in 250 to 500 ml of fluid and erythromycin lactobionate 1 g should be diluted in 100 to 200 ml. Macrolides are excreted in bile, feces, and urine. Because only a small amount is excreted in urine, renal insufficiency is not a contraindication for macrolide use.

Pharmacodynamics

Macrolides suppress bacterial protein synthesis. The onset of action of oral preparations of erythromycin is 1 hour, peak concentration time is 4 hours, and duration of action is 6 hours. New macrolides have a longer half-life and are administered less frequently. Clarithromycin is administered twice a day. Azithromycin (Zithromax) has up to 40- to 68-hours half-life and is prescribed to be taken only once a day for 5 days.

Side Effects and Adverse Reactions

Side effects and adverse reactions to macrolides include GI disturbances such as nausea, vomiting, diarrhea, and abdominal cramping. Allergic reactions to erythromycin are rare. **Hepatotoxicity** (liver toxicity) can occur when erythromycin and azithromycin are taken in high doses with other hepatotoxic drugs, such as acetaminophen (high doses), phenothiazines, and sulfonamides. Erythromycin estolate (Ilosone) appears to have more toxic effects on the liver than the other erythromycins. Liver damage is usually

FIGURE 29–1 The pharmacist discusses the use of azithromycin with the family of an 8-year-old child for whom it was prescribed. What would be the recommended dosage for this child?

Table 29–1

Antibacterials: Macrolides, Lincosamides, Vancomycin, Ketolides, and Lipopeptide

Generic (Brand)	Route and Dosage	Uses and Considerations
Macrolides		
azithromycin (Zithromax)	(Prototype Drug Chart 29–1)	
clarithromycin (Biaxin)	A: PO: 250-500 mg q12h × 7-14 d C: PO: 7.5 mg/kg/d in 2 divided doses	For treatment of upper and lower respiratory infections, skin and soft tissue infections, *Helicobacter pylori* and mycobacterial species, and gram-positive and negative organisms. Report persistent diarrhea. *Pregnancy category*: C; PB: 65%-75%; t½: 3-6 h
erythromycin base (E-Mycin, Ilotycin); erythromycin estolate (Ilosone); erythromycin ethylsuccinate (E.E.S., E-Mycin E, Pediamycin)	A: PO: 250-500 mg q6h C: PO: 30-100 mg/kg/d A, Elderly, & C: IV: 15-20 mg/kg/d; *max*: 4 g/d	For treatment of moderate to severe infections (e.g., pneumococcal pneumonia, acute pelvic inflammatory disease, intestinal amebiasis, Legionnaires' disease, chlamydial infections). Report persistent diarrhea.
erythromycin lactobionate (Erythrocin Lactobionate IV) erythromycin stearate (Erythrocin)		For IV administration. Drug should not be dissolved in solution that contains preservative. *Pregnancy category*: B; PB: 65%; t½: PO: 1-2 h; IV: 3-5 h
Lincosamides		
clindamycin HCl (Cleocin)	A: PO: 150-450 mg q6-8h; *max*: 1800 mg/d	For serious infections. Available in capsule form. Should be taken with full glass of water. Not affected by food. *Pregnancy category*: B; PB: 94%; t½: 2-3 h
clindamycin palmitate (Cleocin Pediatric)	C: PO: 25-40 mg/kg/d in 3-4 divided doses	Available in suspension for children and older adults. *Pregnancy category*: B; PB: 94%; t½: 2-3 h
clindamycin phosphate (Cleocin Phosphate)	A: IM/IV: 300-900 mg q6-8 h; *max*: 2700 mg/d C: IM/IV: 20-30 mg/kg/d in 3-4 divided doses	For treatment of serious infections, such as septicemia, caused by gram-negative organism. Not to be given as a bolus. *Pregnancy category*: B; PB: 94%; t½: 2-3 h
lincomycin (Lincocin)	A: PO: 500 mg q6-8h; *max*: 8 g/d IM: 600 mg daily-q12h IV: 600 mg-1 g q8-12h; dilute in 100 ml of IV fluids C: PO: 30-60 mg/kg/d in 3-4 divided doses IV: 10-20 mg/kg/d in 2-3 divided doses, dilute in IV fluids	In most situations, this drug has been replaced by clindamycin. *Pregnancy category*: B; PB: 70%-75%; t½: 4-6 h
Vancomycin		
vancomycin HCl (Vancocin)	A: IV: 500 mg q6h or 1 g q12h C: IV: 40 mg/kg/d in 4 divided doses; dilute in IV fluids; run for 1-1.5 h	For *S. aureus*-resistant infections and cardiac surgical prophylaxis in clients with penicillin allergy. Adverse reactions include possible ototoxicity, nephrotoxicity, vascular collapse. *Pregnancy category*: C; PB: 10%; t½: 5-11 h
Ketolides		
telithromycin (Ketek)	A: PO: 400 mg twice daily	To treat acute chronic bronchitis, acute bacterial sinusitis, community-acquired pneumonia. *Pregnancy category*: UK; PB: 60%-70%; t½: 10 h
Lipopeptides		
daptomycin (Cubicin)	A: IV: 4 mg/kg/d for 7-14 days	To treat complicated skin and skin structure infections. *Pregnancy category*: B; PB: 92%; t½: 8 h

A, Adult; *C*, child; *d*, day; *h*, hour; *IM*, intramuscular; *IV*, intravenous; *maint*, maintenance; *max*, maximum; *mo*, month; *PB*, protein-binding; *PO*, by mouth; *t½*, half-life; *UK*, unknown; *y*, year.

Prototype DRUG CHART 29–1

AZITHROMYCIN

Drug Class	**Dosage**
Antibacterial macrolide Trade names: Zithromax, AzaSite *Pregnancy Category:* B	**A: PO:** 250-500 mg daily **IV:** 500 mg daily **C: PO:** 5-10 mg/kg/d

Contraindications	**Drug-Lab-Food Interactions**
Hypersensitivity *Caution:* Hepatic dysfunction, lactation, renal dysfunction	***Drug:*** *Increase* effect of digoxin, carbamazepine, theophylline, cyclosporine, warfarin, triazolam; *decrease* effect of penicillins, clindamycin

Pharmacokinetics	**Pharmacodynamics**

Absorption: PO: 37% absorbed
Distribution: PB: 51%
Metabolism: t½: 68 h
Excretion: In bile and small amount in urine
	PO: Onset: 1 h
	  Peak: 2.5-5 h
	  Duration: 24 h
	IV: Onset: UK
	  Peak: UK
	  Duration: UK

Therapeutic Effects/Uses

To treat gram-positive and some gram-negative organisms; for clients who are allergic to penicillin; to treat respiratory infections, gonorrhea, and skin infections. AzaSite is given for bacterial conjunctivitis.
Mode of Action: Inhibition of the steps of protein synthesis; bacteriostatic or bactericidal effect

Side Effects	**Adverse Reactions**
Anorexia, nausea, vomiting, diarrhea, tinnitus, abdominal cramps, pruritus, rash	Superinfections, vaginitis, urticaria, stomatitis, hearing loss ***Life-threatening:*** Hepatotoxicity, anaphylaxis

A, Adult; *C,* child; *d,* day; *h,* hour; *IV,* intravenous; *PB,* protein-binding; *PO,* by mouth; *t½,* half-life; *UK,* unknown.

---

reversible when the drug is discontinued. Erythromycin should not be taken with clindamycin or lincomycin because they compete for receptor sites.

Drug Interactions

Macrolides can increase serum levels of theophylline (bronchodilator), carbamazepine (anticonvulsant), and warfarin (anticoagulant). If these drugs are given with macrolides, their drug serum levels should be closely monitored. To avoid severe toxic effects, erythromycin should not be used with other macrolides. Azithromycin peak levels may be reduced by antacids when taken at the same time.

Extended Macrolide Group

New derivatives of erythromycin have been effective in the treatment of numerous organisms. Like erythromycin, they inhibit protein synthesis. Many of these macrolides have a longer half-life and are administered once a day. The first extended macrolide group developed after the introduction of erythromycin was clarithromycin (Biaxin), which has been effective against many bacterial infections. Clarithromycin is administered twice a day. Another extended macrolide is azithromycin (Zithromax). This drug has a long half-life —up to 40 to 68 hours—therefore it is only prescribed once a day for 5 days.

Elimination of these drugs is via bile and feces. Azithromycin is frequently prescribed for upper and lower respiratory infections, STDs, and uncomplicated skin infections.

When erythromycin is given concurrently with verapamil (Verelan, Isoptin), diltiazem (Cardizem), clarithromycin (Biaxin), fluconazole (Diflucan), ketoconazole (Nizoral), and itraconazole (Sporanox), erythromycin blood concentration and the risk of sudden cardiac death increase (Figure 29–1). Table 29–1 lists the drugs developed from the derivatives of erythromycin.

Common side effects of clarithromycin are nausea, diarrhea, and abdominal discomfort. With azithromycin, the side effects of nausea, diarrhea, and abdominal pain are uncommon.

 Nursing Process

Antibacterials: Macrolides

ASSESSMENT

■ Assess vital signs and urine output. Report abnormal findings.

■ Check laboratory tests (liver enzyme values) to determine liver function. Liver enzyme tests should be periodically ordered for clients taking large doses of azithromycin for a continuous period.

■ Obtain a history of drugs client currently takes. The peak level of azithromycin may be decreased by antacids.

NURSING DIAGNOSES

■ Risk for infection related to invasion of bacteria through broken skin

■ Risk for impaired tissue integrity related to azithromycin side effects

PLANNING

■ Client's infection will be controlled and later eliminated.

NURSING INTERVENTIONS

■ Obtain a sample from infected area and send to laboratory for culture and sensitivity (C & S) test before starting azithromycin therapy. Antibiotic can be initiated after obtaining culture sample.

■ Monitor vital signs, urine output, and laboratory values, especially liver enzymes: alkaline phosphatase, alanine aminotransferase, aspartate aminotransferase, and bilirubin.

■ Monitor client for liver damage resulting from prolonged use and high dosage of macrolides such as azithromycin. Signs of liver dysfunction include elevated liver enzyme levels and jaundice.

■ Administer oral azithromycin 1 hour before or 2 hours after meals. Give with a full glass of water and *not* fruit juice. Give the drug with food if GI upset occurs. Chewable tablets should be chewed and not swallowed whole.

■ For IV azithromycin, dilute in an appropriate amount of solution as indicated in the drug circular.

■ Administer antacids either 2 hours before or 2 hours after azithromycin.

Client Teaching

General

• Instruct client to take the full course of antibacterial agent as prescribed. Drug compliance is most important for all antibacterials (antibiotics).

Side Effects

• Instruct client to report side effects, including adverse reactions. Encourage client to report nausea, vomiting, diarrhea, abdominal cramps, and itching. **Superinfection** (a secondary infection resulting from drug therapy) such as stomatitis or vaginitis may occur.

• Instruct client to report onset of loose stools or diarrhea. Pseudomembranous colitis should be ruled out.

Cultural Considerations ❖

• Recognize that client and family members from various cultural backgrounds may need a written drug schedule as to when the drug should be taken. Have instructions available in the language client speaks or reads most easily, and emphasize reporting possible side effects to health care provider.

EVALUATION

■ Evaluate the effectiveness of azithromycin by determining whether the infection has been controlled or has ceased and that no side effects, including superinfection, have occurred.

Lincosamides

Like erythromycin, lincosamides inhibit bacterial protein synthesis and have both bacteriostatic and bactericidal actions, depending on drug dosage. Clindamycin (Cleocin) and lincomycin (Lincocin) are examples of lincosamides. Clindamycin is more widely prescribed than lincomycin, because it is active against most gram-positive organisms, including *Staphylococcus aureus* and anaerobic organisms. It is not effective against gram-negative bacteria (e.g., *Escherichia coli*, *Proteus*, and *Pseudomonas*). Clindamycin is absorbed better than lincomycin through the GI tract and maintains a higher serum drug concentration. Clindamycin is considered more effective than lincomycin and has fewer toxic effects. Table 29–1 lists the lincosamides.

Side Effects and Adverse Reactions

Side effects and adverse reactions to clindamycin and lincomycin include GI irritation, which may manifest as nausea, vomiting, and stomatitis. Rash may also occur. Severe adverse reactions include colitis and anaphylactic shock.

Drug Interactions

Clindamycin and lincomycin are incompatible with aminophylline, phenytoin (Dilantin), barbiturates, and ampicillin.

Vancomycin

Vancomycin (Vancocin), a glycopeptide bactericidal antibiotic, was widely used in the 1950s to treat staphylococcal infections. Vancomycin is used against drug-resistant *S. aureus* and in cardiac surgical prophylaxis for individuals with penicillin allergies. Serum vancomycin levels should be monitored.

Vancomycin has become ineffective for treating enterococci. Quinupristin/dalfopristin is a combined antibacterial used to treat life-threatening vancomycin-resistant enterococci (VRE) infections. Antibiotic-resistant enterococci can cause staphylococcal endocarditis.

Pharmacokinetics

Vancomycin is given orally for treatment of staphylococcal enterocolitis and antibiotic-associated pseudomembranous colitis due to *Clostridium difficile*. When vancomycin is given orally, it is not absorbed systemically and is excreted in the feces. Vancomycin is given IV for severe infections due to MRSA, septicemia, bone, skin, and lower respiratory tract infections that do not respond or are resistant to other antibiotics. Intermittent vancomycin doses should be diluted in 250 ml of D_5W, NS, or RL and administered at a rate of 10 mg/minute. Vancomycin is excreted in the urine when given IV. It is 30% protein-bound, and the half-life is 6 hours.

Pharmacodynamics

Vancomycin inhibits bacterial cell wall synthesis and is active against several gram-positive microorganisms. The peak action is 30 minutes after the end of the infusion.

Side Effects and Adverse Reactions

Vancomycin may cause nephrotoxicity and ototoxicity. **Ototoxicity** results in damage to the auditory or vestibular branch of cranial nerve VIII. Such damage can result in permanent hearing loss (auditory branch) or temporary or permanent loss of balance (vestibular branch). Side effects may include chills, dizziness, fever, rashes, nausea, vomiting, and thrombophlebitis at the injection site. Too rapid IV injection of vancomycin can cause a condition known as *red man syndrome* or *red neck syndrome*. Characterized by red blotching of the face, neck, and chest, this is a toxic effect rather than an allergic reaction. Severe hypotension, tachycardia, generalized tingling, and, rarely, cardiac arrest are also adverse reactions. Other adverse effects include eosinophilia, neutropenia, and Stevens-Johnson syndrome.

Drug Interactions

Dimenhydrinate (Dramamine), when taken with vancomycin, can mask ototoxicity. The risk of nephrotoxicity and ototoxicity may be potentiated when vancomycin is given with furosemide, aminoglycosides, amphotericin B, colistin, cisplatin, and cyclosporine. Vancomycin may inhibit methotrexate excretion and increase methotrexate toxicity. The absorption of oral vancomycin may be decreased when given with cholestyramine and colestipol.

Ketolides

Ketolides are a new classification of antibiotics, structurally related to macrolides. The first drug in this class is telithromycin (Ketek) used for adults 18 years and older to treat acute chronic bronchitis, acute bacterial sinusitis, and community-acquired pneumonia. These disorders are usually caused by *Streptococcus pneumoniae* and *Haemophilus influenza*.

Pharmacokinetics

Telithromycin is given orally and is well absorbed by the GI tract and not affected by food intake. Telithromycin is excreted in the feces and urine. It is 60% to 70% protein bound and the half-life is 10 hours.

Pharmacodynamics

Telithromycin blocks protein synthesis in microorganisms. The peak action is 1 hour.

Side Effects and Adverse Reactions

Side effects and adverse reactions to telithromycin include visual disturbances, stomatitis, glossitis, gastritis, nausea, vomiting, abdominal distention, flatulence, oral and vaginal candidiasis, constipation, and watery stools. Telithromycin may also lead to an exacerbation of myasthenia gravis.

Drug Interactions

When telithromycin is taken concurrently with antilipidemics (simvastatin, lovastatin, and atorvastatin), class 1A or class III antidysrhythmics, cisapride, or midazolam, the risk of adverse effects are increased. Blood levels of telithromycin are decreased when taken with rifampin, phenytoin, carbamazepine, or phenobarbital, producing a subtherapeutic level. Concurrent use of ketolides (telithromycin) with ergot alkaloid derivatives or macrolides may lead to acute ergot toxicity (severe peripheral vasospasm and impaired sensation).

Tetracyclines

Tetracyclines, isolated from *Streptomyces aureofaciens* in 1948, were the first broad-spectrum antibiotics effective against gram-positive and gram-negative bacteria and many other organisms—mycobacteria, rickettsiae, spirochetes, and chlamydiae, to name a few. Tetracyclines act by inhibiting bacterial protein synthesis and have a bacteriostatic effect.

Tetracyclines are not effective against S. *aureus* (except for the newer tetracyclines), *Pseudomonas*, or *Proteus*. They can be used against *Mycoplasma pneumoniae*. Tetracycline in combination with metronidazole and bismuth subsalicylate is useful in treating *Helicobacter pylori*, a bacterium in the stomach that can cause a peptic ulcer. For years oral and topical tetracycline has been used to treat severe acne vulgaris. Low doses are usually prescribed to minimize the toxic effect of the drug.

Continuous use of tetracyclines has resulted in bacterial resistance to the drugs. Tetracycline resistance has increased in the treatment of pneumococcal and gonococcal infections; therefore tetracyclines are not as useful in treating these infections.

The tetracyclines are frequently prescribed for oral use, although they are also available for IM and IV use (Prototype Drug Chart 29–2). Because IM administration of tetracycline causes pain on injection and tissue irritation, this route of administration is seldom used. The IV route is used to treat severe infections. The newer oral preparations of tetracyclines, doxycycline, minocycline, and methacycline, are more rapidly and completely absorbed. Tetracyclines should not be taken with magnesium and aluminum antacid preparations, milk products containing calcium, or iron-containing drugs, because these substances bind with tetracycline and prevent absorption of the drug. It is suggested that tetracyclines, except for doxycycline and minocycline, be taken on an empty stomach 1

Prototype DRUG CHART 29–2

DOXYCYCLINE

Drug Class

Antibacterial: Tetracycline
Trade names: Adoxa, Doryx, Doxy, Doxycin,
 Vibramycin, Vibra-Tabs, Oracea
Pregnancy Category: D

Contraindications

Hypersensitivity, pregnancy, severe hepatic or
 renal disease
Caution: History of allergies, renal and hepatic
 dysfunction, alcoholism, hypokalemia, antidysrhythmics, significant bradycardia

Dosage

Systemic infection:
A: PO: 100 mg q12h, IV:100-200 mg q24h
C: >8 y: PO: 4.4 mg/kg/d in 1-2 divided doses
C: >8 y: IV: 4.4 mg/kg/d daily or b.i.d.

Drug-Lab-Food Interactions

Drug: May *increase* effects of digoxin; *decrease*
 doxycycline absorption with antacids, iron, and zinc;
 decrease effects of oral contraceptives; may alter
 lithium levels
Lab: *Decrease* serum potassium level
Food: Dairy products (milk, cheese) *decrease* effect

Pharmacokinetics

Absorption: PO: 100% absorbed
Distribution: PB: 25%-93%
Metabolism: t½: 14-24 h
Excretion: Unchanged in the urine

Pharmacodynamics

PO: Onset: 1-2 h
 Peak: 2-4 h
 Duration: 12 h
IV: Onset: Rapid
 Peak: 0.5-1 h
 Duration: 12 h

Therapeutic Effects/Uses

To treat infections caused by uncommon gram-positive and gram-negative organisms, respiratory and skin infections
 or disorders, chlamydial infection, gonorrhea, syphilis, rickettsial infection, and inflammatory papules and pustules associated with rosacea in adults
Mode of Action: Inhibition of the steps of protein synthesis; bacteriostatic or bactericidal

Side Effects

Nausea, vomiting, diarrhea, rash, flatulence,
 abdominal discomfort, headache, photosensitivity,
 pruritus, epigastric distress, heartburn

Adverse Reactions

Superinfections (candidiasis)
Life-threatening: Blood dyscrasias, hepatotoxicity,
 nephrotoxicity, intracranial hypertension, pseudomembranous colitis, CNS toxicity

A, Adult; *b.i.d.,* twice a day; *C,* child; *CNS,* central nervous system; *d,* day; *h,* hour; *IV,* intravenous; *PB,* protein binding; *PO,* by
mouth; *t½,* half life; *y,* year.

hour before or 2 hours after mealtime. The absorption of doxycycline and minocycline is improved with food ingestion. Table 29–2 describes the tetracycline preparations and their dosages, uses, and considerations. The tetracyclines are listed according to short-acting, intermediate-acting, and long-acting.

Although tetracyclines are widely used, they have numerous side effects, adverse reactions, toxicities, and drug interactions.

Side Effects and Adverse Reactions

GI disturbances such as nausea, vomiting, and diarrhea are side effects of tetracyclines. **Photosensitivity** (sunburn reaction) may occur in persons taking tetracyclines, especially demeclocycline (Declomycin). Pregnant women should not take tetracycline during the first trimester of pregnancy because of possible teratogenic effects. Women in the last trimester of pregnancy and children younger than 8 years should *not* take tetracycline

because it irreversibly discolors the permanent teeth. Minocycline (Minocin) can cause damage to the vestibular part of the inner ear, which may result in difficulty maintaining balance. Outdated tetracyclines should always be discarded, because the drug breaks down into a toxic byproduct. **Nephrotoxicity** (kidney toxicity) results when tetracycline is given in high doses with other nephrotoxic drugs. Because tetracycline can disrupt the microbial flora of the body, **superinfection** (a secondary infection resulting from drug therapy) is another adverse reaction that might result.

Drug Interactions

Antacids (Maalox and others) and iron-containing drugs can prevent absorption of tetracycline from the GI tract. Milk and drugs high in calcium can inhibit tetracycline absorption. To avoid drug interaction, these drugs should be taken 2 hours apart from tetracycline. The new lipid-soluble tetracyclines, doxycycline and minocycline, are ac-

Table 29–2

Antibacterials: Tetracyclines and Glycylcyclines

Generic (Brand)	Route and Dosage	Uses and Considerations
Short-Acting Tetracyclines		
tetracycline (Achromycin, Tetracyn, Sumycin, Panmycin)	A: PO: 250-500 mg q6h IM: 250 mg daily C: >8y: PO: 25-50 mg/kg/d in 4 divided doses IM: 15-25 mg/kg/d in 2-3 divided doses; *max:* 250 mg/dose	Used for treatment of infections caused by gram-positive and gram-negative microorganisms, respiratory and skin disorders, chlamydial infection, gonorrhea, syphilis, and rickettsial infections. *Pregnancy category*: D; PB: 30%-60%; $t^{1/2}$: 6-12 h
oxytetracycline HCl (Terramycin)	A: PO: 250-500 mg q6-12h IM: 200-300 mg/d in 2-3 divided doses IV: 250-500 mg in 2 divided doses C: >8 y: PO: 25-50 mg/kg/d in 4 divided doses IM: 15-25 mg/kg/d in 2-3 divided doses; *max:* 250 mg/dose IV: 10-20 mg/kg/d in 2 divided doses	Used for urinary tract infections. Administered primarily by the oral route. *Pregnancy category*: D; PB: 20%-40%; $t^{1/2}$: 6-10 h
Intermediate-Acting Tetracyclines		
demeclocycline HCl (Declomycin)	A: PO: 150 mg q6h or 300 mg q12h C: >8 y: PO: 8-12 mg/kg/d in 2-3 divided doses	Used for gram-positive and gram-negative bacteria. Photosensitivity may occur. *Pregnancy category*: D; PB: 35%-90%; $t^{1/2}$: 10-17 h
Long-Acting Tetracyclines		
doxycycline hyclate (Vibramycin)	(Prototype Drug Chart 29–2)	
minocycline HCl (Minocin)	A: PO/IV: Initially: 200 mg; 100 mg q12h or 50 mg q6h C: >8 y: PO/IV: Initially: 4 mg/kg/d; 2 mg/kg q12h	Effective against bacterial infections and acne. Should not be administered to clients with renal insufficiency. Should take with food. *Pregnancy category*: D; PB: 55%-88%; $t^{1/2}$: 11-20 h
Glycylcyclines		
tigecycline (Tygacil)	A: IV: Initially: 100 mg; then 50 mg q12h for 5-14 days	For treatment of complicated skin and intra-abdominal infections. *Pregnancy category*: D; PB: 71-89%; $t^{1/2}$: 42 h

A, Adult; *C*, child; *d*, day; *h*, hour; *IM*, intramuscular; *IV*, intravenous; *max*, maximum; *PB*, protein-binding; *PO*, by mouth; *t¹/₂*, half-life; *UK*, unknown; *y*, year; *>*, greater than.

tually better absorbed from the GI tract when taken with milk products and food.

The desired action of oral contraceptives can be lessened when taken with tetracyclines. The activity of penicillins given with a tetracycline can be decreased. Tetracyclines could cause a bacterial resistance to the action of penicillin. Administering tetracycline with an aminoglycoside may increase the risk of nephrotoxicity.

Nursing Process

Antibacterials: Tetracyclines

ASSESSMENT

■ Assess vital signs and urine output. Report abnormal findings.
■ Check laboratory results, especially those that indicate renal and liver function (blood urea nitrogen, se-

rum creatinine, aspartate aminotransferase, alanine aminotransferase, bilirubin).
■ Obtain a history of dietary intake and drugs client currently takes. Dairy products, antacids, iron, calcium, and magnesium decrease drug absorption. Digoxin absorption is increased, which may lead to digitalis toxicity.

NURSING DIAGNOSES

■ Risk for infection related to invasion of bacteria into respiratory tract
■ Noncompliance with drug regimen related to denial of illness
■ Risk for impaired skin integrity related to adverse effect of tetracycline (sunburn)

PLANNING

■ Client's infection will be controlled and later eliminated.

NURSING INTERVENTIONS

■ Obtain a sample for culture from the infected area and send to laboratory for culture and sensitivity test. Antibiotic therapy can be started after the culture sample has been taken.

■ Administer tetracycline 1 hour before or 2 hours after meals for optimum absorption.

■ Monitor laboratory values for liver and kidney functions (in particular, liver enzymes, blood urea nitrogen, serum creatinine).

■ Record vital signs and urine output.

Client Teaching

General

• Instruct client to store tetracycline away from light and extreme heat. Tetracycline decomposes in light and heat, causing the drug to become toxic.

• Advise client to check expiration date on the bottle of tetracycline; out-of-date tetracycline can be toxic.

• Inform woman who is contemplating pregnancy and has an infection to tell her health care provider and avoid taking tetracycline because of possible teratogenic effect.

• Warn parents that children less than 8 years old should not take tetracycline; can cause discoloration of permanent teeth.

• Direct client to take the complete course of tetracycline as prescribed.

Side Effects

• Encourage client to use sun block and protective clothing during sun exposure. Photosensitivity is associated with tetracycline.

• Instruct client to report signs of a superinfection (mouth ulcers, anal or genital discharge).

• Advise client to use additional contraceptive techniques and not to rely on oral contraceptives when taking drug, because effectiveness may decrease.

• Teach client to use effective oral hygiene several times a day to prevent or alleviate mouth ulcers (stomatitis).

Diet

• Educate client to avoid milk products, iron, and antacids. Tetracycline should be taken 1 hour before or 2 hours after meals with a full glass of water. If gastrointestinal upset occurs, the drug can be taken with nondairy foods.

Cultural Considerations ❖

• Recognize that client and family members from various cultural backgrounds may need a written drug schedule as to when the drug should be taken. Explain how dairy products should not be taken with specific tetracyclines, but that food helps with the absorption of minocycline and doxycycline.

• Provide a detailed explanation orally or in written form of the possible side effects that should be reported to the health care provider.

EVALUATION

■ Evaluate the effectiveness of tetracycline by determining whether the infection has been controlled or has ceased and that there are no side effects.

Glycylcyclines

Tigecycline (Tygacil) is an antibiotic in a new category called glycylcycline, a synthetic analogue of the tetracyclines. This drug acts by blocking protein synthesis in bacterial cells, resulting in a bacteriostatic action. Indications for use are complicated skin infections and intraabdominal infections, including *Staphylococcus aureus*, *Escherichia coli*, *Streptococcus pyogenes*, *Klebsiella pneumoniae*, and *Clostridium perfringens*.

Pharmacokinetics

Tigecycline is administered IV at an initial loading dose of 100 mg over 30 to 60 minutes, followed by 50 mg q12h. The protein-binding capacity of tigecycline ranges from 71% to 89% and the half-life is 42 hours. The drug is eliminated from the body in bile, feces, and urine, with biliary excretion being the primary route. The pregnancy category is D.

Pharmacodynamics

Tigecycline binds to the 30S ribosomal subunit and causes cell death. It has broad-spectrum activity against gram-positive and gram-negative bacterial pathogens.

Side Effects and Adverse Reactions

Because of their related structural formulas, many side effects of tigecycline are similar to those of tetracycline. The most common side effects of tigecycline involve the gastrointestinal tract and include nausea, vomiting, abdominal pain, and diarrhea. Pseudomembranous colitis may occur but is rare. Other side effects are photosensitivity, headache, dizziness, insomnia, hypertension, hypotension, leukocytosis, and thrombocythemia.

Drug Interactions

Oral contraceptives may be less effective when given concurrently with tigecycline. Warfarin levels may be increased and may lead to bleeding when taken with tigecycline.

Aminoglycosides

Aminoglycosides act by inhibiting bacterial protein synthesis. The aminoglycoside antibiotics are used against gram-negative bacteria such as *E. coli*, *Proteus* spp., and *Pseudomonas* spp. Some gram-positive cocci are resistant to aminoglycosides, so penicillins or cephalosporins may be used.

Streptomycin sulfate, derived from the bacterium *Streptomyces griseus* in 1944, was the first aminoglycoside available for clinical use and was used to treat tuberculosis. Because of its ototoxicity and the bacterial resistance that can develop, it is infrequently used today. Despite its toxicity, streptomycin is the drug of choice to treat tularemia and bubonic pneumonic forms of plague.

Aminoglycosides are for serious infections. Aminoglycosides cannot be absorbed from the GI tract and cannot cross into the cerebrospinal fluid. They cross the blood-brain barrier in children but not in adults. These agents are primarily administered IM and IV, except for a few aminoglycosides (e.g., neomycin, paromomycin) which may be given orally to decrease bacteria and other organisms in the bowel. Neomycin is frequently used as a preoperative bowel antiseptic. Paromomycin is useful in treating intestinal amebiasis and tapeworm infestation.

The aminoglycosides currently used to treat *Pseudomonas aeruginosa* infection include gentamicin (1963), tobramycin (1970), amikacin (1970s), and netilmicin (1980s). Netilmicin is one of the latest aminoglycosides, and the occurrence of toxicities from this drug is not so frequent or intense as with other aminoglycosides. *Pseudomonas aeruginosa* is sensitive to gentamicin. Amikacin (Amikin) may be used when there is bacterial resistance to gentamicin and tobramycin. Prototype Drug Chart 29–3 lists the drug data related to the aminoglycoside gentamicin (Garamycin).

Pharmacokinetics

Gentamicin and netilmicin are administered IM and IV. Both drugs have a short half-life, and the drug dose can be given three to four times a day. Netilmicin has a low protein-binding power. Excretion of these drugs is primarily unchanged in the urine.

Pharmacodynamics

Gentamicin and netilmicin inhibit bacterial protein synthesis and have a bactericidal effect. Although netilmicin is the newer aminoglycoside, its pregnancy category is D, whereas gentamicin has a pregnancy

---

Prototype DRUG CHART 29–3

GENTAMICIN SULFATE

Drug Class

Antibacterial: Aminoglycoside
Trade name: *Garamycin*
Pregnancy Category: C

Dosage

A: **IM:** 3 mg/kg/d in 3-4 divided doses
IV: 3-5 mg/kg/d in 3 divided doses
C: **IM/IV:** 6-7.5 mg/kg q8h
TDM: 5-10 mcg/ml; peak: 10-12 mcg/ml; trough: 0.5-2 mcg/ml

Contraindications

Hypersensitivity, severe renal disease, pregnancy, and breastfeeding
Caution: Renal disease, neuromuscular disorders (myasthenia gravis, parkinsonism), heart failure, elderly, neonates

Drug-Lab-Food Interactions

Drug: Increase risk of ototoxicity with loop diuretics, methoxyflurane; *increase* risk of nephrotoxicity with amphotericin B, polymyxin, cisplatin, furosemide, vancomycin
Lab: Increase BUN, serum AST, ALT, LDH, bilirubin, creatinine; *decrease* serum potassium and magnesium

Pharmacokinetics

Absorption: IM, IV
Distribution: PB: UK
Metabolism: t½: 2 h
Excretion: Unchanged in urine

Pharmacodynamics

IM/IV: Onset: rapid
Peak: 1-2 h
Duration: 6-8 h

Therapeutic Effects/Uses

To treat serious infections caused by gram-negative organisms (e.g., *Pseudomonas aeruginosa, Proteus*); to treat pelvic inflammatory disease; effective against methicillin-resistant *Staphylococcus aureus* infections
Mode of Action: Inhibition of bacterial protein synthesis; bactericidal effect

Side Effects

Anorexia, nausea, vomiting, rash, numbness, visual disturbances, tremors, tinnitus, pruritus, muscle cramps or weakness, photosensitivity

Adverse Reactions

Oliguria, urticaria, palpitation, superinfection
Life-threatening: Ototoxicity, nephrotoxicity, thrombocytopenia, agranulocytosis, neuromuscular blockade, liver damage

A, Adult; *ALT,* alanine aminotransferase; *AST,* aspartate aminotransferase; *BUN,* blood urea nitrogen; *C,* child; *d,* day; *h,* hour; *IM,* intramuscular; *IV,* intravenous; *LDH,* lactic dehydrogenase; *PB,* protein-binding; *t½,* half-life; *TDM,* therapeutic drug monitoring; *UK,* unknown.

category of C. The onset of action for both drugs is similar (rapid or immediate). The peak action for netilmicin is 30 minutes faster than gentamicin.

To ensure a desired blood level, aminoglycosides are usually administered IV. The client's blood levels are drawn periodically to determine the peak blood level (highest concentration) and the drug's trough level (lowest concentration). A therapeutic drug level can be maintained by monitoring the trough level, and peak levels are useful to monitor for toxicity. Many other antibiotics should be monitored as well to maintain effective blood levels.

IV aminoglycosides can be given with penicillins and cephalosporins but should not be mixed together in the same container. When combinations of antibiotics are given IV, the IV line is flushed after each antibiotic has been administered to ensure that the antibiotic was completely delivered.

Side Effects and Adverse Reactions

Serious adverse reactions to aminoglycosides include ototoxicity and nephrotoxicity. Renal function, drug dose, and age are all factors that determine whether a client will de-

velop nephrotoxicity from aminoglycoside therapy. Careful drug dosing is especially important with younger and older clients. The nurse must assess changes in clients' hearing, balance, and urinary output. Prolonged use of aminoglycosides could result in a superinfection. Specific serum aminoglycoside levels should be closely monitored to avoid adverse reactions. Table 29–3 lists the aminoglycosides and their dosages, uses, and considerations.

Drug Interactions

When aminoglycosides are administered concurrently with penicillins, the desired effects of aminoglycosides are greatly decreased. Preferably these drugs should be given several hours apart. The drug action of oral anticoagulants such as warfarin (Coumadin) can increase when taken simultaneously with aminoglycoside administration. The risk of ototoxicity increases when ethacrynic acid and aminoglycoside are given.

Table 29–3

Antibacterials: Aminoglycosides

Generic (Brand)	Route and Dosage	Uses and Considerations
amikacin SO$_4$ (Amikin)	A & C: IM/IV: 15 mg/kg/d in 2 divided doses; *max*: 1.5 g/d C: IV: 5 mg/kg q8h or 7.5 mg/kg q12h TDM: Peak: 15-30 mg/ml; trough: 5-10 mg/ml	Synthetic derivative of kanamycin. Effective against *Pseudomonas* spp. Hearing changes should be monitored. *Pregnancy category*: C; PB: 4%-11%; t½: 2-3 h
gentamicin SO$_4$ (Garamycin)	(Prototype Drug Chart 29–3)	
kanamycin SO$_4$ (Kantrex)	A: PO: 1 g q6h *Hepatic coma*: 8-12 g/d in divided doses IM/IV: 15 mg/kg/d in 2 divided doses C: IV: Same as adult	Used orally for hepatic coma. Effective against gram-negative bacteria with the exception of *Pseudomonas aeruginosa*. Monitor for hearing loss and urinary output. *Pregnancy category*: D; PB: 10%; t½: 2-3 h
neomycin SO$_4$ (Mycifradin)	A: PO: GI surgery: 1 g qh for 4 doses; then 1 g q4h for 5 doses for 24 h or other regimens *Hepatic coma*: 4-12 g/d in divided doses for 5-6 d IM: 15 mg/kg/d in 4 divided doses; *max*: 1 g/d C: PO: 10 mg/kg q4-6h for 3 d	Decreases bacteria in the bowel and is used as a preoperative bowel antiseptic. Also available as a topical antibiotic ointment. *Pregnancy category*: C; PB: 10%; t½: 2-3 h
netilmicin (Netromycin)	A: IM/IV: 3-6.5 mg/kg/d in 3 divided doses C: IM/IV: 2.5-4 mg/kg q12h TDM: Peak: 0.5-10 mcg/ml; trough: < 4 mcg/ml	Used in treating moderate to severe gram-negative infections (e.g., *Enterobacter, Escherichia coli, Klebsiella, Proteus, Pseudomonas, Serratia*). *Pregnancy category*: D; PB: 10%; t½: 2-2.5 h
paromomycin (Humatin)	*Intestinal amebiasis:* A & C: PO: 25-35 mg/kg/d in 3 divided doses for 5-10 d *Hepatic coma:* A: PO: 4 g/d in 2-4 divided doses for 5-6 d	Used in treating hepatic coma and parasitic infections. Hearing changes and urinary output should be monitored. Not systemically absorbed. *Pregnancy category*: C; PB: UK; t½: UK
streptomycin SO$_4$	*Tuberculosis:* A: IM: 1 g daily for 2-3 mo; then 1 g × 3 wk *Endocarditis:* A: IM: 1 g q12h for 1 wk; dose may be decreased	First aminoglycoside. Used with antituberculosis drugs in treatment of tuberculosis. Ototoxicity is a major problem. *Pregnancy category*: C; PB: 30%; t½: 2-3 h
tobramycin SO$_4$ (Nebcin)	A: IM/IV: 3-5 mg/kg/d in 3 divided doses C: IM/IV: 3 mg/kg/d in 3 divided doses TDM: Peak: 10-12 mcg/ml; trough: 0.5-2 mcg/ml	Very effective against *Pseudomonas aeruginosa*. Hearing changes and urinary output should be monitored. Fewer toxic effects than other aminoglycosides. *Pregnancy category*: D; PB: 10%; t½: 2-3 h

A, Adult; *C*, child; *d*, day; *GI*, gastrointestinal; *h*, hour; *IM*, intramuscular; *IV*, intravenous; *max*, maximum; *PB*, protein-binding; *PO*, by mouth; *t*½, half-life; *TDM*, therapeutic drug monitoring; *UK*, unknown; *wk*, week.

Nursing Process

Antibacterials: Aminoglycosides

ASSESSMENT

■ Record vital signs and urine output. Compare these results with future vital signs and urine output. An adverse reaction to most aminoglycosides is nephrotoxicity.

■ Assess laboratory results to determine renal and liver functions, including blood urea nitrogen, serum creatinine, alkaline phosphatase, alanine aminotransferase, aspartate aminotransferase, and bilirubin. Serum electrolytes should also be checked. Aminoglycosides may decrease serum potassium and magnesium levels.

■ Obtain a medical history related to renal or hearing disorders. Large doses of aminoglycosides could cause nephrotoxicity or ototoxicity.

NURSING DIAGNOSES

■ Risk for infection related to an invasion of bacteria

■ Risk for impaired tissue integrity related to aminoglycoside side effect of rash

■ Imbalanced nutrition: less than body requirements related to inability to ingest food

■ Risk for ineffective tissue perfusion: renal related to an aminoglycoside adverse effect of nephrotoxicity

PLANNING

■ Client's infection will be controlled and later eliminated.

NURSING INTERVENTIONS

■ Send sample from infected area to laboratory for culture to determine organism and antibiotic sensitivity before aminoglycoside is started.

■ Monitor intake and output. Urine output should be at least 600 ml/d. Immediately report if urine output is decreased. Urinalysis may be ordered daily. Check results for proteinuria, casts, blood cells, or appearance.

■ Check for hearing loss. Aminoglycosides can cause ototoxicity.

■ Evaluate laboratory results and compare with baseline values. Report abnormal results.

■ Monitor vital signs. Note if body temperature has decreased.

■ For IV use, dilute aminoglycoside in 50-200 ml of normal saline solution or dextrose 5% in water (D₅W) solution and administer over 30-60 minutes.

■ Check that therapeutic drug monitoring (TDM) has been ordered for peak and trough drug levels. The TDM for gentamicin is 5-10 mcg/ml. Blood should be drawn 45-60 minutes after drug has been administered for peak levels and minutes before next drug dosing for trough levels. Drug peak values should be 10-12 mcg/ml, and trough values should be 0.5-2 mcg/ml.

■ Monitor for signs and symptoms of superinfection: stomatitis (mouth ulcers), genital discharge (vaginitis), and anal or genital itching.

Client Teaching

General

• Unless fluids are restricted, encourage client to increase fluid intake.

• Instruct client never to take leftover antibiotics.

Side Effects

• Inform client to report aminoglycoside side effects: nausea, vomiting, tremors, tinnitus, pruritus, and muscle cramps.

• Direct client to use sun block and protective clothing during sun exposure. Photosensitivity can be caused by aminoglycosides.

Cultural Considerations ❖

• Do not give directions such as take one "blue" pill at a specified time. Instead, provide name and dosage of the medication in the language client speaks and reads most easily.

EVALUATION

■ Evaluate the effectiveness of the aminoglycoside by determining whether the infection has ceased and no side effects have occurred.

Fluoroquinolones (Quinolones)

The mechanism of action of fluoroquinolones is to interfere with the enzyme DNA gyrase, which is needed to synthesize bacterial deoxyribonucleic acid (DNA). Their antibacterial spectrum includes both gram-positive and gram-negative organisms. They are bactericidal. Nalidixic acid (NegGram) and cinoxacin (Cinobac) are the earliest derivatives of the fluoroquinolone group, prescribed primarily for urinary tract infection caused by common gram-negative organisms such as *E. coli*. These two drugs are no longer available on the market in the United States. The fluoroquinolones are effective against some gram-positive organisms, such as *Streptococcus pneumoniae*, and against *Haemophilus influenzae*, *P. aeruginosa*, *Salmonella*, and *Shigella*. This group of antibiotics is useful in the treatment of urinary tract, bone, and joint infections; bronchitis; pneumonia; gastroenteritis; and gonorrhea. Table 29–4 lists the various fluoroquinolones.

Ciprofloxacin (Cipro) and norfloxacin (Noroxin) are synthetic antibacterials related to nalidixic acid. These two fluoroquinolones have a broad spectrum of action on gram-positive and gram-negative organisms, including *P. aeruginosa*. Norfloxacin is indicated for urinary tract in-

Table 29–4

Antibacterials: Fluoroquinolones (Quinolones) and Unclassified Drugs

Generic (Brand)	Route and Dosage	Uses and Considerations
Fluoroquinolones		
ciprofloxacin HCl (Cipro)	A: PO: 250-750 mg q12h IV: 200-400 mg q12h	To treat lower respiratory tract, renal, bone and joint, skin infections. *Pregnancy category*: C; PB: 20%-40%; t$^{1/2}$: 4-6 h
gatifloxacin (Tequin)	A: PO/IV: 400 mg/d for 7-10 days	To treat community-acquired pneumonia, acute sinusitis, UTIs. Two to four times more active than levofloxacin against *Streptococcus pneumoniae*. Active against *Legionella pneumophila*, *Mycobacterium tuberculosis*, and *Haemophilus influenzae*. Has similar side effects as other fluoroquinolones. Hypoglycemia and hyperglycemia may occur, therefore contraindicated in clients with diabetes mellitus. *Pregnancy category*: C; PB: UK; t$^{1/2}$: 7-12 h
levofloxacin (Levaquin)	(Prototype Drug Chart 29–4)	
moxifloxacin (Avelox)	A: PO: 400 mg/d for 10 d	Treatment is similar to gatifloxacin. It is 4 to 8 times more active than levofloxacin against *S. pneumoniae*. Side effects similar to other fluoroquinolones. *Pregnancy category*: PB: UK; t$^{1/2}$: 7-12 h
norfloxacin (Noroxin)	A: PO: 400 mg b.i.d., a.c. or p.c. for 1-3 wk	For acute and chronic UTIs. Most potent drug of the fluoroquinolone group. Food may inhibit drug absorption. *Pregnancy category*: C; PB: 10%-15%; t$^{1/2}$: 3-4 h
ofloxacin (Floxin)	A: PO/IV: 200-400 mg q12h 7-10 d	For respiratory and UTIs, prostatitis, skin infections. Not to be taken with meals. Superinfection may result. Avoid excessive sunlight. *Pregnancy category*: C; PB: 20%; t$^{1/2}$: 5-8 h
Unclassified Drugs		
chloramphenicol (Chloromycetin)	A & C: PO/IV: 50 mg/kg/d in 4 divided doses (q6h) NB: 25 mg/kg/d in 4 divided doses (q6h)	For treatment of severe infections. Drug can be toxic. *Pregnancy category*: C; PB: 50%-60%; t$^{1/2}$: 1.5-4 h
quinupristin/dalfopristin (Synercid)	A: IV: 7.5 mg/kg given over 1 h, q8h × 10 days	For treatment of vancomycin-resistant *Enterococcus faecium*. Also effective against skin infected by *Staphylococcus aureus*. Adverse effects at infusion site; pain, inflammation, edema and thrombophlebitis. Central venous line is preferred. *Pregnancy category*: UK; PB: UK; t$^{1/2}$: 1 h
spectinomycin HCl (Trobicin)	A: IM: 2 g as single dose or 2 g q12h for severe infection C: IM: 40 mg/kg as single dose	Has a bacteriostatic effect. Effective against *Neisseria gonorrhoeae*. Ineffective against syphilis. *Pregnancy category*: B; PB: 10%; t$^{1/2}$: 1-3 h

A, Adult; *b.i.d.*, twice a day; *C*, child; *d*, day; *GI*, gastrointestinal; *h*, hour; *IM*, intramuscular; *IV*, intravenous; *max*, maximum; *NB*, newborn; *PB*, protein-binding; *PO*, by mouth; *q.i.d.*, four times a day; *t$^{1/2}$*, half-life; *UK*, unknown; *UTI*, urinary tract infection; *wk*, week; *y*, year.

fections. Ciprofloxacin is approved for use for urinary tract infections; lower respiratory tract infections; and skin, soft tissue, bone, and joint infections.

The use of fluoroquinolones as urinary antibiotics is discussed in Chapter 33. Prototype Drug Chart 29–4 lists the drug data related to levofloxacin. Levofloxacin's use is not limited to urinary tract infections.

The number of new fluoroquinolones has increased in the past few years. Levofloxacin (Levaquin) is used primarily to treat respiratory problems, such as community-acquired pneumonia, chronic bronchitis, acute sinusitis, urinary tract infections, and uncomplicated skin infections.

Gatifloxacin (Tequin) and moxifloxacin (Avelox) received Food & Drug Administration approval in 1999 and are available for once-a-day oral and parenteral dosing. These two drugs are prescribed to treat the same infections other fluoroquinolones are effective against. Gatifloxacin

and moxifloxacin are more active than levofloxacin against *S. pneumoniae*. They are also effective against some strains of *S. aureus* and enterococci but not VRE. The fluoroquinolones are included in Table 29–4.

Pharmacokinetics

Approximately 70% of levofloxacin (Levaquin) is absorbed from the GI tract. It has a low protein-binding effect and a moderately short half-life of 6.5 to 7.5 hours. More than 75% of the drug is excreted unchanged in the urine.

Pharmacodynamics

Levofloxacin inhibits bacterial DNA synthesis by inhibiting the enzyme DNA gyrase. The drug has a high tissue distribution. If possible, it should be taken before meals, because food slows the absorption rate. Antacids also decrease absorption rate. Levofloxacin increases the effect of oral hypoglycemics, theophylline, and caffeine.

Levofloxacin has an average onset of action of 0.5 to 1 hour, and the peak concentration time is 1 to 2 hours. The duration of action is unknown.

Prototype **DRUG CHART 29–4**

LEVOFLOXACIN

Drug Class	**Dosage**
Antibacterials: Quinolone, fluoroquinolone Trade name: Levaquin *Pregnancy Category:* C (X at term, breastfeeding)	A: PO: 500 mg q24h IV: 500 mg q24h, infused over 60 min Moderate to severe infections
Contraindications	**Drug-Lab-Food Interactions**
Severe renal disease, hypersensitivity to other quinolones, pregnancy, and breastfeeding *Caution:* Seizure disorders, renal disorders, children <14 y, elderly, clients receiving theophylline	*Drug:* *Increase* effect of oral hypoglycemics and theo- phylline, caffeine; *decrease* drug absorption with antacids, iron *Lab:* *Increase* AST, ALT
Pharmacokinetics	**Pharmacodynamics**
Absorption: PO: 95%-98% absorbed **Distribution:** PB: 24%-30% **Metabolism:** t½: 6.5-7.5 h **Excretion:** 87% unchanged in urine	**PO:** Onset: 0.5-1 h Peak: 1-2 h Duration: UK

Therapeutic Effects/Uses

To treat lower respiratory tract, renal, bone, and joint infections
Mode of Action: Interference with the enzyme DNA gyrase, which is needed for bacterial DNA synthesis; bactericidal effect

Side Effects	**Adverse Reactions**
Nausea, vomiting, diarrhea, abdominal cramps, flatulence, headache, dizziness, fatigue, restlessness, insomnia, rash, flushing, tinnitus, photosensitivity	Stevens-Johnson syndrome, encephalopathy, seizures, pseudomembranous colitis, dysrhythmias

A, Adult; *ALT,* alanine aminotransferase; *AST,* aspartate aminotransferase; *DNA,* deoxyribonucleic acid; *h,* hour; *IV,* intravenous;
min, minute; *PB,* protein binding; *PO,* by mouth; *t½,* half life; *UK,* unknown; *y,* year; <, less than.

Nursing Process

Antibacterials: Fluoroquinolones

ASSESSMENT

■ Record vital signs and intake and urine output. Compare these results with future vital signs and urine output. Fluid intake should be at least 2000 ml/d.

■ Assess laboratory results to determine renal function:
blood urea nitrogen and serum creatinine.

■ Obtain a drug and diet history. Antacids and iron
preparations decrease absorption of fluoroquinolones
such as levofloxacin (Levaquin). Levofloxacin can increase the effects of theophylline and caffeine. Levofloxacin can increase the effects of oral hypoglycemics.
When levofloxacin is taken with NSAIDs, CNS reactions
including seizures may occur.

NURSING DIAGNOSES

■ Risk for infection related to an invasion of bacteria

■ Risk for impaired tissue integrity related to a fluoroquinolone adverse effect of Stevens-Johnson syndrome
■ Noncompliance with drug regimen related to an un-
caring attitude

PLANNING

■ Client's infection will be controlled and later eliminated.

NURSING INTERVENTIONS

■ Obtain specimen from infected site and send to laboratory for culture and sensitivity before initiating antibacterial drug therapy.

■ Monitor intake and output. Urine output should be
at least 750 ml/d. Client should be well hydrated, and
fluid intake should be >2000 ml/d to prevent crystalluria. Urine pH should be <6.7.

■ Record vital signs. Report abnormal findings.

■ Check laboratory results, especially blood urea nitrogen and serum creatinine. Elevated values may indicate
renal dysfunction.

■ Administer levofloxacin 2 hours before or after antacids and iron products for absorption. Give with a full glass of water. If gastrointestinal distress occurs, drug may be taken with food.

■ For IV levofloxacin, dilute antibiotic in an appropriate amount of solution as indicated in drug circular. Infuse over 60 minutes.

■ Check for signs and symptoms of superinfection: stomatitis (mouth ulcers), furry black tongue, anal or genital discharge and itching.

■ Monitor serum theophylline levels. Levofloxacin can increase theophylline levels. Check for symptoms of central nervous system stimulation: nervousness, insomnia, anxiety, and tachycardia.

■ Monitor blood sugar. Levofloxacin can increase effects of oral hypoglycemics.

Client Teaching

General

• Teach client to drink at least 6 to 8 glasses (8 oz) of fluid daily.

• Encourage client to avoid caffeinated products.

Side Effects

• Direct client to avoid operating hazardous machinery or operating a motor vehicle while taking drug or until drug stability has occurred, because of possible drug-related dizziness.

• Inform client that photosensitivity is a side effect of most fluoroquinolones. Client should use sunglasses, sun block, and protective clothing when in the sun.

• Instruct client to report side effects, such as dizziness, nausea, vomiting, diarrhea, flatulence, abdominal cramps, tinnitus, and rash. Older adults are more likely to develop side effects.

Cultural Considerations ❖

• To establish trust among Hispanics/Latinos and Appalachians, it is necessary to demonstrate an interest in client's family and other personal matters. Drop hints instead of giving orders, and solicit client's opinions and advice.

EVALUATION

■ Evaluate the effectiveness of the fluoroquinolone by determining if the infection has ceased and the body temperature has returned within normal range

Lipopeptides

Daptomycin (Cubicin) is an FDA-approved antibiotic in a new category called lipopeptides. Daptomycin acts by binding to the bacterial membrane and causing rapid depolarization of its membrane potential, inhibiting protein, DNA, and RNA synthesis. This action results in bacterial cell death.

Indications for daptomycin include complicated skin infections due to gram-positive microorganisms, septicemia due to *Staphylococcus aureus* infections, and infective endocarditis due to MRSA.

Pharmacokinetics

Daptomycin is administered IV at a dose of 4 mg/kg/day. The medication is diluted in NS 0.9% or LR solution. However, it *should not* be mixed with dextrose-containing diluents. The protein-binding capacity is 92% with a half-life of 8 hours. Daptomycin is primarily excreted by the kidneys. The pregnancy category is B.

Pharmacodynamics

Daptomycin binds to the bacterial membrane and causes cell death. An effective trough concentration of 5.9 mcg/ml is usually achieved by the third dose.

Side Effects and Adverse Reactions

Side effects that may occur when taking daptomycin include hypertension, hypotension, anemia, numbness, tingling, dizziness, insomnia, pain or burning upon urination, nausea, vomiting, diarrhea, constipation, and pallor. More serious adverse effects that have occurred with daptomycin are chest pain, hypokalemia, hyperkalemia, hyperglycemia, hypoglycemia, bleeding, rhabdomyolysis, and pleural effusion.

Drug Interactions

When daptomycin is given with HMG-CoA reductase inhibitors, the risk of rhabdomyolysis is increased. Daptomycin toxicity may be increased when given concurrently with tobramycin. Warfarin may lead to increased bleeding when taken with daptomycin.

Unclassified Antibacterial Drugs

Several antibacterials, such as chloramphenicol, spectinomycin, and quinupristin/dalfopristin, do not belong to any major drug group. Chloramphenicol (Chloromycetin) was discovered in 1947 and has a bacteriostatic action by inhibiting bacterial protein synthesis. Because of the toxic effects of chloramphenicol, including blood dyscrasias related to bone marrow suppression, it is used only to treat serious infections. It is effective against gram-negative and gram-positive bacteria and many other microorganisms, such as rickettsiae, *Mycoplasmas*, and *H. influenzae*.

Spectinomycin hydrochloride (Trobicin), introduced in 1971, is used against *Neisseria gonorrhoeae*, the microbe that causes gonorrhea. It is also prescribed for persons allergic to penicillins, cephalosporins, or tetracyclines. It is administered IM as a single dose.

Quinupristin/dalfopristin (Synercid) is effective for treating vancomycin-resistant *Enterococcus faecium* (VREF) bacteremia and skin infected by *S. aureus* and *S. pyogenes*. It acts by disrupting the protein synthesis of the organism. When administering the drug through a peripheral IV line, pain, edema, and phlebitis may occur.

Critical Thinking Case Study

AJN, age 46, has a wound infection. The culture report stated that the infection was caused by *Pseudomonas aeruginosa*. AJN's temperature was 104° F (40° C). Amikacin sulfate (Amikin) is to be administered IV in 100 ml of D₅W over 45 minutes every 8 hours. Dosage is 15 mg/kg daily in three divided doses. AJN weighs 165 pounds.

1. What is the drug classification of amikacin? How many milligrams of amikacin should AJN receive every 8 hours?

2. What type of IV infusion should be used? What would be the IV flow rate?

3. When should a wound culture be obtained to determine the appropriate antibacterial agent? Give your rationale.

4. What are the similarities of amikacin to other aminoglycosides such as gentamicin? Would one aminoglycoside be preferred over another one? Explain.

The nurse assessed AJN for hearing and urinary function before and during amikacin therapy.

5. What should a hearing assessment include?

6. AJN's urine output in the last 8 hours was 125 ml. Explain the possible cause for the amount of urine output. What nursing action should be taken?

7. What laboratory tests monitor renal function?

8. The health care provider requests peak and trough serum amikacin levels. When should the blood samples to determine peak serum level and trough serum level be drawn?

NCLEX Study Questions

1. A client is taking azithromycin (Zithromax). The action of this drug is:
   a. inhibition of protein synthesis
   b. alteration of membrane permeability
   c. inhibition of bacterial cell-wall synthesis
   d. alteration of synthesis of bacterial ribonucleic acid

2. A serious adverse effect of lincosamides is:
   a. seizures
   b. ototoxicity
   c. hepatotoxicity
   d. pseudomembranous colitis

3. Which drug is more likely to cause "red man syndrome" with flushing, tachycardia, and severe hypotension following an IV infusion that is too rapid?
   a. tigecycline (Tygacil)
   b. telithromycin (Ketek)
   c. vancomycin (Vancocin)
   d. gentamicin (Garamycin)

4. The nurse is administering tetracycline (Vibramycin) to a client. Which would be appropriate teaching?
   a. Take sunscreen precautions when at the beach.
   b. Take an antacid or milk with the drug to prevent severe GI distress.
   c. Obtain frequent hearing tests for early detection of hearing loss.
   d. Obtain frequent eye checkups for early detection of retinal damage.

5. A client is taking levofloxacin (Levaquin). Which of the following is true regarding this drug?
   a. Administered IV only
   b. May cause hypertension
   c. Classified as an aminoglycoside
   d. Adverse reaction includes dysrhythmias

Answers: 1, a; 2, d; 3, c; 4, a; 5, d.

30
Sulfonamides

ELECTRONIC RESOURCES

Evolve website (http://evolve.elsevier.com/KeeHayes/pharmacology/):
- *Case Studies*
- *Content Updates*
- *Frequently Asked Questions*

Companion CD-ROM:
- *NCLEX Examination Review Questions*
- *Pharmacology Animations*
- *IV Therapy Checklists*
- *Medication Error Checklists*

- *Student Review Activities*
- *WebLinks*
- *Additional Reference Material*

- *Drug Calculation Problems*
- *Electronic Calculators*
- *Top 200 Drugs with Pronunciations*
- *References from the Textbook*

Outline

Objectives

- Differentiate between short-acting and intermediate-acting sulfonamides.
- Describe the uses, side effects, and adverse reactions to all the sulfonamides and co-trimoxazole.
- Explain the pharmacokinetics of sulfonamides.
- Apply the nursing process to the client taking trimethoprim-sulfamethoxazole.

Terms

Sulfonamides are one of the oldest antibacterial agents used to combat infection. When penicillin was initially marketed, the sulfonamide drugs were not widely prescribed, because penicillin was considered the "miracle drug." However, use of sulfonamides has increased as a result of new sulfonamides and the combination drug of sulfonamide with an antibacterial agent in preparations such as trimethoprim-sulfamethoxazole (Bactrim, Septra).

Sulfonamides

Sulfonamides were first isolated from a coal tar derivative compound in the early 1900s and were produced for clinical use against coccal infections in 1935. It was the first group of drugs used against bacteria. Sulfonamides are not classified as an antibiotic, because they were not obtained from biologic substances. The sulfonamides are **bacteriostatic** because they inhibit bacterial synthesis of folic acid, which is essential for bacterial growth. Humans do not synthesize folic acid but acquire it through the diet; therefore sulfonamides selectively inhibit bacterial growth without affecting normal cells. Folic acid (folate) is required by cells for biosynthesis of ribonucleic acid (RNA), deoxyribonucleic acid (DNA), and proteins.

The clinical usefulness of sulfonamides alone, not in combination, has decreased for several reasons. The availability and effectiveness of penicillin and other antibiotics has increased, and bacterial resistance to some sulfonamides can develop. Sulfonamides may be used as an alternative drug for clients allergic to penicillin. They are still used to treat urinary tract and ear infections and may be used for newborn eye prophylaxis. Sulfonamides are approximately 90% effective against *Escherichia coli*; therefore they are frequently a preferred treatment for urinary tract infections, which are often caused by *E. coli*. They are also useful in the treatment of meningococcal meningitis and against the organisms *Chlamydia* and *Toxoplasma gondii*. Sulfonamides are not effective against viruses and fungi.

Pharmacokinetics

Sulfonamide drugs are well absorbed by the gastrointestinal (GI) tract and are well distributed to body tissues and the brain. The liver metabolizes the sulfonamide drug, and the kidneys excrete it.

Pharmacodynamics

Many sulfonamides are for oral administration, because they are absorbed readily by the GI tract. They are also available in solution and ointment for ophthalmic use and in cream form, silver sulfadiazine (Silvadene) and mafenide acetate (Sulfamylon), for burns. Most of the early sulfonamides were highly protein-bound and displaced other drugs by competing for protein sites. The following are two categories of sulfonamides, classified according to their duration of action:

- Short-acting sulfonamides (rapid absorption and excretion rate)
- Intermediate-acting sulfonamides (moderate to slow absorption and slow excretion rate)

Sulfisoxazole (Gantrisin) is a water-soluble sulfonamide that is effective in treating most uncomplicated urinary tract infections. It is also useful, along with sulfadiazine, in prophylactic treatment of streptococcal infections in clients with rheumatic fever who are hypersensitive to penicillin. Sulfadiazine is poorly soluble in urine and can cause crystallization, which could damage the kidneys if there is insufficient fluid and water intake. Sulfamethoxazole (Gantanol), an intermediate-acting sulfonamide, has a longer duration of action than other sulfonamides, but it has poorer water solubility than sulfisoxazole. Table 30–1 lists the protein-binding, half-life, and solubility in urine of most drugs in the sulfonamide group. Sulfisoxazole and sulfamethoxazole are no longer available on the market in the United States.

The only combination of sulfonamides still marketed—but infrequently used—is trisulfapyrimidines. This triple sulfa drug is a combination of low doses of sulfadiazine,

sulfamerazine, and sulfamethazine. The three drugs have an additive effect, increasing the potency of the drug. Trisulfapyrimidines have a longer duration of action than other sulfonamides and are considered poorly soluble in water. With low doses of the three drugs, crystal formation in the urine is less likely to occur. Older sulfonamides (e.g., sulfadiazine) have low solubility and may cause crystallization in the urine. The current sulfonamides have greater water solubility; therefore crystal formations in the urine and renal damage are unlikely. Table 30-2 lists and describes the sulfonamides.

Side Effects and Adverse Reactions

Side effects of sulfonamides may include an allergic response such as skin rash and itching. Anaphylaxis is not common. Blood disorders such as hemolytic anemia, aplastic anemia, and low white blood cell and platelet counts could result from prolonged use and high dosages. GI disturbances (anorexia, nausea, vomiting) may also occur. The early sulfonamides were insoluble in acid urine, and **crystalluria** (crystals in urine) and hematuria were common problems. Crystalluria occurs less commonly with sulfisoxazole (Gantrisin) than it does with sulfadiazine and sulfamethoxazole. Increasing fluid intake dilutes the drug, helping to prevent crystalluria from occurring. **Photosensitivity** (excessive reaction to direct sunlight or ultraviolet light leading to redness and burning of skin) can occur, so the client should avoid sunbathing and excess ultraviolet light. **Cross-sensitivity** (a sensitivity or allergy to one sulfonamide may lead to sensitivity to another sulfonamide) might occur with the different sulfonamides but does not occur with other antibacterial drugs. Sulfonamides should be avoided during the third trimester of pregnancy.

Trimethoprim and Co-Trimoxazole

Trimethoprim (Proloprim, Trimpex) is an antibacterial agent that interferes with bacterial folic acid synthesis just as sulfonamides do. Trimethoprim is classified as a urinary tract antiinfective that may be used alone for uncomplicated urinary tract infections. This drug is effective against the gram-negative bacteria *Proteus* spp., *Klebsiella* spp., and

Table 30–1			
Pharmacokinetics of Selected Sulfonamides			
Drug	**Protein-Binding (%)**	**Half-Life (Hour)**	**Solubility in Urine**
Short-Acting			
sulfadiazine (Microsulfon)	20-60	17	+1
sulfamethizole (Thiosulfil)	90	2.5	+3
sulfisoxazole (Gantrisin)	90	5-7.5	+3
Intermediate-Acting			
sulfamethoxazole (Gantanol)	85-90	11	+1
sulfasalazine (Azulfidine)	99	5-10	+1
trimethoprim-sulfamethoxazole	50-65	8-12	+1-2

Table 30–2

Antibacterials: Sulfonamides

Generic (Brand)	Route and Dosage	Uses and Considerations
Short-Acting		
sulfadiazine (Microsulfon)	A: PO: LD: 2-4 g; then 2-4 g/d in 4-6 divided doses C: >2 mo: PO: LD: 75 mg/kg; then 150 mg/kg/d in 4-6 divided doses	For treatment of systemic infections. Could be classified as a short-immediate-acting sulfonamide. When taking this drug, increase fluid intake to >2000 ml/d. *Pregnancy category: C*; PB: 20%-30%; t½: 8-12 h
sulfamethizole (Sulfasol, Thiosulfil Forte)	A: PO: 0.5-1 g in 3-4 divided doses C: PO: 30-45 mg/kg/d in 4 divided doses	For treatment of urinary tract infections. Highly soluble. Fluid intake should be at least 2000 ml/d. *Pregnancy category: C*; PB: 90%; t½: 1.5 h
sulfisoxazole (Gantrisin)	A: PO: LD: 2-4 g; then 4-8 g/d in 4-6 divided doses C: >2 mo: PO: LD: 75 mg/kg; then 150 mg/kg/d in 4-6 divided doses; *max:* 6 g/d	Popular drug for treating urinary tract infections, because it is more soluble in urine. Rapidly absorbed from GI tract. Used for treatment and prophylaxis of otitis media. Often ordered with a one-time initial loading dose. Fluid intake ≥2000 ml/d. *Pregnancy category: C*; PB: 85%-95%; t½: 4.5-7.5 h
Intermediate-Acting		
sulfamethoxazole (Gantanol)	A: PO: LD: 2 g; then 2-3 g/d in 2-3 divided doses for 7-10 d C: >2 mo: PO: LD: 50-60 mg/kg; then 25-30 mg/kg q12h; *max:* 75 mg/kg/d	For urinary tract infections, otitis media, and meningococcal A strain meningitis prophylaxis. Similar to Gantrisin, except it is absorbed and excreted slowly. Fluid intake should be at least 2000 ml/d. *Pregnancy category: C*; PB: 60%-70%; t½: 7-12 h
sulfasalazine (Azulfidine, Salazopyrin)	A: PO: Initially: 1 g q6-8h; maint: 2 g q6h C: >2 y: PO: Initially: 40-50 mg/kg/d in 4-6 divided doses; *maint:* 20-30 mg/kg/d in 4 divided doses; *max:* 2 g/d	For treatment of ulcerative colitis, Crohn's disease, rheumatoid arthritis (some cases). Take after eating. Side effects include nausea, vomiting, bloody diarrhea. *Pregnancy category: C* (near term: D); PB: 99%; t½: 5.5 h
trimethoprim-sulfamethoxazole: co-trimoxazole (Bactrim, Septra)	(Prototype Drug Chart 30–1)	

A, Adult; *C*, child; *d*, day; *h*, hour; *LD*, loading dose; *maint*, maintenance; *max*, maximum; *mo*, month; *PB*, protein-binding; *PO*, by mouth; *t½*, half-life; *y*, year; >, greater than; ≥, greater than or equal to.

E. coli. In the 1970s it was combined with the sulfonamide sulfamethoxazole (an intermediate-acting sulfonamide) to prevent bacterial resistance to sulfonamide drugs and to obtain a better response against many organisms. Giving both drugs together in one compound form causes bacterial resistance to develop much more slowly than if only one of the drugs is used alone. This combination drug, trimethoprim-sulfamethoxazole (TMP-SMZ) (co-trimoxazole, Bactrim, Septra) is commonly used. The drug ratio is one part trimethoprim to five parts sulfamethoxazole (1:5). The two drugs have a **synergistic effect,** increasing the desired drug response.

Trimethoprim-sulfamethoxazole is effective in treating urinary, intestinal, and lower respiratory tract infections; otitis media; prostatitis; and gonorrhea. It is also used to prevent *Pneumocystis carinii* in clients with acquired immunodeficiency syndrome (AIDS). Increased fluid intake is highly recommended to avoid complications such as crystallization in the urine. Prototype Drug Chart 30–1 describes the pharmacologic behavior of TMP-SMZ.

Pharmacokinetics

TMP-SMZ (Bactrim, Septra) is well absorbed from the GI tract and is moderately protein-bound. Its half-life is 8 to 12 hours; thus it is administered twice a day. It is excreted as unchanged metabolites in the urine.

Pharmacodynamics

The combination drug TMP-SMZ is known generically as *co-trimoxazole* in many countries. Trimethoprim, a nonsulfonamide antibiotic, enhances the activity of the drug combination. Co-trimoxazole blocks steps in bacterial synthesis of protein and nucleic acid, producing a bactericidal effect.

Co-trimoxazole (TMP-SMZ) can be administered orally or intravenously (IV). Orally the drug has a moderately rapid onset of action; drug action is immediate via the IV route. Serum peak concentration time for oral use is 2 to 4 hours and 0.5 to 1 hour for IV use. Co-trimoxazole increases the hypoglycemic response when taken with sulfonylureas (oral hypoglycemic agents). It can also increase the activity of oral anticoagulants.

Side Effects and Adverse Reactions

Side effects of co-trimoxazole may include mild to moderate rashes, anorexia, nausea, vomiting and diarrhea, stomatitis, crystalluria, and photosensitivity. Serious adverse reactions are rare; however, agranulocytosis, aplastic anemia, and allergic myocarditis have been reported as possible life-threatening conditions. Clients with AIDS are more susceptible to TMP-SMZ toxicity.

Topical and Ophthalmic Sulfonamides

Sulfonamides can be administered for topical and ophthalmic uses, but because topical use of sulfonamides can cause hypersensitivity reactions, they are not frequently

Prototype DRUG CHART 30–1

CO-TRIMOXAZOLE/TMP-SMZ

Drug Class

Antibacterial: Sulfonamide
Trade names: Bactrim, Septra
Pregnancy Category: C

Dosage

A: PO: 160/800 mg q12h (160 mg [TMP]/800 mg [SMZ])
IV: 8-10 mg/kg/d in 2-4 divided doses; infuse over 1 to 1.5 h
C: PO: <40 kg: 4 mg/kg/d in 2 divided doses
PO: >40 kg: same as adult
IV: >2 mo: same as adult
NOTE: Sulfa drugs should not be used in infants younger than 2 months.
Dosage may vary according to the severity of the health problem.
Dosing is based on trimethoprim component.

Contraindications

Severe renal or hepatic disease, hypersensitivity to sulfonamides

Drug-Lab-Food Interactions

Drug: *Increase* anticoagulant effect with warfarin; *increase* hypoglycemic effect with an oral hypoglycemic drug
Lab: May *increase* BUN, serum creatinine, AST, ALT, ALP

Pharmacokinetics

Absorption: PO: Well absorbed
Distribution: PB: 50%-65%; crosses placenta
Metabolism: t½: 8-12 h
Excretion: In urine as metabolites

Pharmacodynamics

PO: Onset: 0.5-1 h
Peak: 2-4 h
Duration: UK
IV: Onset: Immediate
Peak: 0.5-1 h
Duration: UK

Therapeutic Effects/Uses

To treat urinary tract infection, otitis media, bronchitis, pneumonia, *Pneumocystis carinii* infection, rheumatic fever, burns
Mode of Action: Inhibition of protein synthesis of nucleic acids; bactericidal effect

Side Effects

Anorexia, nausea, vomiting, diarrhea, rash, stomatitis, fatigue, depression, headache, vertigo, photosensitivity

Adverse Reactions

Life-threatening: Leukopenia, thrombocytopenia, increased bone marrow depression, hemolytic anemia, aplastic anemia, agranulocytosis, Stevens-Johnson syndrome, renal failure

A, Adult; *ALP*, alkaline phosphatase; *ALT*, alanine aminotransferase; *AST*, aspartate aminotransferase; *BUN*, blood urea nitrogen; *C*, child; *d*, day; *h*, hour; *IV*, intravenous; *PB*, protein-binding; *PO*, by mouth; *SMZ*, sulfamethoxazole; *TMP*, trimethoprim; *t½*, half-life; *UK*, unknown; *>*, greater than; *<*, less than.

Preventing MEDICATION ERRORS

Do not confuse...

• **Septra** (an antibacterial) with **Sectral** (a beta-adrenergic antagonist that is used to manage dysrhythmias). These two drugs look alike, but the actions and pharmacology are very different.

used. Mafenide acetate (Sulfamylon) is a sulfonamide derivative prescribed to prevent sepsis in cases of second- and third-degree burns. Silver sulfadiazine (Silvadene) is another topical sulfonamide used to treat burns. Both of these drugs are discussed in more detail in Chapter 48.

Sulfacetamide sodium (AK-Sulf, Cetamide, Isopto Cetamide, Sodium Sulamyd, Sulf-10) is a sulfonamide for ophthalmic and topical uses. In ophthalmic preparations (liquid/drop and ointment) sulfacetamide sodium is used to treat conjunctivitis and corneal ulcers. It is often used as prophylactic treatment after an eye injury or the removal of a foreign body. NOTE: Do not use ointment for the eye unless it has "ophthalmic" printed on the drug label. Sulfacetamide sodium is discussed in more detail in Chapter 48.

Topical sulfacetamide sodium for the skin is an ointment and is used to treat seborrheic dermatitis and secondary bacterial skin infections. This dermatologic form is not used for the eye.

Nursing Process

Antibacterials: Sulfonamides

ASSESSMENT

■ Assess client's renal function by checking urinary output (>600 ml/d), blood urea nitrogen (normal, 8 to 25 mg/dl), and serum creatinine (normal, 0.5 to 1.5 mg/dl).

■ Obtain a medical history from client. Sulfonamides such as co-trimoxazole (trimethoprim-sulfamethoxazole [Bactrim, Septra]) are contraindicated for clients with severe renal or liver disease.

■ Determine whether client is hypersensitive to sulfonamides. An allergic reaction can include rash, skin eruptions, and itching. A severe hypersensitivity reaction includes **erythema multiforme** (erythematous macular, papular, or vesicular eruption; if severe, can cover the entire body) or **exfoliative dermatitis** (desquamation, scaling, and itching of skin).

■ Obtain a history of drugs client currently takes. Oral antidiabetic drugs (sulfonylureas) with sulfonamides increase the hypoglycemic effect; the use of warfarin with sulfonamides increases the anticoagulant effect.

■ Assess baseline laboratory results, especially complete blood count (CBC). Blood dyscrasias may occur as a result of high doses of sulfonamides over a continuous period, causing life-threatening conditions.

NURSING DIAGNOSES

■ Risk for infection related to indwelling catheter
■ Ineffective protection as evidenced by photosensitivity related to sulfonamides
■ Impaired urinary elimination related to prolonged high doses of sulfonamides

PLANNING

■ Client's infection will be controlled and later alleviated.

NURSING INTERVENTIONS

■ Administer sulfonamides with a full glass of water. Extra fluid intake can prevent crystalluria and kidney stone formation.

■ Record client's intake and output. Urine output should be at least 1200 ml/d to decrease the risk of crystalluria. The sulfonamides sulfadiazine and sulfamethoxazole are more likely to cause crystalluria than sulfisoxazole (Gantrisin) and combination drugs. Fluid intake should be at least 2000 ml/d.

■ Monitor vital signs. Note if client's temperature has decreased.

■ Observe client for hematologic reaction that may lead to life-threatening anemias. Early signs are sore throat, purpura, and decreasing white blood cell and platelet counts. Check client's CBC and compare with baseline findings.

■ Check for signs and symptoms of superinfection (secondary infection caused by a different organism than the primary infection). Symptoms include stomatitis (mouth ulcers), furry black tongue, anal or genital discharge, and itching.

Client Teaching

General
• Instruct client to drink several quarts of fluid daily while taking sulfonamides to avoid the complication of crystalluria.
• Advise pregnant woman to avoid sulfonamides during the last 3 months of pregnancy.
• Inform client not to take antacids with sulfonamides, because antacids decrease the absorption rate.
• Warn client who has an allergy to one sulfonamide that all sulfonamide preparations should be avoided, with health care provider's approval, because of the possibility of cross-sensitivity. Observe client for rash or any skin eruptions.

Self-Administration
• Teach client to take the sulfonamide 1 hour before or 2 hours after meals with a full glass of water.

Side Effects
• Direct client to report bruising or bleeding that could be a result of drug-induced blood disorder. Advise client to have blood cell count monitored on a regular basis.
• Advise client to wear sunglasses, avoid direct sunlight, and use sun block and protective clothing to decrease the risk of photosensitive reactions.

Cultural Considerations ❖
• Respect cultural beliefs and values regarding alternative methods for treating infections. Explain the purpose of the drug therapy and how often the drug should be taken.
• Communicate that client should increase fluid intake to 10 to 12 glasses per day. Written instructions in client's own language may be necessary if client's cultural background prevents understanding of the health problem and drug regimen.

EVALUATION

■ Evaluate the effectiveness of the sulfonamide by determining whether the infection has been alleviated and the blood cell count is within normal range.

KEY WEBSITES

Antibacterial Agents—Sulfa Drugs: http://www.elmhurst.edu/~chm/vchembook/653sulfa.html

Co-trimoxazole Oral: http://www.nlm.nih.gov/medlineplus/druginfo/medmaster/a684026.html

Co-trimoxazole Injection: http://www.nlm.nih.gov/medlineplus/druginfo/medmaster/a601165.html

Desensitization to Septra or Bactrim (Trimethoprim-Sulfumethoxazole-TMP/SMX): http://xweb.crha-health.ab.ca/clin/sac/septra.htm

Critical Thinking Case Study

RM, age 46, has a severe urinary tract infection (UTI). She takes TMP-SMZ (co-trimoxazole), 160 mg/800 mg every 6 hours.

1. Is the dose within the recommended drug dose and dosing interval? What is the nurse's responsibility?
2. What are the similarities and differences between trimethoprim-sulfamethoxazole (co-trimoxazole) and sulfisoxazole?
3. What are the signs of thrombocytopenia, hemolytic anemia, and agranulocytosis for clients who take high doses of sulfonamides? Explain the assessment and nursing interventions regarding these severe adverse reactions to sulfonamides.

Client teaching is an important part of nursing interventions. Explain the nurse's role regarding client teaching concerning the following:

4. What is the required amount of daily fluid intake?
5. What are the cross-sensitive effects if a client is allergic to other sulfonamide preparations? What allergic reactions may occur?
6. What time of day should sulfonamides be taken?
7. Why should bruising and bleeding be reported?
8. What protective measures should be taken to prevent possible photosensitive reaction?

RM takes the anticoagulant Coumadin, 7.5 mg a day.

9. What effect does co-trimoxazole have on warfarin (Coumadin), and what is the nursing responsibility? Should RM's Coumadin dosage be increased or decreased? Explain.

NCLEX Study Questions

1. Which of the following are sulfonamides most effective against?
   a. *Escherichia coli* and *Chlamydia*
   b. *Neisseria gonorrhoeae* and *H. influenzae*
   c. *Pseudomonas aeruginosa* and *Helicobacter pylori*
   d. *Enterococcus faecium* and *Staphylococcus aureus*

2. A client is taking sulfasalazine (Azulfidine). The nurse should teach the client to:
   a. drink at least 10 glasses of fluid per day
   b. monitor blood glucose carefully to avoid hyperglycemia
   c. avoid operating a motor vehicle as this drug may cause drowsiness
   d. take this drug with an antacid to decrease the risk of gastrointestinal distress

3. Which of the following is true concerning sulfonamides?
   a. Avoid caffeine during sulfonamide treatment
   b. Administer in 50 ml of fluid over 30 minutes
   c. Avoid sulfonamides during the third trimester of pregnancy
   d. Encourage use of an ultraviolet light to enhance drug effectiveness

4. A client is ordered to take co-trimoxazole/TMP-SMZ. The nurse realizes that _____ is a possible common adverse reaction.
   a. bronchospasm
   b. dysrhythmias
   c. pseudomembranous colitis
   d. Stevens-Johnson syndrome

5. Which of the following is a short-acting sulfonamide?
   a. sulfasalazine (Azulfidine)
   b. sulfisoxazole (Gantrisin)
   c. sulfamethoxazole (Gantanol)
   d. co-trimoxazole/TMP-SMZ (Bactrim)

Answers: 1, a; 2, a; 3, c; 4, d; 5, b.

Unit Ten

Antiinfective Agents

Introduction

Unit X discusses agents prescribed to combat disease-producing microorganisms (pathogens). Included in this unit are antitubercular, antifungal, antiviral, antimalarial, and anthelmintic drugs. Urinary antiseptics and other drugs for urinary tract disorders are also presented.

Infection

Disease-producing organisms may be gram-positive or gram-negative bacteria, viruses, or fungi. The degree to which they are pathogenic depends on the microorganism and its virulence.

The cell walls of bacteria differ in their structure: bacilli are elongated, cocci are spherical, and spirilla are helical.

Viruses are very small organisms that do not have an organized cellular structure. There are numerous families of virus, including herpesviruses, cytomegalovirus, adenovirus, papovavirus, and the human immunodeficiency virus (HIV). HIV agents are discussed in Chapter 34, HIV and AIDS-Related Agents.

The fungi are divided into yeasts and molds. The few fungi that produce disease usually affect the skin and subcutaneous tissues in conditions such as athlete's foot and ringworm. Serious fungal infections are systemic and usually need aggressive drug therapy. Opportunistic fungal infections commonly result from prolonged antibiotic and steroidal therapies and debilitating diseases such as cancer. The yeast *Candida albicans* is a cause of common infections of the mucous membranes of the mouth, gastrointestinal tract, vagina, and skin. Candida, like most fungi, is resistant to penicillin-type antibiotics because of its rigid cell wall structure. Chapter 31, Antituberculars, Antifungals, Peptides, and Metronidazole, describes the variety of topical and systemic drugs used to treat yeast and mold infections.

31

Antituberculars, Antifungals, Peptides, and Metronidazole

ELECTRONIC RESOURCES

Evolve website (http://evolve.elsevier.com/KeeHayes/pharmacology/):
- *Case Studies*
- *Content Updates*
- *Frequently Asked Questions*
- *Student Review Activities*
- *WebLinks*
- *Additional Reference Material*

Companion CD-ROM:
- *NCLEX Examination Review Questions*
- *Pharmacology Animations*
- *IV Therapy Checklists*
- *Medication Error Checklists*
- *Drug Calculation Problems*
- *Electronic Calculators*
- *Top 200 Drugs with Pronunciations*
- *References from the Textbook*

Objectives

- Differentiate between first-line and second-line antitubercular drugs and give examples of each.
- Compare the five groups of antifungal drugs.
- Explain the uses of polyenes.
- Differentiate between the adverse reactions of antitubercular, antifungal, and peptide drugs.
- Apply the nursing process for clients taking antitubercular, antifungal, and peptide drugs.
- Describe the side effects/adverse effects for metronidazole.

Terms

This chapter covers antitubercular drugs, antifungal drugs, peptide drugs, and metronidazole. Although these drug categories differ from each other, they each contain drugs that inhibit or kill organisms that cause disease.

Tuberculosis

Tuberculosis (TB) is caused by the acid-fast bacillus *Mycobacterium tuberculosis*. This pathogen is frequently called the *tubercle bacillus*. Tuberculosis is one of the world's major health problems, killing more persons than any other infectious disease, including **acquired immunodeficiency syndrome (AIDS)** (immune disorder characterized by opportunistic diseases). More than 1.5 billion people in the world have TB, and many are unaware of their infection. Each year more than 8 million new cases of TB are diagnosed. Until the 1980s the incidence of TB had decreased in the United States. The current increase in TB can be attributed, in part, to the increase in persons with AIDS in whom active TB has developed because of compromised immune systems. In addition, the increasing incidence is partly a result of increasingly crowded living conditions in urban areas. Clients more susceptible to TB are those with alcohol addiction, AIDS, and debilitative conditions. Since 1993 the reported number of clients with active TB has declined slightly.

Pathophysiology

Tuberculosis is transmitted from one person to another by droplets dispersed in the air through coughing and sneezing. The organisms are inhaled into the alveoli (air sacs) of the lung. If the body's immune system is strong and intact, phagocytes stop the multiplication of the tubercle bacilli. When the immune system is compromised, however, tubercle bacilli can spread from the lungs to other organs of the body via the blood and lymphatic system. Dissemination of TB bacilli can be found in the liver, kidneys, spleen, and other organs. Symptoms of TB include anorexia, cough and sputum production, increased fever, night sweats, weight loss, and positive acid-fast bacilli in the sputum.

Antitubercular Drugs

Before 1944, many people died from TB because of the absence of drug therapy. Streptomycin, a parenteral antibiotic, was the first drug used to treat TB. Isoniazid (INH), discovered in 1952, was the first oral drug preparation effective against the tubercle bacillus. Isoniazid is a bactericidal drug that inhibits tubercle cell wall synthesis and blocks pyridoxine (vitamin B_6), which is used for intracellular enzyme production. When isoniazid is prescribed, pyridoxine may also be prescribed to avoid deficiency and possible occurrence of peripheral neuropathy. Group names for drugs used to treat TB include *antimycobacterial agents* and **antitubercular drugs** (agents that treat tuberculosis).

Prophylactic antitubercular therapy is suggested for individuals who have been in close contact with persons with TB. Prophylaxis is also recommended for those who test positive for **human immunodeficiency virus (HIV)** (virus causing an infection characterized by profound immunosuppression) and also have a positive TB skin test or are in close contact with someone who has TB. Clients who have converted from a negative to a positive TB skin test should be considered candidates for prophylactic isoniazid therapy. Young children who have been in contact with persons with active TB are at high risk and should receive prophylactic antitubercular therapy. When a person is diagnosed with TB, family members are usually given prophylactic doses of isoniazid for 6 months to 1 year. For HIV-positive clients with positive TB skin tests, a 2-month prophylactic treatment with rifampin and pyrazinamide may be recommended.

Prophylactic therapy is contraindicated for persons with liver disease. Isoniazid is the primary antitubercular drug used and may cause isoniazid-induced liver damage. Other antitubercular drugs may also cause liver damage if given in high doses over an extended period.

Single-drug therapy with isoniazid proved ineffective in treating TB, because resistance to the drug developed in a short time. It was discovered that when a combination of antitubercular drugs was used, bacterial resistance did not occur, and the duration of treatment was reduced from 2 years to 6 to 9 months. Different combinations of drugs can be used: (1) isoniazid and rifampin; (2) isoniazid, rifampin, and ethambutol; or (3) isoniazid, rifampin, and pyrazinamide. Rifampin and ethambutol were discovered in the early 1960s; neither drug is effective against the tubercle bacillus when given alone. In fact, if rifampin is taken alone, bacterial resistance occurs quickly. Prototype Drug Chart 31–1 lists the drug data for isoniazid. Figure 31–1 provides charts used to keep records of clients taking antitubercular drugs.

Multidrug therapy against TB is more effective. The treatment regimen is divided into two phases: the first, or initial, phase lasts 2 months, and the second phase covers the next 4 to 7 months. The total treatment plan is for 6 to 9 months and depends on the response to the antitubercular therapy. Table 31–1 gives examples of various drug regimens to treat TB.

If multidrug resistance to the tubercle bacilli persists, other antibacterial drugs such as the aminoglycosides (streptomycin, kanamycin, amikacin) or the fluoroquinolones (ciprofloxacin, ofloxacin) may be given as part of the multidrug therapy. Susceptibility testing to determine drug resistance should be performed before drug therapy. At times, susceptibility testing of the sputum and antitubercular drugs is performed, but only if the client has not responded to the drug therapy regimen.

Mycobacterium tuberculosis strains that are resistant to streptomycin can be sensitive to kanamycin. An aminoglycoside should not be taken if renal dysfunction is present. When antibacterial agents are used continuously or at high doses, the serum drug level should be closely monitored to avoid drug toxicity.

Prototype DRUG CHART 31–1

ISONIAZID

Drug Class	**Dosage**
Antitubercular	A: PO/IM: 5 mg/kg/d in single dose; *max*: 300 mg/d
Trade names: INH, Nydrazid, Laniazid, ✳Isotamine,	**Prophylaxis:** 300 mg/d
PMS-Isoniazid	C: PO/IM: 10-20 mg/kg/d in single dose; *max*: 300 mg/d
Pregnancy Category: C	**Prophylaxis:** 10 mg/kg/d in a single dose or 15 mg/kg 3×/wk

Contraindications

Severe renal or hepatic disease, alcoholism, diabetic retinopathy

Drug-Lab-Food Interactions

Drug: Increase effect with alcohol, rifampin, cycloserine, and phenytoin; *decrease* GI absorption while taking aluminum antacids
Lab: Increase AST, ALT, bilirubin

Pharmacokinetics

Absorption: PO: Well absorbed
Distribution: PB: 10%
Metabolism: t½: 1-4 h
Excretion: 50% unchanged in urine

Pharmacodynamics

PO: Onset: 0.5 h
 Peak: 1-2 h
 Duration: 6-8 h
IM: Peak: 1-2 h
 Duration: 6 h

Therapeutic Effects/Uses

To treat tuberculosis; prophylactic measure against tuberculosis
Mode of Action: Inhibition of bacterial cell-wall synthesis

Side Effects

Drowsiness, tremors, rash, blurred vision, photosensitivity, tinnitus, dizziness, nausea, vomiting, dry mouth, constipation

Adverse Reactions

Psychotic behavior, peripheral neuropathy, vitamin B_6 deficiency
Life-threatening: Blood dyscrasias, thrombocytopenia, seizures, agranulocytosis, hepatotoxicity

A, Adult; *ALT*, alanine aminotransferase; *AST*, aspartate aminotransferase; *C*, child; *d*, day; *GI*, gastrointestinal; *h*, hour; *IM*, intramuscular; *max*, maximum; *PB*, protein-binding; *PO*, by mouth; *t½*, half-life; *wk*, week; ✳, Canadian drug name.

FIGURE 31–1 When giving multiple drugs for treatment of tuberculosis, such as isoniazid and rifampin, record keeping is essential to ensure that the client is taking the prescribed antituberculin drugs.

Pharmacokinetics

Isoniazid is well absorbed from the gastrointestinal (GI) tract. It can also be administered intramuscularly (IM). It has a very low protein-binding rate (10%), and its half-life is 1 to 4 hours. Isoniazid is metabolized by the liver, and 75% to 95% of the drug is excreted in the urine.

Pharmacodynamics

Isoniazid inhibits cell-wall synthesis of the tubercle bacillus. It is usually prescribed with other antitubercular agents. The onset of action and peak concentration time for oral and IM routes of isoniazid are the same. Peripheral neuropathy is an adverse reaction to isoniazid, so pyridoxine (vitamin B_6) is usually taken with isoniazid to decrease the probability of neuropathy. Alcohol ingestion with the drug can increase the incidence of peripheral neuropathy. If phenytoin is taken with isoniazid, the effect of phenytoin may be decreased. Antacids decrease isoniazid absorption.

Antitubercular drugs are divided into two categories: first-line and second-line drugs. **First-line drugs** (drugs chosen first) (i.e., isoniazid, rifampin, rifabutin, rifapentine, pyrazinamide, ethambutol, and streptomycin) are considered more effective and less toxic than second-line drugs in treating TB. Rifapentine, an analog of rifampin, is the newest first-line drug for treating TB. The client takes it only twice a week, unlike rifampin, which is given daily. To avoid resistance, rifapentine should be combined with another antitubercular drug. **Second-line drugs** (second-choice drugs) (i.e., para-aminosalicylic acid, kanamycin, cycloserine, ethionamide, capreomycin, pyrazinamide, and others) are not as effective as first-line drugs; some can be more toxic. Second-line drugs may be used in combina-

Table 31–1

Possible Drug Regimens for Tuberculosis

Phase	Example I	Example II	Example III	Example IV
First phase (2 mo)*	isoniazid, rifampin	isoniazid, rifampin, pyrazinamide	isoniazid, rifampin, streptomycin	isoniazid, rifampin, pyrazinamide, kanamycin or ciprofloxacin
Second phase (4-7 mo)	isoniazid, rifampin	isoniazid, rifampin, ethambutol	isoniazid, rifampin, capreomycin or cycloserine	isoniazid, rifampin, ethambutol, streptomycin or kanamycin or ciprofloxacin or clarithromycin or capreomycin

mo, Month.

*If there is bacterial resistance to isoniazid, the first phase of the drug regimen may be rifampin, ethambutol, and pyrazinamide. Adjust drug regimen according to drug susceptibility. The health care provider determines which antitubercular drug and how many combinations to use. Symptoms for drug toxicity should be closely monitored. Examples III and IV may be used in various combinations for multidrug resistance.

tion with first-line drugs, especially to treat disseminated TB. First-line drugs and some second-line drugs are described in Table 31–2.

Side Effects and Adverse Reactions

Side effects and adverse reactions differ according to the drug prescribed. For isoniazid, peripheral neuropathy can be a problem, especially for those who are malnourished, have diabetes mellitus, or are alcoholics. This condition can be prevented if pyridoxine (vitamin B_6) is administered. **Hepatotoxicity** (liver toxicity) is an adverse reaction to isoniazid, rifampin, and streptomycin. Clients with liver disorders should not take these drugs unless liver enzymes are closely monitored as liver enzymes may become elevated. The client taking isoniazid, rifampin, and streptomycin may develop headaches, blood dyscrasias, paresthesias, GI distress, and ocular toxicity. Isoniazid may cause hyperglycemia, hyperkalemia, hypophosphatemia, and hypocalcemia. Rifampin turns body fluids orange and soft contact lenses may be permanently discolored. The client taking ethambutol may develop dizziness, confusion, hallucinations, and joint pain. Streptomycin may lead to many adverse effects, such as ototoxicity, optic nerve toxicity, encephalopathy, angioedema, CNS and respiratory depression, nephrotoxicity, and hepatoxicity.

Preventing MEDICATION ERRORS

Do not confuse...

- **rifampin** with other antituberculars, such as **rifabutin** and **rifapentine,** or an antibiotic called **rifaximin,** used to treat diarrhea due to contaminated food or drinking water.

Nursing Process

Antitubercular Drugs

ASSESSMENT

■ Determine a history from client of any past instances of tuberculosis, last purified protein derivative (PPD) tuberculin test and reaction, last chest radiograph and result, and any allergies to antitubercular drugs if taken previously.

■ Obtain a general medical history from client. Most antitubercular drugs are contraindicated if the client has severe hepatic disease.

■ Check laboratory tests for liver enzyme values, bilirubin, blood urea nitrogen (BUN), and serum creatinine. These baseline values can be compared with future laboratory test results.

■ Evaluate client for signs and symptoms of peripheral neuropathy (numbness or tingling of extremities).

■ Assess client for hearing changes if antitubercular drug regimen includes streptomycin. Ototoxicity is an adverse reaction to streptomycin.

NURSING DIAGNOSES

■ Risk for infection related to inadequate primary defenses

■ Disturbed sensory perception related to adverse effects of antituberculars

■ Risk for impaired tissue integrity related to side effects of antituberculars

PLANNING

■ Client's sputum test for acid-fast bacilli will be negative 2 to 3 months after the prescribed antitubercular therapy.

Table 31–2

Antitubercular Drugs

Generic (Brand)	Route and Dosage	Uses and Considerations
First-Line Drugs		
ethambutol HCl (Myambutol)	A: PO: 15 mg/kg as a single dose *Retreatment:* A: PO: 25 mg/kg as a single dose for 2 mo; then decrease to 15 mg/kg/d C: >12 y: same as adult	Used as a combination drug for active TB. Decrease dose if renal insufficiency is present. *Pregnancy category:* C; PB: 10%-20%; $t^{1}/_{2}$: 3-4 h (8 h with renal dysfunction)
isoniazid (INH, Nydrazid)	(Prototype Drug Chart 31–1)	
pyrazinamide (✦ Tebrazid)	A: PO: 20-35 mg/kg/d in 3-4 divided doses; *max:* 3 g/d	Used in combination with other antitubercular drugs for short-term and initial phase of therapy. Promote fluid intake. *Pregnancy category:* C; PB: 10%-20%; $t^{1}/_{2}$: 9.5 h
rifabutin (Mycobutin)	A: PO: 300 mg/d in 1 or 2 divided doses C: PO: 75 mg d	To treat *Mycobacterium tuberculosis* infection; to prevent disseminated *Mycobacterium avium* complex disease in clients with advanced HIV infection. *Pregnancy category:* B; PB: 85%; $t^{1}/_{2}$: 16-69 h
rifampin (Rifadin, Rimactane)	A: PO: 600 mg/d as a single dose C: PO: 10-20 mg/kg/d as a single dose; *max:* 600 mg/d	Used as a combination drug for active TB. For selective gram-positive and gram-negative bacteria, including *Neisseria meningitidis.* Liver enzymes should be monitored. *Pregnancy category:* C; PB: 85%-90%; $t^{1}/_{2}$: 3 h
rifapentine (Priftin)	A: PO: 600 mg × 2 wk for 2 mo, then 600 mg once per wk for 4 mo	To treat TB. Intervals between dose should be at least 72 h. Monitor for toxicity if drug is taken with an anticoagulant, anticonvulsant, or digoxin. Contraindicated with oral contraceptives. *Pregnancy category:* C; PB: 97.7%; $t^{1}/_{2}$: 13.3 h
streptomycin SO$_4$	A: IM: 1 g daily or 7-15 mg/kg/d for 2-3 mo, then 2-3 times per wk C: IM: 20-40 mg/kg/d in divided doses	Used against TB as the third drug with isoniazid and rifampin or with isoniazid and ethambutol. First drug used to treat TB. *Pregnancy category:* C; PB: 30%; $t^{1}/_{2}$: 2-3 h
Second-Line Drugs		
aminosalicylate sodium, P.A.S. sodium	A: PO: 14-16 g/d in 2-3 divided doses C: PO: 275-420 mg/kg/d in 3-4 divided doses; take with food	Second-line antitubercular drug. To treat pulmonary and extrapulmonary TB. Used in combination with other antitubercular drugs. Take after meals to reduce gastric irritation. *Pregnancy category:* C; PB: 15%; $t^{1}/_{2}$: 1 h
capreomycin (Capastat)	A: IM: 1 g/d for 2-4 mo, then 1 g, 2-3 times per wk C: IM: 15 mg/kg/d	Effective against *Mycobacterium tuberculosis,* but should be used in combination with other antitubercular drugs; not effective when used alone. Useful when bacillus is resistant to first-line drug. Hearing loss is an adverse reaction. Client should take supplemental pyridoxine (vitamin B$_6$) to avoid peripheral neuropathy. *Pregnancy category:* C; PB: UK; $t^{1}/_{2}$: 3-6 h
cycloserine (Seromycin)	A: PO: 250 mg q12h for 2 wk; may increase to 500 mg, q12h; *max:* 1 g/d C: PO: 10-20 mg/kg/d in divided doses	Broad-spectrum antimycobacterial drug for the treatment of TB. Second-line drug used when first-line drugs fail. Cycloserine should be used in combination with other antitubercular drugs. *Pregnancy category:* C; PB: UK; $t^{1}/_{2}$: 10 h
ethionamide (Trecator-SC)	A: PO: 250 mg, q8-12h C: PO: 4-5 mg/kg/q8h; *max:* 1 g/d	Like isoniazid, effective against tubercle bacilli. Used when first-line drugs fail. Client should take pyridoxine (vitamin B$_6$) to avoid peripheral neuropathy. Side effects include GI discomfort. **Caution:** Persons with diabetes mellitus, alcoholism, and hepatic disorder should be closely monitored when taking this drug. *Pregnancy category:* D; PB: UK; $t^{1}/_{2}$: 2-3 h

Other Second-Line Drugs

Kanamycin, amikacin, ciprofloxacin, and ofloxacin are effective against tubercle bacilli in combination with antitubercular drugs. Chapter 29 includes more information about aminoglycosides, fluoroquinolones, and other antibacterial drugs.

A, Adult; *C*, child; *d*, day; *GI*, gastrointestinal; *h*, hour; *HIV*, human immunodeficiency virus; *IM*, intramuscular; *max*, maximum; *mo*, month; *PB*, protein-binding; *PO*, by mouth; $t^{1}/_{2}$, half-life; *TB*, tuberculosis; *UK*, unknown; *wk*, week; *y*, year; >, greater than; ✦, Canadian drug.

NURSING INTERVENTIONS

■ Administer the commonly ordered antitubercular drug isoniazid (INH) 1 hour before or 2 hours after meals. Food decreases absorption rate.

■ Give pyridoxine (vitamin B$_6$) as prescribed with isoniazid to prevent peripheral neuropathy.

■ Monitor serum liver enzyme levels, especially if client takes isoniazid, rifampin, or streptomycin. Elevated levels may indicate liver toxicity.

■ Collect sputum specimens for acid-fast bacilli early in the morning. Usually three consecutive morning sputum specimens are sent to the laboratory, and the routine is repeated several weeks later.

■ Have eye examinations performed on clients taking isoniazid and ethambutol, because these antitubercular drugs may cause visual disturbances.

■ Emphasize the importance of complying with the drug regimen.

Client Teaching

General

● Instruct client to take antitubercular drug such as isoniazid 1 hour before meals or 2 hours after meals for better absorption.

● Direct client to take antitubercular drugs as prescribed. Ineffective treatment of tuberculosis might occur if drugs are taken intermittently or discontinued when symptoms are decreased or client is feeling better. *Compliance with the drug regimen is essential.*

● Teach client not to take antacids while taking antitubercular drugs, because they decrease drug absorption. Client should also avoid alcohol, because it may increase risk of hepatotoxicity.

● Advise client to keep medical appointments and participate in sputum testing. Sputum testing is important in evaluating effectiveness of drug regimen.

● Warn women contemplating pregnancy to first check with health care provider about taking the antitubercular drugs ethambutol and rifampin.

Side Effects

● Guide client to report any numbness, tingling, or burning of hands and feet. Peripheral neuritis is a common side effect of isoniazid. Vitamin B$_6$ prevents peripheral neuropathy. Neuritis may not occur if client eats a balanced diet daily.

● Encourage client to avoid direct sunlight to decrease risk of photosensitivity. Client should use sun block while in the sun.

● Inform client taking rifampin that urine, feces, saliva, sputum, sweat, and tears may turn a harmless red-orange color. Soft contact lenses may be permanently stained.

● Alert client receiving ethambutol to take daily single doses to avoid visual problems. Divided doses of ethambutol may cause visual disturbances.

Cultural Considerations ❖

● Increase access to health care. Community involvement and culturally sensitive client education are important. Explain to clients who have active tuberculosis that family members should get a tubercular skin test and may receive a prophylactic drug for 6 months to 1 year. Emphasize the importance of family members seeking medical care.

● Provide a written sheet for drug and treatment regimens in the language client speaks or reads most easily. Explain importance of good hygiene (e.g., discarding tissues that contain sputum, separating dishes, using a dishwasher to clean dishes).

● Understand significance of community if multiple individuals in same community are treated for latent tuberculosis infection. Make all attempts to place on some treatment plan to increase compliance through social support.

EVALUATION

■ Evaluate effectiveness of the antitubercular drugs. Sputum specimen for acid-fast bacilli should be negative after taking antitubercular drugs for several weeks or months.

Antifungal Drugs

An infection caused by a fungus is also called *mycosis*. A fungal or mycotic infection may be superficial or systemic. Superficial fungal infections are acquired via contact with an infected person. Fungi, known as *dermatophytes*, cause superficial fungal infections involving the integumentary system, including mucous membranes, hair, nails, and moist skin areas. An overgrowth of nonsusceptible microorganisms in normal flora following antibiotic treatment may also cause a superficial fungal infection. When *Candida albicans* affects the mouth, it is called *oral candidiasis* or *thrush*. Vaginal candidiasis is common in females who are pregnant, diabetic, or taking antibiotics or oral contraceptives. Systemic fungal infections may involve the lungs, CNS, or abdomen. They are usually transmitted to an individual through inhalation into the lungs from dust, soil, or animal droppings. Fungal infections may be mild, such as tinea pedis (athlete's foot), or severe, such as pulmonary conditions or meningitis.

Fungal infections are also classified as *opportunistic* or *nonopportunistic infections*. **Opportunistic infections** usually occur in the immunocompromised or debilitated population, that is, clients who have cancer, AIDS, or those who are taking antibiotics, corticosteroids, chemotherapy, or other immunosuppressives. Fungi like the *Candida* spp. (yeast) are part of the normal flora of the mouth, skin, intestine, and vagina. An opportunistic infection such as *candidiasis* may occur when the body's defense mechanisms are impaired, allowing overgrowth of the fungus. Other opportunistic infections are *aspergillosis, cryptococcosis,* and *mucormycosis.* Nonopportunistic infections, such as *sporotrichosis, blastomycosis, histoplasmosis,* and *coccidioidomycosis,* can occur in any individual.

Antifungal drugs, also called **antimycotic drugs,** are used to treat fungal infections. Typically antifungals are fungistatic or fungicidal depending upon the susceptibility of the fungus and the dosage. The antifungal drugs are classified into the following groups (Table 31–3):

- Polyenes (e.g., amphotericin B and nystatin)
- Azoles (e.g., ketoconazole)
- Antimetabolites (e.g., flucytosine)
- Echinocandins (e.g., caspofungin)
- Antiprotozoals (e.g., atovaquone)

Polyenes

Amphotericin B

The polyene antifungal drug of choice for treating severe systemic infection is amphotericin B. Introduced in 1956 and used currently with close supervision because of its toxicity, amphotericin B is effective against numerous fungal diseases, including *histoplasmosis, cryptococcosis, coccidioidomycosis, aspergillosis, blastomycosis,* and *candidiasis* (systemic infection). Polyene antifungals act by binding to the fungal cell membrane, forming open channels that increase cell permeability and leakage of intracellular components, especially potassium.

Pharmacokinetics

Amphotericin B is highly protein-bound and has a long half-life. Only 5% of the drug is excreted in the urine. Renal disease does not affect the excretion of amphotericin B.

Pharmacodynamics

Amphotericin B is not absorbed from the GI tract; therefore it is administered IV in low doses for treating systemic fungal infections. Peak effect occurs 1 to 2 hours after IV infusion, and the duration is 20 hours.

Side Effects and Adverse Reactions

Side effects and adverse reactions for amphotericin B include flush, fever, chills, nausea, vomiting, hypotension, paresthesias, and thrombophlebitis. Amphotericin B is considered *highly toxic* and can cause nephrotoxicity and electrolyte imbalance, especially hypokalemia and hypomagnesemia (low serum potassium and magnesium levels). Urinary output, blood urea nitrogen, and serum creatinine levels need to be closely monitored.

Nystatin

Nystatin (Mycostatin), another polyene antifungal drug, is administered orally or topically to treat candidal infection. It is available in suspensions, cream, ointment, and vaginal tablets. Nystatin is poorly absorbed via the GI tract; however, the oral tablet form is used for intestinal candidiasis. The more common use of nystatin is in oral suspension for candidal infection in the mouth. The client is instructed to swish the liquid within the mouth, making contact with the mucous membrane, and then to swallow the liquid after a few minutes. If the throat area is involved, instruct the client to gargle with nystatin after swishing and before swallowing.

Pharmacokinetics

Nystatin is poorly absorbed. Its protein-binding power and half-life are unknown. The drug is excreted unchanged in feces.

Pharmacodynamics

Nystatin increases permeability of the fungal cell membrane, thus causing the fungal cell to become unstable and to discharge its content. This drug has a fungistatic and fungicidal action. The onset of action for both suspension and tablet is rapid. The onset of action for vaginal tablet or cream is approximately 24 or more hours.

Azole Group

The azole group is effective against candidiasis (superficial and systemic), coccidioidomycosis, cryptococcosis, histoplasmosis, and paracoccidioidomycosis. Ketoconazole was the first effective antifungal drug that was orally absorbed. Fluconazole and itraconazole are also azole drugs used to treat systemic fungal infection. These three antifungals can be taken orally, unlike amphotericin B, caspofungin, and voriconazole, which are administered by IV route only. Fluconazole, a systemic azole antifungal agent, is described in Prototype Drug Chart 31–2.

Azoles inhibit cytochrome P_{450} in fungal cells, interfering with the formation of ergosterol. Because ergosterol is a major sterol in the fungal cell membrane, cell permeability and leakage are increased. Numerous azoles are used in topical preparations to treat candidiasis and the tinea infections. These drugs are available in forms of vaginal tablet, cream, ointment, and solution. Topical antifungal agents (azoles and others) are presented in Table 31–4.

Antimetabolite

The antimetabolite flucytosine acts by selectively penetrating the fungal cell, which converts it into fluorouracil, an antimetabolite that disrupts fungal DNA and RNA synthesis. It is well absorbed from the GI tract. Flucytosine is used in combination with other antifungal drugs, such as amphotericin B (Table 31–3).

Echinocandins

The action of echinocandins is to inhibit biosynthesis of essential components of the fungal cell wall, which interferes with growth and reproduction. Caspofungin (Cancidas) is used to treat *Candida* and *Aspergillus* infections. This drug is only administered IV, because it is not absorbed in

Herbal **ALERT 31–1**

When ketoconazole is taken with the herb Echinacea, hepatotoxicity may develop.

Table 31–3

Antifungal Drugs

Generic (Brand)	Route and Dosage	Uses and Considerations
Polyenes		
amphotericin B (Fungizone)	*Test dose:* A: IV: 0.25-1 mg in 20 ml of D_5W infused over 20-30 min A: IV: 0.25-1 mg/kg/d in D_5W or 1.5 mg/kg every other day; *max*: 1.5 mg/kg/d C: IV: Same as adult, except dilution and infusion time differ	For treatment of a variety of systemic fungal (mycotic) infections, such as aspergillosis, blastomycosis, coccidioidomycosis, cryptococcosis, histoplasmosis. Nephrotoxicity may occur when given in high doses. Hypokalemia might occur. *Pregnancy category*: B; PB: 95%; $t^{1/2}$: 24 h
nystatin (Mycostatin)	*Intestinal infections:* A: PO: 500,000-1,000,000 units 3 times/day or q8h *Oral candidiasis:* A: PO: 400,000-600,000 units q6-8h C: PO: 250,000-500,000 units q6h Neonate (<7 d): PO: 100,000 units q6h	To treat *Candida* infections. *Pregnancy category*: C; PB: $t^{1/2}$: UK
Azoles		
fluconazole (Diflucan)	(Prototype Drug Chart 31–2)	Effective against various systemic fungal infections, particularly blastomycosis and histoplasmosis. *Pregnancy category*: C; PB: 99%; $t^{1/2}$: 21-42 h
itraconazole (Sporanox)	A: PO: Loading dose: 200 mg q8h × 3 d; *maint*: 200 mg/d; *max*: 400 mg/d in two divided doses	
ketoconazole (Nizoral)	A: PO: 200-400 mg/d as single dose C: >2 y: PO: 3.3-6.6 mg/kg/d as single dose C: <20 kg: PO: 50 mg/d	For infections by *Candida* spp., histoplasmosis, blastomycosis, and others. Treatment could last 1-6 mo for systemic infections. Take with food to avoid GI discomfort. *Pregnancy category*: C; PB: 95%; $t^{1/2}$: 2-8 h
miconazole nitrate (Monistat, Micatin)	A: IV: 200-3600 mg/d in D_5W in three divided doses; infuse IV over 30-60 min C: IV: 20-40 mg/kg/d in divided doses; *max*: 15 mg/kg per inf A: Supp: 100 mg vaginal at bedtime for 7 d Available: Vaginal cream 2%; lotion	For fungal meningitis and fungal bladder infections. Also for vaginal fungal infections. *Pregnancy category*: B; PB: 92%; $t^{1/2}$: 2-24 h
voriconazole (Vfend)	PO: >40 kg: 400 mg q12h on day 1, then 200 mg q12h, may increase to 300 mg q12h PO: <40 kg: 400 mg q12h on day 1 then 100 mg q12h, may increase to 150 mg q12h A/Elderly: IV: 6 mg/kg q12h day 1 then 4 mg/kg q12h	For treatment of *Aspergillus* infection. *Pregnancy category*: :D; PB: UK; $t^{1/2}$: 6 h-6 d
posaconazole (Noxafil)	A: PO: 200 mg t.i.d.	For prophylactic treatment of invasive *Aspergillus* and *Candida* infections in immunosuppressed clients. *Pregnancy category*: C; PB: 98%; $t^{1/2}$: 35 h
Antimetabolites		
flucytosine (Ancobon)	A: PO: 50-150 mg/kg/d in 4 divided doses C: >50 kg: PO: 50-150 mg/kg/d in 4 divided doses C: <50 kg: PO: 1.5-4.5 g/m^2/d in 4 divided doses Neonate: PO: 50-100 mg/kg/d in 1-2 divided doses	Use with amphotericin B may increase therapeutic action as well as toxicity. Fungal resistance occurs if drug is given alone. *Pregnancy category*: C; PB: UK; $t^{1/2}$: 3-6 h

A, Adult; *b.i.d.*, twice a day; *C*, child; *d*, day; *D_5W*, dextrose 5% in water; *GI*, gastrointestinal; *h*, hour; *inf*, infusion; *IV*, intravenous; *maint*, maintenance; *max*, maximum; *min*, minute; *mo*, month; *PB*, protein-binding; *PO*, by mouth; *supp*, suppository; *$t^{1/2}$*, half-life; *t.i.d.*, three times a day; *UK*, unknown; *y*, year; >, greater than; <, less than.

Continued

Table 31–3

Antifungal Drugs—cont'd

Generic (Brand)	Route and Dosage	Uses and Considerations
Echinocandins		
caspofungin (Cancidas)	*Loading dose:* A: IV: 70 mg *Maintenance dose:* A: IV: 50 mg/d	For treatment of *Aspergillus* infection. *Pregnancy category*: C; PB:UK; t½: 9-11 h
micafungin (Mycamine)	A: PO: 2 g with food in single dose C: >3yr: PO: 50 mg/kg with food in single dose	For treatment of esophageal candidiasis, prevention of *Candida* infection in clients having bone marrow transplantation. May cause GI distress, headache, and elevated liver enzymes. *Pregnancy category*: C; PB: 99%; t½: 12-17 d
anidulafungin (Eraxis)	*Esophageal Candidiasis:* A: IV: 100 mg loading dose on day 1, then 50 mg/d IV for 14 days after last positive culture *Other Candidiasis Infections:* A: IV: 200 mg loading dose on day 1, then 100 mg/d IV for 14 days after last positive culture	For treatment of esophageal candidiasis, candidemia, and other forms of *Candida* infections. *Pregnancy category*: C; PB: 84%; t½: 40-50 h
Antiprotozoals		
atovaquone (Mepron)	A: PO: 750 mg b.i.d. with food × 21 d	For treatment of mild to moderate *Pneumocystis carinii* pneumonia. *Pregnancy category*: C; PB: 99%; t½: 2-3 d
tinidazole (Tindamax)	A: PO: 2 g as single dose with food C: >3 yr: PO: 50 mg/kg as single dose with food, *max:* 2 g	For treatment of giardiasis, intestinal amebiasis, trichomoniasis, and bacterial vaginosis. *Pregnancy category*: C; PB: 12%; t½: 12-14 h
Miscellaneous Antifungals		
griseofulvin (Fulvicin)	A: PO: 500-750 mg microsize/d	For treatment of tinea capitis, tinea corporis, and tinea cruris. *Pregnancy category*: C; PB: UK; t½: 9-24 h

the GI tract. Phlebitis at the IV site and increased AST and ALT are common adverse effects.

Antiprotozoal

Atovaquone (Mepron) is an antiprotozoal agent used to treat mild to moderate *Pneumocystis carinii* pneumonia. This drug acts by disrupting mitochondrial electron transport and inhibiting DNA synthesis.

Nursing Process

Antifungals

ASSESSMENT

■ Obtain a medical history from client of any serious renal or hepatic disorder. Antifungal agents such as amphotericin B, fluconazole (Diflucan), flucytosine (Ancobon), and ketoconazole (Nizoral) are contraindicated if client has a serious renal or liver disease.

■ Check laboratory tests for liver enzyme values (alkaline phosphatase [ALP], alanine aminotransferase [ALT], aspartate aminotransferase [AST], gamma-glutamyl transferase [GGT]), blood urea nitrogen [BUN], bilirubin, and serum creatinine. Elevated levels can indicate liver or renal dysfunction. These test results may be used for future comparisons.

■ Assess prior use of antifungals.

■ Record baseline vital signs for future comparison.

NURSING DIAGNOSES

■ Risk for infection related to poor health practices

■ Risk for impaired urinary elimination related to adverse effects of antifungals

■ Deficient fluid volume related to side effects of antifungals

PLANNING

■ Client's fungal infection will be resolved.

FLUCONAZOLE

Drug Class

Antifungal
Trade name: Diflucan
Pregnancy Category: C

Dosage

Systemic candidiasis:
A: PO/IV: 400 mg/d × 1 then 200 mg/d for 4 wk
C: PO/IV: 3-6 mg/kg/d
Vaginal candidiasis:
A: PO: 150 mg × 1 dose

Contraindications

Hypersensitivity
Caution: Pregnancy

Drug-Lab-Food Interactions

Drug: Increases PT when taking warfarin; increases hypoglycemia when taken with oral sulfonylureas; increases phenytoin, cyclosporine, and haloperidol levels; *decreases* fluconazole level with cimetidine and rifampin

Pharmacokinetics

Absorption: PO: Well absorbed in GI tract
Distribution: PB: 12%
Metabolism: t½: 20-50 h
Excretion: In urine

Pharmacodynamics

PO: Onset: UK
　　Peak: 1-2 h
　　Duration: UK
Vag: Onset: UK
　　Peak: UK
　　Duration: UK

Therapeutic Effects/Uses

To treat *Candida* infections and cryptococcal meningitis
Mode of Action: Increase permeability of the fungal cell membrane

Side Effects

PO: Anorexia, nausea, vomiting, diarrhea (large doses), stomach cramps, rash, headache
Vag: Rash, burning sensation

Adverse Reactions

None known

A, Adult; *C*, child; *d*, day; *GI*, gastrointestinal; *h*, hour; *IV*, intravenous; *PB*, protein-binding; *PO*, by mouth; *PT*, prothrombin time; *t½*, half-life; *UK*, unknown; *vag*, vaginal; *wk*, week.

Table 31-4

Topical Antifungal Agents for Fungal Infections

Tinea Infections

Drug	Drug Form	Candidiasis	Tinea Pedis	Tinea Cruris	Tinea Corporis
Azoles					
butoconazole nitrate (Femstat)	2% vaginal cream	X			
clotrimazole (Femcare, Mycelex, Gyne-Lotrimin)	1% topical cream; vaginal tablet; PO: 1 troche (lozenge)	X	X	X	X
econazole (Spectazole)	1% topical cream	X	X	X	X
miconazole nitrate (Monistat, Micatin)	Vaginal suppository, 2% vaginal cream	X			
oxiconazole (Oxistat)	Cream		X	X	X
sulconazole (Exelderm)	Cream; solution		X	X	X
terconazole (Terazol-3)	Vaginal suppository; 0.4% and 0.8% vaginal cream	X			
Other Topical Antifungals					
ciclopirox olamine (Loprox)	Cream; lotion	X Cutaneous	X	X	X
haloprogin (Halotex)	1% cream; solution		X	X	X
naftifine (Naftin)	1% cream or gel		X	X	X
terbinafine HCl (Lamisil)	1% cream		X	X	X
tolnaftate (Aftate)	1% cream, gel, solution		X	X	X
sertaconazole (Ertaczo)	2% cream	X			

PO, By mouth.

NURSING INTERVENTIONS

■ Obtain a culture to determine fungus type (e.g., *Candida*).

■ Monitor client's urinary output; many antifungal drugs may cause nephrotoxicity.

■ Check laboratory results and compare with baseline findings (i.e., BUN, serum creatinine, ALP, ALT, AST, bilirubin, and electrolytes). Certain antifungals could cause hepatotoxicity as well as nephrotoxicity when taking high doses over a prolonged period.

■ Record vital signs. Compare with baseline findings.

■ Observe for side effects and adverse reactions to antifungal drugs (antimycotics): nausea, vomiting, headache, phlebitis, signs and symptoms of electrolyte imbalance (hypokalemia with amphotericin B).

Client Teaching

General

• Instruct client to take drug as prescribed. *Compliance is of utmost importance, because discontinuing drug too soon may result in relapse.*

• Monitor laboratory testing of serum liver enzymes, BUN, creatinine, and electrolytes.

• Inform client taking ketoconazole not to consume alcohol.

Self-Administration

• Educate client on the administration of nystatin (Mycostatin) suspension: Place the nystatin dose, usually 1 to 2 teaspoons, in the mouth. Swish the solution in the mouth and swallow afterward (swish and swallow).

Side Effects

• Teach client to avoid operating hazardous equipment or a motor vehicle when taking amphotericin B, ketoconazole, or flucytosine, because these drugs may cause visual changes, sleepiness, dizziness, or lethargy.

• Encourage client to report side effects (e.g., nausea, vomiting, diarrhea, dermatitis, rash, dizziness, tinnitus, edema, and flatulence). These symptoms may occur when taking certain antifungal drugs.

Cultural Considerations ❖

• Identify conflicts in values and beliefs because some cultures may not understand the purpose and procedure for the use of vaginal tablets or creams. A detailed explanation may be needed.

• Respect client's apprehensions and fear concerning the use of the topical antifungal drugs and the desire to use alternative methods. Evaluate client's method of topical administration in regard to safe practice. If the method is considered unsafe, explain why and suggest modifications. If appropriate, involve other persons for clarification.

EVALUATION

■ Evaluate the effectiveness of the antifungal (antimycotic) drug by noting the absence of the fungal infection (e.g., decreased itching, redness, and rawness).

Peptides

The two groups of **peptides** used as antibiotics are the polymyxins and bacitracin. Peptides are derived from cultures of *Bacillus subtilis*, and this group appears to interfere with bacterial cell membrane function.

Polymyxins

Polymyxins were one of the early groups of antibacterials, but many of the early drugs were discontinued because they caused nephrotoxicity. Polymyxin B is approved for pharmaceutical use. Polymyxins produce a bactericidal effect by interfering with the cell membrane of the bacterium, thereby causing cell death. They affect most gram-negative bacteria, such as *Pseudomonas aeruginosa*, *Escherichia coli*, *Klebsiella* spp., and *Shigella* spp.

Except for colistin, which exerts action on the colon and is excreted in the feces, the polymyxins are not absorbed through the oral route. Intramuscular injection of polymyxins produces marked pain at the injection site; therefore IV administration of polymyxins at a slow infusion rate is the suggested method. Table 31–5 lists the polymyxins with their dosage and uses.

Severe Adverse Effects

High serum levels of polymyxins can cause nephrotoxicity and neurotoxicity. With nephrotoxicity, the blood urea nitrogen and serum creatinine levels are elevated; however, when the serum drug level decreases, renal toxicity is usually reversed. Signs and symptoms of **neurotoxicity** (toxicity of the nerves) include **paresthesias** (abnormal sensations such as numbness, tingling, burning, and prickling) and dizziness. Neurotoxicity is usually reversible when the drug is discontinued.

Bacitracin

Bacitracin has a polypeptide structure and acts by inhibiting bacterial cell-wall synthesis and damaging the cell-wall membrane. The drug action can be bacteriostatic or bactericidal. Bacitracin is not absorbed by the GI tract and, if given orally, is excreted in the feces. Bacitracin is effective against most gram-positive bacteria and some gram-negative bacteria. Over-the-counter (OTC) bacitracin ointment is available for application to the skin.

Side Effects and Adverse Reactions

The side effects of bacitracin include redness, rash, nausea, and vomiting. Severe adverse reactions are renal damage and ototoxicity. Mild to severe allergic reactions, ranging from hives to anaphylaxis may occur.

Table 31–5

Antibacterials: Peptides

Generic (Brand)	Route and Dosage	Uses and Considerations
bacitracin (Bacitin, Baciquent)	C: <2.5 kg: IM: <900 units/kg/d in 2-3 divided doses C: >2.5 kg: IM: <1000 units/kg/d in 2-3 divided doses. Available in topical and ophthalmic ointment.	Seldom used parenterally except for children. Topical ointment for skin infection and ophthalmic ointment for infections of the eye. *Pregnancy category*: C; PB: <20%; t½: UK
colistimethate sodium (IM/IV) (Coly-Mycin M)	A & C: IM/IV: 2.5-5 mg/kg/d in divided doses	For treating *Pseudomonas aeruginosa* infection. *Pregnancy category*: C; PB: UK; t½: 2-3 h
polymyxin B SO₄ (Aerosporin)	A: IM: 25,000 units/kg/d in 4-6 divided doses IV: 15,000-25,000 units/kg/d in 2 divided doses (q12h) C: >2 y: Same as adult	For systemic use; also available in ointment form. May cause nephrotoxicity if given with aminoglycosides or amphotericin. *Pregnancy category*: B; PB: UK; t½: 4.5-6 h
Additional Antibacterial Agents		
metronidazole (Flagyl, Flagyl-ER, MetroGel, Protostat)	*Amebiasis:* A: PO: 500-750 mg t.i.d. for 5-10 d C: PO: 35-50 mg/kg/d in 3 divided doses *Anaerobic infections:* A: PO: 7.5 mg/kg q6h; *max*: 4 g/d A: IV: 15 mg/kg loading dose, then 7.5 mg/kg q6h *Bacterial vaginosis:* A: PO: ER preparation: 750 mg/d × 7 d *Perioperative prophylaxis:* A: IV: 1 g, 1 h before surgery; 500 mg, 6 and 12 h after first dose *Rosacea:* Thin application twice per day to affected areas Available in vaginal and topical gel	For treatment of intestinal amebiasis, trichomoniasis, inflammatory bowel disease, *H. pylori* infection causing peptic ulcers, bacterial vaginosis, and anaerobic infections and perioperative prophylaxis in colorectal surgery. Side effects may include GI discomfort, headache, depression, although not common. Not recommended during first trimester of pregnancy. *Pregnancy category*: B; PB: UK; t½: 6-8 h

A, Adult; *C*, child; *d*, day; *h*, hour; *IM*, intramuscular; *IV*, intravenous; *PB*, protein-binding; *t½*, half-life; *UK*, unknown; *y*, year; >, greater than; <, less than.

Metronidazole

Metronidazole (Flagyl) acts by impairing DNA function of susceptible bacteria. This drug is used primarily to treat various disorders associated with organisms in the GI tract. It is prescribed to treat intestinal amebiasis, trichomoniasis, inflammatory bowel disease, anaerobic infections, and bacterial vaginosis and is used as perioperative **prophylaxis** (prevention of infection) in colorectal surgery. Metronidazole is commonly used with other agents to treat *Helicobacter pylori*, which is associated with frequent recurrent peptic ulcers. Table 31–5 includes data related to metronidazole. The client taking metronidazole should avoid alcohol and alcohol-containing medications for at least 48 hours after treatment is completed. Drug interaction with alcohol may produce a *disulfiram reaction* (facial flushing, severe headache, tachycardia, palpitations, hypotension, dyspnea, sweating, slurred speech, abdominal cramps, nausea, and vomiting).

Side Effects and Adverse Reactions

The side effects and adverse reactions of metronidazole include dizziness, headache, confusion, depression, irritability, weakness, and insomnia. The client taking high doses of metronidazole may develop dark or reddish brown urine. Dry mouth, metallic or bitter taste, and GI distress may occur. Paresthesias, nasal congestion, decreased libido, dysuria, incontinence, and ECG changes may develop.

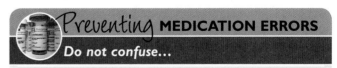

Preventing MEDICATION ERRORS

Do not confuse...

- Flagyl and Flaxedil.

KEY WEBSITES

Information on isoniazid: www.nlm.nih.gov/medlineplus/druginfo/medmaster/a682401.html

Information on amphotericin B: www.nlm.nih.gov/medlineplus/druginfo/uspdi/202032.html

Information on fluconazole: www.hivdent.org/drugs/FLUCONAZOLE.htm

Critical Thinking Case Study

CJ, age 41, has had a constant cough and night sweats for several months. He consumes 1 pint of whiskey per day. Sputum is positive for acid-fast (tubercle) bacillus. The health care provider orders a 6- to 9-month antitubercular drug regimen (time of therapy to be determined according to sputum and radiograph test results). For 2 months, CJ takes isoniazid, rifampin, and pyrazinamide daily. The next 4 to 7 months, CJ takes isoniazid and rifampin biweekly.

1. What could be contributing causes for CJ's contracting tuberculosis? Give other contributing causes for contracting tuberculosis.

2. CJ received first-line antitubercular drugs for treatment of tuberculosis. How can the health professional determine whether the drugs are effective in eradicating the tubercle bacilli? Explain.

3. What is the nurse's role in client teaching concerning the drug regimen?

4. Name at least two serious adverse reactions that can occur when antitubercular drugs are given over an extended period.

5. What laboratory tests should be monitored while CJ takes isoniazid and rifampin? Why?

The health care provider ordered pyridoxine to be given daily.

6. Give your rationale for the use of pyridoxine. What type of drug is it? What is its purpose, and when should it be administered?

7. What health agencies may the nurse suggest that could be helpful to CJ during and after therapy?

NCLEX Study Questions

1. A client is beginning isoniazid and rifampin treatment for tuberculosis. The nurse instructs the client to:
   a. not skip doses
   b. take the drugs t.i.d. with food
   c. take an antacid with the drugs to decrease GI distress
   d. take rifampin initially, then begin isoniazid after two months

2. A client taking isoniazid is worried about the side effects/adverse reactions. The nurse realizes that a common adverse reaction to isoniazid is:
   a. ototoxicity
   b. hepatotoxicity
   c. nephrotoxicity
   d. optic nerve toxicity

3. The nurse teaches the client taking amphotericin B to report signs and symptoms of _____ to the health care provider.
   a. blindness
   b. loss of hearing
   c. nephrotoxicity
   d. Stevens-Johnson syndrome

4. A client with a diagnosis of intestinal amebiasis develops severe nausea, vomiting, fever, facial flushing, slurred speech, tachycardia, hypotension, and palpitations. A beginning assessment reveals that the client has just had several alcoholic beverages. The nurse should obtain a drug history of:
   a. bacitracin (Bacitin)
   b. fluconazole (Diflucan)
   c. metronidazole (Flagyl)
   d. ethambutol (Myambutol)

5. A client has developed *vaginal candidiasis*. The nurse knows that _____ is an appropriate treatment for this condition.
   a. terconazole (Terazol-3)
   b. haloprogin (Halotex)
   c. terbinafine (Lamisil)
   d. tolnaftate (Aftate)

Answers: 1, a; 2, b; 3, a; 4, c; 5, a.

32

Antivirals, Antimalarials, and Anthelmintics

ELECTRONIC
RESOURCES

 evolve

Evolve website (http://evolve.elsevier.com/KeeHayes/pharmacology/):
- *Case Studies*
- *Content Updates*
- *Frequently Asked Questions*
- *Student Review Activities*
- *WebLinks*
- *Additional Reference Material*

Companion CD-ROM:
- *NCLEX Examination Review Questions*
- *Pharmacology Animations*
- *IV Therapy Checklists*
- *Medication Error Checklists*
- *Drug Calculation Problems*
- *Electronic Calculators*
- *Top 200 Drugs with Pronunciations*
- *References from the Textbook*

Objectives

Terms

Viruses
Viral Infections

Vaccines

Diagnostic Tests for Influenza

Antiviral Non-HIV Drugs
Nonclassified Antivirals

Topical Antivirals
Neuraminidase Inhibitors
Gamma Globulin (Immune Globulin)
Purine Nucleosides
Nursing Process: Antiviral: Acyclovir

Antiviral HIV Drugs

Antimalarial Drugs
Nursing Process: Antimalarials

Anthelmintic Drugs
Nursing Process: Anthelmintics

Key Websites

Critical Thinking Case Study

NCLEX Study Questions

- Explain the uses of antiviral and antimalarial drugs.
- Describe the various helminths and the human body sites used for their infestation.
- Describe the action of antivirals, antimalarials, and anthelmintics.
- Compare the side effects and adverse reactions to antiviral, antimalarial, and anthelmintic drugs.
- Apply the nursing process for the client taking antimalarial and anthelmintic drug therapy.

acquired immunodeficiency syndrome (AIDS), p. 476
anthelmintics, p. 482
antimalarial drugs, p. 479
antiviral drugs, p. 474
erythrocytic phase, p. 479
helminthiasis, p. 482
helminths, p. 482
prophylaxis, p. 479
tissue phase, p. 479
trichinosis, p. 482
virus, p. 473

Viruses

Viruses are more difficult to eradicate than most types of bacteria. A **virus** is an obligate intracellular organism that uses the cell to reproduce. Viruses enter healthy cells and use their deoxyribonucleic acid (DNA) and ribonucleic acid (RNA) to generate more viruses. The growth cycle of viruses depends on the host cell enzymes and cell substrates for viral replication. Viruses live and reproduce when they are within living cells.

Viral Infections

Influenza, also called *the flu*, is a highly contagious viral infection that affects the nose, throat, and lungs. This virus is seasonal and more prevalent from December to March. Influenza has three antigen types: A, B, and C. Influenza A causes a moderate to severe infection. Influenza B usually causes mild illness in children. Influenza C is very rare in humans. This viral infection is transmitted easily via contaminated droplets during coughing, sneezing, or talking. Droplets enter into the respiratory tract of the unaffected person and begin replication 24 hours prior to the appearance of symptoms. Usually influenza has an abrupt onset with the first symptom being a fever rising to 104° F. A sore throat, non-productive cough, headache, chills, photophobia, and myalgia may also occur. Following influenza vaccination (flu shot), most individuals develop high antibody titer levels providing protection against similar circulating viral strains.

Herpesviruses are large viruses that cause infections. Among the most familiar are herpes simplex virus type 1 (HSV-1), HSV-2, varicella-zoster viruses (HSV-3, more commonly known as *chickenpox* and *shingles*), Epstein-Barr virus, (HSV-4), and cytomegalovirus (HHV-5, more commonly known as *CMV*). HSV-1 is usually associated with cold sores (vesicular lesions), which grow in neurons. The HSV-1 virus is capable of latency (ability to maintain disease potential without signs and symptoms). HSV-2 is usually associated with genital herpes. The virus in HSV-2 remains dormant by traveling through the peripheral nerves to the sacral dorsal root ganglia. The virus can be transported back the nerve root to the skin for reactivation at any time. While dormant the virus continues to replicate. Both HSV-1 and HSV-2 are capable of causing recurrent infections. Both of these viruses can replicate in mucous membranes and skin of the oropharynx or genitalia. The virus is transmitted by contact with infectious lesions or secretions. HSV-1 is spread by oral secretions from one individual to another. From the mouth, this virus can spread to the genital area by oral intercourse or poor handwashing. HSV-2 is usually spread by intimate sexual contact or an infected mother can transmit this virus to her infant during childbirth. When signs and symptoms are present, they usually include eruption of small pustules and vesicles, fever, headache, malaise, myalgia, as well as tingling, itching, and pain in the genital area.

Cytomegalovirus (CMV or HHV-5) is a very common infectious disease worldwide. It is thought that most adults have had this viral infection at one time and were unaware. Most individuals do not require treatment for CMV unless they are immunocompromised (e.g., babies or individuals who have had organ transplantations). CMV is transmitted via body fluids, especially saliva or urine; by kissing, sexual contact, sharing food; or by pregnant females to their fetus. In susceptible individuals, CMV infection can lead to fatal pneumonia or blindness (due to an infected retina).

Hepatitis B (HBV) is a serious liver infection caused by the hepatitis B virus. The transmission of HBV is usually via a needle-stick, intimate sexual contact, or during childbirth. HBV is found in all body fluids, including blood, semen, and vaginal fluid. The signs and symptoms of HBV include anorexia, vomiting, diarrhea, jaundice, malaise, and myalgia.

A viral infection usually can be detected only after the virus has replicated itself. Viruses can cause mild to severe infections. General signs and symptoms of an acute viral infection include headache, low-grade fever (with a mild viral infection), nausea, vomiting, diarrhea, muscular pain, fatigue, and cough.

Vaccines

Vaccines have been developed to prevent diseases such as smallpox, chickenpox, mumps, rabies, and influenza (see Chapter 35). The influenza virus vaccine may change annually because influenza (flu) virus changes its genetic structure each year. However, the influenza vaccine still promotes the production of antibodies by the immune system, despite the viruses' varying genetic structures. Eggs are used to produce the flu vaccine; therefore any allergies to eggs should be determined before flu vaccine is administered to the client. The success rate of vaccine use to prevent influenza in healthy children and adults is 65% to 90%. In older adults, vaccines are effective 60% of the time, but less than 60% if an older adult has multiple health problems.

Diagnostic Tests for Influenza

Several office laboratory tests can be used to diagnose influenza. The diagnostic test Directigen Flu A has been available for many years to detect influenza A; however, it does not detect influenza B. Flu OIA (Thermo BioStar, Boulder, Colo.), QuickVue Influenza Test (Quidel, San Diego), and ZstatFlu (ZymeTx, Oklahoma City) are new diagnostic tests that identify both influenza A and B. These tests use throat swabs, nasal swabs, or nasal aspiration. Results are available within 10 to 20 minutes. QuickVue tends to be easy and fast for a rapid diagnosis of influenza A and B.

Antiviral Non-HIV Drugs

Antiviral drugs are used to prevent or delay the spread of a viral infection. They inhibit viral replication by interfering with viral nucleic acid synthesis in the cell. There are groups of antiviral drugs effective against various viruses such as influenza A and B, herpes species, cytomegalovirus (CMV), and human immunodeficiency virus (HIV). Drugs for HIV are discussed in Chapter 34. The antiviral non-HIV drugs are listed in Table 32–1. Interferon alfa-2a and 2b are used to treat hepatitis B and C viruses (see Chapter 38).

Table 32–1

Non-HIV Antivirals

Generic (Brand)	Route and Dosage	Uses and Considerations
Systemic Non-HIV Antivirals		
Nonclassified Antivirals		
amantadine HCl (Symmetrel)	*Influenza A:* A: PO: 200 mg/d in 1-2 divided doses C: 1-8 y: PO: 4.4-8.8 mg/kg/d in 2-3 divided doses C: 9-12 y: PO: 100-200 mg/d in 1-2 divided doses	Primary use is prophylaxis against influenza A. Well absorbed by GI tract. *Pregnancy category:* C; PB: UK; t$^{1/2}$: 24 h
cidofovir (Vistide)	A: IV: 5 mg/kg once/wk for 2 wk, then 5 mg/kg every other week. Take probenecid 2 g, 3 h before infusion and 1 g, 8 h after infusion.	For treatment of CMV retinitis, especially in clients with AIDS. Kidney damage may occur; monitor kidney function. *Pregnancy category:* C; PB: UK; t$^{1/2}$: 17-65 h
foscarnet (Foscavir)	*CMV retinitis:* A: IV: Induction: 60 mg/kg infused over 1 h, q8h, for 2 to 3 wk; maint: 90-120 mg/kg/d infused over 2 h *Herpes simplex infections/AIDS:* A: IV: 40-60 mg/kg q8h for 2-3 wk; may include: 50 mg/kg/d for 5 to 7 d/wk up to 15 wk	For treatment of herpesviruses (HSV-1 and HSV-2, VZV) and CMV retinitis. Expensive. Does not cause granulocytopenia or thrombocytopenia. Can cause kidney damage and hyperphosphatemia. Closely monitor kidney function. *Pregnancy category:* C; PB: UK; t$^{1/2}$: 3-4 h
rimantadine HCl (Flumadine)	A: PO: 200 mg/d in 1 or 2 divided doses C: <10 y: PO: 5 mg/kg/d; *max:* 150 mg/d C: >10 y: PO: same as adult	For prophylaxis and treatment against influenza A virus. Drug dose is usually reduced for clients with severe hepatic or renal impairment. *Pregnancy category:* C; PB: 40%; t$^{1/2}$: 33 h
vidarabine monohydrate (Vira-A)	A & C: IV: 10-15 mg/kg/d infused over 12-24 h	Effective against serious HSV-1, herpes zoster, and varicella zoster. *Pregnancy category:* C; PB: 20%-30%; t$^{1/2}$: 1.5-3 h
telbivudine (Tyzeka)	A: PO: 600 mg/d	For treatment of chronic HBV. *Pregnancy category:* B; PB: 3.3%; t$^{1/2}$: 40-49 h.
adefovir dipivoxil (Hepsera)	A: PO: 10 mg qd	For treatment of chronic HBV. *Pregnancy category:* C; PB: UK; t$^{1/2}$: 7.5 h.
entecavir (Baraclude)	A: PO: 0.5-1 mg qd	For treatment of chronic HBV. *Pregnancy category:* C; PB: 13%; t$^{1/2}$: 128-149 h.
Purine Nucleosides		
acyclovir (Zovirax)	(Prototype Drug Chart 32–1)	For treatment of herpes zoster and HSV-1. *Pregnancy category:* C; PB: UK; t$^{1/2}$: 2-3 h
famciclovir (Famvir)	*Herpes zoster:* A: PO: 500 mg q8h × 7 d *Herpes simplex:* A: PO: 500 mg bid × 7 d	
ganciclovir sodium (Cytovene)	A & C: IV: Initially: 5 mg/kg over 1 h q12h × 14-21 d; maint: 5 mg/kg/d over 1 h × 7 d or 6 mg/kg/d over 1 h × 5 d	For treatment of CMV systemic infection in immunocompromised clients. *Pregnancy category:* C; PB: 1%-2%; t$^{1/2}$: 2.5-6 h
ribavirin (Virazole)	A & C: By aerosol inhalation administration	For respiratory syncytial viral infection in infants and children. *Pregnancy category:* X; PB: NA; t$^{1/2}$: 24 h
valacyclovir HCl (Valtrex)	*Herpes zoster:* A: PO: 1 g t.i.d. × 7d *Recurrent genital herpes:* A: PO: 500 mg b.i.d. 5 d *Reduce dosage:* Clients with decreased renal function	Converted to acyclovir during intestinal and liver metabolism. Effective against VZV causing herpes zoster (shingles) and recurrent genital herpes. Monitor kidney function. Encourage client to increase water intake. GI disturbances and headaches are common side effects. *Pregnancy category:* B; PB: 14%-18%; t$^{1/2}$: 2.5-3.5 h
valganciclovir (Valcyte)	A: PO: Induction 900 mg b.i.d. with food for 21 d; maint: 900 mg/d with food	To treat CMV-infected cells of retinitis in AIDS clients. Inhibits viral DNA synthesis. May cause leukopenia, thrombocytopenia, bone marrow depression, and aplastic anemia. *Pregnancy category:* UK; PB: UK; t$^{1/2}$: UK

A, Adult; *AIDS,* acquired immunodeficiency syndrome; *b.i.d.,* twice a day; *C,* child; *CMV,* cytomegalovirus; *d,* day; *DNA,* deoxyribonucleic acid; *GI,* gastrointestinal; *gt,* drop; *gtt,* drops; *h,* hour; *HIV,* human immunodeficiency virus; *HSV,* herpes simplex virus; *IV,* intravenous; *maint,* maintenance; *max,* maximum; *PB,* protein-binding; *PO,* by mouth; *t$^{1/2}$,* half-life; *t.i.d.,* three times a day; *UK,* unknown; *VZV,* varicella-zoster virus; *wk,* week; *y,* year; >, greater than; <, less than.

Continued

Table 32–1

Non-HIV Antivirals—cont'd

Generic (Brand)	Route and Dosage	Uses and Considerations
Neuraminidase Inhibitors		
oseltamivir phosphate (Tamiflu)	A: PO: 75 mg b.i.d. × 5d C: 15-23 kg: PO: 45 mg b.i.d. C: >40 kg: 75 mg/d	For treatment of uncomplicated acute influenza A and B. Treatment should begin within 2 days of flu symptoms. May be taken with or without food. Side effects include transient nausea and vomiting. Dose should be reduced with renal insufficiency. *Pregnancy category:* C; PB: UK, $t^{1/2}$: 6-10 h
zanamivir (Relenza)	A: Inhaler: 10 mg b.i.d. × 5 d	For treatment of influenza A and B. Treatment should begin within 2 days of flu symptoms. Inhaled drug is deposited in oropharynx and throat. Less than 20% absorbed systemically. *Pregnancy category:* C; PB: UK; $t^{1/2}$: 2.5-5 h
Topical Non-HIV Antivirals		
penciclovir (Denavir)	1% cream: apply q2h during the day for 4 d	For treatment of recurrent herpes labialis (cold sores). *Pregnancy category:* B; PB: UK; $t^{1/2}$: UK
trifluridine (Viroptic)	1% ophthalmic solution: 1 gt q2h during the day; *max:* 9 gtt/d	Used primarily for keratoconjunctivitis due to herpes simplex virus. *Pregnancy category:* C; PB: UK; $t^{1/2}$: UK

Nonclassified Antivirals

The first two related antivirals, amantidine hydrochloride (Symmetrel) and rimantadine hydrochloride (Flumadine), were used to treat type A influenza. Both these antivirals are *nonclassified antivirals*. Originally, amantidine was used to treat parkinsonism and only later found to be effective against influenza A. Neither amantidine nor rimantadine are effective against type B influenza. Three other non-classified antivirals are (1) cidofovir, which is used to treat CMV retinitis; (2) foscarnet (Foscavir), which is used to treat HIV retinitis and herpes simplex infection in clients with **acquired immunodeficiency syndrome (AIDS)** (immune disorder characterized by opportunistic diseases); and (3) vidarabine (Vira-A), which is used to treat herpesvirus. In the late 1990s the Food and Drug Administration (FDA) approved two drugs, zanamivir (Relenza) and oseltamivir phosphate (Tamiflu), that inhibit the replication and spread of the influenza virus if given within 48 hours of symptoms; thus early diagnosis of influenza is important.

Vidarabine was first introduced as an antineoplastic drug for the treatment of leukemia. In 1964 it was discovered that vidarabine exerts an antiviral effect against HSV-1, herpes zoster, varicella zoster, and CMV. Although it is not effective against herpes simplex virus type 2 (HSV-2, genital herpes), vidarabine has been used effectively to treat herpes simplex viral encephalitis.

Side Effects and Adverse Reactions

Amantadine and Rimantadine. The side effects and adverse reactions to amantadine include central nervous system (CNS) effects, such as insomnia, depression, anxiety, confusion, and ataxia; orthostatic hypotension; neurologic problems, such as weakness, dizziness, and slurred speech; and gastrointestinal (GI) disturbances, such as anorexia, nausea, vomiting, and diarrhea. The CNS side effects of rimantadine occur less often than with amantadine.

Topical Antivirals

There are three topical antiviral drugs: idoxuridine (Herplex Liquifilm), penciclovir (Denavir), and trifluridine (Viroptic). These topical agents are used to treat herpes simplex viruses.

Neuraminidase Inhibitors

Neuraminidase inhibitors are a group of drugs that decrease the release of the virus from infected cells, thus decreasing viral spread and shortening the duration of flu symptoms. Zanamivir (Relenza) and oseltamivir phosphate (Tamiflu) are two neuraminidase inhibitors approved by the FDA. They should be taken within 48 hours of flu symptoms. These drugs inhibit the activity of neuraminidase, a viral glycoprotein, and are effective against type A and B influenza viruses. Zanamivir and oseltamivir phosphate are not substitutes for the "flu shot."

Gamma Globulin (Immune Globulin)

Gamma globulin (IgG) is rich in antibodies found in the blood. It provides a passive form of immunity to a virus by blocking the penetration of a virus into the host cell. It is administered during the early infectious stage of an illness to prevent a viral invasion in the body.

Human immune globulin (Gamastan) is administered intramuscularly (IM). A single-dose injection protects for approximately 2 to 3 weeks; it then may be repeated in 2 to 3 weeks. For clients who need an immediate increase in immune globulin levels, intravenous (IV) immune globulin (Gamimune N) may be administered.

Purine Nucleosides

The synthetic purine nucleoside antiviral group is effective in interfering with the steps of viral nucleic acid (DNA) synthesis. Drugs in this group of nucleoside analogs include ribavirin (Virazole), acyclovir (Zovirax), famciclovir (Famvir), ganciclovir sodium (Cytovene), and valacyclovir (Valtrex). These drugs are effective in combating herpes simplex viruses (HSV-1, HSV-2), herpes zoster (shingles), varicella-zoster virus (chicken pox), and CMV. Valganciclovir (Valcyte) is a prodrug of ganciclovir and is effective for treating CMV retinitis in clients with AIDS.

The antiviral drug ribavirin was first marketed in 1986. It is used to treat respiratory syncytial virus (RSV) in children and respiratory infections caused by the influenza A and B viruses in older adults. Ribavirin is administered by aerosol.

Acyclovir

Acyclovir was introduced as an antineoplastic drug and later found to be effective against herpesvirus, especially HSV-2, but also against HSV-1, herpes zoster (shingles), and CMV (which can cause congenital defects). There has been reported resistance to acyclovir as a result of the lack of viral-producing enzyme (thymidine kinase) needed to convert the drug to an effective antiviral compound. Prototype Drug Chart 32–1 lists the drug data for acyclovir.

Pharmacokinetics

Acyclovir is slowly absorbed, depending on the dose, and is widely distributed to body and organ tissues. Half the drug passes into the cerebrospinal fluid. The drug is 10% to 30% protein-bound. Its half-life

---

Prototype **DRUG CHART 32–1**

ACYCLOVIR SODIUM

Drug Class	**Dosage**
Antiviral Trade name: Zovirax *Pregnancy Category:* C	*Herpes simplex virus:* **A: PO:** 200 mg q4h, 5 × d; 400 mg t.i.d. for 7-10 d **IV:** 5 mg/kg 5 × d (diluted in D_5W) *Herpes zoster virus:* **A: PO:** 800 mg q4h 5 × d for 5-7 d **C: PO:** 80 mg/kg/d in 5 divided doses *Herpes simplex encephalitis:* **A: IV:** 10-15 mg/kg q8h × 14-21 d **C: IV:** 500 mg/m2 q8h × 7d
Contraindications	**Drug-Lab-Food Interactions**
Hypersensitivity, severe renal or hepatic disease *Caution:* Electrolyte imbalance, nursing mothers, young children	*Drug:* *Increase* nephro-neurotoxicity with aminoglycosides, probenecid, interferon *Lab:* May *increase* AST, ALT, BUN
Pharmacokinetics	**Pharmacodynamics**

Absorption: PO: Slowly absorbed
Distribution: PB: 10%-30%
Metabolism: t½: PO: 2-3 h
Excretion: 95% unchanged in urine
	PO: Onset: UK
	  Peak: 1.5-2 h
	  Duration: 4-8 h
	IV: Onset: Rapid
	  Peak: 1-2 h
	  Duration: 4-8 h

Therapeutic Effects/Uses

To treat HSV-1, HSV-2 (genital)
Mode of Action: Interference with viral synthesis of DNA

Side Effects	**Adverse Reactions**
Nausea, vomiting, diarrhea, headache, tremors, lethargy, rash, pruritus, increased bleeding time, phlebitis at IV site	Urticaria, anemia, gingival hyperplasia *Life-threatening:* Neuropathy, seizures, nephrotoxicity (large doses), bone marrow depression, thrombocytopenia, leukopenia, granulocytopenia

A, Adult; *ALT*, alanine aminotransferase; *AST*, aspartate aminotransferase; *BUN*, blood urea nitrogen; *C*, child; *d*, day; *DNA*, deoxyribonucleic acid; *h*, hour; *HSV*, herpes simplex virus; *IV*, intravenous; *PB*, protein-binding; *PO*, by mouth; *t½*, half-life; *t.i.d.*, three times a day; *UK*, unknown.

is 2 to 3 hours with normal renal function. Acyclovir is excreted unchanged in the urine.

Pharmacodynamics

Acyclovir interferes with the viral synthesis of DNA, thereby short-circuiting its replication. The onset of action for the oral preparation is unknown; for the intravenous (IV) route, the onset is rapid. Peak concentration time is within 2 hours for both routes of administration, and the duration of action for both is similar.

Probenecid can increase the effect of acyclovir. If an aminoglycoside or amphotericin B is taken with acyclovir, the incidence of nephrotoxicity is increased.

Valacyclovir (Valtrex) is converted to acyclovir, which has inhibitory activity against HSV-1, HSV-2, and varicella-zoster virus or herpes zoster. With herpes zoster, valacyclovir offers a greater decrease in pain and an increase in healing time (40 to 43 days) than with acyclovir (59 days).

Famciclovir (Famvir), an antiviral drug developed before valacyclovir, is equally effective as acyclovir for treating acute herpes zoster.

Ganciclovir (Cytovene, Vitrasert) is effective in treating the herpesviruses and CMV. Its primary use is to treat CMV infections. It has serious adverse reactions.

Side Effects and Adverse Reactions

Vidarabine, Acyclovir, and Ganciclovir. The side effects and adverse reactions to vidarabine, acyclovir, and ganciclovir include GI disturbances (e.g., nausea, vomiting, diarrhea). With vidarabine, there might be CNS disturbances such as weakness, malaise, tremors, and confusion. Adverse reactions can include a decrease in hemoglobin, white blood cells, and platelets; liver involvement (transient); and thrombophlebitis.

Acyclovir may cause headache, dizziness, and hematuria. Insomnia, depression, and hypotension, although infrequent, can also occur. Elevated blood urea nitrogen (BUN) and serum creatinine levels can result from renal involvement; such involvement is usually transient.

Ganciclovir can cause thrombocytopenia and granulocytopenia. Because of the possible serious adverse reactions, this drug should be prescribed primarily for severe systemic CMV infections for immunocompromised clients.

Nursing Process

Antiviral: Acyclovir

ASSESSMENT

■ Obtain a medical history from client of any serious renal or hepatic disease.

■ Determine baseline vital signs and a complete blood count (CBC). Use these findings for comparison with future results.

■ Assess baseline laboratory results, particularly blood urea nitrogen (BUN), serum creatinine, liver enzymes, bilirubin, and electrolytes. Use these results for future comparisons.

■ Evaluate baseline vital signs and urine output. Report abnormal findings.

NURSING DIAGNOSES

■ Risk for infection related to insufficient knowledge about avoiding exposure to pathogens

■ Risk for impaired tissue integrity related to adverse effects of antivirals as evidenced by gingival hyperplasia, bone marrow depression

■ Risk for impaired skin integrity related to adverse effects of antivirals as evidenced by rash, pruritus

PLANNING

■ The client's symptoms of viral infections will be eliminated or diminished.

NURSING INTERVENTIONS

■ Check client's CBC. Report abnormal results (leukopenia, thrombocytopenia, low hemoglobin and hematocrit).

■ Monitor other laboratory tests (BUN, serum creatinine, liver enzymes); compare with baseline values.

■ Record client's urinary output. An antiviral drug such as acyclovir can affect renal function.

■ Note vital signs, especially blood pressure. Acyclovir and amantadine may cause orthostatic hypotension.

■ Observe for signs and symptoms of side effects. Most antiviral drugs have many side effects (Prototype Drug Chart 32–1).

■ Check for superimposed infection (superinfection) caused by high dose and prolonged use of an antiviral drug such as acyclovir.

■ Administer oral acyclovir as prescribed. Oral dose can be taken at mealtime.

■ When giving IV, dilute the antiviral drug in an appropriate amount of solution as indicated in the drug circular. Administer IV drug over 60 minutes. Never give acyclovir as a bolus (IV push).

Client Teaching

General

• Advise client to maintain adequate fluid intake to ensure sufficient hydration for drug therapy and increase urine output.

• Instruct client with genital herpes to avoid spreading infection by practicing sexual abstinence or by using condoms. Teach women with genital herpes to have a Pap test done as indicated by health care provider. Cervical cancer is more prevalent in women with genital herpes simplex.

- Direct clients taking zidovudine to have blood cell count monitored.

Side Effects
- Encourage client to perform oral hygiene several times a day. Gingival hyperplasia (red, swollen gums) can occur with prolonged use of antiviral drugs.
- Guide client to report adverse reactions, including decrease in urine output and central nervous system changes such as dizziness, anxiety, or confusion.
- Warn client with dizziness resulting from orthostatic hypotension to arise slowly from a sitting to a standing position.
- Tell client to report any side effects associated with the antiviral drug: nausea, vomiting, diarrhea, increased bleeding time, rash, urticaria, menstrual abnormalities.

Cultural Considerations ❖
- Teach the non-English-speaking client and family members how to use ophthalmic preparations. Pictures may be helpful.

EVALUATION

- Evaluate the effectiveness of the antiviral drug in eliminating the virus or in decreasing symptoms.
- Determine whether side effects are absent.

Antiviral HIV Drugs

The microbe of the human immunodeficiency virus (HIV) is the cause of AIDS. HIV is a *retrovirus*. There are two classes of antiretroviral drugs: (1) reverse transcriptase inhibitors and (2) protease inhibitors. Antiviral drugs classified as reverse transcriptase inhibitors include delavirdine (Rescriptor), didanosine (Videx), lamivudine (Epivir), nevirapine (Viramune), stavudine (Zerit), zalcitabine (Hivid), and zidovudine (Retrovir, AZT). These drugs aid in inhibiting viral replication. Zidovudine was one of the first retroviral drugs approved by the FDA. It inhibits the action of viral reverse transcriptase, thus preventing the synthesis of DNA and allowing the T_4 lymphocytes to increase initially.

The protease inhibitor group includes indinavir (Crixivan), nelfinavir (Viracept), ritonavir (Norvir), and saquinavir (Invirase). This group of antivirals inhibits the replication of retroviruses (HIV-1 and -2). When a protease inhibitor is used in combination with a reverse transcriptase inhibitor, these drugs may greatly reduce the viral level to the point that it is undetectable. The combination of drugs helps decrease HIV drug resistance. Antiviral drugs for suppressing HIV are discussed in Chapter 34.

Antimalarial Drugs

Malaria, caused by the protozoan parasites *Plasmodium* spp. carried by infected *Anopheles* mosquitoes, is still one of the most prevalent protozoan diseases. After the mos-

quito infects the human, the protozoan parasite passes through two phases: the tissue phase and the erythrocytic phase. The **tissue phase** (invasion of body tissue) produces no clinical symptoms in the human, but the **erythrocytic phase** (invasion of the red blood cells) causes symptoms of chills, fever, and sweating. The incubation period is 10 to 35 days, followed by flulike symptoms.

There are approximately 50 species of *Plasmodium*, and 4 types of the species cause malaria: *P. malariae*, *P. ovale*, *P. vivax*, and *P. falciparum*. *P. vivax* is the most prevalent; *P. falciparum* is the most severe. Throughout the world there are about 200 million cases of malaria, but in the United States malaria is confined mainly to persons who enter the country from elsewhere. The incidence of malaria has increased since 1960, primarily because of travel to regions in the world where malaria is endemic and drug-resistant malaria parasites.

Treatment of malaria depends on the type of *Plasmodium* and the organism's life cycle. Quinine was the only antimalarial drug available from 1820 until the early 1940s. Synthetic **antimalarial drugs** have since been developed that are as effective as quinine and cause fewer toxic effects. When drug-resistant malaria occurs, combinations of antimalarials are used to facilitate effective treatment. Chloroquine is a commonly prescribed drug for malaria. If drug resistance to chloroquine occurs, another antimalarial, mefloquine HCl (Lariam), or combinations of antimalarials with or without antibiotics (e.g., tetracycline, doxycycline, clindamycin) may be prescribed.

Three methods used to eradicate malaria are **prophylaxis** (prevention) of malaria, treatment for the acute attack, and prevention of relapse. Many synthetic antimalarials (chloroquine, primaquine, pyrimethamine-sulfadoxine) are used prophylactically. Chloroquine and mefloquine are frequently used to treat an acute malarial attack. Mefloquine HCl and the combination drug atovaquone/proguanil (Malarone) are used to treat chloroquine-resistant *P. falciparum*. Chloroquine and hydroxychloroquine can be toxic to children and may even cause death; therefore the drug dose should be closely monitored. Prototype Drug Chart 32–2 lists the drug data for chloroquine HCl.

The antimalarial drug halofantrine is not available in the United States but is used in countries where acute malaria is prevalent. This drug is effective for treating chloroquine-resistant *P. falciparum*. Clients who have cardiac dysrhythmias should not take it.

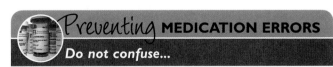

Preventing **MEDICATION ERRORS**

Do not confuse...

- **quinine** (antimalarial) with **quinidine** (antidysrhythmic). These two drugs look alike, but the actions and pharmacology are very different.

Prototype **DRUG CHART 32–2**

CHLOROQUINE HCl

Drug Class	**Dosage**
Antimalarial	*Acute malaria:*
Trade name: Aralen HCl	**A: PO:** 600 mg base/dose; then 6 h later: 300 mg/dose;
Pregnancy Category: C	then at 24 and 48 h: 300 mg/dose
	IM: 200 mg/base q6h, PRN; *max:* 800 mg/d
	C: PO: 10 mg base/kg/dose, then 6 h later: 5 mg base/kg/
	dose; then 5 mg base/kg/d for 2 d
	IM: 5 mg base/kg q12h
	Prophylaxis:
	2 wk before and 6-8 wk after exposure
	A & C: PO: 5 mg/kg/wk; *max:* 300 mg base/wk
Contraindications	**Drug-Lab-Food Interactions**
Hypersensitivity to 4-aminoquinolones; renal	*Drug: Increase* effects of digoxin, anticoagulants,
disease, psoriasis, retinal changes	neuromuscular blocker; *decrease* absorption with
Caution: Alcoholism; liver dysfunction; G-6-PD	antacids and laxatives
deficiency; GI, neurologic, and hematologic	*Lab: Decrease* red blood cell count, hemoglobin,
disorders	hematocrit
Pharmacokinetics	**Pharmacodynamics**
Absorption: Well absorbed from GI tract	**PO:** Onset: Rapid
Distribution: PB: 50%-65%	Peak: 3.5 h
Metabolism: t½: 1.5-2 d	Duration: Days to weeks
Excretion: Excreted slowly in urine	**IM:** Onset: Rapid
	Peak: 0.5 h
	Duration: Days to weeks

Therapeutic Effects/Uses

To treat acute malaria; prophylaxis for malaria
Mode of Action: Increased pH in the malaria parasite inhibits parasitic growth

Side Effects	**Adverse Reactions**
Anorexia, nausea, vomiting, diarrhea, abdominal	ECG changes, hypotension, psychosis
cramps, fatigue, pruritus, nervousness, visual	**Life-threatening:** Agranulocytosis, aplastic anemia,
disturbances (blurred vision)	thrombocytopenia, ototoxicity, cardiovascular collapse

A, Adult; *C*, child; *d*, day; *ECG*, electrocardiogram; *G-6-PD*, glucose-6-phosphate dehydrogenase; *GI*, gastrointestinal; *h*, hour; *IM*,
intramuscular; *IV*, intravenous; *max*, maximum; *PB*, protein-binding; *PO*, by mouth; *PRN*, as needed; *t½*, half-life; *wk*, week.

Pharmacokinetics

Chloroquine HCl is well absorbed from the GI tract. It is moderately protein-binding, and the drug has a long half-life. The first two doses have a loading dose effect. Because of its long half-life, the next dose is given on the second day, and the fourth dose is given on the third day. Chloroquine is metabolized in the liver to active metabolites and excreted in the urine.

Pharmacodynamics

Chloroquine HCl inhibits the malaria parasite's growth by interfering with its protein synthesis. Whether the drug is given orally or IM, the onset of action is rapid. The peak effect is slower when given orally. The duration of effect of the drug is very long—days to weeks.

Side Effects and Adverse Reactions

General side effects and adverse reactions to antimalarials include GI upset, cranial nerve VIII involvement (quinine and chloroquine), renal impairment (quinine), and cardiovascular effects (quinine).

Table 32–2 lists commonly ordered antimalarial drugs and their dosage, uses, and considerations. NOTE: Quinine is an antimalarial drug, and quinidine is an antidysrhythmic drug.

A medication guideline developed by the FDA accompanies mefloquine (Lariam) each time it is dispensed. This type of guideline is used only for drugs that require monitoring for serious adverse effects. Adverse effects that may occur after mefloquine use include severe anxiety, restlessness, disorientation, depression, hallucinations, paranoia, and suicidal thoughts.

Table 32–2

Antimalarials

Generic (Brand)	Route and Dosage	Uses and Considerations
chloroquine HCl (Aralen HCl) hydroxychloroquine SO₄ (Plaquenil SO₄)	(Prototype Drug Chart 32–2) *Acute malaria:* A: PO: 620 mg base or 800 mg, then 310 mg base or 400 mg at 6, 18, and 24 h C: PO: 10 mg base/kg/dose, 6 h: 5 mg base/kg; 5 mg base/kg/d for 2 d *Prophylaxis:* 1 wk before and 6-8 wk after exposure A & C: PO: 5 mg base/kg/wk; *max:* 300 mg base/wk	Alternative to chloroquine. Dosage varies for treating malaria. Can be used adjunctively with primaquine. Give drug with meals to reduce occurrence of GI distress. *Pregnancy category:* C; PB: 55%; $t^{1/2}$: 1.5-2 d
mefloquine HCl (Lariam)	A: PO: Single dose: 1250 mg; then 250 mg q wk × 4 wk; take with plenty of water	Prophylaxis and treatment of acute malaria. *Pregnancy category:* C; PB: 98%; $t^{1/2}$: 10-21 d
primaquine phosphate	*Malaria prophylaxis:* A: PO: 15 mg/d for 14 d (single doses) C: PO: 0.3 mg/kg/d for 14 d (single doses)	Prophylaxis against certain *Plasmodium* spp. (*P. vivax* and *P. ovale*) and for relapse. Can affect white blood cell production (granulocytopenia) and cause acute hemolytic anemia in clients with G-6-PD deficiency. *Pregnancy category:* C; PB: UK; $t^{1/2}$: 3.7-9.6 h
pyrimethamine (Daraprim)	*Malaria prophylaxis:* A & C: >10 y: PO: 25 mg/wk C: <4 y: PO: 6.25 mg/wk C: 4-10 y: PO: 12.5 mg/wk	Prophylaxis use for malaria. For treatment of chloroquine-resistant *Plasmodium falciparum* infections. May be used with quinacrine, quinine, or chloroquine. *Pregnancy category:* C; PB: 80%; $t^{1/2}$: 1.5-2 d
quinacrine HCl (Atabrine HCl)	*Malaria suppression:* A: PO: 100 mg/d C: PO: 50 mg/d	For treating *Plasmodium malariae* and *Plasmodium vivax* infections. *Pregnancy category:* C; PB: UK; $t^{1/2}$: UK
quinine SO₄ (Qualaquin)	*Acute malaria:* A: PO: 650 mg q8h for 3-7 d C: PO: 25 mg/kg/d in 3 divided doses (q8h) for 3-7 d	Used in combination drug therapy or for chloroquine-resistant malaria. Used to treat nocturnal leg cramps. *Pregnancy category:* X; PB: 70%-95%; $t^{1/2}$: 6-14 h
Combination Antimalarial Drugs		
atovaquone/proguanil (Malarone)	A: C >40 kg: PO: 250/100 mg = 1 tab/d for 7 days after exposure C: <40 kg: 62.5/25 to 187.5/75 mg/d	For oral prophylaxis and treatment of malaria. Effective for chloroquine-resistant strains. *Pregnancy category:* C; PB: 99%; $t^{1/2}$: 2-3 d/ 12-20 h

A, Adult; *C*, child; *d*, day; *G-6-PD*, glucose-6-phosphate dehydrogenase; *GI*, gastrointestinal; *h*, hour; *max*, maximum; *PB*, protein-binding; *PO*, by mouth; $t^{1/2}$, half-life; *tab*, tablet; *UK*, unknown; *wk*, week; *y*, year; >, greater than; <, less than.

Nursing Process

Antimalarials

ASSESSMENT

■ Assess client's hearing, especially if receiving quinine or chloroquine. These drugs may affect cranial nerve VIII.
■ Check client for visual changes. Clients who take chloroquine and hydroxychloroquine should have frequent ophthalmic examinations.

NURSING DIAGNOSES

■ Risk for infection related to insufficient knowledge about avoiding exposure to pathogens
■ Risk for impaired skin integrity related to fever and excessive sweating
■ Risk for imbalanced nutrition: less than body requirements related to side effects of vomiting and diarrhea
■ Risk for disturbed sensory perception: visual related to side effects of blurred vision

PLANNING

■ Client will be free of malarial symptoms.

NURSING INTERVENTIONS

■ Monitor client's renal and liver function by checking urine output (>600 ml/d) and liver enzymes. Antimalarial drugs concentrate first in the liver; if client drinks considerable amounts of alcohol or has a liver disorder, liver enzymes require closer monitoring. Renal impairment may occur as an adverse effect of antimalarials.

■ Report if client's serum liver enzymes are elevated or renal function tests are abnormal.

Client Teaching

General

• Advise clients traveling to malaria-infested countries to receive prophylactic doses of antimalarial drug before leaving, during the visit, and upon return.
• Instruct client to take oral antimalarial drugs with food or at mealtime if GI upset occurs.
• Monitor client returning from a malaria-infested area for malarial symptoms.
• Inform client who takes chloroquine or hydroxychloroquine to report vision changes immediately.
• Warn client to avoid consuming large quantities of alcohol.

Side Effects

• Direct client to report signs and symptoms of anorexia, nausea, vomiting, diarrhea, abdominal cramps, pruritus, visual disturbances, and dizziness.

Cultural Considerations ❖

• If client from a malaria-infested country complains of chills, high fever, and profuse sweating, client's serum should be tested for malaria. Client may receive an antimalarial drug as a prophylactic measure or for treatment of an acute attack. Explanation is necessary so client complies with the drug regimen.

EVALUATION

■ Evaluate the effectiveness of the antimalarial drug by determining that client is free of symptoms.

Anthelmintic Drugs

Helminths are large organisms (parasitic worms) that feed on host tissue. The most common site for **helminthiasis** (worm infestation) is the intestine. Other sites for parasitic infestation are the lymphatic system, blood vessels, and liver.

There are four groups of helminths: (1) cestodes (tapeworms), (2) trematodes (flukes), (3) intestinal nematodes (roundworms), and (4) tissue-invading nematodes (tissue roundworms and filariae). The cestodes (tapeworms) are segmented and enter the intestine via contaminated food. There are four species of cestodes: *Taenia solium* (pork tapeworm), *Taenia saginata* (beef tapeworm), *Diphyllobothrium*

latum (fish tapeworm), and *Hymenolepis nana* (dwarf tapeworm). The segmented cestodes have heads and hooks or suckers that attach to the tissue.

The trematodes (flukes) are flat, nonsegmented parasites that feed on the host. Four types of trematodes exist: *Fasciola hepatica* (liver fluke), *Fasciolopsis buski* (intestinal fluke), *Paragonimus westermani* (lung fluke), and *Schistosoma species* (blood fluke).

Five types of nematodes may feed on the intestinal tissue: *Ascaris lumbricoides* (giant roundworm), *Necator americanus* (hookworm), *Enterobius vermicularis* (pinworm), *Strongyloides stercoralis* (threadworm), and *Trichuris trichiura* (whipworm).

Two types of nematodes are tissue-invading: *Trichinella spiralis* (pork roundworm) and *Wuchereria bancrofti* (filariae). The pork roundworm, or *T. spiralis*, can cause **trichinosis** (disease caused by ingestion of raw or inadequately cooked pork that contains larvae of the *T. spiralis* parasite), which can be diagnosed by a muscle biopsy. By thoroughly cooking pork, the roundworm, if present, is destroyed.

Side Effects and Adverse Reactions

The common side effects of **anthelmintics** (agents that destroy worms) include GI distress, which may manifest as anorexia, nausea, vomiting, and occasionally diarrhea and stomach cramps. The neurologic problems associated with anthelmintics are dizziness, weakness, headache, and drowsiness. Adverse reactions do not occur frequently, because the drugs usually are given for a short period (1 to 3 days), with the following exceptions: niclosamide for treatment of dwarf tapeworms, piperazine for treatment of pinworms, and thiabendazole for treatment of threadworms and pork worms. Thiabendazole should be avoided if the client has liver disease.

Table 32–3 lists eight anthelmintic drugs prescribed to treat various types of parasitic worms.

Anthelmintics

ASSESSMENT

■ Obtain a history of foods client has eaten, especially meat and fish, and how food was prepared.
■ Note if any other person in the household has been checked for helminths (worms).
■ Assess client for anal itching.
■ Assess baseline vital signs and collect a stool specimen.

NURSING DIAGNOSES

■ Defensive coping related to the invasion of helminth

Table 32–3

Anthelmintic Drugs

Generic (Brand)	Route and Dosage	Uses and Considerations
bithionol (Actamer)	UK	Effective against flukes. Treatment of *Paragonimus westermani* (lung fluke)
diethylcarbamazine (Hetrazan)	A: PO: 2-3 mg/kg/t.i.d.	Treatment for nematode-filariae
ivermectin (Stromectol)	A & C: >15 kg: PO: 200 mcg/kg/1 dose	A broad-spectrum antiparasitic drug. Causes paralysis to the parasite. Highly active against various mites. *Pregnancy category:* C; PB: UK; t$\frac{1}{2}$: 12-16 h
mebendazole (Vermox)	A: PO: 100 mg b.i.d. × 3 d Repeat in 2-3 wk if necessary C: >2y: PO: same as adult	Treatment for giant roundworm, hookworm, pinworm, whipworm. *Pregnancy category:* C
niclosamide (Niclocide)	A: PO: 2 g, single dose C: >34 kg: PO: 1.5 g, single dose C: 11-34 kg: PO: 1 g, single dose	Treatment for beef and fish tapeworms. *Pregnancy category:* B
oxamniquine (Vansil)	A: PO: 15 mg/kg/ d for 1-2 d C: PO: 10-15 mg/kg/d for 1-2 d	Treatment against mature and immature worms. *Pregnancy category:* C; PB: UK; t$\frac{1}{2}$: 1-2.5 h
piperazine citrate (Antepar)	*Roundworm:* A: PO: 3.5 g/d × 2 d C: PO: 75 mg/kg/d × 2 d; max: 3.5 g/d *Pinworms:* A & C: 65 mg/kg/d × 7 d *max:* 2.5 g/d	Treatment of roundworms and pinworms. *Pregnancy category:* B; PB: UK; t$\frac{1}{2}$: UK
praziquantel (Biltricide)	A & C: PO: 10-20 mg/kg single dose A & C: PO: 20 mg/kg t.i.d. × 1 d A & C: 25 mg/kg t.i.d. 1-2 d	Treatment for beef, pork, and fish tapeworms Treatment for blood flukes Treatment for liver, lung, and intestinal flukes. *Pregnancy category:* B; PB: UK; t$\frac{1}{2}$: 0.8-1.5 h
pyrantel pamoate (Antiminth)	A & C: PO: 11 mg/kg single dose; *max:* 1 g	Treatment of giant roundworm, hookworm, and pinworm. *Pregnancy category:* C; PB: UK; t$\frac{1}{2}$: UK
thiabendazole (Mintezol)	Repeat in 2 wk PRN A: <70 kg: PO: 25 mg/kg 1-2 ×/d for 2 d; repeat in 2 d PRN C: 14-70 kg: PO: 25 mg/kg 1-2 ×/d for 2 d	Treatment of threadworm and pork worm. *Pregnancy category:* C; PB: UK; t$\frac{1}{2}$: UK

A, Adult; *b.i.d.,* two times a day; *C,* child; *d,* day; *h,* hour; *max,* maximum; *PB,* protein-binding; *PO,* by mouth; *PRN,* as needed; *t$\frac{1}{2}$,* half-life; *t.i.d.,* three times a day; *UK,* unknown; *wk,* week; *y,* year; >, greater than; <, less than.

■ Activity intolerance related to dizziness, headache, drowsiness

■ Disturbed body image related to fear of rejection by others

PLANNING

■ Client will be free of helminths.

■ Client will explain how to prepare foods properly to avoid recurrence.

■ Client will describe methods of infection control.

NURSING INTERVENTIONS

■ Collect stool specimen in a clean container. Avoid having stool come in contact with water, urine, or chemicals, which could destroy parasitic worms.

■ Administer prescribed anthelmintics after meals to prevent or minimize occurrence of GI distress.

■ Report to health care provider if client has any side effects.

Client Teaching

• Explain to client the importance of washing hands before eating and after going to the toilet. The parasite can be transferred within the family if proper hygiene is not used.

• Instruct client to take daily showers and not baths.

• Advise client to change sheets, bedclothes, towels, and underwear daily.

• Tell client a second course of anthelmintics may be necessary if helminthiasis persists after therapy.

• Emphasize importance of taking prescribed drug at designated times and keeping health care appointments.

• Instruct client to read all directions regarding over-the-counter drugs prior to use.

• Alert client that drowsiness may occur, and operating a car or machinery should be avoided if this should happen.

• Educate client to report any side effects/adverse reactions to health care provider.

Cultural Considerations ❖

- Obtain an interpreter when necessary; do not rely on family members, who may not fully disclose because of honor and shame.

EVALUATION

- Evaluate the effectiveness of anthelmintic therapy and absence of side effects.
- Determine whether client is using proper hygiene to avoid spread of parasitic worms.

KEY WEBSITES

Acyclovir: http://www.nlm.nih.gov/medlineplus/druginfo/medmaster/a681045.html

Influenza: The Disease: http://www.cdc.gov/flu/about/disease.htm

Malaria: http://www.cdc.gov/malaria/

Critical Thinking Case Study

TP, age 75, has shingles. She complains of pain and blisters (vesicular eruptions), which partially surround her waist. The health care provider prescribed acyclovir, 800 mg, every 4 hours, five times a day for 7 days.

1. When taking the health history, what should the nurse ask TP?
2. How does herpes zoster differ from varicella-zoster virus (VZV)? Explain who would be more susceptible to contracting herpes zoster virus infection.
3. How is acyclovir effective for relieving TP's symptoms?
4. Is the prescribed acyclovir dose correct? If so, why?
5. How does acyclovir differ from famciclovir and amantadine?
6. What comfort measures would you suggest to TP?
7. What should the nurse teach TP about being around other people?

NCLEX Study Questions

1. A client is diagnosed with HSV-3. The nurse understands that this illness is better known as:
   a. chicken pox
   b. hepatitis B
   c. shingles in an adult
   d. cytomegalovirus

2. Zanamivir (Relenza) is ordered for a client. The nurse knows that this drug:
   a. is for the treatment of HSV-2
   b. is taken orally for the treatment of HSV-1
   c. is given for the treatment of varicella-zoster viruses
   d. must be given within 48 hours of onset of symptoms to be effective

3. A client who is taking acyclovir asks the nurse about the drug. Which of the following should the nurse include in client teaching?
   a. restrict fluids to prevent complications
   b. monitor blood pressure for hypertension
   c. Steven's Johnson syndrome is an adverse effect
   d. importance of frequent CBC, BUN, and creatinine tests

4. A client with a history of malaria, presently being treated with chloroquine, is admitted to the hospital. The nurse advises the client to:
   a. get frequent hearing checks
   b. take antimalarials before meals
   c. get stool specimens for frequent testing
   d. check heart rate prior to taking drug to assure at least 60 or above

5. A client is taking thiabendazole. The nurse realizes:
   a. that the drug is given for 7 days
   b. this drug should be avoided if the client has renal disease
   c. other family members should be checked for the same disease
   d. the need to teach proper hygiene to avoid the spread of disease

Answers: 1, c; 2, d; 3, d; 4, a; 5, d.

33

Drugs for Urinary Tract Disorders

ELECTRONIC RESOURCES

Evolve website (http://evolve.elsevier.com/KeeHayes/pharmacology/):
- *Case Studies*
- *Content Updates*
- *Frequently Asked Questions*
- *Student Review Activities*
- *WebLinks*
- *Additional Reference Material*

Companion CD-ROM:
- *NCLEX Examination Review Questions*
- *Pharmacology Animations*
- *IV Therapy Checklists*
- *Medication Error Checklists*
- *Drug Calculation Problems*
- *Electronic Calculators*
- *Top 200 Drugs with Pronunciations*
- *References from the Textbook*

Outline

Objectives

- Compare the groups of drugs that are urinary antiseptics and antiinfectives.
- Describe the side effects and adverse reactions to urinary antiseptics and antiinfectives.
- Differentiate the uses for a urinary analgesic, a urinary stimulant, and a urinary antispasmodic.
- Apply the nursing process, including teaching, to nursing care of the client receiving urinary antiseptic/antiinfective drugs.

Terms

acute cystitis, p. 486
acute pyelonephritis, p. 486
antimuscarinics, p. 491

antispasmodics, p. 491
bactericidal, p. 485
bacteriostatic, p. 485
micturition, p. 490

urinary analgesic, p. 485
urinary antiseptics/ antiinfectives, p. 485

urinary stimulant, p. 485
urinary tract infections (UTIs), p. 485

The largest number of urinary tract disorders are caused by **urinary tract infections** (UTIs; microbial infections of any part of the urinary tract). UTIs may result from an upper UTI, such as pyelonephritis, or a lower UTI, such as cystitis, urethritis, or prostatitis. A group of drugs called **urinary antiseptics/antiinfectives** prevents bacterial growth in the kidneys and bladder, but is not effective for systemic infections. Urinary antiseptics/antiinfectives have a **bacte-riostatic** (inhibit bacterial growth) effect when given in lower dosages. They also have a **bactericidal** (kill bacteria) effect when given in higher dosages.

Urinary antiseptics/antiinfectives, **urinary analgesics** (relieve pain and burning in the urinary tract), **urinary stimulants** (agents that increase muscle tone of urinary muscles), and urinary antispasmodics/antimuscarinics are presented in this chapter. Chapters 28, 29, and 30 present further discussions of antibiotics, fluoroquinolones, and sulfonamides used to treat UTIs. Diuretics are discussed in Chapter 42.

Acute cystitis, a lower UTI, frequently occurs in female clients because of their shorter urethra. It is more common in women of childbearing age, older women, and young girls. Acute cystitis is commonly caused by *Escherichia coli.* Other bacterial causes include the gram-positive *Staphylococcus saprophyticus* and gram-negative *Klebsiella, Proteus,* and *Pseudomonas.* Symptoms of cystitis include pain and burning on urination and urinary frequency and urgency. A urine culture is obtained before the start of any antiinfective/ antibiotic drug therapy. In male clients, a lower UTI is most likely prostatitis with symptoms similar to cystitis.

Acute pyelonephritis, an upper UTI, is commonly seen in women of childbearing age, older women, and young girls. *E. coli* is the most common organism causing pyelonephritis. Symptoms include chills, high fever, flank pain, pain during urination, urinary frequency and urgency, and pyuria. The bacterial count in the urine is greater than 100,000 bacteria/ml. In severe cases, the client may be hospitalized and receive intravenous (IV) antibiotics (e.g., an aminoglycoside, ticarcillin/clavulanic acid, or piperacillin/ tazobactam).

The most commonly used agents for treating UTIs are nitrofurantoin (Furalan, Furadantin, Macrodantin), trimethoprim-sulfamethoxazole (co-trimoxazole, Bactrim, Septra), and fluoroquinolones such as cinoxacin (Cinobac), nalidixic acid (NegGram), norfloxacin (Noroxin), and ciprofloxacin (Cipro). Treatment may consist of a single double-strength dose of the chosen drug, a short-term 3-day course, or the traditional method of 7 to 14 days of drug dosing. Fosfomycin tromethamine (Monurol), a nitrofurantoin prototype drug, is effective for UTIs as a single-dose treatment. Other agents used to treat UTIs include oral amoxicillin/clavulanic acid (Augmentin) and oral third-generation cephalosporins (cefixime, cefpodoxime proxetil, or ceftibuten). With severe UTIs, IV drug therapy followed by oral drug therapy is usually recommended.

Urinary Antiseptics/ Antiinfectives and Antibiotics

Urinary antiseptics/antiinfectives are limited to the treatment of UTIs. Drug action occurs in the renal tubule and bladder, where it is effective in reducing bacterial growth. A urinalysis, as well as a culture and sensitivity test, are usually performed before the initiation of drug therapy. The groups of urinary antiseptics/antiinfectives are nitrofurantoin, methenamine, trimethoprim, and the fluoroquinolones.

Nitrofurantoin

Nitrofurantoin (Furalan, Macrodantin) was first prescribed to treat UTIs in 1953. Nitrofurantoin is bacteriostatic or bactericidal, depending on the drug dosage, and is effective against many gram-positive and gram-negative organisms,

especially *E. coli.* It is used to treat acute and chronic UTIs. The drug data for nitrofurantoin are given in Prototype Drug Chart 33–1.

Pharmacokinetics

Nitrofurantoin is well absorbed from the gastrointestinal (GI) tract. The drug is usually taken with food to decrease GI distress. Decreased absorption occurs when the drug is taken with antacids. Nitrofurantoin is moderately protein-bound. With normal renal function, the drug is rapidly eliminated because of its short half-life of 20 minutes; however, it accumulates in the serum with urinary dysfunction.

Pharmacodynamics

When nitrofurantoin is given in low doses for prophylactic use, the drug has a bacteriostatic effect. High concentration of nitrofurantoin causes a bactericidal effect. Nitrofurantoin is effective against many gram-positive and gram-negative organisms such as *E. coli, Neisseria,* streptococci, *Staphylococcus aureus,* and others. It is not as effective against *Pseudomonas aeruginosa, Proteus* species, and some species of *Klebsiella.* The onset and duration of action are unknown. Peak action occurs 30 minutes after absorption. If sudden onset of dyspnea, chest pain, cough, fever, and chills develops, the client should contact the health care provider. Symptoms resolve after discontinuing the drug.

The nursing process for nitrofurantoin is applicable for the other urinary antiseptics/antiinfectives.

Nursing Process

Urinary Antiinfective: Nitrofurantoin

ASSESSMENT

■ Obtain a history from client of clinical problems with urinary tract infection (UTI), incontinence, or other urinary tract disorders.
■ Check client for signs and symptoms of UTI: pain or burning sensation on urination, frequency and urgency of urination.
■ Evaluate complete blood count (CBC) on clients with long-term therapy; monitor regularly.
■ Check urine culture and sensitivity results.
■ Assess renal and hepatic function.
■ Determine urine pH; 5.5 is desired. However, alkalinization of the urine is not recommended.

NURSING DIAGNOSES

■ Acute pain related to inflammation in the urinary tract.
■ Risk for infection related to insufficient knowledge to avoid invasion of pathogens

PLANNING

■ Client will be free of signs and symptoms of UTI within 10 days.

Prototype **DRUG CHART 33-1**

NITROFURANTOIN

Drug Class
Urinary antiinfective
Trade names: Furalan, Furadantin, Macrodantin,
　✽Apo-Nitrofurantoin, Novofuran
Pregnancy Category: B

Dosage
Initial/recurrent UTI:
A: PO: 50-100 mg q.i.d. with meals and at bedtime; take
　with food
C: 1 mo-12 y: PO: 5-7 mg/kg in 4 divided doses
Long-term prophylaxis:
A: PO: 50-100 mg at bedtime
C: 1 mo-12 y: PO: 1 mg/kg in 1-2 divided doses

Contraindications
Hypersensitivity, moderate to severe renal
　impairment, oliguria, anuria, CL_{cr} <40 ml/min,
　infants <1 mo, term pregnancy, lactation with
　infant suspected of having G-6-PD deficiency
Caution: Vitamin B deficiency, electrolyte imbalance,
　diabetes mellitus

Drug-Lab-Food Interactions
Drug: Decrease effect with probenecid; *decreased*
　absorption with antacids

Pharmacokinetics
Absorption: Well absorbed from GI tract; enhanced
　with food
Distribution: PB: 60%, crosses placenta, excreted in
　breast milk
Metabolism: t½: 20-60 min
Excretion: In urine; small amounts in bile

Pharmacodynamics
PO: Onset: UK
　Peak: 30 min
　Duration: UK

Therapeutic Effects/Uses
To treat acute and chronic UTIs
Mode of Action: Inhibits bacterial enzymes and metabolism

Side Effects
Anorexia, nausea, vomiting, rust/brown discoloration
　of urine, diarrhea, rash, pruritus, dizziness,
　headache, drowsiness

Adverse Reactions
Superinfection, peripheral neuropathy, hemolytic
　anemia, agranulocytosis
Life-threatening: Anaphylaxis, hepatotoxicity, Stevens-
　Johnson syndrome

A, Adult; *C*, child; CL_{cr}, creatinine clearance; *G-6-PD,* glucose-6-phosphate dehydrogenase; *GI*, gastrointestinal; *min,* minute; *mo,*
month; *PB*, protein-binding; *PO,* by mouth; *q.i.d.,* four times a day; *t½,* half-life; *UK,* unknown; *UTI,* urinary tract infection; *y,* year;
<, less than; ✽, Canadian drug name.

NURSING INTERVENTIONS

■ Monitor client's urinary output and urine specific
gravity. Careful attention to output is required when
administering urinary antiseptics to clients with anuria
and oliguria. Report promptly any decrease in urine
output.

■ Obtain urine culture to identify infecting organism
prior to initiation of drug therapy to treat UTI.

■ Observe client for side effects and adverse reactions
to urinary antiseptic drugs. Peripheral neuropathy (tingling, numbness of extremities) may result from renal
insufficiency (inability to excrete drug) or long-term use
of nitrofurantoin. Peripheral neuropathy may be irreversible.

Client Teaching

General
• Teach client not to crush tablets or open capsules.
• Advise client to rinse mouth thoroughly after taking
oral nitrofurantoin. Drug can stain teeth.
• Instruct client to avoid antacids, because they inter-
fere with drug absorption.
• Teach client to shake suspension well before adminis-
tration and protect from freezing.
• Warn client not to drive a motor vehicle or operate
dangerous machinery; drug may cause drowsiness.
• Advise female client to immediately report pregnancy
to health care provider.

Diet
- Inform client to increase fluids and take drug with food to minimize GI upset.

Side Effects
- Alert client that urine may turn a harmless brown color.
- Encourage client to report any signs of secondary fungal or bacterial infection (superinfection), such as stomatitis or anogenital discharge or itching.

Methenamine
- Educate client to drink cranberry juice, eat plums, or take vitamin C (with approval of health care provider) to keep urine acidic. Foods that are alkaline, such as milk and some vegetables, may increase urine pH. Urine pH should be less than 5.5 for the antiseptic to be effective.

Fluoroquinolones
- Warn client to avoid operating hazardous machinery or driving a car while taking drug, especially if dizziness is present.
- Encourage client to take drug with food and avoid antacids, because they interfere with drug absorption.
- Alert client that drug may turn urine a harmless brown color.
- Direct client to report any signs of superinfection or secondary fungal or bacterial infection.
- Tell client to avoid excessive exposure to sunlight.

Cultural Considerations ❖
- Alleviate fear or concerns of client from a different cultural background. Use culturally consistent communication when explaining the treatment regimen for a UTI. An interpreter may be necessary. The use of pamphlets in the language client reads or speaks most easily can facilitate client understanding.
- Provide a detailed explanation of preventive measures of UTIs could be helpful. Proper use of toilet paper after defecation should be emphasized.

EVALUATION

- Evaluate the effectiveness of the urinary antiinfectives in alleviating the UTI. Client is free of side effects and adverse reactions to drug.

Methenamine

Methenamine (Hiprex, Mandelamine) produces a bactericidal effect when the urine pH is less than 5.5. Methenamine is available as mandelate salt (short-acting) and as hippurate salt. It is effective against gram-positive and gram-negative organisms, especially *E. coli* and *P. aeruginosa*. It is used for chronic UTIs. Methenamine should not be taken with sulfonamides, because crystalluria is likely to occur. It is absorbed readily from the GI tract, and approximately 90% of the drug is excreted in the urine unchanged. Methenamine forms ammonia and formaldehyde in acid urine; therefore the urine needs to be acidified to exert a bactericidal action. Cranberry juice (several 8-ounce glasses per day), ascorbic acid, and ammonium chloride can be taken to decrease the urine pH.

Trimethoprim and Trimethoprim-Sulfamethoxazole

Trimethoprim (Proloprim, Trimpex) can be used alone for the treatment of UTIs, although it is usually used in combination with a sulfonamide, sulfamethoxazole (the combined preparation is generically called *co-trimoxazole*, or *TMP/SMZ*), to prevent the occurrence of trimethoprim-resistant organisms. This drug combination produces slow-acting bactericidal effects against most gram-positive and gram-negative organisms. Co-trimoxazole (Bactrim, Septra) is discussed in detail in Chapter 29. Trimethoprim is used in the treatment and prevention of acute and chronic UTIs. The amount of trimethoprim in the prostatic fluid is about two to three times greater than the amount in the vascular fluid. The half-life of trimethoprim is normally 9 to 11 hours, but it is longer in clients with renal dysfunction.

Fluoroquinolones (Quinolones)

Fluoroquinolones are one of the groups of urinary antibacterials that are effective against lower UTIs. Nalidixic acid (NegGram) was developed in 1964, and cinoxacin (Cinobac), norfloxacin (Noroxin), and ciprofloxacin hydrochloride (Cipro) were marketed in the 1980s. Enoxacin was marketed in 1989, ofloxacin in 1990, and lomefloxacin in 1992. The newer fluoroquinolones (norfloxacin, ciprofloxacin, enoxacin, ofloxacin, and lomefloxacin) are effective against a wide variety of UTIs. The drug dosage should be decreased when renal dysfunction is present. The half-lives of these drugs are ordinarily 2 to 4 hours, but are prolonged in clients with renal dysfunction. Table 33–1 lists the urinary antiseptics/antiinfectives and their dosages, uses, and considerations.

Side Effects and Adverse Reactions

The side effects and adverse reactions to urinary antiseptics are listed herein by category.

Nitrofurantoin. Side effects of nitrofurantoin use include (1) GI disturbances such as anorexia, nausea, vomiting, diarrhea, and abdominal pain and (2) pulmonary reactions such as dyspnea, chest pain, fever, and cough.

Methenamine. Methenamine use also has GI side effects, including nausea, vomiting, and diarrhea. There have been allergic reactions to the dye in Hiprex. Bladder irritation and crystalluria (when taken in large doses) may occur.

Trimethoprim. GI symptoms (including nausea and vomiting) and skin problems (including rash and pruritus) can accompany trimethoprim use.

Fluoroquinolones. Nalidixic acid use can have the following side effects: headaches, dizziness, syncope (fainting), peripheral neuritis, visual disturbances, and rash. Nausea, vomiting, diarrhea, headaches, and visual disturbances can occur with cinoxacin and norfloxacin use. Photosensitivity is a common side effect associated with fluoroquinolones.

Table 33–1

Antiseptics and Urinary Antiinfectives

Generic (Brand)	Route and Dosage	Uses and Considerations
fosfomycin tromethamine (Monurol)	A & C: >12 y: PO: 1-3 g packet dissolved in 4 oz water, as a single dose	To treat uncomplicated UTIs in women. Has a bactericidal effect against most gram-negative and gram-positive bacteria. Side effects include headaches and diarrhea. *Pregnancy category*: B; PB: 0; t½: 5.7 h
methenamine mandelate (Mandelamine, Mandameth)	A: PO: 1 g q.i.d. p.c. C: 6-12 y: PO: 0.5 g q.i.d. p.c. or 50 mg/kg in 4 divided doses p.c. C: <6 y: PO: 18.4 mg/kg q.i.d.	For chronic UTIs. Urine pH should be acidic (<5.5). It should not be used with sulfonamides. May cause crystalluria, so push fluids. It can cause GI irritation, so take with meals. *Pregnancy category*: C; PB: UK; t½: 3-6 h
methenamine hippurate (Hiprex, Urex)	A: PO: 1 g b.i.d. C: 6-12 y: PO: 0.5-1 g b.i.d.	Same as above
nitrofurantoin (Furalan, Furadantin, Macrodantin)	(Prototype Drug Chart 33–1)	
trimethoprim (Proloprim, Trimpex)	A: PO: 100 mg q12h or 200 mg q24h; if CL$_{cr}$ (CrCl) is 15-30 ml/min: 50 mg q12h; if CL$_{cr}$ <15 ml/min: do not use	For prevention and treatment of acute and chronic UTIs in both men and women. High doses can cause GI upset. Drug can be combined with sulfamethoxazole (Bactrim). *Pregnancy category*: C; PB: UK; t½: 8-11 h
ertapenem (Invanz)	A: IM/IV: 1 g every day for 10-14 days	To treat complicated UTIs. Effective against gram-positive and gram-negative bacteria. Commonly causes diarrhea, nausea, and headache. *Pregnancy category*: B; PB: 85%-95%; t½: 2-4 h
Sulfonamides		
trimethoprim-sulfamethox-azole (TMP-SMZ, co-trimoxazole, Bactrim, Cotrim, Septra)	(Prototype Drug Chart 30–1)	Effective for serious UTIs and otitis media. *Pregnancy category*: C; PB: 60%-70%; t½: 9 h
Quinolones (Fluoroquinolones)		
cinoxacin (Cinobac)	A: PO: 1 g/d in 2-4 doses for 1-2 wk *Renal dysfunction*: Initially: 500 mg; if CL$_{cr}$ is >80 ml/min: 500 mg b.i.d.; 80-50 ml/min: 250 mg t.i.d.; 50-20 ml/min: 250 mg b.i.d.; <20 ml/min: 250 mg daily Not recommended for infants or prepubertal children.	For acute and chronic UTIs. More effective than nalidixic acid. Absorbed in prostatic tissue. Can cause dizziness and photosensitivity. Avoid excessive exposure to sunlight. *Pregnancy category*: C; PB: 60%-80%; t½: 1.5 h
ciprofloxacin (Cipro)	A: PO: mild to moderate: 250 mg q12h A: PO: severe/complicated: 500-750 mg q12h A: IV: 200-400 mg q12h; dilute and infuse over 1 h *Renal dysfunction*: Decrease dosage *Hemo or peritoneal dialysis*: 250-500 mg q24h after dialysis	Has a broad-spectrum antibacterial effect. For UTI, skin and soft tissue infections, bone and joint infections, and anthrax infection. Antacid inhibits drug absorption. Use with caution in clients with seizure disorders. Can be taken without food. Photosensitivity can occur. Avoid excessive exposure to sunlight. *Pregnancy category*: C; PB: 20%-40%; t½: 4-6 h
enoxacin (Penetrex)	*Uncomplicated UTI*: A: PO: 200 mg q12h for 7 d *Complicated or severe UTI*: A: PO: 400 mg q12h for 14 d If CL$_{cr}$ <30 ml/min, reduce dose by 50%.	Effective against complicated and uncomplicated UTIs. Fluid intake should be increased. Take before or after meals. Phototoxicity may occur. *Pregnancy category*: C (*pregnant*: X); PB: UK; t½: 3-6 h
lomefloxacin (Maxaquin)	A: PO: 400 mg/d × 10 d	For UTIs and transurethral surgery prophylaxis. *Pregnancy category*: C; PB: UK; t½: 6.25-7.75 h

A, Adult; *b.i.d.*, twice a day; *BUN*, blood urea nitrogen; *C*, child; *CL$_{cr}$*, creatinine clearance; *d*, day; *GI*, gastrointestinal; *h*, hour; *IM*, intramuscular; *IV*, intravenous; *min*, minute; *mo*, month; *PB*, protein-binding; *p.c.*, after meals; *PO*, by mouth; *q.i.d.*, four times a day; *t½*, half-life; *t.i.d.*, three times a day; *UK*, unknown; *UTI*, urinary tract infection; *wk*, week; *y*, year; >, greater than; <, less than.   *Continued*

Table 33–1

Antiseptics and Urinary Antiinfectives—cont'd

Generic (Brand)	Route and Dosage	Uses and Considerations
nalidixic acid (NegGram)	A: PO: 1 g q.i.d. for 1-2 wk; 1 g b.i.d. for long-term use C: PO: 55 mg/kg/d in 4 divided doses for 1-2 wk; 33 mg/kg/d for long-term use C: <3 mo: *Do not use*	For acute and chronic UTIs. Resistance to drug may occur. Highly protein-bound. Not distributed in prostatic fluid. Take with food to avoid GI upset. Photosensitivity can occur. Contact health care provider if seizures or severe headaches occur. *Pregnancy category*: B; PB: 93%; t½: 1-2 h (elderly: 12 h)
norfloxacin (Noroxin)	A: PO: 400 mg b.i.d. for 1-2 wk on empty stomach *Uncomplicated cystitis caused by E. coli, K. pneumoniae, P. mirabilis*: 400 mg b.i.d. 3 × d *Uncomplicated UTI caused by any other organism*: 400 mg b.i.d. × 7-10 d *Complicated UTI*: 400 mg b.i.d. × 10-21 d *Renal impairment (CLcr <50 ml/min)*: 400 mg daily	For acute and chronic UTIs. Most potent drug of the quinolone group. Food may inhibit drug absorption. *Pregnancy category*: C; PB: 10%-15%; t½: 3-4 h
ofloxacin (Floxin)	A: PO: IV: 200 mg q12h × 10 d	For UTIs, respiratory tract and skin infections. May cause headaches, dizziness, insomnia. *Pregnancy category*: C; PB: 20%-32%; t½: 5-7.5 h
Other		
aztreonam (Azactam)	A: IM/IV: 500 mg-1 g q8-12h	Treatment of UTIs caused by gram-negative organisms. Also useful for lower respiratory infection and septicemia. *Pregnancy category*: B; PB: 56%-60%; t½: 1.5-2 h
imipenem/cilastatin sodium (Primaxin)	A: IV: 250 mg-1 g q6h; *max*: 4 g/d or 50 mg/kg/d, whichever is the lesser amount C: Safety and efficacy not established Adjust dosing in clients with renal impairment.	Treatment of serious UTIs. Also useful for lower respiratory, bone, and joint infections; septicemia; endocarditis. *Pregnancy category*: C; PB: 20%-40%; t½: 1 h
polymyxin B SO₄ (Aerosporin)	A & C: IV: 15,000-25,000 units/kg/d in divided doses q12h	Effective for UTIs and prevention of bacteruria from indwelling catheter. Can cause nephrotoxicity. Monitor renal function (BUN, serum creatinine). *Pregnancy category*: B; PB: UK; t½: 4-6 h

Drug-Drug Interactions

The following drug-drug interactions can occur with the use of urinary antiseptics/antiinfectives:

* Antacids decrease nitrofurantoin absorption.
* Sodium bicarbonate inhibits the action of methenamine.
* Methenamine taken with sulfonamides increases the risk of crystalluria.
* Nalidixic acid enhances the effects of warfarin (Coumadin).
* Most urinary antiseptics cause false-positive Clinitest results.

Urinary Analgesics

Phenazopyridine

Phenazopyridine hydrochloride (Pyridium), an azo dye, is a urinary analgesic (relieves urinary pain and burning) that has been available for almost 40 years. It is used to relieve the pain, burning sensation, and frequency and urgency of urination that are symptomatic of lower UTIs. The drug can cause GI disturbances, hemolytic anemia, nephrotoxicity, and hepatotoxicity. The urine becomes a harmless reddish orange because of the dye. Phenazopyridine can alter the glucose urine test (Clinitest); therefore a blood test should be used to monitor glucose levels.

Urinary Stimulants

When bladder function is decreased or lost as a result of (1) a neurogenic bladder (a dysfunction caused by a lesion of the nervous system), (2) a spinal cord injury (paraplegia, hemiplegia), or (3) a severe head injury, a parasympathomimetic may be used to stimulate **micturition** (urination). The drug of choice, bethanechol chloride (Urecholine), is a urinary stimulant, also known as a *direct-acting parasympathomimetic* (cholinomimetic). The drug action is to increase bladder tone by increasing tone of the detrusor urinal muscle, which produces a contraction strong enough to stimulate urination. Bethanechol is discussed in detail in Chapter 18.

Urinary Antispasmodics/ Antimuscarinics

Urinary tract spasms resulting from infection or injury can be relieved with **antispasmodics** that have a direct action on the smooth muscles of the urinary tract. This group of drugs (dimethyl sulfoxide [also called *DMSO*], oxybutynin [Ditropan], and flavoxate [Urispas]) is contraindicated for use if urinary or GI obstruction is present or if the client has glaucoma. Antispasmodics have the same effects as **antimuscarinics** (agents that block parasympathetic nerve impulses), parasympatholytics, and anticholinergics (see Chapter 18). Side effects include dry mouth, increased heart rate, dizziness, intestinal distention, and constipation. Tolterodine tartrate (Detrol) is an antimuscarinic/anticholinergic drug used to control an overactive bladder, which causes frequency in urination. This drug also decreases urge urinary incontinence. It has the same side effects as antispasmodics/anticholinergics. The client taking antimuscarinic/anticholinergic drugs

Table 33–2

Urinary Analgesic, Stimulant, and Antispasmodics

Generic (Brand)	Route and Dosage	Uses and Considerations
Urinary Analgesic		
phenazopyridine HCl (Pyridium, Urodine)	A: PO: 100-200 mg t.i.d. p.c. × 2 d C: PO: 12 mg/kg in 3 divided doses	For chronic cystitis to alleviate pain and burning sensation during urination. Urine will be reddish orange. Can be taken concurrently with an antibiotic. Treats only symptoms, not underlying cause. Should not be used long-term for undiagnosed urinary tract pain. *Pregnancy category*: B; PB: UK; t½: UK
Urinary Stimulant		
bethanechol Cl (Urecholine, Duvoid, Urebeth)	A: PO: 10-50 mg t.i.d./q.i.d. 1 h a.c. or 2 h p.c.; *max*: 120 mg/d subQ: 2.5-5 mg t.i.d./q.i.d. PRN C: PO: 0.2 mg/kg t.i.d. or 0.6 mg/m² t.i.d.	For hypotonic or atonic bladder. Should not be taken if peptic ulcer is present. Can cause epigastric distress, abdominal cramps, nausea, vomiting, diarrhea, and flatulence. Can cause dizziness, lightheadedness, and fainting, especially when standing up from lying or sitting position. *Pregnancy category*: C; PB: UK; t½: UK
Urinary Antispasmodics		
dimethyl sulfoxide (DMSO, Rimso-50)	*Bladder instillation:* 50 ml of 50% sol retained for 15 min; repeat q2wk until relief	For cystitis. Administered into the bladder to remain for 15 minutes. Additional effects are antiinflammatory, anesthetic, and bacteriostatic. Can cause a garliclike taste and odor on breath and skin for up to 72 h. *Pregnancy category*: C; PB: UK; t½: UK
flavoxate HCl (Urispas)	A: PO: 100-200 mg t.i.d. or q.i.d.	For urinary tract spasms. To be avoided by persons with glaucoma. Cautious use by older adults. Side effects include nausea, vomiting, dry mouth, drowsiness, blurred vision. *Pregnancy category*: B; PB: UK; t½: UK
oxybutynin Cl (Ditropan)	A: PO: 5 mg b.i.d. or t.i.d. Elderly: PO: 2.5-5 mg b.i.d. C: >5 y: PO: 5 mg b.i.d. C: 1-5 y: PO: 0.2 mg/kg b.i.d.-q.i.d.	For urinary tract spasms and overactive bladder. Contraindicated for persons with cardiac, renal, hepatic, and prostate problems. Side effects include drowsiness, blurred vision, and dry mouth. *Pregnancy category*: B; PB: UK; t½: 1-3 h
Antimuscarinic/Anticholinergic		
tolterodine tartrate (Detrol)	A: PO: 2 mg b.i.d. Decrease to 1 mg b.i.d. with liver or kidney dysfunction	To control overactive bladder by decreasing urinary frequency and urgency. Client with narrow-angle glaucoma should not take this drug. Dry mouth is common. *Pregnancy category*: C; PB: 96%; t½: 2-3.5 h
trospium chloride (Sanctura)	A: PO: 20 mg twice daily	To treat overactive bladder by action of a muscarinic-receptor antagonist. *Pregnancy category*: C; PB: UK; t½: 20 h
solifenacin succinate (VESIcare)	A: PO: 5 mg/d initially; then may be increased to 10 mg/d if tolerated	To treat overactive bladder by action of a muscarinic-receptor antagonist. *Pregnancy category*: C; PB: UK; t½: 45-68 h
darifenacin hydrobromide (Enablex)	A: PO: 7.5-15 mg daily	To treat overactive bladder by action of a muscarinic-receptor antagonist. *Pregnancy category*: C; PB: 98%; t½: 13-19 h

A, Adult; *a.c.*, before meals; *b.i.d.*, twice a day; *C*, child; *d*, daily; *h*, hour; *max*, maximum; *min*, minute; *PB*, protein-binding; *p.c.*, after meals; *PO*, by mouth; *PRN*, as needed; *q.i.d.*, four times a day; *subQ*, subcutaneous; *sol*, solution; *t½*, half-life; *t.i.d.*, three times a day; *UK*, unknown; *wk*, week; *y*, year; *>*, greater than.

should be taught to report urinary retention, severe dizziness, blurred vision, palpitations, and confusion. The client should be warned to use caution in hot environments to avoid heat prostration. Table 32–2 lists drugs that are urinary analgesics, stimulants, and antispasmodics/antimuscarinics.

KEY WEBSITES

Phenazopyridine: www.nlm.nih.gov/medlineplus/druginfo/medmaster/a682231.html

Urecholine: www.rxlist.com/cgi/generic3/bethane.htm

Detrol: www.rxlist.com/cgi/generic/detrol.htm

Critical Thinking Case Study

FL, age 29, is married and has a 3-year-old child. FL complained to her health care provider of painful urinary frequency and urgency. The client has an elevated temperature. A urine specimen indicates that the client has a urinary tract infection (UTI). The health care provider prescribes Co-trimoxazole D.S. tablets (double-strength, T-160 mg/S-800 mg) twice a day for 14 days.

1. What other information should the health care provider obtain from the client?
2. What other dose of co-trimoxazole (TMP-SMZ) could be prescribed? Explain.
3. Explain what the health care provider should discuss with the client in regard to taking the drug and its possible side effects. What other information should FL receive?
4. What preventive measures should be discussed with the client to prevent future occurrences of UTIs?
5. What is the recommended follow-up care for FL?
6. What other drugs might be used instead of co-trimoxazole (TMP-SMZ)? Would one urinary antiinfective drug be more effective than another antiinfective drug? Explain.

NCLEX Study Questions

1. For the client who is taking nitrofurantoin, the nurse should teach the client to:
   a. expect the urine to turn blue
   b. keep urine acid by drinking milk
   c. rinse the mouth after oral nitrofurantoin to avoid teeth staining
   d. take an antacid with oral nitrofurantoin to avoid gastrointestinal distress

2. The client complains about a burning sensation and pain when urinating. The nurse knows that an appropriate urinary analgesic is:
   a. tolterodine (Detrol)
   b. oxybutynin (Ditropan)
   c. bethanechol (Urecholine)
   d. phenazopyridine (Pyridium)

3. A client is taking the urinary antiseptic methenamine mandelate (Mandelamine) for a UTI. The nurse realizes this drug should not be given concurrently with _____ to avoid potential crystalluria.
   a. ertapenem (Invanz)
   b. ciprofloxacin (Cipro)
   c. nalidixic acid (NegGram)
   d. trimethoprim-sulfamethoxazole (Bactrim)

4. A client is receiving solifenacin succinate (VESIcare). The nurse knows that this drug is used to treat:
   a. chronic cystitis
   b. overactive bladder
   c. urinary tract spasms
   d. urinary tract infection

5. The client is taking tolterodine tartrate (Detrol), the nurse should teach the client to report:
   a. alkaline urine
   b. urinary retention
   c. excessive tearing
   d. reddish orange urine

Answers: 1. c; 2. d; 3. d; 4. b; 5. b.

Eleven

Immunologic Agents

Immunity comprises functions that protect people from the effects of invasion of the body by microscopic organisms such as bacteria, viruses, molds, spores, pollens, protozoa, and cells from other persons or animals. A person remains in harmony with these organisms as long as the organisms do not enter the body's internal environment. The body has various defenses (e.g., skin) that prevent microorganisms from gaining access to its internal environment. However, these defenses are not infallible, and invasion of the body's internal environment by microorganisms occurs often. A properly functioning immune system neutralizes, eliminates, or destroys the invading microorganisms. To do this without harming the body, immune system cells use defensive actions against only *nonself* proteins and cells. This means that the immune system cells can differentiate between the body's own healthy *self* cells and other nonself proteins and cells.

Nonself proteins and cells include (1) all foreign cells and microorganisms, (2) infected or debilitated body cells, and (3) self cells that have undergone malignant transformation into cancer cells. This ability to recognize self versus nonself, necessary to prevent healthy body cells from being destroyed along with the invaders, is called *self-tolerance*. The immune system cells are the only body cells capable of recognizing self from nonself.

Unique proteins on the surface of all body cells of each individual serve as a personal identification code for that person. The cell-surface proteins of one person are recognized as "foreign" by the immune system of another person. These are antigens, proteins capable of stimulating an immune response.

Immune function is generally most efficient when people are in their 20s and 30s; it slowly declines with increasing age. Older adults have marginal immune function, causing increased susceptibility to a variety of pathologic conditions.

Immune System Structure

The immune system is not confined to any one organ or body area. Instead, immune system cells originate in the bone marrow. Some of these cells mature in the bone marrow; others leave the bone marrow and mature in different body sites. After maturation most immune system cells are released into the blood, where they circulate throughout the body and exert specific effects.

493

Immune System Function

The three processes necessary for immunity together with the cells involved in these responses can be categorized as inflammation, antibody-mediated immunity (humoral immunity), and cell-mediated immunity. Inflammation is discussed in the introduction to Unit VII. Full immunity, or *immunocompetence*, requires the adequate function and interaction of all three processes, although some functions of each overlap. Long-lasting immune actions are those generated by antibody-mediated immunity and cell-mediated immunity.

Antibody-Mediated Immunity

Antibody-mediated immunity (AMI), also called *humoral immunity*, involves antigen-antibody interactions that neutralize, eliminate, or destroy foreign proteins. Antibodies for these interactions are produced by populations of B lymphocytes.

Antigen-Antibody Interactions

Antigen-antibody interactions occur in the body's internal environment. To make an antibody that can exert its effects on a specific antigen, the body must first be exposed to that antigen to the degree that the antigen enters the body. Even when exposure includes penetration, not all exposures result in the stimulation of antibody production. Invasion by the antigen must occur in such large numbers that some of the antigen either evades detection by the normal nonspecific defenses or overwhelms the abilities of the inflammatory response to neutralize, eliminate, or destroy the invader.

Acquiring Antibody-Mediated Immunity

The two broad categories of immunity are innate immunity and acquired immunity. Innate immunity is a genetically determined characteristic of an individual, group, or species. A person either has or does not have innate immunity. For example, people have many innate immunities to viruses and other microorganisms that cause specific diseases in animals. As a result, humans are not susceptible to such diseases as mange, distemper, hog cholera, or any of a variety of animal afflictions. This type of immunity cannot be developed or transferred from one person to another and is not an adaptive response to exposure or invasion by foreign proteins.

Acquired immunity is the immunity that every person's body makes (or can receive) as an adaptive response to invasion by foreign proteins. Antibody-mediated immunity is an acquired immunity. Acquired immunity occurs either naturally or artificially and can be either active or passive. Active immunity occurs when antigens enter the body and the body responds by making specific antibodies against the antigen. This type of immunity is active because the body takes an active part in making the antibodies. Active immunity can occur under conditions that are either natural or artificial. Natural active immunity occurs when an antigen enters the body without human assistance, and the body responds by actively making antibodies against that antigen (e.g., chickenpox virus). Most of the time the first invasion of the body by this antigen results in the person manifesting signs and symptoms of the disease. However, processes occurring in the body at the same time allow the person to acquire immunity to that antigen so that a second exposure to the same antigen will not cause illness. This type of immunity is the most effective and the longest lasting.

Artificial active immunity is a type of protection developed against illnesses that produce such serious side effects that total avoidance of the disease is most desirable. Small amounts of specific antigens are deliberately placed in the body (as a vaccination) so that the body responds by actively making antibodies against the antigen. Because antigens used for this procedure have been specially processed to make them less likely to proliferate within the body, this exposure does not in itself cause the disease.

Examples of diseases for which artificially acquired active immunity can be obtained include tetanus, diphtheria, measles, smallpox, mumps, and rubella. This type of immunity lasts many years, although repeated but smaller doses of the original antigen are periodically required as a "booster" to maintain complete protection against the antigen.

Passive immunity occurs when antibodies against a specific antigen are in a person's body, but the person did not actively generate these antibodies. Instead, these antibodies are made in the body of another person or animal and then transferred to the body of a specific individual. Because these antibodies are foreign to the individual, the body recognizes the antibodies as nonself and takes steps to eliminate them relatively quickly. For this reason passive immunity can provide only immediate, short-term protection against a specific antigen.

Cell-Mediated Immunity

Cell-mediated immunity (CMI), or cellular immunity, involves many leukocyte actions, reactions, and interactions that range from the simple to the complex. This type of immunity is provided by committed lymphocyte stem cells that mature in the secondary lymphoid tissues of the thymus and pericortical areas of lymph nodes. Certain CMI responses influence and regulate the activities of antibody-mediated immunity and inflammation by producing and releasing cytokines; therefore total immunocompetence relies on optimal CMI function.

The leukocytes playing the most important roles in CMI include several specific T-lymphocyte subsets along with a special population of cells known as *natural killer cells* (NK cells). T lymphocytes further differentiate into a variety of subsets, each of which has a specific function. The three T-lymphocyte subsets crucial to the development and continuation of CMI are helper/inducer T cells, suppressor T cells, and cytotoxic/cytolytic T cells.

Protection Provided By Cell-Mediated Immunity

Specific components of CMI assist in providing protection to the body by their highly developed abilities to differentiate self from nonself. The nonself cells most easily recognized by CMI are those self cells infected by organisms that live within host cells and those self cells mutated at the DNA level and thus abnormal. CMI provides a surveillance system that rids the body of self cells that might potentially harm the body. CMI is critically important in preventing development of cancer and metastasis after exposure to carcinogens.

34

HIV- and AIDS-Related Drugs

Robert Kizior and Lisa Ann Plowfield

ELECTRONIC RESOURCES

Evolve website (http://evolve.elsevier.com/KeeHayes/pharmacology/):
- *Case Studies*
- *Content Updates*
- *Frequently Asked Questions*
- *Student Review Activities*
- *WebLinks*
- *Additional Reference Material*

Companion CD-ROM:
- *NCLEX Examination Review Questions*
- *Pharmacology Animations*
- *IV Therapy Checklists*
- *Medication Error Checklists*
- *Drug Calculation Problems*
- *Electronic Calculators*
- *Top 200 Drugs with Pronunciations*
- *References from the Textbook*

Outline

Objectives

- Describe the life cycle of the human immunodeficiency virus (HIV), and relate it to the actions of pharmacologic agents used in the treatment of HIV disease.

- Describe the four classifications of antiretroviral therapy, and give examples of medications in each group.

- Relate specific issues of medication adherence to the dosing and side effects of antiretroviral agents.

- Explain prophylactic treatment for opportunistic infections.

- Discuss the medical management for preventing mother-to-child transmission of HIV infection during pregnancy.

- Discuss health care workers' exposure risks, and relate the risk and type of exposure to postexposure prophylaxis practices.

- Apply the nursing process, including client teaching, to the care of clients who are infected with HIV; discuss the nurse's role in medication management and issues of adherence.

Terms..

....

Acquired immunodeficiency syndrome (AIDS) was first reported in the United States in 1981 and has spread worldwide to become a major epidemic. The latest data from the World Health Organization estimate that 39.5 million persons worldwide are living with the HIV (human immunodeficiency virus), with 1.2 million residing in the United States. In 2006, about 4.3 million new infections occurred worldwide, 43,000 of which were in the United States.

Highly active antiretroviral therapy (HAART), which consists of at least three agents, has dramatically improved the course of the HIV epidemic. Improvement has been seen in the number of clients attaining undetectable viral loads, improved CD4 counts, and overall survival. No longer does a person diagnosed with HIV receive an early death sentence, but is identified as having a chronic disease. Currently the initial regimen should contain two nucleoside/nucleotide reverse transcriptase inhibitors (NRTI) and either a nonnucleotide reverse transcriptase inhibitor (NNRTI) or a ritonavir-boosted or unboosted protease inhibitor (PI).

Although strides have been made in HIV/AIDS, there are still challenges to be faced. One important negative outcome is increased drug **resistance** to current therapies. The makeup of HIV DNA strands allows the virus to mutate from a drug-sensitive to a drug-resistant form, so clients need to be treated with a combination of medications rather than monotherapy to avert the problem of drug resistance. Of the 1.2 million clients living with HIV in the United States, approximately 40,000 are receiving "salvage therapy" in an effort to stay alive.

Pathology

In 1983 HIV was identified as the causative agent of AIDS. HIV is a retrovirus that causes a gradual deterioration of immune function. The term *AIDS* applies to the most advanced stages of an HIV infection, characterized by profound immunologic deficits, opportunistic infection, secondary infections, and malignant neoplasms.

Once a person is infected with HIV, crucial immune cells called **CD4$^+$ T cells** are disabled and killed. During the course of infection, the numbers of CD4$^+$ T cells progressively decline. CD4$^+$ T cells play a crucial role in the **immune response** (the body's reaction to foreign antigens, neutralized or eliminated), signaling other cells in the **immune system** (lymphatic tissues, organs, and processes that identify foreign antigens and prevent harm to body) to perform their special function.

Transmission of the virus occurs primarily by three modes: (1) sexual contact (includes oral, vaginal, and anal sex); (2) direct blood contact (intravenous drug use with shared needles and blood transfusions [now extremely rare in the United States]); and (3) mother to child (through shared maternal-fetal blood circulation, by direct blood contact during delivery, or in breast milk). Other transmission methods are rare and include accidental needle injury, artificial insemination with donated semen, and organ transplant. HIV is not spread by casual contact (e.g., hugging), by touching items previously touched by a person infected with the virus, or during participation in sports. Those at highest risk include persons engaging in unprotected sex, sexual partners of those who participate in high risk activities (e.g., anal sex), intravenous drug users who share needles, and infants born to mothers with HIV who do not receive HIV therapy during pregnancy.

Classification

HIV disease staging and classification systems are important tools for tracking and monitoring the HIV epidemic and providing the clinician and client with information about HIV disease stage and clinical management.

There are two major classification systems currently in use: the United States Centers for Disease Control and Prevention (CDC) and the World Health Organization (WHO) classification system. The CDC staging system (last revised in 1993), assesses the severity of HIV disease by CD4 cell counts and by the presence of specific HIV related conditions. The CDC system is based on the lowest documented CD4 cell count and on previously diagnosed HIV-related conditions. AIDS is defined as all individuals with CD4 counts of less than 200 cells/mm^3 (or a CD4 percentage less than 14%) as well as clients with certain HIV related conditions and symptoms (Table 34–1).

Laboratory and Diagnostic Tests

Two surrogate markers routinely used for determining initiation of treatment and monitoring the efficacy of therapy are the CD4$^+$ T cell count and the plasma HIV RNA (or

Table 34–1

Classification System for HIV Infection*

	Clinical Categories for Adults		
	(A) Asymptomatic, Acute (Primary) HIV or Persistent Generalized Lymphadenopathy	**(B)** Symptomatic, Not (A) or (C) Conditions	**(C)** AIDS-Indicator Conditions
(1) 500/mcL or greater	A1	B1	C1
(2) 200-499/mcL	A2	B2	C2
(3) less than 200/mcL AIDS-indicator T-cell count	A3	B3	C3

From Department of Health and Human Services, Henry J. Kaiser Family Foundation: *Panel on practices for treatment of HIV infection: guidelines for the use of antiretroviral agents in HIV-infected adults and adolescents*, Dec 1, 1998.

*The revised Centers for Disease Control and Prevention classification system for HIV-infected adolescents and adults categorizes persons on the basis of CD4$^+$ T-lymphocyte counts and clinical conditions associated with HIV infection. The system is based on three ranges of CD4$^+$ T-lymphocyte counts and three clinical categories, represented by a matrix of nine mutually exclusive categories.

CD4$^+$ T-Lymphocyte Categories

HIV-infected persons should be classified based on existing guidelines for the medical management of HIV-infected persons; thus the lowest accurate CD4$^+$ T-lymphocyte count should be used (but not necessarily the most recent) for classification purposes.

Clinical Categories

Category A

Category A consists of one or more of the following conditions in an adolescent or adult (13 years of age or older) with documented HIV infection. Conditions listed in categories B and C must not have occurred.

- Asymptomatic HIV infection
- Persistent generalized lymphadenopathy
- Acute (primary) HIV infection with accompanying illness or history of acute HIV infection

Category B

Category B consists of symptomatic conditions in an HIV-infected adolescent or adult that are not included in category C and are attributed to HIV infection or are considered to have a clinical course complicated by HIV infection. Examples of conditions in category B include, but are not limited to, the following:

- Bacillary angiomatosis
- Candidiasis, oropharyngeal (thrush)
- Candidiasis, vulvovaginal; persistent, frequent, or poorly responsive to therapy
- Cervical dysplasia (moderate or severe)/cervical carcinoma in situ
- Constitutional symptoms, such as fever (38.5° C) or diarrhea lasting >1 month
- Hairy leukoplakia, oral
- Herpes zoster (shingles), involving at least two distinct episodes or more than one dermatome
- Idiopathic thrombocytopenic purpura
- Listeriosis
- Pelvic inflammatory disease, particularly if complicated by tubo-ovarian abscess
- Peripheral neuropathy

For classification purposes, category B conditions take precedence over category A conditions.

Category C

Category C includes the clinical conditions listed in the AIDS surveillance case definition. For classification purposes, once a category C condition occurs, the person remains in category C.

- Bacterial pneumonia, recurrent (2 or more episodes in 12 months)
- Candidiasis of the bronchi, trachea, or lungs
- Candidiasis, esophageal
- Cervical carcinoma, invasive, confirmed by biopsy
- Coccidioidomycosis, disseminated or extrapulmonary
- Cryptococcosis, extrapulmonary
- Cryptosporidiosis, chronic intestinal
- Cytomegalovirus disease
- HIV-related encephalopathy
- Herpes simplex: chronic ulcers or bronchitis, pneumonitis, or esophagitis
- Histoplasmosis, disseminated or extrapulmonary
- Kaposi sarcoma
- Lymphoma, Burkitt, immunoblastic, or primary central nervous system
- Mycobacterium avium complex (MAC) or *M. kansasii*, disseminated or extrapulmonary
- *Mycobacterium tuberculosis*, pulmonary or extrapulmonary
- *Pneumocystis jiroveci* (formerly *carinii*) pneumonia (PCP)
- Progressive multifocal leukoencephalopathy (PML)
- *Salmonella* septicemia, recurrent

viral load [VL, a test to measure the status of person's immune system]).

Also called *T-lymphocytes, T-cells, or T-helper cells,* CD4+ T cells are a type of white blood cell important in fighting infections. CD4+ cells play a crucial role in the client's immune response. A healthy uninfected person usually has 800-1200 CD4+ T cells/mm³. When HIV attacks the CD4+ T cells, this number dramatically decreases in most people who are not receiving treatment for the disease. The CD4+ count helps determine if other infections (opportunistic infections) may occur and over time shows the effect of the virus on the immune system. Adequate treatment response is defined as an increase in CD4+ cell count averaging 100-150 cells/mm³ per year with an accelerated response within the first 3 months.

A viral load test measures how much HIV is in the blood. It is critical for evaluating response to therapy, in that it monitors changes in the HIV infection, guides treatment choices, and monitors how well treatment is working. If the viral load rises, the infection is getting worse; if it drops, the infection is being suppressed. There are three HIV viral load assays approved by the FDA: (1) HIV-1 reverse transcriptase polymerase chain reaction assay, (2) nucleic acid amplification test for HIV RNA, and (3) signal amplification nucleic acid probe assay. One key goal of therapy is a viral load below the limits of detection (less than 50-80 copies/ml, depending on the assay used). This goal should be achieved by 16-24 weeks of therapy.

HIV Life Cycle

HIV is a retrovirus. It uses three different enzymes to genetically encode, replicate, and assemble new virus within the cells (HIV can replicate only inside cells). These three enzymes are reverse transcriptase, integrase, and protease.

The virus enters the cell through the CD4 molecule on the cell surface. The virus uncoats with the help of the **reverse transcriptase (RT)** enzyme, and a single-stranded viral RNA is converted into deoxyribonucleic acid (DNA),
the form in which the cell carries its genes. The viral DNA migrates to the nucleus of the cell, where it is spliced into the host DNA with the help of the second enzyme, **integrase.** Once incorporated, HIV DNA is called the *provirus* and is duplicated together with the cell genes every time the cell divides. **Protease,** the third enzyme, assists in the assembly of newly formed viral particles (Figure 34–1).

Indications for Antiretroviral Therapy

Current guidelines recommend starting therapy for all symptomatic clients with an acquired immunodeficiency syndrome defining illness or severe symptoms of HIV infection regardless of the CD4+ T cell count. Therapy is also recommended for asymptomatic clients with a CD4+ T cell count less than 200. Clients with a CD4+ T cell count between 201 and 350 should be offered treatment. In clients with a CD4+ T cell count above 350 and a viral load greater than 100,000 copies/ml, some clinicians prefer to defer treatment, whereas others will consider starting therapy. Therapy is usually deferred for those with CD4+ T cell counts greater than 350 and a viral load less than 100,000 copies/ml.

If therapy is to be initiated, appropriate agents are selected based on co-morbidities (e.g., liver disease, depression), pregnancy status, **adherence** (to carry out the therapeutic plan) potential (e.g., dosage regimen, pill burden, dosing frequency), food restrictions, side effects, and potential drug-drug interactions.

Combination therapy known as highly active antiretroviral therapy (HAART) is the current treatment recommendation. Medications designed to slow or inhibit the three HIV-related enzymes are called **antiretroviral** (ARV) medications. The goals of HAART include decreasing the VL to undetectable levels, preserving and increasing the number of CD4+ T cells, preventing resistance, having the client in

FIGURE 34–1   The life cycle of the human immunodeficiency virus.

good clinical condition, and preventing secondary infections and cancers. To obtain and maintain the goals of HAART therapy, the client must have excellent adherence/compliance skills. Failure to take combination therapy as directed can lead to resistance to or failure of antiretroviral agents. Clinical management of the HIV/AIDS client must also include measures to minimize associated opportunistic infections and malignancies. Aggressive prophylaxis and treatment of opportunistic infections are suggested. Nutritional therapy, complementary therapy, and supportive care are also necessary.

In addition, treatment should be based on the willingness and readiness of the individual, the degree of existing immunodeficiency, the risk of disease progression, and the likelihood of adherence to the prescribed treatment regimen. Recommendations for offering antiretroviral therapy in asymptomatic clients require analysis of many real and potential risks and benefits. The risks and benefits of early initiation of antiretroviral therapy in the asymptomatic HIV-infected client are listed in Box 34–1.

Antiretroviral Therapy

The goals of antiretroviral therapy are to do the following:
- Suppress viral replication to slow the decline in the number of CD4$^+$ cells
- Suppress viral replication to undetectable levels
- Reduce the incidence and severity of opportunistic infections
- Minimize adverse effects of antiretroviral therapy
- Improve quality of life
- Improve survival and reduce morbidity

Currently **reverse transcriptase inhibitors, protease inhibitors,** and **entry inhibitors** make up the classification of drugs known as *antiretroviral therapy*. Reverse transcriptase inhibitors (RT inhibitors) are further divided into **nucleoside analogues** (inhibit synthesis of HIV by blocking growth of its DNA strand) and **nonnucleoside analogues** (bind to the center of reverse transcriptase and directly inhibit its production). As of 2007 the FDA has approved over 20 different antiretroviral agents. Protease inhibitors have changed the prognosis for millions of clients infected with HIV. Protease inhibitors combined with RT inhibitors can reduce viral plasma levels to undetectable levels, offering significant clinical benefits.

Antiretroviral Agents

Since the 1980s when zidovudine monotherapy showed survival benefits as initial antiretroviral therapy in advanced HIV clients, much progress has been made. Over the past 8 years, newer agents have improved adherence (e.g., fewer pills for more convenient dosing, formulation changes reducing dosing frequency or pill burden, and combination dosage forms with two or three drugs in one convenient pill). Other improvements include increased potency, improved side effect profile (e.g., decreased gastrointestinal effects), and protease-inhibitor boosting with ritonavir.

Box 34–1

Risks and Benefits of Early or Delayed Initiation of Antiretroviral Therapy in the Asymptomatic HIV-Infected Client

Potential Benefits of Early Therapy
- Control of viral replication and mutation; reduction of viral burden
- Prevention of progressive immunodeficiency; potential maintenance or reconstruction of a normal immune system
- Delayed progression to acquired immunodeficiency syndrome and prolongation of life
- Decreased risk of selection of resistant virus
- Decreased risk of drug toxicity
- Possible decreased risk of viral transmission

Potential Risks of Early Therapy
- Reduction in quality of life from adverse drug effects and inconvenience of current maximally suppressive regimens
- Earlier development of drug resistance
- Transmission of drug-resistant virus
- Limitation in future choices of antiretroviral agents as a result of development of resistance
- Unknown long-term toxicity of antiretroviral drugs
- Unknown duration of effectiveness of current antiretroviral therapies

Potential Benefits of Delayed Therapy
- Avoid negative effects of therapy, including quality of life and drug-related adverse effects
- Maintain treatment options
- Delay the development of drug resistance

Potential Risks of Delayed Therapy
- Irreversibly damaging the immune system
- Increased difficulty in suppressing viral replication at a later stage of the disease
- Transmitting HIV during a longer untreated period

From Department of Health and Human Services, Henry J. Kaiser Family Foundation: *Panel on practices for treatment of HIV infection: guidelines for the use of antiretroviral agents in HIV-infected adults and adolescents,* March 23, 2004.

The use of HAART is the present standard of care in the treatment of HIV infection. Combination HAART utilizes two nucleoside reverse transcriptase inhibitors (NRTIs) with either one nonnucleoside reverse transcriptase inhibitor (NNRTI) or one or two protease inhibitors.

Nucleoside/Nucleotide Reverse Transcriptase Inhibitors (NRTIs)

Currently there are seven NRTIs approved for use in the U.S.: zidovudine (Retrovir), didanosine (Videx), stavudine (Zerit), lamivudine (Epivir), abacavir (Ziagen), tenofovir (Viread), and emtricitabine (Emtriva). There are also five fixed-dose combination products available: Combivir (lamivudine/zidovudine), Trizivir (Abacavir/lamivudine/zidovudine), Epzicom (abacavir/lamivudine),

Atripla (efavirenz/emtricitabine/tenofovir), and Truvada (emtricitabine/tenofovir). Of the twelve drugs, Tenofovir (Viread) is the only nucleotide analogue.

Nucleoside/nucleotide reverse transciptase inhibitors, the foundation of HAART, act by blocking the reverse transcriptase enzyme needed for viral replication. Two of these agents are typically included in initial ARV regimens. Most dual NRTI combinations used in clinical practice today consist of a primary NRTI in combination with lamivudine or emtricitabine. The preferred dual NRTIs are zidovudine/lamivudine or tenofovir/emtricitabine.

All NRTIs except didanosine should be taken with food for optimal tolerability. Didanosine should be taken 60 minutes before meals or two hours after meals for optimal absorption. With the exception of abacavir, the NRTIs require dosage adjustment in persons with renal insufficiency (creatinine clearance less than 50 ml/min). Similarly, fixed-dose NRTI combinations should be avoided in clients with renal insufficiency. Gastrointestinal side effects (e.g., nausea, diarrhea, abdominal pain) are transient and improve within the first two weeks of therapy.

As a class the NRTIs are associated with changes in the body's metabolism secondary to mitochondrial toxicity. Complications include lactic acidosis, hepatic steatosis, peripheral neuropathy, myopathy, pancreatitis, and lipoatrophy. Lipoatrophy, or wasting of fat on the extremities, face, and buttocks, is associated with chronic NRTI administration. Fatalities have occurred due to lactic acidosis and hepatic steatosis associated with NRTIs. Drug interactions are uncommon with NRTIs. Gastrointestinal complaints and mitochondrial toxicity are less likely to occur with tenofovir. The major side effect with tenofovir is renal toxicity, occurring rarely (0.3% to 0.5% of users).

Adherence with the NRTIs can be improved with once-daily dosing (currently possible with abacavir, didanosine, emtricitabine, lamivudine, and tenofovir) and with fixed-dosage combination products (e.g., Combivir and Truvada).

Prototype Drug Chart 34–1 presents the pharmacologic data for zidovudine.

Non-Nucleoside Reverse Transcriptase Inhibitors (NNRTIs)

Three NNRTIs are presently in use in the United States: efavirenz (Sustiva), delavirdine (Rescriptor), and nevirapine (Viramune). The NNRTIs prevent viral replication by competing with binding of the reverse transcriptase enzyme at the active site. The primary advantage of using NNRTIs is to reserve a protease-inhibitor-based therapy for future use. In general an NNRTI regimen has lower pill burden compared with most of the PI-based regimens. The major disadvantages are the prevalence of NNRTI-resistant viral strains and the low genetic barrier of NNRTIs for development of resistance. (Resistance testing is recommended for treatment-naïve clients prior to starting therapy.)

Efavirenz is the first-choice drug within the NNRTI class, based on clinical studies supporting its use. It is contrain-

dicated in pregnancy (category D) because neural tube defects have been reported after early human gestational exposure. Central nervous system (CNS) toxicities including dizziness, sedation, nightmares, euphoria, or loss of concentration may occur in up to 50% of clients. Efavirenz should be used cautiously in clients with depression or a history of preexisting psychiatric or mental illness. Efavirenz is optimally administered as a component of Atripla given once daily at bedtime on an empty stomach or with a low-fat meal to prevent excessive drug absorption.

Nevirapine may be used as an alternative in adult females during pregnancy (especially during the first trimester) or in women who are planning to conceive or not using effective and consistent contraception. Nevirapine has a greater risk of severe rash and hepatotoxicity. Delavirdine appears to have the least potent antiviral activity and is not recommended as part of an initial regimen.

Prototype Drug Chart 34–2 presents the pharmacologic data for efavirenz.

Protease Inhibitors (PIs)

Protease-inhibitor-based regimens (1 or 2 PI plus 2 NRTIs) have revolutionized the treatment of HIV infection, leading to sustained viral suppression, improved immunologic function, and prolonged client survival. Currently there are 10 protease inhibitors approved by the FDA: lopinavir/ritonavir (Kaletra), atazanavir (Reyataz), fosamprenavir (Lexiva), amprenavir (Agenerase), tipranavir (Aptivus), darunavir (Prezista), saquinavir (Invirase), indivavir (Crixivan), ritonavir (Norvir), and nelfinavir (Viracept). Unlike the NRTIs and NNRTIs, protease inhibitors act at the end of the HIV life cycle to inhibit the production of infectious HIV viruses. Each PI has its own unique characteristics based on clinical efficacy, side effect profile, and pharmacokinetic properties. Lopinavir/ritonavir is the first-line choice, followed by fosamprenavir or atazanavir "boosted" with ritonavir or as an unboosted regimen.

The selection of a PI-based regimen should consider dosing frequency, food and fluid requirements, pill burden, drug interaction potential, and side effect profile. When initiating therapy with the PIs, gastrointestinal side effects (nausea, vomiting, and diarrhea) can be bothersome and may negatively affect adherence. Metabolic abnormalities, including dyslipidemia, fat maldistribution, and insulin resistance/diabetes are associated with PI use, with each PI differing in its propensity to cause these metabolic complications. Metabolic abnormalities are established risk factors for cardiovascular disease, so lifestyle modifications, weight loss, smoking cessation, exercise, and cardiac risk management are advised for those receiving chronic PI-based therapies.

Ritonavir boosting is a relatively new concept and one of the mainstays of PI therapy. The potent inhibitory effect of ritonavir on the cytochrome P450 3A4 isoenzyme allows the addition of 100-200 mg ritonavir to other PIs as a pharmacokinetic booster to reduce dietary restrictions, increase drug exposure, prolong the half-life of the active PI,

Prototype **DRUG CHART 34–1**

ZIDOVUDINE

Drug Class

Nucleoside reverse transcriptase inhibitor
Trade names: ZDV, AZT, Retrovir
Pregnancy Category: C
FDA approved: 1987
Estimated annual cost: $6550*

Dosage

Prophylaxis vertical transmission HIV:
Maternal therapy: PO: 100 mg 5×/d Initiated at
14-34 wk of gestation through pregnancy
Intrapartum: IV: 2 mg/kg loading dose over 30-60 min
followed by continuous infusion of 1 mg/kg/h until
the cord is clamped
Newborn (syrup): PO: 2 mg/kg q6h; **IV:** 1.5 mg/kg over
30 min q6h
Treatment:
A: PO: 200 mg q8h or 300 mg q12h; **IV:** 1 mg/kg q4h
C: PO: premature birth to 2 wk: 1.5 mg/kg q12h,
increasing to 2 mg/kg q8h after 2 wk of age; neonatal: 2 mg/kg q6h; <12 y: 160 mg/m² q8h; >12 y: adult
dose
C: IV: neonatal: 1.5 mg/kg q6h; <12 y: intermittent infusion: 120 mg/m² q6h; *max:* 160 mg/m² per dose; continuous infusion: 20 mg/m²/h

Contraindications

Life-threatening allergies to zidovudine or
components of preparation
Caution: Bone marrow compromise, renal and
hepatic dysfunction, decreased hepatic blood flow

Drug-Lab-Food Interactions

Drug: Ganciclovir and trimethoprim/sulfamethoxazole
may *increase* risk of neutropenia; probenecid may
increase concentration, risk of toxicity
Lab: May *increase* mean corpuscular volume

Pharmacokinetics

Absorption: PO: 66%-70%
Distribution: PB: 25%-38%, crosses blood-brain barrier,
crosses placenta, peak serum levels: 30-90 min
Metabolism: t½: 60 min; extensive first-pass effect
in liver
Excretion: 63%-95% in urine

Pharmacodynamics

Not applicable

Therapeutic Effects/Uses

Management of clients with HIV infection; prevention of maternal-fetal HIV transmission
Mode of Action: Inhibits viral enzyme reverse transcriptase, an enzyme necessary for viral HIV replication

Side Effects

Numbness, tingling, burning and pain in lower
extremities, abdominal pain, rash, GI intolerance,
fever, sore throat, headache, pruritus, muscle pain,
difficulty swallowing, arthralgia, insomnia, confusion,
mental changes, bluish brown bands on fingernails

Adverse Reactions

Nausea, vomiting, anemia (pale skin, unusual fatigue or
weakness), neutropenia (fever, chills, sore throat),
seizures

A, Adult; *C,* child; *d,* day; *FDA,* Food and Drug Administration; *GI,* gastrointestinal; *h,* hour; *HIV,* human immunodeficiency virus;
IV, intravenous; *max,* maximum; *min,* minute; *PB,* protein-binding; *PO,* by mouth; *t½,* half-life; *wk,* week; *y,* year; >, greater than;
<, less than.
*Estimated average cost as of January 2008.

thus reducing dosing frequency and pill burden. The major drawbacks are the potential for increased risk of hyperlipidemia and increased potential for drug-drug interactions from adding ritonavir.

Prototype Drug Chart 34–3 presents the pharmacologic
data for lopinavir/ritonavir.

Entry Inhibitors

Enfuvirtide (Fuzeon) is the only agent approved in this
class. Enfuvirtide acts by a mechanism that inhibits gp41
fusion to prevent HIV cell entry. This class of agents targets
prevention of the fusion of HIV and CD4 cell and prevents
passing the viral genome to the CD4 cell. Enfuvirtide is

Prototype DRUG CHART 34–2

EFAVIRENZ

Drug Class

Nonnucleoside reverse transcriptase inhibitor
Trade name: Sustiva
Pregnancy Category: C
FDA approved: 1998
Estimated annual cost: $7725*

Dosage

NOTE: Dose given at bedtime to minimize CNS adverse effects
A: PO: 600 mg once daily
C: PO: 10 to <15 kg: 200 mg daily; 15 to <20 kg: 250 mg daily; 20 to <25 kg: 300 mg daily; 25 to <32.5 kg: 350 mg daily; 32.5 kg to <40 kg: 400 mg daily; ≥40 kg: 600 mg daily

Contraindications

Life-threatening allergies to efavirenz or components of preparation; concurrent use of midazolam, triazolam, ergot alkaloids
Caution: History of mental illness/drug abuse; liver impairment

Drug-Lab-Food Interactions

Drug: See contraindications; carbamazepine, nevirapine, phenobarbital, phenytoin, rifampin, St John's wort may *decrease* effect; may *decrease* effect of lopinavir/ritonavir, saquinavir, amprenavir, clarithromycin, methadone, sertraline
Lab: May increase HDL, total cholesterol
Food: Avoid alcohol because of liver/CNS adverse effects; high-fat meals increase absorption

Pharmacokinetics

Absorption: PO: Increased following high fat meal
Distribution: PB: >99%, widely distributed (found in CSF)
Metabolism: t½: 40-55 h; metabolized in liver
Excretion: Feces primarily as unchanged drug (16%-41%); urine primarily as metabolite (14%-34%)

Pharmacodynamics

Not applicable

Therapeutic Effects/Uses

Treatment of HIV-1 infections in combination with at least two other anti-retroviral agents.
Mode of Action: Binds to reverse transcriptase, blocking RNA dependent and DNA dependent DNA polymerase activity including HIV-1 replication.

Side Effects

Rash; CNS effects (dizziness, insomnia, abnormal dreams/thinking, impaired concentration, amnesia, agitation, hallucinations, euphoria, anxiety); nausea, diarrhea

Adverse Reactions

Aggressive reaction, allergic reaction, convulsion, liver failure, neuropathy, suicide, abnormal vision

A, Adult; *C*, child; *CNS*, central nervous system; *CSF*, cerebrospinal fluid; *DNA*, deoxyribonucleic acid; *FDA*, Food and Drug Administration; *h*, hour; *HDL*, high-density lipoprotein; *HIV-1*, human immunodeficiency virus-1; *PB*, protein-binding; *PO*, by mouth; *RNA*, ribonucleic acid; *t½*, half-life; >, greater than; ≥, greater than or equal to; < less than.
*Estimated annual cost as of January 2008.

indicated only in combination with three to five other antiretroviral agents for clients with limited treatment options requiring salvage therapy. It is expensive, and the medication must be taken by subcutaneous injection in a dose of 90 mg twice daily.

Enfuvirtide does not require dosage adjustment in clients with renal failure or hepatic impairment. It is not metabolized by CYP enzymes and is not associated with any CYP mediated drug-drug interactions. Injection site reactions (e.g., subcutaneous nodules, redness) occur in up to 98% of clients. Other side effects reported include rash and diarrhea. Serious allergic reactions, including anaphy-

laxis, fever and hypotension, have occurred in less than 1% of clients.

Summary of Antiretroviral Agents

A list of the antiretroviral agents (nucleoside analogues, nonnucleoside analogues, protease inhibitors, and entry inhibitors) are presented in Table 34–2 with their respective routes, dosages, and considerations. A guide for drug interactions, in the form of multiple charts, is presented at *www.projinf.org/fs/drugin.html*, a website dedicated solely to the treatment of HIV infection. Information on drug interactions is presented in Table 34–3.

Prototype DRUG CHART 34–3

LOPINAVIR/RITONAVIR

Drug Class

Protease inhibitor
Trade name: Kaletra
Pregnancy Category: C
FDA approved: 2000
Estimated annual cost: $11,000*

Dosage

Based on lopinavir:
A & C >12 y: PO: 400 mg b.i.d.
C: 6 mo-12 y: 7 to <15 kg: 12 mg/kg b.i.d.; 15-40 kg:
 10 mg/kg b.i.d.; >40 kg: Same as adult
*Dosage when taken with amprenavir, efavirenz,
 nelfinavir, or nevirapine:*
A & C >12 y: 533 mg b.i.d.
C: 6 mo-12 y: 7 to <15 kg: 13 mg/kg b.i.d.; 15-45 kg:
 11 mg/kg b.i.d.; >45 kg: Same as adult

Contraindications

Life-threatening allergies to lopinavir/ritonavir or
 components of preparations. Ritonavir is
 contraindicated with concurrent use of ergot
 alkaloids, midazolam, triazolam, or pimozide.
Caution: History of pancreatitis, liver impairment

Drug-Lab-Food Interactions

Drug: See contraindications; azole antifungals,
 lovastatin, rifampin, simvastatin, St. John's wort
Lab: May *increase* liver function tests, cholesterol,
 triglycerides
Food: Take with food. If concurrent didanosine, take
 didanosine 1 h before or 2 h after lopinavir/ritonavir

Pharmacokinetics

Absorption: PO: Well absorbed following
 oral administration
Distribution: PB: 98%-99%
Metabolism: t½: 5-6 h. Metabolized in liver
Excretion: Primarily fecal elimination (83%)

Pharmacodynamics

Not applicable

Therapeutic Effects/Uses

Treatment of HIV-1 infection in combination with other antiretroviral agents.
Mode of Action: Inhibits HIV protease, rendering enzyme incapable of processing polyprotease precursors; production of noninfectious immature HIV particles results

Side Effects

Nausea, vomiting, diarrhea, asthenia

Adverse Reactions

Hyperglycemia, diabetes mellitus

A, Adult; *b.i.d.*, twice a day; *C*, child; *FDA*, Food and Drug Administration; *h*, hour; *HIV*, human immunodeficiency virus; *mo*,
month; *PB*, protein-binding; PO, by mouth; *t½*, half-life; *y*, year; >, greater than; <, less than.
*Estimated annual cost as of January 2008.

Table 34–2

Antiretroviral Agents

Name	Availability	Dosage	Comments
Nucleoside Reverse Transcriptase Inhibitors (NRTIs)			
abacavir (ABC) (Ziagen)	Ziagen: 300 mg tablets 20 mg/ml oral solu- tion	Ziagen: 300 mg 2 times/d or 600 mg once daily	Take without regard to meals Metabolized by alcohol dehydrogenase Excreted renally
Trizivir (with ZDC+3TC)	Trizivir: ABC 300 mg, ZDV 300 mg, 3TC 150 mg	Trizivir: 1 tablet 2 times/d	Trizivir and Epzicom not for clients with CL$_{cr}$ <50 ml/min
Epzicom (with 3TC)	Epzicom: ABC 600 mg, 3TC 300 mg	Epzicom: 1 tablet once daily	*Half life:* 1.5 h **Side effects:** hypersensitivity reaction; symptoms may include fever, rash, nausea, vomiting, mal- aise, fatigue, loss of appetite; respiratory symp- toms including sore throat, cough, shortness of breath

d, Day; *GI*, gastrointestinal; *h*, hour; *min*, minute; *subQ*, subcutaneous; *wt*, weight; >, greater than; <, less than.

Table 34–2

Antiretroviral Agents—cont'd

Name	Availability	Dosage	Comments
didanosine (ddI) (Videx EC)	Videx EC: 125 mg, 200 mg, 250 mg, 400 mg	Body wt 60 kg or greater: 400 mg once daily With TDF: 250 mg/d Body wt <60 kg: 250 mg daily With TDF: 200 mg/d	Take ½ h before or 2 h after meal Excreted renally, dosage adjustment in renal insufficiency *Half life:* 1.5 h **Side effects:** pancreatitis, peripheral neuropathy, nausea, lactic acidosis with hepatic steatosis (rare)
emtricitabine (FTC) (Emtriva) Atripla (with EFV+TDF) Truvada (with TDF)	Emtriva: 200 mg capsule 10 mg/ml oral solution Atripla: EFV 600, FTC 200 mg, TDF 300 mg Truvada: FTC 200 mg, TDF 300 mg	Emtriva: 200 mg capsule once daily or 240 mg oral solution once daily Atripla: 1 tablet once daily Truvada: 1 tablet once daily *Half-life:* 10 h Minimal toxicity, hyperpigmentation, skin discoloration	Take without regard to meals Excreted renally, dosage adjustment in renal insufficiency Atripla not for clients with CL_{cr} <50 ml/min; Truvada not for clients with CL_{cr} <30 ml/min **Side effects:** lactic acidosis with hepatic steatosis (rare)
lamivudine (3TC) (Epivir) Combivir (with ZDV) Epizicom (with ABC) Trizivir (with ZDV+ABC)	Epivir: 150 mg, 300 mg tablets 10 mg/ml oral solution Combivir: 3TC 150 mg, ZDV 300 mg Epzicom: ABC 600 mg, 3TC 300 mg Trizivir: ABC 300 mg, ZDV 300 mg, 3TC 150 mg	Epivir: 150 mg 2 times/ d or 300 mg once daily Combivir: 1 tablet 2 times/d Epizicom: 1 tablet once daily Trizivir: 1 tablet 2 times/d	Take without regard to meals Excreted renally, dosage adjustment in renal insufficiency Combivir, Trizivir, Epzicom not for clients with CL_{cr} <50 ml/min *Half-life:* 5-7 h **Side effects:** minimal toxicity, lactic acidosis with hepatic steatosis (rare)
stavudine (d4T) (Zerit)	Zerit: 15 mg, 20 mg, 30 mg, 40 mg capsule 1 mg/ml oral solution	Body wt >60 kg: 40 mg 2 times/d Body wt <60 kg: 30 mg 2 times/d	Take without regard to meals Excreted renally, dosage adjustment in renal insufficiency *Half-life:* 1 h **Side effects:** peripheral neuropathy, lipodystrophy, pancreatitis, hyperlipidemia, rapidly progressive ascending neuromuscular weakness (rare), lactic acidosis with hepatic steatosis (rare)
tenofovir (TDF) (Viread) Atripla (with EFV+FTC) Truvada (with FTC)	Viread: 300 mg tablet Atripla: EFV 600, FTC 200 mg, TDF 300 mg Truvada: FTC 200 mg, TDF 300 mg	Viread: 1 tablet daily Atripla: 1 tablet daily Truvada: 1 tablet daily	Take without regard to meals Excreted renally, dosage adjustment in renal insufficiency Atripla not for clients with CL_{cr} <50 ml/min; Truvada not for clients with CL_{cr} <30 ml/min *Half-life:* 17 h **Side effects:** asthenia, headache, diarrhea, nausea, vomiting, flatulence, renal insufficiency, lactic acidosis with hepatic steatosis (rare)
zidovudine (AZT, ZDV) (Retrovir) Combivir (with ZDV) Trizivir (with ZDV+ABC)	Retrovir: 100 mg capsules 300 mg tablets 10 mg/ml IV solution 10 mg/ml oral solution Combivir: 3TC 150 mg, ZDV 300 mg Trizivir: ABC 300 mg, ZDV 300 mg, 3TC 150 mg	Retrovir: 300 mg 2 times/d or 200 mg 3 times/d Combivir: 1 tablet 2 times/d Trizivir: 1 tablet 2 times/d	Take without regard to meals Excreted renally, dosage adjustment in renal insufficiency Combivir, Trizivir not for clients with CL_{cr} <50 ml/min *Half-life:* 1.1 h **Side effects:** bone marrow suppression, macrocytic anemia, neutropenia, GI intolerance, headache, insomnia, asthenia lactic acidosis with hepatic steatosis (rare)

Continued

Table 34–2

Antiretroviral Agents—cont'd

Name	Availability	Dosage	Comments
Non-Nucleoside Reverse Transcriptase Inhibitors (NNRTIs)			
delavirdine (DLV) (Rescriptor)	Rescriptor: 100 mg, 200 mg tablets	400 mg 3 times/d (100 mg may be mixed with 3 oz water; 200 mg tablets taken as intact tablets)	Take without regard to meals Metabolized by cytochrome P450, excreted in urine/feces *Half-life:* 5.8 h **Side effects:** rash, increased transaminase levels, headaches
efavirenz (EFV) (Sustiva) Atripla (with TDF+FTC)	Sustiva: 50 mg, 100 mg, 200 mg capsules 600 mg tablets Atripla: EFV 600, FTC 200 mg, TDF 300 mg	Sustiva: 600 mg daily on empty stomach, at or before bedtime Atripla: 1 tablet daily	Take on empty stomach, high fat/high caloric meals increase concentration. Metabolized by cytochrome P450 Sustiva: no dosage adjustment in renal insufficiency Atripla not for clients with CL_{cr} <50 ml/min *Half-life:* 40-55 h **Side effects:** rash, increased transaminase levels, CNS symptoms including dizziness, confusion, agitation, hallucinations, euphoria
nevirapine (NVP) (Viramune)	Viramune: 200 mg tablets 50 mg/5ml oral suspension	Viramune: 200 mg daily for 14 d, then 200 mg 2 times/d	Take without regard to meals Metabolized by cytochrome P450 *Half life:* 25-30 h **Side effects:** rash, including Stevens-Johnson syndrome, symptomatic hepatitis
Protease Inhibitors			
amprenavir (APV) (Agenerase)	Agenerase: 50 mg capsules 15 mg/ml oral solution (capsules and oral solution are not interchangeable on a mg-for-mg basis)	Agenerase: 1400 mg 2 times/d	Take without regard to meals (high fat meal should be avoided; can decrease concentration) Cytochrome P450 3A4 inhibitor, inducer and substrate Dosage adjustment in hepatic insufficiency *Half-life:* 7.1-10.6 h **Side effects:** GI intolerance, nausea, vomiting, diarrhea, rash, oral paresthesias, hyperlipidemia, increased transaminase levels, hyperglycemia, fat maldistribution, possible increased bleeding in clients with hemophilia
atazanavir (ATV) (Reyataz)	Reyataz: 100 mg, 150 mg, 200 mg capsules	Reyataz: 400 mg once daily (if taken with efavirenz or tenofovir: RTV 100 mg +ATV 300 mg once daily	Take with food, avoid taking with antacids Cytochrome P450 3A4 inducer and substrate Dosage adjustment in hepatic insufficiency *Half-life:* 7 h **Side effects:** hyperbilirubinemia, prolonged P-R interval (use with caution in clients with underlying conduction defects or concomitant medications that prolong P-R interval), hyperglycemia, fat maldistribution, possible increased bleeding in clients with hemophilia
darunavir (DRV) (Prezista)	Prezista: 300 mg tablets	Prezista: (DRV 600 mg + RTV 100 mg) 2 times/d	Administer with food (increases concentration) Cytochrome P450 3A4 inhibitor and substrate Dosage adjustment in hepatic insufficiency *Half-life:* 15 h **Side effects:** rash, diarrhea, nausea, headache, elevated transaminase levels, hyperglycemia, fat maldistribution, possible increased bleeding in hemophiliacs, hyperlipidemia,
fosamprenavir (fAPV) (Lexiva)	Lexiva: 700 mg tablet	Lexiva: 1400 mg 2 times/d or fAPV 1400 mg + RTV 200 mg daily or fAPV 700 mg + RTV 100 mg 2 times/d	Take with or without food Cytochrome P450 3A4 inhibitor, inducer and substrate Dosage adjustment in hepatic insufficiency *Half-life:* 7.7 h **Side effects:** rash, diarrhea, nausea, vomiting, headache, hyperlipidemia, elevated transaminase levels, hyperglycemia, fat maldistribution, possible increased bleeding in hemophiliacs, hyperlipidemia

Table 34–2

Antiretroviral Agents—cont'd

Name	Availability	Dosage	Comments
indinavir (IDV) (Crixivan)	Crixivan: 200 mg, 333 mg, 400 mg capsules	Crixivan: 800 mg every 8 h With RTV: IDV 800 mg + RTV 100 mg or 200 mg q12h	Unboosted: take 1 hr before or 2 hrs after meals; with RTV: may take with or without meals Cytochrome P450 3A4 inhibitor Dosage adjustment in hepatic insufficiency *Half-life:* 71.5-2 h *Side effects:* nephrolithiasis, GI intolerance, nausea, indirect hyperbilirubinemia, headache, asthenia, blurred vision, dizziness, rash, metallic taste, thrombocytopenia, alopecia, hemolytic anemia, hyperlipidemia, elevated transaminase levels, hyperglycemia, fat maldistribution, possible increased bleeding in clients with hemophilia
lopinavir/ritonavir (LPV/r) (Kaletra)	Kaletra: Tablet: LPV 200 mg and RTV 50 mg Oral solution: LPV 400 mg + RTV 100 mg per 5 ml	Kaletra: LPV 400 mg + RTV 100 mg 2 times/d or LPV 800 mg + RTV 200 mg once daily	May take tablet with or without food; take oral solution with food Cytochrome P450 3A4 inhibitor and substrate *Half-life:* 5-6 h *Side effects:* GI intolerance, nausea, vomiting, diarrhea, asthenia, hyperlipidemia, elevated transaminase levels, hyperglycemia, fat maldistribution, possible increased bleeding in clients with hemophilia
nelfinavir (NFV) (Viracept)	Viracept: 250 mg, 625 mg tablets 50 mg/g oral powder	Viracept: 1250 mg 2 times/d or 750 mg 3 times/d	Take with meal or snack Cytochrome P450 3A4 inhibitor and substrate *Half-life:* 3.5-5 h *Side effects:* diarrhea, hyperlipidemia, elevated transaminase levels, hyperglycemia, fat maldistribution, possible increased bleeding in hemophiliacs
ritonavir (RTV) (Norvir)	Norvir: 100 mg capsules 600 mg/7.5 ml solution	Norvir: 600 mg q12h (when used as only PI) Booster: 100-400 mg in 1-2 divided doses	Take with food if possible Take with meal or snack Cytochrome P450 3A4 potent inhibitor *Half-life:* 3-5 h *Side effects:* GI intolerance, nausea, vomiting, diarrhea, paresthesias, hepatitis, asthenia, taste perversion, hyperlipidemia, hyperglycemia, fat maldistribution, possible increased bleeding in clients with hemophilia
saquinavir (SQV) (Invirase)	Invirase: 200 mg capsules 500 mg tablets	Invirase: SQV 1000 mg + RTV 100 mg 2 times/d	Take within 2 h of a meal Cytochrome P450 3A4 inhibitor and substrate *Half-life:* 1-2 h *Side effects:* GI intolerance, nausea, diarrhea, headache, hyperlipidemia, elevated transaminase levels, hyperglycemia, fat maldistribution, possible increased bleeding in hemophiliacs
tipranavir (TPV) (Aptivus)	Aptivus: 250 mg capsules	Aptivus: TPV 500 mg + RTV 200 mg 2 times/d	Take with food Cytochrome P450 3A4 inducer and substrate *Half-life:* 6 h *Side effects:* hepatotoxicity, rash (has sulfonamide moiety), hyperlipidemia, hyperglycemia, fat maldistribution, possible increased bleeding in clients with hemophilia
Entry Inhibitors			
enfuvirtide (T20) (Fuzeon)	Fuzeon: Injection powder 90 mg/ml after reconstitution	Fuzeon: 90 mg subQ 2 times/d	Store vial at room temperature; following reconstitution, refrigerate and use within 24 h *Half-life:* 3.8 h *Side effects:* local injection site reaction (pain, erythema, induration, nodules, cysts, pruritus, ecchymosis), increased rate of bacterial pneumonia, hypersensitivity reaction (rash, fever, nausea, vomiting, chills, rigors, hypotension, elevated transaminases)

Table 34–3

Interactions

Drug interaction associated with HAART is a challenging issue facing providers treating clients with HIV. Medications used as initial treatment are associated with significant drug interactions. Concurrent treatment of co-morbid disease states and therapies for preventing and/or treating opportunistic infections further increase the risk of drug interactions.

Nucleoside Reverse Transcriptase Inhibitors (NRTIs)

Drug interactions associated with the NRTIs are minimal, because these medications are not metabolized by the CYP450 system. Nevertheless, drug interactions may still occur within the class.

Interaction	Comments
zidovudine-stavudine	Compete for the same site in the growing chain of HIV DNA, resulting in antagonistic effects that lead to treatment failures. Do not combine.
didanosine-tenofovir	Tenofovir increases didanosine concentrations by as much as 68%, resulting in increased toxicity (e.g., pancreatitis, peripheral neuropathy, lactic acidosis) and suppression of CD4 cell counts. When used together, didanosine dose reduced to 250 mg/d ($>$60 kg) or 200 mg/day ($<$60 kg).
tenofovir-atazanavir	Tenofovir reduces atazanavir (Reyataz) concentrations, leading to treatment failure. Addition of 100 mg ritonovir increases concentrations of atazanavir dosed at 300 mg/d.

Non-Nucleoside Reverse Transcriptase Inhibitors (NNRTIs)

Drugs in this class are prone to interactions, because they are extensively metabolized via CYP3A4 and can act as either inducers or inhibitors of CYP3A4. Efavirenz and nevirapine are inducers and delavirdine an inhibitor of the CYP3A4 system.

Interaction	Comments
efavirenz–midazolam	Increased concentration and toxicity of midazolam
efavirenz–ergotamine derivatives	Increased concentration and toxicity of ergotamine derivatives
efavirenz–clarithromycin	Decreased concentration of clarithromycin. Consider changing clarithromycin to azithromycin, which is not CYP3A4. Interactions are unlikely with this medication.
efafirenz–methadone	Methadone withdrawal symptoms may occur due to reduced methadone levels. Full effect of methadone withdrawal may take up to 2 wk.
efavirenz–rifampin	Rifampin reduces concentration of efavirenz. Increase dose of efavirenz to 800 mg daily when using rifampin to treat tuberculosis.
nevirapine–methadone	Methadone withdrawal symptoms may occur due to reduced methadone levels. Full effect of methadone withdrawal may take up to 2 wk.
nevirapine–oral contraceptives	Nevirapine reduces the concentration/effect of oral contraceptives. Alternative method of birth control is recommended.
nevirapine-rifampin	Rifampin reduces concentration of nevirapine. Rifabutin should be given instead of rifampin to minimize the reduction in nevirapine concentration.

Dosing Recommendations When Combining NNRTI and PI

Protease Inhibitor/NNRTI	Dosage Recommendation
indinavir/efavirenz or nevirapine	Standard dose for efavirenz and nevirapine. Indinavir dose increased to 1000 mg every 8 h.
amprenavir/efavirenz or nevirapine	Standard dose for efavirenz and nevirapine. Amprenavir dose increased to 1200 mg 3 times/d.
lopinavir-ritonavir/efavirenz or nevirapine	Standard dose for efavirenz and nevirapine. Increase lopinavir-ritonavir dose to 533 mg/133 mg 2 times/d.
atazanavir/efavirenz	Standard dose for efavirenz. Give atazanavir 300 mg once daily and add ritonavir 100 mg once daily.
fosamprenavir/evavirenz	Standard dose for efavirenz. If using fosamprenavir with ritonavir 2 times/d, give fosamprenavir 700 mg with ritonavir 100 mg 2 times/d. If using fosamprenavir with ritonavir once daily, give fosamprenavir 1400 mg with ritonavir 300 mg once daily.

Protease Inhibitors (PIs)

All protease inhibitors are potent inhibitors of CYP3A4 and result in drug interactions. Levels of medications also metabolized by the same system have the potential to be markedly increased, leading to an increased incidence of adverse effects. The protease inhibitor *ritonavir* is the most potent inhibitor of CYP3A4 in this class.

Interaction	Comments
ergot alkaloids (e.g., ergotamine)	Increased risk of ergot toxicity. Avoid concurrent use. Consider using alternative such as sumatriptan.
HMG CoA reductase inhibitors (lovastatin, simvastatin, high dose atorvastatin)	Increased levels of these HMG CoA reductase inhibitors (statins). Increased risk of myopathy, rhabdomyolysis, possible renal failure. Alternatives include pravastatin, low dose atorvastatin.
carbamazepine, phenytoin, phenobarbital	Potential for increased metabolism of PI, leading to virologic failure. Avoid concurrent use, consider alternative such as levetiracetam, an anticonvulsant that has minimal drug interactions.

d, Day; *h*, hour; *wk*, week.

Table 34–3

Interactions—cont'd

Interaction	Comments
midazolam, triazolam	Midazolam and triazolam concentrations may be markedly increased leading to prolonged sedation. Alternatives may include low dose alprazolam, lorazepam, or temazepam.
St John's wort	Significant decrease in PI levels, potentially leading to virologic failure or resistance. Avoid concurrent use during PI therapy.
rifampin	Significant decrease in PI levels, potentially leading to virologic failure. Consider rifabutin as an alternative.
atazanavir–proton pump inhibitors (e.g., omeprazole)	Significant reductions in atazanavir concentrations. Avoid concurrent use, consider use of an H_2 blocker (e.g., ranitidine) separated by at least 12 h from atazanavir administration.

 Nursing Process

Antiretroviral Therapy

ASSESSMENT

- Assess whether client needs HIV testing.
- Refer as appropriate for anonymous or confidential testing.
- Assess for renal and hepatic disorders; use of oral contraceptives.
- Assess for signs and symptoms related to clinical progression toward a depressed immune system, including profound involuntary weight loss, chronic diarrhea, chronic weight loss, intermittent or constant fever.
- Assess use of other prescription and OTC medications.
- Refer high-risk clients who test negative to counseling.
- Assess physiologic and psychosocial needs; refer to medical care and psychologic support as indicated.
- Obtain client history for clients who test positive for HIV.
- Obtain a medical drug, diet, and herbal history; report probable drug-drug, drug-food, or drug-herb interactions.

NURSING DIAGNOSES

- Ineffective health maintenance related to knowledge deficit about HIV/AIDS
- Fear related to potential outcome of HIV screening, powerlessness, and/or threat to well-being
- Imbalanced nutrition; less than body requirements related to nausea and vomiting
- Ineffective coping and/or compromised family coping related to situational crises (positive HIV screening outcome)
- Risk for infection related to compromised immune system (CD4$^+$ cell count <200)

- Ineffective therapeutic regimen adherence related to difficulty managing medications and lack of knowledge about drug interactions with food
- Readiness for enhanced therapeutic regimen management related to expressed desire to improve knowledge about disease progression and outcomes of care
- Disturbed body image related to excess weight loss
- Deficient knowledge related to medication management
- Impaired memory related to disease progression

PLANNING

- Client's viral load will be undetectable.
- Client's CD4$^+$ count will be as high as possible.
- Client will not experience secondary infections.
- Client will participate in medical treatment and in spiritual and psychologic support that best fits his/her needs and belief system.
- Client will promptly report new onset of symptoms and side effects.
- Client will adhere to medication regimen and/or report difficulties related to adherence.

NURSING INTERVENTIONS

- Promote adherence/compliance to the therapeutic regimen.
- Promote meticulous hand washing; apply standard precautions.
- Administer increased fluids, up to 2400 ml/d unless contraindicated.
- Monitor laboratory reports for indications of decreasing CD4$^+$ T-lymphocyte cell counts; inform primary care provider.
- Refer client for preventive care measures including annual PAP, eye, and dental examinations.
- Refer client for nutritional counseling.
- Refer client for spiritual support.

Client Teaching

General

- Explain how virus may cause severe damage to the immune system.
- Describe modes of transmission of the virus.
- Explain common emotional responses.
- Explain the need for monitoring health practices.
- Emphasize protective precautions to decrease risk of exposure and infection as necessary.
- Advise client not to visit anyone with any type of respiratory infection.
- For women of childbearing age, provide information about managing future pregnancies to reduce risk of HIV transmission to unborn children.
- Provide personal drug therapy plan in writing.
- Inform client that certain foods and herbal products may interact with antiretrovirals.
- Establish client/family partnership in the plan.

Self-Administration

- Assist client to develop a system for taking the correct dose of the correct medications at the correct time. A medication organizer is a practical help to many clients.
- Instruct client in importance of having an adequate supply of medication so there is no interruption in the schedule. Omission of drugs may result in deterioration of client's condition.
- For pediatric clients unable to swallow medications, teach swallowing techniques.

Side Effects

- Advise client about what symptoms to report promptly to health care provider.
- Discuss possible side effects and strategies to manage them.
- Provide suggestions for managing diarrhea.

Diet

- Advise client to eat a variety of foods.
- Advise client how to minimize side effects (e.g., take specific drug with food).
- Discuss BRAT diet (banana, rice, applesauce, and toast) for management of diarrhea.

Cultural Considerations ❖

- Know that there is an oral history that the drug AZT may be harmful to certain groups of people.
- Some cultures pressure women to reproduce regardless of health status and the implications for future generations.
- AIDS is a highly stigmatized disease.
- Some religious and ethnic mores prohibit use of contraception, especially male condom use.
- Ethnic minorities may distrust health care providers and refuse treatment regimens that include research.

- Issues related to adherence and culture for women with HIV is available at *http://hab.hrsa.gov/publications/womencare.htm*.

EVALUATION

- Evaluate the effectiveness of the antiretroviral therapy.
- Determine whether the viral load is undetectable or as low as possible.
- Evaluate medication adherence.

Antiretroviral Therapy: The Nurse's Role

The nurse's role with clients taking complex regimens of antiretroviral medications includes ongoing assessment, analysis, and education. Thorough assessment of the client's physiologic and psychosocial health needs is required initially. Follow-up assessment after therapy begins should include medication side effects, adherence to one's regimen, and issues affecting medication adherence. Clients may confuse medication side effects with a new onset of symptoms. Careful follow-up assessment can detect the need for additional medical care or medication management.

Issues of adherence are common with antiretroviral therapy. Individual assessment of adherence issues with an analysis of the client's lifestyle is essential. Multiple strategies for adherence are available and should be discussed with clients. Medication organizers are commonly used. Due to the high number of pills required with HAART, careful monitoring of administration is desired. A written schedule, medication diary, chalkboard, scheduled pager or cellular telephone messaging systems can be used to help clients maintain accurate administration. For children, parental/guardian support and supervision is needed. Teaching all persons involved in the client's medication management can promote adherence. Friends, family members, and personal support systems can assist clients in adherence to medications. A client information sheet that explains the importance of adherence with HIV disease is available at *http://www.aidsinfonet.org/factsheet_detail.php?fsnumber=405*.

Nurses can facilitate adherence by allowing sufficient time to educate clients about medications, developing a trusting relationship, and building a partnership with the client. Excellent information and strategies for adherence are available at *http://hivinsite.ucsf.edu/InSite?page=kbr-03-02-09*. When simpler regimens are available, nurses can advocate with medical providers for their clients. Therefore the nurse must maintain current knowledge of available regimens and clinical trials. Current open clinical trials may be found at *http://www.aactg.org/clinicaltrials_research.asp*.

In addition to client assessment, education, and advocacy, nurses should identify problems that require additional investigation and research. Because of the individual and lifestyle needs of the diverse HIV/AIDS population, research on strategies to promote adherence will continue to be needed. Best practices for adherence need to be identified.

The nurse's role with research is also needed with clinical trials. Accurate data collection, record keeping, and attention to detail are necessary. Whenever medication regimens change, nurses should contribute to the ongoing evaluation of medication/regimen side effects and adverse event reporting. Adverse events can be reported at *http://www.fda.gov/medwatch/*.

Adherence to Drug Regimen

Adherence to the therapeutic regimen is a major concern and issue with clients receiving antiretroviral therapy. Relative to this, the nurse must be knowledgeable about ways to promote adherence to the regimen. Nonadherence will result in HIV viral replication, increased VLs, deterioration of the immune system, and future medical management problems with medication efficacy and increased potential for drug resistance. Development of resistant viral strains, enhanced with subtherapeutic levels of antiretroviral agents, is a serious current and long-term threat for clients with AIDS. Reasons commonly identified by clients for missing medications include forgetting to take them, feeling too sick, difficulty handling side effects, or not having the medicine with them. In addition, there are public health implications of nonadherence related to the expanding pool of drug-resistant viruses.

The following suggestions are offered to promote client adherence to the therapeutic regimen. Clients' understanding of their drug regimen, including the purpose of each medication, dosage schedule, food and fluid restrictions, recommended food choices, and storage of medications (e.g., refrigeration) is crucial to adherence. Pictorial representation of the medications and a pillbox designed for medications to be taken four times a day may be helpful. Additional helpful hints to promote adherence are associating taking medications with a daily routine, such as brushing the teeth or feeding the pet; having a friend remind the client to take the medication; using a medications calendar to check off medications taken; and using the pharmacist as a resource.

Clients need the telephone number of a contact person to whom they can address questions. Discussion of anticipated side effects of the medications and how to manage their occurrence is necessary. A trusting client-provider relationship is essential. Long-term adherence to the regimen remains a major challenge and requires an interdisciplinary team approach.

Opportunistic Infections

As HIV infection advances, clients are more vulnerable to infections and malignancies, which are called *opportunistic infections* because they take advantage of the opportunity offered by a weakened immune system. Since the introduction of HAART, there has been a dramatic reduction in the incidence of opportunistic infections among HIV-positive clients receiving these medications. However, the prevention and treatment of opportunistic infections remain essential.

The most common HIV-related opportunistic infections/diseases include:

- Bacterial: tuberculosis, MAC, bacterial pneumonia, septicemia
- Protozoal: PCP, toxoplasmosis, cryptosporidiosis, leishmaniasis
- Fungal: candidiasis, cryptococcosis
- Viral: cytomegalovirus, herpes simplex, herpes zoster
- HIV-associated malignancies: Kaposi sarcoma, lymphoma, squamous cell carcinoma

Different conditions typically occur at different stages of HIV infection. Common with CD4$^+$ cell count below 350 cells/ml:

- Herpes simplex virus causes ulcers/vesicles in the mouth or genitals. **Treatment** includes acyclovir, famciclovir, or valacyclovir.
- Herpes zoster virus causes shingles. **Treatment** includes acyclovir, famciclovir, or valacyclovir.
- Both herpes simplex and herpes zoster are also capable of causing retinitis and encephalitis, which can be life-threatening.
- Tuberculosis infection that predominately affects the lungs but can affect other organs, such as the bowel, lining of the heart or lungs, brain, or lining of the central nervous system. **Treatment** includes isoniazid, pyridoxine, rifampin, pyrazinamide.
- Kaposi sarcoma causes dark blue lesions which can occur in a variety of locations, including the skin, mucous membranes, gastrointestinal tract, lungs, or lymph nodes; they usually appear early in the course of HIV infection. **Treatment** depends on the symptoms and location. For local lesions, vinblastine has been used. Radiotherapy has been used in delicate sites such as eyes and face. Chemotherapy is the preferred treatment for severe widespread disease.

Common with CD4$^+$ cell count below 200 cells/ml:

- *Candida* esophagitis, a painful yeast infection of the esophagus
- Bacillary angiomatosis, skin lesions caused by *Bartonella*, usually acquired from cat scratches
- *Pneumocystis carinii* pneumonia (now called *pneumocystic jiroveci* pneumonia) is caused by a parasite that infects the lungs. Symptoms are mainly pneumonia, along with fever and respiratory symptoms such as dry cough, chest pain, and dyspnea. **Treatment** includes TMP-SMX (Bactrim, Septra), clindamycin or oral primaquine.

Common with CD4$^+$ cell count below 100 cells/ml:

- Cryptococcal meningitis infection of the lining of the brain by a yeast
- AIDS dementia
- Toxoplasmosis encephalitis caused by a protozoan found in uncooked meat and cat feces. Infecting the brain, it can cause headache, confusion, motor weakness, and

fever. If left untreated, the disease progression results in seizures, stupor, and coma. **Treatment** includes pyrimethamine, sulfadiazine, clindamycin.

- Progressive multifocal leukoencephalopathy, a viral disease of the brain that results in a severe decline in cognitive and motor functions
- Wasting syndrome causing extreme weight loss and loss of appetite
- Cryptosporidium diarrhea, severe diarrhea caused by parasites

Common with CD4$^+$ cell count below 50 cells/ml:

- Mycobacterium avium complex (MAC) is a blood infection caused by bacteria related to tuberculosis. MAC generally affects multiple organs, with symptoms including fever, night sweats, weight loss, fatigue, diarrhea, abdominal pain. **Treatment** includes clarithromycin, azithromycin, ethambutol, rifabutin.
- Cytomegalovirus infection is a virus infecting the whole body, but most commonly appears as retinitis causing blurred vision; it can lead to blindness. Cytomegalovirus can also affect other organs causing fever, diarrhea, nausea, pneumonia-like symptoms, and dementia. **Treatment** includes ganciclovir, valganciclovir, foscarnet.

End-Stage AIDS

The era of HAART has shown that clients with HIV infection/AIDS are living longer, and the increased survival time of HIV clients has shown an increase of end-stage AIDS conditions. Causes of death have changed from sepsis and opportunistic infections to liver and kidney failure, malignancies, pneumonias, and end-stage AIDS. End-stage AIDS can be manifested by pain, general weight loss, anorexia, neuropathies, dementia, constipation, diarrhea, depression, nausea, and vomiting.

Antiretroviral Therapy in Pregnancy

Optimal drug therapy should be used for women of reproductive age and for those who are pregnant. When initiating antiretroviral therapy for women of reproductive age, the criteria for starting therapy and the goals of treatment are identical to those for other adults and adolescents. Because of considerations related to the prevention of transmission of HIV to the child during pregnancy, the timing of initiation of treatment and the selection of regimens may differ from nonpregnant adults or adolescents.

For women who are pregnant, an additional goal is to prevent mother-to-child transmission, with a goal of viral suppression to less than 1000 copies/ml to reduce the risk of transmission of HIV to the fetus or newborn. A woman infected with HIV can transmit the virus during pregnancy, labor and delivery, and through breastfeeding. If no preventative drugs are taken and breastfeeding is practiced, the chance of the baby becoming infected is 20% to 45%.

Medications, when combined with other interventions (e.g., formula feeding), reduces the risk of transmission to less than 2%.

Antiretroviral therapy is recommended in all pregnant women who test positive for HIV infection, regardless of virologic, immunologic, or clinical parameters for the purpose of preventing mother-to-child transmission of HIV. Zidovudine is often suggested as the medication of choice, because it has been shown to be particularly effective at preventing HIV from being passed from mother to child. The dose for zidovudine is:

- *Maternal:* Oral: 100 mg 5 times/day or 200 mg 3 times/day or 300 mg 2 times/day. Begin at 14-34 weeks gestation and continue until the start of labor. During labor and delivery, administer zidovudine IV at 2 mg/kg as a loading dose followed by a continuous IV infusion of 1 mg/kg/hour until the umbilical cord is clamped.
- *Neonatal:* Oral: 2 mg/kg/dose every 6 hours. If unable to take oral therapy, an IV dose of 1.5 mg/kg/dose every 6 hours is given. Dosing should begin 8-12 hours after birth and continue for the first 6 weeks of life.

Clinicians treating pregnant women infected with HIV are encouraged to report cases of prenatal exposure to antiretroviral drugs to the **Antiretroviral Pregnancy Registry.** The registry collects data regarding antiretroviral exposure during pregnancy to assess potential teratogenicity. The APR telephone number is 910-251-9087 or 1-800-258-4263, and the website is *www.APRegistry.com.*

Postexposure Prophylaxis for Health Care Workers

HIV transmission to health care workers continues to be related to exposure to infectious materials and their sources. *Exposure* is defined as percutaneous injury with a contaminated sharp object or exposure of mucous membranes or nonintact skin (e.g., cut, abraded, chapped, dermatitis) to infectious material. The risk of HIV transmission (without prophylaxis) is 0.3% from percutaneous injury and 0.09% from mucocutaneous exposure. An increased risk of HIV transmission to healthcare workers exists when the worker is exposed to a device (e.g., needle, scalpel) with visible blood, a needle placed in an artery or vein, a deep injury, large volume losses, or exposure to infectious materials containing a high viral load. The majority of HIV exposures will warrant a two-drug regimen (basic regimen). The addition of a third or fourth medication should be considered for exposures posing an increased risk for transmission or involving a source in which antiretroviral drug resistance is likely. The basic and expanded **postexposure prophylaxis (PEP)** (treatment regimens after percutaneous exposure to HIV) regimens are described in Table 34-4, and HIV PEP resources and registries are found in Box 34-2.

Management of a potential HIV exposure needs to be initiated within hours of the event and continued for 4

Table 34–4

Basic and Expanded Post-Exposure Prophylaxis Regimens

Regimen Category	Drug Regimen(s)
Basic	**zidovudine (Retrovir) + lamivudine (Epivir) available as Combivir** zidovudine: 300 mg 2 times/day or 200 mg 3 times/d lamivudine: 300 mg once daily or 150 mg 2 times/d Combivir: one tablet 2 times/d **zidovudine + emtricitabine (Emtriva)** zidovudine: 300 mg 2 times/day or 200 mg 3 times/d emtricitabine: 200 mg once daily **tenofovir (Viread) + lamivudine** tenofovir: 300 mg once daily lamivudine: 300 mg once daily or 150 mg 2 times/d **tenofovir + emtricitabine available as Truvada** tenofovir: 300 mg once daily emtricitabine: 200 mg once daily Truvada: one tablet daily
Expanded	**Basic regimen PLUS lopinavir/ritonavir (Kaletra)** Kaletra: 400/100 = 2 tablets 2 times/d

d, Day.

Box 34-2

HIV Resources

PEPline at *http://www.ucsf.edu/hivcntr/Hotlines*
Telephone: 888-448-4911
HIV Antiretroviral Pregnancy Registry at *http://www. apregistry.com/index.htm*
Telephone: 800-258-4263
FDA at *http://www.fda.gov/medwatch*
Telephone: 800-332-1088
CDC: Telephone: 800-893-0485
HIV/AIDS Treatment Information Service at *http://aidsinfo. nih.gov*

---

weeks. Health care workers taking PEP have reported adverse reactions at rates of 17% to 47%, with the most common reactions being nausea, malaise, and fatigue.

A comprehensive reference for PEP is the "Updated U.S. Public Health Service Guidelines for the Management of Occupational Exposures to HIV and Recommendations for Postexposure Prophylaxis," *MMWR* 54(RR-9): September 30, 2005.

The Future of HIV/ AIDS-Related Agents

Agents Under Investigation

Integrase Inhibitors

Integrase inhibitors block the insertion of HIV DNA into human DNA by attacking the enzyme that allows them to merge. When used with tenofovir and lamivudine (Epivir), the integrase inhibitor has shown comparable viral load reduction to efavirenz, and the reduction occurred more rapidly. In addition, the integrase inhibitor was shown to be effective in those clients who had failed other HIV medication regimens. Integrase inhibitors may not adversely affect serum lipids to the extent of other antiretrovirals. Elvitegravir is currently under clinical trials. Raltegravir (Isentress) was approved by the FDA in late 2007.

CCR5 Entry Inhibitors

CCR5 agents block the receptor responsible for allowing HIV entry into susceptible cells. These medications represent the first attempt to target a cellular structure, rather than the virus, to interfere with viral replication. While CCR5 entry inhibitors look promising, these agents have been associated with isolated cases of severe hepatotoxicity. Vicriviroc (in phase II clinical trials) and maraviroc (Selzentry; approved by the FDA in late 2007) are two CCR5 entry inhibitors.

Maturation Inhibitors

Maturation is the last of 10 steps in HIV replication of the HIV life cycle. Maturation is the step allowing HIV to become infectious. Maturation inhibitors aim to prevent HIV from properly assembling and maturing, forming a protective outer coat or from emerging from human cells. Currently, bevirimat is in clinical trials.

Antisense Drugs

These agents are mirror images of part of the HIV genetic code. These drugs lock onto the virus, preventing it from functioning. At present one antisense drug, HGTV43, is beginning phase II clinical trials.

Two new NNRTIs (rilpivirine and etravirine) and one new PI (brecanavir) are also in phase II or III clinical trials at the present time.

KEY WEBSITES

Drug Adherence in HIV/AIDS: http://hivinsite.ucsf.edu/Insite?page=kbr-03-02-09

HIV/AIDS Bureau—A Guide to the Clinical Care of Women with HIV/AIDS: http://hab.hrsa.gov/publications/womencare.htm

US Food and Drug Administration—HIV and AIDS Activities: www.fda.gov/oashi/aids/hiv.html

Critical Thinking Case Study

At 32 years of age, RS presented with chronic fatigue. Following a medical evaluation, RS was diagnosed with HIV infection and began initial therapy with efavirenz, zidovudine, and lamivudine (with zidovudine and lamivudine coformulated as Combinivir). Two years later, the laboratory reported RS's viral load (VL) at 120,000. At that time, ritonavir was added. The VL decreased to 3500, and the CD4$^+$ T cells increased from 06 mm^3 to 96 mm^3.

Recently RS reports that it is hard to "always be taking medicine" and states, "Now that I'm back to work and going out again, I sometimes forget my pills." RS is experiencing increased fatigue and greater gastric intolerance. VL has increased to 8500, and CD4$^+$ T cells have decreased to 70 mm^3.

It is believed that RS has become resistant to RT inhibitors, so a dual protease inhibitor is started. In 6 weeks, the VL is undetectable and the CD4$^+$ T cells are 85 mm^3.

1. Missing doses of protease inhibitors can be very harmful to the client. Given the client's history, what can the nurse do to assist RS with issues related to adherence/compliance?

2. What is the rationale for including more than one antiretroviral agent in RS's initial therapeutic plan?

3. What actions should the nurse take to facilitate RS's understanding of the consequences of nonadherence to the drug regimen?

4. What are the dangers of missing doses of protease inhibitors?

NCLEX Study Questions

1. A client has been prescribed HAART therapy following a laboratory test that indicated an increasing viral load. The client reports he's glad to have a choice of medications from which to choose. The nurse's response should include:
   a. education about the importance of using multiple medications concurrently
   b. written information about the scheduling of his medications with meals
   c. support and encouragement for the client's readiness for treatment
   d. guidelines for follow-up laboratory monitoring and clinic appointments

2. A client who has been taking antiretroviral treatment for six months indicates increasing difficulty managing the daily dosing and remembering to take the medications at frequent but inconvenient times throughout the day. In discussing the plan of treatment with the health care team, you recommend:
   a. consulting with the dietician to manage food and medication management for greatest efficacy
   b. monitoring the client's laboratory values more frequently
   c. asking the client to bring a significant other to the next appointment to help monitor medication management
   d. using a single daily dose ofcoformulated medication

3. During routine prenatal testing, a client was newly diagnosed with HIV infection. To help prevent perinatal transmission of HIV to the fetus, the nurse should:
   a. provide the parents with contact information for the local AIDS support group
   b. educate the client about the risks of HIV disease to her unborn child
   c. notify the CDC of the client's diagnosis
   d. provide written and oral education about the use of antiretroviral therapy during pregnancy

4. The nurse would expect to find an improvement in which of the blood values as a result of antiretroviral treatment?
   a. serum creatinine level
   b. CD4$^+$ T cell level
   c. lipids
   d. hemoglobin

5. Combivir and Trizivir are fixed combinations of which of the following:
   a. NRTIs
   b. NNRTIs
   c. PIs
   d. NSAIDs

Answers: 1, a; 2, d; 3, d; 4, b; 5, a.

35

Vaccines

Lynette M. Wachholz

ELECTRONIC RESOURCES

Evolve website (http://evolve.elsevier.com/KeeHayes/pharmacology/):
- Case Studies
- Content Updates
- Frequently Asked Questions
- Student Review Activities
- WebLinks
- Additional Reference Material

Companion CD-ROM:
- NCLEX Examination Review Questions
- Pharmacology Animations
- IV Therapy Checklists
- Medication Error Checklists
- Drug Calculation Problems
- Electronic Calculators
- Top 200 Drugs with Pronunciations
- References from the Textbook

Outline

Objectives

- Compare and contrast active and passive immunity.
- Compare and contrast active natural and active acquired immunity.
- Describe infectious diseases for which vaccines are currently available.
- Outline the currently recommended childhood immunization schedule.
- Discuss vaccines routinely administered to adults.
- Discuss contraindications to the administration of recommended immunizations.
- Explain the nursing interventions, including client teaching, related to the administration of vaccines.

Terms

Timely immunizations protect individuals from illness. They can also ultimately lead to the eradication of disease, as was the case with smallpox in 1977. Therefore universal immunization is a national goal. Currently in the United States, just over 80 percent of 19- to 35-month-old children have received all vaccinations in the recommend series.

A recent study suggested that factors such as absence of a two-parent household, large family size, Medicaid enrollment, lack of a usual health care provider, no insurance coverage, or lack of a telephone in the home significantly increased the odds of a child experiencing vaccination delay.

Other studies have looked at racial disparities in immunization rates. One such study noted an increasing gap in coverage rates between white and black children, as well as between white and Hispanic children.

Active Immunity

Active immunity occurs as a part of the human immune response, which is activated when a **pathogen** such as a bacterium or virus invades the body. The body recognizes this pathogen as a foreign substance and promptly begins producing **antibodies** (also called *immunoglobulins*) and other infection-fighting cells whose responsibility it is to rid the body of this foreign substance. On first exposure to the pathogen, the immune response is relatively slow and is typically accompanied by signs and symptoms of disease. However, the immune system retains memory of this pathogen. If this same pathogen invades the body again, the immune response, including the increased production of pathogen-specific antibodies, occurs much more rapidly and generally prevents disease. This active natural immunity may be present for the remaining life of the individual. **Natural immunity** is genetically determined in specific populations or families. Some pathogens cannot infect certain species, because the environment is not suitable (e.g., measles cannot reproduce in dogs; thus, dogs have a natural immunity to measles).

Acquired immunity occurs from exposure to an antigen or from passive injection of immunoglobulins. Active protection against disease may also be provoked by immunization. **Vaccination** involves the administration of a small amount of **antigen,** which although capable of stimulating an immune response does not typically produce disease. The antigen in vaccines may be produced in several ways. Traditional vaccines contain the whole or components of an inactivated (killed) microorganism. Other vaccines are **attenuated viruses** composed of live, attenuated (weakened) microorganisms. **Toxoids** are inactivated toxins, the harmful disease-causing substance produced by some microorganisms.

Some newer vaccines are called **conjugate vaccines.** Such vaccines require a protein or toxoid from an unrelated organism to link to the outer coat of the disease-causing microorganism. This linkage creates a substance that can be recognized by the immature immune system of young infants. *Haemophilus influenzae* type B is an example of a conjugate vaccine.

Recombinant subunit vaccines involve the insertion of some of the genetic material (e.g., deoxyribonucleic acid [DNA]) of a pathogen into another cell or organism, where the antigen is then produced in massive quantities. These antigens are then used as a vaccine in place of the whole pathogen. Hepatitis B is an example of this type of vaccine.

Regardless of the composition of the vaccine, each vaccine is designed to stimulate an immune response against a specific pathogen. Booster doses are sometimes required to maintain sufficient immunity. Because the immune system retains memory, a vaccinated individual who is later exposed to the actual pathogen mounts a rapid immune response, thus preventing disease. This active artificially acquired immunity is the focus of this chapter.

Passive Immunity

Passive immunity occurs when an individual receives antibodies against a particular pathogen from another source. Newborn infants naturally receive passive immunity via the transfer of maternal antibodies across the placenta. Passive immunity may also be acquired through the administration of antibodies pooled from several human or animal sources that have been exposed to disease-causing pathogens. Alternatively, antibodies may be produced using recombinant DNA technology.

Whether natural or acquired, passive immunity is transient, lasting no more than several weeks to a few months. The recipient does not mount his or her own immune response. However, passive immunity is important. It helps young infants who, because of their immature immune systems, are poorly equipped to protect themselves against disease. Acquired passive immunity is important (1) when time does not permit active vaccination alone, (2) when the exposed individual is at high risk for complications of the disease, or (3) when the person suffers from an immune system deficiency that renders that person unable to produce an effective immune response.

Vaccine-Preventable Diseases

In the United States more than 20 infectious diseases may be prevented by active vaccination. Many of these vaccines are routinely administered to healthy children and adults. Others are reserved for special populations, such as military personnel, travelers to certain foreign countries, or the chronically ill. Table 35–1 provides an overview of the disease manifestations and vaccine information, including route of administration and storage temperature. Vaccine-preventable diseases include, but are not limited to, anthrax, diphtheria, *Haemophilus influenzae* type B (Hib), hepatitis A, hepatitis B, human papillomavirus, influenza, Japanese encephalitis, measles, meningococcal disease, mumps, pertussis, pneumococcal disease, poliomyelitis, rabies, rotavirus, rubella, smallpox, tetanus, tuberculosis, typhoid, varicella, yellow fever, and herpes zoster.

Childhood Immunizations

The 2007 Childhood, Adolescent, & Catch-up Immunization Schedules can be found by logging on to the Evolve website. Note that these recommendations change regularly; for the most current information, consult the Centers for Disease Control and Prevention (CDC) website at *www.cdc.gov/vaccines.*

A summary of rules for childhood immunizations is also located at the Immunization Action Coalition's web-

Table 35-1

Vaccine-Preventable Diseases

Disease/Route of Administration and Storage Temperature	Manifestations	Vaccine
Anthrax/subQ	• Spectrum involves three types of infection: *Cutaneous* (malignant pustule): a painless sore that develops at the site of a cut *Inhalational* (wool sorter's disease): severe dyspnea, cyanosis, fever, and death *Gastrointestinal*: abdominal pain, vomiting, bloody diarrhea, toxemia, shock, possibly death • Inhalational form associated with use of bacteria in biologic warfare	• Inactivated bacteria • Administration limited to military personnel
Diphtheria/IM 35°-46° F (2°-8° C)	• Respiratory infection • May result in heart failure or paralysis if left untreated	• Toxoid • Contained in DTaP, Tdap, DT, Td, DTaP-Hib, and DTaP-hepatitis B-polio vaccines
Haemophilus influenzae type B (Hib)/IM 35°-46° F (2°-8° C)	• Causes meningitis, pneumonia, sepsis, arthritis, and skin and throat infections • Most serious in children younger than 1 y	• Bacterial conjugate • Contained in Hib, DTap-Hib, and Hib-hepatitis B vaccines
Hepatitis A/IM 35°-46° F (2°-8° C)	• Fever, malaise, jaundice, anorexia, and nausea • Acute, self-limited illness	• Inactivated viral antigen • Contained in hepatitis A and hepatitis A-hepatitis B vaccines • Administered to children 12-23 mo, high-risk populations, and persons traveling to certain foreign countries
Hepatitis B/IM 35°-46° F (2°-8° C)	• Malaise, anorexia, arthralgias, arthritis, jaundice • Chronic infection can occur, leading to liver cirrhosis, liver cancer, and death	• Recombinant viral antigen • Contained in hepatitis B, Hib-hepatitis B, DTaP-hepatitis B-polio, and hepatitis A-hepatitis B vaccines
Human papillomavirus/IM 35°-46° F (2°-8° C)	• Cervical cancer, genital warts	• Recombinant viral antigen • Administered to females 9-26 y
Influenza/IM, intranasal *Inactivated*: 35°-46° F (2°-8° C) *Live attenuated*: ≤5° F (−15° C)	• Fever, chills, headaches, malaise, myalgias, nasal congestion, and cough • Occasionally causes croup and pneumonia	• Inactivated viral components (IM) or live attenuated virus (intranasal)
Japanese encephalitis/subQ 35°-46° F (2°-8° C)	• Headache, fever, myalgias, encephalitis	• Inactivated virus • Administered to some foreign travelers
Measles/subQ 35°-46° F (2°-8° C), but may be frozen	• Rash, fever, cough, nasal congestion, conjunctivitis, pneumonia • Occasionally results in encephalitis	• Live virus • Contained in measles, MMR, and MMR-varicella vaccines
Meningococcal disease/subQ, IM 35°-46° F (2°-8° C)	• Fever, sepsis, rash, meningitis	• *Old vaccine (MPSV4)*: portions of inactivated bacterial capsule (subQ) *New vaccine (MCV4)*: bacterial conjugate (IM), expected to give better, longer-lasting protection
Mumps/subQ 35°-46° F (2°-8° C), but may be frozen	• Swelling of salivary glands, fever, and headache • Rarely causes encephalitis, inflamed testicles, or permanent hearing loss	• Live attenuated virus • Contained in mumps, MMR, and MMR-varicella vaccines
Pertussis ("whooping cough")/IM	• Severe coughing spasms • Rarely causes pneumonia, seizures, encephalitis, and death • Symptoms more severe in infants and young children	• Antigenic components of inactivated bacteria (acellular) • Contained in DTaP, Tdap, DTaP-Hib, and DTaP-hepatitis B-polio vaccines

BCG, Bacille Calmette-Guérin; *DT*, diphtheria-tetanus; *DTaP*, diphtheria-tetanus-acellular pertussis; *Hib*, *Haemophilus influenzae* type B; *ID*, intradermal; *IM*, intramuscular; *MMR*, measles-mumps-rubella; *mo*, months, *PO*, by mouth; *subQ*, subcutaneous; *Td*, tetanus-diphtheria; *y*, year; >, greater than; ≥, greater than or equal to; <, less than, ≤, less than or equal to.

Continued

Table 35–1

Vaccine-Preventable Diseases—cont'd

Disease/Route of Administration and Storage Temperature	Manifestations	Vaccine
Pneumococcal disease/IM, subQ 35°-46° F (2°-8° C)	• Ear infections, sinus infections, pneumonia • Occasionally causes sepsis and meningitis	• Older polysaccharide vaccine (PPV23) contains portions of 23 serotypes of pneumococcal bacterial capsules (subQ); administered to elderly and certain other high risk populations as long as ≥2 y of age • Newer vaccine (PCV7) is a protein conjugate vaccine containing portions of 7 serotypes of pneumococcal bacterial capsules (IM); recommended for routine administration to children <2 y of age and certain other older high-risk children
Poliomyelitis/subQ, IM 35°-46° F (2°-8° C)	• Mild form causes fever, sore throat, nausea, and headaches • Severe form causes paralysis and death	• Inactivated virus
Rabies/IM 35°-46° F (2°-8° C)	• Anxiety, difficulty swallowing, seizures, almost always progresses to death	• Inactivated virus • Administered to high-risk groups (e.g., veterinarians, animal handlers) and persons traveling to areas where rabies is common
Rotavirus/PO 35°-46° F (2°-8° C)	• Vomiting and diarrhea; may be particularly severe in infants/young children	• Live attenuated virus
Rubella ("German measles")/subQ 35°-46° F (2°-8° C), but may be frozen	• Rash, fever • Birth defects if acquired by pregnant women	• Live attenuated virus • Contained in rubella, MMR, and MMR-varicella vaccines
Smallpox/skin prick 35°-46° F (2°-8° C)	• High fever, severe headache, backache, abdominal pain, and lethargy lasting 2-5 days • Then extensive rash which begins as macules that progress to papules, then firm vesicles, and finally, deep-seated, hard pustules which cause significant scarring • Natural disease eradicated worldwide in 1980 • May be used as a weapon of bioterrorism	• Live virus • Limited immunization program to include military personnel, civilian health care workers, and emergency personnel began in 2002
Tetanus ("lock jaw")/IM 35°-46° F (2°-8° C)	• Headache, irritability, muscle spasms (jaw, neck, arms, legs, back, and abdomen)	• Toxoid • Contained in tetanus, DTaP, DTaP-Hib, DT, DTaP-hepatitis B-polio, Tdap, and Td vaccines
Tuberculosis ("TB")/ID (preferred), subQ 35°-46° F (2°-8° C)	• Highly contagious respiratory infection • May also cause meningitis and bone, joint, and skin infections	• Live attenuated bacteria • Referred to as BCG vaccine • Not routinely administered in the United States • Prevents severe disease but does not prevent infection with the bacterium
Typhoid/subQ, PO 35°-46° F (2°-8° C)	• Fever, headache, anorexia, abdominal pain, enlarged liver and spleen, constipation, and later, diarrhea	• Available as live attenuated bacteria (PO), or inactivated components of typhoid bacterial capsule (subQ) • Recommended only for travelers to certain foreign countries
Varicella ("chickenpox")/subQ ≤5° F (–15° C)	• Fever and rash, consisting of a few to hundreds of itchy, blisterlike lesions • Symptoms more severe in older children and adults • Complications may include encephalitis, bacterial skin infections, pneumonia, Reye syndrome, and death	• Live attenuated virus • Contained in varicella and MMR-varicella vaccines
Yellow fever/subQ 35°-46° F (2°-8° C)	• Fever, jaundice, and gastrointestinal hemorrhage	• Live attenuated virus • Recommended for travelers to foreign countries with high yellow fever rates • Required by international regulations for travel to and from certain countries
Zoster ("shingles")/subQ ≤5° F (–15° C)	• Painful, blisterlike rash in a dermatomal distribution • Occurs due to reactivation of varicella virus • Following resolution of rash, may have prolonged severe pain (postherpetic neuralgia)	• Live attenuated virus • Administered to persons ≥60 y

site at *www.immunize.org/catg.d/rules1.pdf*. Helpful information about each vaccine includes route of administration, schedule for routine vaccine administration, minimum dosing intervals, and contraindications to use. The recommended vaccines are diphtheria-tetanus-pertussis, inactivated polio, varicella, measles-mumps-rubella, *Haemophilus influenzae* type B, hepatitis A, hepatitis B, pneumococcal conjugate, influenza, meningococcal conjugate, human papillomavirus, and rotavirus. Before immunizations are administered, children and their caregivers should be questioned regarding their use of prescription and over-the-counter medications, including herbal preparations, and any food or drug allergies from which they suffer (Herbal Alert 35–1).

Adult Immunizations

While much emphasis is placed on regularly immunizing infants and children, adult immunizations are frequently overlooked. However, they are equally important to the health and well-being of this population. Routine vaccines for adults may include tetanus-diphtheria-pertussis, tetanus-diphtheria, influenza, pneumococcal polysaccharide, human papillomavirus, measles-mumps-rubella, varicella, and zoster. In certain situations, adults may also be immunized with some or all of the following vaccines: hepatitis A, hepatitis B, and meningococcal polysaccharide. The 2006-2007 Adult Immunization Schedule can be found by logging on to the Evolve website. The most current recommendations for adult immunization can be located at *www.cdc.gov/vaccines*. Helpful information for each vaccine includes route of administration, recommended populations, vaccine administration schedules, and contraindications. The CDC suggests review of adult immunization records on decade birthdays (e.g., ages 30, 40, 50 years).

Herbal ALERT 35–1

Vaccines

There are no known interactions between vaccinations and herbal preparations.

Preventing MEDICATION ERRORS

Do not confuse...

- Hepatitis B vaccines have different doses for child/adolescent vs. adult vaccine recipients.
- Hepatitis B vaccines and hepatitis B immunoglobulin (HBIG)
- DTaP and Tdap vaccines contain different amounts of the individual vaccine components and are indicated for different age groups.

Immunization before Foreign Travel

Foreign travel warrants the administration of all routine vaccines indicated based on age or immunization history. Foreign travel also requires consideration of additional vaccines, depending on the client's travel destinations.

Many travelers may need to consider vaccination against typhoid and yellow fever. Typhoid is caused by a bacterium, *Salmonella enterica* typhi, which is generally spread via contaminated food and water (refer to Table 35–1 for disease manifestations). Risk of contracting this infection is greatest for travelers to India, Pakistan, Mexico, Bangladesh, the Philippines, and Haiti. Even stays of less than 2 weeks pose significant risk. Two vaccines are available for use in the United States. The live oral vaccine can be administered to persons 6 years of age and older and consists of four capsules, one taken every 48 hours, with the series completed one week before potential exposure. A booster consisting of the same four-capsule regimen is recommended every 5 years. The polysaccharide vaccine may be administered to travelers 2 years of age and older. It is administered at least 2 weeks before expected exposure as a single, intramuscular (IM) injection. A booster dose is recommended every 2 years.

Yellow fever is a mosquito-borne viral illness. The disease occurs only in sub-Saharan Africa and tropical South America. The vaccine is administered as a single injection; a booster every 10 years is recommended. In the United States, the vaccine is administered only at authorized vaccine centers throughout the country (*www2.ncid.cdc.gov/travel/yellowfever*).

Other vaccines needed for travel may include meningococcal, rabies, and Japanese encephalitis vaccines. A country-specific review of vaccinations is beyond the scope of this chapter. However, current vaccine recommendations and related travel information are available from the CDC at 1-888-232-3299 or *www.cdc.gov/travel*.

Reporting of Diseases and Adverse Reactions

Health care providers are responsible for reporting cases of vaccine-preventable diseases to public health officials, who then make weekly reports to the CDC. These data identify whether an outbreak is occurring and the impact of immunization policies and procedures.

Vaccines are generally safe. Common mild reactions include swelling at the injection site and fever. Awareness of the contraindications for use of vaccines decreases the incidence of serious adverse reactions. Absolute contraindications include **anaphylaxis** (a serious, potentially life-threatening allergic reaction) to a specific vaccine or component of another vaccine or moderate or severe illness. It is important to review vaccine-specific contraindications prior to administering any vaccine. However, in general, vaccines may be given in cases of mild acute illness or convalescent phase of illness; antimicrobial therapy; exposure to infectious disease; or premature birth.

Health care providers must report adverse reactions to the Vaccine Adverse Events Reporting System (VAERS). Information and forms are available at 1-800-822-7967 or *www.vaers.org*. The National Childhood Vaccine Injury Act of 1986 set forth the National Vaccine Injury Compensation Program (NVICP). This program provides compensation for injury or death caused by a vaccination. The NVICP does not require proof of negligence on the part of a health care provider. For more information, call the NVICP at 1-800-338-2382 or visit *www.hrsa.gov/osp/vicp*.

Varicella Vaccine

Prototype Drug Chart 35–1 provides the pharmacologic data for varicella vaccine.

Pharmacokinetics

Biologic products such as vaccines do not undergo the pharmacokinetic processes associated with other drug therapy.

Pharmacodynamics

Seroconversion is the acquisition of detectable levels of antibodies in the bloodstream. In the case of varicella vaccine, seroconversion occurs in more than 98% of 12-month to 12-year-old recipients approximately 6 weeks after receiving a single dose of vaccine. Susceptible clients 13 years of age and older who receive two doses of varicella vaccine 4 to 8 weeks apart show a seroconversion rate of 78% to 82% 4 weeks after the first dose and 99% 4 weeks after the second dose. Despite the high rate of initial seroconversion among children 12 months to 12 years of age, clinical trials have shown that over a 10-year period the vaccine's effectiveness in preventing disease was 94% for children receiving one dose of vaccine and 98% for those who received two doses. Therefore beginning in 2007, a second dose of varicella vaccine was recommended for all susceptible individuals, including children.

Contraindications

Varicella vaccine should be avoided in clients with a history of previous anaphylaxis to this vaccine or to any of its components, including gelatin and neomycin. It is also contraindicated in the presence of moderate to severe acute illness or active untreated tuberculosis.

While varicella infection can cause fetal harm, the possible effects of the vaccine on fetal development are cur-

---

Prototype DRUG CHART 35–1

VARICELLA

Drug Class

Vaccines
Trade name: Varivax
Pregnancy Category: C

Dosage

0.5 ml subQ × 2 doses.
Dose #1: 12-15 mo; dose #2: 4-6 y; catch-up initiated any time after 12-15 mo
<13 y, space doses at least 3 mo apart
≥13 y, space doses 4-8 wk apart

Contraindications

Previous anaphylaxis to this vaccine or to any of its components; pregnancy or possibility of pregnancy within 1 mo; immunocompromised vaccine recipient; presence of moderate to severe acute illness; active untreated tuberculosis

Drug-Lab-Food Interactions

Drug: Separate from MMR vaccine by 4 wk if not given on same day; delay VV for at least 5 mo after blood transfusion or Ig; delay Ig for 2 mo after VV; high dose immunosuppressant medications; avoid salicylates for 6 wk after VV

Pharmacokinetics

Not applicable

Pharmacodynamics

Seroconversion rates:
12 mo-12 y: >98% at 4-6 wk after vaccination
≥13 y: 78%-85% 4 wk after first dose and 99% 4 wk after second dose

Therapeutic Effects/Uses

Prevention of chickenpox. When administered to susceptible individuals, vaccine results in complete protection from chickenpox for the majority. For the minority in whom breakthrough chickenpox develops after vaccination, the disease is typically very mild. The vaccine may also provide prophylaxis protection if administered within 3 to 5 d of exposure to chickenpox.
Mode of Action: Stimulates active immunity against natural disease

Side Effects

Pain and redness at injection site, fever, chickenpox-like rash (generalized or confined to area surrounding injection site)

Adverse Reactions

Anaphylaxis, thrombocytopenia, encephalitis, Stevens-Johnson syndrome

d, Day; *Ig*, immune globulin; *MMR*, measles-mumps-rubella; *mo*, month; *subQ*, subcutaneous; *VV*, varicella vaccine; *wk*, week; *y*, year; <, less than; ≥, greater than or equal to.

rently unknown. Therefore varicella vaccine is contraindicated during pregnancy. Pregnancy should also be avoided for at least 1 month after each dose of the vaccine. NOTE: This recommendation differs from the product package insert, which suggests a 3-month delay in pregnancy.

Clients who are immunocompromised because of malignancies, high-dose systemic steroids, or other immunosuppressive therapy should avoid varicella vaccine. Likewise, the vaccine is generally contraindicated in the presence of primary or acquired immunodeficiencies. However, vaccination may be considered in children with certain classes of human immunodeficiency virus (HIV) infection.

Drug Interactions

Frequently a client is eligible for several immunizations at any given visit. A client receiving varicella vaccine may receive all other vaccines concurrently as long as each is administered at a separate site. If the MMR vaccine is not given the same day as the varicella vaccine, administration of the two vaccines should be separated by at least 4 weeks.

If a client has received a transfusion of blood or blood products, including immune globulin, administration of the varicella vaccine should be deferred at least 5 months. Likewise, such blood products should be avoided for at least 2 months after vaccination if possible. Blood products and immune globulin interfere with the body's production of antibodies specific to chickenpox, thereby decreasing the likelihood that active immunity will develop.

Reye syndrome has occasionally occurred in children following natural chickenpox infection. The majority of these children were also receiving salicylate medications (e.g., aspirin). Therefore it is generally recommended that clients avoid salicylates for 6 weeks after vaccination.

Vaccines

ASSESSMENT

- Identify barriers to timely and complete immunization (e.g., belief that vaccine-preventable diseases no longer exist, misunderstanding of true contraindications to immunization, concerns regarding vaccine safety and efficacy, fear of multiple injections, cost).
- Obtain medical history, including history of malignancy or other immune deficiency.
- Determine history of pregnancy or possible pregnancy within the next month. Many vaccines are contraindicated during pregnancy.
- Obtain drug history, including high-dose immunosuppressants, blood transfusions, and immune globulin.

- Obtain a list of herbal products used by client and/or primary caregiver (in case of breastfed infant).
- Determine complete allergy history, including drugs, vaccines, food, and environmental allergies.
- Assess for adverse reactions (other than allergic) to previous doses of vaccine or any vaccine component.
- Assess for symptoms of moderate to severe acute illness with or without fever.
- Screen for unvaccinated or immunocompromised household contacts.
- Obtain immunization history and history of vaccine-preventable diseases to determine current vaccine needs. For example, a person with a reliable of history of chickenpox or herpes zoster ("shingles") does not need varicella vaccine; natural immunity is assumed.

NURSING DIAGNOSES

- Deficient knowledge related to vaccine-preventable diseases, risks and benefits of vaccination
- Ineffective health maintenance related to non-adherence to recommended immunization schedule
- Health-seeking behavior related to desire to receive recommended vaccines at appropriate intervals
- Readiness for enhanced immunization status related to expressed desire to improve knowledge about vaccines

PLANNING

- Client will adhere to recommended immunization schedule for vaccine-preventable diseases unless contraindications exist.
- Client will be free of adverse reactions.

NURSING INTERVENTIONS

- Strictly adhere to individual vaccine storage requirements to ensure potency of the product.
- Upon preparation, including reconstitution of a given vaccine, administer within time limits stated in package insert to ensure potency.
- At time of visit, administer at separate sites all vaccines for which client is eligible. *Do not* mix vaccines in the same syringe.
- Document in client's record the following data: vaccination date, route, and site; vaccine type, manufacturer, lot number, and expiration date; name, business address, and title of individual administering vaccine.
- Observe clients for signs and symptoms of adverse reactions to vaccines.
- Keep epinephrine readily available for immediate use in case of anaphylactic reaction.
- Provide client with a record of immunizations administered.

Client Teaching

General

- Discuss vaccine-preventable diseases with client and/ or client's family, including manifestations and risk of contracting.
- Answer all questions regarding vaccine safety and efficacy.
- Inform female clients of childbearing age to avoid pregnancy for 1 month, depending on the vaccines to be administered.
- Instruct clients to avoid contact with immunocompromised persons, depending on vaccines to be administered.
- In accordance with federal law, provide client or client's family with current Vaccine Information Statements (VISs), available from the CDC, for each vaccine administered.
- Remind client or client's family to bring immunization record to all visits.
- Provide client or client's family with return date for next vaccination.

Side Effects

- Discuss common side effects of vaccines, such as injection site soreness, fever, and side effects specific to individual vaccines.
- Offer suggestions for management of common side effects (e.g., cold compresses for injection site soreness, acetaminophen for soreness and/or fever).
- Instruct client or client's family to contact the health care provider if signs of a serious reaction are noted.

Cultural Considerations ❖

- Modify communications to meet cultural needs of client/family.
- Do not assume that a positive response means a definite yes.
- Use an interpreter when necessary.
- Vaccine Information Statements (VISs) are available in many languages and can be downloaded from the Immunization Action Coalition's website at *www.immunize.org*.

EVALUATION

- Evaluate client's or client's family's understanding of rationale for immunizations.
- Evaluate client adherence to recommended immunization schedule.

Recent Developments and the Future of Vaccines

A small outbreak of anthrax cases in the United States in 2001 increased the level of awareness of the vaccine for anthrax. As a biologic weapon, anthrax is highly lethal. It is easily produced, stored, and spread over large areas. Proper vaccination is an essential part of protection against this disease. Approved by the FDA in 1970, anthrax vaccine has been routinely and safely administered to laboratory personnel, livestock farmers, veterinarians, and military personnel. The vaccine requires six injections: three given 2 weeks apart followed by three additional doses at 6, 12, and 18 months. No serious side effects have been reported, but the vaccination is contraindicated during pregnancy. An oral anthrax vaccine is on the horizon. The vaccine is derived from a genetically modified plant virus. The virus is introduced into a plant, where it then stimulates the plant to produce new proteins. These proteins are extracted and used to produce a vaccine. When the vaccine is administered to a human, the person's body reacts as if infected with anthrax and creates antibodies against the bacterium. In the event of a bioterrorism attack, large numbers of individuals can be rapidly immunized with an oral vaccine. Additional information is available at *www.anthrax.osd.mil*.

Smallpox was eradicated worldwide by 1980. The United States discontinued routine childhood immunization against smallpox in 1971. However, since the events of September 2001, concern has arisen that the smallpox (or variola) virus could be used as a bioterrorist weapon. Unlike anthrax, smallpox virus is not airborne and is transmitted through human bodily fluids or contaminated materials. A smallpox immunization plan has been implemented in the United States *(www.bt.cdc.gov)*. However, there has been some resistance to vaccination because of a lack of perceived threat and because of the risk of significant side effects from the vaccine. The currently available vaccine is a live virus preparation. It is administered using a bifurcated needle to deliver the vaccine into the epidermis. A skin reaction occurs at the immunization site 3 to 5 days later and eventually leaves a scar. Boosters may be recommended every 10 years.

It has long been known that immunity to pertussis, or "whooping cough," wanes over time and that adolescents and adults are often responsible for transmitting this infection to vulnerable, incompletely immunized infants and young children. While a relatively benign illness in the older population, pertussis in infants is associated with significant morbidity and mortality. In 2005, two products containing tetanus and diphtheria toxoids along with acellular pertussis were licensed for use in older children and adults. Adacel is approved for use in persons 11-64 years old, while Boostrix is approved for use in persons 10-18 years old. Each vaccine contains the same antigens as its respective counterpart administered to young children (DTaP), but with reduced quantities of diphtheria and acellular pertussis (Tdap). Currently it is recommended that for booster immunization, adolescents and adults receive a one-time dose of Tdap in lieu of Td vaccine.

Herpes zoster, commonly known as "shingles" or *zoster*, occurs as the result of reactivation of the varicella virus. Following a primary varicella infection ("chickenpox"), the virus persists but becomes dormant in the body, usually settling in a dorsal root ganglion. Zoster often occurs decades after the primary varicella infection. It appears that development of zoster may be related to a decline in immunity to the varicella-zoster virus (VZV). Zoster is characterized by a painful rash which presents in a dermatomal distribution. Especially in the elderly, resolution of the rash may be followed by a chronic, severe, sometimes debilitating pain, referred to as *postherpetic neuralgia*. In 2006, a live attenuated vaccine, Zostavax, was licensed for use as a one-time injection in adults 60 years of age and over. The vaccine has been shown to boost VZV immunity among vaccine recipients. In clinical trials, Zostavax prevented zoster in about 50 percent of people who received the vaccine. Effectiveness appears to decrease with increasing age of the vaccine recipient. In those who received the vaccine yet went on to develop zoster, the duration of pain was reduced.

Rotavirus is a leading cause of severe acute gastroenteritis in infants and young children. RotaTeq, a live oral vaccine containing five strains of rotavirus, was licensed by the FDA in 2006. It appears to be effective in protecting against severe gastroenteritis and significantly reduces the need for hospitalization among infected children. The vaccine is administered at 2, 4, and 6 months of age.

Gardasil, the human papillomavirus (HPV) vaccine, is being hailed as the first vaccine designed to prevent cancer. It contains four strains of human papillomavirus which account for the vast majority of cases of cervical cancer and genital warts. A recombinant vaccine, it is licensed for use in 9-26 year old females and is administered as a three-shot series given at 0, 2, and 6 months. Since human papillomavirus is sexually-transmitted, Gardasil is most effective if administered prior to initiation of sexual intercourse. Please refer to Chapter 57 for more detailed information about sexually transmitted diseases and the use of this vaccine.

Work continues on new combination vaccines that reduce the number of injections required. Advances are also being made in vaccines against infectious agents such as *Campylobacter jejuni*, parainfluenza virus, respiratory syncytial virus (RSV), *Helicobacter pylori*, and HIV.

New delivery systems for vaccines are currently in development to replace the "needle." Timed-release pills in a one-time dose have the potential to offer lifetime immunity to a targeted disease, eliminating the need for booster vaccination. In addition, skin patches may one day be used to administer tetanus and influenza vaccines.

 Critical Thinking Case Study

JW, a 29-year-old woman, is seen at the immunization clinic with her 2-month-old daughter and her son, who just turned 6 years old last month. She reports they all need shots.

1. JW will soon be returning to work at a long-term care facility for developmentally disabled adults. She reports that her new employer is encouraging her to be immunized against hepatitis B. She wonders how long it will take her to complete the vaccine series. What is your response?

2. You administer JW's first dose of hepatitis B vaccine today. When should she return for the next dose?

3. You ask JW about her vaccine history. She says she does not have an immunization card but remembers last receiving a "booster when I stepped on a nail at my high school graduation picnic." What "booster" did she likely receive? At what point is another booster due? What vaccine should she receive for her next booster?

4. JW says her daughter needs her "regular baby shots." The infant received her first hepatitis B vaccine while in the newborn nursery. Against what vaccine-preventable illnesses will you plan to vaccinate this infant today?

5. When would this infant be due for another series of immunizations?

6. JW asks you about chickenpox vaccine. She would like her daughter to be vaccinated against chickenpox as soon as possible, because she does not want her to suffer through chickenpox as her brother did. What is the earliest age at which her daughter can receive varicella vaccine?

7. JW says she has heard that you can get chickenpox from the vaccination shot. How would you respond to this comment?

8. JW has brought her son's immunization card. It shows he received hepatitis B vaccine at birth, 2 months, and 9 months. He received DTaP, Hib, polio (IPV), and pneumococcal (PCV) vaccines at 2 months, 4 months, and 6 months. She is worried that he will need to start his immunizations over because "he's so far behind." How would you respond to her concern?

9. For what vaccines is he due today?

NCLEX Study Questions

1. Immunity developed in response to immunization best describes this type of immunity:
   a. natural, passive
   b. active, acquired
   c. natural
   d. acquired, passive

2. Attenuated virus vaccines contain:
   a. live, weakened microorganisms
   b. antibodies specific to the virus
   c. inactivated microorganisms
   d. inactivated toxins

3. The correct route of administration for rotavirus vaccine is:
   a. intramuscular (IM)
   b. subcutaneous (subQ)
   c. intradermal (ID)
   d. oral (PO)

4. The following is a contraindication to the use of varicella vaccine:
   a. egg allergy
   b. a sibling currently has chickenpox
   c. pregnancy
   d. a cold (URI)

5. A 2-month-old infant experiences redness and tenderness at the DTaP injection site associated with a fever of 100.8° F. The following vaccine should be administered at the next visit in 6 to 8 weeks:
   a. Td
   b. DTaP
   c. DT
   d. Tdap

Answers: 1. b; 2. a; 3. d; 4. c; 5. b.

Twelve

Antineoplastic Agents

*C*ancer is a leading cause of morbidity and mortality in the United States. The development of cancer is a multistep process that is influenced by environmental hazards (e.g., chemicals, asbestos, radiation), genetic predisposition (e.g., BRCA1 and BRCA2 mutations), lifestyle factors (e.g., smoking, alcohol use), diet (e.g., high fat), infection (e.g., Epstein-Barr, *Helicobacter pylori*, human papillomavirus [HPV]), and immune suppression (e.g., HIV infection, immunosuppressive medications). Cancer (malignant, neoplastic) cells are characterized by unregulated growth, lack of differentiation, and spread (metastasis) to other places in the body. Cancer cells that divide rapidly respond more effectively to anticancer therapy than do slow-growing malignant cells.

Cell Cycle

All cells progress through a distinct cycle that consists of four phases directed toward cell replication and a fifth resting stage. In this way the cell cycles of normal and cancer cells are similar. The first phase of the cell cycle is G_1, the presynthesis phase that prepares the cell for deoxyribonucleic acid (DNA) synthesis. The second phase is the S phase, whereby DNA synthesis occurs. Next is the G_2 postsynthesis phase, in which the cell is prepared for mitosis. Cell division (cytokinesis) occurs in the fourth, or M (mitosis), phase. Cells may immediately progress to the G_1 phase or enter the G_0 or resting phase. Most cells in the human body are in the G_0 stage. Exceptions include metabolically active cells, such as the granulocytes, and epithelial cells found in the gastrointestinal tract. As each cell progresses through the cell cycle, it must pass a number of checkpoints before it can continue its progression through the cell cycle. If a cell is found to be defective at a particular checkpoint, the cell undergoes **apoptosis** (self destruction). The cell cycle is demonstrated in Figure XII–1, and the phases are described in Box XII–1.

Growth Rate

Growth rate *(doubling time)* is defined as the time it takes for a cancerous tumor to double in size. Growth fraction decreases and doubling time increases as the tumor enlarges. Growth rate depends on several factors, including the cell-cycle activity of the proliferating cells in the tumor mass, the number of cells proliferating within the tumor *(growth fraction)* and the rate of cell loss from the tumor. In general, anticancer drugs are more effective against cancer cells that have a high growth fraction. Malignant tumors that have prolonged cell cycles and a slower

FIGURE XII–I Cell division cycle and checkpoints. *CCC,* Cell cycle checkpoint. *G₁ phase (postmitotic gap):* Production of enzyme for DNA synthesis. The G₁ phase lasts 15 to 18 hours. *S phase (synthesis):* The DNA doubles. The S phase lasts 10 to 20 hours. *G₂ phase (premitotic gap):* RNA synthesis for later mitosis. The G₂ phase lasts approximately 3 hours. *M phase (mitosis):* Cell division produces two identical cells. The M phase lasts approximately 1 hour. *G₀ phase (resting):* Cells remain in this phase or return to the cell cycle for cell replication. Cells in this phase are not as sensitive to many antineoplastic drugs. The cells must pass through a series of checkpoints in order to continue through the cycle. Cells that are defective undergo apoptosis (self-destruction).

Box XII–I

Cell Cycle and Phases

1. G₁: enzyme production needed for deoxyribonucleic acid (DNA)
2. S, or synthesis: DNA synthesis and replication
3. G₂: ribonucleic acid (RNA) and protein synthesis
4. M, or mitosis: cell division
5. G₀: resting phase

---

growth rate are more likely to be locally confined and therefore more amendable to surgical excision.

Anticancer Therapy

In the past 3 decades, significant advances have been made in the treatment of malignancies. *Chemotherapy* (chemical treatment) is the use of chemicals to kill cancer cells. Research has led to the use of new anticancer drugs and the development of standard treatment protocols (drug, dose, and schedule) for anticancer drugs to guide therapy. Nurses play a vital role in managing the treatment of those with cancer. This includes the administration of chemotherapy in health care facilities and in the homes of clients. To provide the best possible care, nurses should understand the chemotherapy regimen, contraindications, drug interactions, therapeutic effects, side effects, and adverse reactions of the chemotherapy that clients receive.

Chapter 36 discusses how selected anticancer drugs inhibit or prevent cell reproduction. The anticancer drugs are divided into major classes which include alkylating agents, antimetabolites, antitumor antibiotics, mitotic inhibitors, targeted therapies, and hormonal agents.

Some chemotherapy agents negatively affect cancer cells when they are actively dividing. These are called *cell-cycle specific (CCS) agents. Cell-cycle non-specific (CCNS) drugs* work best in the G₀ (resting) stage to disrupt cancer cells. Chemotherapy usually targets ribonucleic acid (RNA) or deoxyribonucleic acid (DNA) in cancer cells to prevent mitosis or induce apoptosis (self-death). The specific drugs selected are administered based on the type of tumor cells, the rate at which they divide, and the time that the drugs will be most effective. In general, chemotherapy is most effective in destroying cells that are rapidly dividing.

Chapter 37 explores targeted therapies to treat cancer. This modality targets malignant cells and is a recent development. Targeted therapies work by interfering with cancer-cell growth and division in different ways and at various points in the development, growth, and spread of cancer.

Chapter 38, Biologic Response Modifiers, describes the evolving state of biologic response modifiers, which work to (1) enhance host immunologic function, (2) destroy or interfere with tumor activities, and (3) promote differentiation of stem cells.

36

Anticancer Drugs

Paula Klemm

ELECTRONIC RESOURCES

Evolve website (http://evolve.elsevier.com/KeeHayes/pharmacology/):
- *Case Studies*
- *Content Updates*
- *Frequently Asked Questions*
- *Student Review Activities*
- *WebLinks*
- *Additional Reference Material*

Companion CD-ROM:
- *NCLEX Examination Review Questions*
- *Pharmacology Animations*
- *IV Therapy Checklists*
- *Medication Error Checklists*
- *Drug Calculation Problems*
- *Electronic Calculators*
- *Top 200 Drugs with Pronunciations*
- *References from the Textbook*

Outline

Objectives

- Differentiate between cell-cycle specific and cell-cycle nonspecific anticancer drugs.
- Identify general side effects and adverse reactions to anticancer drugs.
- Describe the uses and considerations for alkylating compounds, antimetabolites, antitumor antibiotics, mitotic inhibitors, hormones, and biotherapy agents.
- Describe client education guidelines for administering chemotherapy in the home.
- Identify three ways the nurse can avoid exposure to chemotherapeutic agents.
- Describe the nursing process, including client teaching, related to anticancer drugs.
- Develop client-focused teaching plans related to anticancer drugs.

Terms

The mortality rate from cancer has been slowly declining in the United States since the early 1990s. Even so, cancer-related deaths rank second only to heart disease in this country. One in three women and one in two men will develop cancer over the course of their lifetime. Cancer is the leading cause of death in children between the ages of 1 and 15 years, second only to accidents, which rank first. Excluding skin cancers, the highest incidence rates in men are prostate, lung, and colorectal cancer. In women, breast, lung, and colorectal cancers occur with the highest frequency. Lung cancer remains the leading cause of cancer-related death regardless of gender. Cancer incidence and mortality differ by ethnicity. African-American men have higher incidence and death rates from cancer than do White men. African-American women have a lower incidence of cancer than White women, but a higher mortality rate. Latinos (Hispanic) have a lower incidence than non-Hispanics, except for cancer of the stomach, liver, cervix, and multiple myeloma. Cancer among Asian-Americans has traditionally been lower than other ethnic groups, but incidence increases as immigrants adopt a more westernized lifestyle. The incidence of liver cancer is higher among Asian immigrants secondary to higher rates of chronic hepatitis B in this group.

Cancer is a group of diseases in which abnormal cells grow out of control and may spread to other areas of the body. Deoxyribonucleic acid (DNA) is the genetic substance in the body cells that transfers information necessary for the production of enzymes and protein synthesis. In most cases, cancer is caused by damage to the DNA within the cell. Although some cancers are inherited, most develop when genes in a normal cell become damaged or lost (mutation). More than one mutation is required before a malignancy can develop. Therefore the development of cancer is a multistep process that may take years to complete.

Pharmaceuticals are often used to destroy cancer cells and are called by different names, including *anticancer drugs, cancer chemotherapeutic agents,* **antineoplastic drugs,** or **cytotoxic therapy.** Nitrogen mustard (Mustargen), a derivative of mustard gas employed in warfare, was utilized in the 1940s to treat clients with high white blood counts caused by leukemia and lymphoma. Methotrexate (Rheumatrex, Trexall), cyclophosphamide (Cytoxan), and fluorouracil (5-FU, Adrucil) were introduced soon after and are still used to treat malignancies. In the 1970s the use of two or more chemotherapy agents **(combination chemotherapy)** to treat cancer was adopted and led to improved response rates and increased survival times. Over the years, researchers developed strict guidelines for the administration of anticancer drugs. Chemotherapy may be used as the sole treatment of cancer or in conjunction with other modalities (e.g., radiation, surgery, biologic response modifiers, targeted therapy). Combination chemotherapy has proven effective in curing some cancers (e.g., leukemia, Hodgkin's disease, Wilms tumor). When cancer cannot be cured, anticancer drugs may be given to control the disease for a period of months to years. If the cancer can no longer be controlled, chemotherapy may be used to relieve symptoms associated with the disease. This is called *palliative treatment.*

Genetic, Infective, Environmental, and Dietary Influences

Cancer is a genetic disease. Genes provide the instructions for the production and function of cellular proteins that are essential for normal cellular activities. Genetic defects may occur in a variety of ways, including deletion, translocation, duplication, inversion, or insertion of genetic material. When these defects cannot be effectively repaired, cells exhibit abnormal characteristics and unregulated growth. Over 1600 genes have been causally implicated in the formation of cancer. Cancers that have a proven genetic influence include breast, ovarian, prostate, endometrial, colon, pancreatic, and lung cancers; retinoblastoma; and malignant melanoma. Many more genetic influences are expected to be found. Environment, lifestyle, viruses, and diet can influence the development of these and other types of cancers. Box 36–1 gives examples of types of environmental products, viruses, and foods that have a carcinogenic effect on cancer development in humans.

Table 36-1

Cell-Cycle Nonspecific (CCNS) and Cell-Cycle Specific (CCS) Agents

Type	Drug Group	Cell-Cycle Effect
CCNS	Alkylating drugs	All phases of cell division cycle. Most effective in G_1 and S phases
CCNS	Nitrosoureas	All phases of cell division cycle
CCS	Antimetabolites	S phase
CCNS	Antitumor antibiotics	All phases of cell division cycle
CCS	Vinca alkaloids	M phase
CCS	Taxanes	M phase
CCS	Topoisomerase inhibitors (discussed in Chapter 37)	G_2, S phases

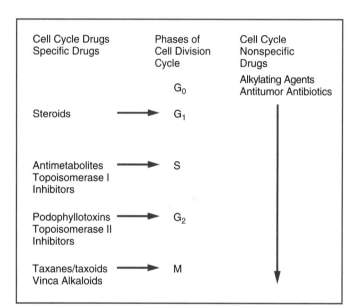

FIGURE 36–1 Cell-cycle nonspecific (CCNS) and cell-cycle specific (CCS) agents.

ing and act to stop the action of oncogenes. If TS genes become lost or dysfunctional, cells could reproduce uncontrollably. Other genes repair damage to DNA. If these DNA-repair genes are damaged, mutations are not mended and are subsequently passed on to the next generation of daughter cells. It may take a long time before sufficient cell mutations take place and cause cancer to develop. As a result cancers more commonly occur in older individuals.

A number of viruses are associated with the development of cancer. The human papillomavirus (HPV) has been found in most women who have invasive cervical cancer. Individuals with human immunodeficiency virus (HIV) may develop lymphomas and anal or genital cancers. The Epstein-Barr virus is found in almost all people with Burkitt's lymphoma in central Africa. This virus has

Genes can cause cells to become cancerous in several ways. *Protooncogenes* are normal genes that are involved in the controlled growth, division and death **(apoptosis)** of cells. An oncogene is a mutation in a protooncogene. An abnormal oncogene can effect cellular growth-control proteins and trigger unregulated cell division. Tumor-suppressor (TS) genes (antioncogenes) signal a cell to cease multiply-been implicated in the development of nasopharyngeal cancer as well. Hepatocellular carcinoma (liver cancer) is linked to the hepatitis B virus. Other viruses that have a link to the development of cancer include human T-cell lymphotropic virus, type 1 (HTLV-1); human T-cell lymphotropic virus, type 2 (HTLV-2); and Kaposi sarcoma-associated herpes virus.

Bacteria can play a role in the development of cancer. The presence of *Helicobacter pylori* in the stomach is associated with an increased risk of developing gastric cancer. Some reports have indicated a link between certain bacteria and cancer of the gallbladder, colon, and lung. However, evidence that supports an association between bacterial infection and other cancers is unclear.

Environmental factors associated with the development of cancer include smoking, diet, infectious diseases, chemicals, and radiation. According to the American Cancer Society (ACS) the use of tobacco, an unhealthy diet, and inadequate physical activity account for 75% of cancer cases and up to two thirds of cancer deaths in the United States.

Cell-Cycle Nonspecific and Specific Anticancer Drugs

The cell cycle for normal and cancer cells, growth fraction, and doubling time are discussed in Unit XII (see Figure XII–1). Refer to the discussion at the beginning of Unit Twelve for clarification of the cell cycle and definitions.

Anticancer drugs cause cell death by interfering with cell replication (see Figure XII-1 in the Unit Twelve opener). **Cell-cycle nonspecific (CCNS) drugs** (also called *cell-cycle independent*) act during any phase of the cell cycle, including the G_0 phase. **Cell-cycle specific (CCS)** drugs exert their influence during a specific phase of the cell cycle. Also called *cell-cycle dependent drugs,* CCS agents are most effective against rapidly growing cancer cells. In general the CCNS drugs include the alkylating drugs (although some alkylating agents are CCS), anti-tumor antibiotics, and hormones. The CCS drugs include antimetabolites and mitotic inhibitors. Table 36–1 and Figure 36–1 list the types of anticancer drugs and the phase of the cell cycle they affect.

Growth fraction and **doubling time** are two factors that play a major role in the response of cancer cells to anticancer drugs. Anticancer drugs are more effective against neoplastic cells that have a high growth fraction. Leukemias and some lymphomas have high growth fractions and thus respond well to anticancer drug therapy. Small and early forming cancer cells and fast-growing tumors respond well to chemotherapy and have a higher cure rate than slow-growing tumors in the advanced stages. When the tumor is 1 cm^3 it is clinically detectable and contains approximately one billion cancer cells, representing 30 doubling times from the initial cancer cell. At that time symptoms may appear.

Solid tumors have a large percentage of their cell mass in the G_0 phase, so they generally have a low growth fraction and are less sensitive to anticancer drugs. High-dose chemotherapy results in better tumoricidal (tumor-killing) effects. Depending on the type of cancer, malignant cell growth is usually faster in the earlier stages of tumor development. As the tumor grows, the blood supply decreases, thereby slowing the growth rate. Anticancer agents are more effective against small tumors with sufficient blood supply. As the tumor enlarges, its growth fraction decreases and its doubling time increases, reducing the effectiveness of anticancer therapy. The vascularization in some solid tumors can be inconsistent. Some areas of tumor may have an adequate blood supply, while other areas are poorly perfused. This characteristic may make some large tumors resistant to anticancer drugs and therefore difficult to treat.

Cancer Chemotherapy

Anticancer drugs are not selective, so both cancer cells and normal cells are affected. The side effects of chemotherapy are largely related to the toxic effects on normal cells. Antineoplastic agents are effective because normal cells are able to repair themselves and continue to grow, whereas cancer cells are less able to do so; thus the side effects of chemotherapy are most often temporary. Chemotherapy is usually administered systemically for cancer that has spread to other parts of the body, for tumors in multiple sites, or for tumors that are too large to be removed through other means (e.g., surgery). The most common route of chemotherapy administration is via intravenous (IV) infusion, although other routes, including oral, intramuscular, subcutaneous, intraperitoneal, intrathecal, intracavitary, intravesical, intraarterial, or topical may be used.

Some types of cancer can be cured with chemotherapy (e.g., Hodgkin's disease, Burkitt's lymphoma, Wilms tumor, testicular cancer). Other types of cancer (e.g., breast cancer, colon cancer) may be treated with surgery first, followed by chemotherapy to eliminate any residual tumor cells (microscopic metastases) that may remain in the body. This is referred to as **adjuvant therapy.** Sometimes **neoadjuvant chemotherapy** may be given first to help shrink a large tumor so that it can be surgically removed. **Palliative chemotherapy** is used to relieve symptoms associated with advanced disease (e.g., pain) and to improve the quality of life.

Chemotherapy administration is guided by specific **protocols** that were developed based on the results of controlled research studies. The length of treatment is determined by the type and extent of the malignancy, type of chemotherapy given, expected side effects of these drugs, and the amount of time that normal cells need to recover. Chemotherapy is usually given in cycles to improve the likelihood that cancer cells will be destroyed and that normal cells can recover. The duration, frequency, and number of cycles of chemotherapy are based on the type and size of the tumor, whether the disease has spread to other areas of the body (metastasis), and the condition of the client. Chemotherapy treatment may consist of one agent or a combination of agents. Combination chemotherapy may be administered on one day or spread out over several days. The duration of each treatment varies from minutes to days and may be repeated weekly, biweekly, or monthly, based on the protocol being followed. Recently, **dose dense chemotherapy** protocols have been administered to treat cancer. In dose dense chemotherapy regimens, the interval between successive doses of chemotherapy is shortened. This has led to improved survival in some cancer patients.

Selected anticancer/antineoplastic drugs are listed in Box 36–2 according to their classification.

Drug Resistance

Malignant tumors often develop resistance to chemotherapeutic agents. This is termed **multidrug resistance (MDR)** and can occur for several reasons. Anticancer drugs may not kill all neoplastic cells, and these cells may mutate and become resistant to the drugs. Some tumor cells have a natural resistance to certain chemotherapy agents, thus making the drugs ineffective. Tumor resistance can occur as a result of *gene amplification*, in which a gene produces many copies of itself. This leads to an overproduction of protein that makes the chemotherapy drug less effective. Some cancer cells develop the ability to repair DNA damage caused by the antineoplastic therapy; others overproduce a P-glycoprotein (P-gp) in the cell membrane that pumps the chemotherapy out of the cells before it can be effective. Understanding, prevention, and reversal of MDR are major foci of cancer research.

Combination Chemotherapy

Single-agent drug therapy is not usually used to treat cancer, because combinations of anticancer agents have demonstrated more effective tumoricidal activity in most cancer patients. Chemotherapy is most effective when it is able to kill cells in all phases of the cell cycle. Using more than one chemotherapy drug at a time (combination chemotherapy) makes this possible.

To maximize cell death CCS and CCNS drugs are often combined. Each individual chemotherapy agent used in combination therapy should have proven tumoricidal activity. Using the drugs together may have a synergistic effect. In addition, each drug should have a different mode of action and different dose-limiting toxicities. The use of a combination of antineoplastic agents has the advantage of decreasing drug resistance and increasing destruction of cancer cells. Some of the combinations of anticancer drugs used in cancer treatment are presented in Table 36–2.

General Side Effects and Adverse Reactions

Anticancer drugs exert adverse effects on rapidly growing normal cells (e.g., skin, hair). These drugs can also affect cells in the gastrointestinal (GI) tract, mucous membranes,

bone marrow, and the reproductive system. Table 36–3 lists the general adverse reactions to anticancer drugs on the fast-growing cells of the body. Selected nursing measures and considerations are included.

Anticancer Therapy in Outpatient Settings and in the Home

The administration of anticancer drugs in outpatient settings is cost-effective and convenient. Although chemotherapy regimens have become increasingly aggressive, most clients are not hospitalized unless they require close monitoring or are very ill. Some chemotherapy agents are administered in the home. Clients receiving highly potent drugs at home may need to be closely monitored for severe adverse reactions or to assure adequate hydration.

When a chemotherapy drug is given in the home, a health care provider qualified to administer anticancer agents follows the policies provided by the oncologist and the home health care agency. Client education guidelines may include the following:

- Assess the learning needs of the client, family members, and caregivers.
- Provide printed information on the chemotherapeutic agents. These materials should be written at an appropriate educational level for the client/family/caregivers (an eighth-grade level or lower is recommended) and in the language the client most easily speaks and reads.
- Provide information in alternative formats when appropriate (e.g., electronic media, CD/DVD, computer programs, illustrations, photos).
- Discuss with the client/family/caregivers the anticancer drug(s) that will be administered, the desired effects, and length of time per administration.
- Discuss the treatment process (i.e., route of administration, schedule of chemotherapy, duration of chemotherapy administration, monitoring side effects, follow-up).
- Discuss potential side effects of chemotherapy and how these will be managed. Include specific information on what is normal and what is not. Be sure the client and caregivers know how to take an oral temperature (rectal temperatures are not done in patients who have low platelet counts).
- Give written instructions regarding diet, medications to control side effects (e.g., antiemetics), and hydration as indicated.
- Emphasize self-care strategies (e.g., mouth care regimen, personal hygiene, exercise, adequate rest).
- Provide written guidelines for calling the physician (e.g., temperature elevation, uncontrolled vomiting, diarrhea, constipation, bleeding, pain, infection).
- Provide written information on the symptoms of infection in a patient with low blood counts (i.e., temperature elevation, chills, shaking, frequent urination and/or pain on urination, and redness, swelling, or pain near a wound or IV site)

Box 36–2

Anticancer Drugs by Classifications

Alkylating Agents

nitrogen mustard (mechlorethamine hydrochloride)
(Mustargen)
chlorambucil (Leukeran)
cyclophosphamide (Cytoxan)
estramustine (Emcyt)
ifosfamide (Ifex)
melphalan (Alkeran)
uracil mustard (Uracil Mustard)
chlorambucil (Leukeran)

Nitrosoureas

carmustine (BiCNU, BCNU, Gliadel)
carmustine with polifeprosan 20 implant (Gliadel Wafer)
lomustine (CeeNU, CCNU)
streptozocin (Zanosar)

Alkylating-Like Agents

altretamine (Hexalen)
carboplatin (Paraplatin)
cisplatin (Platinol)
dacarbazine (DTIC)
oxaliplatin (Eloxatin)
pipobroman (Vercyte)
thiotepa (Thioplex)

Alkyl Sulfonates

busulfan (Myleran)

Antimetabolites

folic acid antagonist
methotrexate (MTX, amethopterin, Folex, Mexate)
pemetrexed disodium (Alimta)

Pyrimidine Analogues

azacitidine (Vidaza)
capecitabine (Xeloda)
cytarabine HCl (Cytosar-U, ARA-C)
floxuridine (FUDR)
fluorouracil (5-FU, Adrucil)
gemcitabine HCl (Gemzar)
procarbazine HCl (Matulane)
nelarabine (Arranon)

Purine Analogues

cladribine (Leustatin)
clofarabine (Clolar)
fludarabine (Fludara)
6-mercaptopurine (6-MP, Purinethol)
thioguanine (Lanvis)

Ribonucleotide Reductase Inhibitors

hydroxyurea (Hydrea)
trimetrexate glucuronate (Neutrexin)
2-deoxycoformycin (Pentostatin, Nipent, DCF)

Enzyme Inhibitors

pentostatin (Nipent)

Mitotic Inhibitors

vinca alkaloids
vinblastine sulfate (Velban)
vincristine sulfate (Oncovin)
vincristine (liposomal) (Marqibo)
vinorelbine (Navelbine)

Antimicrotubules or Taxanes

docetaxel (Taxotere)
paclitaxel (Taxol)

Antitumor Antibiotics

bleomycin sulfate (Blenoxane)
dactinomycin (Actinomycin D, Cosmegen)
daunorubicin HCl (Cerubidine)
daunorubicin (liposomal) (DaunoXome)
doxorubicin (Adriamycin, Rubex)
doxorubicin HCl (liposomal) (Doxil, Caelyx, Myocet)
epirubicin (Ellence)
idarubicin (Idamycin)
mitomycin (Mutamycin)
mitoxantrone (Novantrone)
plicamycin (Mithracin, Mithracin)
valrubicin (Valstar)

Targeted Therapies (see Chapter 37)
Retinoids

bexarotene (Targretin)
thalidomide (Thalomid)
lenalidomide (Revlimid) (derivative of thalidomide)

Hormones, Hormonal Antagonists, and Enzymes
Androgens

testolactone (Teslac)
progesterone (Gesterol 50)

Hormonal Antagonists and Enzymes

aminoglutethimide (Cytadren)
anastrozole (Arimidex)
bicalutamide (Casodex)
exemestane (Aromasin)
flutamide (Eulexin)
fulvestrant (Faslodex)
goserelin acetate (Zoladex)
histrelin acetate implant (Vantas)
letrozole (Femara)
leuprolide acetate (Lupron)
megestrol acetate (Megace)
mitotane (Lysodren)
nilutamide (Nilandron)
polyestradiol phosphate (Estradurin)
raloxifene hydrochloride (Evista)
tamoxifen citrate (Nolvadex) (non-steroidal antiestrogen)
toremifene (Fareston)

Miscellaneous Enzymes

L-asparaginase (Elspar)
pegaspargase (Oncaspar)

Biological Therapies
Cytokines

interferon-alpha-2a, recombinant (Roferon-A, rIFN-A)
interferon-alfa-2b, recombinant (Intron-A, IFN-alpha 2)
interleukin-2 (IL-2), aldesleukin (Proleukin)

Monoclonal Antibodies (see Chapter 37)
Vaccines

Quadrivalent human papillomavirus (Types 6, 11, 16, 18) recombinant vaccine (Gardasil). Approved by FDA in 2006.
Human papillomavirus vaccine, AS04 adjuvant-adsorbed
(Cervarix). Biologics license application submitted to the
FDA in April 2007. If approved, Cervarix will be used to
prevent cervical cancer and precancerous lesions associated with the most common cancer-causing HPV types.

Table 36–2

Selected Combinations of Anticancer Drugs

Drug Name (generic name in lower case; trade name capitalized)	Acronym	Selected Uses
doxorubicin (Adriamycin), bleomycin (Blenoxane), vinblastine (Velban), dacarbazine (DTIC)	ABVD	Hodgkin's lymphoma
cyclophosphamide (Cytoxan), doxorubicin (Adriamycin), fluorouracil (5-FU, Adrucil)	CAF	Breast cancer, prostate cancer
cyclophosphamide (Cytoxan), doxorubicin (Adriamycin), methotrexate (Rheumatrex, Trexall)	CAM	Prostate cancer
cyclophosphamide (Cytoxan), epirubicin (Pharmorubicin), fluorouracil (5-FU, Adrucil)	CEF	Breast cancer
cyclophosphamide (Cytoxan), doxorubicin (Adriamycin), vincristine (Oncovin), prednisone, rituximab (Rituxan)	CHOP + rituximab	Non-Hodgkin's lymphoma
etoposide (VePesid, VP-16), leucovorin, fluorouracil (5-FU, Adrucil)	ELF	Esophageal cancer, stomach cancer
folinic acid (leucovorin), fluorouracil (5-FU, Adrucil), irinotecan (Camptosar)	FOLFIRI	Colorectal cancer
folinic acid (leucovorin), fluorouracil (5-FU, Adrucil), oxaliplatin (Eloxatin)	FOLFOX	Colorectal cancer
gemcitabine (Gemzar), capecitabine (Xeloda)	GEMCAP	Cancer of the pancreas
idarubicin (Idamycin), cytarabine (ARA-C, Cytosar), etoposide (VP-16, VePesid)	ICE	Acute myelogenous leukemia
mechlorethamine (Mustargen), vincristine (Oncovin), procarbazine (Matulane), prednisone	MOPP	Hodgkin's disease
Melphalan (Alkeran), prednisone	MP	Multiple myeloma
mitomycin C (Mutamycin), vinblastine (Velban), cisplatin (Platinol)	MVP	Small cell lung cancer
Paclitaxel (Taxol), carboplatin (Paraplatin)	PC	Non-small cell lung cancer
docetaxel (Taxotere), doxorubicin (Adriamycin), cyclophosphamide (Cytoxan)	TAC	Breast cancer
vinblastine (Velban), bleomycin (Blenoxane), cisplatin (Platinol)	VBP	Testicular cancer

NOTE: Doses of chemotherapy agents vary based on drug protocol, type and stage of cancer, age, weight, functional status, and co-morbid conditions (e.g., heart disease, diabetes, respiratory problems, liver disease, etc.).

- Teach the client/family/caregivers that chemotherapy usually remains in the body for 48 to 72 hours after it is administered and is excreted in urine, stool, emesis, semen, and vaginal secretions. Toilets should be flushed twice when used to dispose of bodily fluids. The use of condoms is recommended for up to seven days after chemotherapy administration to protect sexual partners from exposure to these drugs.
- Teach caregivers (including pregnant caregivers) to wear protective gloves (latex, nitrile, polyurethane, neoprene) when emptying a bedpan, urinal, or emesis basin or when changing soiled bed linens or clothing. Soiled linens should be washed as soon as possible in hot water and kept separate from other laundry. Skin soiled with body waste should be washed immediately with soap and water.
- Provide information on the safe storage of chemotherapy medications that are kept in the home (e.g., keep in a safe place out of reach of children and pets).
- Provide written information on safe handling and disposal of chemotherapy waste.
- Provide information on handling chemotherapy spills in the home.

To reduce the nurse's exposure to chemotherapy drugs during intravenous (IV) administration, the following precautions should be followed:

- Use powder-free gloves (nitrile, polyurethane, neoprene) when handling chemotherapy, regardless of the route of administration.
- Gowns (disposable, impermeable, lint-free) should be worn during the administration of IV chemotherapy.
- A mask is not needed if the drug was prepared by a pharmacist.
- Gloves should be worn when disposing of body fluids (e.g., urine, feces, emesis) of clients who have received chemotherapy in the previous 48 hours.
- A face shield should be used if there is a danger of splashing when administering chemotherapy or disposing of body fluids.
- Change gloves after chemotherapy administration and if they become contaminated or punctured.
- Cytotoxic drugs can be accidentally absorbed by inhalation, contact with skin or mucous membranes, and ingestion. The following guidelines should be followed:
  - Prepare chemotherapy in a separate work area. Use a plastic-backed absorbent pad to contain spills during preparation.
  - Wash hands before and after administration of chemotherapy.
  - Avoid hand-to-mouth or hand-to-eye contact while working with chemotherapy.

Table 36–3

General Adverse Reactions to Anticancer Drugs

Adverse Reactions	Nursing Measures and Considerations
Bone Marrow Suppression	
Low RBC count (anemia)	Assess for fatigue, shortness of breath, low blood pressure, increased heart rate, increased respiratory rate, oliguria, and mental status changes. Anemia may be treated with ferrous sulfate or infusions of RBCs. Assess for cyanosis. Plan rest periods for client. Administer oxygen as prescribed. Elevate head of bed to facilitate breathing. Provide pain mediation if pain is increasing oxygen consumption. Provide assistance to bathroom. Monitor for mental status changes. Erythropoietin may be administered to stimulate production of RBCs.
Low WBC count (neutropenia)	Susceptibility to infections increases as WBCs decrease. Visitors with colds or infections should take precautions (e.g., wear mask) or avoid visiting the client. Fever, chills, upper respiratory infections, or sore throat should be reported to HCP. Health care professionals and visitors should wash hands before and after contact with the client.
	Neutrophils are the primary WBCs that fight infections. Usual signs of infection (pain, swelling, redness, warmth, pus) may be absent or greatly reduced in neutropenic clients. Monitor for increase (or decrease) in body temperature. Elevated temperature should be considered a sign of infection. Temperatures of 38.3° C or above should be reported to HCP immediately. Appropriate cultures (e.g., blood, urine, sputum) are collected and an antibiotic regimen is initiated. Assess for localized infections. Auscultate breath sounds. Monitor WBC.
	Colony-stimulating factors (e.g., filgrastim) may be administered to stimulate production of WBCs.
Low platelet count (thrombo-cytopenia)	Petechiae, bruising, bleeding of gums, and nosebleeds are signs of a low platelet count and should be reported to HCP. Assess for bleeding, petechiae, ecchymoses. Assess for occult bleeding in urine, feces, and emesis. Monitor platelet counts and bleeding time. Apply pressure to injection sites. Platelet transfusions may be needed. Avoid medications that may promote bleeding (e.g., aspirin). Avoid invasive procedures (e.g., injections, indwelling catheters, rectal temperature).
GI Disturbances	
Anorexia	Loss of appetite may be related to anemia, pain, fatigue, or bitter taste caused by some chemotherapy agents. Provide small frequent meals high in calories and protein. Plan for rest periods. Address issues of pain control. Hard candy or ice chips may help relieve bitter taste.
Nausea and vomiting	Antineoplastic drugs often stimulate the chemoreceptor trigger zone (CTZ) leading to nausea and vomiting. Nausea and vomiting may be caused by irritation of GI tract; effects of radiation to chest, abdomen, or brain; anxiety; constipation; pain; electrolyte imbalances; or other medications.
	Provide antiemetics before, during, and after chemotherapy. Assess for GI upset and medicate appropriately. Minimize noise, stimulation, odors. Frequent mouth care is needed.
Diarrhea	Diarrhea may be one of three types: osmotic (absorption defects), secretory (bacterial infection, neoplasm), or exudative (secondary to chemotherapy). Chemotherapeutic agents most commonly associated with diarrhea are alkylating agents, antitumor antibiotics, and antimetabolites. Treatment (medications, diet changes) will depend on cause.
	Diarrhea may be caused by other medications (e.g., antibiotics); comorbid conditions (e.g., Crohn's disease) or enteral feedings (e.g., tube feeding). Assess normal bowel habits, monitor for electrolyte imbalances and dehydration. Administer appropriate antidiarrheal medications (e.g., antibiotics, anticholinergics, antispasmodics, psyllium, kaolin and pectin, octreotide acetate, etc.). Teach client to eat small frequent meals; follow a low residue diet; limit spicy, fatty foods; limit intake of salty foods, whole grains, fresh fruits and vegetables; limit caffeine and carbonated drinks. Client should avoid very hot or very cold foods (may stimulate peristalsis). Monitor intake and output.
Mucositis (stomatitis)	Many antineoplastic agents can cause changes in oral mucosa; generally occur 2 to 14 days after initiation of therapy. Assess for taste changes, tissue swelling, redness, pain, dry mouth, white patches, or a white coating on the oral mucosa. Mucositis ranges from mild to severe.
	Symptomatic treatment may include frequent mouth rinses, topical anesthetics, antibiotics, antifungal medication, saliva substitutes, and pain medication. Client should avoid commercial mouthwash that contains alcohol. A soft toothbrush is recommended. Offer ice chips or ice pops to help relieve pain. Assess intake and output. Evaluate caloric needs.
Alopecia	Not all chemotherapeutic agents cause hair loss. Hair thinning, patchy baldness, or complete alopecia may occur, depending on drug. Hair on all areas of the body is affected. Hair loss may be gradual (progressing with each cycle of chemotherapy) or rapid. Hair regrowth usually occurs once chemotherapy is completed; texture may be somewhat changed. Before therapy, discuss potential hair loss and ways to address problem (wigs, scarves, hats, turbans). Assess for body image changes, concerns.
Fatigue	Fatigue may be caused by chemotherapy, sleep disturbances, emotional distress, depression, bone marrow depression, infection, pain, or electrolyte imbalances.
	Assess fatigue using a visual analogue scale (0 = no fatigue; 10 = worst fatigue). Address conditions that might be contributing to fatigue (e.g., lack of sleep, pain, depression). Plan ways to help client conserve energy. Plan a well-balanced diet. Clients should be encouraged to participate in regular (but *not* strenuous) exercise. Encourage stress reduction measures (e.g., relaxation, guided imagery).
Infertility	If infertility occurs, it may be permanent. Pretreatment counseling is advised.

GI, Gastrointestinal; *HCP*, health care provider; *RBC*, red blood cell; *WBC*, white blood cell.

- Refer to the agency's policies for priming IV tubing and disconnecting tubing after administration.
- Refer to the agency's policies for disposal of used equipment.
- Refer to the agency's policies for chemotherapy spills or exposure.

Alkylating Drugs

One of the largest groups of anticancer drugs is the alkylating compounds. **Alkylating agents** cause cross-linking of DNA strands, abnormal base pairing, or DNA strand breaks, thus preventing the cell from dividing. Drugs in this group belong to the CCNS category and kill cells in various and multiple phases of the cell cycle. However, they are most effective against cells in the G_0 phase. Alkylating agents are effective against many types of cancer, including acute and chronic leukemias, lymphomas, multiple myeloma, and solid tumors (e.g., breast, ovary, uterus, lung, bladder, and stomach). Drugs in this category are classified into several groups: mustard gas derivatives (e.g., cyclophosphamide [Cytoxan]), ethylenimines (e.g., thiotepa [Thioplex]), alkylsulfonates (e.g., busulfan [Myleran]), hydrazines and triazines (e.g., dacarbazine [DTIC]), nitrosoureas (e.g., carmustine [BiCNU]), and metal salts (e.g., cisplatin [Platinol]). Nitrosoureas are unique because they can cross the blood-brain barrier, making them useful in the treatment of brain cancer. Table 36–4 lists the alkylating drugs, uses, and considerations.

The side effects for alkylating drugs include nausea, vomiting, hemorrhagic cystitis, alopecia, anemia, leukopenia, thrombocytopenia, bone marrow suppression (anemia, leukopenia, thrombocytopenia), secondary malignancies and sterility. Major dose-limiting toxicities may occur in the hematopoietic and urinary systems. General adverse reactions to chemotherapeutic drugs are listed in Table 36–3.

Cyclophosphamide (Cytoxan)

Mechlorethamine (nitrogen mustard, [Mustargen]), the first alkylating drug introduced for cancer treatment, became available for clinical use during World War II. Mechlorethamine is administered as part of a chemotherapy regimen to treat Hodgkin's disease, especially if the disease is resistant to other drug combinations. This drug is a severe **vesicant** that can cause tissue necrosis if it infiltrates into the tissues. Cyclophosphamide (Cytoxan), an analogue of nitrogen mustard, may be prescribed orally or IV. The client should be well hydrated while taking this drug to prevent hemorrhagic cystitis (bleeding as a result of severe bladder inflammation). MESNA (2-mercaptoethane sulphonate sodium [MESNEX]) is a **cytoprotectant (chemoprotectant)** drug that is often given with high-dose cyclophosphamide to inactivate urotoxic metabolites in the bladder and minimize damage to this organ. Bone marrow suppression and alopecia are common side effects.

Pharmacokinetics

Cyclophosphamide (Cytoxan) is well absorbed from the GI tract. Its half-life is moderate, and it is moderately protein-bound. The drug is metabolized by the liver, and less than 50% is excreted unchanged in the urine.

Pharmacodynamics

Cyclophosphamide (Cytoxan), an early antineoplastic drug is still prevalent in chemotherapy protocols to treat breast cancer, leukemia, lymphoma, multiple myeloma, ovarian cancer, retinoblastoma neuroblastoma, and sarcoma. The onset of action begins in 2 to 3 hours; however, therapeutic effect may take several days. It is one of the anticancer drugs that can be administered orally.

Several drug interactions may occur with cyclophosphamide. Clients should report all medications they are taking, including over-the-counter (OTC) medicines and herbal supplements. Serious drug interactions can occur when taking cyclophosphamide and aspirin, the gout medication allopurinol, phenobarbital, warfarin, thiazide diuretics, and some psychiatric medications. Herbal Alert 36–1 lists herbal supplements that may also interact with cyclophosphamide.

Side Effects and Adverse Reactions

The side effects of cyclophosphamide (Cytoxan) reflect those seen in this general class of antineoplastic drugs. Hemorrhagic cystitis is a serious problem that can arise when high doses of cyclophosphamide are given. Patients with a high tumor load should be assessed for *syndrome of inappropriate antidiuretic hormone secretion* (SIADH) during treatment with this drug. In addition, cyclophosphamide may cause a change (darkening) in the skin or fingernails. Prototype Drug Chart 36–1 details the pharmacologic behavior of cyclophosphamide.

Preventing MEDICATION ERRORS
Do not confuse...

- **Cytoxan** (cyclophosphamide) with **Cytosar** (cytosine arabinoside)

Herbal ALERT 36–1

Cyclophosphamide (Cytoxan)

Use cautiously with garlic (antiplatelet activity), ginkgo (increased antiplatelet effect), echinacea (decreased effects of immunosuppressive drugs), ginseng (altered bleeding time), St. John's Wort (may interfere with chemotherapy), and kava kava (increased risk of bleeding). Toxicity and actions of both cyclophosphamide and vitamin A are altered if given together. *Do not use with mistletoe,* because it may promote cancer growth.

- Astragalus (Huang-qi [Yellow Leader]; milk vetch root) stimulates the immune system and may help speed recovery from immunosuppressive chemotherapy. Astragalus has blood-clot fighting properties and may increase risk of bleeding when given with cyclophosphamide.

Table 36–4

Antineoplastics: Alkylating Drugs

Generic (Brand)	Uses and Considerations
Nitrogen Mustards	
chlorambucil (Leukeran)	Lymphocytic leukemia, lymphomas, and cancer of the breast and ovaries. Side effects include nausea, vomiting, anorexia, diarrhea, abdominal upset, and leukopenia. *Pregnancy category:* D; PB: 99%; t$^{1/2}$: 1.5 h
cyclophosphamide (Cytoxan)	(Prototype Drug Chart 36–1)
estramustine phosphate sodium (Emcyt)	Progressive carcinoma of prostate. Consists of estrogen and nitrogen mustard. Common side effects include nausea, peripheral edema, thrombophlebitis, and breast tenderness. *Pregnancy category:* X; PB: UK; t$^{1/2}$: 20 h
ifosfamide (Ifex)	Testicular cancer, lymphoma, lung cancer, and sarcomas. Mesna, an uroprotective agent, is added to prevent hemorrhagic cystitis. *Pregnancy category:* D; PB: UK; t$^{1/2}$: 7-15 h (high dose)
mechlorethamine HCl (Mustargen)	Hodgkin's disease, solid tumors, and pleural effusion caused by cancer of the lung. Similar side effects as chlorambucil. *Pregnancy category:* D; PB: UK; t$^{1/2}$: 1 min
melphalan (Alkeran)	Multiple myeloma, melanoma, and cancer of the breast, ovary, and testes. *Pregnancy category:* D; PB: 30%; t$^{1/2}$: 1.5 h
temozolomide (Temodar)	Refractory anaplastic astrocytoma. *Pregnancy category:* UK, PB: UK, t$^{1/2}$: UK
uracil mustard (Uracil Mustard)	Chronic lymphocytic and myelocytic leukemia; non-Hodgkin's; cervix, ovary, and lung cancers. GI distress may occur. *Pregnancy category:* X; PB: UK; t$^{1/2}$: UK
Nitrosoureas	
carmustine (BiCNU)	Hodgkin's disease, multiple myeloma, melanoma, and brain tumors. May be used for cancer of the breast and lung. Nausea, vomiting, and stomatitis may occur. *Pregnancy category:* D; PB: UK; t$^{1/2}$: 15-30 min
carmustine with polifeprosan 20 implant (Gliadel wafer)	Chemotherapeutic wafer implant used in addition to surgery for recurrent glioblastoma multiform to improve survival. Approved by FDA in February 2003.
Lomustine (CeeNu)	Advanced Hodgkin's disease and brain tumors. *Pregnancy category:* D; PB: 50%; t$^{1/2}$: 1-2 d
streptozocin (Zanosar)	Pancreatic islet cell tumor and cancer of the lung. May also be used for Hodgkin's disease and colorectal cancer. Nausea, vomiting, diarrhea, and leukopenia may occur. *Pregnancy category:* C; PB: UK; t$^{1/2}$: 30-45 min
Alkyl Sulfonates	
busulfan (Myleran)	Myelocytic leukemia. WBC should be closely monitored. May be used as preparation agent in bone marrow transplant. *Pregnancy category:* D; PB: UK; t$^{1/2}$: UK
Alkylating-Like Drugs	
altretamine (Hexalen)	Ovarian cancer. Also used for breast, cervix, colon, endometrium, head/neck, and lung cancers; lymphomas. Nausea and vomiting and peripheral neuropathy may occur. *Pregnancy category:* D; PB: 6%; t$^{1/2}$: 13 h
carboplatin (Paraplatin)	Recurrent ovarian cancer. May be used as preparation agent in bone marrow transplant. *Pregnancy category:* D; PB: 0%; t$^{1/2}$: 2-6 h
cisplatin (Platinol, CDDP)	Ovarian and testicular cancer. Used as adjunctive treatment. Has been used for cancer of the bladder, head and neck, and endometrium. Nausea, vomiting, peripheral neuropathy, stomatitis, tinnitus, and blurred vision may occur. Ototoxicity occurs in 30% of clients. *Pregnancy category:* D; PB: >90%; t$^{1/2}$: 58-75 h
oxaliplatin (Eloxatin)	Metastatic colorectal cancer. Used with 5-FU and leucovorin. Ovarian cancer, head and neck cancer, and malignant melanoma. *Pregnancy category:* D; PB: >90%; t$^{1/2}$: 20-40 d
dacarbazine (DTIC)	Metastatic malignant melanoma, sarcomas, neuroblastoma, and refractory Hodgkin's disease. May be given as an IV bolus (push) or by IV infusion. Common side effects are anorexia, nausea, and vomiting. *Pregnancy category:* C; PB: 5%-10%; t$^{1/2}$: 5 h
pipobroman (Vercyte)	Polycythemia and chronic myelocytic leukemia. *Pregnancy category:* D; PB: UK; t$^{1/2}$: UK
thiotepa (Thioplex)	Palliative therapy, especially breast and ovarian cancer. *Pregnancy category:* D; PB: UK; t$^{1/2}$: 1.5-2 h

NOTE: Chemotherapeutic doses and schedules will vary depending on protocol, body surface area (m^2), age, functional status, and comorbid conditions. For a full discussion of body surface area in dosage calculation, see Chapter 4B.

5-FU, Fluorouracil; *d,* day; *FDA,* Food and Drug Administration; *GI,* gastrointestinal; *h,* hour; *IV,* intravenous; *min,* minute; *PB,* protein-binding; *t$^{1/2}$,* half-life; *UK,* unknown; *WBC,* white blood cell; > greater than; < less than.

Prototype **DRUG CHART 36–1**

CYCLOPHOSPHAMIDE (CYTOXAN)

Drug Class

Alkylating drug
Trade names: Cytoxan, Procytox, Endoxan, Neosar
Pregnancy Category: D

Dosage

A: PO: Initially: 1-5 mg/kg over 2-5 d; *maint:* 1-5 mg/kg/d
IV: Initially: 40-50 mg/kg in divided doses over 2-5 d;
   max: 100 mg/d; *maint:* 10-15 mg/kg every 7-10 d
C: PO/IV: Initially: 1-5 mg/kg in divided doses or
   50-150 mg/m^2
If bone marrow depression occurs, dose adjustment is
necessary

Contraindications

Hypersensitivity, severe bone marrow depression
Caution: Pregnancy, liver or kidney disease

Drug-Lab-Food Interactions

Drug: Decreases digoxin level. *Increases* drug action of
barbiturates, chloramphenicol half-life, duration of
leukopenia (if given with thiazide diuretics), and effects of anticoagulant drugs. Potentiates doxorubicin
(Adriamycin) cardiomyopathy. Actions and toxicities
of allopurinol, phenothiazines, potassium iodide,
imipramine, warfarin, succinylcholine, and thiazide diuretics are altered if any of these is given with cyclophosphamide. Toxicity increased if given with corticosteroids, phenytoin, or sulfonamides.
Herb: Use cautiously with garlic, ginkgo, echinacea,
ginseng, St. John's Wort, kava kava, grape seed. Toxicity and actions of both cyclophosphamide and vitamin A are altered if given together. Do not use with
mistletoe. Do not give with Astragalus membranaceus
(Beg Kei, Buck Qi, Huang Chi, Milk Vetch, Yellow
Leader); may decrease effects of chemotherapy
Lab: Suppresses positive reaction to uric acid, purified
protein derivative, mumps, *Candida;* Papanicolaou
test (Pap smear) may cause a false-positive result

Pharmacokinetics

Absorption: PO: Well absorbed
Distribution: PB: 50%
Metabolism: t½: 3-12 h
Excretion: 25%-40% in urine unchanged;
   5%-20% in feces
Nadir: 7-14 d

Pharmacodynamics

PO/IV: Onset: 7 d
   Peak: 10-14 d
   Duration: 21 d

Therapeutic Effects/Uses

Breast, lung, ovarian cancers; Hodgkin's disease; leukemias; lymphomas. An immunosuppressant agent
Mode of Action: Inhibition of protein synthesis through interference with DNA replication by alkylation of DNA

Side Effects

Nausea, vomiting, diarrhea, weight loss, hematuria,
alopecia, impotence, sterility, ovarian fibrosis,
headache, dizziness, dermatitis

Adverse Reactions

Hemorrhagic cystitis, secondary neoplasm, bone marrow
depression
Life-threatening: Leukopenia, thrombocytopenia,
cardiotoxicity (very high doses), hepatotoxicity (long
term)

A, Adult; *C,* child; *d,* day; *DNA,* deoxyribonucleic acid; *h,* hour; *IV,* intravenous; *maint,* maintenance; *max,* maximum; *PB,* protein-
binding; *PO,* by mouth; *t½,* half-life.
NOTE: Chemotherapy drug doses are based on body weight and prescribed either as milligrams per kilogram (mg/kg) or milligrams
per meter squared (mg/m^2). Doses will also vary based on drug protocol, type and stage of cancer, age, functional status, and co-
morbid conditions (e.g., heart disease).

Alkylating Drugs: Cyclophosphamide (Cytoxan)

ASSESSMENT

■ Assess complete blood count (CBC), differential, and platelet count weekly. Drug may be withheld if red blood cell, white blood cell, or platelet counts drop below predetermined levels.
■ Conduct thorough physical assessment; document findings.
■ Assess results of pulmonary function tests, chest radiographs, and renal and liver function studies during therapy.
■ Assess temperature; fever may be an early sign of infection.
■ Monitor for adequate intake and output.

NURSING DIAGNOSES

■ Risk for infection related to bone marrow depression
■ Risk for imbalanced nutrition: less than body requirement related to gastrointestinal (GI) side effects of chemotherapy
■ Risk for impaired urinary elimination related to hemorrhagic cystitis caused by chemotherapy
■ Risk for abnormal bleeding related to effects of chemotherapy on the lining of the bladder and/or bone marrow depression
■ Deficient knowledge (patient/family/caregivers) related to chemotherapeutic protocol
■ Risk for sexual dysfunction related to interference with normal menstrual cycle (in females) or lack of sperm production (in males)
■ Disturbed body image related to hair thinning and/ or loss

PLANNING

■ Client will have white cell, red cell, and platelet counts in the desired range
■ Client will remain free of infection
■ Client will maintain nutritional status (adequate fluid intake and output, sufficient caloric intake, stable weight)
■ Client will maintain adequate urinary output
■ Client will remain free of symptoms of hemorrhagic cystitis
■ Client/family/caregiver will demonstrate understanding of chemotherapeutic protocol (e.g., dose, administration, side effects, adverse reactions)

NURSING INTERVENTIONS

■ Monitor blood counts and laboratory values.

■ Handle drug with care during preparation and administration; avoid direct skin, eye, and mucus membrane contact with anticancer drugs. Follow protocols.
■ Monitor IV site frequently for irritation and phlebitis.
■ Administer antiemetic 30 to 60 minutes before giving drug.
■ Hydrate client with IV and/or oral fluids before chemotherapy is administered.
■ Monitor blood, urea, nitrogen (BUN), and creatinine prior to administration.
■ Assess for signs and symptoms of hematuria, urinary frequency, or dysuria. Teach client to empty bladder every 2 to 3 hours.
■ Increase fluids to 2 to 3 L/day to reduce the risk of hemorrhagic cystitis, urate deposition, or calculus formation.
■ Monitor fluid intake and output and nutritional intake.
■ Maintain strict medical asepsis during dressing changes and invasive procedures.

Client Teaching
General
• Emphasize protective precautions as necessary (e.g., hand washing, personal hygiene).
• Teach client to take cyclophosphamide early in the day to prevent accumulation of drug in the bladder during the night.
• Remind client to consult with a health care provider before administration of any vaccines.
• Advise client that cyclophosphamide is excreted in breast milk. Testicular atrophy and reversible oligospermia/ azoospermia may occur in males.
• Teach importance of using birth control measures as appropriate. Discuss sperm-banking with male clients as appropriate.
• Teach client that pregnancy should be avoided for 3 to 4 months after completing antineoplastic therapy in most situations. Some sources recommend that both men and women avoid conception for 2 years after completion of treatment.
• Advise client not to visit anyone who has a respiratory infection. A decreased WBC count puts client at high risk for acquiring an infection.
• Instruct client to promptly report signs of infection (e.g., elevated temperature, fever, chills, sore throat, frequency and/or burning on urination, redness/ swelling/pain near a wound); bleeding (e.g., bleeding gums, petechiae, bruises, hematuria, blood in the stool); and anemia (e.g., increased fatigue, dyspnea, orthostatic hypotension).

Side Effects
• Instruct client about good oral hygiene with a soft toothbrush for stomatitis; have client use a soft toothbrush when platelet count is <50,000/mm³.

- Remind premenopausal females that they may experience amenorrhea, menstrual irregularities, or sterility; instruct male clients that they may experience impotence.
- Advise client of possible hair loss; recommend a wig, hairpiece, scarf, or turban.
- Assess for use of alternative/complementary therapy that may interact with chemotherapy agent.

Diet
- Advise client to follow a diet low in purines (e.g., organ meats, beans, peas) to alkalize urine.
- Advise client to avoid citric acid.
- Offer client food and fluids that may decrease nausea (e.g., cola, crackers, ginger ale).
- Plan small, frequent meals.

Cultural Considerations ❖

- In some non-Western cultural groups, health care decisions are made by consensus, and the family plays a key role in filtering the information given to a client. Issues related to informed consent and full disclosure of medical information may cause distress in cultural groups who place the needs of the family above the needs of the individual. Interactions should be modified based on family structure, religious values and beliefs, time orientation, cultural health practices, and verbal and nonverbal communication.
- Hyperpigmentation of the tongue and oral mucosa after administration has been reported in African Americans. Incidence rate of high-grade neutropenia may be higher in Asian patients.

EVALUATION

- Client was free of infection.
- Client maintained target weight.
- Client maintained nutritional status.
- Client did not develop hemorrhagic cystitis.
- Client/family/caregiver education needs were met.
- Questions related to sexuality were answered.

Antimetabolites

Antimetabolites resemble natural metabolites which synthesize, recycle, and breakdown organic compounds for use by the body. However, antimetabolites disrupt metabolic processes and can inhibit enzyme synthesis. They are classified as CCS and exert their effects in the S phase (DNA synthesis and metabolism) of the cell cycle. This group is classified according to the substances with which they interfere; they include folic acid (folate) antagonists (e.g., methotrexate [Rheumatrex, Trexall]), pyrimidine antagonists (e.g., fluorouracil [Adrucil]), purine antagonists (e.g., 6-mercaptopurine [Purinethol]), and adenosine deaminase inhibitors (e.g., fludarabine [Fludara]). Antimetabolites are used to treat acute leukemia, breast cancer,

head and neck cancer, lung cancer, osteosarcoma, and non-Hodgkin's lymphoma. Two drugs in this classification, fluorouracil, also known as *5-FU* [Adrucil]), and floxuridine (FUDR) are considered CCNS as well as CCS.

Methotrexate, also designated as *MTX* (Rheumatrex, Trexall), a folic acid antagonist, was discovered in 1948 and is used for the treatment of both cancerous and noncancerous (e.g., rheumatoid arthritis, Crohn's Disease) conditions. Methotrexate acts as a substitute for folic acid, which is needed for the synthesis of proteins and DNA. Cancer clients receiving high doses of MTX must be given leucovorin calcium to "rescue" **(leucovorin rescue)** normal cells from the adverse effects of the drug.

Numerous drug interactions may occur with MTX. Protein-bound drugs (e.g., aspirin, phenytoin) increase the toxicity of MTX. Non-steroidal anti-inflammatory drugs (NSAIDs) increase and prolong MTX levels. Cotrimoxazole (Bactrim) and pyrimethamine (Daraprim) increase MTX levels. Clients who are taking penicillins, cyclooxygenase 2 (COX-2) inhibitors, and OTC herbs should share this information with their physician, because these products interact with MTX. Table 36–5 lists the antimetabolite drugs, uses, and considerations.

The general side effects of antimetabolite drugs include bone marrow suppression (anemia, leukopenia, thrombocytopenia), stomatitis (inflammation of the oral mucosa), nausea, vomiting, alopecia, and hepatic and renal dysfunction. Major dose-limiting toxicities may occur in the hematopoietic and gastrointestinal systems. General adverse reactions to chemotherapeutic drugs are listed in Table 36–3.

Fluorouracil

Fluorouracil (5-FU, Adrucil) received Federal Drug Administration (FDA) approval in 1962 for the treatment of colorectal cancer. Since then it has become a mainstay of treatment for a variety of cancers, including those of the breast, stomach, liver, pancreas, and skin.

Pharmacokinetics

Fluorouracil is administered IV to treat solid tumors and topically for superficial basal cell carcinoma. Less than 10% is bound to protein, and the half-life for the IV route is 10 to 20 minutes. A small amount of the drug is excreted in the urine, and up to 80% is excreted by the lungs as carbon dioxide.

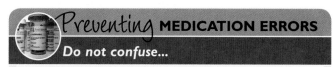

Preventing MEDICATION ERRORS
Do not confuse...

- The fluorouracil (5-FU) drug **Adrucil** with **Efidac** (pseudoephedrine HCl nasal decongestant)

    or

- **fluorouracil** with **flucytosine** (Ancobon systemic antifungal).

Table 36–5

Antineoplastics: Antimetabolites

Generic (Brand)	Uses and Considerations
Folic Acid Antagonist	
methotrexate (Amethopterin, MTX)	Solid tumors, sarcomas, choriocarcinoma, leukemia. At higher doses, clients should be well hydrated; keep urine pH 7.0 for drug solubility for excretion. Higher doses require use of leucovorin as a rescue for normal cells. *Pregnancy category:* D; PB: 50%; t$^{1}/_{2}$: 8-16 h
pemetrexed disodium (Alimta)	A multitargeted antifolate to treat mesothelioma and small cell lung cancer. *Pregnancy category:* D; PB: 81%; t$^{1}/_{2}$: 3 h
Pyrimidine Analogues	
capecitabine (Xeloda)	Solid tumors, sarcomas, choriocarcinoma, leukemia. At higher doses, clients should be well hydrated; keep urine pH 7.0 for drug solubility for excretion. Higher doses require use of leucovorin as a rescue for normal cells. *Pregnancy category:* D; PB: 50%; t$^{1}/_{2}$: 8-16 h
cytarabine HCl (Cytosar-U, ARA-C)	Acute leukemias and lymphomas. Also used as an immunosuppressive drug after organ transplant. May be used in combination with other anticancer drugs. Nausea, vomiting, leukopenia, and thrombocytopenia are common side effects. *Pregnancy category:* D; PB: 15%; t$^{1}/_{2}$: 1-3 h
floxuridine (FUDR)	Metastatic colon cancer and hepatomas. *Pregnancy category:* D; PB: UK; t$^{1}/_{2}$: 20 h
5-Fluorouracil (5-FU, Adrucil)	(Prototype Drug Chart 36–2)
gemcitabine HCl (Gemzar)	Advanced or metastatic adenocarcinoma of the pancreas, non–small-cell lung cancer and bladder cancer. Acts at the S phase of cell cycle. Monitor leukocytes and platelet count; reduce dose if these values are extremely low. *Pregnancy category:* D; PB: UK; t$^{1}/_{2}$: 1-1.5 h
nelarabine (Arranon)	Treatment of refractory or relapsed T-cell lymphoblastic leukemia and T-cell lymphoblastic lymphoma. *Pregnancy category:* D; PB: <25%; t$^{1}/_{2}$: 15 min
procarbazine HCl (Matulane)	Palliative treatment of advanced Hodgkin's disease and for solid tumors. May be used with other anticancer drugs. *Pregnancy category:* D; PB: UK; t$^{1}/_{2}$: 10 min
azacitidine (Vidaza)	Treatment of chronic myelomonocytic leukemia. *Pregnancy category:* D; PB: UK; t$^{1}/_{2}$: 41 min
Purine Analogues	
cladribine (Leustatin)	For treatment of hairy cell leukemia and chronic lymphocytic leukemia. Adverse reactions: bone marrow suppression, fever, nausea, vomiting, diaphoresis. *Pregnancy category:* D; PB: 20%; t$^{1}/_{2}$: 5.4 h
clofarabine (Clolar)	To treat refractory or relapsed acute lymphoblastic leukemia in children. *Pregnancy category:* D; PB: 47%; t$^{1}/_{2}$: 105 min
fludarabine (Fludara)	Chronic lymphocytic leukemia in clients who have not responded to other alkylating drugs; low-grade non-Hodgkin's lymphoma. Anorexia, nausea, diarrhea, fever, and peripheral edema may occur. *Pregnancy category:* D; PB: UK; t$^{1}/_{2}$: 9 h
6-Mercaptopurine (Purinethol)	First used in 1952 for treating acute lymphatic leukemia. Also used as an immunosuppressive drug. Adverse reactions may include hepatoxicity, bone marrow depression, hyperuricemia. *Pregnancy category:* D; PB: 19%; t$^{1}/_{2}$: 45 min
thioguanine (Lanvis)	Acute and chronic myelogenous leukemia. Long duration of action. *Pregnancy category:* D; PB: UK; t$^{1}/_{2}$: 2-11 h
Ribonucleotide Reductase Inhibitor	
hydroxyurea (Hydrea)	Melanoma, resistant chronic myelocytic leukemia, and ovarian cancer. Has a long duration of action. *Pregnancy category:* D; PB: UK; t$^{1}/_{2}$: 3-4 h
trimetrexate glucuronate (Neutrexin)	Alternative drug therapy for *Pneumocystis carinii* pneumonia; treatment for clients with AIDS. May be used for colorectal cancer. CBC should be monitored. *Pregnancy category:* D; PB: 86%-94%; t$^{1}/_{2}$: 11-13 h
Enzyme Inhibitor	
pentostatin (Nipent)	Hairy cell leukemia refractory to alpha-interferon. Has a very long duration of action. *Pregnancy category:* D; PB: UK; t$^{1}/_{2}$: 6 h

NOTE: Chemotherapeutic doses and schedules will vary depending on protocol, body surface area (m^2), age, functional status, and co-morbid conditions. For a full discussion of body surface area in dosage calculation, see Chapter 4B.

5-FU, Fluorouracil; *AIDS*, acquired immunodeficiency syndrome; *CBC*, complete blood cell count; *h*, hour; *min*, minute; *PB*, protein-binding; *t$^{1}/_{2}$*, half-life; *UK*, unknown

Pharmacodynamics

Fluorouracil blocks the enzyme action necessary for DNA and ribonucleic acid (RNA) synthesis. The drug has a low therapeutic index and is used alone or in combination with other anticancer drugs. Fluorouracil can cross the blood-brain barrier. Its duration of action is 30 days.

Side Effects and Adverse Reactions

The side effects of 5-FU (Adrucil) are similar to other anticancer drugs. These include anorexia, nausea, vomiting, diarrhea, stomatitis, alopecia, photosensitivity, increased skin pigmentation, rash, and erythema. Stomatitis is an early sign of toxicity and should be reported to the physician. Bone marrow depression may occur four to eight days after the beginning of drug therapy.

Prototype Drug Chart 36–2 presents the pharmacologic data for 5-FU.

Prototype DRUG CHART 36–2

FLUOROURACIL, 5-FLUOROURACIL, 5-FU (ADRUCIL)

Drug Class

Antimetabolite
Trade names: Adrucil, 5-FU, Efudex (topical)
Pregnancy Category: D

Dosage

A: IV: 12 mg/kg/d × 4 d; *max:* 800 mg/d; repeat with 6 mg/kg on days 6, 8, 10, and 12 or as indicated
Maintenance dose: 10-15 mg/kg/wk as single dose; *max:* 1 g/wk
Topical: 1%-2% sol/cream b.i.d. to head/neck lesions; 5% to other body areas
Refer to specific protocol.

Contraindications

Hypersensitivity, pregnancy, severe infection, myelo-suppression, marginal nutritional status. Reduce dose in clients with impaired hepatic or renal function or malnutrition.

Drug-Lab-Food Interactions

Drug: Bone marrow depressants *increase* chances of toxicity. Avoid live virus vaccines, which may potentiate virus replication. *Increased* 5-FU toxicity with concomitant use of leucovorin calcium. Metronidazole may *increase* 5-FU toxicity (clearance of 5-FU decreased). *Increased* pharmacologic effects of 5-FU when given with cimetidine (Tagamet). Thiazide diuretics *increase* myelosuppression.
Lab: May *decrease* albumin; may *increase* excretion of 5-HIAA in urine
Herb: Use cautiously with ginseng, St. John's Wort, and gingko biloba. Do not use with mistletoe. Topical peppermint oil and eucalyptus oil may increase absorption of topical 5-FU. Avoid simultaneous use.

Pharmacokinetics

Absorption: IV and topical: 5%-10%
Distribution: PB: UK
Metabolism: t½: 10-20 min
Excretion: In urine and expired carbon dioxide
Nadir: 10-14 d

Pharmacodynamics

Effects on blood count:
Peak: 10-14 d
IV: Onset: 1-9 d
       Peak: 9-21 d
       Duration: 30 d
Topical: Onset: 2-3 d
       Peak: 2-6 wk
       Duration: 4-8 wk

Therapeutic Effects/Uses

Cancer of breast, cervix, colon, liver, ovary, pancreas, stomach, and rectum. Given in combination with levamisole after surgical resection in clients with Duke's stage C colon cancer
Mode of Action: Prevention of thymidine synthetase production, thereby inhibiting DNA and RNA synthesis; not phase specific

Side Effects

Stomatitis, nausea, vomiting, diarrhea, alopecia, rash, photosensitivity. Diarrhea may be severe.

Adverse Reactions

Bone marrow depression
Life-threatening: Thrombocytopenia, myelosuppression, hemorrhage, renal failure

5-FU, Fluorouracil; *5-HIAA,* 5-hydroxyindoleacetic acid; *A,* adult; *b.i.d.,* two times a day; *d,* day; *DNA,* deoxyribonucleic acid; *IV,* intravenous; *max,* maximum; *min,* minute; *PB,* protein-binding; *RNA,* ribonucleic acid; *sol,* solution; *t½,* half-life; *UK,* unknown; *wk,* week.

Nursing Process

Antimetabolites: Fluorouracil (5-FU, Adrucil)

ASSESSMENT

- Assess complete blood count (CBC), differential, and platelet count weekly. Chemotherapy may be held if red cell, white cell, or platelet counts drop below predetermined levels.
- Conduct thorough physical assessment; document findings.
- Assess renal function studies before and during drug therapy.
- Assess temperature; fever may be an early sign of infection.

NURSING DIAGNOSES

- Risk for infection related to bone marrow depression
- Risk for imbalanced nutrition: less than body requirements related to GI side effects of chemotherapy
- Risk for acute pain (mucositis/stomatitis) related to GI side effects of chemotherapy
- Risk for impaired perianal skin integrity related to diarrhea caused by chemotherapy
- Deficient knowledge (client/family) related to chemotherapeutic protocol

PLANNING

- Client blood counts will remain in the desired range.
- Client will maintain nutritional status (adequate fluid intake and output, adequate caloric intake, stable weight).
- Client will have adequate pain control.
- Client will limit exposure to sunlight.
- Client/family/caregiver will demonstrate understanding of chemotherapeutic protocol (dose, administration, side effects, and adverse reactions).

NURSING INTERVENTIONS

- Monitor blood counts and laboratory values.
- Handle drug with care during preparation and administration; avoid direct skin contact with anticancer drugs. Follow protocols.
- Monitor IV site frequently. Extravasation produces severe pain. If this occurs, apply ice pack and notify health care provider.
- Administer antiemetic 30 to 60 minutes before drug to prevent vomiting.
- Assess for hyperpigmentation along the vein in which 5-FU was administered.

- Offer client food and fluids that may decrease nausea (e.g., cola, crackers, ginger ale).
- Plan small, frequent meals.
- Maintain strict medical asepsis during dressing changes and invasive procedures.
- Support good oral hygiene; brush teeth with soft toothbrush and use waxed dental floss.
- Encourage mouth rinses every 2 hours with normal saline.
- Monitor fluid intake and output and nutritional intake. GI effects are common on the fourth day of treatment.

Client Teaching

General

- Emphasize protective precautions as necessary (e.g., hand washing, personal hygiene).
- Teach client to examine mouth daily and report signs of stomatitis (soreness, ulcerations, white patches in mouth). Oral hygiene several times a day is essential. If stomatitis occurs, rinse mouth with baking soda or normal saline. Use a soft toothbrush.
- Instruct client to take pain medication as prescribed to relieve mouth pain related to mucositis/stomatitis.
- Advise client to take year-round photosensitivity precautions. Use sunscreen when outdoors.
- Advise client not to visit anyone who has a respiratory infection. A decreased white blood cell (WBC) count puts client at risk for acquiring an infection.
- Teach importance of using birth control measures as appropriate. Discuss sperm-banking with male clients as appropriate.
- Teach client that pregnancy should be avoided for 3 to 4 months after completing antineoplastic therapy in most situations. Some sources recommend that both men and women avoid conception for 2 years after completion of treatment.
- Instruct client to promptly report signs of infection (e.g., fever, sore throat, chills, urinary frequency; burning on urination; redness, swelling, or pain near a wound); bleeding (e.g., bleeding gums, petechiae, bruises, hematuria, blood in the stool); or signs of anemia (e.g., increased fatigue, dyspnea, orthostatic hypotension).

Side Effects

- Instruct client about good oral hygiene with a soft toothbrush for mucositis/stomatitis; have client use a soft toothbrush when platelet count is ≤50,000/mm³. Client should rinse mouth every 2 hours with normal saline and avoid use of commercial mouthwashes that contain alcohol.
- Remind premenopausal females that they may experience amenorrhea, menstrual irregularities, or sterility.

Instruct male clients that they may experience impotence.
- Advise client of possible hair loss; recommend a wig, hairpiece, scarf, or turban.
- Assess for use of alternative/complementary therapy that may interact with chemotherapy agent.

Diet
- Encourage small frequent meals.
- Encourage use of cool, bland foods.
- Offer ice chips or ice pops to help relieve mouth pain.

Cultural Considerations ❖
- In some non-Western cultural groups, health care decisions are made by consensus, and the family plays a key role in filtering information given to the client. Issues related to informed consent and full disclosure of medical information may cause distress in cultural groups who place the needs of the family above the needs of the individual. Interactions should be modified based on family structure, religious values and beliefs, time orientation, cultural health practices, and verbal and nonverbal communication.
- An increased incidence of hyperpigmentation has been reported in dark-skinned people. Hyperpigmentation may be seen on the skin, nails, hair, and oral mucosa. This usually disappears over time.

EVALUATION

- Client was free of infection.
- Oral mucosa was free of erythema and swelling.
- Pain was controlled.
- Skin integrity remained intact.
- Client/family/caregiver education needs were met.
- Questions regarding sexuality were answered.

Antitumor Antibiotics

Antitumor antibiotics (bleomycin [Blenoxane], dactinomycin (actinomycin-D) [Cosmegen], daunorubicin [Cerubidine], doxorubicin [Adriamycin], mitomycin [Mutamycin], and plicamycin [Mithracin]) inhibit protein and RNA synthesis and bind DNA, causing fragmentation. There are several types of antitumor antibiotics, including the anthracyclines (e.g., doxorubicin [Adriamycin], daunorubicin [Cerubidine]), chromomycins (e.g., dactinomycin [Cosmegen], plicamycin [Mithracin]), and miscellaneous drugs (e.g., mitomycin [Mutamycin], bleomycin [Blenoxane]). Except for bleomycin, which has its major effect on the G_2 phase, they are classified as CCNS drugs. Dactinomycin (Cosmegen) was the first antibiotic used in the treatment of tumors in animals in the early 1940s. It was approved by the Federal Drug Administration (FDA) in 1964 for the treatment of cancer in humans. Bleomycin (Blenoxane)

was discovered in 1962 and approved by the FDA for use in cancer patients in 1973. These antitumor antibiotics differ from one another and are used for various cancers, including leukemia and many solid tumors. Table 36–6 lists the antitumor antibiotics, uses, and considerations.

Adverse reactions to the antitumor antibiotics are similar to other antineoplastics and include alopecia, nausea, vomiting, stomatitis, leukopenia, and thrombocytopenia. Antitumor antibiotics are capable of causing **vesication** (blistering of tissue); exceptions to this are bleomycin (Blenoxane) and plicamycin (Mithracin). General adverse reactions to chemotherapeutic drugs are listed in Table 36–3.

Doxorubicin (Adriamycin)

Doxorubicin (Adriamycin) was approved by the FDA over 30 years ago and is used in the treatment of many types of cancer. Doxorubicin is an important prototype drug which has led to the development of many analogs (epirubicin [Ellence], idarubicin [Idamycin]). However, it has severe cardiotoxic side effects and must be given with caution.

Pharmacokinetics

Doxorubicin (Adriamycin) is administered IV and metabolized in the liver to active and inactive metabolites. The various metabolites affect the half-life; the initial phase of doxorubicin is 12 minutes, the intermediate phase is 3.5 hours, and the final phase is 30 hours.

Pharmacodynamics

Doxorubicin (Adriamycin) is prescribed in combination with other anticancer agents for the treatment of cancer of the breast, ovaries, lung, and bladder and also for leukemias and lymphomas. A major concern for clinicians is that doxorubicin can cause cardiac toxicity. Recipients of this drug are limited to a maximum lifetime dose of 550 mg/m². This dose may be lower for individuals who have preexisting cardiac problems, use other cardiac toxic medications, are older, or have received radiation to the chest. Prior to treatment with doxorubicin, the cardiac function of potential recipients is assessed. Dexrazoxane (Zinecard) is a cytoprotective (chemoprotective) agent that may be given to help prevent cardiac toxicities associated with doxorubicin administration.

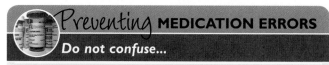

Preventing MEDICATION ERRORS

Do not confuse...

- **doxorubicin** (Adriamycin) with **idarubicin** (Idamycin)

Herbal ALERT 36–3

Doxorubicin (Adriamycin)

🍃 Green tea (*Camellia sinensis*) may enhance antitumor effects of doxorubicin. Report use to the health care provider. Use cautiously with grape seed (inhibits effects of doxorubicin), garlic (anti-clotting properties, may decrease effects of chemotherapy), and St. John's Wort (may decrease effectiveness of chemotherapy). Schizandra Extract (Schisandra, gomishi, Sheng-Mai-San) may decrease the cardiotoxicity associated with doxorubicin. Schizandra stimulates hepatic metabolism and may interfere with doxorubicin, which is excreted through the liver.

Table 36–6

Antineoplastics: Antitumor Antibiotics

Generic (Brand)	Uses and Considerations
bleomycin SO$_4$ (Blenoxane)	Squamous cell carcinomas, testicular tumor (when used with vinblastine and cisplatin), and lymphomas. Low incidence of bone marrow suppression. Lifetime dose is 400 units/m^2. A serious adverse reaction is anaphylaxis. Has a long duration of action. *Pregnancy category:* D; PB: 1%; t^1/$_2$: 2 h
dactinomycin (Actinomycin D, Cosmegen)	Testicular tumors, Wilms tumor, choriocarcinoma, and rhabdomyosarcoma. Nausea and vomiting may occur during the first 24 h. Has a long duration of action. *Pregnancy category:* C; PB: 80%-90%; t^1/$_2$: 36 h
daunorubicin HCl (Cerubidine)	Leukemia, Ewing's sarcoma, Wilms tumor, neuroblastoma, and non-Hodgkin's lymphoma. Has a long duration of action. *Pregnancy category:* D; PB: 80%; t^1/$_2$: 19 h
doxorubicin (Adriamycin)	(Prototype Drug Chart 36–3)
epirubicin (Ellence)	Cancers of breast, lung, lymph system, stomach, and ovaries. Metastatic node-positive breast cancer; adjuvant with anticancer therapy. May be used in combination therapy with cyclophosphamide and fluorouracil (CEF) for breast cancer; improved survival rate over cyclophosphamide, methotrexate, and fluorouracil (CMF). Adverse effects include bone marrow depression, cardiotoxicity (less than doxorubicin), and extravasation necrosis. Less cardiotoxic than doxorubicin; similar efficacy. *Pregnancy category:* D to X; PB: UK; t^1/$_2$: 33 h
idarubicin (Idamycin)	Acute monocytic leukemia and solid tumors. More potent than daunorubicin or doxorubicin. Vesicant, monitor CBC. Urine may be red. *Pregnancy category:* D; PB: 97%; t^1/$_2$: 22 h
mitomycin (Mutamycin)	Disseminated adenocarcinoma of breast, stomach, and pancreas. Also used for cancer of the head, neck, cervix, and lung. Monitor temperature and CBC. *Pregnancy category:* D; PB: UK; t^1/$_2$: 12 min
mitoxantrone (Novantrone)	Acute nonlymphocytic leukemia; may be used for breast cancer. Rash, dyspnea, hypotension, facial swelling, blue urine, sclera, skin hue change may occur. Severe hepatic dysfunction with decreased total body clearance. *Pregnancy category:* D; PB: 95%; t^1/$_2$: 1.5-13 d
plicamycin (Mithracin)	Testicular cancer. May be used to treat hypercalcemia. *Pregnancy category:* X; PB: UK; t^1/$_2$: 2-8 h
valrubicin (Valstar)	Bladder cancer. May cause urinary frequency and urgency, dysuria, hematuria, and bladder pain. *Pregnancy category:* UK; PB: UK; t^1/$_2$: UK

NOTE: Chemotherapeutic doses and schedules will vary depending on protocol, body surface area (m^2), age, functional status, and co-morbid conditions. For a full discussion of body surface area in dosage calculation, see Chapter 4B.
CBC, Complete blood cell count; *d*, day; *h*, hour; *min*, minute; *PB*, protein-binding; *t^1/$_2$*, half-life; *UK*, unknown.

Side Effects and Adverse Reactions

Some antitumor antibiotics can cause organ toxicities. Individuals receiving bleomycin (Blenoxane) may develop pneumonitis that progresses to pulmonary fibrosis. In addition to doxorubicin (Adriamycin), daunorubicin (Cerubidine) and idarubicin (Idamycin) can also cause cardiac toxicity.

Prototype Drug Chart 36–3 presents the pharmacologic data for doxorubicin (Adriamycin).

Antitumor Antibiotics: Doxorubicin (Adriamycin)

Assessment

■ Assess complete blood count (CBC), differential, and platelet count weekly. Drug may be withheld if red blood cell, white blood cell (WBC), or platelet counts drop below predetermined levels.

■ Conduct thorough physical assessment and document findings.
■ Assess temperature; fever may be early sign of infection.
■ Assess plans for pregnancy (if appropriate).

NURSING DIAGNOSES

■ Risk for infection related to bone marrow depression
■ Risk for alteration in cardiac output related to cardiotoxic effects of chemotherapy
■ Risk for impaired skin integrity related to vesicant properties of chemotherapy
■ Deficient knowledge related to antineoplastic therapy

PLANNING

■ Client will maintain blood cell values in the desired range.
■ Client will be free of cardiac dysfunction.
■ Client's skin integrity will remain intact.

- Client/family/caregiver will demonstrate understanding of the chemotherapy regimen, including side effects.
- Assess client/family/caregiver knowledge related to chemotherapeutic protocol.

NURSING INTERVENTIONS

- Monitor blood counts and laboratory values.
- Assess cardiac status.
- Handle drug with care during preparation; avoid direct skin contact with drug.

Prototype DRUG CHART 36–3

DOXORUBICIN (ADRIAMYCIN)

Drug Class
Antitumor antibiotic
Trade name: Adriamycin
Pregnancy Category: D

Dosage
60-75 mg/m^2 as a single dose every 21 days or 30 mg/m^2 IV for 3 days every 4 wk. When used in combination therapy: 40-50 mg/m^2 as a single IV bolus every 21 to 28 days. Safety and efficacy have not been established for children.
Reduce dose with renal impairment.

Contraindications
Pregnancy, severe cardiac disease. Cardiac status and cardiac ejection fraction should be tested before starting doxorubicin therapy. Do not exceed a lifetime cumulative dose of 550 mg/m^2 (450 mg/m^2 if client has had prior chest irradiation or is receiving cyclophosphamide). Dexrazoxane (Zinecard) is used to help prevent or lessen cardiac damage.
Caution: Hepatic and renal impairment

Drug-Lab-Food Interactions
Drug: Calcium channel blockers, paclitaxel (Taxol), and mitomycin increase risk of cardiac toxicity if given with doxorubicin. Doxorubicin may decrease digoxin levels. Doxorubicin decreases levels of phenytoin. Cyclophosphamide (Cytoxan) increases risk of cardiac toxicity and hemorrhage. Increased risk of hepatotoxicity when given with mercaptopurine. Increased plasma clearance of doxorubicin when given with barbiturates. Precipitate will form when doxorubicin is combined with heparin or 5-FU. Decreased metabolic clearance of 5-FU (Adrucil) and increased cytotoxicity when given with Alfa interferon. Prolonged hemotoxic effects may occur if doxorubicin and cyclosporine are given together.
Lab: ECG changes. Increases uric acid.
Herb: Green tea may enhance antitumor effects. Report use to health care provider. Use cautiously with grape seed, garlic, St. John's Wort.

Pharmacokinetics
Absorption: IV
Distribution: PB: 80%-90%
Metabolism: t½: 3-30 h
Excretion: 50% in bile and 5% in urine
Nadir: 10-14 d (doxorubicin)

Pharmacodynamics
IV: Onset: 7-10 d
Peak: 14 d
Duration: 21 d

Therapeutic Effects/Uses
Breast, bladder, ovarian, and lung cancers; leukemias; lymphomas, soft tissue and bone sarcoma
Mode of Action: Inhibits DNA and RNA synthesis; has immunosuppressant activity

Side Effects
Stomatitis, anorexia, nausea, vomiting, diarrhea, rash, alopecia. Doxorubicin is a potent vesicant. May cause a flare reaction. Nausea and vomiting are dose-related and may begin 1-3 h after administration. Causes discolored urine (pink to red) for up to 48 h. May cause "radiation recall" to previously irradiated skin.

Adverse Reactions
Esophagitis; anemia; hyperpigmentation of nails, tongue, and oral mucosa, especially in African Americans. Drug is teratogenic, mutagenic, and carcinogenic.
Life-threatening: Thrombocytopenia, leukopenia, cardiotoxicity, congestive heart failure, electrocardiogram changes, severe myelosuppression, anaphylaxis

5-FU, Fluorouracil; d, day; DNA, deoxyribonucleic acid; ECG, electrocardiogram; h, hour; IV, intravenous; PB, protein-binding; RNA, ribonucleic acid; t½, half-life; wk, week.

■ Monitor IV site frequently. Doxorubicin is a severe vesicant whose effects are not immediately apparent. Give drug through a large bore, quickly running IV infusion.

■ Tissue necrosis may occur 3 to 4 weeks after infiltration into tissue. Extravasation produces severe pain. If this occurs, apply ice pack and notify health care provider.

■ Administer antiemetic 30 to 60 minutes before chemotherapy.

■ Monitor for changes in urine color (pink to red). The drug is red and is excreted in the urine.

■ Offer client food and fluids that may decrease nausea (e.g., cola, crackers, ginger ale).

■ Plan small, frequent meals.

■ Administer prophylactic antibiotics to prevent infection.

■ Offer analgesics for pain as prescribed.

■ Maintain strict medical asepsis during dressing changes and invasive procedures.

■ Support good oral hygiene. Use soft toothbrush. Use waxed dental floss.

■ Monitor fluid intake and output and nutritional intake.

Client (Family Member/Caregiver) Teaching

General

• Emphasize protective precautions (e.g., hand washing, personal hygiene).

• Teach client the signs and symptoms of cardiac dysfunction (shortness of breath, palpitations, edema in extremities) and to report these to health care provider.

• Teach client that complete alopecia occurs with doses >50 mg/m². Teach that hair will begin to regrow within several months after therapy is completed.

• Teach client about "radiation recall" on previously irradiated skin.

• Advise client not to visit anyone who has a respiratory infection. A decreased WBC count puts client at risk for acquiring an infection.

• Teach importance of using birth control measures as appropriate. Discuss sperm-banking with male clients as appropriate.

• Teach client that pregnancy should be avoided for 3 to 4 months after completing antineoplastic therapy in most situations. Some sources recommend that both men and women avoid conception for 2 years after completion of treatment.

• Instruct client to promptly report signs of infection (e.g., fever, sore throat), bleeding (e.g., bleeding gums, petechiae, bruises, hematuria, blood in the stool), and anemia (e.g., increased fatigue, dyspnea, orthostatic hypotension).

Side Effects

• Assess for nausea/vomiting and administer antiemetics as prescribed.

• Teach importance of birth control measures. Discuss sperm banking if appropriate.

• Remind premenopausal females that they may experience amenorrhea, menstrual irregularities, or sterility; instruct male client that he may experience impotence.

• Advise client of possible hair loss; recommend a wig, hairpiece, scarf, or turban.

• Assess for use of alternative/complementary therapies that may interact with chemotherapy agent.

Diet

• Encourage small, frequent meals.

• Encourage eating bland foods.

• Avoid foods with extreme temperatures.

Cultural Considerations ❖

• In some non-Western cultural groups, health care decisions are made by consensus, and the family plays a key role in filtering information given to the client. Issues related to informed consent and full disclosure of medical information may cause distress in cultural groups that place the needs of the family above the needs of the individual. Interactions should be modified based on family structure, religious values and beliefs, time orientation, cultural health practices, and verbal and nonverbal communication.

• Hyperpigmentation of the tongue and oral mucosa has been seen after the administration of doxorubicin in African Americans. Incidence rate of high-grade neutropenia may be higher in Asian patients.

EVALUATION

■ Client was free of infection.
■ Cardiac function was maintained.
■ Client and family education needs were met.
■ Side effects of therapy were controlled.
■ Client/family/caregiver education needs were met.

Mitotic Inhibitors (Plant Alkaloids)

Mitotic inhibitors are plant alkaloids and other compounds derived from natural products that are CCS and block cell division at the M phase of the cell cycle. The **vinca alkaloids** (e.g., vinblastine [Velban], vincristine [Oncovin], and vinorelbine [Navelbine]) are obtained from the periwinkle plant. The antimicrotubules or taxanes group (e.g., docetaxel [Taxotere] and paclitaxel [Taxol]) were originally procured from the needles and bark of the yew tree, which only grows in the Pacific Northwest. Due to the scarcity of this natural resource, a semisynthetic form of paclitaxel was developed and approved by the FDA. Docetaxel (Taxotere) is a semisynthetic analogue of paclitaxel. Table 36–7 lists the mitotic inhibitors and their uses and considerations.

Adverse reactions to mitotic inhibitors include leukopenia, allergic reactions, partial-to-complete alopecia, constipation, nausea, vomiting, diarrhea, and phlebitis. The plant alkaloids damage peripheral nerve fibers and may cause reversible or irreversible neurotoxicity. Signs and symptoms of neurotoxicity include a decrease in muscular strength, numbness, tingling of fingers and toes ("stocking/glove" syndrome), constipation, and motor instability. Other adverse effects of the mitotic inhibitors include loss of deep tendon reflexes, muscle weakness, joint pain and bone marrow depression. Docetaxel may cause fluid retention. General adverse reactions to chemotherapeutic drugs are listed in Table 36–3.

Vincristine (Oncovin)

Vincristine (Oncovin), developed from the periwinkle plant, was originally approved by the FDA in the 1960s to treat Wilms tumor in children.

Pharmacokinetics

Vincristine (Oncovin) is given IV. Its half-life is between 5 minutes and 85 hours, and it is primarily protein-bound. The drug is extensively metabolized by the liver.

Pharmacodynamics

Vincristine (Oncovin) is used in chemotherapy protocols to treat acute leukemia, Hodgkin's disease, non-Hodgkin's lymphoma, neuroblastoma, rhabdomyosarcoma, Ewing's sarcoma, Wilms tumor, multiple myeloma, chronic leukemia, thyroid cancer, and brain tumors. The onset of action begins in a few minutes; however, therapeutic effect may take several days. *Vincristine is an anticancer drug that is only administered IV.*

Side Effects and Adverse Reactions

Several drug interactions may occur with vincristine (Oncovin). The patient should report all medications that he or she is taking, including OTC medicines and herbal supplements. Serious drug interactions can occur when taking vincristine (Oncovin) and L-asparaginase (Elspar), the cardiac medication digoxin (Lanoxin), phenobarbital (Solfoton), calcium channel blockers, and mitomycin (Mutamycin).

Prototype Drug Chart 36–4 details the pharmacologic behavior of vincristine (Oncovin).

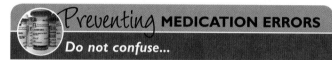

Preventing MEDICATION ERRORS

Do not confuse...

- **Oncovin** (vincristine) with **Oncaspar** (pegaspargase)

Preventing MEDICATION ERRORS

Do not confuse...

- **vincristine** (Oncovin) with **vinblastine** (Velban)

Table 36–7	
Antineoplastics: Mitotic Inhibitors	
Generic (Brand)	**Uses and Considerations**
Mitotic Inhibitors	
vinblastine SO₄ (Velban)	Cancer of the testes, breast, and kidney and for treatment of lymphomas, lymphosarcomas, and neuroblastomas. Nausea, vomiting, and alopecia are common side effects. Check CBC before dosing. *Pregnancy category:* D; PB: 75%; t½: 25 h
vincristine SO₄ (Oncovin)	Cancer of the breast, lungs, and cervix; multiple myelomas, sarcomas, lymphomas, Wilms tumor. Neurologic difficulties should be assessed. Used for treating Hodgkin's disease in combination therapy, MOPP (mechlorethamine, vincristine, procarbazine, and prednisone). Never should be given intrathecally. *Pregnancy category:* D; PB: 75%; t½: triphasic 2-85 h (Prototype Drug Chart 36–4)
vinorelbine (Navelbine)	First-line treatment for ambulatory clients with advanced, unresectable non-small cell lung cancer (NSCLC). May be used alone or in combination with cisplatin for stage IV NSCLC and in combination with cisplatin for stage III NSCLC. *Pregnancy category:* D; PB: UK; t½: UK
Antimicrotubules/Taxanes	
docetaxel (Taxotere)	Advanced or metastatic breast cancer. Inhibits mitosis in cells. Has greater antitumor activity with lower toxicity effect than paclitaxel (Taxol). Monitor WBC and platelet count; if low, dose may need to be decreased. *Pregnancy category:* D; PB: UK; t½: 11.1 h
paclitaxel (Taxol)	Metastatic ovarian and breast cancer. Monitor vital signs and electrocardiogram. Has a long duration of action (3 wk). Peak action is 11 d. *Pregnancy category:* D; PB: 80%-90%; t½: 5-17 h

NOTE: Chemotherapeutic doses and schedules will vary depending on protocol, body surface area (m²), age, functional status, and comorbid conditions. For a full discussion of body surface area in dosage calculation, see Chapter 4B.
CBC, Complete blood cell count; *d,* day; *h,* hour; *PB,* protein-binding; *t½,* half-life; *UK,* unknown; *WBC,* white blood cell; *wk,* week.

Prototype **DRUG CHART 36–4**

VINCRISTINE (ONCOVIN)

Drug Class

Mitotic inhibitor/plant alkaloid
Trade name: Oncovin
Pregnancy Category: D

Dosage

A: IV: use only via free flowing IV catheter. 1.4 mg/m², weekly.
C: IV: use only via free flowing IV catheter. 2 mg/m². For children ≤10 kg, starting dose is 0.05 mg/kg, weekly
If peripheral neuropathies occur, reduction or discontinuance of therapy may be needed.

Contraindications

FATAL if given intrathecally.
Do not give to patients receiving radiation therapy through ports into the liver
Hypersensitivity
Do not give to patients with Charcot-Marie-Tooth Syndrome
Caution: Pregnancy, liver or kidney disease, neuromuscular disease, or infection

Drug-Lab-Food Interactions

Drug: Vincristine should be given 12 to 24 hours prior to L-asparaginase to minimize toxicity.
Acute life-threatening bronchospasm may occur, especially if drug is given with mitomycin (Mutamycin).
L-asparaginase (Elspar) may reduce hepatic clearance of vincristine.
Vincristine *decreases* digoxin effects. Monitor digoxin levels.
Vincristine *decreases* phenytoin effects. Monitor patient for seizure activity.
Do not dilute in solutions that increase or decrease pH outside a range of 3.5 to 5.5.
Mix only with normal saline or glucose in water.
Herb: Use cautiously with bromelain (pineapple extract).
Cantharanthus Roseus (periwinkle) may increase risk of bone marrow depression when given with vincristine.
Lab: May cause hyponatremia, hyperuricemia, anemia, leukopenia, thrombocytopenia.

Pharmacokinetics

Absorption: IV
Distribution: PB: 75%
Metabolism: Liver t½: first phase, 5 min; second phase, 2¼ h; terminal phase, 85 h
Excretion: 80% feces; 10%-20% in urine
Nadir: 7-10 d

Pharmacodynamics

Effects on blood count: Decreased
IV: Onset: 7 d
  Peak: 10-14 d
  Duration: 21 d

Therapeutic Effects/Uses

Acute leukemia, Hodgkin's Disease, non-Hodgkin's lymphoma, neuroblastoma, rhabdomyosarcoma, Ewing's sarcoma, Wilms tumor, multiple myeloma, chronic leukemia, thyroid cancer, brain tumors
Mode of Action: Affects cells in the M phase of the cell cycle and inhibits mitosis

Side Effects

Peripheral neuropathy, loss of deep tendon reflexes, phlebitis, constipation, cramps, nausea, vomiting, muscle weakness, reversible alopecia

Adverse Reactions

Sensory loss, hypotension, visual disturbances, ptosis, ileus, SIADH, hyponatremia, hyperuricemia, severe local reaction with extravasation, fever
Life-threatening: intestinal necrosis, seizures, coma, acute bronchospasm, bone marrow depression

d, Day; *h,* hour; *IV,* intravenous; *PB,* protein-binding; *SIADH,* syndrome of inappropriate antidiuretic hormone secretion; *t½,* half-life; ≤, less than or equal to.

Nursing Process

Mitotic Inhibitors/Plant (Vinca) Alkaloids: Vincristine (Oncovin)

ASSESSMENT

- Assess baseline condition of patient before and during chemotherapy treatment.
- Assess complete blood count (CBC), differential, and platelet count weekly.
- Monitor bilirubin levels. Dose may be reduced if bilirubin levels are >1.5 mg/dl.
- Conduct thorough physical assessment and document findings. Be especially aware of evidence of neurotoxicity, because this is a dose-limiting toxicity.
- Assess for signs of peripheral neuropathy (numbness or tingling in fingers or toes), loss of deep tendon reflexes, foot drop, slapping gait, difficulty walking.
- Monitor bowel function. Autonomic neuropathy may lead to constipation and paralytic ileus. The use of vincristine (Oncovin) and narcotic analgesics may increase the risk of constipation.
- Assess temperature; fever may be early sign of infection.
- Monitor for acute bronchospasm.
- Assess plans for pregnancy (if appropriate).
- Evaluate patient/family/caregiver knowledge of drug therapy.

NURSING DIAGNOSES

- Risk for infection related to bone marrow depression
- Risk for constipation related to neuropathic side effects of chemotherapy
- Risk for injury related to neuropathic side effects of chemotherapy
- Deficient knowledge related to antineoplastic therapy

PLANNING

- Client will maintain blood cell values in the desired range.

- Client will maintain adequate bowel function.
- Client will be free of neuropathic dysfunction.
- Client/family/caregiver will demonstrate understanding of the chemotherapy regimen, including side effects.

NURSING INTERVENTIONS

- Monitor blood counts and laboratory values.
- Assess bowel function.
- Administer stool softener or laxative as prescribed.
- Monitor for signs of peripheral neuropathy (numbness and/or tingling in hands and/or feet), sensory loss, loss of deep tendon reflexes, paresthesia, foot drop, wrist drop, ataxia).
- Assess IV site carefully. Vincristine (Oncovin) is a severe vesicant whose effects are not immediately apparent. Give drug through a large bore, quickly running IV infusion over 1 minute.
- Tissue necrosis may occur 3 to 4 weeks after infiltration into tissue. Extravasation produces severe pain. If extravasation occurs, stop infusion immediately. Notify health care provider. Apply heat intermittently every two hours for 24 hours. Give hyaluronidase into the infiltrated area, per physician order.
- Administer antiemetic 30 to 60 minutes before chemotherapy, or as prescribed.
- Monitor fluid intake and output and nutritional intake.
- Maintain strict medical asepsis during dressing changes and invasive procedures.

Client (Family Member/Caregiver) Teaching
General
- Emphasize protective precautions (e.g., hand washing, personal hygiene) as necessary.
- Teach client the signs and symptoms of neurotoxicity (numbness and/or tingling in hands and/or feet, sensory loss, loss of deep tendon reflexes, paresthesia, foot drop, wrist drop, ataxia). Inability to button clothes or to close zippers may be an early sign of peripheral neuropathy.
- Teach patient signs of "stocking/glove" syndrome (numbness/tingling of hands and feet). This may last as long as a year or may never completely resolve.
- Teach client that complete alopecia may occur. Teach that hair will begin to regrow within several months after therapy is completed.
- Advise client not to visit anyone who has a respiratory infection. A decreased WBC count puts client at risk for acquiring an infection.
- Teach importance of using birth control measures as appropriate. Discuss sperm-banking with male clients as appropriate.
- Teach client that in most situations pregnancy should be avoided for 3 to 4 months after completing anti-

neoplastic therapy. Some sources recommend that both men and women avoid conception for 2 years after completion of treatment.
- Instruct client to promptly report signs of infection (e.g., fever, sore throat), bleeding (e.g., bleeding gums, petechiae, bruises, hematuria, blood in the stool), and anemia (e.g., increased fatigue, dyspnea, orthostatic hypotension).

Side Effects
- Teach patient the signs of peripheral neuropathy.
- Teach patient to report constipation and abdominal pain.
- Assess for nausea, vomiting; administer antiemetics as prescribed.
- Advise patient of possible hair loss; recommend a wig, hairpiece, scarf, or turban.
- Teach importance of birth control measures. Discuss sperm banking if appropriate.
- Remind premenopausal females that they may experience amenorrhea, menstrual irregularities, or sterility; instruct male client that he may experience impotence.
- Assess for use of alternative/complementary therapy that may interact with chemotherapy agent.

Diet
- Encourage bulky high-fiber foods, adequate fluid intake, and moderate exercise to reduce risk of constipation.

Cultural Considerations ❖
- In some non-Western cultural groups, health care decisions are made by consensus, and the family plays a key role in filtering information given to the client. Issues related to informed consent and full disclosure of medical information may cause distress in cultural groups that place the needs of the family above the needs of the individual. Interactions should be modified based on family structure, religious values and beliefs, time orientation, cultural health practices, and verbal and nonverbal communication.
- Asians may be at increased risk for hyponatremia and syndrome of inappropriate antidiuretic hormone secretion (SIADH)

EVALUATION
- Client was free of infection.
- Bowel function was maintained.
- Peripheral neuropathy did not occur.
- Side effects of therapy were controlled.
- Extravasation and tissue necrosis did not occur.
- Client/family/caregiver education needs were met.

Targeted Therapies

Chapter 37 provides in-depth information on this treatment modality.

Liposomal Chemotherapy

A recent change in the delivery of chemotherapy involves the use of anticancer drugs that have been packaged inside synthetic fat globules called *liposomes*. The fatty coating helps the chemotherapy drug remain in the system longer, decreases side effects (e.g., hair loss, nausea, vomiting, cardiac toxicity) and increases the duration of therapeutic effects. Encapsulated forms of doxorubicin (Doxil, Caelyx, Myocet), daunorubicin (DaunoXome), and vincristine (ONCO-TCS, Marqibo) are examples of liposomal chemotherapy.

Hormonal Agents

Although **hormones** are not considered true chemotherapeutic agents, several classes of hormonal agents are used in the treatment of cancer. These include corticosteroids, sex hormones, antiestrogens, aromatase inhibitors, gonadotropin-releasing hormone analogues, and antiandrogens.

Corticosteroids

Corticosteroids (glucocorticoids) are antiinflammatory agents that suppress the inflammatory process that occurs as a result of tumor growth. Although the exact mechanism of action is unknown, these agents may block steroid-specific receptors on the surface of cells. This blocking action slows the growth fraction of the tumor, thus retarding its growth. Prednisone (Cordrol, Deltasone), dexamethasone (Cortastat, Dalalone), and hydrocortisone (Hydrocortone, Solu-Cortef) can help decrease cerebral edema caused by a malignant brain tumor. Cortisone drugs give the client a sense of well-being and varying degrees of euphoria. Cortisone derivatives taken internally produce many adverse side effects, including fluid retention, potassium loss, increased risk of infection, increase in blood sugar, increased fat distribution, muscle weakness, increased bleeding tendency, and euphoria.

Sex Hormones

The sex hormones (e.g., estrogen, androgen) or hormone-like agents are used to slow the growth of hormone-dependent tumors (e.g., prostate cancer, breast cancer). Estrogen therapy is a palliative treatment used to decrease the progression of prostatic cancer in men and to slow the growth of hormone-dependent breast cancer in women. Estrogen preparations suppress tumor growth, and these drugs may induce remission of the cancer for up to a year. Examples of this group of drugs are diethylstilbestrol (DES, Stilbestrol), ethinyl estradiol (Estinyl), chlorotrianisene (TACE), and conjugated estrogens (Premarin).

Progestins may be prescribed to treat breast cancer, endometrial carcinoma, and renal cancer. These drugs (e.g., hydroxyprogesterone caproate [Duralutin]), medroxyprogesterone acetate [Depo-Provera], and megestrol acetate [Megace]) act by shrinking the cancer tissues. Adverse reactions include fluid retention and thrombotic (clot) disorders.

Androgens are given to treat advanced breast cancer in premenopausal women. This male hormone promotes regression of tumors. If androgen therapy is used over a long period of time, masculine secondary sexual characteristics, such as body hair growth, lowering of the voice, and muscle growth, will occur. Antiestrogens such as tamoxifen [Nolvadex] and fulvestrant [Faslodex] are used to treat breast cancer tumors that are estrogen-receptor positive (ER+). Tamoxifen has shown proven efficacy in preventing tumor recurrence in both pre- and postmenopausal women, but it has a number of side effects associated with it. These include hot flashes, irregular menses, fatigue, headaches, nausea, and vomiting. Men who take tamoxifen may experience headaches, impotence, and a decreased interest in sexual activity. Tamoxifen increases a woman's risk of developing cancer of the uterus.

Other drugs called *selective estrogen receptor modulators* (SERM) act like antiestrogens to slow tumor growth, but have fewer side effects than tamoxifen. SERM drugs currently in use include raloxifene (Evista) and toremifene (Fareston). A new generation of SERM drugs (e.g., bazedoxifene, arzoxifene, lasofoxifene, ospemifene) is currently being evaluated to determine effects on preventing recurrent breast cancer, decreasing postmenopausal bone loss, and reducing the risk of cardiovascular disease.

Gonadotropin-Releasing Hormone Analogues

Luteinizing hormone-releasing hormone (LH-RH) agonists (e.g., leuprolide [Lupron], goserelin [Zoladex]) suppress the secretion of follicle-stimulating hormone and luteinizing hormone from the pituitary gland. Initially an increase in testosterone levels is seen. However, with continued use the pituitary becomes insensitive to this stimulation, leading to a reduction in the production of androgens and estrogens.

Antiandrogens

Antiandrogens (e.g., flutamide [Eulexin], nilutamide [Nilandron], bicalutamide [Casodex]) are useful in treating men with hormone-responsive prostate cancer that has metastasized. These agents work by binding to androgen receptors and blocking the effects of dihydrotestosterone on the prostate cancer cells.

Aromatase Inhibitors

In postmenopausal females, the ovaries no longer produce estrogen, but androgen is converted to estrogen in this group of women. The aromatase inhibitors block the peripheral conversion of androgens to estrogens, thus suppressing the postmenopausal synthesis of estrogen and slowing tumor growth. Aromatase inhibitors are used in the treatment of hormonally sensitive breast cancer in postmenopausal women or premenopausal women who have had their ovaries removed. Anastrozole (Arimidex), letrozole (Femara), and exemestane (Aromasin) are examples of aromatase inhibitors currently in use. Increas-

ingly these agents are being used before tamoxifen in postmenopausal women with hormonally responsive metastatic breast cancer. Table 36-8 lists hormonal agents, uses, and considerations.

Miscellaneous Chemotherapy Agents

This category includes a number of antineoplastic agents in which the mechanism of action is unclear. Table 36-8 describes two: L-asparaginase (Elspar) and pegaspargase (Oncaspar).

Biotherapy Agents

The immune system plays a critical role in preventing sickness and fighting diseases such as cancer. **Biotherapy (immunotherapeutic) agents,** developed to augment the natural ability of the immune system, have become a focus of cancer treatment over the past 20 years. Antitumor biotherapy is divided into three general categories that include cytokines, monoclonal antibodies, and vaccines (Table 36-9). Cytokines are proteins in cells that use chemical signals to mediate immunity, inflammation, and hematopoiesis. Examples of cancer-fighting cytokines include interferon (Roferon-A, Intron-A), interleukin (Proleukin), and tumor necrosis factors. Cytokines are made by recombinant DNA technology that uses genetically engineered *E. coli* bacteria containing DNA that code for human protein. Although the mechanism of action is not clear, these agents provide antiviral, antiproliferative, and immunomodulatory effects that are used to combat cancer.

Monoclonal antibodies (MoAbs, mAbs) (e.g., trastuzumab [Herceptin], lapatinib [Tykerb]) are agents that recognize proteins on specific cancer cells (e.g., breast cancer). For more information on these agents, see Chapter 37.

Vaccines used to prevent cancer include the hepatitis B vaccine, given to prevent infection with the hepatitis B virus, which can cause liver cancer. Quadrivalent human papillomavirus (Types 6, 11, 16, 18) recombinant vaccine (Gardasil) and Cervarix (an experimental human papillomavirus [HPV]) are used to prevent human papillomavirus infection that can cause cervical cancer. Chapter 38 provides in-depth information on biotherapy agents. Approval of Gardasil was given in 2006 by the FDA. Approval of Cervarix was expected in May 2007. An experimental vaccine has shown promise in the treatment of prostate cancer.

Summary

Many antineoplastic drugs act to disrupt cancer cells in one (CCS) or more than one (CCNS) phase of the cell cycle. These agents include the alkylating compounds, antimetabolites, antitumor antibiotics, mitotic inhibitors, targeted therapy, hormones, and hormone antagonists. Newer chemotherapy agents designed to target specific enzymes

Table 36–8

Antineoplastics: Hormones, Hormone Antagonists, and Enzymes

Generic (Brand)	Uses and Considerations
Androgens	
testolactone (Teslac)	Palliative treatment of breast carcinoma in postmenopausal women. Serum calcium levels should periodically be checked. Voice may deepen and facial hair may increase. *Pregnancy category:* D; PB: UK; t½: UK
progesterone (Gesterol 50)	Palliative treatment of endometrial and breast carcinoma. *Pregnancy category:* X; PB: UK; t½: 5 min
Hormonal Antagonists	
aminoglutethimide (Cytadren)	Adrenal carcinoma, ectopic adrenocorticotropic hormone (ACTH)-producing tumors. Suppresses adrenal activity. May be used in breast cancer therapy. Treatment typically used for 3 months. *Pregnancy category:* D; PB: 20%-25%; t½: 7-15 h
anastrozole (Arimidex)	Advanced breast cancer in postmenopausal women. Diarrhea, headache, hot flashes, pain, hypertension, and dyspnea might occur. *Pregnancy category:* D; PB: 40%; t½: 50 h
bicalutamide (Casodex)	Advanced metastatic prostatic carcinoma. *Pregnancy category:* X; PB: UK; t½: 5.8 d
exemestane (Aromasin)	
flutamide (Eulexin)	Advanced breast cancer in postmenopausal women. Prostatic cancer. *Pregnancy category:* D; PB: UK; t½: 24 h
fulvestrant (Faslodex)	Metastatic prostatic carcinoma, usually in combination with other anticancer drugs. *Pregnancy category:* D; PB: 95%; t½: 5–10 h
goserelin acetate (Zoladex)	Treatment of hormone-receptor positive metastatic breast cancer in postmenopausal women whose disease has progressed after antiestrogen therapy. *Pregnancy category:* D; PB: 99%; t½: 40 d
histrelin acetate implant (Vantas)	Treatment of advanced prostate cancer. A small, thin implant is placed under the skin of the arm. The drug works for 12 months, then the implant needs to be replaced. *Pregnancy category:* X
letrozole (Femara)	Metastatic prostatic carcinoma. Drug is a synthetic luteinizing hormone-releasing analogue. May also be used in breast cancer and endometriosis. Gynecomastia, breast swelling, and hot flashes may occur. *Pregnancy category:* X; PB: UK; t½: 4-6 h
leuprolide (Lupron)	Advanced breast cancer in postmenopausal women. Decreases estrogen biosynthesis. May be more effective than megestrol acetate and aminoglutethimide. *Pregnancy category:* UK; PB: UK; t½: 2 d Used to slow the growth of prostate cancer. Can be given daily (Lupron) or at 3- or 4-month intervals (Lupron Depot). May be used to treat endometriosis. Hypersensitivity reactions may occur in people with allergy to benzyl alcohol. Pregnant women should not take this drug (high risk of fetal damage). *Pregnancy category:* X; PB: 49%; t½: 3 h
megestrol acetate (Megace)	Palliative treatment of advanced carcinoma of breast and endometrium. May promote weight gain by increasing appetite. *Pregnancy category:* X; PB: UK; t½: 15-20 h
mitotane (Lysodren)	Palliative treatment of inoperable adrenal cortical carcinoma. Adverse reactions include hemorrhagic cystitis, hypouricemia, and hypercholesterolemia. Monitor vital signs. *Pregnancy category:* C; PB: UK; t½: 20-160 d
nilutamide (Nilandron)	Prostatic carcinoma. Loss of libido and sexual potency may occur. Monitor liver function. *Pregnancy category:* C: PB: UK: t½: 24-72 h
polyestradiol PO4 (Estradurin)	Palliative treatment of inoperable prostatic carcinoma. Estrogen derivative. Side effects may include fluid retention, nausea, vomiting, hypertension, weight change, and thromboembolic disorders. *Pregnancy category:* X; PB: UK; t½: UK
tamoxifen citrate (Nolvadex)	Palliative treatment of advanced breast carcinoma with positive lymph nodes in postmenopausal women. Competes with estradiol at estrogen receptor sites. Decreases DNA synthesis. Reduces risk of breast cancer in postmenopausal women. *Pregnancy category:* D; PB: UK; t½: 7 d
raloxifene (Evista)	Selective estrogen receptor modulator (SERM) originally approved to fight osteoporosis in postmenopausal women. Reduces risk of breast cancer with fewer side effects than tamoxifen. *Pregnancy category:* X; PB: 95%; t½: 27 h
toremifene citrate (Fareston)	Advanced breast cancer in postmenopausal women. An antiestrogen drug. *Pregnancy category:* D; PB: >99%; t½: 5 d
Miscellaneous Enzymes	
L-asparaginase (Elspar)	Acute lymphocytic leukemia. Used in combination with another anticancer drug. Common side effects include nausea, vomiting, anorexia, leukopenia, and impaired pancreatic function. *Pregnancy category:* C; PB: 30%; t½: 8–30 h (IV)
pegaspargase (Oncaspar)	Acute lymphoblastic leukemia. A CCS agent affecting G₁ phase of the cell cycle. Interferes with DNA, RNA, and protein synthesis. *Pregnancy category:* C; PB: UK; t½: 1.4 to 5.2 d

NOTE: Chemotherapeutic doses and schedules will vary depending on protocol, body surface area (m²), age, functional status, and comorbid conditions. For a full discussion of body surface area in dosage calculation, see Chapter 4B.

CCS, Cell-cycle specific; *d*, day; *DNA*, deoxyribonucleic acid; *h*, hour; *IV*, intravenous; *min*, minute; *PB*, protein-binding; *RNA*, ribonucleic acid; *t½*, half-life; *UK*, unknown; > greater than.

Table 36–9

Biologic Therapies

Generic (Brand)	Uses and Considerations
Cytokines	
interferon alfa-2a (Roferon-A)	Multiple myeloma, chronic myelogenous leukemia, hairy cell leukemia, malignant melanoma, AIDS-related Kaposi sarcoma. Common side effects include irritation at injection site, flulike syndrome, fatigue, dizziness, anorexia, nausea, vomiting, diarrhea, alopecia, depression, low blood counts. *Pregnancy category:* C; $t^{1/2}$: 3.7 to 8.5 h (IV); 3.7 h (IM) and 7.3 h (SQ)
interferon alfa-2b (Intron-A, IFN-alpha 2)	Hairy cell leukemia, AIDS-related Kaposi sarcoma, malignant melanoma. Common side effects include flulike syndrome, fatigue, GI symptoms (nausea, vomiting, diarrhea), depression, alopecia, low blood counts. *Pregnancy category:* C; $t^{1/2}$: 2-2 h IM or SQ; IV 2 h
interleukin-2, aldesleukin (Proleukin)	Metastatic myeloma, metastatic kidney cancer. Common side effects include capillary leak syndrome, renal insufficiency, cardiac dysrhythmias, flushing, erythema, rash, pruritus, thrombocytopenia, mental status changes. *Pregnancy category:* C; $t^{1/2}$: 13 min IV or SQ
Vaccines	
Hepatitis B (Engerix-B, Recombivax HB)	First anticancer vaccine. Prevents hepatitis B disease and its serious consequences like hepatocellular carcinoma (liver cancer).
Gardasil (quadrivalent human papillomavirus [types 6, 11, 16, 18] recombinant vaccine)	Licensed by the FDA in 2006 for vaccination of females 9 to 26 years of age for prevention of the following diseases caused by human papillomavirus (HPV) types 6, 11 (genital warts) 16, and 18 (cervical cancer).
Cervarix	Application for license by FDA applied for in 2007. If approved, Cervarix will be given to prevent cervical cancer and precancerous lesions associated with the most common cancer-causing HPV types.

IV, intravenous; *SQ*, subcutaneous; *min*, minute; $t^{1/2}$, half-life; *UK*, unknown;

or proteins in cancer cells are in use or being evaluated for clinical efficacy (see Chapter 37). Drugs designed to block growth factors on the surface of cancer cells, deliver toxic therapy directly to tumors, or block the growth of blood vessels that supply tumors, have been approved by the FDA or are being evaluated in clinical trials.

Nurses play an important role in helping people understand the process of chemotherapy administration. Client/family/caregiver education is critical. Nurses will often review treatment protocols and provide information in verbal, written, or other formats regarding the chemotherapeutic agents that will be given. Clients require information about the side effects that can be expected, how these will be managed, and when to call their health care provider. Chemotherapy drugs are highly toxic. Nurses should provide information to clients, family, and caregivers about the safe handling and disposal of these agents if they are to be administered in the home environment.

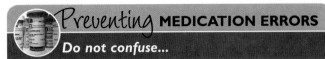

Preventing MEDICATION ERRORS

Do not confuse...

- **5-fluorouracil** (5-FU) with **5-fluorocytosine** (cytosine arabinoside)

- **Alkeran** (melphalan) with **Leukeran** (chlorambucil)

- **busulfan** (Myleran) with **Buscopan** (scopolamine butylbromide)

- **carmustine** (Gliadel, BiCNU) with **lomustine, CCNU** (CeeNU)

- **cisplatin** (Platinol) with **carboplatin** (Paraplatin)

- **Cytoxan** (cyclophosphamide) with **Cytosar** (cytosine arabinoside)

- **Adriamycin** (doxorubicin) with **Idamycin** or **Idarubicin**

- **Taxotere** (docetaxal) with **Taxol** (paclitaxel)

- **eloxatin** (Oxaliplatin) with **Elixomin** (theophylline)

- **floxuridine** (FUDR) with **Floxin** (ofloxacin)

- **gemcitabine** (Gemzar) with **capecitabine** (Xeloda)

- **Gliadel** (carmustine) with **Gleevec** (imatinib mesylate, a targeted therapy [see Chapter 37])

- **hydroxyurea** (Hydrea) with **hydroxyzine** hydrochloride (Atarax)

- **interferon-alpha-2a** (Roferon-A) with **interleukin-2** (IL-2)

- **mitomycin** (Mutamycin) with **mitotane** (Lysodren)

- **Myleran** (busulfan) with **Mylicon** (simethicone, an antiflatulent)

- **Oxaliplatin** (eloxatin) with **oxaprozin** (Daypro)

- **topotecan** (Hycamtin) with **Toposar** (etoposide)

- **Velban** (vinblastine) with **Velcade** (borezomib, a targeted therapy [see Chapter 37])

- **Xeloda** (capecitabine) with **Xenical** (orlistat, a weight loss drug)

KEY WEBSITES

Agency for Healthcare Research and Quality: http://www.ahrq.gov/
National Cancer Institute: http://www.nci.nih.gov/
    cancertopics/chemotherapy-and-you
Oncolink: http://www.oncolink.org/

Critical Thinking Case Study

Your client, a 61-year-old Caucasian woman, was recently diagnosed with breast cancer. She is scheduled to receive combination chemotherapy consisting of IV cyclophosphamide (Cytoxan), doxorubicin (Adriamycin), and fluorouracil (5-FU, Adrucil). This therapy is designated by the acronym *CAF.*

Her treatment regimen consists of the following:

cyclophosphamide (Cytoxan)	500 mg/m^2	IV	Day 1
doxorubicin (Adriamycin)	50 mg/m^2	IV	Day 1
fluorouracil (5-FU, Adrucil)	500 mg/m^2	IV	Day 1

This cycle is to be repeated every 21 days for six cycles.

1. Differentiate the drug actions of cyclophosphamide (Cytoxan), fluorouracil (5-FU, Adrucil), and doxorubicin (Adriamycin).
2. What side effects and adverse reactions should the nurse assess for during therapy? Why would assessment of the cardiac, GI, and genitourinary systems be important with this drug regimen?
3. What is the maximum lifetime dose for doxorubicin (Adriamycin)? Why is this so important?
4. Describe the early signs of cardiac toxicity that you might see days to months after the administration of doxorubicin (Adriamycin).
5. Briefly explain why hydration would be important during this drug regimen.
6. What nursing interventions would be appropriate when caring for this client?
7. Describe the teaching you would provide to the client and her family.
8. After two cycles of chemotherapy, the client complains that her mouth feels sore, and it hurts to eat. Which chemotherapy agent is most likely responsible for this finding? What nursing interventions would you initiate to address this problem?
9. Analyze protective measures necessary to avoid accidental exposure to chemotherapy agents during administration.
10. The client calls you at the clinic and tells you that she has a temperature of 38.3° C. What actions would you take?

NCLEX Study Questions

1. Your male patient is to receive three different anticancer drugs to treat his cancer. He asks the nurse why he needs so much chemotherapy. The nurse's BEST response would be that combination chemotherapy:
   a. works in just one phase of the cell cycle
   b. increases tumor cell kill
   c. uses drugs that work the same way
   d. has no dose-limiting toxicities

2. Your client is scheduled to receive chemotherapy drugs that will cause myelosuppression. Which of the following nursing actions would be the MOST important to carry out?
   a. monitor for a change in temperature
   b. evaluate gastrointestinal function
   c. assess for evidence of cardiac compromise
   d. question client about changes in sense of taste

3. Your client has low platelet counts secondary to the administration of chemotherapy. Which of the following nursing actions would be MOST appropriate?
   a. assess for diarrhea; provide small frequent meals
   b. assess intake and output; help client conserve energy
   c. assess for localized infections; monitor breath sounds
   d. assess for occult bleeding; apply pressure to injection sites

4. Your client is to receive a chemotherapeutic drug that often causes nausea and vomiting. Which of the following nursing actions would be MOST appropriate in this situation?
   a. be prepared to administer antiemetics before, during, and after chemotherapy
   b. tell client not to eat the day before chemotherapy is administered
   c. tell client to drink plenty of fluids to prevent dehydration
   d. wait until client vomits before administering an antiemetic

5. A client in the outpatient oncology clinic complains of fatigue after her chemotherapy. Which of the following would be the MOST appropriate nursing intervention?
   a. assess for other things that might be contributing to her fatigue (e.g. pain, sleep disturbances)
   b. plan a high-protein, high-calorie diet with client
   c. suggest that client participate in daily strenuous exercise
   d. encourage client to sleep as much as possible during the day if she cannot sleep at night

6. You are teaching your client about alopecia, which is one of the side effects of the chemotherapy drugs she is to receive. Which of the following statements, made by your client, indicates that she needs ADDITIONAL teaching about alopecia?
   a. "I've heard the hair on all areas of my body will be affected."
   b. "I've heard my hair won't grow back after chemotherapy is completed."
   c. "A nurse told me the extent of my hair loss will depend on the chemotherapy drugs I get."
   d. "A nurse told me the texture of my hair may be different when it grows back."

7. A client in the outpatient oncology clinic has developed mucositis after receiving fluorouracil (Adrucil, 5-FU). Which of the following statements made by the client would indicate the need for ADDITIONAL teaching about mucositis?
   a. "I'm supposed to frequently rinse out my mouth with normal saline."
   b. "I'm supposed to try using ice pops or ice chips to help relieve my mouth pain."
   c. "I'm going to use a mouthwash with an alcohol base to get my mouth cleaner."
   d. "I'm going to use a soft toothbrush."

8. Your client is scheduled to receive high-dose cyclophosphamide (Cytoxan) via IV infusion as treatment for cancer. Which of the following would you include when teaching your client about cyclophosphamide (Cytoxan)?
   a. an indwelling urinary catheter will be placed
   b. drink 2 to 3 L of fluid a day
   c. empty bladder every 4 to 6 hours
   d. limit fluid intake during chemotherapy

9. Your client is scheduled to receive MVP: mitomycin C (Mutamycin), vincristine (Oncovin), and cisplatin (Platinol) as treatment for her lung cancer. She asks you what side effects she can expect. An appropriate nursing diagnosis would be:
   a. anxiety related to a diagnosis of cancer
   b. knowledge deficit related to side effects of chemotherapy
   c. potential for bleeding related to chemotherapy administration
   d. risk for alteration in nutrition related to the side effects of chemotherapy

10. You are administering doxorubicin (Adriamycin) to a client in the outpatient oncology clinic. You would be sure to include which of the following in your client teaching?
    a. blood counts will most likely remain normal
    b. complete alopecia rarely occurs with this drug
    c. report any shortness of breath, palpitations, or edema to your doctor
    d. tissue necrosis usually occurs 2 to 3 days after administration

Answers: 1, b; 2, a; 3, d; 4, a; 5, a; 6, b; 7, c; 8, b; 9, b; 10, c.

37
Targeted Therapies to Treat Cancer

Objectives

- Describe the rationale, uses, and considerations for targeted therapy.
- Identify general side effects and adverse reactions common to targeted anticancer therapy.
- Describe client education guidelines for self-administration of oral anticancer targeted agents at home.
- Describe the nursing process, including client teaching, related to targeted anticancer drugs.

Terms

angiogenesis, p. 564
angiogenesis inhibitors, p. 564
apoptosis, p. 556
cytochrome P450 system, p. 562

ligand, p. 556
monoclonal antibodies, p. 566
multikinase inhibitors (MKIs), p. 562

protein tyrosine kinases (PTKs), p. 557
proteasome inhibitors, p. 562
targeted cancer therapies, p. 556

topoisomerase inhibitors, p. 557
tyrosine kinase inhibitors (TKIs), p. 557

Targeted cancer therapies are a new approach in cancer treatment. They work by interfering with cancer cell growth and division in different ways and at various points in the development, growth, and spread of cancer. These therapies may interfere with proteins or enzymes in cancer cells, leading to **apoptosis** (programmed cell death). By blocking the signals that tell cancer cells to grow and di-vide uncontrollably, **targeted cancer therapies** can help stop the growth and division of cancer cells. Transmission of these signals may be initiated from outside the cell as a **ligand** (growth factor protein) binds to a receptor activating it or intracellularly, where kinase (transfer enzyme) activity takes place. This is referred to as *downstream signal transduction*. Targeted therapies inhibit signal transduction by blocking a receptor or blocking tyrosine kinase activity. These agents may be used as monotherapy (as a single agent), in combination regimens with other anti-cancer medications, sequentially, and/or with concurrent radiotherapy. Oral targeted therapies that are self-administered at home are convenient for clients and have predictable toxicity profiles that can be managed proactively.

Controversies over these treatments often lie within the socioeconomic burden that may be placed on the client and family for such costly (yet effective) treatments. Treatments can range in cost up to as much as $30,000 per dose. Not all clients and families are able to afford such therapies, and many insurance companies will not cover the expense. Some clinical trials are available, but expenditures may not be covered in part or at all.

Some of the novel targets for cancer therapy include:
- EGF: Epidermal growth factor/receptor (EGFR)
- PDGF: Platelet derived growth factor/receptor (PDGFR)
- bFGF: Basic fibroblast growth factor/receptor (bFGFR)
- EGF: Epidermal growth factor/receptor (EGFR)
- VEGF: Vascular endothelial growth factor/receptor (VEGFR)
- mTOR: Mammalian target of rapamycin
- HER2/neu protein/receptor (EGFR2)
- EGF/c-kit

The targeted therapies that will be discussed in this chapter include topoisomerase I and II inhibitors, small molecule tyrosine kinase inhibitors, multikinase inhibitors (MKIs), angiogenesis inhibitors, and monoclonal antibodies.

Topoisomerase I and II Inhibitors

Topoisomerase inhibitors are nuclear enzymes that alter the shape of DNA coils, which are responsible for DNA replication and repair. There are two types of topoisomerase, I and II, that destroy the replication of DNA and cell structure.

Topoisomerase I affects the S phase of the cell cycle of the cancer cell, inhibiting cellular reproduction. The two drugs classified as Topoisomerase I inhibitors are topotecan (Hycamtin) and irinotecan (Camptosar). Topotecan is primarily prescribed for small cell lung cancer and metastatic cancer of the ovaries refractory to previous chemotherapy. Usually four courses of treatment with topotecan are prescribed for 5 consecutive days, with 16 days between each course of treatment. Irinotecan is for metastatic colorectal cancer. It may be administered once a week for 4 weeks.

The topoisomerase II inhibitors work on the G_2 phase of cellular reproduction of the cancer and can also act on the S phase, which is the DNA synthesis phase. Two drugs, etoposide (VePesid, VP-16, Etopophos) and teniposide (Vumon, VM-26), are examples of topoisomerase II inhibitors. Etopo-

side (VePesid) is mainly given for small cell cancer of the lung and testicular cancer. Teniposide (Vumon) is an analog of etoposide and is indicated for acute lymphoblastic leukemia occurring in childhood. Prototype Drug Chart 37–1 provides data related to etoposide (VePesid), and Table 37–1 lists the two topoisomerase I and II inhibitors along with their route, dosage, uses, and considerations.

Pharmacokinetics

The topoisomerase II inhibitor etoposide (VePesid) can be given orally or intravenously. Low concentration can be found in the cerebrospinal fluid (CSF). It is highly protein-bound. The half-life is 3 to 12 hours. Etoposide is excreted in the urine. The dose should be reduced with renal impairment.

Pharmacodynamics

Etoposide is an epipodophyllotoxin, and it interferes with the action of topoisomerase enzymes, destroying the structure of DNA for replication. The recommended dose of oral etoposide should be approximately twice the IV dose. The intravenous dose should be slowly infused in 250 ml of IV fluids.

Side Effects and Adverse Reactions

The side effects and adverse reactions of topoisomerase I inhibitors include alopecia, constipation, nausea, vomiting, and peripheral neuropathy. With topotecan (Hycamtin) stomatitis, abdominal pain, and headaches might occur. Irinotecan (Camptosar) has been known to cause diarrhea.

The side effects of topoisomerase II inhibitors include alopecia, nausea, vomiting, and flushing. Adverse reactions of etoposide can be leukopenia and thrombocytopenia, and of teniposide, bone marrow depression and anemia.

Tyrosine Kinase Inhibitors (Small Molecule)

Protein tyrosine kinases (PTKs) are a family of proteins that regulate cellular growth, proliferation, and angiogenesis. These protein kinase enzymes mediate signal transmission within human cells. Their receptors are on the suface of endothelial cells and tumor cells. These proteins are involved in both normal and malignant cell growth and development; however, higher tyrosine kinase activity is seen in cancer cells and correlates with the degree of malignant transformation and disease prognosis.

Several small molecule **tyrosine kinase inhibitors (TKIs)** have been developed. These agents act on the tumor and tumor vasculature, blocking receptor tyrosine kinase activity and signaling pathways that are critical for tumor growth and progression. This may be done by blocking the ligand from binding to a receptor at the cell surface or by blocking tyrosine kinase activation and intracellular signal transduction. The tyrosine kinase domain is on the cytoplasmic side of the cell membrane and transmits growth and activation signals through a number of pathways to the nucleus of the cell. This is known as *downstream signal transduction*.

Prototype **DRUG CHART 37–1**

ETOPOSIDE

Drug Class

Topoisomerase II inhibitor
Trade names: VePesid, VP-16
Pregnancy Category: D

Dosage

Testicular cancer:
A: IV: 50-100 mg/m^2 day for 5 consecutive days every
    2 ½ to 4 wk for 3 to 4 courses of treatment
A: PO: 2 × IV dose
Small cell lung cancer:
A: IV: 35 to 50 mg/m^2/d for 4 consecutive days every
    3 to 4 wk
A: PO: 2 × IV dose

Contraindications

Severe bone marrow depression, severe renal or
    hepatic impairment, severe viral and bacterial
    infections, pregnancy and lactation.

Drug-Lab-Food Interactions

Drug: Increased bleeding with anticoagulants,
    antiplatelet drugs, aspirin, NSAIDs
Bone marrow depressants can *decrease* bone marrow
    production

Pharmacokinetics

Absorption: Approximately 50% absorbed from
    the GI tract
Distribution: PB: 97%
Metabolism: t½: 3 to 12 h
Elimination: 45% to 60% in urine, 2% to 15% in
    feces; within 3 days

Pharmacodynamics

IV: Not applicable
PO: Onset: 30 min
    Peak: 1 to 1½ h
    Duration: UK

Therapeutic Effects/Uses

To treat testicular cancer. Other uses not yet approved are for Hodgkin's, non-Hodgkin's, and acute myelogenous
    lymphomas.
Mode of Action: To arrest S phase and G$_2$ phase of the cell cycle

Side Effects

Nausea, vomiting, anorexia, diarrhea, stomatitis,
    weakness, abdominal cramps, transient hypotension,
    reversible alopecia, rash, chills

Adverse Reactions

Bronchospasm, leukopenia, thrombocytopenia,
    anemia, myelosuppression, anaphylactic reaction,
    tachycardia

A, Adult; *PO*, by mouth; *IV*, intravenous; *UK*, unknown; *PB*, protein-binding; PO, by mouth; *t½,* half-life.

Table 37–1

Targeted Therapies to Treat Cancer

Generic (Brand)	Route and Dosage	Uses and Considerations
Topoisomerase I Inhibitors		
irinotecan HCl (Camptosar)	A: IV: 125 mg/m^2 infused over 90 min q week × 4 wk	Advanced and metastatic carcinoma of colon and rectum. Inhibits topoisomerase enzyme needed for DNA and RNA synthesis. Increased fluid intake is necessary. Monitor WBC count. *Pregnancy category:* D; PB: UK; t$^{1/2}$: 6-10 h
topotecan HCl (Hycamtin)	A: IV: 1.5 mg/m^2 by IVF over 30 minutes daily × 5 d starting on day 1 of a 21-day course. In absence of tumor progression, recommend minimum of 4 courses, because tumor response may be delayed	Advanced and metastatic carcinoma of ovary. Used when other anticancer therapy fails. Inhibits topoisomerase I enzyme required for DNA replication. Monitor WBCs. *Pregnancy category:* D; PB: 35%; t$^{1/2}$: 2-3 h

NOTE: Targeted therapies to be administered under the supervision of qualified physician/health care provider qualified in the use of chemotherapeutic agents. Assure adequate treatment facilities are readily available for management and complications of therapy.
A, Adult; *C,* child; *CML,* chronic myelogenous leukemia; *d,* day; *DNA,* deoxyribonucleic acid; *GIST,* gastrointestinal stroma tumor; *h,* hour; *IV,* intravenous; *maint,* maintenance; *max,* maximum; *min,* minute; *PB,* protein-binding; *PO,* by mouth; *t$^{1/2}$,* half-life; *wk,* week.

Table 37–1

Targeted Therapies to Treat Cancer—cont'd

Generic (Brand)	Route and Dosage	Uses and Considerations
Topoisomerase II Derivatives		
etoposide (VePesid, VP-16, Toposar, Etopophos)	*For testicular tumors in combination therapy:* A: IV range: 50-100 mg/m²/d on days 1-5 to 100 mg/m²/d on days 1, 3, and 5 *Small cell lung cancer:* A: IV range: 35 mg/m²/d × 4 d to 50 mg/m²/d × 5 d A: PO: Twice the IV dose rounded to nearest 50 mg	Refractory testicular tumors and small cell lung carcinoma. Monitor CBC before, during, and after each cycle. Has standard chemotherapy side effects. Has a long duration of action. Most reactive cells are in S and G_2 phase. Transient hypotension with rapid IV infusion. *Pregnancy category:* D; PB: 97%; t½: 4-11 h
teniposide (Vumon, VM-26)	A: IV: Based on body weight; infused over 30-60 min	Acute lymphoblastic leukemia (ALL) in children. Used in combination with other anticancer drugs. Severe adverse reactions include bone marrow depression and anaphylaxis. *Pregnancy category:* D; PB: 99%; t½: 5 h
Tyrosine Kinase Inhibitors (TKIs)		
erlotinib (Tarceva)	A: PO: 50 mg daily between meals at least 1 hour before or 2 hours after eating	For treatment of clients with locally advanced or metastatic non-small cell lung cancer (NSCLC) after failure of at least one prior chemotherapy regimen. In clinical trials of first line NSCLC clients, erlotinib showed no clinical benefit given with concurrent administration of chemotherapy. Infrequent reports of serious interstitial lung disease (IDL) in clients taking erlotinib. Women should be advised to avoid becoming pregnant and breastfeeding. *Pregnancy category:* D; t½: UK (Prototype Drug Chart 37–1)
gefitinib (Iressa)		
imatinib mesylate (Gleevec)	*For (CML):* A: PO: recommended starting dose is 400 mg/d for chronic phase and 600 mg/d for accelerated phase or blast crisis. Dose increases to *max* of 800 mg (given as 400 mg twice daily); may be considered if tolerated for accelerated phase or blast crisis *For GIST:* A: PO: recommended starting dose is 400 mg/d	Approved in 2001 to treat chronic myeloid leukemia (CML) and approved in February 2002 for metastatic malignant gastrointestinal stromal tumors (GIST). Avoid pregnancy and breastfeeding. Take with meal and large glass of water to minimize gastric irritation. *Pregnancy category:* D; PB: 95%; t½: 18-40 h
Proteasome Inhibitors		
bortezomib (Velcade)		(Prototype Drug Chart 37–2)
Multikinase Inhibitors (MKIs)		
sorafenib (Nexavar, BAY 43-9006)	A: PO: 400 mg twice daily, continuous. If poorly tolerated, dose adjustments are 400 mg once daily, then 400 mg every other day. Dose interruptions and reductions are not uncommon.	First approved MKI for treatment of metastatic renal cell cancer (December 2005). Hand-foot skin reaction & rash are most common adverse reactions. Hypertension occurs in about 30% of clients within a few weeks of starting treatment. BP should be monitored closely, especially during first 6 weeks of therapy; may require initiation or adjustment of antihypertensive therapy. *Pregnancy category:* D; t½: 25-48 h
sunitinib (Sutent)	A: PO: 50 mg daily for 4 wk followed by 2 wk off therapy. Dose increases or reductions in 12.5 mg increments is recommended, based on individual safety and tolerability	Sunitinib approved for advanced (RCC) renal cell carcinoma and (GIST) gastrointestinal stromal tumor January 2006. Co-administration of sunitinib with strong CYP 3A4 inducers/inhibitors may affect sunitinib plasma concentrations. Take with or without food. Women should be advised to avoid becoming pregnant or breastfeeding while taking sunitinib. *Pregnancy category:* D; t½: 40-60 h drug (80-110 h metabolite)

Continued

Table 37–1

Targeted Therapies to Treat Cancer—cont'd

Generic (Brand)	Route and Dosage	Uses and Considerations
temsirolimus, CCI-779	A: IV: 25 mg IV infused over 30 to 60 min weekly via peripheral or central venous catheter. Prophylactic premedication with IV diphenhydramine 25 mg to 50 mg, 30 min prior to each dose	Newly FDA approved May 2007 for advanced/poor risk RCC and MCL. An mTOR inhibitor, temsirolimus has been in clinical trials for clients with RCC, breast cancer, prostate cancer, and other solid tumors. Avoid co-administration with inducers or inhibitors of the CYP3A4 isoenzyme. Grapefruit juice and St. John's wort may alter exposure of temsirolimus and its metabolite sirolimus. *Pregnancy category:* D; $t^1/_2$: UK
Angiogenesis Inhibitors		
bevacizumab (Avastin)		(Prototype Drug Chart 37–3)
Monoclonal Antibodies		
alemtuzumab (Campath)	A: PO: Initial 3 mg in 2 h IV daily. When tolerated, titrate up to 10 mg; then up to 30 mg maint dose & administer 3 ×/wk on alternate days (M-W-F) for up to 12 wk	Approved by the FDA May 2001 to treat B-cell chronic lymphocytic leukemia (B-CLL). Binds to CD52 surface antigen, resulting in cell lysis. Do NOT administer IV push or bolus Generally premedicate with diphenhydramine and acetaminophen. Dose modification related to toxicities. *Pregnancy category:* C; $t^1/_2$: 12 d
cetuximab (Erbitux)	A: IV: Loading dose: 400 mg/m² in 2 h infusion at 5 mL/min *Maint:* 250 mg/m² infused over 1 hr; *max 5 ml/min*	Metastatic colorectal cancer. Approved by FDA February 2004. Binds to human epidermal growth factor (EGFR) and blocks activation of receptor-associated kinases. Used alone or in combination with irinotecan (Camptosar). Premedication with diphenhydramine recommended. Must use low protein-binding 0.22 micrometer in-line filter. Observation postinfusion for 1 h recommended. *Pregnancy category:* C; $t^1/_2$: 114 h
gemtuzumab ozogamicin (Mylotarg)	A: IV: 9 mg/m² as 2 h infusion. 2 doses with 14 d between doses	Relapsed acute myeloid leukemia (AML) for selected clients age 60 and older. Premedicate 1 h prior with diphenhydramine 50 mg and acetaminophen 650-1000 mg. Monitor vital signs during and 4 h postinfusion. *Pregnancy category:* D; PB: UK; $t^1/_2$: 72 h
lapatinib (Tykerb)	A: O: 1250 mg daily, continuously In combination with Capecitabine 2000 mg/m²/d on days 1-14 of repeating 21-d cycle	Prolongs time to progression in women with heavily pretreated advanced breast cancer. Used in combination with capecitabine (Xeloda). Most common adverse effects with combination therapy: GI and cutaneous. *Pregnancy category:* D; $t^1/_2$ 24h
panitumumab (Vectibix)	A: IV: 6 mg/kg IV infusion over 60 min every 14 d. Doses >1000 mg: administer over 90 min. Use low protein-binding in-line filter	To treat metastatic EGRF-expressing colorectal cancer. Monitor for hypomagnesemia and hypocalcemia. Dermatologic, mucosal, and ocular toxicities. *Pregnancy category:* C; $t^1/_2$ 7.5 d
rituximab (Rituxan)		(Prototype Drug Chart 37–4)
trastuzumab (Herceptin)	A: IV: loading dose 4 mg/kg IV administered over 90 min, followed by maint dose of 2 mg/kg IV on a weekly basis until disease progression or intolerance. Alternative is a loading dose of 8 mg/kg IV administered over 90 min, followed by maint dose of 6 mg/kg IV every 3 wk. Maint doses are administered over 30 min as tolerated. Not to be given IV push.	Metastatic breast cancer with tumors that overexpress the HER2 (human epidermal growth factor receptor 2) protein. Used in combination with paclitaxel for first-line therapy or as a single agent in second- and third-line therapy. Clinical trials are under way to determine usefulness of trastuzumab in treatment of osteosarcoma and cancers of lung, pancreas, salivary gland, colon, prostate, endometrium, and bladder. *Pregnancy category:* B; $t^1/_2$: 1.7-12 d

The three TKIs currently prescribed are erlotinib (Tarceva), gefitinib (Iressa) and imatinib mesylate (Gleevec). Table 37–1 lists the TKIs, their dosages, routes, uses, and considerations. Prototype Drug Chart 37–2 lists the drug data related to the TKI gefitinib (Iressa).

Pharmacokinetics

Gefitinib (Iressa) is absorbed slowly in the gastrointestinal tract, with 60% reaching systemic circulation. It is metabolized mainly in the liver by the CP3A4 enzyme. Gefitinib has a long half-life (2 days). Eighty-six percent is excreted in feces; renal elimination accounts for less than 4% of an administered dose.

Prototype DRUG CHART 37–2

GEFITINIB

Drug Class

Tyrosine kinase inhibitor (TKI)
Trade name: Iressa
Pregnancy Category: D

Dosage

A: PO: 250 mg per day

Contraindications

Hypersensitivity to gefitinib and clients who are
   pregnant or breastfeeding

Drug-Lab-Food Interactions

Drug: Drugs that inhibit the liver microsomal CYP 3A4
   enzyme (ketoconazole, erythromycin, and others)
   decrease rate of metabolism of gefitinib, resulting in
   potential for increased toxicity.
Drugs that stimulate the liver microsomal CYP 3A4
   enzyme, including carbamepazine, rifampin, phenobarbital, and St. John's wort *increase* the rate of metabolism of gefitinib, resulting in its inactivation.
Coagulation PT/INR should be closely monitored when
   clients are receiving warfarin; gefitinib inhibits metabolism of warfarin by the liver P450 system.
Lab: May alter liver transaminases
Food: None known

Pharmacokinetics

Absorption: Bioavailability is about 60%
Distribution: 90% PB with extensive tissue distribution;
   steady state drug concentration 7-10 d
Metabolism: Metabolized mainly in the liver by the
   CYP 3A4 enzyme; t½: 48 hours
Excretion: Mainly hepatic with excretion in the feces;
   renal elimination accounts for <4% of an
   administered dose

Pharmacodynamics

Oral absorption is relatively slow and not affected by
food

Therapeutic Effects/Uses

To treat non-small cell lung cancer that is refractory to platinum-based chemotherapy and/or second-line docetaxel
   chemotherapy
Mode of Action: Selectively inhibit the kinase domain of the epidermal growth factor receptor, thus blocking the
   downstream kinase pathway. Turning off this signal inhibits mitogenic and antiapoptotic signals involved in proliferation, growth, metastases, angiogenesis, and response to chemotherapy and/or radiation therapy. Clinical responses may be seen within the first week of therapy, as evidenced by improvement in symptoms.

Side Effects

Hypertension, pruritus, dry skin with a pustular
   acneiform rash, elevations in serum transaminases
   (usually transient and asymptomatic), asthenia,
   anorexia, mild nausea and vomiting, mucositis,
   conjunctivitis, blepharitis, and corneal erosions
   (rare) with abnormal eyelash growth

Adverse Reactions

Hemoptysis (rare) and GI hemorrhage

A, Adult; *d*, day; *PB*, protein-binding; *PO*, by mouth; *t½*, half-life, <, less than.

Pharmacodynamics

Oral absorption of gefitinib is relatively slow and not affected by food.
Peak plasma levels occur 3 to 7 hours after dosing. Gefitinib has a long
half-life.

Herbal ALERT 37–1

Gefitinib

🌿 The herb St. John's wort increases the rate of metabolism of gefitinib, resulting in its inactivation.

Side Effects and Adverse Reactions

Side effects of gefitinib include hypertension, pruritus, dry
skin with a pustular acneiform rash, elevations in serum
transaminases (usually transient and asymptomatic), asthenia, anorexia, mild nausea and vomiting, mucositis,
conjunctivitis, blepharitis, and corneal erosions (rare)
with abnormal eyelash growth. Adverse reactions include
hemoptysis (rare), GI hemorrhage, and interstitial lung
disease.

Drug-Lab-Herb Interactions

1. Drugs that *inhibit* the liver microsomal CYP 3A4 enzyme (ketoconazole, erythromycin, and others) decrease the rate of metabolism of gefitinib, resulting in the potential for increased toxicity.

2. Drugs that *stimulate* the liver microsomal CYP 3A4 enzyme (carbamepazine, rifampin, phenobarbital, and the herb St. John's wort) increase the rate of metabolism of gefitinib, resulting in its inactivation.

3. Gefitinib inhibits the metabolism of warfarin by the liver P450 system (Box 37-1), so coagulation PT/INR should be closely monitored in clients receiving gefitinib concomitantly with warfarin.

Proteasome Inhibitors

Proteasome inhibitors are intracellular multienzyme complexes that degrade proteins to eliminate the cells of proteins that are not needed. Such proteins regulate transcription, cell adhesion, apoptosis (programmed cell death), cell cycle progression, and mitosis. Cancer may develop when these processes become abnormal.

Box 37-1

THE CYTOCHROME P450 SYSTEM

The **cytochrome P450 system** is a family of isoenzymes involved in drug metabolism and drug-drug interaction in humans. Becoming familiar with the role of various CYP450 enzymes in drug metabolism can help predict drug-drug interactions due to inhibition or induction of these enzymes. The CYP 3A4 subfamily is the most abundant isoenzyme of the CYP 450 family and metabolizes the greatest number of drugs in humans. It is found mostly in the liver and intestines.

Drugs that are inhibitors of the CYP3A4 isoenzyme can be expected to decrease metabolism of drugs metabolized by CYP3A4 and in general lead to increased drug exposure which may require a dose reduction. Drugs that are inducers of the CYP3A4 isoenzyme are expected to increase the metabolism of drugs metabolized by CYP3A4 and generally lead to decreased drug effect, requiring a dose increase.

Caution: The oral targeted agents (TKIs) discussed in this chapter are metabolized by the CYP3A enzyme and inhibit the metabolism of **warfarin** by the liver. Warfarin dose requires careful monitoring when taken concurrently with these agents. Low-molecular-weight heparin may be considered for some clients requiring anticoagulation.

Herb-Drug Interaction: **Grapefruit and grapefruit juice** may increase plasma concentration of TKIs (CYP3A4 inhibitors). **St. John's wort** (a CYP3A4 inducer) increases the rate of metabolism of the TKI, resulting in its inactivation.

Examples of CYP3A4 inhibitors include ketoconazole, itraconazole, itraconazole, clarithromycin, atazanavir, indinavir, nefazodone, nelfinavir, ritonavir, saquinavir, telithromycin, and voriconazole. Grapefruit may also increase plasma concentrations.

Examples of CYP3A4 inducers include dexamethasone, phenytoin, carbamazepine, rifampin, rifabutin, rifapentine, phenobarbital • and St. John's wort.

Proteasome inhibitors disrupt aspects of cellular structure, promoting apoptosis. Bortezomib (Velcade), approved in 2004, inhibits a specific (26 S) proteasome, altering proteins that regulate cellular growth and division. This drug has been approved for treatment of multiple myeloma and has also been used to treat colorectal and lung cancers. Cancer cells are more sensitive to proteasome inhibitors than normal cells. At present, bortezomib (Velcade) is the only proteasome inhibitor available.

Table 37-1 lists the proteasome inhibitor bortezomib (Velcade) with route, dosage, use, and considerations information. Prototype Drug Chart 37-3 lists the drug data related to bortezomib.

Pharmacokinetics

Bortezomib (Velcade) is administered intravenously; the absorption rate has not been determined. It has a moderately high (83%) protein-binding effect and an average half-life of 9 to 15 hours. No pharmacokinetic studies were conducted with clients having hepatic or renal impairment. Elimination pathways have not been determined.

Pharmacodynamics

Bortezomib (Velcade) is administered as an IV bolus (direct IV). It is administered twice a week for 2 weeks, then followed by a 10-day rest period. The peak and duration of action is unknown.

Side Effects and Adverse Reactions

Common side effects include malaise, fatigue, nausea, vomiting, anorexia, diarrhea, and constipation. Less frequent side effects are headaches, insomnia, leg pain, edema, and rash. Adverse reactions include thrombocytopenia (occurring in about 40% of clients), neutropenia, peripheral neuropathies, pyrexia, and hypotension.

Multikinase Inhibitors (MKIs)

Because multiple pathways may be used for tumor angiogenesis, blockade of more than one pathway is thought to be more effective and is the reasoning behind some of the antiangiogenic combinations. As the result of clinical trial findings, the newest classification of targeted therapies for cancer, **multikinase inhibitors (MKIs),** was developed in December 2005. Each of the MKIs has its own unique dosing and formulation. Toxicities are mostly dose-related and may require interruption and/or dose reduction. Toxicities usually resolve within a few days of stopping the drug. The drug can then be restarted at a reduced dose or slowly titrated upward as tolerated by the client. Side effects are predictable and can be managed proactively.

Advanced renal cell cancer (RCC) has a poor prognosis, and the standard of care has long been cytokine therapy

---

Herbal ALERT 37-2

Temsirolimus

Grapefruit juice and St. John's Wort may alter exposure of temsirolimus and its metabolite sirolimus.

Prototype **DRUG CHART 37–3**

BORTEZOMIB

Drug Class
Proteasome inhibitor
Trade name: Velcade
Pregnancy Category: D

Dosage
A: IV: 1.3 mg/m² IVP over 3 to 5 seconds followed by a saline flush. One 21-day cycle consists of 2 doses given twice weekly for 2 weeks out of 3 (days 1, 4, 8, 11) followed by a 10-day rest period before beginning the next cycle. At least a 72-h rest period between doses is required. Dose reduction may be required for toxicity.

Contraindications
Clients with hypersensitivity to bortezomib, boron, or mannitol
Caution: Concomitant use of meds related to peripheral neuropathy and with decrease in blood pressure. Bortezomib is a cytotoxic agent, and safe-handling precautions should be observed. (See Chapter 36.)

Drug-Lab-Food Interactions
Drug: No formal interaction studies
Lab: May alter blood glucose levels of diabetics
Food: None known

Pharmacokinetics
Absorption: UK
Distribution: PB 83%
Metabolism: t½ 9-15 h
Excretion: UK

Pharmacodynamics
IV: Not applicable

Therapeutic Effects/Uses
To treat clients with multiple myeloma who have received at least two prior therapies and have had disease progression on the last therapy. Newly approved second-line therapy for mantle cell lymphoma. Drug is cytotoxic to a variety of cancer cell types and causes a delay in tumor growth (cytostatic activity). Drug has shown a synergistic effect when given with other chemotherapy and/or other novel agents; optimal combinations for a variety of cancers are under investigation.
Mode of Action: A reversible inhibitor of 26S proteasome, resulting in changes of protein concentration responsible for cell growth and division regulation. Drug is cytotoxic in vitro to variety of cancer cell types and causes tumor growth delay in vivo.

Side Effects
Fatigue, dizziness, hypotension

Adverse Reactions
Asthenia (malaise, fatigue, weakness), nausea, diarrhea, decreased appetite/anorexia, vomiting, constipation, peripheral neuropathies, thrombocytopenia , pyrexia, neutropenia, and hypotension

A, Adult; *d,* day; *h,* hour; *IV,* intravenous; *PB,* protein-binding; *t½,* half-life, *UK,* unknown.

(high dose IL-2 and/or interferon), which is highly toxic. Sorafenib (2005) and sunitinib (2006) were the first new drugs approved for the treatment of RCC in 13 years and offer new treatment options for RCC clients. Sunitinib has also been approved for gastrointestinal stromal tumors. Temsirolimus, an investigational mTOR inhibitor, was approved by the FDA in May 2007 as an MKI. It has been used in clinical trials to treat clients with RCC, breast cancer, prostate cancer, and other solid tumors. The MKIs are under investigation as monotherapy or in combination regimens with cytokines or other targeted therapy for cancers that may be responsive to them.

Table 37–1 lists examples of MKIs, along with routes, dosages, uses, and considerations.

Pharmacokinetics

Oral sorafenib is rapidly absorbed, but should be taken 1 hour before or 2 hours after a meal. Absorption of sunitinib occurs in 6 to 12 hours. Temsirolimus is administered intravenously. Sorafenib and sunitinib have long half-lives and the protein-binding effects are very long.

Side Effects and Adverse Reactions

The common side effects of MKIs are nausea, vomiting, diarrhea, taste disturbance, stomatitis, hair thinning or alopecia, rash, and thickened or cracking skin on palms and soles (hand-foot skin reaction). An adverse reaction of sorafenib (Nexavar) is hypertension, occurring in 30% of clients during the first 6 weeks of treatment. Adverse effects of sunitinib (Sutent) include electrolyte disturbances, neu-

Prototype DRUG CHART 37–4

BEVACIZUMAB

Drug Class

Angiogenesis inhibitor; recombinant humanized
   monoclonal antibody
Trade name: Avastin
Pregnancy Category: C

Dosage

A: IV: Recommended 5 mg/kg every 14 days for CRC;
   7.5 mg/kg every 3 weeks in combination with
   capecitabine-based regimens for advanced CRC;
   15 mg/kg every 3 weeks for advanced NSCLC

Contraindications

Clients with hypersensitivity to bavacizumab

Drug-Lab-Food Interactions

Drug: UK
Lab: UK
Food: none known

Pharmacokinetics

Absorption: UK
Distribution: UK
Metabolism: t½ 20 d
Excretion: UK

Pharmacodynamics

IV: Not applicable

Therapeutic Effects/Uses

Metastatic colorectal cancer in combination with any IV 5-fluorouracil-based chemotherapy as first-line therapy, and
   in combination with FOLFOX-4 in second-line therapy. Approved for non-squamous, non-small cell lung cancer in
   combination with carboplatin/paclitaxel. Treatment of renal cell cancer and breast cancer remains investigational.
Mode of Action: Binds to all forms of VEGF, preventing its interaction with its receptor (VEGFR) on the surface of
   endothelial cells and tumors, thus inhibiting VEGFR signaling. VEGF is a proangiogenic growth factor overexpressed in a number of human cancers. Immunologic antitumor activity may also be involved, including recruitment of antibody-dependent cell cytotoxicity and/or complement-mediated cell lysis.

Side Effects

Diarrhea, dizziness, headache, decreased appetite,
   asthenia, epistaxis

Adverse Reactions

GI perforation, impaired wound healing, pulmonary
   hemorrhage, thromboembolism, hypertensive crisis

A, Adult; *d*, day; *GI*, gastrointestinal; *h*, hour; *IV*, intravenous; *PB*, protein-binding; *t½*, half-life, *UK*, unknown.

tropenia, and thrombocytopenia. Twenty-five percent of clients taking temsirolimus may have dyspnea, cough, fever, and abnormal laboratory values (e.g., hyperlipidemia and hyperglycemia).

Angiogenesis Inhibitors

Angiogenesis is the process of new capillary formation from existing blood vessels. This is a physiologic process required for maintenance of normal tissue (e.g., fetal growth and development, menstruation, and wound healing). Angiogenesis is also critical for tumor growth and metastases and has become an important target in anticancer therapy. A positive correlation has been shown between tumor angiogenesis and tumor stage. Angiogenesis occurs when there is an imbalance of proangiogenic signals, stimulated by the absence of normal regulatory processes and hypoxia. This is called the *angiogenic switch* and may happen when the tumor has outgrown its blood supply. Uncontrolled angiogenesis is a pathologic process that leads to cancer and other diseases such as macular degeneration.

Angiogenesis inhibitors are a class of drugs that inhibit the formation of blood vessels needed for tumor growth and metastasis. At present there is only one angiogenesis inhibitor, bevacizumab (Avastin). It is used primarily for metastatic carcinoma of the colon and rectum. Bevacizumab can be combined with other chemotherapy drugs for the treatment of breast, prostate, and renal cell cancers.

Vascular endothelial growth factor (VEGF) is the most important ligand involved in angiogenesis and the one most studied. VEGF and vascular endothelial growth factor receptor (VEGFR) are both produced by tumor cells and are among the main drivers of angiogenic activity.

Table 37–1 lists bevacizumab (Avastin), the angiogenesis inhibitor, along with its route, dosage, uses, and considerations. Prototype Drug Chart 37–4 includes the drug data related to bevacizumab (Avastin), the first approved antineoplastic agent that specifically targets all known isoforms of the vascular endothelial growth factor.

Pharmacokinetics

The half-life of bevacizumab (Avastin) is extremely long, 11 to 50 days. Clients should be monitored for cumulative effects.

Prototype **DRUG CHART 37-5**

RITUXIMAB

Drug Class	**Dosage**

Drug Class

Monoclonal antibody, biologic response modifier
Trade name: Rituxan
Pregnancy Category: C

Dosage

A: IV: Recommended dose is 375 mg/m^2 IV weekly for 4 or 8 weeks

Monitor for infusion reaction, usually seen and most severe with first infusion and within first 30 to 120 minutes. Infusion should be stopped immediately for signs or symptoms of HSR (hypotension, angioedema, bronchospasm, hypoxia). Administer supportive medications as indicated, including diphenhydramine, bronchodilators, acetaminophen, corticosteroids, IVFs, or vasopressors. Have resuscitation equipment readily available. Most often infusion can be restarted at 50% rate after symptoms have completely resolved. NOTE: Rituximab should not be given by IV push. Client monitoring should continue 2-4 hours after completion of infusion.

Monitor for tumor lysis syndrome in clients with a high tumor burden or high number of circulating cells (>25,000/mm^3).

Contraindications

Known hypersensitivity or anaphylactic reactions to murine proteins or any component of this product; breastfeeding should be avoided

Drug-Lab-Food Interactions

Drug: No formal drug interaction studies.
Lab: Monitor CBC and platelet counts at regular intervals, more frequently in those with cytopenias.
Food: None known

Pharmacokinetics

Absorption: UK
Distribution: PB UK
Metabolism: t½: 60 h after first infusion; 175 h after fourth infusion
Excretion: UK

Pharmacodynamics

Duration: May be detected in serum for 3-6 months

Therapeutic Effects/Uses

To treat client with relapsed or refractory, low-grade or follicular, CD20-positive, B-cell non-Hodgkin's lymphoma (NHL)

Mode of Action: CD20 is expressed on greater than 90% of all B-cell NHLs and leukemias. Binding of antibodies to CD20 induces the transmembrane signal that blocks cell activation and cell cycle progression. Rituximab is used as a single agent or in combination regimens such as EPOCH or CHOP.

Side Effects

Nausea, vomiting, anorexia, headaches, vertigo, fatigue, fever, chills

Adverse Reactions

Most serious include: transfusion reactions, tumor lysis syndrome, mucocutaneous reactions, hypersensitivity reactions, cardiac arrhythmias, angina, renal failure, leukopenia, thrombocytopenia, neutropenia

A, Adult; *h*, hour; *IV*, intravenous; *PB*, protein-binding; *t½*, half-life; *UK*: unknown; >, greater than.

Pharmacodynamics

Bevacizumab blocks the proliferation of new blood vessels in tumor cells, thus inhibiting the progression of metastatic cancer. It is given intravenously in 100 ml of normal saline solution over 90 minutes (NOT dextrose solution). Second dose can be given in 60 minutes. The duration of bevacizumab would be very long.

Side Effects and Adverse Reactions

Side effects of bevacizumab may include pain, headache, hypertension, diarrhea, nausea, vomiting, anorexia, stomatitis, constipation, upper respiratory infection, nosebleed, dyspnea, exfoliative dermatitis, and proteinuria with nephritic syndrome in 5% of clients.

Adverse reactions include leukopenia, hypertension, bleeding, wound-healing complications, GI perforation, arterial thrombolic events, reversible posterior encephalopathy syndrome, and nasal septum perforation. Fatal hemoptysis has occurred in non-small cell lung cancer (NSCLC) clients receiving bevacizumab.

Monoclonal Antibodies

Monoclonal antibodies (MoAbs, mAbs) are produced in the laboratory and designed to recognize and bind to specific antigens expressed on the surface of cancer cells. They work by blocking the growth of the tumor and/or alerting the body's immune system to attack the cancer cells. They also inhibit the human epidermal growth factor receptors 1 and 2 (EGFR1 and EGFR2) that are attached to the protein. These agents can be used as monotherapy, in combination with chemotherapy or other targeted agents, or as vehicles to deliver drugs, toxins, or radioactive material to tumor sites (conjugated).

Three types of engineered monoclonal antibodies include chimeric, humanized, and fully human antibodies. Drug names for the chimeric antibodies have a suffix of "-ximab"; humanized antibodies carry the suffix "-zumab"; and fully human antibodies, "-umab." Examples of monoclonal antibodies include cetuximab (Erbitux), rituximab (Rituxan), alemtuzumab (Campath), gemtuzumab ozogamicin (Mylotarg), trastuzumab (Herceptin), panitumumab (Vectibix), and lapatinib (Tykerb),

Each of the monoclonal antibodies is targeted for specific cancers. Cetuximab is used in the treatment of metastatic colorectal cancer and can be used in combination with other chemotherapeutic drugs. Gemtuzumab ozogamicin is frequently prescribed for acute myeloid leukemia. Rituximab is used for the treatment of B cell non-Hodgkin's lymphoma. Trastuzumab is used in the treatment of breast cancer.

Monoclonal antibodies had been classified as *biologic response modifiers* (BRMs); however, this group specifically targets cancer cells and have been reclassified under *targeted therapies (agents)* for the treatment of cancer. Chapter 38 provides in-depth information on biologic response modifiers.

Table 37–1 lists examples of monoclonal antibodies, along with routes, dosages, uses, and considerations. Prototype Drug Chart 37–5 includes drug data related to the monoclonal antibody rituximab (Rituxan).

Pharmacokinetics

The half-life of rituximab (Rituxan) is long following the first infusion. After the fourth infusion, the half-life can be greater than 175 hours or up to 8 days. Protein-binding percent and elimination is not known; however, with a long half-life, cumulative effects should be monitored.

Pharmacodynamics

Rituximab is primarily prescribed for refractory CD 20 positive, B-cell non-Hodgkin's lymphoma. Duration of rituximab is 3 to 6 months (detected in client's serum).

Side Effects and Adverse Reactions

Side effects for most monoclonal antibodies are nausea, vomiting, anorexia, diarrhea, headaches, and vertigo. Other side effects may include fever, chills, pain, difficulty in breathing, and rashes.

Adverse reactions can vary among the monoclonal antibodies and commonly include leukopenia, thrombocytopenia, neutropenia, and anemia. Anaphylaxis, urticaria, bronchospasm, and angioedema may occur with trastuzumab. With cetuximab, pulmonary embolism and kidney failure are rare, but could occur. Elevated liver enzymes, blood sugar elevation, and electrolyte imbalances might occur with gemtuzumab ozogamicin.

Nursing considerations for clients on targeted therapies include the following (see the Nursing Process section for further details):

- Client/family education
- Understanding the mechanism of action
- Self-administration drug issues
- Access to therapy
- Side effect management
- Reproductive issues
- Quality of life
- Financial implications (e.g., drug assistance programs)

Nursing Process

Targeted Therapies to Treat Cancer

ASSESSMENT

- Conduct a thorough physical assessment and document findings.
- Assess laboratory studies, including CBC with differential, hepatic and renal studies, electrolytes, and urinalysis. Treatment may be interrupted or dose reduction may occur if laboratory findings are not at acceptable levels.
- Conduct a comprehensive medication history including prescription medicines, herbals, dietary supplements, and vitamins.
- Assess client's access to the drug (oral agents), as well as any financial needs.
- Assess client and family knowledge related to therapeutic regimen.

NURSING DIAGNOSES

- Risk for infection related to bone marrow suppression
- Risk for decreased cardiac output related to cardiotoxic effects of therapy
- Risk for impaired skin integrity related to dermatologic effects of therapy

---

Preventing MEDICATION ERRORS

Do not confuse:

- **etoposide** with **teniposide**
- **sunitinib** with **sorafenib**
- **bevacizumab** with **bortezomib**

- Deficient knowledge (client and family) related to treatment regimen
- Imbalanced nutrition: less than body requirements related to GI effects of targeted therapy
- Risk for deficient fluid volume related to GI effects of therapy
- Diarrhea related to GI effects of therapy

PLANNING

- Client will have laboratory values in desired range.
- Client will be free of cardiac dysfunction.
- Client's skin toxicities will be minimized.
- Client will maintain adequate GI function (nutrition, hydration, and elimination).
- Client and family will demonstrate understanding of treatment regimen, including schedule, dose, side effects, and knowledge of who and when to call.

NURSING INTERVENTIONS

- Monitor blood counts and laboratory values.
- Handle IV drugs with care, following Oncology Nursing Society (ONS) and Occupational Health and Safety Administration (OSHA) guidelines.
- Closely monitor client for infusion reactions during monoclonal antibody therapy.
- Administer premedications as ordered 30 to 60 minutes before infusion.
- Offer client food and fluids that may decrease nausea (cola, crackers, ginger ale).
- Plan small, frequent meals.
- Offer analgesics for pain as prescribed.
- Maintain strict medical asepsis.
- Monitor weight, fluid intake and output, and nutritional intake.

Client Teaching

General
- Moisturize skin regularly and start early; hypoallergenic and fragrance-free moisturizers and colloidal oatmeal lotions are recommended. Avoid hot water and harsh detergents.
- Use oral or topical antihistamines for pruritus; topical steroidals are generally not recommended.
- Treatment for acnelike rash (not really acne) to be determined by health care provider; OTC products not recommended. Use water-based makeup if desired.
- Avoid sun exposure to reduce dryness and erythema. Use SPF 15 or higher and avoid tanning salons.
- Consider a dermatology consult, if appropriate, through a referral from oncology physician.
- Teach client that hair loss is variable. Discuss the use of a wig, scarf, or turban. Refer to "Look Good . . . Feel Better" service (available through the American Cancer Society) and other support services as appropriate.

- Teach client to call early about hand-foot skin reaction before it becomes too painful. Observe for swelling, erythema, pain, peeling, cracking of palms and soles, and signs of infection. Suggest cotton socks and gel soles.
- Consider OTC foot care products that help exfoliate the hard outer skin layer. Pedicures are not indicated or appropriate in the immunocompromised client with thrombocytopenia and at risk for bleeding.

Side Effects
Dermatologic
- Teach client that dry skin and rash are the earliest side effects of targeted therapies. Rashes vary and may be surrogate markers for response to therapy.

Gastrointestinal
- Assess for nausea and vomiting; administer antiemetics as prescribed.
- Encourage small, frequent meals.
- Teach client to perform oral inspection and to be alert to changes.
- Encourage good oral hygiene and use of a soft toothbrush, waxed dental floss, or dental tape; frequent mouth rinses with plain water, salt water, or baking soda and water. Commercial mouthwashes that contain alcohol should be avoided.
- Teach client about use of appropriate mouth care products or pain reliever for stomatitis as ordered by health care provider.
- Assess for diarrhea, which can be a dose-limiting toxicity of TKIs; stress importance of early treatment.
- Teach client appropriate use of OTC antidiarrheal. If diarrhea persists with OTC product use, consult physician to rule out GI infection. More potent medication may be indicated upon physician recommendation.
- Assess any medication that could worsen diarrhea: potassium supplements, artificial sweeteners such as sorbitol, antibiotics, quinine-containing medications, and some herbal preparations.
- Advise client to avoid caffeine; carbonated, greasy, or spicy foods; raw fruits and vegetables; whole grains; gas-forming foods and drinks; and lactose products.
- Encourage the BRAT diet (bananas, rice, applesauce, and toast).
- Assess for dehydration and encourage increased fluid intake.
- Instruct client to call HCP for persistent diarrhea, fever of 38° C or higher, black tarry stools, and an inability to take in fluids. Arrange for evaluation of dehydration; may need IVF.

Home Care
- Include family members when teaching client.
- Explain rationale for cancer therapy and how it works.
- Teach client and family how and when to take oral targeted therapy (e.g., with or without food, dose, and

schedule), and counsel on potential drug and herbal interactions.

- Discuss potential side effects of therapy and how to manage them. Emphasize self-care strategies.
- Provide written as well as oral instructions (at a fourth-grade level).
- Instruct client to check blood pressure as directed (including how, when, and where).
- Provide a drug/symptom/BP diary for client/family to record at home.
- Provide written guidelines for when to call the health care provider (e.g., temperature, uncontrolled diarrhea or nausea, hand-foot skin reaction). If client does not read, provide illustrations or audiotaped instructions.
- Teach client energy-conserving strategies.

Cardiovascular Toxicity
- Confirm that client has stable blood pressure prior to beginning treatment.
- Teach client the importance of monitoring and recording blood pressures; hypertension is a known side effect of TKIs and may require an interruption in therapy.
- Assess client's access to monitoring equipment at home, a local office, or perhaps a nurse relative or neighbor. Provide a BP diary.
- Give client clearly written instructions for when to report hypertension.
- Review client's medication profile for cardiac medication.
- Teach client to check weight daily and monitor for swelling, ascites, shortness of breath, cough, palpitations, hypotension, chest pain, and increased fatigue. If present, instruct client to report them promptly to health care provider.

Infection Prevention
- Emphasize protective precautions (e.g., hand-washing, personal hygiene) as necessary.
- Advise client not to visit anyone who has a respiratory infection. A decreased WBC count puts client at risk for acquiring an infection.
- Teach client to perform good perirectal care and report pain or perirectal bleeding.

Blood Dyscrasias
- Instruct client to promptly report signs of infection (e.g., fever, sore throat, dysuria, cough), bleeding, dizziness, increased fatigue, petechiae (bleeding gums, fatigue, anemia, and exertional shortness of breath can also be toxicities of cancer therapy), dyspnea, and orthostatic hypotension. If any of these signs are present, the client should be assessed.

Reproductive
- Teach client that pregnancy should be avoided for 3 to 4 months after completing antineoplastic therapy. Some sources recommend that both men and women

avoid conception for 2 years after completion of treatment.
- Teach the importance of birth control measures. Discuss sperm banking if appropriate.
- Remind the premenopausal female that she may experience amenorrhea, menstrual irregularities, or sterility. Instruct the male client that he may experience impotence.
- Refer to resources such as *www.fertilehope.com* when appropriate

EVALUATION

- Client is free of infection.
- Cardiac function is maintained.
- Client and family education needs have been met.
- Side effects of therapy are manageable.

Summary

Newer chemotherapy agents designed to target specific enzymes or proteins in cancer cells continue to be developed and evaluated for clinical efficacy and safety. These agents include topoisomerase inhibitors, tyrosine kinase inhibitors, proteasome inhibitors, and others. Numerous drugs designed to block growth factors on the surface of cancer cells, interrupt cytoplasmic tyrosine kinase activity, deliver toxic therapy directly to tumors, or block the growth of blood vessels that supply tumors are in use or being tested in clinical trials (e.g., monoclonal antibodies, angiogenesis inhibitors). Targeted therapy is changing the way cancer is treated. Because these drugs are target-specific, there may be fewer toxic effects than those seen with conventional chemotherapy, but they do have their own side-effect profiles.

Nurses play a critical role in helping people understand cancer treatment regimens and administration. Client and family education is essential. Nurses need to explain the treatment protocol to clients and provide verbal and written information on the agents that will be administered. Clients require information about what side effects can be expected, how these will be addressed, and when to call their health care provider. Targeted antineoplastic drugs, although oral and given at home, are powerful agents and can be highly toxic. This must be understood by both client and caregiver. Telephone triage nursing has evolved into a valuable role that provides much-needed guidance to clients receiving oral targeted therapy at home. Treatment-related side effects are expected and usually seen within the first week or two of beginning these agents. With proactive management—including drug interruption and/or dose reduction—drug toxicities can be minimized and clients may safely continue on therapy.

KEY WEBSITES

Cancer treatment information: www.oncolink.com/treatment

Advances in Targeted Cancer Therapies journal: www.targetedtherapies.org

Targeted therapy information: www.chemocare.com/whatis/targeted_therapy.asp

Critical Thinking Case Study

SH is a 45-year-old university faculty member under medical care for multiple myeloma refractory to prior therapy. She calls the office nurse after her fourth infusion of bortezomib (Velcade) to report fatigue and weakness and asks about "rest periods" in therapy.

1. What would be an appropriate response by the nurse?

The client reports she has nutrition questions, because she does not feel like eating and has diarrhea.

2. What advice might the nurse offer SH?
3. Identify two potential diagnoses for SH.
4. Describe at least four nursing interventions to review with SH.
5. Identify at least three evaluation criteria for SH.

NCLEX Study Questions

1. The client is receiving gefitinib (Iressa), and the nurse reviews his other medications. Which of the following medications *decrease* the rate of drug metabolism, resulting in the potential for increased toxicity?
   a. ketoconazole
   b. fluoroquinolones
   c. digoxin
   d. warfarin

2. The client is receiving gefitinib. The nurse assesses for common side effects of this drug including:
   a. hypotension
   b. hand-foot skin reaction
   c. urinary retention
   d. hypertension

3. The client has canal cell carcinoma and is receiving temsirolimus. Common side effects with this medication include:
   a. severe headache
   b. lab abnormalities
   c. urinary retention
   d. hand-foot skin reaction

4. The client is receiving a targeted therapy. The nurse instructs the client to avoid which food item?
   a. nuts
   b. pickles
   c. caffeine
   d. grapefruit juice

5. What are the earliest side effects of targeted therapies?
   a. nausea and vomiting
   b. dry skin and rashes
   c. hand-foot skin reaction
   d. pharyngitis and hoarseness

6. Swelling, erythema, pain, peeling, and cracking of palms and soles are clinical manifestations of which of the following adverse reactions?
   a. Stevens-Johnson syndrome
   b. allergic reaction
   c. abnormal lab results
   d. hand-foot skin reaction

7. The nurse is caring for a client receiving bevacizumab (Avastin). Which clinical manifestations would alert the nurse to an adverse reaction?
   a. hypertension and stomatitis
   b. leukopenia and diarrhea
   c. wound-healing complications
   d. urinary retention and double vision

Answers: 1, a; 2, d; 3, b; 4, c; 5, b; 6, d; 7, a.

38

Biologic Response Modifiers

Margaret Barton-Burke and Gail Wilkes

ELECTRONIC RESOURCES

Evolve website (http://evolve.elsevier.com/KeeHayes/pharmacology/):
- *Case Studies*
- *Content Updates*
- *Frequently Asked Questions*
- *Student Review Activities*
- *WebLinks*
- *Additional Reference Material*

Companion CD-ROM:
- *NCLEX Examination Review Questions*
- *Pharmacology Animations*
- *IV Therapy Checklists*
- *Medication Error Checklists*
- *Drug Calculation Problems*
- *Electronic Calculators*
- *Top 200 Drugs with Pronunciations*
- *References from the Textbook*

Outline

Objectives

- Discuss the actions of drugs classified as *biologic response modifiers.*
- Describe two client populations that may benefit from the use of biologic response modifiers.
- Discuss three common side effects of interferons, colony-stimulating factors, and interleukin-2.
- Distinguish anaphylaxis reactions from the anaphylactoid reactions caused by the administration of monoclonal antibody therapy.
- Describe the nursing process, including client teaching, when caring for clients who receive biologic response modifiers.

Terms

absolute neutrophil count (ANC), p. 578
biologic response modifiers (BRMs), p. 571
colony-stimulating factors (CSFs), p. 574
epidermal growth factor receptor (EGFR), p. 585
erythropoietin (EPO), p. 575

erythropoietin stimulating agents (ESAs), p. 575
granulocyte, p. 577
granulocyte colony-stimulating factor, p. 577
granulocyte macrophage colony-stimulating factor, p. 579

human epidermal growth factor receptor 2 (HER2), p. 585
hybridoma technology, p. 571
interferons (IFNs), p. 571
interleukins, p. 582
keratinocyte growth factor, p. 584

lymphokines, p. 582
macrophages, p. 572
myelosuppression, p. 575
nadir, p. 577
neutrophils, p. 575
pegylation, p. 579
recombinant DNA, p. 571
thrombocytopenia, p. 573

Biologic response modifiers (BRMs) are a class of pharmacologic agents used to enhance the body's immune system. (Another group of immunostimulants are monoclonal antibodies, considered targeted therapy agents and discussed in Chapter 37.) **Recombinant DNA** (the genetic engineering process that produces mass quantities of human proteins) and **hybridoma technology** (the process that uses mice to mass-produce monoclonal antibodies) are two advances that have led to commercial mass production of BRMs (Figure 38–1). Interferons (α, β, γ), colony-stimulating factors, interleukins, and monoclonal antibodies are some currently known BRMs. With the exception of monoclonal antibodies, BRMs are complex proteins produced by the cells of the immune system (Figure 38–2). Individuals taking BRMs are immune-compromised and should be counseled on concurrent drug and herb use (Herbal Alert 38–1).

The following three BRM functions have been identified:

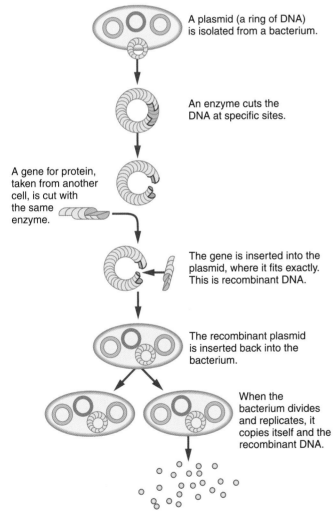

A plasmid (a ring of DNA) is isolated from a bacterium.

An enzyme cuts the DNA at specific sites.

A gene for protein, taken from another cell, is cut with the same enzyme.

The gene is inserted into the plasmid, where it fits exactly. This is recombinant DNA.

The recombinant plasmid is inserted back into the bacterium.

When the bacterium divides and replicates, it copies itself and the recombinant DNA.

The new gene directs the bacterium to make a new protein product, such as interferon.

FIGURE 38–1   Recombinant DNA. (Redrawn from *Understanding the immune system*, NIH Pub No 88-529, Bethesda, MD, 1991, National Institutes of Health, p. 29.)

- Enhance host immunologic function (immunomodulation)
- Destroy or interfere with tumor activities (cytotoxic/cytostatic effects)
- Promote differentiation of stem cells (other biologic effects) (Table 38–1)

While many BRMs have clinical indications, others are under investigation. Erythropoietin-stimulating agents (darbepoetin [Aranesp], epoetin-alfa [Procrit]), granulocyte colony-stimulating factors (GCSF) (filgrastim [Neupogen], pegfilgrastim [Neulasta]), granulocyte macrophage colony-stimulating factor (GMCSF) (sargramostim [Leukine]), thrombopoietic growth factor (oprelvekin [Neumega]), interferons (interferon alfa-2a [Roferon A], interferon alfa-2b [Intron A], interferon gamma [Actimmune]), and interleukin-2 (aldesleukin [Proleukin]) are approved by the Food and Drug Administration (FDA) and commercially available. A number of monoclonal antibodies have been approved by the FDA (see Chapter 37). Interferons, interleukins, and colony-stimulating factors are discussed in this chapter.

Interferons

Interferons (IFNs) are a family of naturally occurring proteins that were first discovered in the 1950s. Three major types of IFNs have been identified: alpha (α) IFN, beta (β) IFN, and gamma (γ) IFN. Each type is produced by a different cell within the immune system. All three types can be manufactured using recombinant DNA technology. Type I IFNs include IFNs-α and -β, which bind selectively to either α- or β-cell surface receptors on effector cells. Interferon gamma (IFN-γ) is a type II IFN and binds to a

Table 38–1

Action of Biologic Response Modifiers

Biologic Response Modifier	Action
Interleukins	I
Interferons	I, C
Monoclonal antibodies	C
Tumor necrosis factor	C
Colony-stimulating factors	O

C, Cytotoxic/cytostatic; *I*, immunomodulation; *O*, other biologic activity.

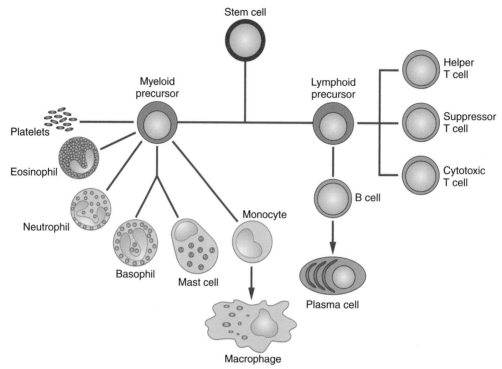

FIGURE 38–2 Cells of the immune system. (Redrawn from *Understanding the immune system,* NIH Pub No 88-529, Bethesda, MD, 1991, National Institutes of Health, p. 5.)

different cell surface receptor. Common to both Type I and II IFNs are their abilities to (1) regulate the immune system to improve resistance to invading micro-organisms and (2) reduce cell proliferation. However, each IFN group has specific functionality as well.

Interferon-α

Interferon alpha (IFN-α) is produced by B cells, T cells, **macrophages** (type of monocyte—the major phagocytic cells of the immune system), and null cells in response to the presence of viruses or tumor cells. This interferon has been shown to have antiviral, antiproliferative, and immunomodulatory effects, which means that IFN-α inhibits intracellular replication of viral DNA, interferes with tumor cell growth, and enhances natural killer (NK) cell (antitumor) activity. Recombinant IFN-α is manufactured as Roferon-A (alfa-2a) and Intron A (alfa-2b).

Roferon-A is approved by the FDA for the treatment of (1) hairy cell leukemia in patients 18 years and older; (2) minimally pretreated patients with chronic-phase Philadelphia chromosome positive chronic myelogenous leukemia (CML) within 1 year of diagnosis, and (3) non-malignant condition-chronic hepatitis C. Intron A is FDA approved for the treatment of patients with (1) malignant melanoma (adjuvant), (2) hairy cell leukemia, (3) follicular non-Hodgkin's lymphoma (NHL), (4) AIDS-related Kaposi sarcoma, and (5) non-malignant condition-chronic hepatitis B and C and condylomata acuminata. Clinically IFN-α has been used to treat non-Hodgkin's lymphoma (intermediate grade), cutaneous T-cell lymphoma, multiple myeloma, renal cell carcinoma, malignant melanoma, bladder cancer,

and carcinoid (a type of cancer-like disease). Intravesical administration of IFN-α has proved successful for low-grade bladder tumors; intraperitoneal administration of IFN-α has been used to treat ovarian cancer; and intralesional application of IFN-α has been used to treat melanoma and basal cell carcinoma. IFN-α-n3 is a human leukocyte-derived interferon which binds to the same receptors as IFN-α-2b. It is FDA approved for intralesional treatment of refractory or recurring external condylomata acuminata in patients 18 years of age or older.

Interferon Beta (IFN-β)

IFN-β (Betaseron, IFN-β-1b) is FDA indicated for the treatment of multiple sclerosis. Specifically this interferon (1) enhances the activity of suppressor T-cells (thymocyte-dependent lymphocytes that turn off an immune reaction—an active part of the cell-mediated immune system), (2) reduces the production of proinflammatory cytokines, (3) reduces antigen-presentation (recruiting members of the immune system to start an immune reaction), and (4) inhibits the movement of lymphocytes in the central nervous system.

Interferon Gamma

IFN-γ (Actimmune, IFN-γ-1b) is FDA indicated for (1) delaying time to disease progression in patients with severe malignant osteopetrosis, and (2) reducing the frequency and severity of serious infections related to chronic granulomatous disease. IFN-γ-1b has been shown to: (1) enhance oxidative metabolism of macrophages, (2) enhance antibody-dependent cell cytotoxicity (ADCC), (3) activate natural killer (NK) cells, and (4) enhance the Fc receptors (on antibody) and major histocompatibility antigens (HLA). Malignant osteopetrosis is a congenital disorder hallmarked by two characteristic defects: a defect in osteoclasts that causes bone overgrowth and a defect in phagocyte oxidative metabolism, which can be improved with IFN-γ-1b. Chronic granulomatous disease (CGD) is an inherited error in leukocyte function related to enzyme defects that are responsible for killing invading microorganisms (phagocyte superoxide generation).

Pharmacokinetics

IFN-α is metabolized by the liver and filtered by the kidneys. However, the body absorbs approximately 80% of the dose. Peak serum concentrations are reached 4 to 8 hours after administration. IFN-α can be administered subcutaneously (subQ), intramuscularly (IM), and intravenously (IV), although subQ or IM administration are the preferred routes of administration; subQ administration is recommended for clients with platelet counts below 50,000. Interferons-α-n3, -β and -γ will not be discussed further, since they are not used as antineoplastic agents.

Side Effects and Adverse Reactions

The major side effect of IFN-α is a flulike syndrome. Other effects occur in the gastrointestinal (GI), neurologic, cardiopulmonary, renal, hepatic, hematologic, and dermatologic systems.

The flulike syndrome is characterized by chills, fever, fatigue, malaise, and myalgias. Chills can occur 3 to 6 hours after IFN-α administration and may progress to rigors. A fever as high as 101° F to 104° F (39° C to 40° C) may occur within 30 to 90 minutes after the onset of chills and last 24 hours. Fatigue, malaise, and myalgias are cumulative side effects; fatigue is the dose-limiting toxicity (i.e., the side effect that necessitates a decrease in dose or discontinuation of the drug).

GI side effects include nausea, diarrhea, vomiting, anorexia, taste alterations, and xerostomia (dry mouth). These side effects are mild; anorexia is considered the dose-limiting toxicity for this system.

Neurologic side effects are reversible (after the drug is stopped) and occur in 70% of clients who receive IFN-α. These effects are manifested by mild confusion, somnolence (sleepiness), irritability, poor concentration, seizures, transient aphasia (temporary loss of ability to speak), hallucinations, paranoia, and psychoses. Depression, suicidal ideation and suicide attempts have occurred in clients taking IFN-α, requiring drug discontinuance.

Cardiopulmonary side effects are dose-related and occur more frequently in older adults and clients with underlying cardiac disease. Side effects include tachycardia, pallor, cyanosis, tachypnea, nonspecific electrocardiographic changes, rare myocardial infarction, and orthostatic hypotension.

Renal and hepatic effects are dose-dependent and usually result in few or no symptoms. The effects are manifested by increased blood urea nitrogen (BUN) and creatinine levels, proteinuria, and elevated transaminases.

Hematologic effects are reversible and dose-limiting. Neutropenia (decreased number of neutrophils in the blood) and **thrombocytopenia** (decreased number of thrombocytes in the blood) are manifestations of such effects. Neutropenia is usually rare and does not predispose the client to infection. Thrombocytopenia is more common in clients with hematopoietic (affecting the formation of blood cells) diseases than in those with solid tumors.

Maculopapular rashes of the trunk and extremities, pruritus, irritation at the injection site, desquamation (shedding of epithelial cells of the skin), and alopecia are dermatologic effects of IFN-α. Alopecia can occur after more than 4 months of therapy.

Dosing and Preparation

Roferon-A is supplied in prefilled syringes containing 3 million International Units per 0.5 ml, 6 million International Units per 0.5 ml, and 9 million International Units per 0.5 ml. All prefilled syringes should be refrigerated at 36° F to 46° F (2° C to 8° C). The syringes should not be frozen or shaken and should be protected from light.

Intron A is supplied as single-use vials (either powder or liquid), multidose vials, and multidose pens. The lyophilized powder is for single-dose use, and available in 10, 18, and 50 million International Units. The powder is reconstituted with 1 ml of the provided diluent (sterile water for injection) and gently swirled to dissolve. Final vial concentrations are 10 million International Units/ml, 18 million International Units/ml, and 50 million International Units/ml. The single-dose solution vial for injection is available as 10 million International Units (10 million International Units/ml), and multidose vials are available as 18 million International Units (3 million International Units/0.5 ml) and 25 million International Units (5 million International Units/0.5 ml). The multidose pens for injection are available as pens containing 3 million International Units (with a concentration of 22.5 million International Units/1.5 ml delivering 3 million International Units/0.2 ml, and containing 6 doses), 5 million Units (concentration 37.5 million International Units, with each dose of 5 million International Units/0.2 ml, containing 6 doses), and 10 million International Units (concentration 75 million International Units, with each dose of 10 million International Units /0.2 ml, containing 6 doses). Multidose solutions and pens should be stored at 36° F to 46° F (2° C to 8° C). The IFN alphas are listed in Table 38–2 with their dosages, uses, and considerations.

Administration

The administration of IFN-α is contraindicated in clients with known hypersensitivity to IFN-α, mouse immunoglobulin, or any component of the product. It should be used cautiously in clients with severe cardiac, renal, or hepatic disease and in those with seizure disorders or central nervous system dysfunction. Manufacturers recommend administering the agent to persons 18 years or older only under the supervision of a qualified physician. There have been no studies demonstrating the safety and effectiveness of IFN-α in pregnant women, nursing mothers, or children. Women of childbearing age should use contraceptives while receiving IFN-α because of the agent's effects on serum estra-

Table 38–2

Biologic Response Modifiers: Interferons

Generic (Brand)	Route and Dosage	Uses and Considerations
interferon alfa-2a (Roferon-A)	*Hairy-cell leukemia:* A: subQ /IM: 3 million international units daily for 16-24 wk, then maintenance dose 3 million international units subQ /IM 3 times wk *Chronic myelogenous leukemia:* A: subQ: 9 million international units daily (gradually increase initial dose of 3 million international units daily for 3 days to 6 million for 3 days, and then increasing to final 9 million international units dose	For treating hairy-cell leukemia, chronic myelogenous leukemia, condyloma acuminata, and AIDS-related Kaposi sarcoma. Flulike symptoms such as fatigue, aches, pain, fever, chills, headaches may occur. *Pregnancy category:* C; PB: UK; $t^{1/2}$: 2-3 h
interferon alfa-2b (Intron A)	*Hairy cell leukemia:* A: Subcutaneous/IM: 2 million international units/m² 3 times a wk for up to 6 months *Kaposi sarcoma:* A: IM/subQ: Initially: 30 million international units three times a week until severe intolerance or maximal response at 16 wk; use only 50-million international units strength; 50% dose reduction for severe side effects *Malignant melanoma:* A: Induction: 20 million international units/m² IV over 20 min daily for 5 consecutive days per wk, × 4 wk. Maint: 10 million international units/m² subQ 3 times wk for 48 wk *Follicular lymphoma:* A: 5 million international units subQ 3 times wk for up to 18 mo, together with anthracycline-containing chemotherapy regimen and then alone after chemotherapy is completed	Hairy-cell leukemia, adjuvant to surgical resection of malignant melanoma, follicular non-Hodgkin's lymphoma, condyloma acuminata, AIDS-related Kaposi sarcoma, and chronic hepatitis B and non-A hepatitis. Flulike symptoms may occur. Monitor CBC, AST, ALT, ALP, LDH. *Pregnancy category:* C; PB: UK; $t^{1/2}$: 2 h
interferon gamma-1b (Actimmune)	*Body surface area:* >0.5 m²: A: subQ: 50 mcg/m² 3 × wk *Body surface area:* <0.5 m²: A & C: >1 y: subQ: 1.5 mcg/kg 3 × wk	For treating chronic granulomatous disease. Flulike symptoms may occur. *Pregnancy category:* C; PB: UK; $t^{1/2}$: 0.5-6 h
interferon alfa-n3 (Alferon N)	*Condylomata acuminata:* A: Inject into wart: 250,000 units (0.05 ml) twice weekly; *max:* 8 wk Do not repeat for >3 mo after end of therapy	For treating recurring condylomata acuminata (genital venereal warts). Flulike symptoms may occur. Monitor CBC, AST, ALT, ALP, LDH. *Pregnancy category:* C; PB: UK; $t^{1/2}$: 6-8 h
interferon beta-1b (Betaseron)	Reduce number of clinical exacerbations of multiple sclerosis: A: >18 y: subQ: 8 million units every other day C: Not recommended	For treating multiple sclerosis (MS). Flulike symptoms may occur. *Pregnancy category:* C; PB: UK; $t^{1/2}$: 8 min-4.3 h

A, Adult; *AIDS,* acquired immunodeficiency syndrome; *ALT,* alanine aminotransferase; *ALP,* alkaline phosphatase; *AST,* aspartate aminotransferase; *C,* child; *CBC,* complete blood count; *h,* hour; *IM,* intramuscular; *IV,* intravenous; *LDH,* lactate dehydrogenase; *maint,* maintenance; *max,* maximum; *min,* minute; *mo,* month; *PB,* protein-binding; *subQ,* subcutaneous; $t^{1/2}$, half-life; *UK,* unknown; *wk,* week; *y,* year; >, greater than; <, less than.

diol and progesterone concentrations. Studies have not demonstrated fertility or teratogenic effects in men.

It is recommended that baseline and periodic complete blood counts (CBCs) and liver function tests be performed during the course of IFN therapy. Manufacturers suggest that clients undergo IFN therapy for at least 6 months before a decision is made whether to continue treatment in those who respond or discontinue treatment in those who do not; optimal treatment duration has not been determined. Patients should be well hydrated during IFN therapy, especially during treatment for malignant melanoma, because this minimizes severe side effects. Dose reductions of 50% or drug discontinuation should be considered if severe adverse reactions occur. Concurrent or prior treatment with chemotherapeutic agents or radiation therapy may increase the effectiveness and toxicity of IFN-α.

Colony-Stimulating Factors

Hematopoietic **colony-stimulating factors (CSFs)** are proteins that stimulate or regulate the growth, maturation, and differentiation of bone marrow stem cells. The CSFs are manufactured through recombinant DNA techniques.

Although CSFs are not directly tumoricidal, they are useful in cancer treatment, because they do the following:

- Decrease the length of posttreatment neutropenia (the length of time **neutrophils** (a type of white blood cell) are decreased secondary to chemotherapy), thereby reducing the incidence and duration of infection
- Permit the delivery of higher doses of drugs. **Myelosuppression** (suppression of bone marrow activity) is often a dose-limiting toxicity of chemotherapy. Higher, possibly tumoricidal, doses of drugs cannot be administered because of potentially life-threatening side effects. Colony Stimulating Factors can minimize the myelosuppressive toxicity, thus allowing the delivery of higher doses of drugs.
- Reduce bone marrow recovery time after bone marrow transplantation
- Enhance macrophage or granulocyte tumor-, virus-, and fungus-destroying ability
- Prevent severe thrombocytopenia after myelosuppressive chemotherapy

Colony stimulating factors have been used to treat clients with neutropenia secondary to disease or treatment and can be administered both IV and subQ. The CSFs that are FDA approved for clinical use are erythropoietin stimulating agents, granulocyte colony-stimulating factor (G-CSF), granulocyte macrophage colony-stimulating factor (GM-CSF), and thrombopoietic growth factor.

Erythropoietin Stimulating Agents

Erythropoietin stimulating agents (ESAs) include epoetin alfa (Procrit) and darbepoetin alfa (Aranesp). **Erythropoietin** is a glycoprotein produced by the kidney; it stimulates red blood cell production in response to hypoxia (decreased oxygen to body tissues). Specifically erythropoietin stimulates the division and differentiation of committed red blood cell progenitors (parent cells destined to become circulating red blood cells) in the bone marrow. Recently, ESAs have undergone close scrutiny as data from clinical trials reveal more deaths in cancer patients receiving ESAs as compared to patients receiving red blood cell transfusions. Therefore ESAs should be used cautiously and only as indicated, because of the increased risk for death and serious cardiovascular events when administered to increase hemoglobin levels to greater than 12 g/dl. Procrit is currently FDA approved for treatment of clients with anemia secondary to chronic renal failure (CRF), zidovudine (AZT)-treated human immunodeficiency virus (HIV) infections, cancer chemotherapy, and anemic patients who are undergoing surgery. Aranesp is FDA approved for treatment of anemia resulting from chronic renal failure and for use with chemotherapy treatment of nonmyeloid malignancies. The use of ESAs in clients with anemia may decrease the need for and frequency of red cell transfusion.

Pharmacokinetics

Erythropoietin Stimulating Agents can be administered IV (IV push) or subQ. According to the manufacturer, ESAs administered by IV are eliminated at a rate consistent with first-order kinetics (process by which the drug is eliminated in part by hepatic and renal blood flow). It has a circulating half-life ranging from approximately 4 to 13 hours in clients with CRF. Plasma levels of Procrit have been detected for at least 24 hours. After subQ administration of Procrit to CRF clients, peak serum levels are achieved within 5 to 24 hours. The half-life of IV-administered Procrit is approximately 20% shorter in normal clients without CRF than in clients with CRF. (Pharmacokinetic studies have not been done with HIV-infected clients.) Prototype Drug Chart 38–1 details the characteristics of this biologic response modifier.

Side Effects and Adverse Reactions

It is imperative that the target hemoglobin never exceed 12 g/dl, because the risks of death, serious cardiovascular events, and tumor progression increase at greater values. Close monitoring of hemoglobin response to the ESA and possible dose modification are essential to safe therapy.

The side effects of erythropoietin include hypertension, headache, arthralgias (joint pain), nausea, edema, fatigue, diarrhea, vomiting, chest pain, injection site skin reaction, asthenia (weakness), dizziness, seizures, thrombosis (clots), and allergic reactions. Studies demonstrate that ESA administration is usually well tolerated, and there have been no reports of serious allergic reactions or anaphylaxis. Rare transient skin reactions have been reported. Blood pressure may increase in clients with CRF who receive ESA during the early phase of treatment when the hematocrit (Hct) is on the rise. About 25% of clients with CRF who receive dialysis may require initiation of or increase in antihypertensive therapy. It is postulated that increases in blood pressure may relate to increases in Hct; therefore it is recommended that the dose of ESA be decreased if the Hct increase exceeds four points in any 2-week period. Similarly an increase in Hct may cause increased vascular access clotting (clots in the blood vessel at the connection site of the artificial kidney) in hemodialysis clients. Clients may require increased heparinization during ESA therapy to prevent clotting of the artificial kidney. Seizures occurred in clients with CRF who received ESA during clinical trials; activity was particularly evident during the first 90 days of therapy.

Dosing

Procrit should be administered at starting doses of 50 to 100 units/kg three times a week for clients with CRF. For clients receiving cancer chemotherapy the dose should be 150 units/kg three times a week or 40,000 units per week given subQ. The dose should be reduced by 25% when the Hgb approaches 12 g/dl or increases greater than 1 g/dl in any 2 weeks. The dose should be held if the Hgb exceeds 12 g/dl until the Hgb falls below 11 g/dl and then restarted at 25% below the previous dose. Aranesp dose is 2.25 mcg/kg subQ every week or 500 mcg subQ every 3 weeks. If the rate of Hgb increase is greater than 1 g/dl in 2 weeks or if the Hgb is greater than 11 g/dl, the dose should be reduced by 40% of the prior dose. If the Hgb is greater than 12 g/dl, the dose should be held until the Hgb is less than 11g/dl, and the dose should be restarted at 40% of the previous dose.

Prototype DRUG CHART 38–I

EPOETIN ALFA (ERYTHROPOIETIN)

Drug Class

Biologic response modifier
Trade names: Epogen, Procrit, ✦Eprex
Pregnancy Category: C

Dosage

A: Modify dose to keep target hemoglobin ≤12 g/dl
CRF: 50-100 units/kg 3 × wk,
Cancer Chemotherapy: 150 units/kg 3 × wk or
    40,000 units/wk
IV: Dialysis clients
IV/subQ: Nondialysis, CRF clients
IV/subQ: 100 U/kg 3 × wk for 8 wk in AZT-treated HIV-
    infected clients
Initial dose to those with EPO levels <500 mU/ml and
    receiving <4200 mg of AZT/wk. Clients with EPO level
    >500 mU/ml are unlikely to respond to EPO therapy.
subQ: Cancer chemotherapy

Contraindications

Uncontrolled hypertension, hypersensitivity to
    mammalian cell-derived products or human albumin
Caution: Pregnancy, lactation, porphyria; safety in
    children not known; increased mortality and/or
    tumor progression, serious cardiovascular and
    thromboembolic events if target hemoglobin of
    12 g/dl exceeded.

Drug-Lab-Food Interactions

Drug: None known
Lab: Increase hematocrit, *decrease* plasma volume
Clients with serum ferritin <100 mcg/L, or serum
    transferring saturation <20% should receive
    supplemental iron therapy
Food: None known

Pharmacokinetics

Absorption: subQ, IV
Distribution: PB: UK
Metabolism: t½: 4-13 h in clients with CRF;
    20% less in those with normal renal function
Excretion: In urine

Pharmacodynamics

IV: Onset: 7-10 d
    Peak: 2-4 wk
    Duration: UK
subQ: Onset: 7-10 d
    Peak: 5-24 h
    Duration: UK

Therapeutic Effects/Uses

To treat anemia secondary to CRF or AZT (zidovudine) treatment of HIV infections. Use in clients with anemia sec-
    ondary to cancer chemotherapy
Mode of Action: Increased production of RBCs triggered by hypoxia or anemia

Side Effects

Sense of well-being, hypertension, arthralgias,
    nausea, edema, fatigue, injection site reaction,
    rash, diarrhea, shortness of breath

Adverse Reactions

Seizures, hyperkalemia
Life-threatening: Cerebrovascular accident, myocardial
    infarction

A, Adult; *CRF,* chronic renal failure; *d,* day; *EPO,* erythropoietin; *h,* hour; *HIV,* human immunodeficiency virus; *IV,* intravenous; *PB,*
protein-binding; *RBC,* red blood cell; *subQ,* subcutaneous; *t½,* half-life; *UK,* unknown; *wk,* week; <, less than; >, greater than;
✦, Canadian drug name.

According to the manufacturer the following situations must be considered and evaluated if a client does not respond to an ESA or maintain a response:

1. Iron deficiency
2. Underlying infections, inflammatory or malignant processes
3. Occult blood loss
4. Underlying hematologic disease
5. Folic acid or vitamin B_{12} deficiency
6. Hemolysis
7. Aluminum intoxication

8. Osteitis fibrosa cystica (fibrous degeneration with formation of cysts and nodules secondary to hyperparathyroidism)

Administration

Erythropoietin stimulating agent administration is contraindicated in clients with (1) uncontrolled hypertension, (2) known hypersensitivity to mammalian cell-derived products, and (3) known hypersensitivity to human albumin or polysorbate. Evaluation of iron stores should occur during erythropoietin therapy. Transferrin saturation should be at least 20% and ferritin should be at least 100 ng/ml. Iron supplements may be used to increase and maintain transferrin saturation to support erythropoietin stimulated erythropoiesis.

The safety and effectiveness of ESA therapy in pregnant women, nursing mothers, and children have not been established. There are no known ESA drug interactions.

Preparation

The following are the manufacturer's preparation and administration recommendations for Procrit:

1. Do not shake, because shaking may denature the glycoprotein, rendering it biologically inactive.
2. Use only one dose per vial. Do not reenter the vial. Discard any unused portion, because the vial contains no preservatives.
3. Store the 2000-, 3000-, 4000-, 10,000-, 20,000-, or 40,000 unit vials at 36° F to 46° F (2° C to 8° C). Do not freeze.
4. Warm the vial to room temperature before subQ administration.
5. Use the smallest volume of erythropoietin per injection (1 ml or less per injection) to decrease injection site discomfort.
6. Use ice to numb the injection site.
7. Do not use the same needle to draw medication into the syringe and to inject the medication. Use a new needle to inject medication.

The single-dose vial contains no preservative; the multidose vial contains preservatives and must be stored at 36° F to 46° F (2° C to 8° C) between doses; discard 21 days after initial access.

Aranesp is available in 1 ml single-dose polysorbate preserved vials OR 1 ml single-dose, albumin containing vials (200 mcg/ml, 300 mcg/ml, 500 mcg/ml); single-dose prefilled syringes (with either polysorbate or albumin) in 200 mcg/0.4 L, 300 mcg/0.6 ml, or 500 mcg/1 ml doses with 27 gauge ^{1}/$_2$ inch needle (SingleJect); single-dose prefilled SureClick autoinjector (with either polysorbate or albumin) in 25 mcg/0.42 ml, 40 mcg/0.4 ml, 60 mcg/0.3 ml, 100 mcg/0.5 ml, 150 mcg/0.3 ml, 200 mcg/0.4 ml, 300 mcg/0.6 ml, and 500 mcg/1 ml. All forms of the drug should be stored at 36° F to 46° F (2° C to 8° C), protected from freezing, shaking, and from light.

Granulocyte Colony-Stimulating Factor

Filgrastim (Neupogen) and pegfilgrastim (Neulasta) are human **granulocyte** (type of white blood cell [WBC] responsible for fighting infection) colony-stimulating factors (G-CSF) produced by recombinant DNA technology. **Granulocyte colony-stimulating factor** is a glycoprotein produced by monocytes (a type of WBC), fibroblasts (immature fiber-producing cells), and endothelial cells (cells that line the heart cavity and blood and lymph vessels). It regulates the production of neutrophils (granular leukocytes, WBCs) within the bone marrow. It is FDA approved and commercially available for the following indications to decrease the incidence of infections in clients: (1) receiving myelosuppressive cancer chemotherapy, (2) receiving induction or consolidation chemotherapy for acute myeloid leukemia, (3) receiving bone marrow transplantation for cancer, (4) undergoing peripheral blood progenitor cell collection and therapy (mobilization of stem cells for rescue), and (5) with severe, chronic neutropenia. Granulocyte colony-stimulating factor has been evaluated as an adjunct to chemotherapy for both solid tumor and hematologic malignancies and has been evaluated in studies using a number of different chemotherapy regimens. Filgrastim and pegfilgrastim are commercially available forms of G-CSF. Prototype Drug Chart 38–2 gives the drug data for filgrastim and pegfilgrastim.

Filgrastim

Pharmacokinetics

Filgrastim administration results in a two-phase neutrophil response. An early response is seen within 24 hours of administration, and then following the chemotherapy-induced **nadir** (lowest value of formed blood cells) there is a second peak in circulating neutrophils. The proliferation-induced increase in neutrophils usually begins 4 to 5 days after administration is initiated, but timing may vary based on the type and dose of myelosuppressive therapy, the client's underlying disease, and prior treatment history. The elimination half-life of G-CSF in both normal clients and those with cancer is 3.5 hours. Clearance rates are approximately 0.5 to 0.7 ml/min/kg.

Side Effects and Adverse Reactions

The side effects of filgrastim therapy include nausea, vomiting, skeletal pain, alopecia, diarrhea, neutropenia, fever, mucositis, fatigue, anorexia, dyspnea, headache, cough, skin rash, chest pain, generalized weakness, sore throat, stomatitis, constipation, and pain of unspecified origin. Of these reactions bone pain is the only consistently observed reaction attributed to G-CSF therapy, and this relates to the expanding bone marrow. Bone pain was of mild to moderate severity and well controlled with nonopioid analgesia. It occurs more frequently in clients receiving higher (20 to 100 mcg/kg daily) IV doses than in clients receiving lower (3 to 10 mcg/kg daily) subcutaneous doses. Rarely splenic rupture may occur, and clients who complain of left upper abdominal pain and/or shoulder tip pain, should be evaluated for an enlarged spleen or splenic rupture. The drug may rarely cause adult respiratory distress syndrome in neutropenic patients who are septic and may cause sickle cell crisis in patients with sickle cell disease.

Dosing

Granulocyte colony-stimulating factor should not be administered 24 hours before or after the administration of chemotherapy agents, because of the potential sensitivity of rapidly dividing myeloid cells to chemotherapy. It may stimulate the proliferation of rapidly dividing cells that may be destroyed by chemotherapy drugs. Granulocyte colony-stimulating factor can be administered subQ and by IV infusion. The recommended starting dose of G-CSF for patients receiving myelosuppressive cancer chemotherapy is 5 mcg/kg daily subQ or IV infusion over 15-30

Prototype DRUG CHART 38–2

FILGRASTIM

Drug Class

Granulocyte colony-stimulating factor (G-CSF)
Trade names: Neupogen; long-acting pegylated form
is Neulasta
Pregnancy Category: C

Contraindications

Hypersensitivity to *Escherichia coli*-derived proteins;
24 hours before or after cytotoxic chemotherapy
Caution: Pregnancy, lactation; safety in children
not known

Dosage

A: IV inf/subQ: 5 mcg/kg/d
C: 5-10 mcg/kg/d
Neulasta: 6 mg subQ × 1 during chemotherapy cycle
Refer to specific protocols

Drug-Lab-Food Interactions

Drug: None known
Lab: Increase lactic acid, LDH, alkaline phosphatase;
transient *increase* in neutrophils
Food: None known

Pharmacokinetics

Absorption: subQ: Well absorbed
Distribution: PB: UK
Metabolism: t½: 2-3.5 h; Neulasta: 15-80 h
Excretion: Probably in urine

Pharmacodynamics

IV/subQ: Onset: 24 h
Peak: 3-5 d
Duration: 4-7 d

Therapeutic Effects/Uses (Neupogen)

To decrease incidence of infection in clients receiving myelosuppressive chemotherapeutic agents, including clients
with AML undergoing induction or consolidation therapy, and clients undergoing bone marrow transplant; adjunct to chemotherapy for both solid tumor and hematologic malignancies; and for mobilization of progenitor
stem cells used in autologous transplant; also for the treatment of clients with severe, chronic neutropenia.
Mode of Action: Increases production of neutrophils and enhances their phagocytosis

Side Effects

Nausea, vomiting, skeletal pain, alopecia, diarrhea,
fever, skin rash, anorexia, headache, cough, chest
pain, sore throat, constipation

Adverse Reactions

Neutropenia, dyspnea, splenomegaly, psoriasis,
hematuria
Life-threatening: Thrombocytopenia, myocardial infarction, adult respiratory distress syndrome in clients
with sepsis, splenic rupture

A, Adult; *C*, child; *d*, day; *h*, hour; *IV*, intravenous; *LDH*, lactate dehydrogenase; *PB*, protein-binding; *subQ*, subcutaneous; *t½*, half-
life; *UK*, unknown.

---

minutes. Doses may be increased in 5-mcg/kg increments
for each chemotherapy cycle, according to the duration
and severity of the absolute neutrophil count nadir. The
absolute neutrophil count (ANC) is determined using the
following equation:

$$ANC = \text{Total white blood cell count (WBC)} \times \text{percentage}$$
$$\text{of neutrophils} + \text{percentage of bands}$$

Granulocyte colony-stimulating factor causes a transient increase in neutrophil counts 1 to 2 days after initiation of therapy. However, to achieve a sustained therapeutic response, G-CSF therapy should be continued until
postchemotherapy nadir ANC is 10,000/mm³. Premature
discontinuation of G-CSF therapy before expected ANC
recovery is not recommended.

The dose of G-CSF given for bone marrow transplantation is 10 mcg/kg/day IV infusion over 4 hours or as a
continuous IV infusion over 24 hours. The first dose must
be given at least 24 hours after cytotoxic chemotherapy
and at least 24 hours after bone marrow infusion. Subse-

quent dosing is determined by the ANC. The dose of G-
CSF for stem cell mobilization (progenitor cell collection)
is 10 mcg/kg/day subQ or IV as a bolus or continuous infusion. It is given for at least 4 days prior to the first leukapheresis procedure and is continued until the last leukapheresis. Monitor the ANC closely and modify the dose if
the WBC is greater than 100,000/mm³.

Administration

Granulocyte colony-stimulating factor administration has
no demonstrable effects on fertility in male and female
rats. Its carcinogenic potential is not known. Caution
should be used when G-CSF is given to pregnant women
and nursing mothers. The manufacturer recommends that
the benefits justify the potential risks.

Filgrastim's efficacy has not been demonstrated in children, although safety data indicate that it does not cause
any greater toxicity in children than in adults.

There has been no evidence of other drug interaction
with filgrastim, but its administration is contraindicated in

clients with known hypersensitivity to *Escherichia coli*-derivant proteins.

Preparation

Neupogen is supplied either as 1-ml vials containing 300 mcg of filgrastim or as 1.6-ml vials containing 480 mcg of filgrastim or prefilled syringes (SingleJect with UltraSafe needle guard) containing 300 mcg of filgrastim in 0.5 ml (600 mcg/ml), or 480 mcg in 0.8 ml (600 mcg/ml). Both the vials and prefilled syringes are preservative-free, therefore the manufacturer recommends that the vials and syringes be used one time only and any vials left at room temperature for longer than 6 hours be discarded. Filgrastim should be stored in a refrigerator at 36° F to 46° F (2° C to 8° C). Do not freeze or shake the vials or syringes.

Pegfilgrastim

Pharmacokinetics

Filgrastim is eliminated via the kidneys. Pegfilgrastim is a pegylated (**pegylation** is the process of adding a polyethylene glycol [PEG] molecule to another molecule) form of filgrastim. Pegfilgrastim therefore becomes a larger substance and as a result is not as easily eliminated from the body via the kidneys. The decreased rate of urinary excretion keeps this G-CSF in the body longer, thereby reducing the frequency of injections. Filgrastim requires daily IV or subcutaneous injections for up to 2 weeks to be effective, whereas pegfilgrastim only requires a once per chemotherapy cycle injection to be effective. For clients and their families, this reduction in dosing frequency alleviates the burden of daily clinic trips for injections.

Pegfilgrastim is FDA indicated to decrease the incidence of infections and febrile neutropenia in clients with nonmyeloid malignancies receiving chemotherapy associated with clinically significant febrile neutropenia.

Side Effects and Adverse Reactions

Side effects are similar to those of filgrastim with the most frequently reported adverse event being bone pain. This bone pain is effectively reduced with acetaminophen 650 mg or ibuprofen 400 mg by mouth every 4 to 6 hours.

Dosing and Administration

The recommended dose is 6 mg of pegfilgrastim administered as a single subcutaneous injection given at least 24 hours after chemotherapy once per chemotherapy cycle. The drug should not be administered in the period between 14 days before and 24 hours after administration of cytotoxic chemotherapy.

Preparation, Storage, and Handling

Pegfilgrastim is supplied in prefilled syringes containing 6 mg in 0.6 ml. This colorless, preservative-free medication should be protected from light and refrigerated at 2° C to 8° C. Only one injection is to be given, and any unused pegfilgrastim must be discarded.

Granulocyte-Macrophage Colony-Stimulating Factor

Granulocyte-macrophage colony-stimulating factor (GM-CSF), or sargramostim, belongs to a group of growth factors that support survival, clonal expression, and differentiation (maturation) of hematopoietic progenitor cells. It induces partially committed progenitor (parent) cells to divide and differentiate in the granulocyte macrophage (a type of WBC responsible for recognizing and destroying bacteria through phagocytosis) pathway. Granulocyte-macrophage colony-stimulating factor, unlike G-CSF, is a multilineage factor, promoting proliferation of myelomonocytic, megakaryocytic, and erythroid progenitors. Activated T cells, endothelial cells, and fibroblasts produce GM-CSF in vivo. Commercial production of GM-CSF is accomplished through recombinant DNA technology and is FDA approved for use to induce and support myeloid reconstitution (1) after induction chemotherapy in acute myelogenous leukemia (AML), (2) in both autologous and allogeneic bone marrow transplant (BMT), (3) for the mobilization of autologous peripheral blood progenitor cells, and (4) in BMT failure or delayed engraftment. Sargramostim (GM-CSF) is commercially available as Leukine. Prototype Drug Chart 38–3 presents the drug data for sargramostim.

Pharmacokinetics

Granulocyte-Macrophage Colony-Stimulating Factor has been found to effectively accelerate myeloid engraftment (growth and development of bone marrow and subsequent circulating blood cell activity) in autologous BMT. After autologous BMT in clients with non-Hodgkin's lymphoma, acute lymphoblastic leukemia, or Hodgkin's disease, GM-CSF administration resulted in accelerated myeloid engraftment, decreased duration of antibiotic use, reduced duration of infectious episodes, and shortened hospitalizations.

Side Effects and Adverse Reactions

Side effects of GM-CSF administration include fever, mucous membrane disorder, asthenia, malaise, sepsis, nausea, diarrhea, vomiting, anorexia, liver damage, alopecia, rash, peripheral edema, dyspnea, blood dyscrasias, renal dysfunction, and central nervous system disorder. This drug should be administered with caution to clients with preexisting pleural or pericardial effusions, because it may increase fluid retention. Sequestration of granulocytes in the pulmonary circulation has been seen with GM-CSF administration. The phenomenon results in dyspnea and suggests that special attention be given to respiratory symptoms during or immediately following GM-CSF infusions, a caution that is especially important for clients with underlying pulmonary disease. The GM-CSF infusion should be reduced by half or discontinued if client experiences dyspnea.

Supraventricular dysrhythmia has been observed during GM-CSF infusion, suggesting cautious administration in clients with preexisting cardiac disease. Renal and hepatic dysfunction, as indicated by elevated serum creatinine, bilirubin, and liver function tests, have occurred with GM-CSF administration. If these values become elevated, GM-CSF dosage should be reduced or therapy interrupted.

Granulocyte macrophage-colony stimulating factor therapy is contraindicated in clients with excessive leukemia myeloid blast cells in the bone marrow or peripheral blood (greater than 10%) and in clients with known hypersensitivity to GM-CSF, yeast-derived products, or any component

Prototype **DRUG CHART 38–3**

SARGRAMOSTIM

Drug Class

Granulocyte macrophage colony-stimulating factor (GM-CSF)
Trade name: Leukine
Pregnancy Category: C

Contraindications

Within 24 h of chemotherapy administration or within 12 h after last dose of radiation therapy; excessive leukemia myeloid blast cells in bone marrow; hypersensitivity to GM-CSF, yeast-derived products
Caution: Pregnancy, lactation, heart failure; safety in children not established; not FDA approved for children

Dosage

A: IV: 250 mcg/m^2/d as a 2-h infusion for 21 d after autologous BMT; a maximum tolerated dose has not been determined
Some protocols use subQ administration.

Drug-Lab-Food Interactions

Drug: Lithium and steroids may increase effect
Lab: Increase in WBC and platelet counts, bilirubin, creatinine, and liver enzymes
Food: None known

Pharmacokinetics

Absorption: IV: Essentially complete
Distribution: PB: UK
Metabolism: t½: 2 h
Excretion: Probably in urine

Pharmacodynamics

IV: Onset: 7-14 d
  Peak: UK
  Duration: Baseline WBCs by 1 wk after administration

Therapeutic Effects/Uses

To accelerate growth and development of bone marrow and circulating blood cell activity in autologous BMT
Mode of Action: Increased production and functional activity of eosinophils, macrophages, monocytes, and neutrophils

Side Effects

Generally well tolerated; diarrhea, fatigue, chills, weakness, local irritation at injection site; peripheral edema, rash

Adverse Reactions

Pleural/pericardial effusion, rigors, GI hemorrhage, dyspnea

A, Adult; *BMT*, bone marrow transplant; *d*, day; *FDA*, Food and Drug Administration; *GI*, gastrointestinal; *h*, hour; *IV*, intravenous; *PB*, protein-binding; *subQ*, subcutaneous; *t½*, half-life; *UK*, unknown; *WBC*, white blood cell; *wk*, week.

---

of the product. Because of the sensitivity of rapidly dividing hematopoietic progenitor cells to cytotoxic chemotherapy or radiologic therapy, GM-CSF should not be administered within 24 hours before or after chemotherapy or within 12 hours before or after radiation therapy.

It should be administered to pregnant women or nursing mothers only if clearly indicated (i.e., if the benefits outweigh the risks). Efficacy in the pediatric population has not been established.

Carcinogenic, mutagenic, or fertility effects have not been determined. A full evaluation of drug interactions has not been conducted, but drugs that may potentiate the myeloproliferative effects of GM-CSF, such as lithium and corticosteroids, should be used with caution.

Dosing

The recommended dose of GM-CSF is 250 mcg/m^2/day for 21 days as a 2-hour infusion beginning 2 to 4 hours after autologous bone marrow infusion; or on day 11 (4 days after the completion of induction chemotherapy for AML)

until the ANC is greater than 1500 cells/mm^3. When used for stem cell mobilization, the dose is given daily prior to and through the period of stem cell collection; when used after stem cell reinfusion, the drug should be administered daily until the ANC is greater than 1500 cells/mm^3. When used for bone marrow transplant graft failure or delay, the drug is given daily for 14 days followed by an assessment of the response.

Administration

Granulocyte-macrophage colony-stimulating factor is administered IV over 2 to 4 hours or subQ. The drug should not be administered within 24 hours of chemotherapy administration or within 12 hours before or after radiation therapy. Manufacturers recommend dose reduction or discontinuation in the presence of a severe adverse reaction, appearance of blast cells (immature, possibly malignant cells), or disease progression. To avoid potential complications associated with leukocytosis, therapy should be stopped if the ANC is greater than 20,000 cells/mm^3.

Preparation

Leukine is available as lyophilized Leukine (250 mcg), a sterile, white, preservative-free powder that requires reconstitution, or as Liquid Leukine (500 mcg). The powder is reconstituted with 1 ml of sterile water for injection. During reconstitution the diluent should be directed at the side of the vial and the contents gently swirled but not shaken. Further dilution with 0.9% sodium chloride only is done in preparation for the 2-hour IV infusion. The final concentration of solution should be greater than 10 mcg/ml. The infusion should be completed within 6 hours of preparation to ensure stability and potency. Sargramostim powder, reconstituted vials, and diluted solution should be refrigerated at 36° F to 46° F (2° C to 8° C). The liquid sargramostim vials can be stored at 36° F to 46° F (2° C to 8° C) for up to 20 days once the vial has been entered.

Thrombopoietic Growth Factor

Oprelvekin is recombinant human interleukin-11, a platelet growth factor available commercially as Neumega. This product can potentially prevent recurrent severe chemotherapy-induced thrombocytopenia. According to the manufacturer, Oprelvekin stimulates megakaryocyte and thrombocyte production. This effect results in functionally and morphologically normal circulating platelets. Neumega is marketed as a much needed option in clients who are receiving myelosuppressive chemotherapy. Neumega is indicated to prevent severe thrombocytopenia and to reduce the need for platelet transfusions following myelosuppressive chemotherapy in adult patients with nonmyeloid malignancies who are at high risk of severe thrombocytopenia. Neumega is not indicated following myeloablative (transplant) chemotherapy. It has the potential to prevent severe thrombocytopenia and to reduce the need for platelet transfusions following myelosuppressive chemotherapy. Efficacy is most evident in those who experience severe thrombocytopenia following the previous chemotherapy cycle. However, in clinical practice the potential side effect of severe fluid retention limits its use.

Pharmacokinetics

Product dosing should begin 6 to 24 hours after the completion of chemotherapy. Studies have shown that daily subQ dosing for 14 days increased the platelet count in a dose-dependent way. Platelet counts begin to increase between 5 and 9 days after the start of Neumega administration. After administration of the product stops, the platelet count continues to rise for up to 7 days, returning to baseline within 14 days.

Animal studies demonstrate that Neumega is cleared rapidly from the serum and distributed to highly perfused organs. The kidney is the primary route of elimination, although most of the product is metabolized before excretion. Neumega is contraindicated in clients with a history of hypersensitivity to the product or any of its components and should be used cautiously in patients with heart failure.

Side Effects and Adverse Reactions

The side effects of Neumega include serious fluid retention, cardiovascular events, ophthalmologic events, and severe hypersensitivity reactions. Fluid retention as evidenced by peripheral edema, exertional dyspnea, and worsening of preexisting pleural effusions, ascites, and pericardial effusions is reversible within several days once the product is discontinued. Transient atrial arrhythmias (fibrillation or flutter) have occurred in approximately 10% of clients and postmarketing reports have indicated ventricular arrhythmias occur as well. These arrhythmias may be related to fluid retention, advanced age, or underlying cardiac disease. Papilledema and transient visual blurring have been reported in about 1.5% of clients. Postmarketing reports also indicate that hypersensitivity reactions including anaphylaxis have occurred, and the drug should be discontinued if there is evidence of symptomatic bronchospasm or anaphylaxis.

Drug interactions include Neumega and diuretics, which may increase the risk of hypokalemia. Laboratory abnormalities include a decrease in hemoglobin related to increased plasma volume (fluid retention), decreased serum proteins (albumin, transferrin, gamma globulins), and elevated plasma fibrinogen. No studies have been done to assess the carcinogenic potential of the product, and no studies have determined its safety and effectiveness in children, pregnant women, or nursing mothers. Use in these situations should be evaluated carefully.

Dosing

The recommended dose of Neumega in adults is 50 mcg/kg given once daily. It should be administered subQ as a single injection in the thigh, abdomen, hip, or upper arm. If the client has severe renal impairment (creatinine clearance less than 30 ml/min), the dose is reduced to 25 mcg/kg. Safety and efficacy in pediatric patients has not been established. The first dose of Neumega should be given 6 to 24 hours after the completion of chemotherapy. Platelet counts should be monitored to determine the duration of Neumega therapy.

Administration

Administration should continue until the post-nadir count is greater than 50,000 cells/μl. Dosing beyond 21 days is not recommended. Neumega should be discontinued at least 2 days before chemotherapy is begun.

Preparation

Neumega is available for subQ administration in single-use vials containing 5 mg of oprelvekin as a sterile, lyophilized powder. When reconstituted with 1 ml of sterile water for injection the resulting solution has a pH of 7.0 and a concentration of 5 mg/ml. Reconstituted Neumega is a clear, colorless, isotonic solution with a pH of 7.0. During reconstitution avoid excessive shaking of the vial; sterile water for injection USP should be directed at the side of the vial and contents swirled gently. Do not reenter or reuse a single-dose vial. The parenteral drug product should be visually inspected and discarded if there is discoloration or visible particulate matter.

Neumega should be used within 3 hours of reconstitution whether it has been stored refrigerated at 36° F to 46° F (2° C to 8° C) or at room temperature up to 77° F (25° C). Do not freeze and do not shake the reconstituted product.

Client Information

Self-administration of Neumega should not be attempted until the client fully understands the health care provider's instructions about its preparation, correct dose, and proper method for injection. The injection site should not be rubbed. The dose should be given at the same time each day. If a dose is missed the next scheduled dose should be taken.

NOTE: Clients can safely receive concurrent doses of ESA, G-CSF, and Neumega. Different injection sites should be used for each agent.

Interleukin-2

Interleukins are a group of proteins produced by the body's WBCs—the lymphocytes. Because interleukins are hormone-like glycoproteins manufactured by the lymphocytes, they are sometimes called **lymphokines.** One of the most widely studied interleukins is interleukin-2 (IL-2).

First defined in 1976 this substance was found to have antitumor activities, particularly in renal cell carcinoma and malignant melanoma. Interleukin-2 is produced commercially through recombinant DNA technology as aldesleukin (Proleukin). Proleukin is FDA-indicated for the treatment of metastatic renal cell carcinoma and metastatic melanoma.

Pharmacokinetics

Proleukin, administered either by IV infusion or subQ injection, is rapidly distributed to the extravascular, extracellular space and eliminated from the body by the kidney. The serum half-life of IL-2 is short, and because of this rapid clearance, IL-2 is administered frequently in short infusions.

Side Effects and Adverse Reactions

Proleukin should be administered only to patients with normal cardiac and pulmonary function, because side effects may be severe. The principal serious side effects are capillary leak syndrome and infection. *Capillary leak syndrome* is characterized by loss of vascular tone with leakage of plasma fluids into the extravascular space, including the lungs. This can cause hypotension and decreased blood circulation to vital organs, resulting in angina, myocardial infarction, respiratory distress, gastrointestinal bleeding, and mental status changes. Infection may result from alteration in neutrophil function, with the most severe infection being sepsis and bacterial endocarditis. Many clients with cancer are at risk for gram-negative infections related to their indwelling central lines, and they may benefit from prophylactic antibiotic therapy. The most frequent side effects reported as a result of IL-2 use include hypotension, nausea, vomiting, diarrhea, mental status changes, oliguria/anuria, anemia, thrombocytopenia, fever, chills, sinus tachycardia, pulmonary congestion, dyspnea, pain at injection site, fatigue, weakness, malaise, and elevated liver function tests. Table 38–3 lists adverse events/effects of IL-2. According to the manufacturer, Proleukin should be dis-

Table 38–3

Incidence of Adverse Events to Interleukin-2

Events by Body System	% of Clients	Events by Body System	% of Clients
Cardiovascular		**Gastrointestinal**	
Hypotension	85	Nausea and vomiting	87
(requiring pressors)	71	Diarrhea	76
Sinus tachycardia	70	Stomatitis	32
Arrhythmias	22	Anorexia	27
Atrial	8	Gastrointestinal bleeding	13
Supraventricular	5	(requiring surgery)	2
Ventricular	3	Dyspepsia	7
Junctional	1	Constipation	5
Bradycardia	7	Intestinal perforation/ileus	2
Premature ventricular contractions	5	Pancreatitis	1
Premature atrial contractions	4		
Myocardial Ischemia	3	**Neurologic**	
Myocardial infarction	2	Mental status changes	73
Cardiac arrest	2	Dizziness	17
Congestive heart failure	1	Sensory dysfunction	10
Myocarditis	1	Special sensory disorders (vision, speech, taste)	7
Stroke	1		
Gangrene	1	Syncope	3
Pericardial effusion	1	Motor dysfunction	2
Endocarditis	1	Coma	1
Thrombosis	1	Seizure (grand mal)	1

From *Proleukin: aldesleukin for injection,* Emeryville, CA, 2000, Chiron Corp.

continued permanently if certain organ system toxicities occur (Table 38–4) and should be held and restarted under specific parameters for other toxicities (Table 38–5).

Preparation

Proleukin is supplied in single-use vials, each containing 22×10^6 units of Proleukin. Unreconstituted vials should be stored refrigerated at 36° F to 46° F (2° C to 8° C). After aseptic reconstitution with 1.2 ml of sterile water for injection (*not* bacteriostatic water), each vial contains 18 million International Units (1.1 mg) of Proleukin. Inject the sterile water into the vial and swirl gently; do not shake. The resulting solution should be a clear, colorless to pale yellow liquid. Withdraw the indicated dose of Proleukin from the vial and dilute in a 50-ml 5% dextrose IV bag. If not used immediately the IV bag can be stored for 48 hours in a refrigerator. Infuse over a 15-minute period through nonfiltered IV tubing. Discard any unused portion

Table 38–4

Organ System Toxicities with Interleukin-2

Organ System	Permanently Discontinue Treatment for the Following Toxicities
Cardiovascular	Sustained ventricular tachycardia (5 beats) Cardiac rhythm disturbances not controlled or unresponsive to management Recurrent chest pain with electrocardiographic changes, documented angina, or myocardial infarction Pericardial tamponade
Pulmonary	Intubation required >72 h
Renal	Renal dysfunction requiring dialysis >72 h
Central nervous system	Coma or toxic psychosis lasting >48 h Repetitive or difficult-to-control seizures
Gastrointestinal	Bowel ischemia/perforation/gastrointestinal bleeding requiring surgery

From *Proleukin: aldesleukin for injection*, Emeryville, CA, 2000, Chiron Corp.
h, Hour; >, greater than.

Table 38–5

Interleukin-2 Dose Held and Given

Organ System	Hold Dose For:	Subsequent Doses May be Given If:
Cardiovascular	Atrial fibrillation, supraventricular tachycardia, or bradycardia that requires treatment or is recurrent or persistent Systolic BP <90 mmHg with increasing requirements for pressors Any ECG change consistent with MI or ischemia with or without chest pain; suspicion of cardiac ischemia	Client is asymptomatic with full recovery to normal sinus rhythm Systolic BP 90 mmHg and stable or improving requirements for pressors Client is asymptomatic, MI has been ruled out, clinical suspicion of angina is low
Pulmonary	O_2 saturation <94% on room air or <90% with 2 L O_2 by nasal prongs	O_2 saturation 94% on room air or 90% with 2 L O_2 by nasal prongs
Central nervous system	Mental status changes, including moderate confusion or agitation	Mental status changes completely resolved
Systemic	Sepsis syndrome, client is clinically unstable	Sepsis syndrome has resolved, client is clinically stable, infection is under treatment
Renal	Serum creatinine 4.5 mg/dl or a serum creatinine of 4 mg/dl in the presence of severe volume overload, acidosis, or hyperkalemia Persistent oliguria, urine output of 10 ml/h for 16 to 24 h with rising serum creatinine	Serum creatinine <4 mg/dl and fluid and electrolyte status is stable Urine output >10 ml/h with a decrease of serum creatinine 1.5 mg/dl or normalization of serum creatinine
Hepatic	Signs of hepatic failure, including encephalopathy, increasing ascites, liver pain, hypoglycemia	All signs of hepatic failure have resolved*
Gastrointestinal	Stool guaiac repeatedly >3-4+	Stool guaiac negative
Skin	Bullous dermatitis or marked worsening of preexisting skin condition (avoid topical steroid therapy)	Resolution of all signs of bullous dermatitis

From *Proleukin: aldesleukin for injection*, Emeryville, CA, 2000, Chiron Corp.
BP, Blood pressure; *ECG*, electrocardiographic; *h*, hour; *MI*, myocardial infarction; O_2, oxygen; >, greater than; <, less than.
*Discontinue all further treatment for that course. Consider starting a new course of treatment at least 7 weeks after cessation of adverse event and hospital discharge.

of the reconstituted drug. Table 38–6 presents route, dosage, use, and considerations information.

Keratinocyte Growth Factor

Keratinocyte growth factor (palifermin) is available commercially as Kepivance and is indicated for decreasing the incidence and duration of severe oral mucositis in patients with hematologic malignancies receiving myelotoxic therapy requiring hematologic stem cell support. There is no evidence at this time as to its safety (may stimulate growth of tumors dependent upon this growth factor) or efficacy in clients receiving chemotherapy for solid tumors. The drug is contraindicated in patients with hypersensitivity to *E. coli*-derived therapy or to palifermin.

Pharmacokinetics

Kepivance binds to the keratinocyte growth factor receptor on epithelial cells, such as those of the oral mucosa, and initiates proliferation, differentiation, and migration of the epithelial cells. Thicker buccal mucosa is laid down, and in clinical trials this led to a significantly reduced incidence of grade 3/4 oral mucositis, a decreased duration of oral mucositis, and less opioid use for oral mucositis in transplant clients.

Side Effects and Adverse Reactions

The most common side effects of Kepivance are skin toxicities (rash, erythema, edema, pruritus) and oral toxicities (tongue thickening, oral/perioral dysesthesia [distorted sensation], tongue discoloration, and taste alteration). Other side effects are hypertension and transient increases in serum lipase and serum amylase. The most concerning potential adverse reaction is the possible stimulation of tumor growth, in that some solid tumors are composed of epithelial cells, which are stimulated to grow when Kepivance stimulates keratinocyte growth receptors. For this reason the drug is approved only in hematologic malignancies treated with myelotoxic chemotherapy requiring stem cell support.

Drug Interactions

Kepivance binds to heparin, so lines containing heparin should be flushed with normal saline prior to the infusion of Kepivance and following the infusion of Kepivance.

Dosing and Administration

Kepivance must not be administered within 24 hours of, during, or within 24 hours after the administration of myelotoxic chemotherapy. Kepivance is administered in a dose of 60 mcg/kg/day as an IV bolus for three consecutive days *before* and three consecutive days *after* myelotoxic chemotherapy, for a total of six doses. The third dose must be administered 24 to 48 hours before chemotherapy. The fourth dose is given on the same day as, but after, stem cell reinfusion and at least four days after the third dose of Kepivance. Flush central lines with normal saline prior to and following the administration of Kepivance if heparin has been used in the line.

Preparation, Storage, and Handling

Kepivance is available as a white lyophilized powder for IV injection, which is reconstituted with 1.2 ml Sterile Water for Injection, USP, yielding a clear, colorless solution with a Kepivance concentration of 5 mg/ml. Do not shake or vigorously agitate the vial to mix. The reconstituted solu-

Preventing MEDICATION ERRORS

Do not confuse...

- **epoetin alfa (Epogen, Procrit)** and **darbepoetin (Aranesp)** with **Neupogen**

- **filgrastim (Neupogen)** with **Epogen, Aranesp,** or **Nutramigen**

- **sargramostim (Leukine)** with **Leukeran**

- **interferon alfa-2a (Roferon-A)** with **interferon alfa-2b**

- **interferon alfa-2b (Intron-A)** with **interferon alfa-2a**

- **interferon beta-1a (Avonex, Rebif)** with **interferon beta-1b (Avelox)**

- **interferon beta-1b (Betaseron)** with **interferon beta-1a**

- **interleukin-2 (IL-2, Proleukin)** with **interferon 2**

Table 38–6		
Interleukin*		
Generic (Brand)	**Route and Dosage**	**Uses and Considerations**
Interleukin-2 (Proleukin)	Two 5-day treatment periods separated by a rest period A: IV: 600,000 International Units/kg (0.037 mg/kg) by a 15-min IV infusion q8h for a maximum of 14 doses. Following 9 days of rest, the schedule is repeated for another 14 doses, for a maximum of 28 doses per course	For treating metastatic renal cancer and metastatic melanoma. DO NOT give dexamethasone during treatment unless absolutely necessary; it may negate the effects of Proleukin,

A, Adult; *d*, day; *h*, hour; *IV*, intravenous; *min*, minute; *wk*, week.
*Clients receiving IL-2 by any route, in any dose, and in any setting—inpatient or outpatient—should be monitored closely for signs of toxicity.

tion remains stable refrigerated in its carton at 36° F to 46° F (2° C to 8° C) for up to 24 hours. Prior to administration remove the reconstituted vial from the refrigerator and bring it to room temperature for up to one hour, while keeping it protected from light in its carton. If the vial is out of the refrigerator for more than one hour, it must be discarded. Also discard any remaining drug after the dose is withdrawn. Do not freeze or filter the drug.

Monoclonal Antibodies

Monoclonal antibodies are engineered in the laboratory for the specific purpose of targeting antigens and receptors that are expressed most frequently on cancer cells. Because of the specificity of the monoclonal antibody targets, their use has become known as *targeted therapy*. The human **epidermal growth factor receptor (EGFR)** contains two important receptors that are overexpressed or "turned on" in cancer: EGFR1 and EGFR2. EGFR2 is also known as **human epidermal growth factor 2 (HER2).** Overexpression of EGFR1 results in: (1) increased cell proliferation, (2) avoidance of programmed cell death or apoptosis, (3) increased cell invasiveness leading to metastasis, and (4) release of vascular endothelial growth factor (VEGF). Because a tumor cannot grow beyond 1-2 mm (the diffusion distance of oxygen) without a new blood supply, VEGF has become an important target. Inhibition of VEGF leads to prevention of new blood vessel formation and possibly normalization of malignant blood vessels. Drugs inhibiting these important receptors are discussed in Chapter 37.

Refer to Table 38–7 for information on additional monoclonal antibodies (targeted therapies) and the Preventing Medication Errors box for a safety alert related to BRMs.

Table 38–7

Additional Monoclonal Antibodies (Targeted Therapies)

Drug	Indications	Adverse Reactions
gemtuzumab ozogamicin (Mylotarg)	Humanized MAb conjugated with antitumor antibiotic calicheamicin. Treatment of CD33 positive AML in clients over 60 y in first relapse or not eligible for other chemo; 30% remission rate.	Severe bone marrow suppression in all clients due to CD33 antigen on normal cells. Other serious events are hypersensitivity reactions (anaphylaxis, hepatotoxicity, tumor lysis syndrome). Reactions are most severe in clients with WBC >30,000 cells/mm³, so they may require lowering of WBC by chemotherapy or leukapheresis prior to receiving Mylotarg. Give acetaminophen and diphenhydramine before infusion to reduce infusion reactions that usually occur within 24 h. Closely monitor vital signs, especially if WBC >30,000 cells/mm³. Corticosteroids and meperidine may also be needed. Monitor electrolytes, CBC, platelets, and liver enzymes.
alemtuzumab (Campath)	Humanized MAb for treatment of B-cell CLL for those treated with alkylating agents and refractory to fludarabine.	Hematologic toxicity, opportunistic infections, infusion reactions. Premedicate and titrate dose slowly. Prophylaxis for *Pneumocystis carinii* and herpes is recommended. Monitor CBC and CD4 counts.
ibritumomab tiuxetan (Zevalin)	Radiolabeled MAb for B-cell non-Hodgkin's lymphoma as part of regimen after administration of rituximab (follow premed guidelines)	Severe, prolonged, and delayed bone marrow suppression. Monitor CBC and platelet count. Requires institutional certification in procedure.
tositumomab and iodine-131 tositumomab (Bexxar)	Mouse-derived MAb for CD20-positive, follicular non-Hodgkin's lymphomas refractory to rituximab with relapse.	Severe and prolonged neutropenia, thrombocytopenia, and anemia. Need thyroid protective medications (start 1 d before and continue for 14 d after). Monitor CBC and serum creatinine. Iodine-131 contraindicated in pregnancy. Requires institutional certification in procedure.
cetuximab (Erbitux)	Chimeric MAb, binds to EGRF; for advanced metastatic colorectal cancer (mCRC) in combination with irinotecan (Camptosar).	May get infusion reactions, usually with first treatment; mild to severe. Pretreat with diphenhydramine. Rash can be severe; correlates with response in clients with mCRC.
panitumumab (Vectibix)	Human MAb, binds to EGFR; for clients with advanced mCRC who have progressed on prior chemotherapy	
bevacizumab (Avastin)	Humanized MAb, angiogenesis inhibitor. First-line treatment for metastatic colorectal cancer in combination with 5-FU.	GI perforation, hemorrhage, impaired wound healing. Also proteinuria and CHF, HTN. Monitor BP, serial urinalysis (do 24-hour urine for creatinine clearance, and hold drug if 24-h urine protein is >2 g).

AML, Acute monocytic leukemia; *BP,* blood pressure; *CBC,* complete blood cell count; *CHF,* chronic heart failure; *CLL,* chronic lymphocytic leukemia; *d,* day; *EGRF,* epidermal growth factor receptor; *5-FU,* fluorouracil; *g,* gram; *GI,* gastrointestinal; *h,* hour; *HTN,* hypertension; *MAb,* monoclonal antibody; *y,* year; *>,* greater than.

Nursing Process

Biologic Response Modifiers

ASSESSMENT

■ Obtain a drug and herbal supplement history from client.

■ Obtain baseline information about client's physical status. This should include height, weight, vital signs, laboratory values (complete blood count [CBC], uric acid, electrolytes, blood urea nitrogen [BUN], creatinine, and liver function tests), cardiopulmonary assessment, intake and output, skin assessment, daily activities status (i.e., ability to perform activities of daily living, sleep-rest cycle), nutritional status, presence or absence of underlying symptoms of disease, and the use of current or past medication and treatment.

■ Assess CBC (with filgrastim, pegfilgrastim, sargramostim, and oprelvekin) before therapy and biweekly throughout therapy to avoid leukocytosis and thrombocytosis. Assess renal and hepatic function tests in clients with dysfunction (liver enzymes, BUN, serum creatinine). With erythropoietin stimulating agents, assess hematocrit and hemoglobin, serum ferritin and serum iron transferring saturation. Most clients will need supplemental iron. Desired levels are >100 ng/ml for serum ferritin and >20% for serum iron transferrin saturation. Assess blood pressure before start of and, especially, early in therapy.

■ Obtain baseline data regarding client's psychosocial status, including educational level, ability and desire to learn, support systems, past coping strategies, presence or absence of emotional difficulties, and self-care abilities.

■ Assess client for signs and symptoms associated with biologic response modifiers (BRMs), such as fatigue, chills, diarrhea, and weakness. With filgrastim be alert to changes in clients with preexisting cardiac conditions. With oprelvekin assess for peripheral edema and impact on cardiopulmonary system. With aldesleukin assess for signs and symptoms of capillary leak syndrome, including hypotension and respiratory distress.

■ Assess client's and family's ability to administer subcutaneous BRMs.

■ Determine client's and family's understanding of BRMs and related side effects.

NURSING DIAGNOSES

■ Imbalanced nutrition: less than body requirements related to the side effects of biologic response modifier therapy

■ Risk for infection related to the side effects of cancer chemotherapy treatments and disease condition

■ Risk for deficient fluid volume related to the side effects of cancer therapy

■ Impaired oral mucous membrane related to the side effects of cancer chemotherapy and disease condition

■ Fatigue related to the side effects of biologic response modifier therapy

■ Disturbed body image related to cancer treatment

■ Anxiety related to the diagnosis of cancer and the unknown outcomes of treatment

■ Fear related to the cancer diagnosis

■ Risk for caregiver role strain related to the cancer diagnosis, treatment, and care responsibilities

PLANNING

■ Client and family will verbalize an understanding of the importance of reporting BRM-related side effects.

■ Client and family will demonstrate correct and safe BRM administration.

■ Client and family will identify strategies to deal with BRM-related side effects.

■ Client will remain free of infection (filgrastim and sargramostim).

■ Client will remain free of hemorrhage.

NURSING INTERVENTIONS

■ Monitor client's temperature at the onset of chills.

■ Administer prescribed meperidine 25 mg to 50 mg intravenously to decrease rigors.

■ Premedicate client with acetaminophen to reduce chills and fever and with diphenhydramine to reduce nausea.

■ Cover client with blankets to promote warmth during chills.

■ Encourage client to rest when tired and to notify health care provider if profound fatigue or anorexia occurs.

■ Encourage client to drink at least 2 L of fluid a day to promote excretion of cellular breakdown products. Assess need for IV hydration especially during IFN-α therapy.

■ Administer an antiemetic as necessary. Premedicate client with antiemetic and administer antiemetic around the clock for 24 hours after BRM administration to further delay nausea or vomiting.

■ Consult dietitian, social worker, and physical or occupational therapist as necessary.

■ Provide client and family the opportunity to discuss the effect of BRM therapy on the quality of life.

■ Refer client and family to a financial counselor if reimbursement of BRM therapy is problematic.

■ Administer BRM at bedtime to decrease the consequences of fatigue.

■ Continue with the same brand of BRM and notify the health care provider if considering changing the brand.

■ Remember to use only one dose per vial when administering sargramostim; be alert for expiration date. Avoid shaking vial. Reconstituted solutions are clear; use within 6 hours and discard unused portion. Recall that albumin may be added, depending on drug concentration, to prevent adsorption of drug to components of the drug delivery system.

■ Remember that drug vials are for one-time use when administering filgrastim; any vial left at room temperature for more than 6 hours should be discarded. Drug vials are preservative-free. Store in refrigerator at 36° F to 46° F (2° C to 8° C). Avoid shaking vials.

■ Remember to avoid excessive agitation during preparation with oprelvekin. Use only one dose per vial. Inspect the parenteral product and discard if it is discolored or has particulate matter. Use within 3 hours of reconstitution if stored at 36° F to 46° F (2° C to 8° C). Avoid freezing or shaking the drug.

■ Remember that palifermin binds with heparin, so if the patient has a central line, it must be flushed with normal saline prior to and after administration of palifermin.

Client Teaching

General

• Explain to client and family the rationale for BRM therapy.
• Explain the frequency and rationale for studies and procedures during BRM therapy.
• Inform client and family that most BRM side effects disappear within 72 to 96 hours after discontinuation of therapy.
• Instruct clients of childbearing age to use contraceptives during BRM therapy and for 2 years after completion of therapy.
• Provide client with information regarding the effect of BRM-related fatigue on activities of daily living (ADLs), including sexuality.
• Explain to client that concurrent use of herbal products with BRM therapy is not recommended (Herbal Alert 38–1).

Side Effects

• Advise client to report episodes of difficulty in concentration, confusion, or somnolence.
• Report weight loss.
• Report dyspnea, palpitations, and signs of infection or bleeding.

Self-Administration

• Demonstrate correct drug administration techniques.
• Provide client and family with written or video instructions regarding BRM self-administration.

Cultural Considerations ❖

• Obtain an interpreter when necessary; do not rely on family members who may not fully disclose because of cultural norms.

EVALUATION

■ Evaluate client's and family's education strategies by asking them to discuss the potential effect of BRM therapy on the quality of life.

■ Evaluate client's and family's BRM self-administration technique if appropriate.
■ Periodically evaluate client's and family's management of BRM-related side effects.
■ There will be a decreased incidence of infection in clients after autologous bone marrow transplantation.
■ There will be a decreased incidence of thrombocytopenia in clients after chemotherapy administration.

Summary

BRM therapy is growing rapidly. As clinical trial results yield more information about BRM activity and clinical efficacy, indications for the use of BRMs will expand. As more is learned about the effect of BRMs on the quality of client life, attention will be directed toward side effect management and symptom prevention. Nurses play a key role in both the identification and management of BRM-related toxicities. Through assessment of clients receiving BRMs and a knowledge of BRM activity, nurses can develop a plan of care that will result in clients receiving BRM therapy in a safe and comfortable manner.

KEY WEBSITES

Biological Response Modifiers: www.oncolink.com/treatment/article.cfm?c52&s59&id554

Biologic Response Modifier: What is It?: http://arthritis.about.com/cs/enbrel/a/biologics.htm

Biological Response Modifiers in Cancer: www.medscape.com/viewarticle/545538

 Critical Thinking Case Study

JW, age 55, has metastatic non–small cell cancer of the lung. His past treatment regimen included external-beam chest irradiation and combination chemotherapy. Two weeks before hospitalization JW received a course of carboplatin and paclitaxel as an outpatient. He was admitted to the hospital with neutropenia, thrombocytopenia, and anemia. Upon assessment JW was cachectic, weak, and able to perform activities of daily living only with assistance. Admitting laboratory data were Hgb (hemoglobin) 6.9, Hct (hematocrit) 20.6, platelets 16,000, and WBC 600 with ANC of 96. JW was started on Neupogen 480 mcg subQ daily; Procrit 40,000 U subQ once a week; and Neumega 50 mcg/kg subQ daily. Parenteral antibiotic therapy was also initiated. Nursing diagnoses for JW included a potential for infection related to neutropenia, bleeding related to thrombocytopenia, fatigue related to anemia, and anxiety related to hospitalization.

Nursing interventions included the following:

1. Maintaining scrupulous hand washing and hand hygiene before and after client contact
2. Allowing no one with cold or infection to enter client's room

3. Obtaining vital signs and pulmonary assessment every 4 hours
4. Inspecting all sites associated with a risk for infection (e.g., venipuncture sites, oral cavity, perirectal area) every shift
5. Protecting the skin and mucosal surfaces to prevent the entry of microorganisms by not using suppositories, enemas, or urinary catheters, by avoiding IM injections, and by obtaining no rectal temperatures
6. Monitoring laboratory values daily

LAB TESTS	DAY 1	DAY 2	DAY 3	DAY 4	DAY 5
Hgb	6.9	6.5	7.1	7.8	7.9
Hct	20.6	19.4	21.6	22.9	22.9
Platelets	16,000	15,000	16,000	20,000	30,000
WBC/ANC	600/96	1000/0	1200/168	9400/4700	31,500/18,270

7. Providing bedside range-of-motion exercises and physical therapy
8. Giving emotional support to client and family
9. Instructing client and family in giving subQ injections and self-assessment of the signs and symptoms of infection and bleeding

JW continued therapy with filgrastim (Neupogen), oprelvekin (Neumega), and erythropoietin (EPO). The following laboratory data were obtained:

Neupogen was discontinued on day 5 and antibiotics were discontinued on day 4, but Procrit and Neumega were continued. JW's physical therapy was continued in the physical therapy department. JW refused red blood cell transfusion on the basis of religious beliefs and was discharged to home (day 5) on Procrit 40,000 units subQ once a week and Neumega 50 mcg/kg subQ daily for 7 days.

1. Why were Neupogen, Neumega, and Procrit indicated?
2. What is an often overlooked side effect of Procrit? Based on this side effect, what should be closely monitored in a client receiving this agent? Why was the client receiving this agent on days 1 to 4, and what risk does this pose?

MJ, age 38, has stage IV breast cancer that was diagnosed 3 years ago. When first diagnosed she underwent lumpectomy, axillary node dissection, and breast irradiation. She recently was seen by her medical oncologist because she was experiencing lower back pain and dyspnea at rest. Magnetic resonance imaging (MRI) identified bone metastasis in the thoracic and lumbar spine, and chest radiographs revealed a large left-sided pleural effusion. MJ has a history of atrial fibrillation. She takes MS Contin and MSIR (morphine sulfate) for back pain. She receives radiation to her lower thoracic and lumbar spine. She will begin receiving a bisphosphonate pamidronate (Aredia), an inhibitor of cancer-related bone loss. She has also received two courses of chemotherapy. She tolerated the first course without incident. However, ten days after the second course of chemotherapy she was seen at the emergency department with shortness of breath, fever, chills, weakness, and a 2-day history of epistaxis and bruising. Laboratory results are Hb 9.5, WBC 1000 with 30% neutrophils, 50% lymphocytes, 5% bands, platelet count 9000. She is admitted to the oncology unit with orders for IV fluid, empiric antibiotics, Neupogen, and Neumega. MJ is a single mother who lives at home with her two children, a 10-year-old son and a 6-year-old daughter.

1. Why are Neupogen and Neumega indicated? What is the client's ANC?
2. How would the products be ordered?
3. What are the expected side effects of these agents?
4. What are the nursing interventions for the client while hospitalized and postdischarge?
5. How long should Neupogen and Neumega be administered?
6. Discuss the use of trastuzumab (Herceptin) in this client's situation.

NCLEX Study Questions

1. The three functions of BRMs include:
   a. enhance immune function, WBC production, antigen/antibody reaction
   b. cause allergic reactions, RBC production, interferon production
   c. immunomodulation, cytotoxic/cytostatic effects, differentiate stem cells
   d. cytokine production, interleukin production, fight infection

2. The side effects of interferon-a include:
   a. increase of WBCs
   b. increase of RBCs
   c. a flulike syndrome
   d. other stem cell effects

3. Platelet production can be stimulated with which of the following drugs?
   a. epoetin alfa (EPO)
   b. filgrastim
   c. interleukin-11
   d. sargramostim

4. The following drug is administered by IV infusion:
   a. Procrit or Aranesp
   b. interleukin-2
   c. G-CSF
   d. GM-CSF

5. Mrs. A lives 120 miles from her medical oncologist's office and relies on her working daughter for transportation there and back. The best reason pegfilgrastim would be most appropriate for her is because:
   a. filgrastim is eliminated via the kidneys
   b. pegfilgrastim is a pegylated filgrastim
   c. pegfilgrastim is not as easily eliminated from the body
   d. pegfilgrastim requires a once per chemotherapy cycle injection

Answers: 1, a; 2, c; 3, d; 4, b; 5, d.

THIRTEEN

Respiratory Agents

T he respiratory tract is divided into two major parts: (1) the upper respiratory tract, which consists of the nares, nasal cavity, pharynx, and larynx, and (2) the lower respiratory tract, which consists of the trachea, bronchi, bronchioles, alveoli, and alveolar-capillary membrane. Air enters through the upper respiratory tract and travels to the lower respiratory tract, where gas exchanges occur. Figure XIII–1 illustrates these components.

Ventilation and *respiration* are distinct terms and should not be used interchangeably. Ventilation is the movement of air from the atmosphere through the upper and lower airways to the alveoli. *Respiration* is the process whereby gas exchange occurs at the alveolar-capillary membrane. Respiration has three phases: ventilation, perfusion, and diffusion.

1. Ventilation is the phase in which oxygen passes through the airways. With every inspiration air is moved into the lungs, and with every expiration air is transported out of the lungs.
2. Perfusion involves blood flow at the alveolar-capillary bed. *Perfusion* is influenced by alveolar pressure. For gas exchange to occur, the perfusion of each alveolus must be matched by adequate ventilation. Factors such as mucosal edema, secretions, and bronchospasm increase resistance to airflow and decrease ventilation and diffusion of gases.
3. Diffusion (molecules move from higher concentration to lower concentration) of gases takes place when oxygen passes into the capillary bed to be circulated, and carbon dioxide leaves the capillary bed and diffuses into the alveoli for ventilatory excretion.

The chest cavity is a closed compartment bounded by 12 ribs, the diaphragm, thoracic vertebrae, sternum, neck muscles, and intercostal muscles between the ribs. The pleura are membranes that encase the lungs. The lungs are divided into lobes; the right lung has three lobes, and the left lung has two lobes. The heart, which is not attached to the lungs, lies on the midleft side in the chest cavity.

Lung Compliance

Lung compliance is the lung volume based on the unit of pressure in the alveoli. This volume determines the lung's ability to stretch. Factors that influence lung compliance include (1) connective tissue (collagen and elastin) and (2) surface tension in the alveoli, controlled by surfactant. Surfactant lowers the surface tension in the alveoli and prevents interstitial fluid from entering. Increased lung compliance is present with chronic obstructive pulmonary disease (COPD), and decreased lung compliance occurs with restrictive pulmonary disease. With low compliance there is decreased lung volume, resulting from increased connective tissue or in-

FIGURE XIII–I   Basic structures of the respiratory tract.

FIGURE XIII–2 The bronchial smooth muscle fibers become more closely spaced as they near the alveoli.

creased surface tension. The lungs become "stiff," and it takes greater than normal pressure to expand lung tissue.

Control of Respiration

Oxygen (O_2), carbon dioxide (CO_2), and hydrogen (H^+) ion concentration in the blood influence respiration. Chemoreceptors are sensors that are stimulated by changes in these gases and ion. The central chemoreceptors, located in the medulla near the respiratory center and cerebrospinal fluid, respond to an increase in carbon dioxide and a decrease in pH by increasing ventilation. However, if the carbon dioxide level remains elevated, the stimulus to increase ventilation is lost.

Peripheral chemoreceptors, located in the carotid and aortic bodies, respond to changes in oxygen (Po_2) levels. A low blood oxygen level ($Po_2 < 60$ mmHg) stimulates the peripheral chemoreceptors, which in turn stimulate the respiratory center in the medulla, and ventilation is increased. If oxygen therapy increases the oxygen level in the blood, the Po_2 may be too high to stimulate the peripheral chemoreceptors, and ventilation will be depressed.

Bronchial Smooth Muscle

The tracheobronchial tube is composed of smooth muscle whose fibers spiral around the tracheobronchial tube, becoming more closely spaced as they near the terminal bronchioles (Figure XIII–2). Contraction of these muscles constricts the airway. The sympathetic and parasympathetic nervous systems affect the bronchial smooth muscle in opposite ways. The vagus nerve (parasympathetic nervous system) releases acetylcholine, which causes bronchoconstriction. The sympathetic nervous system releases epinephrine, which stimulates the beta$_2$ receptor in the bronchial smooth muscle, resulting in bronchodilation. These two nervous systems counterbalance each other to maintain homeostasis.

Cyclic adenosine monophosphate (cyclic AMP) in the cytoplasm of bronchial cells increases bronchodilation by relaxing the bronchial smooth muscles. The pulmonary enzyme phosphodiesterase can inactivate cyclic AMP. Drugs of the methylxanthine group (theophylline) inactivate phosphodiesterase, thus permitting cyclic AMP to function.

This unit includes Chapter 39, Drugs for Upper Respiratory Disorders, and Chapter 40, Drugs for Lower Respiratory Disorders. Chapter 39 discusses drugs used to relieve cold symptoms, such as antihistamines, decongestants, antitussives, and expectorants. Drugs used to alleviate and control airway obstruction are presented in Chapter 40. These include the sympathomimetics (adrenergics), particularly the beta$_2$ adrenergics, the methylxanthines such as theophylline, leukotriene receptor antagonists, glucocorticoids, cromolyn sodium, and mucolytics.

39

Drugs for Upper Respiratory Disorders

Outline

Objectives

- Compare antihistamine, decongestant, antitussive, and expectorant drug groups.
- Differentiate between rhinitis, sinusitis, and pharyngitis.
- Describe the side effects of nasal decongestants and how they can be avoided.
- Apply the nursing process for drugs used to treat the common cold.

Terms

Upper respiratory infections (URIs) include the common cold, acute rhinitis, sinusitis, and acute pharyngitis. The **common cold** is the most prevalent type of URI. Adults have an average of two to four colds per year, and children have an average of 4 to 12 colds per year. Incidence is seasonally variable, with approximately 50% of the population experiencing a winter cold and 25% experiencing a summer cold. Normally a cold is not considered a life-threatening illness; however, it causes physical and mental discomfort and loss of time at work and school. The common cold is an expensive illness in the United States—more than $500 million is spent each year on over-the-counter (OTC) cold and cough preparations.

Common Cold, Acute Rhinitis, and Allergic Rhinitis

The common cold is caused by the rhinovirus and affects primarily the nasopharyngeal tract. Acute rhinitis (acute inflammation of the mucous membranes of the nose) usually accompanies the common cold. **Acute rhinitis** is not the same as **allergic rhinitis**, often called *hay fever*, which is caused by pollen or a foreign substance (e.g., animal dander). Nasal secretions increase in both acute rhinitis and allergic rhinitis.

A cold is most contagious 1 to 4 days before the onset of symptoms (the incubation period) and during the first 3 days of the cold. Transmission occurs more frequently from touching contaminated surfaces and then touching the nose or mouth than it does from viral droplets released by sneezing.

Home remedies for a cold include rest, chicken noodle soup, hot toddy (sugar, alcohol, and tea), vitamin C (which is debatable), and megadoses of vitamins (which is controversial). The four groups of drugs used to manage cold symptoms are antihistamines (H_1 blocker), decongestants (sympathomimetic amines), antitussives, and expectorants. These drugs can be used singly or in combination preparations.

Symptoms of the common cold include **rhinorrhea** (watery nasal discharge), nasal congestion, cough, and increased mucosal secretions. If a bacterial infection secondary to the cold occurs, infectious rhinitis may result, and nasal discharge becomes tenacious, mucoid, and yellow or yellow-green. The nasal secretions are discolored by white blood cells and cellular debris that are byproducts of the fight against the bacterial infection. Antibiotics used to treat bacterial respiratory infections are discussed in Chapters 28, 29, and 30.

Antihistamines

Antihistamines, H_1 blockers or H_1 antagonists, compete with histamine for receptor sites, preventing a histamine response. The two types of histamine receptors, H_1 and H_2, cause different responses. When the H_1 receptor is stimulated, the extravascular smooth muscles, including those lining the nasal cavity, are constricted. With stimulation of the H_2 receptor an increase in gastric secretions occurs, which is a cause of peptic ulcer (see Chapter 47). These two types of histamine receptors should not be confused. Antihistamines decrease nasopharyngeal secretions by blocking the H_1 receptor.

Although antihistamines are commonly used as cold remedies, these agents can also treat allergic rhinitis. However, the antihistamines are not useful in an emergency situation such as anaphylaxis. Most antihistamines are rapidly absorbed in 15 minutes, but they are not potent enough to combat anaphylaxis.

First-Generation Antihistamines

The antihistamine group can be divided into first and second generations. Most first-generation antihistamines cause drowsiness, dry mouth, and other anticholinergic symptoms, whereas second-generation antihistamines have fewer anticholinergic effects and a lower incidence of drowsiness. Many OTC cold remedies contain a first-generation antihistamine, which can cause drowsiness; therefore clients should be alerted not to drive or operate dangerous machinery when taking such medications. The anticholinergic properties of most antihistamines cause dryness of the mouth and decreased secretions, making them useful in treating rhinitis caused by the common cold. Antihistamines also decrease the nasal itching and tickling that cause sneezing.

The first-generation antihistamine diphenhydramine (Benadryl) has been available for years and is frequently combined with other ingredients in cold remedy preparations. Its primary use is to treat rhinitis. Prototype Drug Chart 39–1 lists the pharmacologic behavior of diphenhydramine.

Second-Generation Antihistamines

The second-generation antihistamines are frequently called *nonsedating antihistamines*, because they have little to no effect on sedation. In addition, these antihistamines cause fewer anticholinergic symptoms. Although a moderate amount of alcohol and other central nervous system (CNS) depressants may be taken with second-generation antihistamines, many clinicians advise against such use.

The second-generation antihistamines cetirizine (Zyrtec), fexofenadine (Allegra), and loratadine (Claritin) have half-lives between 7 to 15 hours. Azelastine (Astelin, Optivar) is a second-generation antihistamine that has a half-life of 22 hours and is administered by nasal spray. Table 39–1 lists the first- and second-generation antihistamines used to treat rhinitis.

Pharmacokinetics

Diphenhydramine can be administered orally, intramuscularly (IM), or intravenously (IV). It is well absorbed from the gastrointestinal (GI) tract, but systemic absorption from topical use is minimal. It is highly protein-bound (98%) and has an average half-life of 2 to 7 hours. Diphenhydramine is metabolized by the liver and excreted as metabolites in the urine.

Pharmacodynamics

Diphenhydramine blocks the effects of histamine by competing for and occupying H_1-receptor sites. It has anticholinergic effects and should not be used by clients with narrow-angle glaucoma. Drowsiness is a major side effect of the drug; in fact, it is sometimes used in sleep-aid products. Diphenhydramine is also used as an antitussive (i.e., it alleviates cough). Its onset of action can occur in as few as 15 minutes when taken orally and IM. IV administration results in an immediate onset of action. The duration of action is 4 to 8 hours.

Diphenhydramine can cause CNS depression if taken with alcohol, narcotics, hypnotics, or barbiturates.

Side Effects of Most First-Generation Antihistamines

The most common side effects of first-generation antihistamines are drowsiness, dizziness, fatigue, and disturbed coordination. Skin rashes and anticholinergic symptoms (e.g., dry mouth, urine retention, blurred vision, wheezing) may also occur.

Prototype DRUG CHART 39–1

DIPHENHYDRAMINE

Drug Class

Antihistamine
Trade names: Benadryl, ✦Allerdryl
Pregnancy Category: B

Dosage

A: PO: 25-50 mg q6-8h
A: IM/IV: 10-50 mg as single dose, q4-6h; *max:* 400 mg/d
C: PO/IM/IV: 5 mg/kg/d in 4 divided doses; *max:*
   300 mg/d

Contraindications

Acute asthmatic attack, severe liver disease, lower
   respiratory disease, neonate; MAOIs
Caution: Narrow-angle glaucoma, benign prostatic
   hypertrophy, pregnancy, newborn or premature
   infant, breastfeeding, urinary retention

Drug-Lab-Food Interactions

Drug: Increase CNS depression with alcohol, narcotics,
   hypnotics, barbiturates; avoid use with MAOIs

Pharmacokinetics

Absorption: PO: Well absorbed
Distribution: PB: 98%
Metabolism: $t\frac{1}{2}$: 2-7 h
Excretion: In urine as metabolites

Pharmacodynamics

PO: Onset: 15-45 min
   Peak: 1-4 h
   Duration: 4-8 h
IM: Onset: 15-30 min
   Peak: 1-4 h
   Duration: 4-7 h
IV: Onset: Immediate
   Peak: 0.5-1 h
   Duration: 4-7 h

Therapeutic Effects/Uses

To treat allergic rhinitis, itching; to prevent motion sickness; sleep aid; antitussive
Mode of Action: Blocks histamine$_1$ thereby decreasing allergic response; affects respiratory system, blood vessels,
   and GI system

Side Effects

Drowsiness, dizziness, fatigue, nausea, vomiting,
   urinary retention, constipation, blurred vision,
   dry mouth and throat, reduced secretions,
   hypotension, epigastric distress, hearing
   disturbances; excitation in children; photosensitivity

Adverse Reactions

Life-threatening: Agranulocytosis, hemolytic anemia,
   thrombocytopenia

A, Adult; *C*, child; *CNS*, central nervous system; *d*, day; *GI*, gastrointestinal; *h*, hour; *IM*, intramuscular; *IV*, intravenous; *MAOI*,
monoamine oxidase inhibitor; *max*, maximum; *min*, minute; *PB*, protein-binding; *PO*, by mouth; *t½*, half-life; ✦, Canadian drug
name.

Nursing Process

Antihistamine: Diphenhydramine

ASSESSMENT

■ Determine baseline vital signs.
■ Obtain drug history; report if drug-drug interaction is probable.
■ Assess for signs and symptoms of urinary dysfunction, including retention, dysuria, and frequency.
■ Note complete blood count (CBC) during drug therapy.
■ Assess cardiac and respiratory status.

■ If allergic reaction, obtain history of environmental exposures, drugs, recent foods eaten, and stress.

NURSING DIAGNOSES

■ Ineffective airway clearance related to nasal congestion
■ Risk for imbalanced fluid volume related to excessive sweating and loss of fluids
■ Sleep deprivation related to frequent coughing

PLANNING

■ Client will have decreased nasal congestion, mucosal secretions, and cough.
■ Client will sleep 6 to 8 hours per night.

Table 39–1

Antihistamines for Treatment of Allergic Rhinitis

Generic (Brand)	Route and Dosage	Uses and Considerations
First-Generation Antihistamines		
Alkylamine Derivatives		
brompheniramine maleate (Lodrane, Bromfenex, Dimetapp, Dimetane)	A: PO: 4 mg q4-6h or SR: 8 mg q8-12h; *max:* 24 mg/d IM/IV/subQ: 10 mg q8-12h; *max:* 40 mg/d C: 6-12 y: PO: 2 mg q4-6h; *max:* 12 mg/d	For allergies. Also present in various cough and decongestant formulas. *Pregnancy category:* C; PB: UK; t^{1}/$_{2}$: 25-36 h
chlorpheniramine maleate (Chlor-Trimeton, Phenetron, Telechlor, Teldrin)	A: PO: 2-4 mg q4-6h; *max:* 24 mg/24 h SR: 8-12 mg q8-12 h C: 6-12 y: PO: 2 mg q4-6h; *max:* 12 mg/d	For allergies including allergic rhinitis. May be used in combination with nasal decongestant. *Pregnancy category:* C; PB: 72%; t^{1}/$_{2}$: 20-24 h
dexchlorpheniramine maleate (Tanafed, Polaramine)	A: PO: 2 mg q4-6h or SR: 4-6 mg q8-12h or at bedtime C: >6 y: PO: 1 mg q4-6h or SR: 4 mg at bedtime	Relief of allergic rhinitis. May be used with epinephrine to treat anaphylactic reaction. *Pregnancy category:* B; PB: UK; t^{1}/$_{2}$: UK
Ethanolamine Derivatives		
clemastine fumarate (Tavist)	A: PO: 1.34-2.68 mg b.i.d./t.i.d.; *max:* 8 mg/d C: <12 y: PO: 0.67-1.34 mg b.i.d.	For relief of allergic rhinitis and urticaria. *Pregnancy category:* C; PB: UK; t^{1}/$_{2}$: UK
diphenhydramine (Benadryl)	(Prototype Drug Chart 39–1)	
Ethylenediamines		
tripelennamine (PBZ)	A: PO: 25-50 mg q4-6h or 100 mg sustained release q8-12h, *max:* 600 mg/d C: PO: 5 mg/kg/d in 4-6 divided doses, *max:* 300 mg/d	For relief of symptoms of allergic conditions. *Pregnancy category:* B; PB: UK; t^{1}/$_{2}$: UK
Piperidine Derivatives		
azatadine maleate (Trinalin)	A: PO: 1-2 mg b.i.d./t.i.d. C: <12 y: PO: not recommended	Relief of allergic rhinitis and chronic urticaria. Drowsiness, dizziness, and hypotension may occur. *Pregnancy category:* B; PB: UK; t^{1}/$_{2}$: 9-12 h
cyproheptadine HCl (Periactin)	A: PO: 4-20 mg/d in divided doses; *max:* 0.5 mg/kg/d C: >6 y: PO: 4 mg q8-12h; *max:* 16 mg/d C: 2-6 y: PO: 2 mg q8-12h	For allergies (rhinitis, conjunctivitis, pruritus). Common side effects include drowsiness, dry mouth, dizziness, and epigastric distress. *Pregnancy category:* B; PB: UK; t^{1}/$_{2}$: UK
phenindamine (Nolahist)	A, C: >12 y: PO: 25 mg q4-6h, *max:* 150 mg/d C: <12 y: 12.5 mg q4-6h, *max:* 75 mg/d	For temporary relief of allergic rhinitis. *Pregnancy category:* B; PB: UK; t^{1}/$_{2}$: UK
Other Antihistamines		
triprolidine and pseudoephedrine (Actifed)	A: PO: 1 tab q4-6h; *max:* 4 tab/d C: >6 y: PO: ½ tab q6-8h; *max:* 2 tab/d	For rhinitis. Combination of an antihistamine and decongestant. *Pregnancy category:* B; PB: UK; t^{1}/$_{2}$: 3 h
triprolidine HCl (Zymine, Myidil)	A: PO: 2.5 mg b.i.d., t.i.d.; *max:* 10 mg/d C: 6-12 y: PO: 1.25 mg b.i.d., t.i.d.; *max:* 5 mg/d C: 2-5 y: PO: 0.6 mg t.i.d./q.i.d.; *max:* 2.5 mg/d C: 4 mo-2 y: PO: 0.3 mg t.i.d./q.i.d.; *max:* 1.25 mg/d	For allergies. Similar effects as other antihistamines. Has a low incidence of drowsiness. *Pregnancy category:* C; PB: UK; t^{1}/$_{2}$: UK
Second-Generation Antihistamines		
azelastine (Astelin)	*Nasal Spray* A, C: >12 y, and elderly: 1-2 sprays in each nostril q12h	For allergic rhinitis. May cause headaches, mild sedation, and bitter taste. *Pregnancy category:* UK; PB: UK; t^{1}/$_{2}$: UK
cetirizine (Zyrtec)	A: 5-10 mg/d	For allergic rhinitis and urticaria. Has few anticholinergic effects. *Pregnancy category:* C; PB: 93%; t^{1}/$_{2}$: 8 h
fexofenadine (Allegra) with pseudoephedrine (Allegra-D)	A, C: >12 y, and elderly: PO: 60 mg q12h	To treat allergic rhinitis and rhinorrhea. Has less sedative effect. *Pregnancy category:* C; PB: UK; t^{1}/$_{2}$ 14.4 h
loratadine (Claritin)	A, C: >6 y: PO: 10 mg/d	Relief of allergic rhinitis and urticaria. Long-acting H$_1$ blocking effect. *Pregnancy category:* B; PB: UK; t^{1}/$_{2}$: 3-20 h; metabolite: 28 h
desloratadine (Clarinex)	A: PO: 5 mg daily	For relief of allergic rhinitis. *Pregnancy category:* C; PB: 85%-89%; t^{1}/$_{2}$: 27 h

A, Adult; *b.i.d.*, twice a day; *C*, child; *d*, day; *h*, hour; *IM*, intramuscular; *IV*, intravenous; *max*, maximum; *mo*, month; *PB*, protein-binding; *PO*, by mouth; *q.i.d.*, four times a day; *subQ*, subcutaneous; *SR*, sustained-release; *t^{1}/$_{2}$*, half-life; *tab*, tablet; *t.i.d.*, three times a day; *UK*, unknown; *y*, year; >, greater than; <, less than.

NURSING INTERVENTIONS

- Give oral form with food to decrease gastric distress.
- Administer IM form in large muscle. *Avoid subQ injection.*

Client Teaching

General

- Encourage client to avoid driving a motor vehicle and performing other dangerous activities if drowsiness occurs or until stabilized on drug.
- Avoid alcohol and other central nervous system depressants.
- Instruct client to take drug as prescribed. Notify health care provider if confusion or hypotension occurs.
- Take drug at least 30 minutes before offending event and also before meals and at bedtime during the event for prophylaxis of motion sickness.
- Inform the breastfeeding mother that small amounts of drug pass into the breast milk. Because children are more susceptible to the side effects of antihistamines (e.g., unusual excitement or irritability), breastfeeding is not recommended while using these drugs.

Side Effects

- Advise family members or parents that children are more sensitive to the effects of antihistamines. Nightmares, nervousness, and irritability are more likely to occur in children.
- Inform older adults that they are more sensitive to the effects of antihistamines. Confusion; difficult or painful urination; dizziness; drowsiness; feeling faint; and dryness of the mouth, nose, or throat are more likely to occur in older clients.
- Suggest using sugarless candy or gum, ice chips, or a saliva substitute for temporary relief of mouth dryness.

Cultural Considerations ❖

- Decrease language barriers by decoding the jargon of health care environment for those with language difficulties and for those who are not in the health care field.

EVALUATION

- Evaluate effectiveness of drug in relieving allergic symptoms or as a sleep aid.

Nasal and Systemic Decongestants

Nasal congestion results from dilation of nasal blood vessels caused by infection, inflammation, or allergy. With this dilation, there is a transudation of fluid into the tissue spaces, resulting in swelling of the nasal cavity. Nasal **decongestants** (sympathomimetic amines) stimulate the alpha-adrenergic receptors, producing vascular constriction (vasoconstriction) of the capillaries within the nasal mucosa. The result is shrinking of the nasal mucous membranes and a reduction in fluid secretion (runny nose).

Nasal decongestants are administered by nasal spray or drops or in tablet, capsule, or liquid form. Frequent use of decongestants, especially nasal spray or drops, can result in tolerance and rebound nasal congestion (rebound vasodilation instead of vasoconstriction). **Rebound nasal congestion** is caused by irritation of the nasal mucosa.

Systemic decongestants (alpha-adrenergic agonists) are available in tablet, capsule, and liquid form and are used primarily for allergic rhinitis, including hay fever and acute coryza (profuse nasal discharge). Examples of systemic decongestants are ephedrine (Ephedrine), phenylephrine (Neo-Synephrine), and pseudoephedrine (Sudafed). In the past, phenylpropanolamine was used in many cold remedies; however, the Food and Drug Administration (FDA) ordered its removal from OTC cold remedies and weight-loss aids because of reports that suggested the drug might cause stroke, hypertension, renal failure, and cardiac dysrhythmias. Ephedrine, phenylephrine, and pseudoephedrine are frequently combined with an antihistamine, analgesic, or antitussive in oral cold remedies. The advantage of systemic decongestants is that they relieve nasal congestion for a longer period than nasal decongestants; however, currently there are long-acting nasal decongestants. Nasal decongestants usually act promptly and cause fewer side effects than systemic decongestants. Table 39–2 lists nasal and systemic decongestants and their dosages, uses, and considerations.

Side Effects and Adverse Reactions

The incidence of side effects is low with topical preparations such as nose drops. Decongestants can make a client jittery, nervous, or restless. These side effects decrease or disappear as the body adjusts to the drug.

Usage of nasal decongestants for longer than 5 days could result in rebound nasal congestion. Instead of the nasal membranes constricting, vasodilation occurs, causing increased stuffy nose and nasal congestion. The nurse should emphasize the importance of limiting the use of nasal sprays and drops.

As with any alpha-adrenergic drug (e.g., decongestants), blood pressure and blood glucose levels can increase. These drugs are contraindicated or to be used with extreme caution in clients with hypertension, cardiac disease, hyperthyroidism, and diabetes mellitus.

Drug Interactions

When using decongestants with other drugs, drug interactions can occur. Pseudoephedrine may decrease the effect of beta-blockers. Taken together with monoamine oxidase (MAO) inhibitors, decongestants may increase the possibility of hypertension or cardiac dysrhythmias. The client should also avoid large amounts of caffeine (coffee, tea), because it can increase restlessness and palpitations caused by decongestants.

Table 39-2

Systemic and Nasal Decongestants (Sympathomimetic Amines)

Generic (Brand)	Route and Dosage	Uses and Considerations
ephedrine SO$_4$ (Efedron)	A: PO: 25-50 mg t.i.d./q.i.d. PRN; *max:* 150 mg/d subQ/IM/IV: 12.5-25 mg; may repeat; *max:* 150 mg/24 h C: 6-12 y: 6.25-12.5 mg q4h; *max:* 75 mg/d	Relief of allergic rhinitis, nasal congestion, sinusitis, mild acute and chronic asthma; improves narcotic-impaired respiration; corrects hypotension. Alpha- and beta-adrenergic agonist. OTC drug used alone or in combination. *Pregnancy category:* C; PB: UK; t$^{1/2}$: 3-6 h
naphazoline HCl (Allerest, Privine)	A & C: >12 y: 2 gtt or 0.05% spray in each nostril; q3-6h, 5 d C: 6-12 y: 0.025%, 1-2 gtt in each nostril	Relief of nasal congestion, allergic rhinitis. Can cause rebound congestion, transient hypertension, bradycardia, and cardiac dysrhythmias. Use only 3-5 d. *Pregnancy category:* C; PB: UK; t$^{1/2}$: UK
oxymetazoline HCl (Afrin)	A & C: >6 y: 0.05% gtt or spray; 2-3 gtt or 1-2 sprays in each nostril b.i.d. C: 2-5 y (0.025% gtt only): 2-3 gtt b.i.d. (q10-12h)	Long-acting decongestant. Taken twice a day, morning and evening. Can cause rebound congestion. Use only 3-5 d. *Pregnancy category:* C; PB: UK; t$^{1/2}$: UK
phenylephrine HCl (Neo-Synephrine, Sinex)	A: Sol (0.25%-1%): 2-3 gtt or 1-2 sprays in each nostril q4h C: 6-12 y: Sol (0.25%): 1-2 gtt or sprays in each nostril q4th C: 6 mo-5 y: Sol (0.125%-0.16%): 1-2 gtt in each nostril q4h	For rhinitis. Less potent than epinephrine. Can cause transient hypertension and headaches. Do not use for longer than 3-5 d. *Pregnancy category:* C; PB: UK; t$^{1/2}$: 2.5 d
pseudoephedrine (Novafed, Sudafed)	A: PO: 60 mg q4-6h; 120 mg SR q12h; *max:* 240 mg/d C:6-12 y: 30 mg q4-6h; *max:* 120 mg/d C: 2-5 y: 15 mg q4-6h; *max:* 60 mg/d	For rhinitis. Less CNS stimulation and hypertension than ephedrine. *Pregnancy category:* C; PB: UK; t$^{1/2}$: 9-15 h
tetrahydrozoline (Tyzine)	A & C: >6 y: Nasal: 2-4 drops of 0.1% sol or spray in each nostril q3h PRN C: 2-6 y: Nasal: 2-4 drops of 0.5% sol or spray in each nostril q3h PRN	For relief of nasopharyngeal congestion. *Pregnancy category:* C; PB: UK; t$^{1/2}$: UK
xylometazoline (Otrivin, Neo-Synephrine II)	A: Nasal: 1-2 sprays or 1-2 drops of 0.1% sol in each nostril q8-10h, *max:* 3 doses/d C: 6-12 y: Nasal: 1 spray or 2-3 drops of 0.05% sol in each nostril q8-10h, *max:* 3 doses/d C: <6 mo: Nasal: 1 drop of 0.05% sol in each nostril q6h, *max:* 3 doses/d	For temporary relief of nasal congestion associated with the common cold, sinusitis, acute and chronic rhinitis, hay fever, and other allergies. *Pregnancy category:* C; PB: UK; t$^{1/2}$: UK

A, Adult; *b.i.d.*, twice a day; *C*, child; *CNS*, central nervous system; *d*, day; *gtt*, drops; *h*, hour; *IM*, intramuscular; *IV*, intravenous; *max*, maximum; *OTC*, over-the-counter; *PB*, protein-binding; *PO*, by mouth; *PRN*, as necessary; *q.i.d.*, four times a day; *subQ*, subcutaneous; *sol*, solution; *SR*, sustained release; *t$^{1/2}$*, half-life; *t.i.d.*, three times a day; *UK*, unknown; *y*, year; *>*, greater than; *<*, less than.

Herbal ALERT 39-1

Decongestant

🌿 Peppermint may be used as a nasal decongestant.

Intranasal Glucocorticoids

Intranasal glucocorticoids or steroids are effective for treating allergic rhinitis. Because these agents are steroids, they have an antiinflammatory action, thus decreasing the allergic rhinitis symptoms of rhinorrhea, sneezing, and congestion. The following are six examples of intranasal steroids:

- beclomethasone (Beconase, Vancenase, Vanceril)
- budesonide (Rhinocort)
- dexamethasone (Decadron)
- flunisolide (Nasalide)
- fluticasone (Flonase)
- triamcinolone (Nasacort)

These drugs may be used alone or in combination with an H$_1$ antihistamine. With continuous use, dryness of the nasal mucosa may occur.

It is rare for systemic effects of steroids to occur, but they are more likely to result with the use of intranasal dexamethasone, which should not be used for longer than 30 days. The other intranasal glucocorticoids undergo rapid deactivation after absorption. Most allergic rhinitis is seasonal; therefore the drugs are for short-term use unless otherwise indicated by the health care provider. Table 39-3 lists the intranasal glucocorticoids and their dosages, uses, and considerations.

Table 39–3

Intranasal Glucocorticoids

Generic (Brand)	Route and Dosage	Uses and Considerations
beclomethasone (Beconase, Vancenase, Vanceril)	A: 1-2 puffs/sprays, b.i.d. to q.i.d. C: 6-12 y: 1-2 sprays b.i.d. to q.i.d.	To treat seasonal allergic rhinitis and bronchial asthma. Not for acute asthma. *Pregnancy category:* C; PB: UK; t½: 3-15 h
budesonide (Pulmicort, Rhinocort)	A & C: >6 y: 2 sprays b.i.d. or 4 sprays in the morning	For seasonal rhinitis in adults and children. May be used in maintenance therapy for asthma. *Pregnancy category:* C; PB: UK; t½: 2.5-3 h
dexamethasone (Decadron)	A: 2 sprays b.i.d. or t.i.d. C: 6-12 y: 1-2 sprays b.i.d.	Administered orally, intravenously, ophthalmically, topically, and intranasally. A potent steroid used for short-term therapy. May have a systemic effect. *Pregnancy category:* C; PB: UK; t½: 3-4.5 h
flunisolide (AeroBid, Nasalide)	A: 2 sprays b.i.d. to t.i.d. C: 6-14 y: 1 spray t.i.d. or 2 sprays b.i.d.	For seasonal rhinitis for adults and children. May be used for steroid-dependent asthma. *Pregnancy category:* C; PB: UK; t½: 1-2 h
fluticasone (Flonase, Flovent)	A: 2 sprays daily or 1 spray b.i.d. C: >6 y: 1 spray daily	For seasonal allergic rhinitis. When symptoms have decreased, reduce dose to 1 spray daily. *Pregnancy category:* C; PB: UK; t½: 3.1 h
mometasone furoate (Nasonex)	A: 2 sprays daily	For seasonal allergic rhinitis. *Pregnancy category:* C; PB: UK; t½: UK NOTE: Direct spray away from nasal septum; gently sniff.
triamcinolone (Nasacort)	A: 1-2 sprays daily	For allergic rhinitis. Has many uses, such as an immunosuppressant. *Pregnancy category:* C; PB: UK; t½: 2-5 h

A, Adult; *b.i.d.*, twice a day; *C*, child; *h*, hour; *PB*, protein-binding; *q.i.d.*, four times a day; *t½*, half-life; *t.i.d.*, three times a day; *UK*, unknown; *y*, year; >, greater than.

Antitussives

Antitussives act on the cough-control center in the medulla to suppress the cough reflex. The cough is a naturally protective way to clear the airway of secretions or any collected material. A sore throat may cause coughing that increases throat irritation. If the cough is nonproductive and irritating, an antitussive may be taken. Hard candy may decrease the constant, irritating cough. Dextromethorphan, a nonnarcotic antitussive, is widely used in OTC cold remedies. Prototype Drug Chart 39–2 lists the drug data related to dextromethorphan (Benylin).

The three types of antitussives are nonnarcotic, narcotic, or combination preparations. Antitussives are usually used in combination with other agents (Table 39–4).

Pharmacokinetics

Dextromethorphan is available in numerous cold and cough remedy preparations in syrup or liquid form, chewable capsules, and lozenges. Brand name formulations include Robitussin DM, Romilar, PediaCare, Contac Cold Formula, Sucrets cough formulas, and many others. The drug is rapidly absorbed and exerts its effects 15 to 30 minutes after oral administration. Its protein-binding percentage and half-life are unknown. Dextromethorphan is metabolized by the liver and excreted in the urine.

Pharmacodynamics

Dextromethorphan, a nonnarcotic antitussive, suppresses the cough center in the medulla but does not depress respiration. It causes neither physical dependence nor tolerance. If the cough lasts longer than 1 week and a fever or rash is present, medical care should be sought. Clients with underlying medical conditions should seek prompt medical attention.

The onset of action for dextromethorphan is relatively fast, and its duration is 3 to 6 hours. Usually preparations containing dextromethorphan can be used several times a day. CNS depression may occur if the drug is used with alcohol, narcotics, sedative-hypnotics, barbiturates, or antidepressants.

Expectorants

Expectorants loosen bronchial secretions so they can be eliminated by coughing. They can be used with or without other pharmacologic agents. Expectorants are found in many OTC cold remedies along with analgesics, antihistamines, decongestants, and antitussives. The most common expectorant in such preparations is guaifenesin. Hydration is the best natural expectorant. Table 39–4 lists the drug data for antitussives and expectorants.

Nursing Process

Common Cold

ASSESSMENT

■ Determine whether there is a history of hypertension, especially if a decongestant is an ingredient in the cold remedy.

■ Note baseline vital signs. An elevated temperature of 99° F to 101° F (37.2° C to 38.3° C) may indicate a viral infection caused by a cold.

■ Obtain drug history; report if drug-drug interaction is probable. Dextromethorphan HCl given with MAOIs, narcotics, sedative-hypnotics, barbiturates, antidepressants, and alcohol may increase toxicity.

Prototype DRUG CHART 39–2

DEXTROMETHORPHAN HYDROBROMIDE

Drug Class	**Dosage**
Antitussive Trade names: Robitussin DM, Romilar, Sucrets Cough Control, PediaCare, Benylin DM, and others; ✹Balminil DM, Neo-DM, Ornex DM *Pregnancy Category:* C	**A: PO:** 10-20 mg q4-8h; *max:* 120 mg/24 h **C: 6-12 y: PO:** 5-10 mg q4-6h; *max:* 60 mg/d **C: 2-5 y: PO:** 2.5-5.0 mg q4-8h; *max:* 30 mg/d *Sustained action liquid (Delsym):* **A:** 60 mg q12h **C: 6-12 y:** 30 mg q12h **C: 2-5 y:** 15 mg q12h
Contraindications	**Drug-Lab-Food Interactions**
Chronic obstructive pulmonary disease, chronic productive cough, hypersensitivity; MAOIs	*Drug: Increase* effect/toxicity with MAOIs, narcotics, sedative-hypnotics, barbiturates, antidepressants, alcohol
Pharmacokinetics	**Pharmacodynamics**
Absorption: PO: Rapidly absorbed **Distribution:** PB: UK **Metabolism:** t½: UK **Excretion:** In urine	**PO:** Onset: 15-30 min Peak: UK Duration: 3-6 h

Therapeutic Effects/Uses

To provide temporary suppression of a nonproductive cough; to reduce viscosity of tenacious secretions
Mode of Action: Inhibition of the cough center in the medulla

Side Effects	**Adverse Reactions**
Nausea, dizziness, drowsiness, sedation	Hallucinations at high doses *Life-threatening:* None known

A, Adult; *C*, child; *d*, day; *h*, hour; *MAOIs*, monoamine oxidase inhibitors; *max*, maximum; *min*, minute; *PB*, protein-binding; *PO*, by mouth; *t½*, half-life; *UK*, unknown; *y*, year; ✹, Canadian drug name.

■ Assess cardiac and respiratory status.

NURSING DIAGNOSES

■ Ineffective airway clearance related to nasal congestion
■ Risk for imbalanced fluid volume related to excessive sweating and loss of fluids
■ Sleep deprivation related to chronic coughing
■ Fatigue related to sleep deprivation
■ Risk for infection related to insufficient knowledge to avoid exposure to pathogens

PLANNING

■ Client will be free of nonproductive cough. A secondary bacterial infection does not occur.
■ Client will be free of a secondary bacterial infection.

NURSING INTERVENTIONS

■ Monitor vital signs. Blood pressure can become elevated when a decongestant is taken. Dysrhythmias can also occur.
■ Observe color of bronchial secretions. Yellow or green mucus is indicative of a bronchial infection. Antibiotics may be needed.

■ Be aware that codeine preparations for cough suppression can lead to tolerance and physical dependence.

Client Teaching

General
• Tell client that hypotension and hyperpyrexia may occur when dextromethorphan is taken with MAOIs.
• Instruct client on proper use of a nasal spray and proper use of "puff" or squeeze products. Instruct client not to use more than one or two puffs, four to six times a day, for 5 to 7 days. Rebound congestion can occur with overuse.
• Advise client to read the label on OTC drugs and to check with the health care provider before taking cold remedies. This is especially important when taking other drugs or when client has a major health problem such as hypertension or hyperthyroidism.
• Inform client that antibiotics are not helpful in treating common cold viruses. However, they may be prescribed if a secondary infection occurs.
• Encourage older client with heart disease, asthma, emphysema, diabetes mellitus, or hypertension to contact the health care provider concerning the selection of drug, including OTC drugs.

Table 39–4

Antitussives and Expectorants

Generic (Brand)	Route and Dosage	Uses and Considerations
Narcotic Antitussives		
codeine CSS II	A: PO: 10-20 mg q4-6h; *max:* 120 mg/d C: 6-12 y: PO: 5-10 mg q4-6h; *max:* 60 mg/d C: 2-5 y: PO: 2.5-4.5 mg q4-6h; *max:* 18 mg/d	Schedule II drug. Can be a Schedule V drug when combined in cough syrup. Usually mixed with an antihistamine, decongestant, and/or expectorant. Can cause drowsiness, dizziness, nausea, constipation, and respiratory depression. *Pregnancy category:* C; PB: 7%; t^1/$_2$: 2.5-4 h
guaifenesin and codeine (Cheracol, Robitussin A-C) CSS V	*Temporary relief of cough caused by minor irritation:* A: PO: 5-10 ml q6-8h C: 2-6 y: PO: 2.5 ml q6-8h PRN	An expectorant combined with a narcotic antitussive. Also to control a cough caused by the common cold or bronchitis. *Pregnancy category:* C; PB: UK; t^1/$_2$: UK
hydrocodone bitartrate (Hycodan) CSS III	A: PO: 5-10 mg q4-6h; *max:* 15 mg/d C: PO: 1.25 mg q4-6h; 0.6 mg/kg/d in 3-4 divided doses, not to exceed 10 mg/single dose	Relief of cough and pain. Has similar side effects as codeine. *Pregnancy category:* C; PB: UK; t^1/$_2$: 3-4 h
Nonnarcotic Antitussives		
benzonatate (Tessalon)	*Relief of nonproductive cough:* A: PO: 100 mg t.i.d. or q4h; *max:* 600 mg/d C: <10 y: PO: 8 mg/kg/d in 3-6 divided doses	Relief of cough. Does not depress the respiratory center. Has few side effects. *Pregnancy category:* C; PB: UK; t^1/$_2$: UK
Dextromethorphan hydrobromide (Benylin)	(Prototype Drug Chart 39–2)	
promethazine with dextromethorphan	A: PO: 5 ml q4-6h; *max:* 30 ml/d C: 6-12 y: PO: 2.5-5 ml q4-6h; *max:* 20 ml/d C: 2-6 y: PO: 1.25-5 ml, q4-6h	For cough. Combination of a phenothiazine and a nonnarcotic antitussive. *Pregnancy category:* C; PB: UK; t^1/$_2$: UK
Expectorants		
guaifenesin (Robitussin, Anti-Tuss, Glycotuss)	A: PO: 200-400 mg q4h; *max:* 2.4 g/d C: 6-12 y: PO: 100-200 mg q4h; *max:* 1.2 g/d C: 2-5 y: PO: 50-100 mg q4h; *max:* 600 mg/d	For dry, unproductive cough. Can cause nausea and vomiting. Can be combined with other cold remedies. Take with glass of water to loosen mucus. *Pregnancy category:* C; PB: UK; t^1/$_2$: UK
Antitussive/Expectorant		
guaifenesin and dextromethorphan (Robitussin-DM)	A: PO: 10 ml q6-8h C: 6-12 y: PO: 5 ml q6-8h C: 2-5 y: PO: 2.5 ml q6-8h	For nonproductive cough. *Pregnancy category:* C; PB: UK; t^1/$_2$: UK

A, Adult; *C*, child; *CSS*, Controlled Substances Schedule; *d*, day; *h*, hour; *max*, maximum; *PB*, protein-binding; *PO*, by mouth; *PRN*, as necessary; *t^1/$_2$*, half-life; *t.i.d.*, three times a day; *UK*, unknown; *y*, year; <, less than.

- Direct client not to drive during initial use of a cold remedy containing an antihistamine, because drowsiness is common.
- Instruct client to maintain adequate fluid intake. Fluids liquefy bronchial secretions to ease elimination with coughing.
- Teach client not to take a cold remedy before or at bedtime. Insomnia may occur if it contains a decongestant.
- Encourage client to get adequate rest.
- Inform client that common cold and flu viruses are transmitted frequently by hand-to-hand contact or touching a contaminated surface. Cold viruses can live on the skin for several hours and on hard surfaces for several days.
- Instruct client to avoid environmental pollutants, fumes, smoking, and dust to lessen irritating cough.

- Teach client to perform three effective coughs before bedtime to promote uninterrupted sleep.
- Direct client and parents to store the drug out of reach of small children; request childproof caps.
- Advise client to contact the health care provider if cough persists for more than 1 week or is accompanied by chest pain, fever, or headache.

Self-Administration

- Instruct client about self-administration of medications such as nose drops and inhalants.
- Encourage client to cough effectively, to take deep breaths before coughing, and to be in the upright position.

Cultural Considerations ❖

- Allow client's traditional remedies for treating the common cold to be incorporated into prescribed

Western medical practices if they are harmless. Discuss practices that could cause bodily harm.

- Identify conflicts in values and beliefs in treatment of the common cold.
- Respectfully present treatment methods to care for the common cold for clients from various cultural backgrounds, such as increasing fluid intake, getting adequate rest, and using disposable tissues to remove nasal and bronchial secretions. Advise client to contact a health professional if the cold persists and if the body temperature is greater than 101° F (38.3° C).

EVALUATION

■ Evaluate the effectiveness of the drug therapy. Determine that client is free of a nonproductive cough, has adequate fluid intake and rest, and is afebrile.

Sinusitis

Sinusitis is an inflammation of the mucous membranes of one or more of the maxillary, frontal, ethmoid, or sphenoid sinuses. A systemic or nasal decongestant may be indicated. Acetaminophen, fluids, and rest may also be helpful. For acute or severe sinusitis, an antibiotic may be prescribed.

Acute Pharyngitis

Acute pharyngitis (inflammation of the throat, or "sore throat") can be caused by a virus, beta-hemolytic streptococci (strep throat), or other bacteria. It can occur alone or with the common cold and rhinitis or acute sinusitis. Symptoms include elevated temperature and cough. A throat culture should be obtained to rule out beta-hemolytic streptococcal infection. If the culture is positive for beta-hemolytic streptococci, a 10-day course of antibiotics is often prescribed. Saline gargles, lozenges, and increased fluid intake are usually indicated. Acetaminophen may be taken to decrease an elevated temperature. Antibiotics are not effective for viral pharyngitis.

KEY WEBSITES

Cetirizine: http://www.nlm.nih.gov/medlineplus/druginfo/medmaster/a698026.html

Sinusitis: http://www.nlm.nih.gov/medlineplus/sinusitis.html

Loratadine: www.medicinenet.com/loratadine/article.htm

Critical Thinking Case Study

GH, age 35, has allergic rhinitis. Her prescriptions include loratadine (Claritin), 5 mg per day, and fluticasone, two nasal inhalations per day. Previously she had taken OTC drugs and asked whether she should continue to take the OTC drug with her prescriptions. She has never used a nasal inhaler.

Critical Thinking Case Study

1. What additional information is needed from GH concerning her health problem?
2. What is your response to GH concerning the use of OTC drugs with her prescription drugs?
3. How would you instruct GH to use a nasal inhaler? Explain. (You may consult Chapter 3.)
4. What are the similarities and differences between loratadine and diphenhydramine? Could one of these antihistamines be more effective than the other? Explain.
5. Design a client teaching plan for GH in regard to medications and environmental allergens.
6. What could you suggest to decrease allergens (e.g., dust mites) in the home?

NCLEX Study Questions

1. A client tells the nurse that he has started to take an over-the-counter antihistamine, diphenhydramine. In teaching him about side effects, it is most important for the nurse to tell the client:
   a. not to take this drug at bedtime to avoid insomnia
   b. to avoid driving a motor vehicle until stabilized on the drug
   c. that nightmares and nervousness are more likely in an adult
   d. to limit use to 1-2 puffs/sprays 4-6 times per day to avoid rebound congestion

2. The client complains of a sore throat and has been told it is due to beta-hemolytic streptococcal infection. The nurse realizes this condition is called acute:
   a. rhinitis   c. pharyngitis
   b. sinusitis   d. rhinorrhea

3. A client is prescribed the decongestant oxymetazoline (Afrin) nasal spray. The nurse should teach the client:
   a. to take this drug at bedtime as a sleep aid
   b. to directly spray away from the nasal septum and gently sniff
   c. that this drug may be used in maintenance treatment for asthma
   d. that limiting the drug to 5 days of use should prevent rebound nasal congestion

4. The goal of care for a client is to loosen bronchial secretions so they can be eliminated by coughing. The nurse knows that the best drug for this condition is:
   a. benzonatate (Tessalon)
   b. guaifenesin (Robitussin)
   c. hydrocodone (Hycodan)
   d. phenylephrine (Neo-Synephrine)

5. Beclomethasone (Beconase) has been prescribed for a client with allergic rhinitis. The nurse teaches the client that the most common side effect from continuous use is:
   a. dizziness   c. hallucinations
   b. rhinorrhea   d. dry nasal mucosa

40

Drugs for Lower Respiratory Disorders

ELECTRONIC RESOURCES

evolve

Evolve website (http://evolve.elsevier.com/KeeHayes/pharmacology/):
- *Case Studies*
- *Content Updates*
- *Frequently Asked Questions*
- *Student Review Activities*
- *WebLinks*
- *Additional Reference Material*

Companion CD-ROM:
- *NCLEX Examination Review Questions*
- *Pharmacology Animations*
- *IV Therapy Checklists*
- *Medication Error Checklists*
- *Drug Calculation Problems*
- *Electronic Calculators*
- *Top 200 Drugs with Pronunciations*
- *References from the Textbook*

Outline

Objectives

- Compare chronic obstructive pulmonary disease (COPD) and restrictive lung disease.
- Differentiate the drug groups used to treat COPD and asthma and the desired effects of each.
- Describe the side effects of beta$_2$-adrenergic agonists and methylxanthines.
- Describe the therapeutic serum or plasma theophylline level and the toxic level.
- Contrast the therapeutic effects of leukotriene antagonists, glucocorticoids, cromolyn, antihistamines, and mucolytics for COPD and asthma.
- Apply the nursing process for the client taking drugs commonly used for COPD, including asthma, and restrictive lung disease.

Terms

Chronic obstructive pulmonary disease (COPD) and restrictive pulmonary disease are the two major categories of lower respiratory tract disorders. COPD is caused by airway obstruction with increased airway resistance of airflow to lung tissues. Four major pulmonary disorders cause COPD: chronic bronchitis, bronchiectasis, emphysema, and asthma. Chronic bronchitis, bronchiectasis, and emphysema frequently result in irreversible lung tissue damage. The lung tissue changes resulting from an acute asthmatic attack are normally reversible; however, if the asthma attacks are frequent and asthma becomes chronic, irreversible changes in the lung tissue may result. Clients with COPD usually have a decrease in forced expiratory volume in 1 second (FEV_1) as measured by pulmonary function tests.

Restrictive lung disease is a decrease in total lung capacity as a result of fluid accumulation or loss of elasticity of the lung. Pulmonary edema, pulmonary fibrosis, pneumonitis, lung tumors, thoracic deformities (scoliosis), and disorders affecting the thoracic muscular wall (e.g., myasthenia gravis) are among the types and causes of restrictive pulmonary disease.

Drugs discussed in this chapter are primarily used to treat COPD, particularly asthma. These drugs include **bronchodilators** (sympathomimetics [primarily beta$_2$-adrenergic agonists], methylxanthines [xanthines]), leukotriene antagonists, glucocorticoids, cromolyn, anticholinergics, and mucolytics. Some of these drugs may also be used to treat restrictive pulmonary diseases.

Chronic Obstructive Pulmonary Disease

Asthma is an inflammatory disorder of the airway walls associated with a varying amount of airway obstruction. This disorder is triggered by stimuli such as stress, allergens, and pollutants. When activated by stimuli, the bronchial airways become inflamed and edematous, leading to constriction of air passages. Inflammation aggravates airway hyperresponsiveness to stimuli, causing bronchial cells to produce more mucous, which obstructs air passages. This obstruction contributes to wheezing, coughing, dyspnea (breathlessness), and tightness in the chest, particularly at night or early morning.

Bronchial asthma, one of the COPD lung diseases, is characterized by bronchospasm (constricted bronchioles), wheezing, mucus secretions, and dyspnea. There is resistance to airflow caused by obstruction of the airway. In acute and chronic asthma, minimal to no changes are seen in the structure and function of lung tissues when the disease process is in remission. In chronic bronchitis, emphysema, and bronchiectasis, there is permanent, irreversible damage to the physical structure of lung tissue. Symptoms are similar to those of asthma in these three pulmonary disorders, except wheezing does not occur. Figure 40–1 displays the overlapping symptoms of COPD conditions.

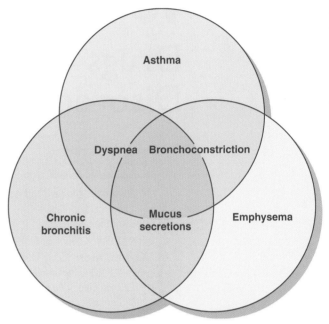

FIGURE 40–1 Overlapping signs and symptoms of chronic obstructive pulmonary disease (COPD) conditions.

Frequently there is a steady deterioration over a period of years.

Chronic bronchitis is a progressive lung disease caused by smoking or chronic lung infections. Bronchial inflammation and excessive mucous secretion result in airway obstruction. Productive coughing is a response to excess mucus production and chronic bronchial irritation. Inspiratory and expiratory rhonchi may be heard on auscultation. Hypercapnia (increased carbon dioxide retention) and hypoxemia (decreased blood oxygen) lead to respiratory acidosis.

In **bronchiectasis** there is abnormal dilation of the bronchi and bronchioles secondary to frequent infection and inflammation. The bronchioles become obstructed by the breakdown of the epithelium of the bronchial mucosa. Tissue fibrosis may result.

Emphysema is a progressive lung disease caused by cigarette smoking, atmospheric contaminants, or lack of the alpha$_1$-antitrypsin protein that inhibits proteolytic enzymes that destroy alveoli (air sacs). Proteolytic enzymes are released in the lung by bacteria or phagocytic cells. The terminal bronchioles become plugged with mucus, causing a loss in the fiber and elastin network in the alveoli. Alveoli enlarge as many of the alveolar walls are destroyed. Air becomes trapped in the overexpanded alveoli, leading to inadequate gas (oxygen and carbon dioxide) exchange.

Cigarette smoking is the most common risk factor for COPD, especially with chronic bronchitis and emphysema. There is no cure for COPD at this time; however, it remains preventable in most cases. Because cigarette smoking is the most directly related cause, not smoking significantly prevents COPD from developing. Quitting smoking will slow the disease process.

Medications frequently prescribed for COPD include the following:

- Bronchodilators such as sympathomimetics (adrenergics), parasympatholytics (anticholinergic drug, Atrovent), and methylxanthines (caffeine, theophylline) are used to assist in opening narrowed airways.
- Glucocorticoids (steroids) are used to decrease inflammation.
- Leukotriene modifiers reduce inflammation in the lung tissue, and cromolyn and nedocromil act as antiinflammatory agents by suppressing the release of histamine and other mediators from the mast cells.
- Expectorants are used to assist in loosening mucus from the airways.
- Antibiotics may be prescribed to prevent serious complications from bacterial infections.

The website, *https://health.live.com/article.aspx?id=articles%2fmlp%2fpages%2f2%2fSmoking_Cessation.htm&qu=Smoking+Cessation* provides links to recommended methods of smoking cessation. One site is the American Academy of Family Physicians (December, 2006) entitled *Smoking: Steps to Help You Break the Habit*, which suggests nicotine products as well as bupropion (Zyban) and varenicline (Chantix).

Bronchial Asthma

Bronchial asthma is a COPD characterized by periods of bronchospasm resulting in wheezing and difficulty breathing. **Bronchospasm**, or bronchoconstriction, results when the lung tissue is exposed to extrinsic or intrinsic factors that stimulate a bronchoconstrictive response. Factors that can trigger an asthmatic attack (bronchospasm) include humidity; air pressure changes; temperature changes; smoke; fumes (exhaust, perfume); stress; emotional upset; exercise; and allergies to animal dander, dust mites, food, and drugs (e.g., aspirin, ibuprofen, beta-adrenergic blockers). Reactive airway disease (RAD) is a cause of asthma resulting from sensitivity stimulation from allergens, dust, temperature changes, and cigarette smoking.

Pathophysiology

Mast cells, found in connective tissue throughout the body, are directly involved in the asthmatic response, particularly to extrinsic factors. Allergens attach themselves to mast cells and basophils, resulting in an antigen-antibody reaction on the mast cells in the lung; thus the mast cells stimulate the release of chemical mediators such as histamines, cytokines, serotonin, eosinophil chemotactic factor of anaphylaxis (ECF-A), and leukotrienes. Eosinophil counts are usually elevated during an allergic reaction, which indicates that an inflammatory process is occurring. These chemical mediators stimulate bronchial constriction, mucous secretions, inflammation, and pulmonary congestion. Histamine and ECF-A are strong bronchoconstrictors. Bronchial smooth muscles are wrapped spirally around the bronchioles and contract as they are stimulated by these mediators. Exposure to an allergen results in

bronchial hyperresponsiveness, epithelial shedding of the bronchial wall, mucous gland hyperplasia and hypersecretion, leakage of plasma leading to swelling, and bronchoconstriction.

Figure 40–2 shows the factors contributing to bronchoconstriction. Cyclic adenosine monophosphate (cyclic AMP, or cAMP), a cellular signaling molecule, is involved in many cellular activities and responsible for maintaining bronchodilation. When histamine, ECF-A, and leukotrienes inhibit the action of cAMP, bronchoconstriction results. The sympathomimetic (adrenergic) bronchodilators and methylxanthines increase the amount of cAMP in bronchial tissue cells.

In an acute asthmatic attack, the short-acting sympathomimetics (beta$_2$-adrenergic agonists) are the first line of defense. They promote cAMP production and enhance bronchodilation. Long-acting sympathomimetics are used for maintenance. Sympathomimetics (adrenergics) are also discussed in Chapter 17.

Sympathomimetics: Alpha- and Beta$_2$-Adrenergic Agonists

Sympathomimetics increase cAMP, causing dilation of the bronchioles. In an acute bronchospasm caused by anaphylaxis from an allergic reaction, the nonselective sympathomimetic epinephrine (Adrenalin), which is an alpha$_1$, beta$_1$, and beta$_2$ agonist, is given subcutaneously to promote bronchodilation and elevate blood pressure. Epinephrine is administered in emergency situations to restore circulation and increase airway patency (see Chapter 58).

For bronchospasm associated with chronic asthma or COPD, selective beta$_2$-adrenergic agonists are given by aerosol or as a tablet. These drugs act primarily on the beta$_2$ receptors; therefore the side effects are less severe than those of epinephrine, which acts on alpha$_1$, beta$_1$, and beta$_2$ receptors.

Albuterol

The newer beta-adrenergic drugs for asthma are more selective for beta$_2$ receptors. High doses or overuse of the beta$_2$-adrenergic agents for asthma may cause some degree of beta$_1$ response such as nervousness, tremor, and increased pulse rate. The ideal beta$_2$ agonist is one that has a rapid onset of action, longer duration of action, and few side effects. Albuterol (Proventil, Ventolin) is a selective beta$_2$ drug that is effective for treatment and control of asthma by causing

Preventing **MEDICATION ERRORS**

Do not confuse...

- **albuterol** (beta$_2$-adrenergic) with **Accupril** (cardiovascular agent). The names look alike, but the class and action are very different.

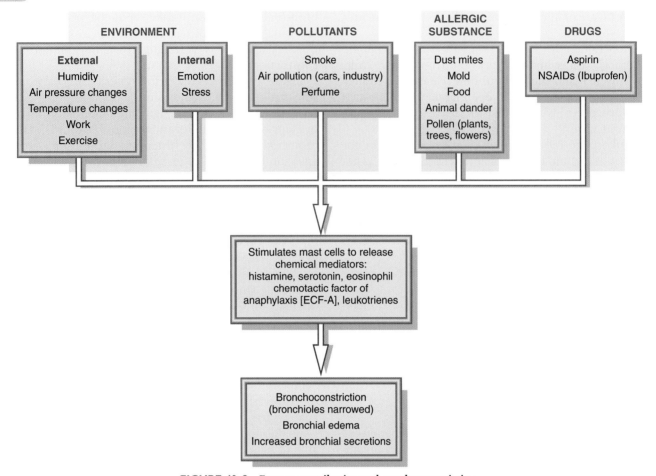

FIGURE 40–2   Factors contributing to bronchoconstriction.

bronchodilation with long duration of action. See Prototype Drug Chart 17–2 for drug data related to albuterol.

Metaproterenol

The second beta-adrenergic agent is metaproterenol (Alupent, Metaprel), which was first marketed in 1961. It has some beta$_1$ effect but is primarily used as a beta$_2$ agent. It can be administered orally or by inhalation with a metered-dose inhaler or a nebulizer.

For long-term asthma treatment, beta$_2$-adrenergic agonists are frequently administered by inhalation. This route of administration usually delivers more of the drug directly to the constricted bronchial site. The effective inhalation drug dose is less than it would be by the oral route, and there are also fewer side effects using this route. The

onset of action of the drug is more rapid (1 minute) by inhalation than orally (15 minutes). Prototype Drug Chart 40–1 lists the pharmacologic behavior of metaproterenol.

Pharmacokinetics

Metaproterenol is well absorbed from the GI tract. Its protein-binding percentage and half-life are unknown. It is metabolized by the liver and excreted in the urine.

Pharmacodynamics

Metaproterenol reverses bronchospasm by relaxing bronchial smooth muscle. The drug acts on the beta$_2$ receptor, promoting bronchodilation, and increases cAMP.

The onset of action for oral and inhalational metaproterenol is fast, and its duration is short. Excessive use of the drug by inhalation may cause tolerance and paradoxic bronchoconstriction. Because it has some beta$_1$ properties, it can cause tremor, nervousness, heart palpitations, and increased heart rate when taken in large doses. A few drug interactions need to be considered. When metaproterenol is taken with a beta-adrenergic blocker, its effects are decreased. Other sympathomimetic agents increase the effects of metaproterenol.

Isoproterenol

The first beta-adrenergic agent used for bronchospasm was isoproterenol (Isuprel), introduced in 1941. It has no alpha-agonist properties, but it is considered a nonselective beta agonist because it stimulates both beta$_1$ and beta$_2$ re-

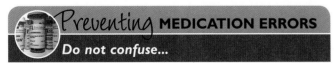

Preventing MEDICATION ERRORS

Do not confuse...

• **Alupent** (beta-adrenergic) with **Atrovent** (another beta-adrenergic bronchodilator). These beta-adrenergic drugs may look alike, but their pharmacology (e.g., interactions, side effects, adverse effects) is different.

Prototype DRUG CHART 40–1

METAPROTERENOL

Drug Class	**Dosage**

Bronchodilator: adrenergic beta$_2$ and some beta$_1$
Trade names: Alupent, Metaprel
Pregnancy Category: C
	A & C >9 y and >27 kg: PO: 20 mg q6-8h
	C 6-9 y or >27 kg: PO: 10 mg q6-8h
	A & C >12 y: MDI 2-3 inhalations as single dose; wait
	  2 min before second dose, if necessary; use only q3-4h
	  to *max:* 12 inhalations/d

Contraindications	**Drug-Lab-Food Interactions**

Hypersensitivity, cardiac dysrhythmias
Caution: Narrow-angle glaucoma, cardiac disease,
  hypertension
	Drug: *Increase* action with sympathomimetics; *decrease*
	  with beta blockers
	Lab: *Decreased* serum potassium

Pharmacokinetics	**Pharmacodynamics**

Absorption: PO: Well absorbed
Distribution: PB: UK
Metabolism: t½: UK
Excretion: In urine as metabolites
	PO: Onset: 15-30 min
	  Peak: 1 h
	  Duration: 4 h
	subQ: Onset: 1-5 min
	  Peak: 1 h
	  Duration: 3-4 h

Therapeutic Effects/Uses

To treat bronchospasm, asthma; to promote bronchodilation
Mode of Action: Relaxation of smooth muscle of bronchi

Side Effects	**Adverse Reactions**

Nervousness, tremors, restlessness, insomnia,
  headache, nausea, vomiting, hyperglycemia,
  muscle cramping in extremities
	Tachycardia, palpitations, hypertension
	Life-threatening: Cardiac dysrhythmias, cardiac arrest,
	  paradoxical bronchoconstriction

A, Adult; *C,* child; *h,* hour; *MDI,* metered-dose inhaler; *min,* minute; *PB,* protein-binding; *PO,* by mouth; *subQ,* subcutaneous; *t½,*
half-life; *UK,* unknown; *y,* year; *>,* greater than; *<,* less than.

---

ceptors. Because the beta$_1$ receptors are stimulated, the heart rate increases, and tachycardia may result. Beta$_2$ stimulation promotes bronchodilation. Isoproterenol is administered by inhalation, using an aerosol inhaler or nebulizer, or intravenously (IV) for severe asthmatic attacks. Its duration of action is short. Because of its severe side effects from beta$_1$ response, it is seldom prescribed.

Use of an Aerosol Inhaler

If the beta$_2$ agonist is given by a metered-dose inhaler (MDI) or dry powdered inhaler (DPI), correct use of the inhaler and dosage intervals need to be explained to the client. If the client does not receive effective relief from the inhaler, either the technique is faulty or the canister is empty (see Chapter 3, Figure 3–16, for how to determine the amount of drug left in the canister). A spacer device may be attached to the inhaler to improve drug delivery to the lung with less deposition in the mouth (see Chapter 3, Figure 3–15). If the client does not use the inhaler properly to deliver the drug dose, the medication may be trapped in the upper airways. Because of drug inhalation, mouth dryness and throat irritation could result. The correct method of using the inhaler is described in the *Nursing Process* box for the bronchodilator Alupent. Chapter 3 also offers a detailed discussion of the proper use of aerosol inhalers.

Excessive use of the aerosol drug can lead to tolerance and loss of drug effectiveness. Occasionally severe paradoxical airway resistance (bronchoconstriction) develops with repeated, excessive use of sympathomimetic oral inhalation. Frequent dosing can cause tremors, nervousness, and increased heart rate. Table 40–1 lists the sympathomimetics used as bronchodilators.

Preventing MEDICATION ERRORS

Do not confuse...

- **Isuprel** (beta-adrenergic) with **Isordil** (nitrate vasodilator). The names look alike, but the class and action are very different.

Table 40–1

Adrenergic Bronchodilators and Anticholinergics

Generic (Brand)	Route and Dosage	Uses and Considerations
Alpha- and Beta-Adrenergic		
ephedrine SO$_4$ (Ephedsol) Alpha$_1$, beta$_1$, beta$_2$	A: PO: 25-50 mg q3-4h; *max:* 150 mg/d PRN; subQ/IM/IV: 12.5-25 mg PRN C: >2 y: PO: 2-3 mg/kg/d in 4-6 divided doses C: 6-12 y: PO: 6.25-12.5 mg q4h; *max:* 75 mg	Relief of allergic rhinitis and sinusitis; improves respiration caused by narcotic excess; corrects hypotensive state. Nervousness, tachycardia, and insomnia could occur. *Pregnancy category:* C; PB: UK; t$^{1/2}$: 3-6 h
epinephrine (Adrenalin, Primatene Mist, Bronkaid Mist) Alpha$_1$, beta$_1$, beta$_2$	A: subQ: 0.1-0.5 mg or ml of 1:1000 sol; may repeat q10-15min PRN C: subQ: 0.01 mg or ml of 1:1000 sol; may repeat q20min-4h PRN Inhal: 1-2 puffs of 1:100 q15min × 2 doses, then q3h	For relief of acute bronchoconstriction and to combat anaphylactic reaction. Nonselective (alpha, beta$_1$, and beta$_2$) adrenergic drug. Used frequently by nebulizer. Side effects include nervousness, tremors, dizziness, palpitations, tachycardia, and other cardiac dysrhythmias. *Pregnancy category:* C; PB: UK; t$^{1/2}$: UK
Beta-Adrenergic		
albuterol (Proventil, Ventolin) Beta$_2$	A & C: >6 y: inhal MDI: 1-2 puffs q4-6h or 2 puffs 15 min before exercise A: PO: 2-4 mg t.i.d. or q.i.d.; *max:* 8 mg q.i.d. SR: 4-8 mg q12h C: 6-12 y: PO: 2 mg t.i.d./q.i.d. C: 2-6 y: PO: 0.1 mg/kg t.i.d.; *max:* 4 mg/dose	Treatment of acute and chronic asthma, bronchitis, and exercise-induced bronchospasm. Onset of action orally is 30 minutes and duration of action is 4-6 hours; SR: 8-12 hours. *Pregnancy category:* C; PB: UK; t$^{1/2}$:4-5 h
bitolterol mesylate (Tornalate) Beta$_1$ (some), beta$_2$	A: inhal MDI: 2 puffs (1-3 min apart), q4-6h; *max:* 12 inhal/d	Treatment of asthma and acute bronchitis. Can be used as single-treatment therapy or in combination with theophylline or corticosteroid. Tremors and nervousness may occur. Has a longer duration of action than many other adrenergics (5-8 hours) by inhalation. *Pregnancy category:* C; PB: UK; t$^{1/2}$: 3 h
isoetharine HCl (Bronkosol) Beta$_1$ (some), beta$_2$	Inhal: 1-2 puffs A: IPPB: 0.5-1.0 ml of 5% sol or 0.5 ml of 1% sol diluted in 3 ml of NSS	For bronchoconstriction and reversible obstructive pulmonary disease. Rapid onset (1-5 min); short duration of action (1-4 hours). *Pregnancy category:* C; PB: UK; t$^{1/2}$: UK
isoproterenol (Isuprel) Beta$_1$ and beta$_2$	A & C: inhal: 1-2 puffs q4-6h	For bronchoconstriction. Nonselective (beta$_1$ and beta$_2$). Beta$_1$ effect causes heart rate to increase. Monitor heart rate and blood pressure. Absorption of sublingual drug can be variable and unpredictable. *Pregnancy category:* C; PB: UK; t$^{1/2}$: 2-5 min
levalbuterol (Xopenex) Beta$_2$	A & C: >12 y: nebulizer 0.63-1.25 mg/ 3 ml q6-8h PRN	Treatment of acute bronchospasm and prevention of exercise-induced asthma. Product from albuterol derivative. Expensive. Rapid absorption and short acting. Side effects are nervousness and tremors. *Pregnancy category:* UK; PB: UK; t$^{1/2}$: UK
metaproterenol sulfate (Alupent, Metaprel) Beta$_1$ (some) and beta$_2$	(Prototype Drug Chart 40–1)	
pirbuterol acetate (Maxair) Beta$_2$	*Prevention:* A & C: >12 y: inhal MDI: 2 puffs q4-6h *Bronchospasm:* A & C: >12 y: inhal MDI: 2 puffs (1-3 min apart) followed by 1 puff; not to exceed 12 inhal/d	Treatment of asthma. Moderate duration of action (5 hours). *Pregnancy category:* C; PB: UK; t$^{1/2}$: 2-3 h
formoterol fumarate (Foradil Aerolizer)	A & C: >5 y: inhal: Inhale contents of 1 capsule q12h	Treatment of asthma and prevention of exercise-induced asthma. *Pregnancy category:* C; PB: UK; t$^{1/2}$: 10 h

A, Adult; *C,* child; *COPD,* chronic obstructive pulmonary disease; *d,* day; *h,* hour; *IM,* intramuscular; *inhal,* inhalation; *IPPB,* intermittent positive-pressure breathing; *IV,* intravenous; *max,* maximum; *MDI,* metered dose inhaler; *min,* minute; *NSS,* normal saline solution; *PB,* protein-binding; *PO,* by mouth; *PRN,* as needed; *q.i.d.,* four times a day; *subQ,* subcutaneous; *sol,* solution; *SR,* sustained-release; *t$^{1/2}$,* half-life; *t.i.d.,* three times a day; *UK,* unknown; *y,* year; *>,* greater than.

Table 40–1

Adrenergic Bronchodilators and Anticholinergics—cont'd

Generic (Brand)	Route and Dosage	Uses and Considerations
tiotropium (Spiriva)	A: inhal: Inhale contents of 1 capsule daily	Treatment of bronchospasm associated with chronic obstructive pulmonary disease (COPD). First long-acting inhaled anticholinergic drug for treatment of COPD. *Pregnancy category*: UK; PB: UK; $t^{1/2}$: 5-6 days
salmeterol (Serevent) Beta$_2$	*Maintenance bronchodilation*: A & C: >12 y: Inhal MDI: 2 puffs q12h *Prevention of exercise-induced broncho-spasm*: A & C: >12 y: Inhal MDI: 2 puffs 30-60 min before exercise	Treatment for chronic asthma and exercise-induced bronchospasm. Not effective for treating acute bron-chospasms. Has a long duration of action (12 h). *Pregnancy category*: C; PB: 94%-98%; $t^{1/2}$: 5.5 h
terbutaline SO$_4$ (Brethine, Bricanyl) Beta$_2$	Inhal MDI: 1-2 puffs q4-6h A: PO: 2.5-5 mg t.i.d.; subQ: 0.25-0.5 mg q8h IV: 10 mcg/min, gradually increase; *max*: 80 mcg/min C: >12 y: PO: 2.5 mg t.i.d.	To treat reversible airway obstruction caused by asthma, bronchitis, and emphysema. May cause ner-vousness, tremors, lightheadedness, palpitations, or tachycardia if taken in excess. Slow to moderate on-set (15-30 min); long oral duration (4-8 h) and moderate inhaled duration (3-6 h). *Pregnancy cate-gory*: B; PB: 25%; $t^{1/2}$: 3-11 h
arformoterol tartrate (Brovana) Beta$_2$	A: inhal nebulizer: 15 mcg bid; *max*: 30 mcg/d	For long-term, maintenance treatment of COPD. Not effective for treating acute bronchospasms. Has a long duration of action. *Pregnancy category*: C; PB: 52%-65%; $t^{1/2}$: 26 h
Anticholinergics		
ipratropium bromide (Atrovent)	*COPD*: A: inhal MDI: 2 puffs t.i.d., q.i.d., >4 h intervals; *max*: 12 inhal/d	To treat bronchospasm associated with COPD, includ-ing asthma. Use with caution in clients with nar-row-angle glaucoma. *Pregnancy category*: B; PB: UK; $t^{1/2}$: 1.5-2 h
ipratropium with albuterol (Combivent)	A: inhal MDI: 2 puffs t.i.d., q.i.d.	Anticholinergic agent combines with beta$_2$-adrenergic agonist to increase bronchodilation. With use of this combination of drugs, duration of action is pro-longed. *Pregnancy category*: UK; PB: UK; $t^{1/2}$: UK

Side Effects and Adverse Reactions

The side effects and adverse reactions of epinephrine include tremors, dizziness, hypertension, tachycardia, heart palpitations, cardiac dysrhythmias, and angina. The client needs to be closely monitored when epinephrine is administered.

The side effects associated with beta$_2$-adrenergic drugs (e.g., albuterol, terbutaline) include tremors, headaches, nervousness, increased pulse rate, and palpitations (high doses). The beta$_2$ agonists may increase blood glucose levels, so clients with diabetes should be taught to closely monitor their serum glucose levels. Side effects of beta$_2$ agonists may diminish after a week or longer. The bron-chodilating effects may decrease with continued use. It is believed that tolerance to these drugs can develop; if this occurs, the dose may need to be increased. Failure to re-spond to a previously effective dose may indicate worsen-ing asthma that requires reevaluation before increasing the dose.

Anticholinergics

Recently a new anticholinergic drug, ipratropium bromide (Atrovent), was introduced to treat asthmatic conditions by dilating the bronchioles. Unlike other anticholinergics,

ipratropium has few systemic effects. It is administered by aerosol.

Clients who use a beta-agonist inhalant should admin-ister it 5 minutes before using ipratropium. When using the anticholinergic agent in conjunction with an inhaled glucocorticoid (steroid) or cromolyn, the ipratropium should be used 5 minutes before the steroid or cromolyn. This causes the bronchioles to dilate so the steroid or cro-molyn can be deposited in the bronchioles.

The combination of ipratropium bromide with alb-uterol sulfate (Combivent) is used to treat chronic bron-chitis. The combination is more effective and has a longer duration of action than if either agent is used alone. These two agents combined increase the FEV$_1$, the index used to evaluate asthma and obstructive lung disease and the cli-ent's response to bronchodilator therapy. Table 40–2 lists the inhalants for asthma control.

Methylxanthine (Xanthine) Derivatives

The second major group of bronchodilators used to treat asthma is the methylxanthine (xanthine) derivatives, which include aminophylline, theophylline, and caffeine. Xan-

Table 40–2

Inhalants for Asthma Control

Categories	Inhalant Agents
Adrenergics	
Beta$_1$ and beta$_2$	isoproterenol (Isuprel)
Beta$_2$ and some beta$_1$	bitolterol mesylate (Tornalate)
	isoetharine HCl (Bronkosol)
	metaproterenol sulfate (Alupent, Metaprel)
Beta$_2$	albuterol (Proventil, Ventolin)
	pirbuterol acetate (Maxair)
	salmeterol (Serevent)
	terbutaline sulfate (Brethine, Brethaire)
	arformoterol tartrate (Brovana)
Anticholinergics	ipratropium bromide (Atrovent)
	ipratropium and albuterol (Combivent)
Antiinflammatory Drugs	
cromolyn and nedocromil	cromolyn (Intal)
	nedocromil (Tilade)
glucocorticoids (corticosteroids)	beclomethasone (Beclovent, Vanceril)
	budesonide (Rhinocort)
	dexamethasone (Decadron)
	flunisolide (Nasalide)
	fluticasone (Flonase)
	mometasone furoate (Nasonex)
	triamcinolone (Nasacort)

thines also stimulate the central nervous system (CNS) and respiration, dilate coronary and pulmonary vessels, and cause diuresis. Because of their effect on respiration and pulmonary vessels, xanthines are used in the treatment of asthma.

Theophylline

The first theophylline preparation, aminophylline, was produced in 1936. Theophylline relaxes the smooth muscles of the bronchi, bronchioles, and pulmonary blood vessels by inhibiting the enzyme phosphodiesterase, resulting in an increase in cAMP, which promotes bronchodilation.

Theophylline has a low therapeutic index and a narrow therapeutic range (10 to 20 mcg/ml). The serum or plasma theophylline concentration level should be monitored frequently to avoid severe adverse effects. Toxicity is likely to occur when the serum level is greater than 20 mcg/ml. Certain theophylline preparations can be given with sympathomimetic (adrenergic) agents, but the dose may need to be adjusted.

Theophylline was once used as the first-line drug for treating clients with chronic asthma and other COPDs. However, theophylline use has declined sharply, because there is a potential danger of serious adverse effects (e.g.,

dysrhythmias, convulsions, cardiorespiratory collapse), and efficacy has not been found to be greater than beta agonists or glucocorticoids. Because of its numerous adverse reactions, drug-drug interactions, and narrow therapeutic drug range, it is prescribed mostly for maintenance therapy in clients with chronic stable asthma and other COPDs. Theophylline drugs are NOT prescribed for clients with seizure disorders or cardiac, renal, or liver disease. Clients who receive theophylline preparations need to be closely monitored for serious side effects and drug interactions.

Table 40–3 lists the theophylline preparations and their dosages, uses, and considerations.

Pharmacokinetics

Theophylline is usually well absorbed after oral administration, but absorption may vary according to the specific dosage form. Theophylline is also well absorbed from oral liquids and uncoated plain tablets. Sustained-release dosage forms are slowly absorbed. Food and antacids may decrease the rate but not the extent of absorption; large volumes of fluid and high-protein meals may increase the rate of absorption. The dose size can also affect the rate of absorption: larger doses are absorbed more slowly. Theophylline can also be administered in IV fluids.

The theophylline drugs are metabolized by liver enzymes, and 90% of the drug is excreted by the kidneys. Tobacco smoking increases metabolism of theophylline drugs, thereby decreasing the half-life of the drug. The half-life is also shorter in children. With a short half-life, theophylline is readily excreted by the kidneys, so the drug dose may need to be increased to maintain therapeutic serum/plasma range. In nonsmokers and older adults, the average half-life of theophylline is 7 to 9 hours, and the dose requirements may be decreased. However, in smokers and children, the half-life is 4 to 5 hours, and the dose requirement may be increased. In premature infants, the half-life is 15 to 55 hours. In clients with heart failure (HF), cor pulmonale, COPD, or liver disease, the half-life is 12 hours. Kidney function may be decreased in older adults, so to avoid drug toxicity, caution should be used regarding the theophylline dosage.

Pharmacodynamics

Theophylline increases the level of cAMP, resulting in bronchodilation. The average onset of action for oral theophylline preparations is 30 minutes; for sustained-release capsules, it is 1 to 2 hours. The duration of action for the sustained-release form is 8 to 24 hours and approximately 6 hours for other oral and IV theophylline preparations.

Side Effects and Adverse Reactions

Side effects and adverse reactions to theophylline include anorexia, nausea and vomiting, gastric pain caused by increased gastric acid secretion, intestinal bleeding, nervousness, dizziness, headache, irritability, cardiac dysrhythmias, tachycardia, palpitations, marked hypotension, hyperreflexia, and seizures. Adverse CNS reactions (e.g., headaches, irritability, restlessness, nervousness, insomnia, dizziness, seizures) are often more severe in children than in adults. To decrease the potential for side effects, clients should not take other xanthines while taking theophylline.

Theophylline toxicity is most likely to occur when serum concentrations exceed 20 mcg/ml. Theophylline can cause hyperglycemia, decreased clotting time, and, rarely, increased white blood cell count (leukocytosis). Because of the diuretic effect of xanthines, including theophylline, clients should avoid caffeinated products (e.g., coffee, tea, colas, chocolate) and increase their fluid intake.

Table 40-3

Theophylline Preparations

Generic (Brand)	Route and Dosage	Uses and Considerations
aminophylline—theophylline ethylenediamine (Somophyllin)	A: PO: LD 400 mg; then increase dose according to body weight; *max*: 24 mg/kg/d IV: LD: 6 mg/kg over 30 min; then 0.2-0.9 mg/kg/h C: PO: LD: 7.5 mg/kg; then 3-6 mg/kg q6-8h IV: LD 6 mg/kg then 1 mg/kg/h **Caution:** Individual titration is based on serum theophylline levels.	IV for acute asthmatic attack. For IV use, drug must be diluted. Oral preparations are tablets or elixirs. For oral use, give with food to avoid GI distress. Side effects include restlessness, syncope, palpitation, tachycardia, hyperventilation, and cardiac dysrhythmias. *Pregnancy category*: C; PB: UK; t$\frac{1}{2}$: 4-9 h
dyphylline—dihydroxypropyl theophylline-like (Dilor, Lufyllin)	A: PO: 15 mg/kg q.i.d. A: IM: 250-500 mg q6h C: >6 y: PO: 4-7 mg/kg/d in 4 divided doses Therapeutic serum theophylline range: 10-20 mcg/ml	Treatment of asthma, chronic bronchitis, and emphysema. One tenth as potent as theophylline. Structure is similar to that of theophylline, but it does not convert to theophylline in the body. *Pregnancy category*: C; PB: UK; t$\frac{1}{2}$: 2 h
oxtriphylline—choline theophyllinate (Choledyl)	A: PO: 200 mg q8h C: 2-12 y: PO: 4 mg/kg q6h Therapeutic serum theophylline range: 10-20 mcg/ml	Relief of asthma and COPD. Useful for long-term therapy. Drug tolerance is infrequent. Contains 64% theophylline. *Pregnancy category*: C; PB: UK; t$\frac{1}{2}$: 3-13 h
theophylline (Theo-Dur and others)	Dose individualized according to serum theophylline levels *Initially*: A: PO: 16 mg/kg/d; *max*: 300 mg/d C: >45 kg: PO: 300 mg/d divided q8-12h C: <45 kg: PO: 12-14 mg/kg/d Premature neonates: >24 h postnatal age: 1.5 mg/kg q12h Premature neonates: <24 h postnatal age: 1 mg/kg q12h May increase in 25% increments after 3 days as tolerated until dose effective	To promote bronchodilation and treat asthma and chronic obstructive pulmonary disease

A, Adult; *C*, child; *COPD*, chronic obstructive pulmonary disease; *d*, day; *GI*, gastrointestinal; *h*, hour; *IM*, intramuscular; *IV*, intravenous; *LD*, loading dose; *max*, maximum; *min*, minute; *PB*, protein-binding; *PO*, by mouth; *q.i.d.*, four times a day; *t$\frac{1}{2}$*, half-life; *UK*, unknown; *y*, year; . >, greater than; <, less than.

Rapid IV administration of aminophylline (a theophylline product) can cause dizziness, flushing, hypotension, severe bradycardia, and palpitations. To avoid severe adverse effects, IV theophylline preparations MUST be administered slowly via an infusion pump.

Drug Interactions

Beta-blockers, cimetidine (Tagamet), propranolol (Inderal), and erythromycin decrease the liver metabolism rate and increase the half-life and effects of theophylline; barbiturate and carbamazepine decrease its effects. In both situations, the theophylline dosage would need adjustment. Theophylline increases the risk of digitalis toxicity and decreases the effects of lithium. Phenytoin decreases theophylline levels. If theophylline and a beta-adrenergic agonist are given together, a synergistic effect can occur; cardiac dysrhythmias may result.

Nursing Process

Bronchodilators

ASSESSMENT

■ Obtain a medical and drug history; report probable drug-drug interactions.

■ Note baseline vital signs for abnormalities and future comparisons.

■ Assess for wheezing, decreased breath sounds, cough, and sputum production.

■ Assess sensorium for confusion and restlessness caused by hypoxia and hypercapnia.

■ Determine hydration; diuresis may result in dehydration in children and older adults.

■ Assess serum theophylline levels. Toxicity occurs at a higher frequency with levels greater than 20 mcg/ml.

NURSING DIAGNOSES

■ Ineffective breathing pattern related to fatigue
■ Ineffective airway clearance related to retained secretions in the bronchi
■ Impaired gas exchange related to ineffective airway clearance
■ Noncompliance with drug therapy related to inadequate financial resources
■ Activity intolerance related to fatigue and an imbalance between oxygen supply and demand

PLANNING

■ Client will be free of wheezing, and lung fields will be clear within 2 to 5 days.
■ Client will self-administer oral drugs and inhaler as prescribed.

NURSING INTERVENTIONS

■ Monitor vital signs. Blood pressure and heart rate can increase greatly. Check for cardiac dysrhythmias.
■ Provide adequate hydration. Fluids aid in loosening secretions.
■ Monitor drug therapy. Observe for side effects.
■ Administer medication after meals to decrease gastrointestinal distress.
■ Administer medication at regular intervals around the clock to have a sustained therapeutic level.
■ Do *not* crush enteric-coated or sustained-released (SR) tablets or capsules.
■ Check serum theophylline levels (normal level is 10 to 20 mcg/ml).

Client Teaching

General

• Teach client to monitor pulse rate.
• Encourage client to monitor amount of medication remaining in the canister.
• Advise client not to take OTC preparations without first checking with health care provider. Some OTC products may have an additive effect.
• Encourage client contemplating pregnancy to seek medical advice before taking a theophylline preparation.
• Instruct client to avoid smoking. Avoid marked sudden changes in smoking amounts, which could affect theophylline blood levels. Smoking increases drug elimination, which may require an increased drug dose.
• Discuss ways to alleviate anxiety, such as relaxation techniques and music.
• Advise client having asthma attacks to wear an ID bracelet or MedicAlert tag.
• Inform client that certain herbal products may interact with theophylline (Herbal Alert 40–1).

Self-Administration

• Teach client to correctly use inhaler or nebulizer. Caution against overuse, because side effects and tolerance may result.
• Instruct client to monitor pulse rate and report to health care provider any irregularities in comparison with baseline.

Diet

• Advise client that a high-protein, low-carbohydrate diet increases theophylline elimination. Conversely, a low-protein, high-carbohydrate diet prolongs the half-life; dosage may need adjustment.

Correct Use of Metered-Dose Inhaler to Deliver Beta$_2$ Agonist:

• Insert medication canister into plastic mouthpiece.
• Shake inhaler well *before* using. Remove cap from mouthpiece.
• Breathe *out* through the mouth. Open mouth wide and hold mouthpiece 1 to 2 inches from mouth or place inhaler mouthpiece in mouth. A spacer may be used. Discuss technique with health care provider.
• Open mouth, take a *slow deep* breath through the mouth, and at same time push the top of the medication canister once.
• Hold breath for a few seconds; exhale slowly through pursed lips.
• Wait 2 minutes if a second dose is required, then repeat the procedure by first shaking the inhaler with the mouthpiece cap in place.
• Do a "test spray" before administering the metered dose of a new inhaler or when the inhaler has not been used recently.
• Self-administer a bronchodilator first when taken at the same time as a steroid, then *wait 5 minutes* for optimal bronchodilator effect before using the steroid.

Cultural Considerations ❖

• Respect cultural beliefs and practices concerning alternative ways to treat asthma or other chronic obstructive pulmonary disease, and incorporate them into client care if they are harmless. If traditional practices/medicines are unsafe, explain in terms that can be understood.
• If client from a different cultural background does not comply with drug regimen, the health care provider might consult a health care provider of similar background and provide a written plan in the language client speaks and reads most easily.

EVALUATION

■ Evaluate the effectiveness of the bronchodilator. Client is breathing without wheezing and without side effects of the drug.
■ Determine serum theophylline levels to assure therapeutic range.

Table 40–4

Antiinflammatory Drugs for Chronic Obstructive Pulmonary Disease

Generic (Brand)	Route and Dosage	Uses and Considerations
Leukotriene Modifiers (Do Not Administer for Acute Asthmatic Attack)		
Leukotriene Receptor Antagonists		
zafirlukast (Accolate)	A: PO: 20 mg b.i.d. 1 h before or 2 h after meals C: >12 y: PO: same as adults C: 7-12 y: PO: 10 mg b.i.d.	For prophylaxis and maintenance therapy for chronic asthma. Reduces inflammation within bronchial tubes and airways. *Pregnancy category*: B; PB: .99%; t$^{1/2}$: 10 h
montelukast (Singulair)	(Prototype Drug Chart 40–2)	
Leukotriene Synthesis Inhibitors		
zileuton (Zyflo)	A: PO: 600 mg q.i.d. C: >12 y: PO: 600 mg q.i.d.	For prophylaxis and maintenance therapy for chronic asthma. Reduces inflammation in airways and decreases bronchoconstriction. Hepatotoxicity may result; liver enzymes should be closely monitored. *Pregnancy category*: C; PB: 93%; t$^{1/2}$: 2.5 h
Glucocorticoids (Corticosteroids)		
Intranasal Spray (see Chapter 39, Table 39–3)		
beclomethasone (Beconase, Vancenase)		
budesonide (Pulmicort, Rhinocort)		
dexamethasone (Decadron)		
flunisolide (AeroBid, Nasalide)		
fluticasone (Flonase, Flovent)		
mometasone furoate (Elocon, Nasonex)		
triamcinolone (Nasacort)		
Aerosol Inhalation (see Chapter 50, Table 50–5)		
beclomethasone (Beconase, Vanceril)		
dexamethasone (Decadron)		
flunisolide (AeroBid, Nasalide)		
triamcinolone (Azmacort, Kenalog, Nasacort)		
Oral and Intravenous Administration (see Chapter 50, Table 50–5)		
betamethasone (Celestone)		
cortisone acetate (Cortone Acetate, Cortistan)		
dexamethasone (Decadron)		
fludrocortisone acetate (Florinef acetate)		
hydrocortisone (Cortef, Hydrocortone)		
methylprednisolone (Medrol, Solu-Medrol, Depo-Medrol)		
paramethasone acetate (Haldrone)		
prednisolone (Delta-Cortef, Hydeltrasol)		
prednisone		
triamcinolone (Aristocort)		
Combination Drug: Glucocorticoid and Beta$_2$ Agonist		
fluticasone propionate (Flonase) and salmeterol (Serevent) (Advair Diskus 100 mcg/50 mcg)	A & C: >12 y: DPI Diskus inhal: 1 puff b.i.d.	For asthma; not to treat acute asthmatic attacks. If insufficient response, fluticasone dose may be increased.
Cromolyn and Nedocromil (Do Not Use for Acute Asthmatic Attack)		
cromolyn sodium (Intal)	A & C: >6 y: Inhal MDI: 1 puff q.i.d.; available: oral solution and powder, intranasal	For chronic asthma and prophylactic use. Suppresses inflammation in bronchial tubes; does not have bronchodilating effects. Prevents release of histamine. *Pregnancy category*: B; PB: UK; t$^{1/2}$: 80 min
nedocromil sodium (Tilade)	A & C: >6 y: Inhal MDI: 2 puffs, q.i.d.; may decrease to b.i.d. to t.i.d.	For maintenance therapy for mild to moderate asthma. Has antiinflammatory effect. Suppresses release of histamine. *Pregnancy category*: B; PB: UK; t$^{1/2}$: 1.5-3 h

A, Adult; *b.i.d.*, twice a day; *C*, child; *DPI*, dry powdered inhaler; *h*, hour; *inhal*, inhalation; *MDI*, metered dose inhaler; *min*, minute; *PB*, protein-binding; *PO*, by mouth; *q.i.d.*, four times a day; *t$^{1/2}$*, half-life; *t.i.d.*, three times a day; *UK*, unknown; *y*, year; >, greater than.

Prototype DRUG CHART 40–2

MONTELUKAST

Drug Class Bronchodilator: Leukotriene receptor antagonist Trade name: Singulair *Pregnancy Category:* B	**Dosage** A: PO: 10 mg daily at bedtime C: 6-14 y: PO: 5 mg daily at bedtime C: 2-5y: 4 mg daily at bedtime
Contraindications Hypersensitivity, severe asthma attack, status asthmaticus *Caution:* Severe liver disease	**Drug-Lab-Food Interactions** *Lab:* Abnormal liver function tests (ALT, AST)

Pharmacokinetics
 	
Absorption: Well absorbed
Distribution: PB: 99%
Metabolism: t½: 2.7-5.5 h
Excretion: Feces
	Pharmacodynamics
	
	PO: Onset: UK
	  Peak: 3-4 h
	  Duration: UK

Therapeutic Effects/Uses

For the prevention and maintenance treatment of asthma
Mode of Action: Binds with leukotriene receptors to inhibit smooth muscle contraction and bronchoconstriction

Side Effects	**Adverse Reactions**
Fever, headache, dizziness, fatigue, nasal congestion, cough, sore throat, dental pain, influenza, dyspepsia, abdominal pain, rash	None known *Life-threatening:* None known

A, Adult; *ALT,* alanine aminotransferase; *AST,* aspartate aminotransferase; *C,* child; *h,* hour; *PB,* protein-binding; *PO,* by mouth; *t½,* half-life; *UK,* unknown; *y,* year.

Leukotriene Receptor Antagonists and Synthesis Inhibitors

Leukotriene (LT) is a chemical mediator that can cause inflammatory changes in the lung. The cysteinyl leukotrienes promote an increase in eosinophil migration, mucus production, and airway wall edema, which result in bronchoconstriction. LT receptor antagonists and LT synthesis inhibitors, called *leukotriene modifiers*, are effective in reducing the inflammatory symptoms of asthma triggered by allergic and environmental stimuli. These drug groups are not recommended for the treatment of an acute asthma attack. They are used for exercise-induced asthma. Three leukotriene modifiers—zafirlukast (Accolate), zileuton (Zyflo), and montelukast sodium (Singulair)—are available in the United States. These drugs are listed in Table 40–4.

Zafirlukast (Accolate) was the first drug in the class of leukotriene modifiers. It acts as an LT receptor antagonist, reducing the inflammatory process and decreasing bronchoconstriction. It is administered orally and absorbed rapidly. It has a moderate to moderately long half-life and is given twice a day. Zileuton (Zyflo) is an LT synthesis inhibitor. It decreases the inflammatory process and bron-

choconstriction. Zileuton has a short half-life and is given four times a day. Zafirlukast and zileuton are for adults and children older than 12 years. Montelukast (Singulair) is a newer LT receptor antagonist (Prototype Drug Chart 40–2). It has a short half-life of 2.5 to 5.5 hours and is considered safe for use in children 6 years and older.

This category of drugs is the newest group used to control asthma. Again, LT receptor antagonists and synthesis inhibitors should NOT be used during an acute asthmatic attack. They are only for prophylactic and maintenance drug therapy for chronic asthma.

Nursing Process

Leukotriene Receptor Antagonists

ASSESSMENT

■ Obtain a medical, drug, and herbal history; report probable drug-drug or drug-herb interactions.
■ Note baseline vital signs for identifying abnormalities and for future comparisons.

■ Assess for wheezing, decreased breath sounds, cough, and sputum production.

■ Assess sensorium for confusion and restlessness caused by hypoxia and hypercapnia.

■ Assess for a history of phenylketonuria when montelukast is prescribed, because children's chewable tablets contain phenylalanine.

■ Determine hydration; diuresis may result in dehydration in children and older adults.

NURSING DIAGNOSES

■ Ineffective airway clearance related to retained secretions in the bronchi

■ Activity intolerance related to an imbalance between oxygen supply and demand

■ Deficient knowledge of OTC drug interaction related to lack of exposure to information

PLANNING

■ Client will be free of wheezing or significantly improved.

■ Client's lung fields will be clear within 2 to 5 days.

■ Client will take medications as prescribed.

NURSING INTERVENTIONS

■ Monitor respirations for rate, depth, rhythm, and type.

■ Monitor lung sounds for rhonchi, wheezing, or rales.

■ Observe lips and fingernails for cyanosis.

■ Monitor drug therapy for effectiveness. Observe for side effects.

■ Provide adequate hydration. Fluids aid in loosening secretions.

■ Monitor liver function tests; AST and ALT may be elevated with zafirlukast and montelukast.

■ Provide pulmonary therapy by chest clapping and postural drainage, as appropriate.

Client Teaching

General

• Advise client that if allergic reaction occurs (i.e., rash, urticaria), drug should be discontinued and health care provider should be notified.

• Monitor periodic liver function tests.

• Direct client not to take St. John's wort without first checking with health care provider, because this herb may decrease montelukast concentration.

• Warn client that black or green tea and guarana with montelukast and zafirlukast may cause increased stimulation.

• Encourage client to stop smoking.

• Discuss ways to alleviate anxiety (relaxation techniques, music).

• Advise client having frequent or severe asthma attacks to wear an ID bracelet or MedicAlert tag.

• Encourage client contemplating pregnancy to seek medical advice before taking montelukast.

• Tell client or significant other that oral granule packets should not be opened until ready for use. After opening the packet, the dose must be administered within 15 minutes. If mixed with baby formula or approved food (applesauce, carrots, rice, or ice cream), it must not be stored for future use.

• Advise client with known aspirin sensitivity to avoid a bronchoconstrictor response by avoiding aspirin and NSAIDs while taking montelukast.

Self-Administration

• Teach client not to use montelukast for reversal of an acute asthmatic attack, because it is only recommended for prevention of acute attacks and treatment of chronic asthma.

• Advise client to continue to use their usual regimen of inhaled prophylaxis and short-acting rescue medication for exercise-induced bronchospasm.

• Encourage client to inform health care provider if short-acting inhaled bronchodilators are needed more often than usual with montelukast.

• Instruct client to comply with medication regimen even in symptom-free periods.

• Advise client (especially children) that chewable tablets are to be chewed thoroughly because swallowing whole may alter absorption.

Diet

• Tell client to take leukotriene receptor antagonists in the evening for maximum effectiveness.

Cultural Considerations ❖

• When offering a prescription, instructions, or pamphlets to Asian and Pacific Islanders, use both hands to show respect.

EVALUATION

■ Evaluate the effectiveness of the bronchodilators. Client is breathing without wheezing and without side effects of the drug.

■ Evaluate tolerance to activity.

Glucocorticoids (Steroids)

Glucocorticoids, members of the corticosteroid family, are used to treat respiratory disorders, particularly asthma. These drugs have an antiinflammatory action and are indicated if asthma is unresponsive to bronchodilator therapy or if the client has an asthma attack while on maximum doses of theophylline or an adrenergic drug. It is thought that glucocorticoids have a synergistic effect when given with a beta$_2$ agonist.

Glucocorticoids can be given using the following methods:

• *MDI inhaler:* beclomethasone (Vanceril, Beclovent)

- *Tablet:* triamcinolone (Aristocort), dexamethasone (Decadron), prednisone, prednisolone, and methylprednisolone
- *Intravenous:* dexamethasone (Decadron), hydrocortisone

Inhaled glucocorticoids are not helpful in treating a severe asthma attack, because it may take 1 to 4 weeks for an inhaled steroid to reach its full effect. When maintained on inhaled glucocorticoids, asthmatic clients demonstrate an improvement in symptoms and a decrease in asthma attacks. Inhaled glucocorticoids are more effective for controlling symptoms of asthma than beta$_2$-agonists, particularly in the reduction of bronchial hyperresponsiveness. The use of an oral inhaler minimizes the risk of adrenal suppression associated with oral systemic glucocorticoid therapy. Inhaled glucocorticoids are preferred over oral preparations unless they fail to control the asthma.

Clients with acute asthma exacerbations are usually given systemic glucocorticoids (i.e., IV) for rapid effectiveness in large doses (40-60 mg prednisone for 5 days; 1-2 mg/kg/day for children for 3-5 days). An additional week with a reduced dose may be needed. With a single dose or short term use, glucocorticoids may be discontinued abruptly after symptoms are controlled. Suppression of adrenal function does not usually occur within 1-2 weeks.

When severe asthma requires prolonged glucocorticoid therapy, weaning or tapering of the dose may be necessary to prevent an exacerbation of asthma symptoms and suppression of adrenal function. Previously, alternate-day therapy (ADT) with oral prednisone was used in some asthmatic clients. Currently, inhaled glucocorticoids are thought to be preferable in the treatment of most clients with asthma. Glucocorticoid preparations are discussed in detail in Chapter 50.

Glucocorticoids can irritate the gastric mucosa and should be taken with food to avoid ulceration. A combination drug containing the glucocorticoid fluticasone propionate 100 mcg and salmeterol 50 mcg (Advair Diskus 100/50) is effective in controlling asthma symptoms. Advair is used every day, but requires only one inhalation in the morning and one at night. This drug does not replace fast-acting inhalers for sudden symptoms. The purpose of Advair is to alleviate airway constriction and inflammation.

Side Effects and Adverse Reactions

Side effects associated with orally inhaled glucocorticoids are generally local (e.g., throat irritation, hoarseness, dry mouth, coughing) rather than systemic. Oral, laryngeal, and pharyngeal fungal infections have occurred but can be reversed with discontinuation and antifungal treatment. *Candida albicans* oropharyngeal infections may be prevented by using a spacer with the inhaler to reduce drug deposits in the oral cavity, rinsing the mouth and throat with water after each dose, and washing the apparatus (cap and plastic nose or mouthpiece) daily with warm water.

Oral and injectable glucocorticoids have many side effects when used long-term, but short-term use usually causes no significant side effects. Most adverse reactions are seen within 2 weeks of glucocorticoid therapy and are usually reversible. Side effects that may occur include headache, euphoria, confusion, sweating, insomnia, nausea, vomiting, weakness, and menstrual irregularities. Adverse effects may include depression, peptic ulcer, loss of bone density and development of osteoporosis, and psychosis.

When oral and IV steroids are used for prolonged periods, electrolyte imbalance, fluid retention (puffy eyelids, edema in the lower extremities, moon face, weight gain), hypertension, thinning of the skin, purpura, abnormal subcutaneous (fat) distribution, hyperglycemia, and impaired immune response are likely to occur.

Cromolyn and Nedocromil

Cromolyn sodium (Intal) is used for prophylactic treatment of bronchial asthma and must be taken daily. It is not used for acute asthmatic attacks. Cromolyn does not have bronchodilator properties, but instead acts by inhibiting the release of histamine to prevent an asthma reaction. Its most common side effects are cough and a bad taste. These effects can be decreased by drinking water before and after using the drug.

Cromolyn is administered by inhalation. It can be used with beta adrenergics and xanthine derivatives. Rebound bronchospasm is a serious side effect of cromolyn. The drug should not be discontinued abruptly, because a rebound asthma attack can result.

Action and uses of nedocromil sodium are similar to those of cromolyn sodium. It has an antiinflammatory effect and suppresses the release of histamine, leukotrienes, and other mediators from the mast cells. Like cromolyn, it should not be used during an acute asthma attack, but instead to prevent bronchospasm and acute asthma attack. The inhalation may cause an unpleasant taste. Nedocromil is believed to be more effective than cromolyn.

Table 40–4 lists the antiinflammatory drugs for COPD, which include LT receptor antagonists, LT synthesis inhibitors, glucocorticoids (intranasal spray, aerosol, inhalation, oral, intramuscular, and intravenous), and cromolyn sodium and nedocromil sodium.

Drug Therapy for Asthma According to Severity

Chronic asthma may be controlled through a long-term drug treatment program and by a quick-relief program during an acute phase. A list of steps for controlling and

---

Herbal ALERT 40–1

Lower Respiratory Disorders

Ephedra may increase the effect of the theophylline group and may cause theophylline toxicity.

treating chronic asthma according to the severity of the asthma is presented in Figure 40–3. This treatment regimen was developed by the National Asthma Education and Prevention Program of the National Heart, Lung, and Blood Institute in Bethesda, Maryland, in 1997 and updated in 2007. The long-term drug treatment program may vary according to the symptoms of the asthma and its severity. The quick-relief drug therapy is the same for all classes of asthma.

Key: **Alphabetical order is used when more than one treatment option is listed within either preferred or alternative therapy.** ICS, inhaled corticosteroid; LABA, long-acting inhaled beta$_2$-agonist; LTRA, leukotriene receptor antagonist; SABA, inhaled short-acting beta$_2$-agonist

Notes:
• The stepwise approach is meant to assist, not replace, the clinical decisionmaking required to meet individual patient needs.
• If alternative treatment is used and response is inadequate, discontinue it and use the preferred treatment before stepping up.
• Zileuton is a less desirable alternative due to limited studies as adjunctive therapy and the need to monitor liver function. Theophylline requires monitoring of serum concentration levels.
• In step 6, before oral corticosteroids are introduced, a trial of high-dose ICS + LABA + either LTRA, theophylline, or zileuton may be considered, although this approach has not been studied in clinical trials.
• Step 1, 2, and 3 preferred therapies are based on Evidence A; step 3 alternative therapy is based on Evidence A for LTRA, Evidence B for theophylline, and Evidence D for zileuton. Step 4 preferred therapy is based on Evidence B, and alternative therapy is based on Evidence B for LTRA and theophylline and Evidence D zileuton. Step 5 preferred therapy is based on Evidence B. Step 6 preferred therapy is based on (EPR—2 1997) and Evidence B for omalizumab.
• Immunotherapy for steps 2–4 is based on Evidence B for house-dust mites, animal danders, and pollens; evidence is weak or lacking for molds and cockroaches. Evidence is strongest for immunotherapy with single allergens. The role of allergy in asthma is greater in children than in adults.
• Clinicians who administer immunotherapy or omalizumab should be prepared and equipped to identify and treat anaphylaxis that may occur.

FIGURE 40–3 Stepwise approach for managing asthma in clients 11 years of age and older. (From the National Asthma Education and Prevention Program Expert Panel Report 3: *Guidelines for the diagnosis and management of asthma* [NIH Publication Number 08-5845]. Washington, DC, National Heart, Lung, and Blood Institute, U.S. Department of Health and Human Services. Accessed May 13, 2008, at *http://www.nhlbi.nih.gov/guidelines/asthma/asthsumm.pdf.*)

Drug Therapy for Asthma According to Age

Young Children

Cromolyn and nedocromil are drugs used to treat the inflammatory effects of asthma in children. Oral glucocorticoids may be prescribed for the young child to control a moderate to severe asthmatic state. An inhalation dose of a glucocorticoid should be about 400 to 800 mcg/daily. If the condition is severe, selected young children may be ordered an oral beta$_2$-adrenergic agonist.

Older Adults

Drug selection and dosage need to be considered for the older adult with an asthmatic condition. Beta$_2$-adrenergic agonists and methylxanthines (e.g., theophylline) can cause tachycardia, nervousness, and tremors in older adults, especially those with cardiac conditions. Frequent use of glucocorticoids can increase the risk of the client developing cataracts, osteoporosis, and diabetes mellitus. If a theophylline drug is ordered, dosages of glucocorticoids are normally decreased.

Mucolytics

Mucolytics act like detergents to liquefy and loosen thick mucous secretions so they can be expectorated. Acetylcysteine (Mucomyst) is administered by nebulization. *The drug should not be mixed with other drugs.* When clients with asthma or hyperactive airway disease produce increased secretions that obstruct bronchial airways, acetylcysteine may be administered as an adjunct to a bronchodilator (not mixed together). The bronchodilator should be given 5 minutes before the mucolytic. Side effects include nausea and vomiting, stomatitis (oral ulcers), and "runny nose."

Acetylcysteine (Mucomyst) can be used as an antidote for acetaminophen overdose if given within 12 to 24 hours after the overdose ingestion. It can be given orally, diluted in juice or soft drinks.

Dornase alfa (Pulmozyme) is an enzyme that digests deoxyribonucleic acid (DNA) in thick sputum secretions of clients with cystic fibrosis (CF). This agent helps reduce respiratory infections and improves pulmonary function. Improvement usually occurs in 3 to 7 days with its use. Side effects include chest pain, sore throat, laryngitis, and hoarseness.

Antimicrobials

Antibiotics are used only if a bacterial infection results from retained mucus secretions. Trimethoprim-sulfamethoxazole is effective for the treatment of mild to moderate acute exacerbations of chronic bronchitis (AECB) from infectious causes.

 Critical Thinking Case Study

MA, age 55, was recently diagnosed with bronchial asthma. Her mother and three brothers also have asthma. In the past year, MA has had three asthmatic attacks that were treated with prednisone and albuterol (Proventil) inhaler. At an office visit today, prednisone was prescribed for 4 weeks, and the order was written as follows: day 1, one tablet four times that day; day 2, one tablet three times that day; day 3, one tablet two times that day; day 4, one tablet in the morning; day 5, one-half tablet in the morning.

1. Explain the purpose for the use of prednisone during an asthmatic attack. Explain why the dosage is decreased (tapered) over a period of 5 days.
2. Can cromolyn sodium be substituted for prednisone during an asthmatic attack? Explain.
3. MA is prescribed albuterol. What effect does albuterol have on controlling asthma?
4. Albuterol is administered by an inhaler. For each drug dose, MA is to take two puffs. What instructions should she be given concerning the use of the inhaler?

To minimize the frequency of MA's asthmatic attacks, the health care provider prescribed Theo-Dur 200 mg b.i.d. The albuterol inhalation is to be taken as needed. Nursing interventions include client history of asthmatic attacks and physical assessment.

5. What should the nurse include when taking the client's history concerning asthmatic attacks? What physical assessment would suggest an asthmatic attack?
6. What type of drug is Theo-Dur? Why should the nurse ask MA whether she smokes?
7. What are the side effects, adverse reactions, and drug interactions related to Theo-Dur?
8. What nonpharmacologic measures can the nurse suggest that may decrease the frequency of asthmatic attacks?

NCLEX Study Questions

1. A client is diagnosed with a pulmonary disorder that causes COPD. Lung tissue changes are normally reversible with this condition. The nurse understands that the client's diagnosis is most likely:
   a. asthma
   b. emphysema
   c. bronchiectasis
   d. chronic bronchitis

2. A client with COPD has an acute bronchospasm. The nurse knows that the best medication for this emergency situation is:
   a. zafirlukast (Accolate)
   b. epinephrine (Adrenalin)
   c. dexamethasone (Decadron)
   d. oxtriphylline-theophyllinate (Choledyl)

3. A client is taking aminophylline–theophylline ethylenediamine (Somophyllin). The nurse should monitor the client for:
   a. drowsiness
   b. hypoglycemia
   c. increased heart rate
   d. decreased white blood cell count

4. A client is prescribed theophylline to relax the smooth muscles of the bronchi. The nurse monitors the client's theophylline serum levels to maintain a therapeutic range of:
   a. 1 to 10 mcg/ml
   b. 10 to 20 mcg/ml
   c. 20 to 30 mcg/ml
   d. 30 to 40 mcg/ml

5. A client with COPD is taking a leukotriene antagonist, montelukast (Singulair). The nurse is aware that this medication is given for:
   a. maintenance treatment of asthma
   b. treatment of an acute asthma attack
   c. reversing bronchospasm associated with COPD
   d. treatment of inflammation in chronic bronchitis

Answers: 1, a; 2, b; 3, c; 4, b; 5, a.

FOURTEEN

Cardiovascular Agents

The cardiovascular system includes the heart, blood vessels (arteries and veins), and blood. Blood rich in oxygen (O_2), nutrients, and hormones moves through vessels called *arteries*, which narrow to arterioles. Capillaries transport rich, nourished blood to body cells and absorb waste products, such as carbon dioxide (CO_2), urea, creatinine, and ammonia. The deoxygenated blood returns to the circulation by the venules and veins to be eliminated by the lungs and kidneys with other waste products (Figure XIV-1).

The heart's pumping action serves as the energy source that circulates blood to body cells. Blockage of vessels can inhibit blood flow.

Heart

The heart is composed of four chambers: the right and left atria and the right and left ventricles (Figure XIV-2). The right atrium receives deoxygenated blood from the circulation, and the right ventricle pumps blood through the pulmonary artery to the lungs for gas exchange (carbon dioxide for oxygen). The left atrium receives oxygenated blood, and the left ventricle pumps the blood into the aorta for systemic circulation.

The heart muscle, called the *myocardium*, surrounds the ventricles and atria. The ventricles are thick-walled (especially the left ventricle) to achieve the muscular force needed to pump blood to the pulmonary and systemic circulations. The atria are thin-walled, have less pumping action, and serve as receptacles for blood from the circulation and lungs.

The heart has a fibrous covering called the *pericardium*, which protects it from injury and infection. The *endocardium* is a three-layered membrane that lines the inner part of the heart chambers. Four valves—two atrioventricular (tricuspid and mitral) and two semilunar (pulmonic and aortic)—control blood flow between the atria and ventricles and between the ventricles and the pulmonary artery and the aorta. There are two coronary arteries. The right coronary artery supplies blood to the right atrium and ventricle of the heart, and the left coronary artery supplies blood to the left atrium and ventricle of the heart. The left coronary artery divides near its origin to form the left circumflex artery and the anterior descending artery. Blockage to one of these arteries can result in a myocardial infarction (MI), or heart attack.

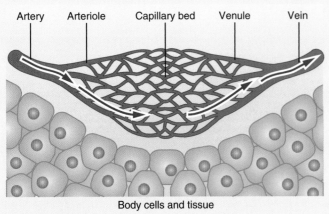

FIGURE XIV-I   Basic structures of the vascular system.

Conduction of Electrical Impulses

The myocardium is capable of generating and conducting its own electrical impulses. The cardiac impulse usually originates in the *sinoatrial (SA) node* located in the posterior wall of the right atrium. The SA node is frequently called the *pacemaker,* because it regulates the heartbeat (firing of cardiac impulses), which is approximately 60 to 80 beats/min in the normal adult. The *atrioventricular (AV) node,* located in the posterior right side of the interatrial septum, has a continuous tract of fibers called the *bundle of His,* or the AV bundle. The AV node is called the *functional pacemaker,* having an adult rate of 40 to 60 beats/min. If the SA node fails, the AV node takes over, thus causing a slower heart rate. The AV node sends impulses to the ventricles. These two conducting systems (SA node and AV node) can act independently of each other. The ventricle can contract independently 30 to 40 times per minute.

Drugs that affect cardiac contraction include calcium, digitalis preparations, and quinidine and its related preparations. The autonomic nervous system (ANS) and the drugs that stimulate or inhibit it influence heart contractions. The sympathetic nervous system and the drugs that stimulate it *increase* heart rate; the parasympathetic nervous system and the drugs that stimulate it *decrease* heart rate.

Regulation of Heart Rate and Blood Flow

The heart beats approximately 60 to 80 times per minute in an adult, pumping blood into the systemic circulation. As blood travels, resistance to blood flow develops and arterial pressure increases. The average systemic arterial pressure, known as *blood pressure,* is 120/80 mmHg. Arterial blood pressure is determined by peripheral resistance and *cardiac output,* the volume of blood expelled from the heart in 1 minute, which is calculated by multiplying the heart rate by the stroke volume:

$$CO \text{ (Cardiac Output)} = HR \text{ (Heart Rate)} \times SV \text{ (Stroke Volume)}$$

FIGURE XIV-2   Anatomy of the heart. *AV node,* Atrioventricular node; *SA node,* sinoatrial node.

The average cardiac output is 4 to 8 L/min. *Stroke volume,* the amount of blood ejected from the left ventricle with each heart beat, is approximately 70 ml/beat.

Three factors—preload, contractility, and afterload—determine the stroke volume (Figure XIV-3). *Preload* refers to the blood flow force that stretches the ventricle. However, an increase in preload can increase stroke volume, and a decrease in preload can decrease stroke volume. *Contractility* is the force of ventricular contraction, and afterload is the resistance to ventricular ejection of blood, which is caused by opposing pressures in the aorta and systemic circulation. If afterload increases, stroke volume will decrease, and if afterload decreases, stroke volume will increase.

Specific drugs can increase or decrease preload and afterload, affecting both stroke volume and cardiac output. Most vasodilators decrease preload and afterload, thus decreasing arterial pressure and cardiac output.

Circulation

There are two types of circulation—pulmonary and systemic, or peripheral. With pulmonary circulation, the heart pumps deoxygenated blood from the right ventricle through the pulmonary artery to the lungs. In this situation the artery carries blood that has a high concentration of carbon dioxide. Oxygenated blood returns to the left atrium by the pulmonary vein.

With systemic or peripheral circulation, the heart pumps blood from the left ventricle to the aorta and into the general circulation. Arteries and arterioles carry the blood to capillary beds. Nutrients in the capillary blood are transferred to cells in exchange for waste products. Blood returns to the heart through venules and veins.

FIGURE XIV–3 Cardiac output and stroke volume.

Blood

Blood is composed of plasma, red blood cells (erythrocytes), white blood cells (leukocytes), and platelets. Plasma, made up of 90% water and 10% solutes, constitutes 55% of the total blood volume. The solutes in plasma include glucose, protein, lipids, amino acids, electrolytes, minerals, lactic and pyruvic acids, hormones, enzymes, oxygen, and carbon dioxide.

The major function of blood is to provide nutrients, including oxygen, to body cells. Most of the oxygen is carried on the hemoglobin of red blood cells (RBCs). White blood cells (WBCs) are the major defense mechanism of the body and act by engulfing microorganisms. They also produce antibodies. The platelets are large cells that cause blood to coagulate. RBCs have a life span of approximately 120 days, whereas the life span of a WBC is only 2 to 24 hours.

Unit XIV, Cardiovascular Agents, is composed of five chapters dealing with drugs for cardiac disorders, diuretics and antihypertensive drugs, and drugs for circulatory disorders. Cardiac glycosides, antianginals, and antidysrhythmics are described in Chapter 41. Chapter 42 discusses the five categories of diuretics. Five major categories of antihypertensive agents are presented in Chapter 43. The five groups of drugs covered in Chapters 44 and 45 are the anticoagulants, antiplatelets, thrombolytics, antilipidemics, and peripheral vasodilators.

41

Cardiac Glycosides, Antianginals, and Antidysrhythmics

ELECTRONIC RESOURCES

evolve

Evolve website (http://evolve.elsevier.com/KeeHayes/pharmacology/):
- *Case Studies*
- *Content Updates*
- *Frequently Asked Questions*
- *Student Review Activities*
- *WebLinks*
- *Additional Reference Material*

Companion CD-ROM:
- *NCLEX Examination Review Questions*
- *Pharmacology Animations*
- *IV Therapy Checklists*
- *Medication Error Checklists*
- *Drug Calculation Problems*
- *Electronic Calculators*
- *Top 200 Drugs with Pronunciations*
- *References from the Textbook*

Outline

Objectives

- Explain the actions related to cardiac glycosides, antianginal drugs, and antidysrhythmic drugs.
- Describe the signs and symptoms of digitalis toxicity.
- Identify the side effects and adverse reactions of nitrates, beta-blockers, calcium channel blockers, quinidine, and procainamide.
- Explain the nursing process, including client teaching, related to cardiac glycosides, antianginal drugs, and antidysrhythmic drugs.

Terms

afterload, p. 629
angina pectoris, p. 628
antianginal drugs, p. 628
antidysrhythmic (antiarrhythmic) drugs, p. 635
atrial fibrillation, p. 623
atrial flutter, p. 623
beta-blockers, p. 630
bradycardia, p. 624

calcium channel blockers, p. 632
cardiac dysrhythmia (arrhythmia), p. 634
cardiac glycosides, p. 623
chronotropic, p. 623
congestive heart failure (CHF), p. 623

depolarization, p. 635
dromotropic, p. 623
heart failure, p. 623
hypercapnia, p. 634
hypokalemia, p. 625
hypoxia, p. 634
inotropic, p. 623
myocardial ischemia, p. 630

nitrates, p. 629
preload, p. 629
repolarization, p. 634
tachycardia, p. 634
therapeutic serum level, p. 624

Three groups of drugs—cardiac glycosides, antianginals, and antidysrhythmics—are discussed in this chapter. Drugs in these groups regulate heart contraction, heart rate and rhythm, and blood flow to the myocardium (heart muscle).

Cardiac Glycosides

Digitalis began being used as early as 1200 AD, making it one of the oldest drugs. It is still used in a purified form. Digitalis is obtained from the purple and white foxglove plant, and it can be poisonous. In 1785, William Withering of England used digitalis to alleviate "dropsy," edema of the extremities caused by kidney and cardiac insufficiency. Withering and his medical colleagues did not realize that dropsy was the result of heart failure, however. Digitalis preparations have come to be known for their effectiveness in treating heart failure (HF), also known as *cardiac failure (CF)*, and previously referred to as **congestive heart failure (CHF)**. When the heart muscle *(myocardium)* weakens and enlarges, it loses its ability to pump blood through the heart and into the systemic circulation. This is called **heart failure**, or pump failure. When compensatory mechanisms fail and the peripheral and lung tissues are congested, the condition is CHF. The causes of heart failure include chronic hypertension, myocardial infarction (MI), coronary artery disease (CAD), valvular heart disease, congenital heart disease, and the aging heart.

Heart failure can be left-sided or right-sided. The client has left-sided heart failure when the left ventricle does not contract sufficiently to pump the blood returned from the lungs and left atrium out through the aorta into the peripheral circulation; this causes excessive amounts of blood to back up into the lung tissue. Usually the client has shortness of breath (SOB) and dyspnea. Right-sided heart failure occurs when the heart does not sufficiently pump the blood returned into the right atrium from the systemic circulation. As a result, the blood and its constituents are backed up into peripheral tissues, causing peripheral edema. One type of heart failure can lead to the other. Myocardial hypertrophy resulting in *cardiomegaly* (increased heart size) can be a major problem associated with progressive heart failure.

In the cardiac physiology of heart failure, there is an increase in *preload* and *afterload*. The increase in preload results from an increase in blood in the ventricle at the end of diastole. This occurs because of a pathologic increase in the elasticity of the ventricular walls associated with a weakened heart. With an increased afterload, there is an increased pressure or force in the ventricular wall caused by increased resistance in the aorta which must be overcome to open the aortic valve so blood can be injected into the circulation. In 2001 the American College of Cardiology (ACC) and the American Heart Association (AHA), (ACC/AHA), classified heart failure in stages according to its severity. Table 41–1 lists the stages of heart failure according to ACC/AHA. In the early stage of heart failure,

there are no symptoms and no structural heart damage. Detailed information related to the staging process of heart failure can be found on the Internet at *www.acc.org/clinical/guidelines/failure/hf_index.htm* and *www.americanheart.org/presenter.jhtml?identifier=11841*.

Naturally occurring **cardiac glycosides** are found in a number of plants, including *Digitalis*. Also called *digitalis glycosides*, they are a group of drugs that inhibit the sodium-potassium pump, resulting in an increase in intracellular sodium. This increase leads to an influx of calcium, causing the cardiac muscle fibers to contract more efficiently. Digitalis preparations like digoxin have three effects on heart muscle: (1) a positive **inotropic** action (*increases* myocardial contraction stroke volume), (2) a negative **chronotropic** action (*decreases* heart rate), and (3) a negative **dromotropic** action (*decreases* conduction of the heart cells). The increase in myocardial contractility increases cardiac, peripheral, and kidney function by increasing cardiac output, decreasing preload, improving blood flow to the periphery and kidneys, decreasing edema, and increasing fluid excretion. As a result, fluid retention in the lung and extremities is decreased. Digoxin does not prolong life. It acts by increasing the force and velocity of myocardial systolic contraction.

Today the cardiac glycoside digoxin is a secondary drug for heart failure. First-line drugs used to treat acute heart failure include inotropic agents (dopamine and dobutamine) and phosphodiesterase inhibitors (inamrinone, formerly known as *amrinone*, and milrinone [Primacor]). Other drugs prescribed for heart failure include diuretics, beta blockers, ACE inhibitors, angiotensin-receptor blockers (ARBs), calcium channel blockers, and vasodilators, all of which are discussed in this chapter.

Cardiac glycosides are also used to correct **atrial fibrillation** (cardiac dysrhythmia with rapid uncoordinated contractions of atrial myocardium) and **atrial flutter** (cardiac dysrhythmia with rapid contractions of 200 to 300 beats per minute [bpm]). This is accomplished by the negative chronotropic effects (decreases heart rate) and negative dromotropic effects (decreases conduction through the atrioventricular [AV] node).

Table 41–1	
ACC/AHA Stages of Heart Failure (HF)	
Stage	**Characteristics According to Stages**
1 (A)	High risk for HF without symptoms or structural heart disease
2 (B)	Some level of cardiac changes, e.g., decreased ejection fraction without symptoms of heart failure.
3 (C)	Structural heart disease with symptoms of heart failure, i.e., fatigue, shortness of breath, edema, and decrease in physical activity.
4 (D)	Severe structural heart disease and marked symptoms of heart failure at rest.

ACC, American College of Cardiology; AHA, American Heart Association.

Digoxin does not convert atrial fibrillation to normal heart rhythm. For management of atrial fibrillation, a calcium channel blocker (e.g., verapamil [Calan]) may be prescribed. To prevent thromboemboli resulting from atrial fibrillation, warfarin (Coumadin) is prescribed concurrently with other drug therapy. Warfarin is discussed in Chapter 44.

Nonpharmacologic Measures to Treat Heart Failure

Nondrug therapy is an integral part of the regimen for controlling heart failure. The nondrug component of the regimen should be tailored to meet the needs of each client, but the following are some general recommendations. The client should limit salt intake to 2 g daily, which is approximately 1 teaspoon. Alcohol intake should be either decreased to one drink per day or completely avoided, because excessive alcohol use can lead to cardiomyopathy. Smoking should be avoided, because it deprives the heart of oxygen (O_2). Obesity increases cardiovascular problems; thus obese clients should decrease fat and caloric intake. Mild exercise such as walking or bicycling is recommended.

Laboratory Tests

Atrial Natriuretic Hormone or Peptide

Reference value: 20-77 pg/ml; 20-77 ng/l (SI units). An elevated atrial natriuretic hormone (ANH) or peptide (ANP) may confirm HF. ANH is secreted from the atria of the heart and acts as an antagonist to renin and aldosterone. It is released during expansion of the atrium, produces vasodilation, and increases glomerular filtration rate.

Brain Natriuretic Peptide

Reference values: Desired value: less than 100 pg/ml; positive value: greater than 100 pg/ml. The brain natriuretic peptide (BNP) test aids in the diagnoses of heart failure. Diagnosing heart failure is difficult in persons with lung disease who are experiencing dyspnea and in those who are obese or elderly. Frequently the BNP is higher than 100 pg/ml in women 65 years or older. An 80-year-old woman's BNP may be 160 pg/ml; however, with heart failure, the BNP is markedly higher, as high as 400 pg/ml. BNP is considered a more sensitive test than ANP for diagnosing heart failure. Today there is a bedside/emergency department machine to measure BNP.

Digoxin

Prototype Drug Chart 41–1 gives the pharmacologic data for digoxin, a cardiac glycoside.

Pharmacokinetics

The absorption rate of digoxin in oral tablet form is greater than 70%. The rate is 90% in liquid form and 90% to 100% in capsule form. The protein-binding power for digoxin is low; however, its half-life is 36 hours. Because of its long half-life, drug accumulation can occur. Side effects should be closely monitored to detect digitalis toxicity. Clients should be made aware of side effects that need to be reported to the health care provider. Serum digoxin levels are most commonly drawn when actual digitoxicity is suspected. This allows the health care provider to ascertain the extent of such toxicity and to confirm elimination of the drug after it is stopped or decreased in dosage (see Digitalis Toxicity).

Thirty percent of digoxin is metabolized by the liver, and 70% is excreted by the kidneys mostly unchanged. Kidney dysfunction can affect the excretion of digoxin. Thyroid dysfunction can alter the metabolism of cardiac glycosides. For clients with hypothyroidism, the dose of digoxin should be decreased; in hyperthyroidism, the dose may need to be increased.

Digitoxin is a potent cardiac glycoside that has a very long half-life and is highly protein-bound. This drug is seldom prescribed. The names *digoxin* and *digitoxin* are very similar, so the nurse must be extremely careful to administer the correct drug. The client should consistently take the same brand of digoxin to avoid unnecessary side effects or adverse reactions.

Pharmacodynamics

In clients with a failing heart, cardiac glycosides increase myocardial contraction, which increases cardiac output and improves circulation and tissue perfusion. Because these drugs decrease conduction through the AV node, the heart rate decreases.

The onset and peak actions of oral and intravenous (IV) digoxin vary. The **therapeutic serum level** is 0.5 to 2.0 ng/ml for digoxin. To treat HF, the lower serum therapeutic levels should be obtained, and for atrial flutter or fibrillation, the higher therapeutic serum levels are required.

Of these two drugs, digoxin is more frequently used. It can be administered orally or IV. Table 41–2 lists the drug data for digitalis preparations.

Digitalis (Digoxin) Toxicity

Overdose or accumulation of digoxin causes digitalis toxicity. Signs and symptoms include anorexia, diarrhea, nausea and vomiting, **bradycardia** (pulse rate below 60 bpm), premature ventricular contractions, cardiac dysrhythmias, headaches, malaise, blurred vision, visual illusions (white, green, yellow halos around objects), confusion, and delirium. Older adults are more prone to toxicity.

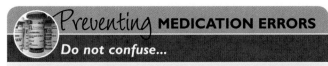

Preventing **MEDICATION ERRORS**

Do not confuse...

- **digoxin** with **digitoxin.** Both drugs are cardiac glycosides. **Digoxin** (Lanoxin) is usually the first-choice drug, because its half-life is 36 hours, whereas the half-life of digitoxin is 4 to 9 days. **Digitoxin** is rarely prescribed.

Right Drug, Right Dose
Maintenance dose for **digoxin** is 0.125 to 0.5 mg/dl. For older adults, dose is usually 0.125 mg/dl.

Right Assessment
Check for digoxin or digitalis toxicity. Pulse rate (heart rate) should be above 60 bpm. Other signs and symptoms are discussed under chapter heading. Monitor serum level of digoxin (therapeutic range: 0.5 to 2 ng/ml). Digoxin can have a cumulative effect under certain circumstances.

Prototype DRUG CHART 41–1

DIGOXIN (LANOXIN)

Drug Class

Cardiac glycoside
Trade name: Lanoxin
Pregnancy Category: C

Dosage

A: PO: 0.5-1 mg initially in 2 divided doses
  (digitalization); *maint:* 0.125-0.5 mg/daily
IV: Same as PO dose but given over 5 min
Elderly: 0.125 mg/daily
C: PO: 1 mo-2 y: 0.01–0.02 mg/kg in 3 divided doses;
  maint: 0.012 mg/kg/daily in 2 divided doses
IV: Dosage varies
C: PO: 2-10 y: 0.012-0.04 mg/kg in divided doses
Pediatric doses are usually ordered in mcg in elixir form.

Contraindications

Ventricular dysrhythmias, second- or third-degree
  heart block
Caution: AMI, renal disease, hypothyroidism,
  hypokalemia

Drug-Lab-Food Interactions

Drug: Increase digoxin serum level with quinidine,
  flecainide, verapamil; *decrease* digoxin absorption
  with antacids, colestipol; *increase* risk for digoxin
  toxicity with thiazide diuretics, loop diuretics
Lab: Hypokalemia, hypomagnesemia, hypercalcemia
  can increase digitalis (digoxin) toxicity

Pharmacokinetics

Absorption: PO tablet: 60%-70%; PO liquid: 90%;
  PO capsule: 90%-100%
Distribution: PB: 25%
Metabolism: t½: 30-45 h
Excretion: 70% in urine; 30% by liver metabolism

Pharmacodynamics

PO: Onset: 1-5 h
  Peak: 6-8 h
  Duration: 2-4 d
IV: Onset: 5-30 min
  Peak: 1-5 h
  Duration: 2-4 d

Therapeutic Effects/Uses

To treat HF, atrial tachycardia, flutter, or fibrillation
Mode of Action: Inhibits sodium-potassium ATPase, promoting increased force of cardiac contraction, cardiac output, and tissue perfusion; decreases ventricular rate

Side Effects

Anorexia, nausea, vomiting, headache, blurred vision
  (yellow-green halos), diplopia, photophobia,
  drowsiness, fatigue, confusion

Adverse Reactions

Bradycardia, visual disturbances
Life-threatening: Atrioventricular block, cardiac
  dysrhythmias

A, Adult; *AMI,* acute myocardial infarction; *ATPase,* adenosine triphosphatase; *C,* child; *d,* day; *HF,* heart failure; *h,* hour; *IV,* intravenous; *maint,* maintenance; *min,* minute; *mo,* month; *PB,* protein-binding; *PO,* by mouth; *t½,* half-life; *y,* year.

Cardiotoxicity is a serious adverse reaction to digoxin; ventricular dysrhythmias result. Three cardiac-altered functions can contribute to digoxin-induced ventricular dysrhythmias: (1) suppression of AV conduction, (2) increased automaticity, and (3) a decreased refractory period in ventricular muscle. The antidysrhythmics phenytoin and lidocaine are effective in treating digoxin-induced ventricular dysrhythmias.

Antidote for Cardiac/Digitalis Glycosides

Digoxin immune Fab (ovine, Digibind) may be given to treat severe digitalis toxicity. This agent binds with digoxin to form complex molecules that can be excreted in the urine; thus digoxin is unable to bind at the cellular site of action. Signs and symptoms of digoxin toxicity should be reported promptly to the health care provider. Serum di-

goxin levels should be closely monitored. Digitalis toxicity may result in first-degree, second-degree, or complete heart block.

Drug Interactions

Drug interaction with digitalis preparations can cause digitalis toxicity. Many of the potent diuretics, such as furosemide (Lasix) and hydrochlorothiazide (HydroDIURIL), promote the loss of potassium from the body. The resultant **hypokalemia** (low serum potassium level) increases the effect of digoxin at its myocardial cell site of action, resulting in digitalis toxicity. Cortisone preparations taken systemically promote sodium retention and potassium excretion or loss and can also cause hypokalemia. Clients who take digoxin along with a potassium-wasting diuretic or a cortisone drug should consume foods rich in potas-

Table 41–2

Cardiac Glycosides and Inotropic Agents

Generic (Brand)	Route and Dosage	Uses and Considerations
Rapid-Acting Digitalis		
digoxin (Lanoxin)	(Prototype Drug Chart 41-1)	
Long-Acting Digitalis		
digitoxin (Crystodigin)	A: PO/IV: LD: 0.8-1.2 mg; maint: PO: 0.05-3 mg/d	For HF. Serum therapeutic level: 15-30 ng/ml. Because of its long half-life, this drug is seldom given. *Pregnancy category*: C; PB: 97%; $t^{1/2}$: 7-8 h
Phosphodiesterase Inhibitors (Positive Inotropic Bipyridines)		
amrinone lactate (Inocor)	A: IV: LD: 0.75 mg/kg bolus over 2-3 min; *maint*: IV inf: 5-10 mcg/kg/min; *max*: 10 mcg/kg/d	For HF, amrinone may be prescribed when digoxin and diuretics have not been effective. May be used in conjunction with diuretic, but is incompatible with furosemide. Drug is for short-term use. *Pregnancy category*: C; PB: 10%-50%; $t^{1/2}$: 3.5-7 h
milrinone lactate (Primacor)	A: IV: Initially: 50 mcg/kg/over 10 min *Continuous infusion*: 0.375-0.75 mcg/ kg/min with 0.45%-0.9% saline	For short-term treatment of HF. May be given before heart transplantation. Heart rate and blood pressure should be closely monitored. *Pregnancy category*: C; PB: 70%; $t^{1/2}$: 1.5-2.5 h
Atrial Natriuretic Peptide Hormone		
nesiritide (Natrecor)	A: IV bolus: 2 mcg/kg, followed by 0.01 mcg/kg/min, by IV infusion	To treat acute HF by increasing sodium loss. Useful in managing dyspnea at rest. Causes vasodilation. Contraindicated for clients with systolic BP less than 90 mm Hg. *Pregnancy category*: C; PB: UK; $t^{1/2}$: 18-22 min
Antidote for Digitalis Toxicity		
digoxin immune Fab (ovine, Digibind)	Dose varies. Use manufacturer's dosing guidelines. Approx 760 mg, IV diluted in 50 ml of NSS. Infuse over 30 min.	To correct serious digitalis toxicity. Agent binds with digoxin to form complex molecules. (A serum digoxin level >2 ng is indicative of digitalis toxicity.) Onset of action: 30 min; duration of action: 3-4 d. *Pregnancy category*: C; PB: UK; $t^{1/2}$: 15-20 h

A, Adult; *BP*, blood pressure; *d*, day; *HF*, heart failure; *inf*, infusion; *IV*, intravenous; *LD*, loading dose; *maint*, maintenance; *min*, minute; *NSS*, normal saline solution; *PB*, protein-binding; *PO*, by mouth; $t^{1/2}$, half-life; *UK*, unknown; >, greater than.

sium or take potassium supplements to avoid hypokalemia and digitalis toxicity. Antacids can decrease digitalis absorption if taken at the same time. To prevent this problem, doses should be staggered.

Cardiac Glycosides: Digoxin

ASSESSMENT

■ Obtain a drug and herbal history. Report if a drug-drug or drug-herb interaction is probable. If client is taking digoxin and a potassium-wasting diuretic or cortisone drug, hypokalemia might result, causing digitalis toxicity. A low serum potassium level enhances the action of digoxin. A client taking a thiazide and/or cortisone with digoxin should take a potassium supplement.

■ Obtain a baseline pulse rate for future comparisons. Apical pulse should be taken for a full minute and should be greater than 60 bpm.

■ Assess for signs and symptoms of digitalis toxicity. Common symptoms include anorexia, nausea, vomiting, bradycardia, cardiac dysrhythmias, and visual disturbances. Report symptoms immediately to the health care provider.

NURSING DIAGNOSES

■ Decreased cardiac output related to heart failure
■ Ineffective tissue perfusion (cardiopulmonary, cerebral) related to heart failure because of the inability of the heart to contract adequately
■ Anxiety related to cardiac problem

PLANNING

■ Client checks pulse rate daily before taking digoxin. Client will report pulse rate of less than 60 bpm or a marked decline in pulse rate.
■ Client eats foods rich in potassium to maintain a desired serum potassium level (see Client Teaching, Diet).

NURSING INTERVENTIONS

■ Do *not* confuse *digoxin* with *digitoxin.* Read the drug labels carefully. Digoxin has a long half-life and digitoxin has a VERY long half-life.

■ Check the apical pulse rate before administering digoxin. Do *not* administer if pulse rate is less than 60 bpm.

■ Determine the signs of peripheral and pulmonary edema, which indicate heart failure is present. With pulmonary edema, heart failure may be referred to as *congestive heart failure* (CHF).

■ Check the serum digoxin level. The normal therapeutic drug range for digoxin is 0.5 to 2 ng/ml. A serum digoxin level of greater than 2 ng/ml is indicative of digitalis toxicity. Check serum potassium level (normal range, 3.5 to 5.3 mEq/l) and report if hypokalemia (less than 3.5 mEq/l) is present.

Client Teaching

General

- Explain to client the importance of compliance with drug therapy. A visiting nurse may ensure that the medications are properly taken.
- To avoid adverse drug interactions, advise client not to take OTC drugs without first consulting the health care provider.
- Keep drugs out of reach of small children. Request childproof bottles.
- Instruct client or parent of child to check pulse rate before administering the drug.
- Inform client of possible herb-drug interactions. (Herbal Alert 41–1)

Self-Administration

- Instruct client how to check the pulse rate before taking digoxin and to call the health care provider for pulse rate less than 60 bpm or irregular pulse.

Side Effects

- Instruct client to report side effects: pulse rate less than 60 bpm, nausea, vomiting, headache, and visual disturbances, including diplopia.

Diet

- Advise client to eat foods rich in potassium: fresh and dried fruits, fruit juices, and vegetables, including potatoes.

Cultural Considerations ❖

- Identify conflicts in values and beliefs, and use culturally consistent communication practices. It is essential that clients taking digoxin, diuretics, and potassium supplements for heart failure do not miss doses of their medication. Client should be fully aware of adverse effects and readily report them to the health care provider.
- Speak clearly and slowly; allow time for client to respond.

- Be certain that client understands the purposes for taking these drugs. The Amish respect authority and usually follow orders without question, but the family must be involved in decision making.

EVALUATION

■ Evaluate the effectiveness of digoxin by noting client's response to the drug (decreased heart rate, decreased chest rales) and the absence of side effects. Continue monitoring the pulse rate.

Herbal ALERT 41–1

Cardiac Glycosides: Digoxin

- *Ginseng* may falsely elevate digoxin levels.
- *St. John's wort* decreases absorption of digoxin and thus decreases serum digoxin level.
- *Psyllium* (Metamucil) may decrease digoxin absorption.
- *Hawthorn* may increase the effect of digoxin.
- *Licorice* can potentiate the effect of digoxin. It promotes potassium loss (hypokalemia), which increases the effect of digoxin. It may cause digitalis toxicity.
- *Aloe* may increase the risk of digitalis toxicity. It increases potassium loss, which increases the effect of digoxin.
- *Ma-huang* or ephedra increases the risk of digitalis toxicity.
- *Goldenseal* may decrease the effects of cardiac glycosides and increase the effects of antidysrhythmics.

Phosphodiesterase Inhibitors

The phosphodiesterase inhibitors are another positive inotropic group of drugs given to treat acute HF or when there is no response to the use of other agents. This drug group inhibits the enzyme phosphodiesterase, promoting a positive inotropic response and vasodilation. The two drugs in this group are inamrinone lactate (Inocor) and milrinone lactate (Primacor). These drugs increase stroke volume and cardiac output and promote vasodilation. They are administered IV for no longer than 48 to 72 hours. Severe cardiac dysrhythmias might result from the use of phosphodiesterase inhibitors, so the client's electrocardiogram (ECG) and cardiac status should be closely monitored.

Other Agents Used to Treat Heart Failure

Vasodilators, angiotensin-converting enzyme (ACE) inhibitors, angiotensin II receptor antagonists (blockers), diuretics (thiazides, furosemide), spironolactone (Aldactone), and some beta-blockers are other drug groups prescribed to treat heart failure.

Vasodilators can be used to treat heart failure. The vasodilators decrease venous blood return to the heart; thus there is a decrease in cardiac filling, ventricular stretching (preload), and oxygen demand on the heart. The arteriolar dilators act in three ways: (1) to reduce cardiac afterload, which increases cardiac output; (2) to dilate the arterioles of the kidneys, which improves renal perfusion and increases fluid loss; and (3) to improve circulation to the skeletal muscles.

ACE inhibitors are usually prescribed for heart failure. ACE inhibitors dilate venules and arterioles, improving renal blood flow and decreasing blood fluid volume. They also moderately decrease the release of aldosterone, which in turn reduces sodium and fluid retention.

ACE inhibitors can increase potassium levels, so serum potassium levels should be monitored, especially if potassium-sparing diuretics (e.g., spironolactone [Aldactone]) are being taken concomitantly. Angiotensin II receptor blocker (ARB) agents such as valsartan (Diovan) and candesartan (Atacand) have been approved for HF in clients who cannot tolerate an ACE inhibitor. ACE inhibitors and ARBs are discussed Chapter 43.

Diuretics are the first-line drug treatment for reducing fluid volume and are frequently prescribed with digoxin or other agents.

Spironolactone (Aldactone), a potassium-sparing diuretic, is used in treating moderate to severe HF. Aldosterone secretions are increased in HF; this promotes body loss of potassium and magnesium needed by the heart and increases sodium and water retention. Spironolactone blocks the production of aldosterone. This drug improves heart rate variability and decreases myocardial fibrosis. The recommended dose is 12.5 to 25 mg per day. Occurrence of hyperkalemia (excess serum potassium) is rare unless the client is receiving 50 mg daily and has renal insufficiency. However, the serum potassium level should be closely monitored.

Certain beta-blockers are usually contraindicated for clients with heart failure, because this drug class reduces cardiac contractility. However, with chronic heart failure certain beta-blockers (carvedilol [Coreg] and metoprolol tartrate [Toprol-XL]) have been shown to improve cardiac performance. Nonetheless, other beta-blockers are not recommended for clients with class IV heart failure. Beta blockers are discussed in Chapters 17 and 43.

Nesiritide (Natrecor) is an atrial natriuretic peptide hormone that inhibits antidiuretic hormone (ADH) by increasing urine sodium loss. Its effect in correcting HF is achieved by promoting vasodilation, natriuresis, and diuresis. It is useful for treating clients who have acute decompensated HF with dyspnea at rest or who have dyspnea with little physical exertion.

BiDil, a combination of hydralazine (for blood pressure) and isosorbide dinitrate (a dilator to relieve heart pain) received FDA approval in 2005 for treating heart failure, especially in African Americans. African Americans have more than twice the rate of heart failure as whites, and a research study has shown this drug to be effective in treating heart failure in the African-American population.

Antianginal Drugs

Antianginal drugs are used to treat **angina pectoris.** This is a condition of acute cardiac pain caused by inadequate blood flow to the myocardium due to either plaque occlusions within or spasms of the coronary arteries. With decreased blood flow there is a decrease in O_2 to the myocardium, which results in pain. Anginal pain is frequently described by the client as tightness, pressure in the center of the chest, and pain radiating down the left arm. Referred pain felt in the neck and left arm commonly occurs with severe angina pectoris. Anginal attacks may lead to myocardial infarction (MI), or *heart attack.* Anginal pain usually lasts for only a few minutes. Stress tests, echocardiogram, cardiac profile laboratory tests, and cardiac catheterization may be needed to determine the degree of blockage in the coronary arteries.

Types of Angina Pectoris

The frequency of anginal pain depends on many factors, including the type of angina. There are three types of angina:

- *Classic (stable):* Occurs with stress or exertion
- *Unstable (preinfarction):* Occurs frequently over the course of a day with progressive severity
- *Variant (Prinzmetal, vasospastic):* Occurs during rest

The first two types are caused by a narrowing or partial occlusion of the coronary arteries; variant angina is caused by vessel spasm (vasospasm). It is common for a client to have both classic and variant angina. Unstable angina often indicates an impending MI. This is an emergency that needs immediate medical intervention.

Nonpharmacologic Measures to Control Angina

A combination of pharmacologic and nonpharmacologic measures is usually necessary to control and prevent anginal attacks. Nonpharmacologic ways of decreasing anginal attacks are to avoid heavy meals, smoking, extremes in weather changes, strenuous exercise, and emotional upset. Proper nutrition, moderate exercise (only after consulting with a health care provider), adequate rest, and relaxation techniques should be used as preventive measures.

Types of Antianginal Drugs

Antianginal drugs increase blood flow either by increasing oxygen supply or by decreasing oxygen demand by the myocardium. Three types of antianginals are nitrates, beta-blockers, and calcium channel blockers. The major systemic effect of nitrates is a reduction of venous tone, which decreases the workload of the heart and promotes vasodilation. Beta-blockers and calcium channel blockers decrease the workload of the heart and decrease oxygen demands.

Nitrates and calcium channel blockers are effective in treating variant (vasospastic) angina pectoris. Beta-blockers are not effective for this type of angina. With stable angina, beta-blockers can effectively be used to prevent

Table 41–3		
Effects of Antianginal Drug Groups on Angina		
Drug Group	**Variant (Vasospastic) Angina**	**Classic (Stable) Angina**
Nitrates	Relaxation of coronary arteries, which decreases vasospasms and increases O_2 supply	Dilation of veins, which decreases preload and decreases O_2 demand
Beta-blockers	Not effective	Decreases heart rate and contractility, which decreases O_2 demand
Calcium channel blockers	Relaxation of coronary arteries, which decreases vasospasms and increases O_2 supply	Dilation of arterioles, which decreases afterload and decreases O_2 demand. Verapamil and diltiazem decrease heart rate and contractility.

Modified from Lehne RA: *Pharmacology for nursing care*, ed 6, St. Louis, 2007, Elsevier.
O_2, Oxygen.

angina attacks. Table 41–3 lists the effects of antianginal drug groups on angina.

With unstable angina, immediate medical care is necessary. Nitrates are usually given subcutaneously and intravenously as needed. If the heart pain continues, a beta blocker is given intravenously, and if the client is unable to tolerate beta blockers, a calcium blocker may be substituted.

Nitrates

Nitrates, developed in the 1840s, were the first agents used to relieve angina. They affect coronary arteries and blood vessels in the venous circulation. Nitrates cause generalized vascular and coronary vasodilation, thus increasing blood flow through the coronary arteries to the myocardial cells. This group of drugs reduces myocardial ischemia but can cause hypotension.

The sublingual (SL) nitroglycerin tablet, absorbed under the tongue, comes in various dosages, but the average dose prescribed is 0.4 mg or gr $^1/_{150}$ following cardiac pain, repeated every 5 minutes for a total of three doses. The effects of SL nitroglycerin last for 10 minutes. The SL tablets decompose when exposed to heat and light, so they should be kept in their original airtight glass containers. The tablets themselves are normally dispensed in these original glass containers, which have screw-cap tops that are not childproof. This facilitates emergency use by older adults who may have reduced manual dexterity and are experiencing an anginal attack. After a dose of nitroglycerin the client may experience dizziness, faintness, or headache as a result of the peripheral vasodilation. If pain persists, the client should immediately call for medical assistance.

Sublingual (SL) nitroglycerin is the most commonly used nitrate. It is not swallowed, because it undergoes first-pass metabolism by the liver, which decreases its effectiveness. Instead, it is readily absorbed into the circulation through the SL vessels. Nitroglycerin is also available in other forms: topical (ointment, transdermal patch), buccal extended-release tablet, oral extended-release capsule and tablet, aerosol spray (inhalation), and IV. Prototype Drug Chart 41–2 summarizes the action of nitroglycerin (nitrates).

There are various types of organic nitrates. Isosorbide dinitrate (Isordil, Sorbitrate) can be administered in SL

Preventing MEDICATION ERRORS
Do not confuse...

- **Nitrostat** and **Nystatin**. **Nitrostat** is a nitroglycerin drug that promotes coronary vasodilation and thus increases blood flow to the coronary arteries. **Nystatin** is an antifungal antibiotic that has fungistatic and fungicidal activity against yeasts and fungi.

tablet form and is also available as chewable tablets, immediate-release tablets, and sustained-release tablets and capsules. Isosorbide mononitrate (Monoket, Imdur) can be given orally in immediate-release and sustained-release tablets.

Pharmacokinetics

Nitroglycerin, taken SL, is absorbed rapidly and directly into the internal jugular vein and the right atrium. Approximately 40% to 50% of nitrates absorbed through the gastrointestinal (GI) tract are inactivated by liver metabolism (first-pass metabolism in the liver). The nitroglycerin in Nitro-Bid ointment and in the Transderm-Nitro patch is absorbed slowly through the skin. It is excreted primarily in the urine.

Pharmacodynamics

Nitroglycerin acts directly on the smooth muscle of blood vessels, causing relaxation and dilation. It decreases cardiac **preload** (the amount of blood in the ventricle at the end of diastole) and **afterload** (peripheral vascular resistance) and reduces myocardial O_2 demand. With dilation of the veins, there is less blood return to the heart, and with dilation of the arteries, there is less vasoconstriction and resistance.

The onset of action of nitroglycerin depends on the method of administration. With SL and IV use, the onset of action is rapid (1 to 3 minutes); it is slower with the transdermal method (30 to 60 minutes). The duration of action of the transdermal nitroglycerin patch is approximately 24 hours. Because Nitro-Bid ointment is effective for only 6 to 8 hours, it must be reapplied three to four times a day. The use of Nitro-Bid ointment has declined since the advent of the transdermal nitroglycerin patch, which is applied only once a day. It is important to note that the patch should be removed nightly to allow for an 8- to 12-hour nitrate-free interval. This is also true for most other forms of nitroglycerin. This is necessary to avoid tolerance associated with uninterrupted use or continued dosage increases of nitrate preparations. Table 41–4 lists the drug data for the nitrates.

Prototype **DRUG CHART 41–2**

NITROGLYCERIN

Drug Class	**Dosage**

Antianginal
Trade names: Nitrostat, Nitro-Bid, Transderm-Nitro
    patch, NTG, ✤Nitrogard SR, Nitrol Nitrate
Pregnancy Category: C
	A: PO/SL: 0.3, 0.4, 0.6 mg; repeat q5min × 3 as needed;
	    SR: 2.5-26 mg, 2-4 × d
	IV: Initially: 5 mcg/min; dose may be increased
	Oint: 2% 1-2 inch to chest or thigh area
	Patch: 2.5-15 mg/d to chest or thigh area

Contraindications	**Drug-Lab-Food Interactions**

Marked hypotension, AMI, increased intracranial
    pressure, severe anemia
Caution: Severe renal or hepatic disease, early MI
	Drug: Increase effect with alcohol, beta-blockers,
	    calcium channel blockers, antihypertensives; *decrease*
	    effects of heparin

Pharmacokinetics	**Pharmacodynamics**

Absorption: SL: greater than 75% absorbed; oint.
    and patch: slow absorption
Distribution: PB: 60%
Metabolism: t½: 1-4 min
Excretion: Liver and urine
	SL: Onset: 1-3 min
	    Peak: 4 min
	    Duration: 20-30 min
	SR Cap: Onset: 20-45 min
	    Duration: 3-8 h
	Oint: Onset: 20-60 min
	    Peak: 1-2 h
	    Duration: 6-8 h
	Patch: Onset: 30-60 min
	    Peak: 1-2 h
	    Duration: 20-24 h
	IV: Onset: 1-3 min
	    Duration: 3-5 min

Therapeutic Effects/Uses

To control angina pectoris (anginal pain)
Mode of Action: Decreases myocardial demand for oxygen; decreases preload by dilating veins, indirectly decreasing
    afterload

Side Effects	**Adverse Reactions**

Nausea, vomiting, headache, dizziness, syncope,
    weakness, flush, confusion, pallor, rash, dry mouth
	Hypotension, reflex tachycardia, paradoxical
	    bradycardia
	Life-threatening: Circulatory collapse

A, Adult; *AMI,* acute myocardial infarction; *cap,* capsule; *d,* day; *h,* hour; *IV,* intravenous; *MI,* myocardial infarction; *min,* minute;
NTG, nitroglycerin; *PB,* protein-binding; *PO,* by mouth; *SL,* sublingual; *SR,* sustained-release; *t½,* half-life; ✤, Canadian drug name.

Side Effects and Adverse Reactions

Headaches are one of the most common side effects of nitroglycerin, but they may become less frequent with continued use. Otherwise acetaminophen may provide some relief. Other side effects include hypotension, dizziness, weakness, and faintness. When nitroglycerin ointment or transdermal patches are discontinued, the dose should be tapered over several weeks to prevent the rebound effect of severe pain caused by **myocardial ischemia** (lack of blood supply to the heart muscle). In addition *reflex tachycardia* may occur if the nitrate is given too rapidly; the heart rate increases greatly because of overcompensation of the cardiovascular system.

Drug Interactions

Beta-blockers, calcium channel blockers, vasodilators, and alcohol can enhance the hypotensive effect of nitrates. IV nitroglycerin may antagonize the effects of heparin.

Beta-Blockers

Beta-adrenergic blockers block the beta₁- and beta₂-receptor sites. **Beta-blockers** decrease the effects of the sympathetic nervous system by blocking the action of the catecholamines epinephrine and norepinephrine, thereby decreasing the heart rate and blood pressure. They are used as antianginal, antidysrhythmic, and antihypertensive drugs. Beta-blockers are effective as antianginals because by decreasing the heart rate and myocardial contractility, they reduce the need for oxygen consumption and consequently reduce anginal pain. These drugs are most useful for classic (stable) angina.

Beta-blockers should not be abruptly discontinued. The dose should be tapered over a specified number of days to avoid reflex tachycardia and recurrence of anginal pain. A client who has decreased heart rate and blood pressure usually can not take beta-blockers. Clients who have second or third degree AV block should not take beta-blockers.

Table 41–4

Antianginals

Generic (Brand)	Route and Dosage	Uses and Considerations
Nitrates		
Short Acting		
nitroglycerin (Nitrostat, Nitro-Bid, Transderm-Nitro)	(Prototype Drug Chart 41-2)	
Long Acting		
isosorbide dinitrate (Isordil, Sorbitrate)	A: SL: 2.5-10 mg q.i.d. Chewable: 5-10 mg PRN PO: 2.5-30 mg q.i.d. a.c. and bedtime SR: 40 mg q6-12h	To prevent anginal attacks. Drug can lower blood pressure. Tolerance builds up over time. Headaches, dizziness, light-headedness, and flush may occur. *Pregnancy category:* B; PB: UK; t$\frac{1}{2}$: 1-4 h
isosorbide mononitrate (Imdur)	A: PO: SR: 30-60 mg q morning; *max:* 240 mg/d	To prevent anginal attacks. Sustained-release form provides controlled delivery and a 6-hour drug-free period. By allowing a drug-free period, tolerance to nitrates is reduced; effectiveness is increased. *Pregnancy category:* C; PB: 5%; t$\frac{1}{2}$: 6.6 h
Beta-Adrenergic Blockers		
atenolol (Tenormin) (beta$_1$)	A: PO: 25-100 mg/d; *max:* 200 mg/d	To control angina pectoris. Also effective in managing hypertension. Blood pressure and heart rate should be closely monitored. Cardioselective drug, blocks beta$_1$. Can be used by clients with asthma. *Pregnancy category:* C; PB: 5%-15%; t$\frac{1}{2}$: 6-7 h
metoprolol tartrate (Lopressor) Toprol XL (beta$_1$)	A: PO: 50-100 mg in 2 divided doses; may increase to 100-400 mg/daily Elderly: PO 25 mg/daily. May increase dose A: IV: 5 mg q 2 min	Similar to atenolol in blocking beta$_1$. High doses of metoprolol can effect beta$_2$ and could cause bronchoconstriction. Can reduce cardiac oxygen demand, which decreases heart rate and contractility. *Pregnancy category:* C; PB: 12%; t$\frac{1}{2}$: 3-7 h
nadolol (Corgard) (beta$_1$ and beta$_2$)	A: PO: 40 mg/d; dose may be increased; *max:* 240-320 mg/d in divided doses	To treat angina pectoris and hypertension. *Pregnancy category:* C; PB: 28%; t$\frac{1}{2}$: 10-24 h (renal disease: 45 h)
propranolol HCl (Inderal) (beta$_1$ and beta$_2$)	A: PO: Initially: 10-20 mg t.i.d.-q.i.d.; *maint:* 20-60 mg t.i.d.-q.i.d.; *max:* 320 mg/d SR: 80-160 mg/d	First beta-blocker; blocks beta$_1$ and beta$_2$. No longer drug of choice to prevent angina because of risk of bronchospasm. Heart rate, blood pressure, and respiratory status should be monitored. *Pregnancy category:* C; PB: 90%; t$\frac{1}{2}$: 3-6 h
Calcium Channel Blockers		
amlodipine (Norvasc)	A: PO: Initially: 10 mg; *maint:* 2.5-10 mg/d Elderly: Initially: 2.5 mg/d	Management of angina pectoris and hypertension. May be given with another antianginal or antihypertensive drug. *Pregnancy category:* C; PB: 95%; t$\frac{1}{2}$: 30-50 h
bepridil HCl (Vascor)	A: PO: Initially 200 mg × 10 d; *maint:* 300 mg/day; *max:* 400 mg/d	Treatment of angina pectoris. May be used as single drug or in combination with nitrates. Given as a single dose. *Pregnancy category:* C; PB: 99%; t$\frac{1}{2}$: 2-24 h
diltiazem HCl (Cardizem)	A: PO: 30-60 mg q.i.d.; may increase to 360 mg/d in 4 divided doses SR: 60 mg q12h; *max:* 360 mg/daily CD: 120-180 mg/d; *max:* 360 mg/daily	For angina pectoris. Hypotensive effect is not as severe as with nifedipine. Kidney function should be monitored. *Pregnancy category:* C; PB: 70%-85%; t$\frac{1}{2}$: 3.5-9 h
felodipine (Plendil)	A: PO: Initially: 5 mg/d single dose; *maint:* 2.5-10 mg/d Elderly: Initially: 2.5 mg/daily	To treat chronic angina pectoris and manage hypertension. Reduces O$_2$ demand by the heart. Potent peripheral vasodilator; increases heart rate and myocardial contractility. *Pregnancy category:* C; PB: >99%; t$\frac{1}{2}$: 10-16 h
isradipine (DynaCirc)	A: PO: 2.5-7.5 mg t.i.d.	Primary use is to treat hypertension. Also can be given for angina pectoris. *Pregnancy category:* C; PB: 99%; t$\frac{1}{2}$: 5-11 h

A, Adult; *a.c.*, before meals; *b.i.d.*, twice a day; *CD*, controlled delivery; *d*, day; *h*, hour; *HF*, heart failure; *IV*, intravenous; *maint*, maintenance; *max*, maximum; *MI*, myocardial infarction; *min*, minute; *O$_2$*, oxygen; *PB*, protein-binding; *PO*, by mouth; *PRN*, as necessary; *q.i.d.*, four times a day; *SL*, sublingual; *SR*, sustained-release; *t.i.d.*, three times a day; *t$\frac{1}{2}$*, half-life; *UK*, unknown; *>*, greater than.

Continued

Table 41–4

Antianginals—cont'd

Generic (Brand)	Route and Dosage	Uses and Considerations
nicardipine HCl (Cardene, Cardene SR)	A: PO: 20 mg t.i.d.; *maint:* 20-40 mg t.i.d. SR: 30 mg b.i.d.; *maint:* 30-60 mg b.i.d.	Used for angina pectoris. May be used alone or in combination with other antianginals. Also used for hypertension. Peripheral edema, headache, dizziness, and light-headedness may occur. *Pregnancy category:* C; PB: 95%; $t^{1/2}$: 5 h
nifedipine (Procardia, Adalat)	A: PO: 10-30 mg q6-8h; *max:* 180 mg/daily	For angina pectoris. Blood pressure should be closely monitored, especially if client is taking nitrates or beta-blockers. Is a potent calcium blocker. *Pregnancy category:* C; PB: 92%-98%; $t^{1/2}$: 2-5 h
nisoldipine (Sular, Nisocor)	A: PO: Initially: 20 mg/d; *maint:* 10-40 mg/d in 2 divided doses Elderly: A: PO: 10-20 mg/daily	To treat angina pectoris and hypertension. Suppresses contraction of cardiac and vascular smooth muscle. Increases heart rate and cardiac output. Decreases blood pressure. *Caution:* Clients with heart disease are prone to MI and HF. *Pregnancy category:* C; PB: >99%; $t^{1/2}$: 7-12 h
verapamil HCl (Calan, Isoptin, Verelan)	A: PO: 40-120 mg t.i.d.; *max:* 480 mg/daily IV: 5-10 mg over 2 min; may repeat if needed in 15-30 min	Treatment of angina pectoris, cardiac dysrhythmias, and hypertension. Peripheral edema, constipation, dizziness, headache, and hypotension may occur. *Pregnancy category:* C; PB: 90%; $t^{1/2}$: 3-8 h

Beta-blockers, discussed in detail in Chapter 17, are subdivided into nonselective beta-blockers (blocking beta$_1$ and beta$_2$) and selective (cardiac) beta-blockers (blocking beta$_1$).

Examples of nonselective beta-blockers are propranolol (Inderal), nadolol (Corgard), and pindolol (Visken). These drugs decrease the heart rate and can cause bronchoconstriction. The cardioselective beta-blockers act more strongly on the beta$_1$ receptor, thus decreasing the heart rate but avoiding bronchoconstriction because of their relative lack of activity at the beta$_2$ receptor. Examples of selective beta-blockers are atenolol (Tenormin) and metoprolol (Lopressor, Toprol-XL). Selective beta-blockers are the group of choice for controlling angina pectoris. Table 41–4 lists the beta-blockers most frequently used for angina.

Pharmacokinetics

Beta-blockers are well absorbed orally. Absorption of sustained-release capsules is slow. The half-life of propranolol (Inderal) is 3 to 6 hours. Of the selective beta-blockers, atenolol (Tenormin) has a half-life of 6 to 7 hours, and metoprolol (Lopressor) has a half-life of 3 to 7 hours. Propranolol and metoprolol are metabolized and excreted by the liver. Half an *oral* dose of atenolol is absorbed from the GI tract, the remainder excreted unchanged in feces; 85% of an IV dose is excreted in urine within 24 hours.

Pharmacodynamics

Because beta-blockers decrease the force of myocardial contraction, oxygen demand by the myocardium is reduced, and the client can tolerate increased exercise with less oxygen requirement. Beta-blockers tend to be more effective for classic (stable) angina than for variant (vasospastic) angina.

The onset of action of the nonselective beta-blocker propranolol is 30 minutes, its peak action is reached in 1 to 1.5 hours, and its duration is 4 to 12 hours. For the cardioselective beta-blockers, the onset of action of atenolol is 60 minutes, its peak action occurs in 2 to 4 hours, and its duration of action is 24 hours; the onset of action of metoprolol is reached in 15 minutes, and the duration of action is 6 to 12 hours.

Side Effects and Adverse Reactions

Both nonselective and selective beta-blockers cause a decrease in heart rate and blood pressure. For the nonselective beta-blockers, bronchospasm, behavioral or psychotic response, and impotence (with use of Inderal) are potential adverse reactions.

Vital signs need to be closely monitored in the early stages of beta-blocker therapy. When discontinuing use, the dosage should be tapered for 1 or 2 weeks to prevent a rebound effect like reflex tachycardia or life-threatening cardiac dysrhythmias.

Calcium Channel Blockers

Calcium channel blockers, or *calcium blockers,* were introduced in 1982 for the treatment of stable and variant angina pectoris, certain dysrhythmias, and hypertension. Calcium activates myocardial contraction, increasing the workload of the heart and the need for more oxygen. Calcium blockers relax coronary artery spasm (variant angina) and relax peripheral arterioles (stable angina), decreasing cardiac oxygen demand. They also decrease cardiac contractility (negative inotropic effect that relaxes smooth muscle), decrease afterload, decrease peripheral resistance, and reduce the workload of the heart, thus decreasing the need for oxygen. Calcium channel blockers achieve their effect in controlling variant (vasospastic) angina by relaxing coronary arteries and in controlling classic (stable) angina by decreasing oxygen demand. Figure 41–1 shows the suggested steps for treating classic and variant angina pectoris. Table 41–4 presents the drug data for the calcium blockers used to treat angina.

FIGURE 41–1 Suggested steps for treating classic and variant angina pectoris.

Pharmacokinetics

Three calcium blockers—verapamil (Calan), nifedipine (Procardia), and diltiazem (Cardizem)—have been effectively used for the long-term treatment of angina. Eighty to ninety percent of calcium channel blockers are absorbed through the GI mucosa. However, first-pass metabolism by the liver decreases the availability of free circulating drug, and only 20% of verapamil, 45% to 65% of diltiazem, and 35% to 40% of nifedipine are bioavailable. All three drugs are highly protein-bound (80%-90%), and their half-lives are 2 to 6 hours.

Several other calcium blockers are available: nicardipine HCl (Cardene), amlodipine (Norvasc), bepridil HCl (Vascor), felodipine (Plendil), and nisoldipine (Sular). All are highly protein-bound (greater than 95%). Nicardipine has the shortest half-life at 5 hours. Bepridil is used for angina pectoris.

Pharmacodynamics

Bradycardia is a common problem with the use of verapamil, the first calcium blocker. Nifedipine, the most potent of the calcium blockers, promotes vasodilation of the coronary and peripheral vessels, and hypotension can result. The onset of action is 10 minutes for verapamil and 30 minutes for nifedipine and diltiazem. Verapamil's duration of action is 3 to 7 hours when given orally and 2 hours when given IV; for nifedipine and diltiazem, the duration of action is 6 to 8 hours.

Side Effects and Adverse Reactions

The side effects of calcium blockers include headache, hypotension (more common with nifedipine and less common with diltiazem), dizziness, and flushing of the skin. Reflex tachycardia can occur as a result of hypotension. Calcium blockers can cause changes in liver and kidney function, and serum liver enzymes should be checked periodically. Calcium blockers are frequently given with other antianginal drugs such as nitrates to prevent angina.

Nifedipine, in its immediate-release form (10- and 20-mg capsules), has been associated with an increased incidence of sudden cardiac death, especially when prescribed in high doses for outpatients. This is not true of the sustained-release preparations (Procardia XL, Adalat CC). For this reason, immediate-release nifedipine is usually prescribed only as needed in the hospital setting for acute rises in blood pressure.

Nursing Process

Antianginals

ASSESSMENT

■ Obtain baseline vital signs for future comparisons.
■ Obtain health and drug histories. Nitroglycerin is contraindicated for marked hypotension or acute myocardial infarction (AMI).

NURSING DIAGNOSES

■ Decreased cardiac output related to poor myocardial perfusion
■ Anxiety related to cardiac problems
■ Acute pain related to anginal pain due to inadequate coronary perfusion and lack of oxygen
■ Activity intolerance related to lack of oxygen due to poor blood perfusion to the heart and lungs

PLANNING

■ Client takes nitroglycerin or other antianginals and angina pain is controlled.

NURSING INTERVENTIONS

■ Monitor vital signs. Hypotension is associated with most antianginal drugs.

■ Have client sit or lie down when taking a nitrate for the first time. After administration, check the vital signs while client is lying down and then sitting up. Have client rise slowly to a standing position.

■ Offer sips of water before giving sublingual (SL) nitrates; dryness may inhibit drug absorption.

■ Monitor effects of IV nitroglycerin. Report angina that persists.

■ Apply Nitro-Bid ointment to the designated mark on paper. Do *not* use fingers because the drug can be absorbed; use a tongue blade or gloves. For the Transderm-Nitro patch, do not touch the medication portion.

■ Do *not* apply the Nitro-Bid ointment or the Transderm-Nitro patch in any area on the chest in the vicinity of defibrillator-cardioverter paddle placement. Explosion and skin burns may result.

Client Teaching

General

• A SL nitroglycerin tablet is used if chest pain occurs. Repeat in 5 minutes if pain has not subsided and again in another 5 minutes if it persists. Do *not* give more than three tablets. If chest pain persists longer than 15 minutes, immediate medical help is necessary. *Call 911.*

• To avoid hypotension, weakness, and faintness instruct client not to ingest alcohol while taking nitroglycerin.

• Tolerance to nitroglycerin can occur. If client's chest pain is not completely alleviated, client should notify health care provider.

Beta-Blockers and Calcium Blockers

• Inform client not to discontinue these drugs without the health care provider's approval. Withdrawal symptoms (reflex tachycardia and pain) may be severe.

Self-Administration

• Demonstrate how (SL) nitroglycerin tablets are taken. The tablet is placed under the tongue for quick absorption. A stinging or biting sensation indicates the tablet is fresh; however, with the newer SL nitroglycerin tablets, the biting sensation may not be present. The medication bottle must be stored away from light and kept dry. Keep drug in original screw-cap, amber glass bottle. The amber color of the glass provides light protection and the screw-cap closure protects from moisture in the air, which can easily reduce the potency of the tablets.

• Instruct client about the Transderm-Nitro patch. Apply once a day, usually in the morning. Rotation of skin sites is necessary. The patch is usually applied to the chest wall, but thighs and arms may also be used. Avoid hairy areas.

Side Effects

• Headaches commonly occur when first taking nitroglycerin products and last about 30 minutes. Acetaminophen is suggested for relief.

• If hypotension results from SL nitroglycerin, place client in supine position with legs elevated.

Beta-Blockers and Calcium Blockers

• Instruct client how to take a pulse rate. Advise client to call health care provider if dizziness or faintness occurs; this may indicate hypotension.

Cultural Considerations ❖

• Address cultural issues directly, especially in matters concerning dietary contributors to cardiac conditions. Family and community are important resources for promoting adherence to medication regimens and lifestyle changes.

• Discuss with clients from various cultures the importance of the drug regimen. Provide printed materials in the language client speaks and reads most easily. An interpreter may be necessary to establish a sound, trusting relationship and ensure compliance with drug and diet regimens.

EVALUATION

■ Evaluate client's response to nitrate product for relieving anginal pain. Note headache, dizziness, or faintness.

Antidysrhythmic Drugs

Cardiac Dysrhythmias

A **cardiac dysrhythmia (arrhythmia)** is defined as any deviation from the normal rate or pattern of the heartbeat. This includes heart rates that are too slow (bradycardia), too fast **(tachycardia)**, or irregular. The terms *dysrhythmia* (disturbed heart rhythm) and *arrhythmia* (absence of heart rhythm) are used interchangeably, despite the slight difference in meaning.

The ECG identifies the type of dysrhythmia. The P wave of the ECG reflects atrial activation, the QRS complex indicates ventricular depolarization, and the T wave reflects ventricular **repolarization** (return of cell membrane potential to resting after depolarization). The P-R interval indicates AV conduction time, and the Q-T interval reflects ventricular action potential duration. Atrial dysrhythmias prevent proper filling of the ventricles and decrease cardiac output by one third. Ventricular dysrhythmias are life-threatening, because ineffective filling of the ventricle results in decreased or absent cardiac output. With ventricular tachycardia, ventricular fibrillation is likely to occur, followed by death. Cardiopulmonary resuscitation (CPR) is necessary to treat these clients.

Cardiac dysrhythmias frequently follow an MI (heart attack) or can result from **hypoxia** (lack of oxygen to body tissues), **hypercapnia** (increased carbon dioxide in the blood), thyroid disease, coronary artery disease, cardiac surgery, excess catecholamines, or electrolyte imbalance.

Cardiac Action Potentials

Electrolyte transfer occurs through the cardiac muscle cell membrane. When sodium and calcium enter the cardiac cell, **depolarization** (myocardial contraction) occurs. Sodium enters rapidly to start the depolarization, and calcium enters later to maintain it. Calcium influx leads to an increased release of intracellular calcium from the sarcoplasmic reticulum, resulting in cardiac contraction. In the presence of myocardial ischemia, the contraction can be irregular.

Cardiac action potentials are transient depolarizations followed by repolarizations of myocardial cells. Figure 41–2 illustrates the action potential of a ventricular cardiac cell (myocyte) during the course of a heartbeat. There are five phases. Phase 0 is the rapid depolarization caused by an influx of sodium ions. Phase 1 is initial repolarization, which coincides with termination of sodium ion influx. Phase 2 is the plateau and is characterized by the influx of calcium ions, which prolong the action potential and pro-

mote atrial and ventricular muscle contraction. Phase 3 is rapid repolarization caused by influx of potassium ions. Phase 4 is the resting membrane potential between heartbeats. It is normally flat in ventricular muscle, but begins to rise in the cells of the sinoatrial (SA) node as they slowly depolarize toward the threshold potential just before depolarization occurs, initiating the next heartbeat.

Types of Antidysrhythmic Drugs

The desired action of **antidysrhythmic (antiarrhythmic) drugs** is to restore the cardiac rhythm to normal. Box 41–1 describes the various mechanisms by which this is accomplished.

The antidysrhythmics are grouped into four classes: (1) fast (sodium) channel blockers IA, IB, and IC; (2) beta-blockers; (3) drugs that prolong repolarization; and (4) slow (calcium) channel blockers. Table 41–5 lists the classes, actions, and indications for cardiac antidysrhythmic drugs. Table 41–6 lists the drug data for the commonly administered antidysrhythmics.

FIGURE 41–2   Action potential of the ventricular myocyte.

Box 41-1

Pharmacodynamics of Antidysrhythmics

Mechanisms of Action

- Block adrenergic stimulation of the heart
- Depress myocardial excitability and contractility
- Decrease conduction velocity in cardiac tissue
- Increase recovery time (repolarization) of the myocardium
- Suppress automaticity (spontaneous depolarization to initiate beats)

Table 41-5

Classes and Actions of Antidysrhythmic Drugs

Classes	Actions	Indications
Class I		
Sodium Channel Blockers		
IA	Slow conduction and prolong repolarization	Atrial and ventricular dysrhythmias, paroxysmal atrial tachycardia (PAT), supraventricular dysrhythmias
IB	Slow conduction and shorten repolarization	Acute ventricular dysrhythmias
IC	Prolong conduction with little to no effect on repolarization	Life-threatening ventricular dysrhythmias
Class II		
Beta-blockers	Reduce calcium entry Decrease conduction velocity, automaticity, and recovery time (refractory period)	Atrial flutter and fibrillation, tachydysrhythmias, ventricular and supraventricular dysrhythmias
Class III		
Drugs that prolong repolarization	Prolong repolarization during ventricular dysrhythmias Prolong action potential duration	Life-threatening atrial and ventricular dysrhythmias resistant to other drugs
Class IV		
Calcium channel blockers	Block calcium influx Slow conduction velocity Decrease myocardial contractility (negative inotropic) Increase refraction in the AV node	Supraventricular tachydysrhythmias; prevention of paroxysmal supraventricular tachycardia (PSVT)

AV, Atrioventricular.

Table 41-6

Antidysrhythmics

Generic (Brand)	Route and Dosage	Uses and Considerations
Class I		
Sodium Channel Blockers IA		
disopyramide phosphate (Norpace, Napamide)	A: PO: 100-200 mg q6h CR: 300 mg q12h C: 4-12 y: PO: 10-15 mg/kg/d in divided doses 13-18 y: PO: 6-15 mg/kg/d in divided doses	Prevention and suppression of unifocal and multifocal premature ventricular contractions (PVCs). For ventricular dysrhythmias. May cause anticholinergic symptoms. Serum therapeutic level: 3-8 mcg/ml. *Pregnancy category:* C; PB: 50%-66%; $t^1/_2$: 4-10 h
procainamide HCl (Procanbid, Pronestyl)	A: PO: 250-500 mg q3-4h SR: 250 mg-1 g q12h or q6 h IM: 50 mg/kg/d in 4 divided doses IV: Inf: 20 mg/min for 25-30 min (500-600 mg) C: PO: 40-60 mg/kg/d in 4 divided doses TDM: 4-8 mcg/ml	Controls dysrhythmias (PVCs), ventricular tachycardia. Depresses myocardial excitability by slowing down conductivity of cardiac tissue. *Pregnancy category:* C; PB: 20%, $t^1/_2$: 3-4 h
quinidine sulfate, quinidine polygalacturonate, quinidine gluconate (Quinidex, Cardioquin)	A: PO: 200-300 mg t.i.d.-q.i.d. C: PO: 30 mg/kg or 900 mg/m² in 5 divided doses	For atrial, ventricular, and supraventricular dysrhythmias. Nausea, vomiting, diarrhea, abdominal pain, or cramps are common side effects. If given with digoxin, can increase digoxin concentration. Serum therapeutic level: 2-6 mcg/ml. *Pregnancy category:* C; PB: 80%; $t^1/_2$: 6-7 h
Sodium Channel Blockers IB		
lidocaine (Xylocaine)	A: IV: 50-100 mg bolus in 2-3 min; then IV inf: 20-50 mcg/kg/min	For acute ventricular dysrhythmias following MI and cardiac surgery. Serum therapeutic range: 1.5-6 mcg/ml. *Pregnancy category:* B; PB: 60%-80%; $t^1/_2$: 1.5-2 h
mexiletine HCl (Mexitil)	A: PO: 200-400 mg q8h	Analogue of lidocaine. Treatment for acute and chronic ventricular dysrhythmias. Take with food to decrease GI distress. Common side effects: nausea, vomiting, heartburn, tremor, dizziness, nervousness, lightheadedness. Serum therapeutic range: 0.5-2 mcg/ml. *Pregnancy category:* C; PB: 50%-60%; $t^1/_2$: 10-12 h
tocainide HCl (Tonocard)	A: PO: LD: 600 mg. PO: 400 mg q8h; *max:* 2.4 g/day	For ventricular dysrhythmias, especially PVCs. Similar to lidocaine except in oral form. Serum therapeutic level: 4-10 mcg/ml. *Pregnancy category:* C; PB: 10%-20%; $t^1/_2$: 10-17 h
Sodium Channel Blockers IC		
flecainide (Tambocor)	A: PO: Initial: 50-100 mg q12h Increase by 50 mg q12h q4d; *maint:* 150 mg q12h; *max:* 300 mg/day	For life-threatening ventricular dysrhythmias; prevention of paroxysmal supraventricular tachycardia (PSVT) and paroxysmal atrial fibrillation or flutter (PAF). Avoid use in cardiogenic shock, second- or third-degree heart block, or right bundle branch block. *Pregnancy category:* C; PB: 40%-50%; $t^1/_2$: 12-27 h
propafenone HCl (Rythmol)	A: PO: 150-300 mg q8h; *max:* 900 mg/d	Treatment of life-threatening ventricular dysrhythmias. Avoid use if cardiogenic shock, uncontrolled HF, heart block, severe hypotension, bradycardia, and bronchospasms occur. *Pregnancy category:* C; PB: 97%; $t^1/_2$: 5-8 h
Other Class I		
moricizine (Ethmozine)	A: PO: Initially: 200-300 mg q8h; *maint:* 300 mg q8h; decrease dose for clients with liver and kidney disease	To treat life-threatening ventricular dysrhythmias. Blocks sodium channels, decreases conduction velocity in atria and ventricles, prolongs refractory period in the AV node. May cause bradycardia, heart block, and HF in high doses. *Pregnancy category:* B; PB: UK; $t^1/_2$: 1.5-3.5 h

A, Adult; *AV,* atrioventricular; *b.i.d.,* two times a day; *BP,* blood pressure; *C,* child; *CR,* controlled release; *d,* day; *FDA,* Food and Drug Administration; *h,* hour; *HF,* heart failure; *GI,* gastrointestinal; *IM,* intramuscular; *inf,* infusion; *IV,* intravenous; *LD,* loading dose; *maint,* maintenance; *max,* maximum; *MI,* myocardial infarction; *min,* minute; *PAT,* paroxysmal atrial tachycardia; *PB,* protein-binding; *PO,* by mouth; *q.i.d.,* four times a day; *SR,* sustained release; $t^1/_2$, half-life; *t.i.d.,* three times a day; *UK,* unknown; *y,* year; >, greater than; <, less than.

Table 41–6

Antidysrhythmics—cont'd

Generic (Brand)	Route and Dosage	Uses and Considerations
Class II		
Beta-Adrenergic Blockers		
acebutolol HCl (Sectral) (beta₁ blocker)	A: PO: 200 mg b.i.d.; may increase dose	Management of ventricular dysrhythmias. Also used for angina pectoris and hypertension. Primarily for PVCs. Affects cardiac beta₁ receptors. Can cause bradycardia and decrease cardiac output. *Pregnancy category:* B; PB: 26%; $t^{1/2}$: 3-13 h
esmolol (Brevibloc) (beta₁ blocker)	A: IV: LD: 500 mcg/kg over 1 min; *maint:* 50-100 mcg/kg/min; *max:* 200 mcg/kg/min	To control atrial flutter and fibrillation. For short-term use only. Mainly for clients having dysrhythmias during surgery. May cause bradycardia, heart block, and HF. *Pregnancy category:* C; PB: 55%; $t^{1/2}$: 9 min
propranolol HCl (Inderal) (beta₁ and beta₂ blocker)	A: PO: 10-30 mg t.i.d.-q.i.d. A: IV bolus: 0.5-3 mg at 1 mg/min	For ventricular dysrhythmias, PAT, and atrial and ventricular ectopic beats. Clients with asthma should not use drug. *Pregnancy category:* C; PB: 90%; $t^{1/2}$: 3-6 h
sotalol HCl (Betapace) (beta₁ and beta₂ blocker; also Class III)	A: PO: 80 mg b.i.d.; *max:* 240-320 mg/day in divided doses Increase dose interval with renal dysfunction	For ventricular dysrhythmias. Avoid if bronchial asthma or heart block is present. *Pregnancy category:* B; PB: 0%; $t^{1/2}$: 12 h
Class III		
Drugs That Prolong Repolarization		
adenosine (Adenocard)	A: IV: Initially, 6 mg rapid IV bolus (1-2 sec) Repeat if necessary: 12 mg rapid IV bolus × 2 doses	Treatment of PSVT, Wolff-Parkinson-White syndrome. Avoid if second- or third-degree AV block or atrial flutter or fibrillation is present. *Pregnancy category:* C; PB: UK; $t^{1/2}$: <10 sec
amiodarone HCl (Cordarone)	A: PO: LD: 400-1600 mg/d in divided doses; *maint:* 200-600 mg/d; dose may be individualized	For life-threatening ventricular dysrhythmias. Initially dosage is greater then decreases over time. Therapeutic serum level: 1-2.5 mcg/ml. *Pregnancy category:* D; PB: 96%; $t^{1/2}$: 7 to 50 d
bretylium tosylate (Bretylol)	A: IM: 5-10 mg/kg q6-8h IV: 5-10 mg/kg; may repeat in 15-30 min, IV drip or IV bolus	For ventricular tachycardia and fibrillation (to convert to normal sinus rhythm). Used when lidocaine and procainamide are ineffective. *Pregnancy category:* C; PB: UK; $t^{1/2}$: 4-17 h
dofetilide (Tikosyn)	PO: 250-1000 mcg/d in 2 divided doses Dose is based on calculated creatinine clearance	A selective potassium-channel blocker that prolongs repolarization. Prescribed for atrial flutter and fibrillation. Renal function should be monitored. *Pregnancy category:* C; PB: 60%-70%; $t^{1/2}$: 10 h
ibutilide (Corvert)	A: >60 kg: IV: 0.1 mg/kg or 1 mg (1 vial) over 10 min; may repeat in 10 min. A: < 60 kg: IV: 0.01 mg/kg given over 10 min	Prolongs action potential and increases atrial and ventricular refractories; prolongs Q-T interval. May be given to convert atrial flutter and fibrillation to normal sinus rhythm. Pregnancy category: C; PB 40%; $t^{1/2}$: 6 h
sotalol (Betapace)	A: PO: Same as Class II (*See sotalol in Class II*)	Beta-blocker. Can be classified as Class II or III. To treat life-threatening ventricular dysrhythmias (ventricular tachycardia). Slows heart rate, decreases AV conduction, increases AV refractory period, and decreases systolic and diastolic BP. *Caution:* second- and third-degree heart block. (*See sotalol in Class II.*)
Class IV		
Calcium Channel Blockers		
verapamil HCl (Calan, Isoptin)	A: PO: 240-480 mg/d in 3-4 divided doses IV: 5-10 mg IV push	For supraventricular tachydysrhythmias, prevention of PSVT. Also used for angina pectoris and hypertension. Avoid use if cardiogenic shock, second- or third-degree AV block, severe hypotension, severe HF occur. Serum therapeutic level: 80-300 ng/ml or 0.08-0.3 mcg/ml. *Pregnancy category:* C; PB: 90%; $t^{1/2}$: 3-8 h
diltiazem (Cardizem)	A: IV: 0.25 mg/kg IV bolus over 2 min, or 5-10 mg/hours in IV infusion	For PSVT and atrial flutter or fibrillation. Avoid use if second- or third-degree AV block or hypotension occurs. *Pregnancy category:* C; PB: 70%-80%; $t^{1/2}$: 3-8 h
Others		
phenytoin (Dilantin)	A: IV: 100 mg q5-10min until dysrhythmia ceases; *max:* 1000 mg	Treatment of digitalis-induced dysrhythmias. Not approved as dysrhythmic drug by FDA. Serum level <20 mcg/ml. *Pregnancy category:* D; PB: 95%; $t^{1/2}$: 22 h
digoxin (Lanoxin)	A: IV: LD: 0.6-1 mg/d in 24 h C: >10 yr: IV: LD: 8-12 mcg/kg	For atrial flutter or fibrillation; to prevent recurrence of paroxysmal atrial tachycardia. *Pregnancy category:* C; PB: 20%-25%; $t^{1/2}$: >36 h

Class I: Sodium Channel Blockers

A sodium channel blocker decreases sodium influx into cardiac cells. Responses to the drug are decreased conduction velocity in cardiac tissues; suppression of automaticity, which decreases the likelihood of ectopic foci; and increased recovery time (repolarization or refractory period). There are three subgroups of sodium channel blockers: IA slows conduction and prolongs repolarization (quinidine, procainamide, disopyramide); IB slows conduction and shortens repolarization (lidocaine, mexiletine HCl); and IC prolongs conduction with little to no effect on repolarization (flecainide).

Lidocaine, an IB sodium channel blocker, was used in the 1940s as a local anesthetic and is still used for that purpose. It was later discovered to have antidysrhythmic properties as well. Lidocaine is still used by some cardiologists to treat acute ventricular dysrhythmias. It slows conduction velocity and decreases action potential amplitude. Onset of action (IV) is rapid. About one third of lidocaine reaches the general circulation. A bolus of lidocaine is short-lived. Other IB sodium channel blockers are mexiletine and tocainide.

Class II: Beta-Blockers

The drugs in the second class, beta-blockers, decrease conduction velocity, automaticity, and recovery time (refractory period). Examples are propranolol (Inderal), acebutolol (Sectral), esmolol (Brevibloc), and sotalol (Betapace). Beta-blockers are more frequently prescribed for dysrhythmias than sodium channel blockers.

Class III: Drugs That Prolong Repolarization

Drugs in the third class prolong repolarization and are used in emergency treatment of ventricular dysrhythmias when other antidysrhythmics are ineffective. These drugs, bretylium (Bretylol) and amiodarone (Cordarone), increase the refractory period (recovery time) and prolong the action potential duration (cardiac cell activity).

Class IV: Calcium Channel Blockers

The fourth class consists of the calcium channel blockers verapamil (Calan, Isoptin) and diltiazem (Cardizem). Verapamil is a slow (calcium) channel blocker that blocks calcium influx, thereby decreasing the excitability and contractility (negative inotropic) of the myocardium. It increases the refractory period of the AV node, which decreases ventricular response. Verapamil is contraindicated for clients with AV block or heart failure.

Prototype Drug Chart 41–3 provides information about the beta-blocker acebutolol HCL (Sectral), which can be prescribed to treat recurrent stable ventricular dysrhythmias.

Pharmacokinetics

The cardioselective beta drug acebutolol (Sectral) is well absorbed in the GI tract. It is metabolized in the liver to active metabolites; 50% to 60% of the drug is eliminated in the bile via feces, and 30% to 40% is excreted in the urine. The half-life for the drug is 3 to 4 hours, but the half-life for the metabolites is 8 to 13 hours.

Pharmacodynamics

Acebutolol is prescribed for ventricular dysrhythmias as well as for angina pectoris and hypertension. As an antidysrhythmic drug, the onset of action is 1 hour; peak time is 4 to 6 hours, and duration of action is 10 hours. To treat hypertension, the duration of action is 20 to 24 hours.

Side Effects and Adverse Reactions for Antidysrhythmic Drugs

Quinidine, the first drug used to treat cardiac dysrhythmias, has many side effects (e.g., nausea, vomiting, diarrhea, confusion, and hypotension). It can also cause heart block and neurologic and psychiatric symptoms. Procainamide causes less cardiac depression than quinidine.

High doses of lidocaine can cause cardiovascular depression, bradycardia, hypotension, seizures, blurred vision, and double vision. Less serious side effects may include dizziness, light-headedness, and confusion. The use of lidocaine is contraindicated in clients with advanced AV block. It should also be used with caution in clients with liver disorder and heart failure. Mexiletine and tocainide have side effects similar to lidocaine. They are contraindicated for use in clients with cardiogenic shock or in those with second- or third-degree heart block.

Side effects of beta-blockers are bradycardia and hypotension. Bretylium and amiodarone can cause nausea, vomiting, hypotension, and neurologic problems. Side effects of calcium blockers include nausea, vomiting, hypotension, and bradycardia.

It should be noted that *all* antidysrhythmic drugs are potentially prodysrhythmic. This is because of both the pharmacologic activity of the drug on the heart and the inherently unpredictable activity of a diseased heart, with or without the use of drugs. In some cases life-threatening ventricular dysrhythmias can result from appropriate and skillful attempts at drug therapy to treat clients with heart disease. For these reasons antidysrhythmic drug therapy is often initiated during continuous cardiac monitoring of the client's heart rhythm in a hospital setting.

Nursing Process

Antidysrhythmics

ASSESSMENT

■ Obtain health and drug histories. The history may include shortness of breath (SOB), heart palpitations, coughing, chest pain (type, duration, and severity), previous angina or cardiac dysrhythmias, and drugs client currently takes.

Prototype DRUG CHART 41–3

ACEBUTOLOL HCl

Drug Class	**Dosage**
Beta$_1$ blocker, cardioselective beta-adrenergic antagonist Trade names: Sectral, Monitan *Pregnancy Category:* B	*Ventricular dysrhythmia:* **A: PO:** 200 mg b.i.d. q12h May increase to 600-1200 mg in two divided doses. Not for children under 12 years of age
Contraindications	**Drug-Lab-Food Interactions**
Second- and third-degree heart block, severe bradycardia, severe HF, cardiogenic shock *Caution:* Undergoing major surgery, renal and hepatic impairment, labile mellitus	***Drug:*** *Increase* effects with diuretics; prolong hypoglycemic effects of insulin and oral antidiabetics; antagonist effect with albuterol, metaproterenol, terbutaline. ***Lab:*** May *increase* ALT, AST, ALP, ANA titer, BUN, lipoproteins, potassium.
Pharmacokinetics	**Pharmacodynamics**

Absorption: Well absorbed
Distribution: PB: UK
Metabolism: t½: 3-4 h; metabolites: 8-13 h
Excretion: 90%-100% in bile/feces and urine
	Ventricular dysrhythmias:
	PO: Onset: 1 h
	  Peak: 4-6 h
	  Duration: 10 h

Therapeutic Effects/Uses

To aid in the treatment of recurrent stable ventricular dysrhythmias, angina pectoris, and hypertension.
Mode of Action: Drug blocks beta$_1$-adrenergic receptors in cardiac tissues.

Side Effects	**Adverse Reactions**
Dizziness, nausea, headache, hypotension, diaphoresis, fatigue, constipation, diarrhea, occasionally impotence	Palpitations with abrupt withdrawal *Life-threatening:* agranulocytosis, bronchospasm with high doses

A, Adult; *ALT,* alanine aminotransferase; *AST,* aspartate aminotransferase; *ALP,* alkaline phosphatase; *ANA,* antinuclear antibodies; *b.i.d.,* twice a day; *BUN,* blood urea nitrogen; *h,* hour; *HF,* heart failure; *PB,* protein-binding; *PO,* by mouth; *UK,* unknown; *t½,* half-life.

■ Obtain baseline vital signs and electrocardiogram (ECG) for future comparisons.
■ Check early cardiac enzyme results (aspartate aminotransferase, lactate dehydrogenase, creatine phosphokinase), and troponins (cardiac-specific) to compare with future laboratory results.

NURSING DIAGNOSES

■ Decreased cardiac output related to cardiac dysrhythmia
■ Anxiety related to irregular heartbeat
■ Risk for activity intolerance related to lack of oxygen because of irregular heart rate

PLANNING

■ Client will no longer experience abnormal sinus rhythm.
■ Client will comply with the antidysrhythmic drug regimen.

NURSING INTERVENTIONS

■ Monitor vital signs. Hypotension can occur.
■ Administer drug by IV push or bolus over a period of 2 to 3 minutes or as prescribed.
■ Monitor ECG for abnormal patterns and report findings such as premature ventricular contractions (PVCs), increased P-R and Q-T intervals, and/or widening of QRS complex. Increased Q-T interval is a risk factor for *torsades des pointes.*

Client Teaching

General
• Instruct client to take prescribed drug as ordered. Drug compliance is essential.
• Provide specific instructions for each drug (e.g., photosensitivity for amiodarone).

Side Effects
• Instruct client to report side effects and adverse reactions to the health care provider. These can include dizziness, faintness, nausea, and vomiting.

- Advise client to avoid alcohol, caffeine, and tobacco. Alcohol can intensify the hypotensive reaction; caffeine increases the catecholamine level; and tobacco promotes vasoconstriction.

Cultural Considerations ❖

- For some people of African-American and Hispanic descent, food is a symbol of health and wealth and is used to celebrate special events. Being overweight, compared with the dominant U.S. culture's view of what constitutes normal weight, is often seen as healthy. Client education may need to focus on the relationship between certain dietary habits and cardiac disease.
- Discuss the importance of the drug regimen in terms that directly address cultural issues and accommodate family values. An interpreter may be necessary to ensure client's understanding and compliance with drug and diet regimens.

EVALUATION

■ Evaluate the effectiveness of the prescribed antidysrhythmic by comparing heart rates with the baseline heart rate and assessing client's response to the drug. Report side effects and adverse reactions. The drug regimen may need to be adjusted. A proarrhythmic effect may occur, which may require discontinuation of the drug.

 Critical Thinking Case Study

ST, age 64, has heart failure (HF) which has been controlled with digoxin, furosemide (Lasix), and a low-sodium diet. She is taking potassium chloride (KCl) 20 mEq orally per day. Three days ago ST had flulike symptoms of anorexia, lethargy, and diarrhea. Her fluid and food intake was diminished. She refused to take the KCl, stating that the drug makes her sick. She has taken the digoxin and furosemide daily.

The nurse's assessment during the home visit includes poor skin turgor, poor muscle tone, irregular pulse rate, and decreased bowel sounds. The nurse obtained a blood sample for serum electrolytes; results indicated potassium (K) 2.9 mEq/l, sodium (Na) 137 mEq/l, and chloride (Cl) 96 mEq/l.

1. List reference values for serum potassium (K), serum sodium (Na), and serum chloride (Cl). Are ST's electrolytes within normal range? Explain.
2. Match ST's physical findings with the corresponding electrolyte imbalance.
3. What are the reasons for the electrolyte imbalance?
4. ST said she was not taking KCl because the drug makes her sick. What information can you give her concerning the administration of potassium?
5. What is the effect of furosemide on digoxin when there is a potassium deficit? Explain.
6. The nurse should assess ST for digitalis toxicity. Why? List the signs and symptoms of digitalis toxicity.

ST was referred to the health care provider because of her serum potassium deficit and its effect on digoxin. A repeat serum potassium determination was taken and the result was 2.8 mEq/l. A liter of dextrose 5% in water with KCl 40 mEq/l was administered over 4 hours.

7. How many milliequivalents of KCl per hour would ST receive? Does this amount constitute an acceptable dosage?
8. Why is it important that the nurse monitor the rate of intravenous fluids containing potassium, the hourly urine output, and vital signs?
9. Because of the low serum potassium level, what other electrolyte value should be checked and why?

After ST's serum electrolytes returned to normal, the health care provider instructed her to continue taking the prescribed KCl dosage daily with her other medications.

10. ST asks you why she has to continue taking these drugs. What should be your response?
11. The nurse instructs ST to eat foods rich in potassium. Which foods are the richest sources of potassium?

DK, age 72, had a myocardial infarction (MI) 5 years ago. He has been having angina attacks at night and at rest while watching television. He complains of stabbing pain in the chest that lasts 5 minutes. Pain does not radiate to the arm. DK is prescribed propranolol (Inderal), 20 mg q.i.d. His vital

Critical Thinking Case Study

signs are: blood pressure, 108/58; pulse, 56 (at times irregular); respirations, 28. His clinical history indicates that he has mild asthma.

1. What other clinical information is needed in regard to DK's health problem and drug?
2. Of the various types of angina, DK's angina occurrence may indicate which type? Explain.
3. What assessments should the nurse make while DK is taking propranolol? Is propranolol an appropriate anginal drug for DK? Explain.
4. What client teaching should be included for DK in regard to his health history and drug?

DK notified the health care provider that he was having "dizzy spells." His blood pressure was 86/50, pulse 46, and respirations 30. His propranolol was stopped, and diltiazem (Cardizem), 30 mg q.i.d., was ordered. He is experiencing an increasing amount of wheezing.

5. What are the correlations between DK's dizziness, wheezing, and vital signs and propranolol?
6. Is the diltiazem ordered for DK within the therapeutic dosage range? In what ways could this drug benefit DK?
7. List the side effects of diltiazem that should be included in client teaching. What other pertinent information should the nurse include in the teaching data for DK?
8. What other drug regimen might be helpful to DK?

NCLEX Study Questions

1. Mrs. AJ takes digoxin 0.25 mg per day. What is the serum therapeutic range for digoxin?
   a. 0.1 to 1.5 ng/ml
   b. 0.5 to 2.0 ng/ml
   c. 1.0 to 2.5 ng/ml
   d. 2.0 to 4.0 ng/ml

2. Mrs. AJ's serum digoxin level is 3.0 ng/ml. Her serum digoxin level would be:
   a. high (elevated) range
   b. low (decreased) range
   c. within normal range
   d. low average range

3. You are assessing Mrs. AJ for possible digitalis toxicity. Signs and symptoms of digitalis toxicity include:
   a. fast pulse (heart) rate of 100 bpm
   b. pulse of 72 with an irregular rate
   c. pulse greater than 60 bpm and irregular rate
   d. pulse below 60 bpm and irregular rate

4. Mrs. AJ is also taking a diuretic that decreases her potassium level. A low potassium level (hypokalemia) could have what effect on the digoxin?
   a. Increases the serum digoxin sensitivity level
   b. Decreases the serum digoxin sensitivity level
   c. Does not have any effect on the serum digoxin sensitivity level
   d. Causes a low average serum digoxin sensitivity level

5. When a client first takes a nitrate, a common symptom that often occurs is:
   a. nausea and vomiting
   b. headaches
   c. stomach cramps
   d. irregular pulse rate

6. Beta blockers are effective as antianginals because they:
   a. increase oxygen to the systemic circulation
   b. maintain heart rate and blood pressure
   c. decrease heart rate and decrease myocardial contractility
   d. decrease heart rate and increase myocardial contractility

7. What instruction should the client receive when discontinuing a beta blocker?
   a. The beta blocker should be abruptly stopped when another cardiac drug is prescribed.
   b. The beta blocker should NOT be abruptly stopped; the dose should be tapered down.
   c. The beta blocker dose should be maintained while taking another antianginal drug.
   d. Half the beta blocker dose should be taken for the next several weeks.

8. The beta blocker acebutolol (Sectral) is prescribed for dysrhythmias. The primary purpose of the drug is to:
   a. increase the $beta_1$ and $beta_2$ receptors in the cardiac tissues
   b. increase the flow of oxygen to the cardiac tissues
   c. block the $beta_1$ adrenergic receptors in the cardiac tissues
   d. block the $beta_2$ adrenergic receptors in the cardiac tissues

Answers: 1, b; 2, a; 3, d; 4, a; 5, b; 6, c; 7, b; 8, c.

42

Diuretics

Outline

Objectives

- Explain the action and uses of diuretics.
- Identify the various groups of diuretics.
- Describe several side effects and adverse reactions related to thiazide, loop, and potassium-sparing diuretics.
- Explain the nursing interventions, including client teaching, related to diuretics, especially thiazide, loop, and potassium-sparing diuretics.

Terms

Diuretics are used for two main purposes: to decrease hypertension (lower blood pressure) and to decrease edema (peripheral and pulmonary) in heart failure (HF) and renal or liver disorders. **Hypertension** is an elevated blood pressure. Diuretics discussed in this chapter are used either alone or in combination to decrease blood pressure and edema.

Diuretics produce increased urine flow **(diuresis)** by inhibiting sodium and water reabsorption from the kidney tubules. Most sodium and water reabsorption occurs throughout the renal tubular segments (proximal, loop of Henle [descending loop and ascending loop], and collecting tubule). Diuretics can affect one or more segments of the renal tubules. Figure 42–1 illustrates the renal tubule along with the normal process of water and electrolyte reabsorption and diuretic effects on the tubules.

Every 1.5 hours, the total volume of the body's extracellular fluid (ECF) goes through the kidneys (glomeruli) for

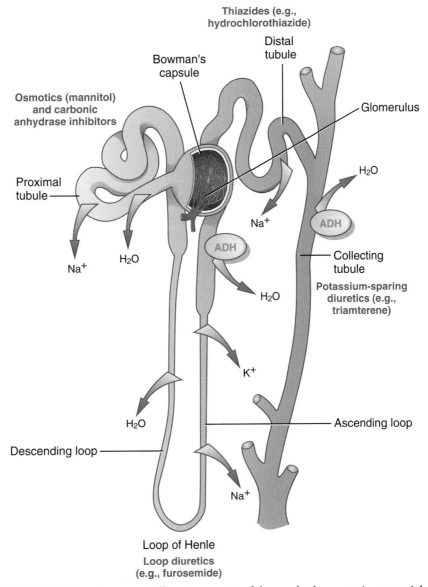

FIGURE 42–1 Diuretics act on different segments of the renal tube: osmotic, mercurial, and carbonic anhydrase inhibitor diuretics affect the proximal tubule; loop (high-ceiling) diuretics affect the loop of Henle; thiazides affect the distal tubule; and potassium-sparing diuretics act primarily on the collecting tubules.

cleansing; this is the first process for urine formation. Small particles such as electrolytes, drugs, glucose, and waste products from protein metabolism are filtered in the glomeruli. Larger products such as protein and blood cells are not filtered with normal renal function, and they remain in the circulation. Sodium and water are the largest filtrate substances.

Normally 99% of the filtered sodium that passes through the glomeruli is reabsorbed. From 50% to 55% of sodium reabsorption occurs in the proximal tubules, 35% to 40% in the loop of Henle, 5% to 10% in the distal tubules, and less than 3% in the collecting tubules. Diuretics that act on the tubules closest to the glomeruli have the greatest effect in causing **natriuresis** (sodium loss in the urine). A classic example is the osmotic diuretic mannitol. The diuretic ef-

fect depends on the drug reaching the kidneys and its concentration in the renal tubules.

Diuretics have an **antihypertensive** effect because they promote sodium and water loss by blocking sodium and chloride reabsorption. This causes a decrease in fluid volume, lowering blood pressure. With fluid loss, edema (fluid retention in body tissues) should decrease, but if sodium is retained, water is also retained, and blood pressure increases.

Many diuretics cause the loss of other electrolytes, including potassium, magnesium, chloride, and bicarbonate. The diuretics that promote potassium excretion are classified as **potassium-wasting diuretics**, and those that promote potassium retention are called **potassium-sparing diuretics**.

The following five categories of diuretics are effective in removing water and sodium:

- Thiazide and thiazide-like
- Loop or high-ceiling
- Osmotic
- Carbonic anhydrase inhibitor
- Potassium-sparing

The thiazide, loop or high-ceiling, and potassium-sparing diuretics are most frequently prescribed for hypertension and for edema associated with HF. Except for those in the potassium-sparing group, all diuretics are potassium-wasting.

Combination diuretics that contain both potassium-wasting and potassium-sparing drugs have been marketed primarily for the treatment of hypertension. Combinations have an additive effect in reducing blood pressure and are discussed in more detail in the section on potassium-sparing diuretics. Chapter 43 offers a closer look at the combinations of antihypertensive agents with hydrochlorothiazide.

Thiazides and Thiazide-Like Diuretics

The first thiazide, chlorothiazide, was marketed in 1957 and followed a year later by hydrochlorothiazide. There are numerous thiazide and thiazide-like preparations. Thiazides act on the distal convoluted renal tubule, beyond the loop of Henle, to promote sodium, chloride, and water excretion. Thiazides are used to treat hypertension and peripheral edema. They are not effective for immediate diuresis and should not be used to promote fluid loss in clients with severe renal dysfunction. Table 42–1 lists the drugs, dosages, uses, and considerations for the thiazide and thiazide-like diuretics. Drug dosages for hypertension and edema are similar.

Table 42–1		
Diuretics: Thiazides		
Generic (Brand)	**Route and Dosage**	**Uses and Considerations**
Short-Acting		
chlorothiazide (Diuril)	*Hypertension:* A: PO: 250-500 mg/d or b.i.d. *Edema:* A: PO: 500-1000 mg/d A: IV: 250-1000 mg/d in 1-2 divided doses C: >1 y: PO: 20 mg/kg/d in 2 divided doses C: <6 mo: PO: 10-30 mg/kg/d in divided doses	For hypertension and peripheral edema. Adults may be given IV chlorothiazide, but it is *not* recommended for infants and children. *Pregnancy category:* B; PB: 20%-80%; t½: 1-2 h
hydrochlorothiazide (HydroDIURIL, HCTZ)	(Prototype Drug Chart 42–1)	
Intermediate-Acting		
bendroflumethiazide (Naturetin)	A: PO: 2.5-20 mg/d C: PO: *maint:* 0.05-0.1 mg/kg/d or 1.5-3 mg/m²/d or in divided doses	Treatment of hypertension and edema associated with HF and cirrhosis. Has similar effects as the prototype drug HCTZ. Hypokalemia, hyperglycemia, and hyperuricemia may occur. *Pregnancy category:* UK; PB: 94%; t½: 3-4 h
benzthiazide (Exna)	*Hypertension:* A: PO: 25-100 mg/d or 25-100 mg in divided doses *Edema:* A: PO: 25-200 mg/d C: PO: 1-4 mg/kg/d in 3 divided doses	Similar to hydrochlorothiazide. *Pregnancy category:* D; PB: UK; t½: UK
hydroflumethiazide (Saluron, Diucardin)	*Hypertension:* A: PO: 50-100 mg/d *Edema:* A: PO: 25-200 mg/d C: PO: 1 mg/kg/d	Similar to hydrochlorothiazide, its effects, side effects, adverse reactions, and abnormal laboratory results. *Pregnancy category:* C; PB: 74%; t½: 17 h
Long-Acting		
methyclothiazide (Aquatensen, Enduron)	*Hypertension/edema:* A: PO: 2.5-10 mg/d C: PO: 0.05-0.1 mg/kg/d	For hypertension and edema associated with HF and renal or liver dysfunction. Side effects and drug interactions are similar to those of HCTZ. Has a long duration of action. *Pregnancy category:* C; PB: UK; t½: UK

A, Adult; *b.i.d.*, twice a day; *C*, child; *d*, day; *h*, hour; *HF*, heart failure; *IV*, intravenous; *maint*, maintenance; *max*, maximum; *mo*, month; *PO*, by mouth; *PB*, protein-binding; *t½*, half-life; *UK*, unknown; *wk*, week; *y*, year; >, greater than; <, less than.

Table 42–1

Diuretics: Thiazides—cont'd

Generic (Brand)	Route and Dosage	Uses and Considerations
polythiazide (Renese-R)	*Hypertension:* A: PO: 2-4 mg/d *Edema:* A: PO: 1-4 mg/d C: PO: 0.02-0.08 mg/kg/d	Similar to hydrochlorothiazide. *Pregnancy category:* D; PB: 84%; t½: 25 h
trichlormethiazide (Diurese Metahydrin, Naqua)	*Hypertension:* A: PO: 2-4 mg/d in 1-2 divided doses *Edema:* A: PO: 1-4 mg/d or b.i.d. C: PO: 0.07 mg/kg/d in divided doses	Similar to HCTZ. Has a long duration of action (24 h). *Pregnancy category:* B; PB: UK; t½: 2.5-7 h
Thiazide-Like Diuretics *(Similar to but not exactly like HCTZ effects)* chlorthalidone (Hygroton)	*Hypertension:* A: PO: 12.5-50 mg/d *Edema:* A: PO: 25-100 mg/d; *max:* 200 mg/d C: PO: 2 mg/kg/3 × wk	For hypertension and edema associated with HF and renal or liver dysfunction. Has a very long duration of action (24-72 h). *Pregnancy category:* C; PB: 75%; t½: 40-54 h
indapamide (Lozol)	*Hypertension/edema:* A: PO: 2.5 mg/d; may increase to 5 mg/d	For hypertension and edema. Long-acting diuretic. May be classified as a loop diuretic. *Pregnancy category:* B; PB: 75%; t½: 14-18 h
metolazone (Zaroxolyn)	*Hypertension:* A: PO: 2.5-5.0 mg/d *Edema:* A: PO: 5-20 mg/d	For hypertension and edema. Intermediate-acting diuretic. More effective than thiazides in clients with decreased renal function. *Pregnancy category:* D; PB: 33%; t½: 8-14 h
quinethazone (Hydromox)	A: PO: 50-100 mg/d; *max:* 200 mg/d in divided doses	For edema. Intermediate-acting diuretic. *Pregnancy category:* D; PB: UK; t½: UK

Thiazide diuretics are used primarily for clients with normal renal function. If the client has a renal disorder and creatinine clearance is less than 30 ml/min, the effectiveness of the thiazide diuretic is greatly decreased. Thiazides cause a loss of sodium, potassium, and magnesium, but they promote calcium reabsorption. **Hypercalcemia** (calcium excess) may result, and the condition can be hazardous to the client who is digitalized or has cancer that causes hypercalcemia. Thiazides affect glucose tolerance, so hyperglycemia can also occur. Thiazides should be used cautiously in clients with diabetes mellitus. Laboratory test results (e.g., electrolytes, glucose) need to be monitored.

The thiazide drug hydrochlorothiazide has been combined with selected angiotensin-converting enzyme (ACE) inhibitors, beta-blockers, alpha-blockers, angiotensin II blockers, and centrally acting sympatholytics to control hypertension. Prototype Drug Chart 42–1 outlines the pharmacologic data for hydrochlorothiazide.

Pharmacokinetics

Thiazides are well absorbed from the gastrointestinal (GI) tract. Hydrochlorothiazide has a moderate protein-binding power. The half-life of the thiazide drugs is longer than that of the loop diuretics. For this reason, thiazides should be administered in the morning to avoid nocturia (nighttime urination) and sleep interruption.

Pharmacodynamics

Thiazides act directly on arterioles to cause vasodilation, which can lower blood pressure. Other action includes the promotion of sodium chloride and water excretion, resulting in a decrease in vascular fluid volume and a concomitant decrease in cardiac output and blood pressure. The onset of action of hydrochlorothiazide occurs within 2 hours. Peak concentration times are long (3 to 6 hours). Thiazides are divided into three groups, according to their duration of action: short-acting (duration less than 12 hours), intermediate-acting (duration 12 to 24 hours), and long-acting (duration more than 24 hours).

Side Effects and Adverse Reactions

Side effects and adverse reactions of thiazides include electrolyte imbalances (hypokalemia, hypercalcemia, hypomagnesemia, and bicarbonate loss), **hyperglycemia** (elevated blood sugar), **hyperuricemia** (elevated serum uric acid level), and hyperlipidemia (elevated blood lipid level). Signs and symptoms of hypokalemia should be assessed, and serum potassium levels must be closely monitored. Potassium supplements are frequently needed. Serum calcium and uric acid levels should be checked, because thiazides block calcium and uric acid excretion. Thiazides affect the metabolism of carbohydrates, and hyperglycemia can result, especially in clients with high to high-normal blood sugar levels. Thiazides can increase serum choles-

Prototype DRUG CHART 42–1

HYDROCHLOROTHIAZIDE

Drug Class

Thiazide diuretic
Trade names: HydroDIURIL, HCTZ, Esidrix, Oretic,
  ✚Apo-Hydro, Urozide
Pregnancy Category: B

Contraindications

Renal failure with anuria, electrolyte depletion
Caution: Hepatic cirrhosis, renal dysfunction,
  diabetes mellitus, gout, systemic lupus erythematosus

Dosage

A: PO: Hypertension; 12.5-50 mg/d
Edema: Initially: 25-200 mg in divided doses; *maint:*
  25-100 mg/day
C: PO: 1-2 mg/kg/d in divided doses
C: <6 mo: PO: 1-3 mg/kg/d in divided doses

Drug-Lab-Food Interactions

Drug: Increase digitalis toxicity with digitalis and
  hypokalemia; *increase* potassium loss with steroids;
  potassium loss; *decrease* antidiabetic effect; *decrease*
  thiazide effect with cholestyramine and colestipol
Lab: Increase serum calcium, glucose, uric acid; *decrease*
  serum potassium, sodium, magnesium

Pharmacokinetics

Absorption: Readily absorbed from the GI tract
Distribution: PB: 65%
Metabolism: t½: 6-15 h
Excretion: In urine

Pharmacodynamics

PO: Onset: 2 h
  Peak: 3-6 h
  Duration: 6-12 h

Therapeutic Effects/Uses

To increase urine output; to treat hypertension, edema from HF, hepatic cirrhosis, renal dysfunction
Mode of Action: Action is on the renal distal tubules, promoting sodium, potassium, and water excretion and decreasing preload and cardiac output; also decreases edema; acts on arterioles, causing vasodilation, thus decreasing blood pressure

Side Effects

Dizziness, vertigo, weakness, nausea, vomiting,
  diarrhea, hyperglycemia, constipation, rash,
  photosensitivity

Adverse Reactions

Severe dehydration, hypotension
Life-threatening: Severe potassium depletion, marked
  hypotension, uremia, aplastic anemia, hemolytic
  anemia, thrombocytopenia, agranulocytosis

A, Adult; *C,* child; *d,* day; *GI,* gastrointestinal; *h,* hour; *HF,* heart failure; *maint,* maintenance; *mo,* month; *PB,* protein-binding; *PO,*
by mouth; *t½,* half-life; *,<* less than; ✚, Canadian drug name.

terol, low-density lipoprotein, and triglyceride levels. A drug may be ordered to lower blood lipids. Other side effects include dizziness, headaches, nausea, vomiting, constipation, urticaria (hives) (rare), and blood dyscrasias (rare). Table 42–2 summarizes the serum chemistry abnormalities that can occur with thiazide use.

Contraindications

Thiazides are contraindicated for use in renal failure. Symptoms of severe kidney impairment or shutdown include **oliguria** (marked decrease in urine output), elevated blood urea nitrogen (BUN), and elevated serum creatinine.

Drug Interactions

Of the numerous thiazide drug interactions, the most serious occurs with digoxin. Thiazides can cause **hypokalemia**, which enhances the action of digoxin, and digitalis toxicity can occur. Potassium supplements are frequently prescribed, and serum potassium levels are monitored.

Thiazides also induce hypercalcemia, which enhances the action of digoxin, resulting in possible digitalis toxicity. Signs and symptoms of digitalis toxicity (bradycardia, nausea, vomiting, visual changes) should be reported. Thiazides enhance the action of lithium, and lithium toxicity can occur. Thiazides potentiate the action of other antihypertensive drugs, which may be used to advantage in combination drug therapy for hypertension.

 Nursing Process

Diuretics: Thiazides

ASSESSMENT

■ Assess vital signs, weight, urine output, and serum chemistry values (electrolytes, glucose, uric acid) for baseline levels.

Table 42–2

Serum Chemistry Abnormalities Associated with Thiazides

Serum Chemistry Parameter	Abnormal Results
Electrolytes, Normal Levels	
Potassium, 3.5-5-3 mEq/l	Hypokalemia (low serum potassium). Potassium is excreted from the distal renal tubule.
Magnesium, 1.8-3.0 mg/dl	Hypomagnesemia (low serum magnesium). Potassium and sodium loss prompt magnesium loss.
Calcium, 4.5-5.5 mEq/l	Hypercalcemia (elevated serum calcium). Thiazides may block calcium excretion.
Chloride, 95-105 mEq/l	Hypochloremia (low serum chloride). Sodium and potassium losses produce chloride loss.
Bicarbonate, 24-28 mEq/l	Minimal bicarbonate loss from proximal tubule.
Uric acid, 2.8-8.0 mg/dl	Hyperuricemia (elevated uric acid). Thiazides can block uric acid excretion.
Blood sugar, 70-110 mg/dl	Hyperglycemia (increased blood sugar). Thiazides increase fasting blood sugar levels and those of prediabetic state.
Blood Lipids	
Cholesterol: less than 200 mg/dl	Cholesterol, LDLs, and triglycerides can be elevated.
LDL: less than 100 mg/dl	
Triglyceride: 10-190 mg/dl	

LDL, Low-density lipoprotein.

■ Check peripheral extremities for presence of edema. Note pitting edema.

■ Obtain a history of drugs and herbal supplements taken daily. Review for drugs and herbals that may cause drug interaction (digoxin, corticosteroids, antidiabetics, ginkgo, licorice).

NURSING DIAGNOSES

■ Risk for deficient fluid volume related to use or overuse of thiazides

■ Impaired urinary elimination related to kidney dysfunction

■ Excess fluid volume related to body fluid retention

PLANNING

■ Client's blood pressure will be decreased and/or return to normal value.

■ Client's edema will be decreased.

■ Client's serum chemistry levels remain within normal ranges.

NURSING INTERVENTIONS

■ Monitor vital signs and serum electrolytes, especially potassium, glucose, uric acid, and cholesterol levels. Report changes. If client is taking digoxin and hypokalemia occurs, digitalis toxicity frequently results.

■ Observe for signs and symptoms of hypokalemia (muscle weakness, leg cramps, cardiac dysrhythmias).

■ Check client's weight daily or when specified. Weight gain of 2.2 pounds is equivalent to an excess liter of body fluids.

■ Monitor urine output to determine fluid loss or retention.

Client Teaching

General

● Emphasize the need for compliance. Client may not "feel better" for some time or may not "feel worse" if treatment is missed or discontinued.

● Suggest that client take hydrochlorothiazide in early morning to avoid sleep disturbance resulting from nocturia.

● Keep drugs out of reach of small children. Request childproof bottle.

● Inform client that certain herbal products may interact with thiazide diuretics (Herbal Alert 42–1).

Self-Administration

● Instruct client or family member how to take and record blood pressure. Record daily results.

Side Effects

● Instruct client to slowly change positions from lying to standing, because dizziness may occur as a result of orthostatic (postural) hypotension.

● Advise client who may be prediabetic to have blood sugar checked periodically, because large doses of hydrochlorothiazide increase blood glucose levels.

● Suggest that client use sun block when in direct sunlight.

Diet

● Instruct client to eat foods rich in potassium (fruits, fruit juices, and vegetables). Potassium supplements may be ordered.

● Advise client to take drugs with food to avoid gastrointestinal upset.

Cultural Considerations ❖

● Respect cultural beliefs and values. If client from a foreign background tells the health care provider that she or he only eats pasta and does not eat fruits and vegetables, the nurse may have two options: to encourage client to eat fruits and vegetables or to contact the health care provider so that an adequate potassium supplement would be prescribed to overcome potassium loss. An interpreter may be necessary.

- Emphasize the importance of client taking a potassium supplement with the potassium-wasting diuretic. In addition, advise client of consequences and dangers of not taking potassium supplements or lack of appropriate diet while taking potassium-wasting diuretics. Serum potassium values should be monitored.

EVALUATION

■ Evaluate the effectiveness of drug therapy. Client's blood pressure and edema will be reduced, and blood chemistry will remain within normal range.

■ Determine the absence of side effects and adverse reactions to therapy.

Loop (High-Ceiling) Diuretics

The loop, or high-ceiling, diuretics act on the thick ascending loop of Henle to inhibit chloride transport of sodium into the circulation (inhibit passive reabsorption of sodium). Sodium and water are lost, together with potassium, calcium, and magnesium. Loop diuretics can affect blood sugar and increase uric acid levels. Drugs in this group are extremely potent and cause marked depletion of water and electrolytes. This high diuretic potential is the reason they are often called *high-ceiling diuretics*. The effects of loop diuretics are dose-related (i.e., increasing the dose increases the effect and response of the drug). More potent than thiazides for promoting diuresis (inhibiting reabsorption of sodium two to three times more effectively), loop diuretics are less effective as antihypertensive agents.

Loop (high-ceiling) diuretics should not be prescribed if a thiazide could alleviate body fluid excess. If furosemide (Lasix) alone is not effective in removing body fluid, a thiazide may be added, but furosemide should never be combined with another loop diuretic. Furosemide is usu-

---

Herbal ALERT 42–1

Diuretics

- *Aloe* can decrease the serum potassium level, thereby causing hypokalemia, when taken with a potassium-wasting diuretic such as a thiazide.
- *Uva ursi* may increase the effects of diuretics. It may cause electrolyte imbalance.
- *Gingko* may increase blood pressure when taken with thiazide diuretics.
- *Licorice* can increase potassium loss, leading to hypokalemia.

---

ally administered as an oral dose in the morning or intravenously when the client's condition warrants immediate removal of body fluid, for example, in cases of acute heart failure or pulmonary edema.

Loop diuretics can increase renal blood flow up to 40%. Furosemide is a frequently prescribed diuretic for clients whose creatinine clearance is less than 30 ml/min and for those with end-stage renal disease. This group of diuretics causes excretion of calcium, unlike thiazides, which inhibit calcium loss.

The first loop diuretic marketed was ethacrynic acid (Edecrin) in the late 1950s, followed by furosemide (Lasix) in 1960. Approved by the FDA in 1983, bumetanide (Bumex) is more potent than furosemide on a per milligram-for-milligram basis. Furosemide and bumetanide are derivatives of sulfonamides. Ethacrynic acid, a phenoxyacetic acid derivative, is a seldom-chosen loop diuretic. It is usually reserved for clients allergic to sulfa drugs. Prototype Drug Chart 42–2 lists the drug data for the loop diuretic furosemide.

Pharmacokinetics

Loop diuretics are rapidly absorbed by the GI tract. These drugs are highly protein bound with half-lives that vary from 30 minutes to 1.5 hours. Loop diuretics compete for protein-binding sites with other highly protein-bound drugs.

Pharmacodynamics

Loop diuretics have a great **saluretic** (sodium-chloride–losing) or **natriuretic** (sodium-losing) effect and can cause rapid diuresis, decreasing vascular fluid volume and causing a decrease in cardiac output and blood pressure. Because furosemide is a more potent diuretic than thiazide diuretics, it causes a vasodilatory effect; thus renal blood flow increases before diuresis. Furosemide is used when other conservative measures, such as sodium restriction and use of less potent diuretics, fail. The oral dose of furosemide is usually twice that of an intravenous (IV) dose.

The onset of action of loop diuretics occurs within 30 to 60 minutes. The onset of action for IV furosemide is 5 minutes. Duration of action is shorter than that of the thiazides.

Side Effects and Adverse Reactions

The most common side effects of loop diuretics are fluid and electrolyte imbalances such as hypokalemia, hyponatremia, hypocalcemia, hypomagnesemia, and hypochloremia. Hypochloremic metabolic alkalosis may result, which can worsen hypokalemia. Orthostatic hypotension can occur. Thrombocytopenia, skin disturbances, and transient deafness are rarely seen. Prolonged use of loop diuretics could cause thiamine deficiency. Table 42–3 lists the physiologic and laboratory changes associated with loop diuretics.

Drug Interaction

The major drug interaction is with digitalis preparations. If the client takes digoxin with a loop diuretic, digitalis toxicity can result. Hypokalemia enhances the action of digoxin and increases the risk of digitalis toxicity. The client needs potassium replacement with food or supplements. Serum potassium levels should be closely monitored, especially when the client is taking high dosages of loop diuretics. Table 42–4 lists the data for the four loop (high-ceiling) diuretics.

Prototype DRUG CHART 42–2

FUROSEMIDE

Drug Class

Loop (high ceiling) diuretic
Trade names: Lasix, ♣Fumide, Furomide
Pregnancy Category: C

Dosage

A: PO: 20-80 mg single dose/d; may increase in
   6-8 h, 20-40 mg; *max:* 600 mg/d
IM/IV: 20-40 mg single dose over 1-2 min IV; repeat
   20 mg in 2 h
C: PO: 2 mg/kg single dose; repeat in 6-8 h *max:*
   6 mg/kg/d
IM/IV: 1 mg/kg single dose; repeat 1 mg/kg in 2 h

Contraindications

Presence of severe electrolyte imbalances, hypovolemia,
   anuria, hypersensitivity to sulfonamides,
   hepatic coma

Drug-Lab-Food Interactions

Drug: Increase orthostatic hypotension with alcohol;
   increase ototoxicity with aminoglycosides; *increase*
   bleeding with anticoagulants; *increase* potassium loss
   with steroids; *increase* digitalis toxicity and cardiac
   dysrhythmias with digoxin and hypokalemia; *increase*
   lithium toxicity; increase amphotericin B ototoxicity
   and nephrotoxicity
Lab: Increase BUN, blood/urine glucose, serum uric acid,
   ammonia; *decrease* potassium, sodium, calcium, magnesium, chloride serum levels

Pharmacokinetics

Absorption: PO: Readily absorbed from GI tract
Distribution: PB: 95%
Metabolism: t½: 30-50 min
Excretion: In urine, some in feces; crosses placenta

Pharmacodynamics

PO: Onset: less than 60 min
   Peak: 1-4 h
   Duration: UK
IV: Onset: 5 min
   Peak: 20-30 min
   Duration: 2 h

Therapeutic Effects/Uses

To treat fluid retention/fluid overload caused by HF, renal dysfunction, cirrhosis; hypertension; acute pulmonary
   edema
Mode of Action: Inhibition of sodium and water reabsorption from the loop of Henle and distal renal tubules; potassium, magnesium, and calcium also may be excreted

Side Effects

Nausea, diarrhea, electrolyte imbalances, vertigo,
   cramping, rash, headache, weakness, ECG changes,
   blurred vision, photosensitivity

Adverse Reactions

Severe dehydration; marked hypotension
Life-threatening: Renal failure, thrombocytopenia,
   agranulocytosis

A, Adult; *BUN*, blood urea nitrogen; *C*, child; *d*, day; *ECG*, electrocardiogram; *GI*, gastrointestinal; *h*, hour; *HF*, heart failure; *IM*, intramuscular; *IV*, intravenous; *max*, maximum; *min*, minute; *PB*, protein-binding; *PO*, by mouth; *t½*, half-life; ♣, Canadian drug name.

Nursing Process

Diuretics: Loop (High-Ceiling)

ASSESSMENT

■ Obtain a history of drugs that are taken daily. Note
whether client is taking a drug that may interact with
the loop diuretic (alcohol, aminoglycosides, anticoagulants, corticosteroids, lithium, amphotericin B, digitalis). Recognize that furosemide is highly protein-
bound and can displace other protein-bound drugs
such as warfarin (Coumadin).

■ Assess vital signs, serum electrolytes, weight, and
urine output for baseline levels.

■ Compare client's drug dose with recommended dose
and report discrepancy.

■ Note whether client is hypersensitive to sulfonamides.

NURSING DIAGNOSES

■ Risk for deficient fluid volume related to fluid loss
with excessive use of loop diuretics

Table 42–3

Physiologic and Laboratory Changes Associated with Loop Diuretics

Physiologic/Laboratory Changes	Possible Effects of Loop (High-Ceiling) Diuretics
Physiologic Changes	
Hypotension	Postural (orthostatic) hypotension can result because of ECFV deficit.
Ototoxicity	Hearing impairment, although rare, may occur. It is more common with use of ethacrynic acid. Diuretics in other categories are not considered ototoxic. Caution: Avoid taking a loop diuretic with a drug that can be ototoxic, such as an aminoglycoside.
Skin disturbances	Pruritus, urticaria, exfoliative dermatitis, and purpura may occur in some persons allergic to the drug or when taking the loop diuretic in high doses over a long period.
Photosensitivity	When exposed to sun or sunlamp for a prolonged time, severe sunburn could result. The client should use sun block and avoid long sun exposure.
Hypovolemia	Excess extracellular fluid is lost through increased urine excretion.
Laboratory Changes	
Hypokalemia, hypomagnesemia, hyponatremia, hypocalcemia, hypochloremia	Potassium, magnesium, sodium, calcium, and chloride are lost from the body from increased urine excretion. Chloride, an anion, is attached to the cations potassium and sodium; thus chloride is lost along with potassium and sodium.
Hyperglycemia	Increased glycogenolysis may contribute to an elevated blood sugar level. Clients with diabetes should closely monitor their blood glucose levels when taking a loop diuretic.
Hyperuricemia	Elevated uric acid levels are common in clients susceptible to gout.
Elevated BUN and creatinine	These elevations may result from ECFV loss. Hemoconcentration can cause elevated BUN and creatinine levels, which are reversible when fluid volume returns to normal levels.
Thrombocytopenia, leukopenia	Decreases in platelet and white blood cell counts are rare, but they should be closely monitored.
Elevated lipids	Loop diuretics can decrease high-density lipoproteins (HDL) and increase low-density lipoproteins (LDL). Clients with elevated cholesterol levels should have their levels of HDL and LDL checked. Regardless of the lipid effects, loop diuretics are useful for clients with serious fluid retention caused by a cardiac condition such as HF.

BUN, Blood urea nitrogen; *HF,* heart failure; *ECFV,* extracellular fluid volume.

■ Risk for potassium deficit related to excessive use of loop diuretics

PLANNING

■ Client's edema and/or hypertension will be decreased.
■ Client's serum chemistry levels will remain within normal ranges.

NURSING INTERVENTIONS

■ Check the half-life of furosemide. With a short half-life, the drug can be repeated or given more than once a day.
■ Check onset of action for furosemide, orally and IV. If the drug is given IV, the urine output should increase in 5 to 20 minutes. If urine output does not increase, notify the health care provider. Severe renal disorder may be present.
■ Monitor urinary output to determine body fluid gain or loss. Urinary output should be at least 25 ml/hour or 600 ml/24 hour.
■ Check client's weight to determine fluid loss or gain. A loss of 2.2 pounds is equivalent to a fluid loss of 1 liter.

■ Monitor vital signs. Be alert for marked decrease in blood pressure.
■ Administer IV furosemide slowly; hearing loss may occur if rapidly injected.
■ Observe for signs and symptoms of hypokalemia (less than 3.5 mEq/L), such as muscle weakness, abdominal distention, leg cramps, and/or cardiac dysrhythmias.
■ Monitor serum potassium levels, especially when a client is taking digoxin. Hypokalemia enhances the action of digitalis, causing digitalis toxicity.

Client Teaching

General
• To prevent sleep disturbance and nocturia, instruct client to take furosemide in the morning and *not* in the evening.

Side Effects
• Instruct client to rise slowly from lying or sitting to standing to prevent dizziness resulting from fluid loss.

Diet
• Suggest taking furosemide at mealtime or with food to avoid nausea.

Table 42–4

Diuretics: Loop (High-Ceiling), Osmotics, and Carbonic Anhydrase Inhibitors

Generic (Brand)	Route and Dosage	Uses and Considerations
Loop (High-Ceiling)		
bumetanide (Bumex)	A: PO: 0.5-2.0 mg/d; *max:* 10 mg/d IV: 0.5-1 mg/dose; repeat in 2-4 h C: PO: 0.015 mg/kg/d	Treatment of renal disease and hypertension and edema associated with HF. Similar effects as furosemide. *Pregnancy category:* C; PB: 95%; t½: 1-1.5 h
ethacrynic acid (Edecrin)	A: PO: 50-100 mg/d or b.i.d.; *max:* 400 mg/d IV: 0.5-1 mg/kg/dose or 50-100 mg/d C: PO: 1 mg/kg/d	For severe edema (pulmonary and peripheral). Potent diuretic with rapid action. Also used for hypercalcemia. Moderate to high doses may cause ototoxicity. *Pregnancy category:* B; PB: 95%; t½: 1-1.5 h
furosemide (Lasix)	(Prototype Drug Chart 42–2)	
torsemide (Demadex)	*Hypertension:* A: PO/IV: Initially: 5 mg/d; *maint:* PO: 5-10 mg/d; IV: in 2 min *HF:* A: PO/IV: 10-20 mg/d; *max:* 200 mg/d	Similar to furosemide. *Pregnancy category:* C; PB: greater than 97%; t½: 2-4 h
Osmotics	**ICP/IOP:**	
mannitol	A: IV: 1.5-2.0 mg/kg; 15%-25% sol infused over 30-60 min Edema, ascites, or oliguria: A: IV: 50-100 g; 10%-20% sol infused over 90 min to 6 h	For oliguria and decreasing ICP. To prevent acute renal failure. Used in narrow-angle glaucoma for reducing IOP. Client should have effective renal function. Potent diuretic. *Pregnancy category:* C; PB: UK; t½: 1.5 h
urea (Ureaphil)	A: IV: 1-1.5 g/kg of 30% sol, inf over 1-2.5 h; *max:* 120 g/d C: >2 y: IV: 0.5-1.5 g/kg of 30% sol, inf over 1-2.5 h	Same uses as mannitol. Not the drug of choice. Used during prolonged surgery to prevent acute renal failure. *Pregnancy category:* C; PB: UK; t½: 1 h
Carbonic Anhydrase Inhibitors		
acetazolamide (Diamox)	A: PO/IV: 250 mg q12h; dose may vary A: SR: 500 mg/d or b.i.d. C: PO: 10-15 mg/kg/d in divided doses C: IV: 5-10 mg/kg/d; dose may vary	For edema, treating absence (petit mal) seizures, and open-angle glaucoma. May cause hyperglycemia, hyperuricemia, and hypercalcemia. Metabolic acidosis can result. *Pregnancy category:* C; PB: 90%; t½: 2.5-5.5 h
dichlorphenamide (Daranide, Oratrol)	A: PO: 100 mg q12h; *maint:* 25-50 mg/d t.i.d.	Treatment of open-angle glaucoma by reducing the IOP and for narrow-angle glaucoma before surgery. *Pregnancy category:* C; PB: UK; t½: UK
methazolamide (Neptazane)	A: PO: 50-100 mg b.i.d.-t.i.d.	Similar to dichlorphenamide. *Pregnancy category:* C; PB: 50%-60%; t½: 14 h

A, Adult; *b.i.d.*, twice a day; C, child; *d*, day; *h*, hour; *HF*, heart failure; *ICP*, intracranial pressure; *inf*, infusion; *IOP*, intraocular pressure; *IV*, intravenous; *maint*, maintenance dose; *max*, maximum; *min*, minute; *PB*, protein-binding; *PO*, by mouth; *sol*, solution; *SR*, sustained-release; *t½*, half-life; *t.i.d.*, three times a day; *UK*, unknown; *y*, year; >, greater than.

Cultural Considerations ❖

- Respect cultural beliefs and values. If client from a foreign background tells the health care provider that she or he only eats pasta and does not eat fruits and vegetables, the nurse may have two options: to encourage the client to eat fruits and vegetables or to contact the health care provider so that an adequate potassium supplement would be prescribed to overcome potassium loss. An interpreter may be necessary.
- Emphasize the importance of client taking a potassium supplement with the potassium-wasting diuretic. In addition, advise client of consequences and dangers of not taking potassium supplements or lack of appropriate diet while taking potassium-wasting diuretics.

EVALUATION

- Evaluate the effectiveness of drug action: decreased fluid retention or fluid overload, decreased respiratory distress, increased cardiac output.
- Check for side effects and increase in urine output.

Osmotic Diuretics

Osmotic diuretics increase the **osmolality** (concentration) and sodium reabsorption in the proximal tubule and loop of Henle. Sodium, chloride, potassium (to a lesser degree), and water are excreted. This group of drugs is used to prevent kidney failure, to decrease intracranial pressure (ICP) (e.g., in cerebral edema), and to decrease intraocular pressure (IOP) (e.g., in glaucoma). Mannitol is a potent osmotic potassium-wasting diuretic frequently used in emergency situations such as ICP and IOP. In addition, mannitol can be used with cisplatin and carboplatin in cancer chemotherapy to induce a frank diuresis and decreased side effects of treatment.

Mannitol is the most frequently prescribed osmotic diuretic, followed by urea. Diuresis occurs within 1 to 3 hours after IV administration. Table 42–4 describes the two osmotic diuretics.

Side Effects and Adverse Reactions

The side effects and adverse reactions of mannitol include fluid and electrolyte imbalance, pulmonary edema from rapid shift of fluids, nausea, vomiting, tachycardia from rapid fluid loss, and acidosis. Crystallization of mannitol in the vial may occur when the drug is exposed to a low temperature. The vial should be warmed to dissolve the crystals. The mannitol solution should not be used for IV infusion if crystals are present and have not been dissolved.

Contraindications

Mannitol must be given with extreme caution to clients who have heart disease and HF. It should be immediately discontinued if the client develops HF or renal failure.

Carbonic Anhydrase Inhibitors

The carbonic anhydrase inhibitors acetazolamide, dichlorphenamide, ethoxzolamide, and methazolamide block the action of the enzyme *carbonic anhydrase*, which is needed to maintain the body's acid-base balance (hydrogen and bicarbonate ion balance). Inhibition of this enzyme causes increased sodium, potassium, and bicarbonate excretion. With prolonged use, metabolic acidosis can occur.

This group of drugs is used primarily to decrease IOP in clients with open-angle (chronic) glaucoma. These drugs are not used in narrow-angle or acute glaucoma. Other uses include diuresis, management of epilepsy, and treatment of high-altitude or acute mountain sickness. Table 42–4 presents the drug data for carbonic anhydrase inhibitor diuretics. The drug may also be used for a client in metabolic alkalosis who needs a diuretic. Carbonic anhydrase inhibitors may be alternated with a loop diuretic.

Side Effects and Adverse Reactions

Acetazolamide can cause fluid and electrolyte imbalance, metabolic acidosis, nausea, vomiting, anorexia, confusion, orthostatic hypotension, and crystalluria. Hemolytic anemia and renal calculi can also occur. These drugs are contraindicated during the first trimester of pregnancy.

Potassium-Sparing Diuretics

Potassium-sparing diuretics, which are weaker than thiazides and loop diuretics, are used as mild diuretics or in combination with another diuretic (e.g., hydrochlorothiazide or antihypertensive drugs). Continuous use of potassium-wasting diuretics requires a daily oral potassium supplement, because the kidneys excrete potassium,

sodium, and body water. However, potassium supplements are *not* used when the client takes a potassium-sparing diuretic; in fact, serum potassium excess, called **hyperkalemia**, results when a potassium supplement is taken with a potassium-sparing diuretic. The serum potassium should be periodically monitored when the client continuously takes a potassium-sparing diuretic. If the serum potassium level is greater than 5.3 mEq/L, the client should discontinue the potassium-sparing diuretic and restrict foods high in potassium (see Chapter 15).

Potassium-sparing diuretics act primarily in the collecting duct renal tubules and late distal tubule to promote sodium and water excretion and potassium retention. The drugs interfere with the sodium-potassium pump controlled by the mineralocorticoid hormone aldosterone (sodium retained and potassium excreted).

Spironolactone (Aldactone), an aldosterone antagonist discovered in 1958, was the first potassium-sparing diuretic. Aldosterone is a mineralocorticoid hormone that promotes sodium retention and potassium excretion. Spironolactone blocks the action of aldosterone and inhibits the sodium-potassium pump (i.e., potassium is retained and sodium is excreted). Spironolactone (Aldactone) has been prescribed by cardiologists for clients with cardiac disorders because of its potassium-retaining effect. As a result of the action of spironolactone, the heart rate is more regular, and the possibility of myocardial fibrosis is decreased. The effects of spironolactone may take 48 hours.

Amiloride, triamterene, and eplerenone are three additional potassium-sparing diuretics commonly prescribed. Amiloride (Midamor) and eplerenone (Inspra) are effective as antihypertensive agents. Triamterene (Dyrenium) is useful in the treatment of edema caused by HF or cirrhosis of the liver. Low doses of spironolactone and eplerenone are effective for chronic HF. Spironolactone (Aldactone), amiloride (Midamor), triamterene (Dyrenium), and eplerenone (Inspra) should not be taken with ACE inhibitors and angiotensin II receptor blockers (ARBs), because they can also increase serum potassium levels. Prototype Drug Chart 42–3 provides the pharmacologic data for triamterene.

When potassium-sparing diuretics are used alone, they are less effective than when used in combination to reduce body fluid and sodium. These drugs are usually combined with a potassium-wasting diuretic, primarily hydrochlorothiazide or a loop diuretic. The combination of potassium-sparing and potassium-wasting diuretics intensifies the diuretic effect and prevents potassium loss. The common combination diuretics contain spironolactone and hydrochlorothiazide (Aldactazide), amiloride and hydrochlorothiazide (Moduretic), and triamterene and hydrochlorothiazide (Dyazide, Maxzide). Table 42–5 lists the potassium-sparing diuretics and the combination potassium-wasting and potassium-sparing diuretics.

Side Effects and Adverse Reactions

The main side effect of these drugs is hyperkalemia. Caution must be used when giving potassium-sparing diuretics to a client with poor renal function, because the kidneys

Prototype **DRUG CHART 42–3**

TRIAMTERENE

Drug Class	Dosage
Potassium-sparing diuretic Trade name: Dyrenium *Pregnancy Category:* B	**A: PO:** Edema: 100 mg/d in 2 divided doses, p.c.; not to exceed 300 mg/d **C: PO:** 2-4 mg/kg/d in divided doses
Contraindications	**Drug-Lab-Food Interactions**
Severe kidney or hepatic disease, severe hyperkalemia *Caution:* Renal or hepatic dysfunction, diabetes mellitus	***Drug:*** *Increase* serum potassium level with potassium supplements; *increase* effects of antihypertensives and lithium; **life-threatening:** hyperkalemia if given with ACE inhibitor ***Lab:*** *Increase* serum potassium level; may *increase* BUN, AST, alkaline phosphatase levels; *decrease* serum sodium, chloride

Pharmacokinetics	Pharmacodynamics
Absorption: PO: Rapidly absorbed from GI tract **Distribution:** PB: 67% **Metabolism:** t½: 1.5-2.5 h **Excretion:** In urine, mostly as metabolites and bile	**PO:** Onset: 2-4 h Peak: 6-8 h Duration: 12-16 h

Therapeutic Effects/Uses

To increase urine output; to treat fluid retention/overload associated with HF, hepatic cirrhosis, or nephrotic syndrome
Mode of Action: Acts on distal renal tubules to promote sodium and water excretion and potassium retention

Side Effects	Adverse Reactions
Nausea, vomiting, diarrhea, rash, dizziness, headache, weakness, dry mouth, photosensitivity	***Life-threatening:*** Severe hyperkalemia, thrombocytopenia, megaloblastic anemia

A, Adult; *ACE,* angiotensin-converting enzyme; *AST,* aspartate aminotransferase; *BUN,* blood urea nitrogen; *C,* child; *d,* day; *GI,* gastrointestinal; *h,* hour; *HF,* heart failure; *PB,* protein-binding; *p.c.,* after meals; *PO,* by mouth; *t½,* half-life.

excrete 80% to 90% of potassium. Urine output should be at least 600 ml per day. Clients should *not* use potassium supplements while taking potassium-sparing diuretics, unless the serum potassium level is low. If a potassium-sparing diuretic is given with antihypertensive ACE inhibitors, hyperkalemia could become severe or life-threatening, because both drugs retain potassium. Monitoring serum potassium levels is essential to safe drug therapy. GI disturbances (anorexia, nausea, vomiting, diarrhea, and numbness and tingling of the hands and feet) can occur.

Nursing Process

Diuretics: Potassium-Sparing

ASSESSMENT

■ Obtain a history of drugs taken daily. Note whether client is taking a potassium supplement or using a salt substitute.
■ Assess vital signs, serum electrolytes, weight, and urinary output for baseline levels.

■ Compare client's drug dose with the recommended dose and report any discrepancy.

NURSING DIAGNOSES

■ Risk for deficient fluid volume related to fluid loss with excessive use of the potassium-sparing diuretic
■ Risk for potassium excess related to the excessive use of the potassium-sparing diuretic

PLANNING

■ Client's fluid retention and blood pressure will be decreased.
■ Client's serum electrolytes remain within their normal values.

NURSING INTERVENTIONS

■ Check the half-life of triamterene. With a long half-life, drug dose is usually administered once a day, sometimes twice a day.
■ Monitor urinary output. Urine output should increase. Report if urine output is less than 30 ml/hour or less than 600 ml/day.

Table 42–5

Diuretics: Potassium-Sparing

Generic (Brand)	Route and Dosage	Uses and Considerations
Single Agents		
amiloride HCl (Midamor)	A: PO: 5 mg/d; may increase to 10-20 mg/d in 1-2 divided doses	For diuretic-induced hypokalemia; used for hypertension, HF, and cirrhosis of the liver. Serum potassium level should be monitored to detect hyperkalemia. *Pregnancy category:* B; PB: 23%; $t^{1/2}$: 6-9 h
eplerenone (Inspra)	A: PO: 25 mg; increase to 50 mg/d. May increase 50 mg b.i.d. or 100 mg	For hypertension or chronic HF post MI. Approved in 2002. Also classified as a selective aldosterone receptor blocker. Serum potassium should be monitored to detect hyperkalemia. *Pregnancy Category:* B ; PB: 50%; $t^{1/2}$: 4-6 h
spironolactone (Aldactone)	*Hypertension:* A: PO: 25-100 mg/d in 1-2 divided doses *Edema:* A: PO: 25-200 mg/d in divided doses C: PO: 3.3 mg/kg/d in divided doses	For edema and hypertension. Dosage for hypertension is usually slightly lower than for edema. Has a long duration of action. *Pregnancy category:* C; PB: 98%; $t^{1/2}$: 1.5-2 h
triamterene (Dyrenium)	(Prototype Drug Chart 42–3)	
Combinations		
amiloride HCl and hydrochlorothiazide (Moduretic)	A: PO: 1-2 tab (amiloride 5 mg/hydrochlorothiazide 50 mg)	Combinations contain potassium-wasting and potassium-sparing diuretics. Drugs are to control hypertension and edema. They are used to prevent the occurrence of hypokalemia.
spironolactone and hydrochlorothiazide (Aldactazide)	A: PO: 25/25 and 50/50 mg tab	Same as Moduretic.
triamterene and hydrochlorothiazide (Dyazide, Maxzide)	A: PO: 1-2 cap b.i.d., p.c. (Dyazide: triamterene 50 mg/hydrochlorothiazide 25 mg)	Dyazide: each tablet contains triamterene 50 mg and hydrochlorothiazide 25 mg. Maxzide comes in two strengths: triamterene 37.5 mg or 75 mg and hydrochlorothiazide 50 mg or 75 mg. *Pregnancy category:* B; PB: UK; $t^{1/2}$: UK

A, Adult; *b.i.d.,* twice a day; *C,* child; *cap,* capsule; *d,* day; *h,* hour; *HF,* heart failure; *PB,* protein-binding; *p.c.,* after meals; *PO,* by mouth; $t^{1/2}$, half-life; *tab,* tablet; *UK,* unknown.

■ Monitor vital signs. Report abnormal changes.

■ Observe for signs and symptoms of hyperkalemia (serum potassium greater than 5.3 mEq/L). Nausea, diarrhea, abdominal cramps, numbness and tingling of the hands and feet, tachycardia and later bradycardia, peaked narrow T wave on electrocardiogram, or oliguria may signal hyperkalemia.

■ To avoid nocturia, administer triamterene in the morning and not in the evening.

Client Teaching

General

• Instruct client to take triamterene with or after meals to avoid nausea.

• Drug must not be discontinued without consulting health care provider.

Side Effects

• Instruct client to avoid exposure to direct sunlight, because drug can cause photosensitivity.

• Advise client to report possible side effects of drug: rash, dizziness, weakness, GI upset.

Diet

• Advise clients with high average serum potassium levels to avoid foods rich in potassium when taking potassium-sparing diuretics.

EVALUATION

■ Evaluate effectiveness of the potassium-sparing diuretic (e.g., triamterene). Fluid retention (edema) should be decreased or absent.

■ Determine whether urine output has increased and serum potassium level is within normal range.

Critical Thinking Case Study

JQ, age 58, has recently been diagnosed with hypertension. His resting blood pressure is 158/92. He has been prescribed hydrochlorothiazide (HydroDIURIL), 50 mg daily, and told to eat foods rich in potassium.

1. How does hydrochlorothiazide differ from furosemide? What are their similarities and differences?
2. Why is it necessary for JQ to eat foods rich in potassium when taking hydrochlorothiazide? Explain.
3. What are the nursing interventions that should be considered while JQ takes HydroDIURIL?

After a month on hydrochlorothiazide therapy, JQ became weak and complained of nausea and vomiting. His muscles were "soft." His serum potassium level was 3.3 mEq/L. JQ's diuretic was changed to triamterene/hydrochlorothiazide (Dyazide). Again he is advised to eat foods rich in potassium. (Refer to Chapter 15 as needed.)

4. Explain the rationale for changing JQ's diuretic.
5. Should JQ receive a potassium supplement? Explain.
6. What nursing interventions should be followed for JQ?
7. What care plan should the nurse develop for JQ in relation to client teaching?
8. What medical follow-up care is needed for JQ?

NCLEX Study Questions

1. TS is taking hydrochlorothiazide 50 mg daily and digoxin 0.25 mg daily. What type of electrolyte imbalance can occur?
   a. Hypocalcemia
   b. Hypokalemia
   c. Hyperkalemia
   d. Hypermagnesemia

2. TS's electrolyte imbalance would be because of:
   a. high dose of digoxin
   b. digoxin taken daily
   c. hydrochlorothiazide
   d. low dose of hydrochlorothiazide

3. MR has diabetes mellitus and is taking hydrochlorothiazide, 50 mg. Concerning the hydrochlorothiazide, client teaching should include monitoring:
   a. hemoglobin and hematocrit
   b. serum blood urea nitrogen (BUN)
   c. blood gases
   d. serum glucose (sugar) levels

4. CP has heart failure and is prescribed Lasix. What type of diuretic is furosemide (Lasix)?
   a. Thiazide diuretic
   b. Osmotic diuretic
   c. High-ceiling (loop) diuretic
   d. Potassium-sparing diuretic

5. What type of electrolyte imbalance could occur when taking furosemide?
   a. Hypokalemia
   b. Hyperkalemia
   c. Hypoglycemia
   d. Hypermagnesemia

6. Why would a diuretic combination such as triamterene and hydrochlorothiazide be prescribed?
   a. To decrease the serum potassium level
   b. To increase the serum potassium level
   c. To decrease the glucose level
   d. To increase the glucose level

Answers: 1. b; 2. c; 3. d; 4. c; 5. a; 6. b.

43
Antihypertensives

ELECTRONIC RESOURCES

Evolve website (http://evolve.elsevier.com/KeeHayes/pharmacology/):
- *Case Studies*
- *Content Updates*
- *Frequently Asked Questions*
- *Student Review Activities*
- *WebLinks*
- *Additional Reference Material*

Companion CD-ROM:
- *NCLEX Examination Review Questions*
- *Pharmacology Animations*
- *IV Therapy Checklists*
- *Medication Error Checklists*
- *Drug Calculation Problems*
- *Electronic Calculators*
- *Top 200 Drugs with Pronunciations*
- *References from the Textbook*

Outline

Objectives

- Identify the categories of antihypertensive drugs, along with the stepped-care approach and the modified pharmacologic approach to antihypertensive drugs.

- Explain the pharmacologic action of the individual groups of antihypertensive drugs.

- Describe the side effects and adverse reactions to sympatholytics (beta-blockers, centrally acting and peripherally acting alpha-blockers, alpha- and beta-blockers), direct-acting vasodilators, and angiotensin antagonists.

- Explain the nursing interventions, including client teaching, related to antihypertensives.

- Give the blood pressure guidelines for determining hypertension.

Terms

Hypertension

Hypertension is an increase in blood pressure such that the systolic pressure is greater than 140 mmHg and the diastolic pressure is greater than 90 mmHg. **Essential hypertension** is the most common type, affecting 90% of persons with high blood pressure. The exact origin of essential hypertension is unknown; however, contributing factors include: (1) a family history of hypertension, (2) hyperlipidemia, (3) African American background, (4) diabetes, (5) obesity, (6) aging, (7) stress, and (8) excessive smoking and alcohol ingestion. Ten percent of hypertension cases are related to renal and endocrine disorders and are classified as **secondary hypertension.**

Selected Regulators of Blood Pressure

The kidneys and blood vessels strive to regulate and maintain a "normal" blood pressure. The kidneys regulate blood pressure via the renin-angiotensin-aldosterone system. The process is illustrated in Figure 43–1. Renin (from the renal cells) stimulates production of angiotensin II (a potent vasoconstrictor), which causes the release of aldosterone (adrenal hormone that promotes sodium retention and thereby water retention). Retention of sodium and water causes fluid volume to increase, elevating blood pressure.

The baroreceptors in the aorta and carotid sinus and the vasomotor center in the medulla also assist in the regulation of blood pressure. Catecholamines such as norepinephrine, released from the sympathetic nerve terminals, and epinephrine, released from the adrenal medulla, increase blood pressure through vasoconstriction activity.

Other hormones that contribute to blood pressure regulation are the antidiuretic hormone (ADH), atrial natriuretic peptide (hormone) (ANP), and brain natriuretic peptide (BNP). ADH is produced by the hypothalamus and is stored and released by the posterior pituitary gland (neurohypophysis). This hormone stimulates the kidneys to conserve and retain water when there is a fluid volume deficit. When there is a fluid overload, ADH secretion is inhibited, and the kidneys then excrete more water.

Physiologic Risk Factors

Certain physiologic risk factors contribute to hypertension. A diet with excess fat and carbohydrates can increase blood pressure. Carbohydrate intake can affect sympathetic nervous activity. Alcohol increases renin secretions, causing the production of angiotensin II. Obesity affects the sympathetic and cardiovascular systems by increasing cardiac output, stroke volume, and left-ventricular filling. Two thirds of hypertensive persons are obese. Normally weight loss can decrease hypertension, as can mild to moderate sodium restriction.

Cultural Responses to Antihypertensive Agents

African Americans are more likely to develop hypertension at an earlier age than white Americans. They also have a higher mortality rate from hypertension than the white population.

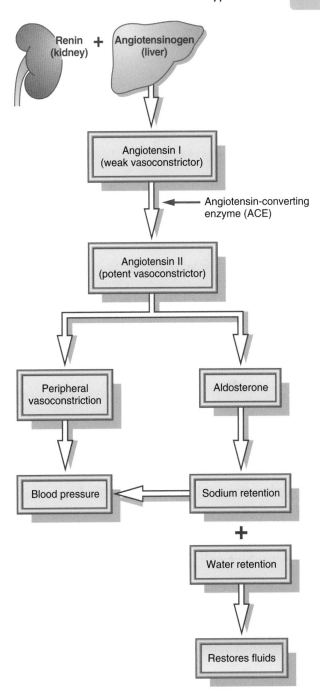

FIGURE 43–1 Renin-angiotensin-aldosterone system (RAAS). Renin, an enzyme located in the juxtaglomerular cells of the kidney, is released when blood pressure decreases. This diagram shows how the RAAS restores fluid balance and stabilizes blood pressure.

The use of beta-adrenergic blockers (beta-blockers) and angiotensin-converting enzyme (ACE) inhibitors is less effective for the control of hypertension in African Americans unless the drug is combined or given with a diuretic. This group is susceptible to low-renin hypertension, therefore they do not respond well to beta-blockers and ACE inhibitors. The antihypertensive drugs that are effective for African Americans are the alpha$_1$ blockers and calcium channel blockers (calcium blockers). African American clients do respond to diuretics as the initial monotherapy for controlling hypertension. White clients usually have high-renin hypertension and respond well to all antihypertensive agents.

Asian Americans are twice as sensitive as whites to beta-blockers and other antihypertensives. A reduction in antihypertensive dosing is frequently needed. American Indians have a reduced or lower response to beta-blockers compared with whites. Monitoring blood pressure and drug dosing should be an ongoing assessment for these cultural groups.

Hypertension in Older Adults

By the age of 65, 26% of males and 30% of females are hypertensive. Between 65 and 75 years of age, 30% of males and 45% of females are hypertensive. Both systolic and diastolic hypertension are associated with increased cardiovascular morbidity and mortality. With antihypertensive therapy, the greatest decrease in cardiovascular disorders is 34% for stroke and 19% for coronary heart disease.

One of the troublesome side effects of the use of antihypertensive agents in older adults, especially frail or institutionalized persons, is orthostatic hypotension. If orthostatic hypotension occurs, the antihypertensive drug dose may need to be decreased or another antihypertensive drug used. Older adults with hypertension should be instructed to modify their lifestyle activities. This includes restricting dietary sodium to 2.4 g (2400 mg) daily, avoiding tobacco, and losing weight if obese.

Nonpharmacologic Control of Hypertension

A sufficient decrease in blood pressure can be accomplished by nonpharmacologic methods. There are many nonpharmacologic ways to decrease blood pressure, but if the systolic pressure is greater than 140 mmHg, **antihypertensive** drugs are generally ordered. Nondrug methods to decrease blood pressure include: (1) stress-reduction techniques, (2) exercise (increases high-density lipoproteins [HDL]), (3) salt restriction, (4) decreased alcohol ingestion, and (5) weight reduction (Figure 43–2).

When hypertension cannot be controlled by nonpharmacologic means, antihypertensive drugs are prescribed. However, nonpharmacologic methods should be combined with antihypertensive drugs to control hypertension.

Guidelines for Hypertension

Blood pressure guidelines for determining hypertension have been revised and are contained in the Seventh Report of the Joint National Committee on Prevention, Detection, Evaluation, and Treatment of High Blood Pressure, or JNC 7. The purpose of these guidelines is to decrease the risk of cardiovascular disease (CVD) in the American population. The guideline for normal blood pressure is less than 120/80 mmHg. *Prehypertension* is the second category, defined as a systolic blood pressure (SBP) 120 to

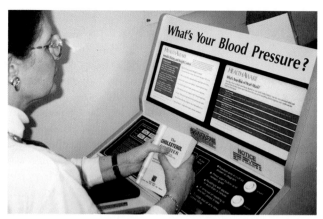

FIGURE 43–2 Blood pressure should be charted at specific intervals, especially if the client has an elevated cholesterol level or borderline hypertension.

139 and a diastolic blood pressure (DBP) 80 to 89. No longer is normal blood pressure equal to or less than 140/90. A decade ago, if a client's blood pressure were 130/85 it fell within the range of acceptable, but now it is considered prehypertension. Stage 1 hypertension falls between 140/90 and 159/99, and stage 2 hypertension is greater than 160/100. Table 43–1 lists the JNC 7 guidelines for hypertension.

Two out of three clients with hypertension have uncontrolled blood pressure or are not optimally treated. The SBP is more important than the DBP as a CVD risk for clients 50 years or older. According to the JNC 7, if the blood pressure is greater than 20/10 mmHg above goal, a drug regimen should be started. CVD risk doubles with each increase of 20/10 mmHg, starting at 115/75 mmHg.

Pharmacologic Control of Hypertension

An individualized approach to the treatment of hypertension is used by many health care providers. All drugs are considered *initial agents* when first prescribed for hypertension. Reduction of other cardiovascular risk factors and the use of fewer drugs (i.e., substituting instead of adding drugs) at the lowest effective doses are emphasized. It has been suggested that after a client has taken an antihyper-

Table 43–1

Guidelines for Determining Hypertension

Category	Systolic Pressure (mmHg)	Diastolic Pressure (mmHg)
Normal	Less than 120	Less than 80
Prehypertension	120-139	80-89
Stage 1 hypertension	140-159	90-99
Stage 2 hypertension	Greater than 160	Greater than 100

tensive drug for a year, the drug dose and its effect on blood pressure should be evaluated.

In 1993 the JNC 5 classified treatment for elevated SBP hypertension into four stages: stage 1, SBP 140 to 160; stage 2, SBP 160 to 180; stage 3, SBP 180 to 200; and stage 4, SBP greater than 200. As a result of staging, the **stepped-care hypertension approach** to treatment was developed. It included a single drug stepped up to multiple drugs, depending upon severity of disease. Under the current guidelines (JNC 7) there are three classifications for defining an elevated SBP: *prehypertension*, SBP 120 to 139; stage 1, SBP 140 to 160; and stage 2, SBP greater than 160. JNC-7 combines prior stages 2, 3, and 4 into the present stage 2, stating that drug management of the former three groups is the same as that for the present stage 2.

If the systolic blood pressure is stage 2 and the diastolic blood pressure is below 90 mmHg, the staging would be known as *2 isolated systolic hypertension, or 2 ISH.* When the systolic blood pressure (SBP) is in stage 1 or 2 and the diastolic blood pressure (DBP) is normal or prehypertensive, the staging would be assigned according to SBP and would be known as *isolated systolic hypertension,* or 1 or 2 ISH. For example, if the SBP is 175 mmHg (stage 2) and the DSP is 85 mmHg (prehypertensive), the stage would be considered 2 ISH. Most clients may need two or more antihypertensive drugs to achieve goal blood pressure. A thiazide diuretic may be the first antihypertensive drug prescribed.

Antihypertensive drugs, used either singly or in combination with other drugs, are classified into six categories: (1) diuretics, (2) sympatholytics (sympathetic depressants), (3) direct-acting arteriolar vasodilators, (4) ACE inhibitors, (5) angiotensin II receptor blockers (ARBs), and (6) calcium channel blockers.

Diuretics

Diuretics promote sodium depletion, which decreases extracellular fluid volume (ECFV). Diuretics are effective as first-line drugs for treating mild hypertension. Hydrochlorothiazide (HydroDIURIL), is the most frequently prescribed diuretic for controlling mild hypertension. It can be used alone for recently diagnosed or mild hypertension or with other antihypertensive drugs. Many antihypertensive drugs can cause fluid retention; therefore diuretics are often administered together with antihypertensive agents. The various types of diuretics are discussed in Chapter 42.

Thiazide diuretics should not be used for clients with renal insufficiency (creatinine clearance less than 30 ml/min). The loop (high-ceiling) diuretics such as furosemide (Lasix) are usually recommended, because they do not depress renal blood flow. Diuretics are not used if hypertension is the result of renin-angiotensin-aldosterone system involvement, because they tend to elevate the serum renin level.

Instead of a single thiazide drug, a combination of potassium-wasting and potassium-sparing diuretics may be useful; less potassium excretion would occur. In addition, thiazides can be combined with other antihypertensive drugs to increase their effectiveness. Box 43–1 lists the combina-

---

Box 43–1

Combination of Thiazides with Antihypertensive Drugs and other Combinations

Thiazide with Potassium-Sparing Diuretics
- hydrochlorothiazide with spironolactone (Aldactazide)
- hydrochlorothiazide with amiloride (Moduretic)
- hydrochlorothiazide with triamterene (Dyazide, Maxzide)

Thiazide with Beta-Blockers
- hydrochlorothiazide with bisoprolol fumarate (Ziac)
- hydrochlorothiazide with metoprolol (Lopressor HCT)
- bendroflumethiazide with nadolol (Corzide)
- hydrochlorothiazide with propranolol (Inderide)
- hydrochlorothiazide with timolol (Timolide)
- chlorthalidone (thiazide-like diuretic) with atenolol (Tenoretic)

Thiazide with ACE Inhibitors
- hydrochlorothiazide with benazepril (Lotensin HCT)
- hydrochlorothiazide with captopril (Capozide)
- hydrochlorothiazide with enalapril maleate (Vaseretic)
- hydrochlorothiazide with fosinopril (Monopril HCT)
- hydrochlorothiazide with lisinopril (Prinzide, Zestoretic)
- hydrochlorothiazide with moexipril (Uniretic)
- hydrochlorothiazide with quinapril (Accuretic)

Thiazide with Angiotensin II Antagonists
- hydrochlorothiazide with candesartan (Atacand HCT)
- hydrochlorothiazide with eprosartan (Teveten HCT)
- hydrochlorothiazide with irbesartan (Avalide)
- hydrochlorothiazide with losartan (Hyzaar)
- hydrochlorothiazide with olmesartan medoxomil (Benicar HCT)
- hydrochlorothiazide with telmisartan (Micardis HCT)
- hydrochlorothiazide with valsartan (Diovan HCT)

Thiazide with Centrally Acting Alpha$_2$ Agonist
- chlorthalidone with clonidine (Combipres)
- hydrochlorothiazide with methyldopa (Aldoril)

Thiazide with Alpha-Blocker
- polythiazide with prazosin (Minizide)

Combination of ACE Inhibitors with Calcium-Channel Blocker
- See Table 43–4

Combination of a Calcium-Channel Blocker with a Statin Drug
- amlodipine with atorvastatin (Caduet)

ACE, Angiotensin-converting enzyme; *HCT,* hydrochlorothiazide.

---

tions of thiazides with other drugs. Many drug products on the market include combinations of thiazide diuretics and potassium-sparing diuretics, beta-blockers, ACE inhibitors, or angiotensin II receptor blockers. ACE inhibitors tend to increase serum potassium (K) levels, so when they are combined with a thiazide diuretic, serum potassium loss is minimized.

Sympatholytics (Sympathetic Depressants)

The **sympatholytics** comprise five groups of drugs: (1) beta-adrenergic blockers, (2) centrally acting alpha$_2$-agonists, (3) alpha-adrenergic blockers, (4) adrenergic neuron blockers (peripherally acting sympatholytics), and (5) alpha$_1$ and beta$_1$ adrenergic blockers. Beta-adrenergic blockers block the beta receptors, and alpha-adrenergic blockers block the alpha receptors.

Beta-Adrenergic Blockers

Beta-adrenergic blockers, frequently called *beta-blockers*, are used as antihypertensive drugs or in combination with a diuretic. Beta-blockers are also used as antianginals and antidysrhythmics and discussed in that context in Chapter 41.

Beta (β_1 and β_2)-adrenergic blockers reduce cardiac output by diminishing the sympathetic nervous system response to decrease basal sympathetic tone. With continued use of beta-blockers, vascular resistance is diminished, and blood pressure is lowered. Beta-blockers reduce heart rate, contractility, and renin release. There is a greater hypotensive response in clients with higher renin levels.

African American hypertensive clients do not respond well to beta-blockers for the control of hypertension. Instead, hypertension can be controlled by combining beta-blockers with diuretics.

There are numerous types of beta-blockers. Nonselective beta-blockers such as propranolol (Inderal) inhibit beta$_1$ (heart) and beta$_2$ (bronchial) receptors. Heart rate slows (blood pressure decreases secondary to the decrease in heart rate), and bronchoconstriction occurs because of unopposed parasympathetic tone. Cardioselective beta-blockers are preferred, because they act mainly on the beta$_1$ rather than the beta$_2$ receptors and bronchoconstriction is less likely to occur. Acebutolol (Sectral), atenolol (Tenormin), betaxolol (Kerlone), bisoprolol (Zebeta), and metoprolol (Lopressor) are cardioselective beta-blockers that block beta$_1$ receptors.

Cardioselectivity does not confer absolute protection from bronchoconstriction. In tests measuring forced expiratory volume in 1 second (FEV$_1$) as a measure of β_2 reactivity, only atenolol demonstrated true protection. Other cardioselective beta-blockers were only partially effective. Studies also show that at the upper end of the dosage range, cardioselectivity is less effective. In clients with preexisting bronchospasms or other pulmonary disease, beta-blockers, even those considered cardioselective, should be used with caution. Some experts regard this as a relative contraindication. The real value of beta selectivity is in maintaining renal blood flow and minimizing the hypoglycemic effects of beta blockade.

The combination of beta-blockers with hydrochlorothiazides is packaged together in tablet form (see Box 43–1). Usually the hydrochlorothiazide dose is 12.5 to 25 mg, approximately half the average dose.

Again, beta-blockers tend to be more effective in lowering blood pressure in clients who have an elevated serum renin level. The cardioselective prototype drug metoprolol (Lopressor) is presented in Prototype Drug Chart 43–1.

Beta-blockers should not be used by clients with second- or third-degree atrioventricular (AV) block or sinus bradycardia. A noncardioselective beta-blocker such as propranolol (Inderal) should not be given to a client with chronic obstructive pulmonary disease (COPD).

Pharmacokinetics

Metoprolol is well absorbed from the gastrointestinal (GI) tract. Its half-life is short and its protein-binding power is low.

Pharmacodynamics

Cardioselective beta-adrenergic blockers block beta$_1$ receptors, thereby decreasing heart rate and blood pressure. The nonselective beta-blockers block beta$_1$ and beta$_2$ receptors, which can result in bronchial constriction. Beta-blockers cross the placental barrier and are excreted in breast milk.

The onset of action of oral beta-blockers is usually 30 minutes or less, and the duration of action is 6 to 12 hours. When beta-blockers are administered intravenously (IV), the onset of action is immediate, peak time is 20 minutes (compared with 1.5 hours orally), and duration of action is 4 to 10 hours.

Side Effects and Adverse Reactions

Side effects and adverse reactions include decreased pulse rate, markedly decreased blood pressure, and (with noncardioselective beta$_1$ and beta$_2$ blockers) bronchospasm. Beta-blockers should not be abruptly discontinued, because rebound hypertension, angina, dysrhythmias, and myocardial infarction can result. Beta-blockers can cause insomnia, depression, nightmares, and sexual dysfunction. Other side effects are discussed in Chapter 41. Table 43–2 presents the drug data for beta-blockers commonly used to treat hypertension.

Noncardioselective beta-blockers inhibit the liver's ability to convert glycogen to glucose in response to hypoglycemia. Because of this side effect, beta-blockers should be used with caution in clients with diabetes mellitus. In addition, the depression of heart rate masks the symptom (tachycardia) of hypotension.

Nursing Process

Antihypertensives: Beta-Blockers

ASSESSMENT

■ Obtain a medication and herbal history from client. Report if a drug-drug or drug-herbal interaction is probable.

■ Obtain vital signs. Report abnormal blood pressure. Compare vital signs with baseline finding.

■ Check laboratory values related to renal and liver function. An elevated blood urea nitrogen (BUN) and serum creatinine may be caused by beta-blockers or

Prototype DRUG CHART 43–1

METOPROLOL

Drug Class

Antihypertensive: Beta$_1$-blocker
Trade names: Lopressor, ✤Betaloc, Apo-Metoprolol, Toprol SR
Pregnancy Category: C; D (second and third trimester)

Dosage

Hypertension:
A: PO: 50-100 mg/d in 1-2 divided doses; *maint:* 100-450 mg in divided doses; *max:* 450 mg/d in divided doses
Elderly: PO: 25 mg/day; *maint:* 25-300 mg/d
SR: 50-100 mg/day; *max:* 450 mg/d
Myocardial infarction:
A: PO: 100 mg b.i.d.
IV: 5 mg q2min × 3 doses

Contraindications

Second- and third-degree heart block, cardiogenic shock, HF, sinus bradycardia. NOTE: metoprolol and carvedilol may be prescribed for early use in management of chronic HF
Caution: Hepatic, renal, or thyroid dysfunction; asthma; peripheral vascular disease; type 1 diabetes mellitus

Drug-Lab-Food Interactions

Drug: Increase bradycardia with digitalis; *increase* hypotensive effect with other antihypertensives, alcohol, anesthetics

Pharmacokinetics

Absorption: PO: 95%
Distribution: PB: 12%
Metabolism: t½: 3-7 hours
Excretion: In urine

Pharmacodynamics

PO: Onset: 15 min
Peak: 1.5 h
Duration: 10-19 h
IV: Onset: Immediate
Peak: 20 min
Duration: 5-10 h

Therapeutic Effects/Uses

To control hypertension
Mode of Action: Promotion of blood pressure reduction via beta$_1$-blocking effect

Side Effects

Fatigue, weakness, dizziness, nausea, vomiting, diarrhea, mental changes, nasal stuffiness, impotence, decreased libido, depression

Adverse Reactions

Bradycardia, thrombocytopenia
Life-threatening: Complete heart block, bronchospasm, agranulocytosis

A, Adult; *b.i.d.,* twice a day; *d,* day; *h,* hour; *HF,* heart failure; *IV,* intravenous; *maint,* maintenance; *max,* maximum; *min,* minute; *PB,* protein-binding; *PO,* by mouth; *SR,* sustained release; *t½,* half-life; ✤, Canadian drug name.

---

cardiac disorder. Elevated cardiac enzymes, such as aspartate transaminase (AST) and lactate dehydrogenase (LDH), could result from use of a beta-blocker or from a cardiac disorder.

NURSING DIAGNOSES

■ Decreased cardiac output related to hypertension
■ Noncompliance with drug regimen related to multiple drugs ordered
■ Sexual dysfunction related to beta blockers (a side effect)

PLANNING

■ Client's blood pressure will be decreased or will return to normal value.

■ Client takes the medication as prescribed.

NURSING INTERVENTIONS

■ Monitor vital signs, especially blood pressure and pulse.
■ Monitor laboratory results, especially BUN, serum creatinine, AST, and LDH.

Client Teaching

General

● Instruct client to comply with drug regimen; abrupt discontinuation of the antihypertensive drug may cause rebound hypertension.
● Inform client that herbs can interfere with beta-blockers (Herbal Alert 43–1).

Table 43–2

Antihypertensives: Beta-Blockers and Central Alpha₂ Agonists

Generic (Brand)	Route and Dosage	Uses and Considerations
Beta-Adrenergic Blockers		
acebutolol HCl (Sectral) Cardioselective beta₁	A: PO: 400-800 mg/d in 1 or 2 divided doses; *max:* 1200 mg/d	For hypertension and cardiac dysrhythmia. May be used alone or in combination with a diuretic. Side effects include dizziness, fatigue, hypotension, bradycardia, constipation/diarrhea. Vital signs should be closely monitored. *Pregnancy category:* B; PB: 26%; $t^{1/2}$: 6-7 h
atenolol (Tenormin) Cardioselective beta₁	A: PO: 25-100 mg/d	For hypertension and angina. Similar side effects as acebutolol. *Pregnancy category:* C; PB: 6%-16%; $t^{1/2}$: 6-7 h
betaxolol HCl (Kerlone) Cardioselective beta₁	A: PO: 10-20 mg/d; also for ophthalmic use (glaucoma)	For hypertension and glaucoma. Ophthalmic preparation is used to decrease IOP. *Pregnancy category:* C; PB: UK; $t^{1/2}$: 14-22 h
bisoprolol fumarate (Zebeta) Beta₁-blocker	A: PO: Initially: 5 mg/d; *maint:* 2.5-20 mg/d	For hypertension and angina pectoris. Long-acting beta₁ blocker. Heart rate and blood pressure may be decreased. *Pregnancy category:* C; PB: <30%; $t^{1/2}$: 9-12 h
carteolol HCl (Cartrol) Nonselective beta₁ and beta₂	A: PO: 2.5-5.0 mg/d	For hypertension and glaucoma. Should be avoided for clients who have asthma because of its beta₂-blocker effect. May be used in combination with a thiazide diuretic. *Pregnancy category:* C; PB: 23%-30%; $t^{1/2}$: 4-6 h
carvedilol (Coreg) alpha-blocker; nonselective beta₁ and beta₂	A: PO: Initially: 3.125-6.25 mg, b.i.d.; may increase after 1-2 wk; *max:* 50 mg/d Elderly: Same as adult	For treating essential hypertension. Contraindicated for decompensated cardiac failure bronchial asthma, bronchospastic conditions, severe bradycardia. Food delays absorption. *Pregnancy category:* C; PB: 98%; $t^{1/2}$: 7-10 h
metoprolol (Lopressor) Cardioselective beta₁	(Prototype Drug Chart 43–1)	
nadolol (Corgard) Nonselective beta₁ and beta₂	A: PO: 40-80 mg/d; *max:* 320 mg/d	For hypertension and angina pectoris. Similar to carteolol HCl. *Pregnancy category:* C; PB: 30%; $t^{1/2}$: 10-24 h
penbutolol SO₄ (Levatol) Nonselective beta₁ and beta₂	A: PO: 10-20 mg/d; *max:* 80 mg/day	Treatment of stage 1 and 2 hypertension. Clients with asthma should avoid taking drug. *Pregnancy category:* C; PB: 80%- 98%; $t^{1/2}$: 5 h
pindolol (Visken) Nonselective beta₁ and beta₂	A: PO: 5 mg b.i.d.-t.i.d.; *maint:* 10-30 mg in divided doses; *max:* 60 mg/d in divided doses	For hypertension. May be used alone or in combination with thiazide diuretic. Also may be used for angina pectoris. *Pregnancy category:* B; PB: 50%; $t^{1/2}$: 3-4 h
propranolol (Inderal) Nonselective beta₁ and beta₂	A: PO: Initially: 40 mg b.i.d.; SR: 80 mg/d; *maint:* 120-240 mg/d in divided doses; *max:* 480 mg/d C: PO: Initially 1 mg/kg/d in 2 divided doses; *maint:* 2 mg/kg/d	For hypertension, angina, and cardiac dysrhythmias. First beta-blocker. May cause bronchospasm because of beta₂-blocker effect. *Pregnancy category:* C; PB: 90%; $t^{1/2}$: 3-6 h
timolol maleate (Blocadren) Nonselective beta₁ and beta₂	A: PO: Initially: 10 mg b.i.d.; *maint:* 20-40 mg/d in 2 divided doses; *max:* 60 mg/d; also for ophthalmic use (glaucoma)	For hypertension, angina pectoris, and glaucoma. Used as step 1 antihypertensive, like most of the beta-blockers. Similar to propranolol. *Pregnancy category:* C; PB: 60%; $t^{1/2}$: 3-4 h
Central Alpha₂ Agonists		
clonidine HCl (Catapres)	A: PO: Initially: 0.1 mg b.i.d.; *maint:* 0.2-1.2 mg/d in divided doses; *max:* 2.4 mg/d A: Transdermal patch: 100 mcg (0.1 mg)/q7d 200 mcg (0.2 mg)/q7d 300 mcg (0.3 mg)/q7d	For hypertension. Long-acting. Well absorbed from GI tract. Can be taken with a diuretic. Decreases sympathetic effect. Drowsiness, dizziness, and dry mouth may occur. *Pregnancy category:* C; PB: 20%-40%; $t^{1/2}$: 6-20 h
guanabenz acetate (Wytensin)	A: PO: 4 mg b.i.d.; may increase to 4-8 mg/d; *max:* 32 mg b.i.d.	For hypertension and tachycardia. Can be taken with a thiazide diuretic. Intermediate acting. May cause drowsiness, dizziness, headache, fatigue, and dry mouth. If GI distress occurs, take with food. *Pregnancy category:* C; PB: 90%; $t^{1/2}$: 4-14 h
guanfacine HCl (Tenex)	A: PO: 1 mg/d at bedtime; may increase to 2-3 mg/d	For hypertension. Long acting. May be taken alone or with a thiazide diuretic. *Pregnancy category:* B; PB: 70%; $t^{1/2}$: >17 h
methyldopa (Aldomet)	A: PO: 250-500 mg b.i.d.; *max:* 3 g/d IV: 250-500 mg q6h; *max:* 1 g q6h C: PO: 10 mg/kg/d in 2-4 divided doses	For stage 1 to 3 hypertension. May be used alone or in combination with a diuretic. Long acting. Can be given IV. If GI upset occurs, take with food. *Pregnancy category:* C; PB: ,15%; $t^{1/2}$: 1.7 h

A, Adult; *b.i.d.*, twice a day; *C*, child; *d*, day; *GI*, gastrointestinal; *h*, hour; *IOP*, intraocular pressure; *IV*, intravenous; *maint*, maintenance; *max*, maximum; *PB*, protein-binding; *PO*, by mouth; *SR*, sustained release; $t^{1/2}$, half-life; *t.i.d.*, three times a day; *UK*, unknown; *wk*, week; > greater than; < less than.

- Suggest that client avoid OTC drugs without first checking with health care provider. Many OTC drugs carry warnings against use in the presence of hypertension or against use concurrently with antihypertensives.
- Suggest that client wear a MedicAlert bracelet or carry a card indicating the health problem and prescribed drugs.
- Instruct client in a trauma situation to inform health care provider of drugs taken daily (such as a beta-blocker). Beta-blockers block the compensatory effects of the body to the shock state. Glucagon may be needed to reverse the effects so client can be resuscitated.

Self-Administration

- Instruct client or family member how to take a radial pulse and blood pressure. Advise client to report abnormal findings to health care provider.

Side Effects

- Advise client that antihypertensives may cause dizziness (orthostatic hypotension). Instruct client to rise slowly from a lying or sitting to a standing position.
- Instruct client to report dizziness, slow pulse rate, changes in blood pressure, heart palpitation, confusion, or gastrointestinal upset to health care provider.
- Alert client with diabetes mellitus to possible hypoglycemic symptoms.
- Inform client that antihypertensives may cause sexual dysfunction (e.g., impotence).

Diet

- Teach client and family members nonpharmacologic methods to decrease blood pressure, such as a low-fat and low-salt diet, weight control, relaxation techniques, exercise, smoking cessation, and decreased alcohol ingestion (1 to 2 oz daily).
- Advise client to report constipation. Foods high in fiber, a stool softener, and increased water intake (except in clients with heart failure) are usually indicated.

Cultural Considerations ❖

- For African-American clients, monotherapy with beta-blockers is generally less effective in controlling their hypertension. However, taking a diuretic together with a beta-blocker can increase the effectiveness of therapy.

EVALUATION

- Evaluate the effectiveness of the drug therapy (i.e., decreased blood pressure, absence of side effects).
- Determine that client adheres to the drug regimen.

Herbal ALERT 43–1

Antihypertensives

- *Ma-huang* and *ephedra* decrease or counteract the effect of antihypertensive drugs. When taken with beta-blockers, hypertension may continue or increase.
- *Ephedra* increases hypertension when taken with beta-blockers.
- *Black cohosh* increases the hypotensive effect of antihypertensive drugs.
- *Hawthorn* may increase the effects of beta-blockers and angiotensin-converting enzyme (ACE) inhibitors.
- *Licorice* antagonizes the effects of antihypertensive drugs.
- *Goldenseal* may increase the effects of antihypertensives.
- *Parsley* may increase the cause of hypotension when taken with an antihypertensive drug.

Centrally Acting Alpha$_2$ Agonists

Centrally acting alpha$_2$ agonists decrease the sympathetic response from the brainstem to the peripheral vessels. They stimulate the alpha$_2$ receptors, which in turn decreases sympathetic activity; increases vagus activity; decreases cardiac output; and decreases serum epinephrine, norepinephrine, and renin release. All these actions result in reduced peripheral vascular resistance and increased vasodilation. This group of drugs has minimal effects on cardiac output and blood flow to the kidneys. Beta-blockers are not given with centrally acting sympatholytics, because accentuation of bradycardia during therapy and rebound hypertension on discontinuing therapy can occur.

Drugs in this group include methyldopa, clonidine, guanabenz, and guanfacine. Methyldopa (Aldomet) was one of the first drugs widely used to control hypertension. In high doses methyldopa and clonidine can cause sodium and water retention. Frequently methyldopa and clonidine are administered with diuretics. Clonidine is available in a transdermal preparation that provides a 7-day duration of action. Transdermal patches are replaced every 7 days and may be left on while bathing. Skin irritations have occurred in approximately 20% of clients. Guanabenz and guanfacine are newer centrally acting alpha$_2$ agonists with effects similar to clonidine. Guanfacine has a long half-life and usually is taken once a day. Table 43–2 lists the centrally acting alpha$_2$ agonists along with the beta-blockers.

Side Effects and Adverse Reactions

Side effects and adverse reactions of alpha$_2$ agonists include drowsiness, dry mouth, dizziness, and slow heart rate (bradycardia). Methyldopa should not be used in clients with impaired liver function, and serum liver enzymes should be monitored periodically in all clients. This group of drugs must not be abruptly discontinued, because a rebound hypertensive crisis can result. If the drug needs to be stopped immediately, another antihypertensive drug is usually prescribed to avoid rebound hypertensive symptoms (e.g., restlessness, tachycardia, tremors, headache, and increased blood pressure). Rebound hypertension is less likely to occur with guanabenz and guanfacine. The nurse should emphasize the need to take the medication as prescribed. This group of drugs can cause sodium and water retention, resulting in peripheral edema. A diuretic may be ordered with methyldopa or clonidine to decrease water and sodium retention (edema). Clients who are pregnant or contemplating pregnancy should avoid clonidine. Methyldopa is frequently used to treat chronic or pregnancy-induced hypertension; however, it crosses the placental barrier, and small amounts may enter the breast milk of a lactating client.

Alpha-Adrenergic Blockers

This group of drugs blocks the alpha-adrenergic receptors (alpha-blockers), resulting in vasodilation and decreased blood pressure. They help maintain the renal blood flow rate. Alpha-blockers are useful in treating hypertension in clients with lipid abnormalities. They decrease the very-low-density lipoproteins (VLDL) and the low-density lipoproteins (LDL) that are responsible for the buildup of fatty plaques in the arteries (atherosclerosis). In addition, they increase high-density lipoprotein (HDL) levels ("friendly" lipoprotein). Alpha-blockers are safe for clients with diabetes, because they do not affect glucose metabolism. They also do not affect respiratory function.

The selective alpha$_1$-adrenergic blockers—prazosin, terazosin, and doxazosin—are used mainly to reduce blood pressure and can be used to treat benign prostatic hypertrophy (BPH). Prazosin is a commonly prescribed drug. Terazosin and doxazosin have longer half-lives than prazosin, and they are normally given once a day. When prazosin is taken with alcohol or other antihypertensives, the hypotensive state can be intensified. These drugs, like the centrally acting alpha$_2$ agonists, cause sodium and water retention with edema; therefore diuretics are frequently given concomitantly to decrease fluid accumulation in the extremities.

The more potent alpha-blockers—phentolamine, phenoxybenzamine, and tolazoline—are used primarily for hypertensive crisis and severe hypertension resulting from catecholamine-secreting tumors of the adrenal medulla (pheochromocytomas).

Pharmacokinetics

Prazosin is absorbed through the GI tract, but a large portion of prazosin is lost during hepatic first-pass metabolism. The half-life is short, so the drug should be administered twice a day. Prazosin is highly protein-bound, and when it is given with other highly protein-bound drugs, the client should be assessed for adverse reactions.

Pharmacodynamics

Selective alpha-adrenergic blockers dilate the arterioles and venules, decreasing peripheral resistance and lowering blood pressure. With prazosin, the heart rate is only slightly increased, whereas with non-selective alpha-blockers such as phentolamine and tolazoline, the blood pressure is greatly reduced, and reflex tachycardia can occur. Nonselective alpha-blockers are more effective for acute hypertension; selective alpha-blockers are more useful for long-term essential hypertension.

The onset of action of prazosin occurs between 30 minutes and 2 hours. The duration of action of prazosin is 10 hours. Table 43–3 presents the drug data for selective and nonselective alpha-blockers.

Table 43–3		
Antihypertensives: Sympatholytics: Alpha Adrenergic and Peripherally Acting Blockers and Direct Acting Vasodilators		
Generic (Brand)	**Route and Dosage**	**Uses and Considerations**
Selective Alpha-Adrenergic Blockers		
doxazosin mesylate (Cardura)	A: PO: Initially:1 mg/day; *maint:* 2-4 mg/day; *max:* 16 mg/d	For stage 1 or 2 hypertension. May be used alone or with another antihypertensive. May cause orthostatic hypotension, headache, dizziness, and GI upset. *Pregnancy category:* B; PB: 98%; t$^{1/2}$: 22 h
prazosin HCl (Minipress)	(Prototype Drug Chart 43–2)	
tamsulosin (Flomax)	A: PO: 0.4 mg/d	Blocks alpha$_1$ receptors. Not too effective for hypertension, and has been approved for BPH. Should not be combined with other antihypertensive drugs; not to be taken with sildenafil (Viagra), can increase the hypotensive state. Pregnancy category: B; PB: 94-98 %; t$^{1/2}$: 9-13 h
terazosin HCl (Hytrin)	A: PO: Initially: 1 mg at bedtime; *maint:* 1-5 mg/d; *max:* 20 mg/d	For stage 1 or 2 hypertension. May be used alone or with another antihypertensive drug. Dizziness and headache may occur. *Pregnancy category:* C; PB: 95%; t$^{1/2}$: 9-12 h

A, Adult; *b.i.d.*, twice a day; *C*, child; *d*, day; *GI*, gastrointestinal; *h*, hour; *IM*, intramuscular; *IV*, intravenous; *maint*, maintenance; *MAO*, monoamine oxidase; *max*, maximum; *min*, minute; *NB*, newborn; *PB*, protein-binding; *PO*, by mouth; *PRN*, as needed; *q.i.d.*, four times a day; *sec*, second; *t$^{1/2}$*, half-life; *t.i.d.*, three times a day; *UK*, unknown; *wk*, week.

Table 43–3

Antihypertensives: Sympatholytics: Alpha Adrenergic and Peripherally Acting Blockers and Direct Acting Vasodilators—cont'd

Generic (Brand)	Route and Dosage	Uses and Considerations
Nonselective Alpha-Adrenergic Blockers		
phenoxybenzamine HCl (Dibenzyline)	A: PO: Initially: 10 mg/d at bedtime; *maint:* 20-40 mg b.i.d./t.i.d. C: PO: 0.2 mg/kg/d in 1-2 divided doses; may increase dose by 0.2 mg	For hypertension related to adrenergic excess, pheochromocytoma. Lowers peripheral resistance. Has a long action. *Pregnancy category:* C; PB: UK; t$\frac{1}{2}$: 24 h
phentolamine (Regitine)	A: IM/IV: 2.5-5 mg; repeat q5min until controlled; then q2-3h PRN C: IM/IV: 0.05-0.1 mg/kg; repeat if needed	For hypertensive crisis caused by pheochromocytoma, MAO inhibitors, or clonidine withdrawal. Potent antihypertensive drug. In heart failure, decreases afterload and increases cardiac output. For hypertension, antagonizes effects of epinephrine and norepinephrine, causing vasodilation. *Pregnancy category:* C; PB: UK; t$\frac{1}{2}$: 20 min
tolazoline HCl (Priscoline HCl)	NB: IV: Initially: 1-2 mg/kg; followed by 1-2 mg/kg/h for 24-48 h; expected effect within 30 min of initial dose A: IM/IV: 10-50 mg q.i.d.	For pulmonary hypertension of newborn and for peripheral vasospastic disorders. *Pregnancy category:* C; PB: UK; t$\frac{1}{2}$: 3-10 h
Adrenergic Neuron Blockers (Peripherally Acting Sympatholytics)		
guanadrel sulfate (Hylorel)	A: PO: Initially: 5 mg b.i.d.; *maint:* 20-75 mg/d in divided doses	For moderate to severe hypertension. Intermediate-acting duration. Rapid onset. *Pregnancy category:* B; PB: 20%; t$\frac{1}{2}$: 10-12 h
guanethidine monosulfate (Ismelin)	A: PO: Initially: 10 mg/d; *maint:* 25-50 mg/d; *max:* 3 mg/kg/d C: PO: 0.2 mg/kg/d; *max:* 1-1.6 mg/kg/d	For severe hypertension. Long acting. Can be taken with a diuretic. Potent antihypertensive drug. May cause marked orthostatic hypotension, edema, weight gain, diarrhea, and bradycardia. *Pregnancy category:* C; PB: UK; t$\frac{1}{2}$: 5 d
reserpine (Serpasil, Serpalan)	A: PO: Initially: 0.25-0.5 mg/d for 1-2 wk; *maint:* 0.1-0.25 mg/d	One of the early antihypertensives. For hypertension. Not frequently used. May cause nightmares and vivid dreams. Pregnancy category: C; PB: 90%; t$\frac{1}{2}$: 4.5-11 h
Alpha$_1$- and Beta$_1$-Adrenergic Blockers		
carteolol HCl (Cartrol, Ocupress)	A: PO: Initially: 2.5 mg/d.; *maint:* 2.5-5 mg/d.; *max:* 10 mg/d	To treat hypertension. May be used alone or in combination with other antihypertensive agents. Not for hypertensive crisis or client with open-angle glaucoma. *Pregnancy category:* C; PB: 20%-30%; t$\frac{1}{2}$: 4-6 h
labetalol HCl (Trandate, Normodyne)	A: PO: Initially: 100 mg b.i.d.; *maint:* 200-800 mg/d in 2 divided doses; *max:* 1200-2400 mg/d A: IV: 20 mg over 2 min; continuous infusion: 2 mg/min; *max:* 300 mg as total dose	For stage 1 or 2 hypertension. May be used alone or with a thiazide diuretic. May cause orthostatic hypotension, palpitation, and syncope. *Pregnancy category:* C; PB: 50%; t$\frac{1}{2}$: 4-8 h
Direct-Acting Vasodilators		
diazoxide (Hyperstat, Proglycem)	A & C: IV: 1-3 mg/kg in bolus (30 sec); repeat in 5-15 min PRN; *max:* 150 mg	For hypertensive emergency. Dose may be repeated in 5-15 min until adequate decrease in blood pressure is achieved. Oral antihypertensive drugs may follow. *Pregnancy category:* C; PB: 90%; t$\frac{1}{2}$: 20-45 h
hydralazine HCl (Apresoline HCl)	A: PO: Initially: 10 mg q.i.d.; *maint:* 25-50 mg q.i.d. *Severe hypertension:* IM-IV: 10-40 mg, repeat PRN C: PO: 0.1-0.2 mg/kg/dose	For hypertension. Short-acting duration. Can be taken with diuretic to decrease edema and beta-blocker to prevent tachycardia. Dizziness, tremors, headaches, tachycardia, and palpitation may occur. Vital signs should be closely monitored. *Pregnancy category:* C; PB: 87%; t$\frac{1}{2}$: 2-6 h
minoxidil (Loniten, Rogaine)	A: PO: Initially: 5 mg/d; *maint:* 10-40 mg/d in single or divided doses; *max:* 100 mg/d C: PO: Initially: 0.2 mg/kg/d; *max:* 5 mg/day; *maint:* 0.25-1 mg/kg/d in divided doses; *max:* 50 mg/d *Topical for alopecia:* 2% sol b.i.d.	For hypertension. Can be taken with a diuretic to reduce edema and with a beta-blocker to prevent tachycardia. Long-acting effect. When discontinuing drug, it should be slowly decreased to avoid rebound hypertension; should not be abruptly withdrawn. Vital signs should be closely monitored. *Pregnancy category:* C; PB: 0%; t$\frac{1}{2}$: 3.5-4 h
sodium nitroprusside (Nipride, Nitropress)	A: IV: 1-3 mcg/kg/min in D$_5$W; *max:* 10 mcg/kg/min	For hypertensive crisis. Potent antihypertensive drug. Drug decomposes in light; container must be wrapped in aluminum foil. Good for 24 h. Drug should be discarded if red or blue. Can cause cyanide toxicity. Measure cyanide and thiocyanate levels. May cause profound hypotension. *Pregnancy category:* C; PB: UK; t$\frac{1}{2}$: 10 min

Prototype DRUG CHART 43-2

PRAZOSIN (HCL)

Drug Class	**Dosage**
Antihypertensive: Alpha-adrenergic blocker	**A: PO:** 1 mg b.i.d.-t.i.d.; *maint:* 3-15 mg/d; *max:*
Trade name: Minipress	20 mg/d in divided doses
Pregnancy Category: C	
Contraindications	**Drug-Lab-Food Interactions**
Renal disease	*Drug: Increased* hypotensive effect with other antihypertensives, nitrates, alcohol

Pharmacokinetics	**Pharmacodynamics**
Absorption: GI: 60% (5% to circulation)	**PO:** Onset: 0.5-2 h
Distribution: PB: 95%	Peak: 2-4 h
Metabolism: t½: 3 hours	Duration: 10 h
Excretion: In bile and feces; 10% in urine	

Therapeutic Effects/Uses

To control hypertension, refractory HF; to treat benign prostatic hypertrophy
Mode of Action: Dilation of peripheral blood vessels via blocking the alpha-adrenergic receptors

Side Effects	**Adverse Reactions**
Dizziness, drowsiness, headache, nausea, vomiting, diarrhea, impotence, vertigo, urinary frequency, tinnitus, dry mouth, incontinence, abdominal discomfort	Orthostatic hypotension, palpitations, tachycardia, pancreatitis

A, Adult; *b.i.d.,* twice a day; *d,* day; *h,* hour; *HF,* heart failure; *GI,* gastrointestinal; *maint,* maintenance; *max,* maximum; *PB,* protein-binding; *PO,* by mouth; *t½,* half-life; *t.i.d.,* three times a day.

Side Effects and Adverse Reactions

The side effects of prazosin, doxazosin, and terazosin include orthostatic hypotension (dizziness, faintness, light-headedness, increased heart rate, which may occur with first dose), nausea, drowsiness, nasal congestion caused by vasodilation, edema, and weight gain.

Side effects of phentolamine include hypotension, reflex tachycardia caused by the severe decrease in blood pressure, nasal congestion caused by vasodilation, and GI disturbances.

Drug Interactions

Drug interactions occur when alpha-adrenergic blockers are taken with antiinflammatory drugs and nitrates (e.g., nitroglycerin for angina). Peripheral edema is intensified when prazosin and an antiinflammatory drug are taken daily. Nitroglycerin taken for angina lowers blood pressure. If prazosin is taken with nitroglycerin, syncope (faintness) caused by a decrease in blood pressure can occur. The selective alpha-adrenergic blocker prazosin is shown in Prototype Drug Chart 43-2.

Nursing Process

Antihypertensives: Alpha-Adrenergic Blockers

ASSESSMENT

■ Obtain a medication history from client, including current drugs. Report if a drug-drug or drug-herbal interaction is probable. Prazosin is highly protein-bound and can displace other highly protein-bound drugs.
■ Obtain baseline vital signs and weight for future comparisons.
■ Check urinary output. Report if it is decreased (less than 600 ml/day), because drug is contraindicated if renal disease is present.

NURSING DIAGNOSES

■ Risk for activity intolerance related to drug regime and/or cardiac status

■ Deficient knowledge related to drug regimen related to drug regime
■ Ineffective sexuality pattern related to beta blocker or other drug therapy

PLANNING

■ Client's blood pressure will decrease.
■ Client will follow proper drug regimen.

NURSING INTERVENTIONS

■ Monitor vital signs. The desired therapeutic effect of prazosin may not fully occur for 4 weeks. A sudden marked decrease in blood pressure should be reported.
■ Check daily for fluid retention in the extremities. Prazosin may cause sodium and water retention.

Client Teaching

General

• Instruct client to comply with drug regimen. Abrupt discontinuation of the antihypertensive drug may cause rebound hypertension.
• Inform client that orthostatic hypotension may occur. Explain that before rising, client should sit and dangle the feet.

Self-Administration

• Instruct client or family member how to take a blood pressure reading. A record for daily blood pressures should be kept.

Side Effects

• Caution client that dizziness, light-headedness, and drowsiness may occur, especially when the drug is first prescribed. If these symptoms occur, the health care provider should be notified.
• Inform male client that impotence may occur if high doses of the drug are prescribed. This problem should be reported to the health care provider.
• Instruct client to report if edema is present in the morning. Water retention is a problem with alpha-blockers.
• Inform client not to take cold, cough, or allergy OTC medications without first contacting the health care provider.

Diet

• Encourage client to decrease salt intake unless otherwise indicated by the health care provider.

Cultural Considerations ❖

• African-American clients with hypertension can take alpha-adrenergic blockers and calcium channel blockers but should avoid taking beta-blockers, because these agents are not generally effective in controlling their hypertension. However, taking a diuretic together with a beta-blocker increases the effectiveness for these clients.
• Asians are twice as sensitive to the effects of propranolol on the blood pressure and heart rate, so the dose should be decreased or another antihypertensive drug may be given.
• Obtain an interpreter when necessary.

EVALUATION

■ Evaluate the effectiveness of the drug in controlling blood pressure; side effects should be absent.
■ Evaluate client's adherence to medication schedule.

Adrenergic Neuron Blockers (Peripherally Acting Sympatholytics)

Adrenergic neuron blockers are potent antihypertensive drugs that block norepinephrine release from the sympathetic nerve endings, causing a decrease in norepinephrine release that results in a lowering of blood pressure. There is a decrease in both cardiac output and peripheral vascular resistance. Reserpine, guanethidine, and guanadrel (the three most potent drugs) are used to control severe hypertension. Orthostatic hypotension is a common side effect, so the client should be advised to rise slowly from a reclining or sitting position. The adrenergic neuron blockers are considered the last choices for treatment of chronic hypertension, because these drugs can cause orthostatic (postural) hypotension. Use of reserpine may cause vivid dreams, nightmares, and suicidal intention. The drugs in this group can cause sodium and water retention. These drugs can be taken alone or with a diuretic to decrease peripheral edema.

Alpha$_1$- and Beta$_1$-Adrenergic Blockers

This group of drugs blocks both the alpha$_1$ and beta$_1$ receptors. Labetalol (Normodyne) and carteolol (Cartrol) are examples of alpha-/beta-blockers. Blocking the alpha$_1$-receptor causes vasodilation, decreasing resistance to blood flow. The effect on the alpha-receptor is stronger than the effect on the beta-receptor; therefore blood pressure is lowered and pulse rate is moderately decreased. By blocking the cardiac beta$_1$-receptor, both heart rate and atrioventricular (AV) contractility are decreased. Large doses of alpha-/beta-blockers could block beta$_2$-adrenergic receptors, thus increasing airway resistance. Clients who have severe asthma should not take large doses of labetalol or carteolol. Table 43–3 lists these two alpha-/beta-blockers.

Common side effects of these drugs include orthostatic (postural) hypotension, GI disturbances, nervousness, dry mouth, and fatigue. Large doses of labetalol or carteolol may cause AV heart block.

Direct-Acting Arteriolar Vasodilators

Vasodilators are potent antihypertensive drugs. Direct-acting vasodilators act by relaxing the smooth muscles of the blood vessels, mainly the arteries, causing vasodilation. Vasodilators promote an increase in blood flow to the brain and kidneys. With vasodilation, the blood pressure decreases and sodium and water are retained, resulting in peripheral edema. Diuretics can be given with a direct-acting vasodilator to decrease the edema.

Two of the direct-acting vasodilators, hydralazine and minoxidil, are used for moderate to severe (dose related) hypertension. These two drugs cause little orthostatic (postural) hypotension, because of the minimum dilation of the arterioles. However, reflex tachycardia and release of renin can occur secondary to vasodilation and decreased blood pressure. Beta-blockers are frequently prescribed with arteriolar vasodilators to decrease the heart rate; this counteracts the effect of reflex tachycardia.

Nitroprusside and diazoxide are prescribed for acute hypertensive emergency. The latter two drugs are very potent vasodilators that rapidly decrease blood pressure. Nitroprusside acts on both arterial and venous vessels, diazoxide acts on arterial vessels only. Table 43–3 lists direct-acting vasodilators.

Side Effects and Adverse Reactions

The effects of hydralazine are numerous and include tachycardia, palpitations, edema, nasal congestion, headache, dizziness, GI bleeding, lupuslike symptoms, and neurologic symptoms (tingling, numbness). Minoxidil has similar side effects, as well as tachycardia, edema, and excess hair growth. It can precipitate an anginal attack.

Nitroprusside and diazoxide can cause reflex tachycardia, palpitations, restlessness, agitation, nausea, and confusion. Hyperglycemia can occur with diazoxide, because the drug inhibits insulin release from the beta cells of the pancreas. Nitroprusside and diazoxide are discussed in greater detail in Chapter 58.

Angiotensin-Converting Enzyme [ACE] Inhibitors

Drugs in this group inhibit ACE, which in turn inhibits the formation of angiotensin II (vasoconstrictor) and blocks the release of aldosterone. Aldosterone promotes sodium retention and potassium excretion. When aldosterone is blocked, sodium is excreted along with water, and potassium is retained. ACE inhibitors cause little change in cardiac output or heart rate, and they lower peripheral resistance. Figure 43–1 illustrates the renin-angiotensin-aldosterone system (RAAS). These drugs can be used in clients who have elevated serum renin levels.

The ACE inhibitors are used primarily to treat hypertension; some of these agents are also effective in treating heart failure. The first ACE inhibitor, captopril (Capoten), became available in the early 1970s. By the mid-1990s there were five ACE inhibitors, and in the late 1990s there were 10. These 10 ACE inhibitors include benazepril (Lo-tensin), captopril (Capoten), enalapril maleate (Vasotec), fosinopril (Monopril), lisinopril (Prinivil, Zestril), moexipril (Univasc), perindopril (Aceon), quinapril (Accupril), ramipril (Altace), and trandolapril (Mavik), which are all presented in Table 43–4. These drugs can be used for first-line antihypertensive therapy, but thiazide diuretics are recommended by the JNC 7.

African Americans and older adults do not respond to ACE inhibitors with the desired reduction in blood pressure, but when taken with a diuretic, blood pressure usually will be lowered. ACE inhibitors should not be given during pregnancy, because they reduce placental blood flow.

For clients with renal insufficiency, reduction of the drug dose (except for fosinopril [Monopril]), is necessary.

With the exception of moexipril (Univasc), which should be taken on an empty stomach for maximum effectiveness, ACE inhibitors can be administered with food.

Side Effects and Adverse Reactions

The primary side effect of ACE inhibitors is a constant, irritated cough. Other side effects include nausea, vomiting, diarrhea, headache, dizziness, fatigue, insomnia, serum potassium excess (hyperkalemia), and tachycardia. The major adverse effects are first-dose hypotension and hyperkalemia. Hypotension results because of the vasodilating effect. First-dose hypotension is more common in clients also taking diuretics.

Contraindications

ACE inhibitors should not be given during pregnancy; harm to the fetus due to reduction in placental blood flow could occur. This group of drugs should not be taken with potassium-sparing diuretics such as spironolactone (Aldactone) or salt substitutes that contain potassium, because of the risk of hyperkalemia (serum potassium excess).

Nursing Process

Antihypertensives: Angiotensin Antagonist (ACE) Inhibitors

ASSESSMENT

■ Obtain a drug and herbal history from client of current drugs that are taken. Report if a drug-drug or drug-herbal interaction is probable.

■ Obtain baseline vital signs for future comparisons.

■ Check laboratory values for serum protein, albumin, blood urea nitrogen (BUN), creatinine, and white blood cell (WBC) count, and compare with future serum levels.

Table 43–4

Antihypertensives: ACE Inhibitors and Angiotensin II Receptor Blockers

Generic (Brand)	Route and Dosage	Uses and Considerations
Angiotensin Antagonists (ACE Inhibitors)		
benazepril HCl (Lotensin)	A: PO: Initially: 10 mg/d; *maint:* 20-40 mg/d in 2 divided doses	Management of stage 1 and 2 hypertension. Headache, dizziness, hypotension, nausea, diarrhea, or constipation may occur. *Pregnancy category:* C and D; PB: 97%; t$^{1}/_{2}$: 10 h
captopril (Capoten)	A: PO: Initially: 12.5-25 mg, b.i.d.-t.i.d.; *maint:* 25-100 mg, b.i.d.-t.i.d.; *max:* 450 mg/d	To reduce blood pressure and to control HF. Inhibits angiotensin I conversion to angiotensin II. Irritating cough is a side effect; retains potassium. *Pregnancy category:* C and D (second and third trimester); PB: 25%-30%; t$^{1}/_{2}$: 2-3 h with normal renal function
enalapril maleate (Vasotec)	A: PO: Initially: 5 mg/d; *maint:* 10-40 mg/d in 1-2 divided doses IV: 1.25 mg q6h infuse in 5 min *Hypertensive emergencies:* IV: 5 mg q6h as needed	For hypertension and HF. Similar to captopril and benazepril. Has a long duration of action (orally). *Pregnancy category:* C and D (second and third trimester); PB: 50%-60%; t$^{1}/_{2}$: 1.5-2 h
fosinopril (Monopril)	A: PO: 5-40 mg/d; *max:* 80 mg/d	To treat hypertension and heart failure. Reduces peripheral resistance (afterload) and improves cardiac output. Dose does not have to be reduced because of renal insufficiency. *Pregnancy category:* C and D (second and third trimester); PB: 97%; t$^{1}/_{2}$: 3-4 h; 12 h active metabolite
lisinopril (Prinivil, Zestril)	A: PO: Initially: 10 mg/d; *maint:* 20-40 mg/d; *max:* 80 mg/d	For hypertension and HF. Usually given in combination with a diuretic. Has a long duration of action (24 hours). Monitor vital signs. *Pregnancy category:* D; PB: 0%; t$^{1}/_{2}$: 12 h
moexipril (Univasc)	A: PO: 7.5 mg/d; *max:* 30 mg/d in divided doses	For treatment of hypertension. Reduce dose with renal insufficiency; creatinine clearance <40 ml/min. May increase serum lithium levels and cause toxicity. *Pregnancy category:* C and D (second and third trimester); PB: 50%; t$^{1}/_{2}$: 2-9 h
perindopril (Aceon)	A: PO: 2-8 mg/d	To treat mild to moderate hypertension. Reduces vasoconstriction. Common side effect of ACE inhibitors is cough. *Pregnancy category:* C and D (second and third trimester); PB: 10%-60%; t$^{1}/_{2}$: 1.5-3 h (parent drug); 25-30 h
quinapril HCl (Accupril)	A: PO: 10-20 mg/d; *max:* 80 mg/d in divided doses Elderly: A: PO: 2.5-5 mg/d	To treat hypertension and heart failure. A potent, long-acting, second-generation ACE inhibitor. Reduces systemic vascular resistance and increases cardiac output. *Pregnancy category:* D; PB: 97%; t$^{1}/_{2}$: 2 h
ramipril (Altace)	A: PO: 2.5-5 mg/d; *max:* 20 mg/d	Treatment of stage 1 and 2 hypertension and HF. Similar to captopril. Has a long duration of action (24 hours). *Pregnancy category:* D; PB: 97%; t$^{1}/_{2}$: 2-3 h
trandolapril (Mavik)	A: PO: 1 mg/d; may increase weekly to 2-4 mg/d; *max:* 8 mg/d	To treat hypertension. May be used alone or combined with other antihypertensives. Diuretics should be discontinued 2 to 3 days before taking trandolapril. Reduce dose if client has renal (creatinine clearance <30 ml/min) or hepatic insufficiency. African Americans respond to trandolapril, including those with low-renin hypertension. *Pregnancy category:* C and D; PB: 80%; t$^{1}/_{2}$: 6 h
Combinations of ACE Inhibitors with Calcium Blockers		
benazepril with amlodipine (Lotrel)	A: PO: amlodipine/benazepril 2.5/10 mg; 5/10mg; 5/20 mg/d	For hypertension
enalapril with diltiazem (Teczem)	A: PO: enalapril/diltiazem ER: 5/180 mg/d	For hypertension
enalapril with felodipine (Lexxel)	A: PO: felodipine/enalapril 5/5 mg; 2.5/5 mg/d	For hypertension
trandolapril with verapamil (Tarka)	A: PO: trandolapril/verapamil SR: 2/180 mg; 1/240 mg; 2/240 mg; 4/240 mg	For hypertension

A, Adult; *ACE*, angiotensin-converting enzyme; *b.i.d.*, two times a day; *d*, day; *h*, hour; *HF*, heart failure; *IV*, intravenous; *maint*, maintenance; *max*, maximum; *min*, minute; *PB*, protein-binding; *PO*, by mouth; *t$^{1}/_{2}$*, half-life; *t.i.d.*, three times a day; *UK*, unknown; >, greater than; <, less than.

Continued

Table 43–4

Antihypertensives: ACE Inhibitors and Angiotensin II Receptor Blockers—cont'd

Generic (Brand)	Route and Dosage	Uses and Considerations
Angiotensin II Receptor Blockers (ARBs)		
candesartan (Atacand)	A: PO: 16 mg/d; *maint:* 8-32 mg/d	For treating hypertension. May be used when client does not respond or cannot tolerate ACE inhibitors. May be combined with the calcium blocker amlodipine for a more effective response in decreasing high blood pressure. Can be used for HF. *Pregnancy category:* C and D (second and third trimester); PB: >99%; $t^{1/2}$: 9 h
eprosartan (Teveten)	A: PO: Initially: 200 mg/d; 400-800 mg/d or in 2 divided doses	To treat mild to moderate hypertension. Does not cause irritating cough that ACE inhibitors do. Food can cause a slight delay in drug absorption. *Pregnancy category:* C and D (second and third trimester); PB: 98%; $t^{1/2}$: 5-9 h
irbesartan (Avapro)	A: PO: 150 mg/d; *maint:* 150-300 mg/d	For treating hypertension. May be used alone or in combination with other antihypertensive drugs. *Pregnancy category:* C and D (second and third trimester); PB: 90%; $t^{1/2}$: 11-15 h
losartan potassium (Cozaar)	A: PO: 25-50 mg/d, in single dose or in 2 divided doses; *max:* 100 mg/d	For treating hypertension. May be used alone or in combination with other antihypertensive drugs. *Pregnancy category:* C and D (second and third trimester); PB: 95%; $t^{1/2}$: 1.5-2 h
olmesartan medoxomil (Benicar)	A: PO: 20 mg/d; may increase 40 mg/d Elderly: Same as adult	Inhibits binding angiotensin II to AT_1 receptors. Promotes vasodilation and decreases peripheral resistance. Not to be given if client is volume-depleted. *Pregnancy category:* C and D (second and third trimester); PB: UK; $t^{1/2}$: 13 h
telmisartan (Micardis)	A: PO: 40-80 mg/d	To treat mild to moderate hypertension. Does not cause cough associated with ACE inhibitors. Angioedema has been reported, but rare. *Pregnancy category:* C and D (second and third trimester); PB: 99.5%; $t^{1/2}$: 24 h
Valsartan (Diovan)	A: PO: 80 mg/d; *max:* 320 mg/d	For treating hypertension. Similar action to candesartan, irbesartan, and losartan. Can also be used for HF. *Pregnancy category:* C and D (second and third trimester); PB: 99%; $t^{1/2}$: 6 h
Others **Aldosterone Receptor Antagonist**		
eplerenone (Inspra)	A: PO: 50 mg/d; may increase to 50 mg b.i.d.	Binds aldosterone at the mineralocorticoid receptor. Contraindications: serum potassium >5.5 mEq/L, creatinine clearance <50 ml/min, type 2 diabetes, and taking potassium-sparing diuretics. Drug is used to treat hypertension and HF postmyocardial infarction. *Pregnancy category:* B; PB: UK; $t^{1/2}$: UK
Direct Renin Inhibitor		
aliskiren (Tekturna)	A: PO: 150-300 mg/d	First direct renin inhibitor for treatment of mild to moderate hypertension. Used either as monotherapy or in combination with an antihypertensive drug such as ARB valsartan (Diovan). Hyperkalemia uncommon for monotherapy. *Pregnancy category:* D or X; PB: UK; $t^{1/2}$: 24 h

NURSING DIAGNOSES

- Deficient knowledge related to drug regimen
- Anxiety related to hypertensive state

PLANNING

- Client's blood pressure will be within desired range.
- Client is free of moderate to severe side effects.

NURSING INTERVENTIONS

- Monitor laboratory tests related to renal function (BUN, creatinine, protein) and blood glucose levels. Caution: Watch for hypoglycemic reaction in clients with diabetes mellitus. Urine protein may be checked in the morning using a dipstick.
- Report to the health care provider occurrences of bruising, petechiae, and/or bleeding. These may indi-

cate a severe adverse reaction to an angiotensin antagonist such as captopril.

Client Teaching
General
- Instruct client not to abruptly discontinue use of captopril without notifying the health care provider. Rebound hypertension could result.
- Inform client not to take OTC drugs (e.g., cold or allergy medications) without first contacting the health care provider (see Herbal Alert 43–1).
- Instruct client who is pregnant or contemplating becoming pregnant not to take any ACE inhibitors or ARBs; they can cause harm to the fetus.

Self-Administration
- Teach client how to take and record blood pressure. A blood pressure chart should be established, and blood pressure changes should be reported.

Side Effects
- Explain to client that dizziness and/or light-headedness may occur during the first week of captopril therapy. If dizziness persists, health care provider should be notified.
- Instruct client to report any occurrence of bleeding.

Diet
- Instruct client to take captopril 20 minutes to 1 hour before a meal. Food decreases 35% of captopril absorption.
- Inform client that the taste of food may be diminished during the first month of drug therapy.

Cultural Considerations ❖
- African Americans do not respond well to angiotensin-converting enzyme (ACE) inhibitors unless the drug is taken with a diuretic.

EVALUATION

■ Evaluate the effectiveness of the drug therapy (i.e., absence of severe side effects, blood pressure return to desired range).

Angiotensin II Receptor Blockers (ARBs)

Angiotensin II receptor blockers or ARBs are another group of antihypertensive drugs. These agents are similar to ACE inhibitors, in that they prevent the release of aldosterone (sodium-retaining hormone). They act on the renin-angiotensin-aldosterone system (RAAS). The difference between ARBs and ACE inhibitors is that ARBs block angiotensin II from the AT_1 receptors found in many tissues, whereas ACE inhibitors inhibit the angiotensin-converting enzyme in the formation of angiotensin II. The ARBs cause vasodilation and decrease peripheral resistance. They do not cause the constant, irritated cough ACE inhibitors can.

Like ACE inhibitors, ARBs should not be taken during pregnancy.

Losartan (Cozaar), valsartan (Diovan), irbesartan (Avapro), candesartan cilexetil (Atacand), eprosartan (Teveten), olmesartan medoxomil (Benicar), and telmisartan (Micardis) are examples of ARBs. These agents block the vasoconstrictor effects of angiotensin II at the receptor site. The Food and Drug Administration (FDA) approves them for the treatment of hypertension. The combination of losartan potassium and hydrochlorothiazide tablets and valsartan and hydrochlorothiazide tablets and others should not cause serum potassium excess or loss. ARBs may be used as a first-line treatment for hypertension.

Prototype Drug Chart 43–3 gives the pharmacologic data related to losartan potassium (Cozaar).

Pharmacokinetics

Losartan potassium (Cozaar) is prescribed primarily to manage hypertension. The combination drug Hyzaar contains losartan potassium plus a low dose of hydrochlorothiazide. It is rapidly absorbed in the GI tract and undergoes first-pass metabolism in the liver to form active metabolites. It is highly protein-bound and should not be given during pregnancy, especially the second and third trimester. The half-life is 1.2 to 2 hours, and the half-life of the metabolite is 6 to 9 hours. The drug is excreted in urine and feces.

Pharmacodynamics

Losartan potassium is a potent vasodilator. It blocks the binding of angiotensin II to the AT_1 receptors found in many tissues. Its peak time is 6 hours, and it has a long duration of action: 24 hours.

Like ACE inhibitors, the ARBs are less effective for treating hypertension in African Americans. In addition ARBs, like ACE inhibitors, may cause angioedema. These agents can be taken with or without food and are suitable for clients with mild hepatic insufficiency.

Direct Renin Inhibitor

The first FDA-approved direct renin inhibitor for treating hypertension is aliskiren (Tekturna). Aliskiren binds with renin, causing a reduction of angiotensin I, angiotensin II, and aldosterone levels (see Figure 43–1). It is effective for mild and moderate hypertension. Aliskiren can be used alone or with another antihypertensive agent. It has an additive effect in reducing blood pressure when combined with a thiazide diuretic or an ARB.

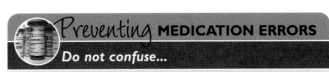
Preventing MEDICATION ERRORS
Do not confuse...

- **Diovan** and **Dioval**; they sound alike and look alike. Diovan (valsartan) is an angiotensin II receptor blocker, or ARB, an antihypertensive drug. Dioval is an estradiol, an estrogen hormone. If both drugs are in the home, caution must be taken to select the *correct* drug, especially by the male taking Diovan and the female taking Dioval.

Prototype DRUG CHART 43–3

LOSARTAN POTASSIUM

Drug Class

Antihypertensive: angiotensin II receptor blocker
Trade names: Cozaar; also Hyzaar (hydrochlorothiazide
  with losartan potassium)
Pregnancy Category: C (first trimester); D (second
  and third trimesters)

Contraindications

Pregnancy, breastfeeding
Caution: Renal and hepatic impairments

Dosage

Hypertension:
A: **PO:** 25-50 mg/d in single or 2 divided doses;
  max: 100 mg/d
C: Safety not established

Drug-Lab-Food Interactions

Drug: Phenobarbital *decreases* effects of losartan and
  its metabolites.
Lab: May *increase* AST, ALT, ALP, bilirubin, BUN,
  creatinine, Hct, Hgb

Pharmacokinetics

Absorption: Rapidly absorbed, 25-30 in
  blood circulation
Distribution: PB: 90%-95%
Metabolism: t½: 1.2-2 h; metabolite: 6-9 h
Excretion: 35% in urine and 60% in bile/feces

Pharmacodynamics

PO: Onset: less than 1 h
  Peak: 6 h
  Duration: 24 h

Therapeutic Effects/Uses

To treat hypertension
Mode of Action: Potent vasodilator; inhibits the binding of angiotensin II

Side Effects

Dizziness, diarrhea, insomnia, and occasional cough

Adverse Reactions

Upper respiratory infection

A, Adult; *ALP*, alkaline phosphatase; *ALT*, alanine aminotransferase; *AST*, aspartate aminotransferase; *BUN*, blood urea nitrogen;
C, child; *d*, day; *h*, hour; *Hct*, hematocrit; *Hgb*, hemoglobin; *max*, maximum; *PO*, by mouth; *PB*, protein-binding; *t½*, half-life.

This drug, when used as monotherapy, has not proven to be as effective in reducing blood pressure in the African American population.

Calcium Channel Blockers

Slow calcium channels are found in the myocardium (heart muscle) and vascular smooth muscle (VSM) cells. Free calcium increases muscle contractility, peripheral resistance, and blood pressure. Calcium channel blockers, also called *calcium antagonists* and *calcium blockers,* block the calcium channel in the VSM, promoting vasodilation. The large central arteries are not as sensitive to calcium blockers as coronary and cerebral arteries and the peripheral vessels. Calcium blockers are highly protein-bound but have a short half-life. Slow-release preparations decrease frequency of administration. Table 43–5 lists the calcium blockers in 3 groups: diphenylalkylamine (verapamil), benzothiazepines (diltiazem), and dihydropyridine (amlodipine and others). Calcium blockers are also discussed in Chapter 41.

Verapamil (Calan) is used to treat chronic hypertension, angina pectoris, and cardiac dysrhythmias. Verapamil and diltiazem act on the arterioles and the heart. The dihydropyridines are the largest group of calcium channel blockers

and consist of seven drugs; six of these are used to control hypertension. The calcium blocker nimodipine is used to prevent ischemic brain injury due to vasospasm that often accompanies subarachnoid hemorrhage.

Nifedipine (Procardia) was the first drug in this group. Nifedipine decreases blood pressure in older adults and in those with low serum renin values. Nifedipine and verapamil are potent calcium blockers. Nifedipine, in its immediate-release form (10- and 20-mg capsules), has been associated with an increased incidence of sudden cardiac death, especially when prescribed for outpatients at high doses. This is not true of the sustained-release preparations (i.e., Procardia XL, Adalat CC). For this reason, immediate-release nifedipine is usually prescribed for acute rises in blood pressure only on an "as needed" basis in the hospital setting. Like the vasodilators, calcium-channel blockers can cause reflex tachycardia; it is more prevalent with nifedipine.

Prototype Drug Chart 43–4 gives the pharmacologic data related to amlodipine (Norvasc).

Pharmacokinetics

Amlodipine (Norvasc), like other calcium blockers, is highly protein-bound. It is gradually absorbed via the GI tract. Because the half-life of

Table 43–5

Antihypertensives: Calcium Channel Blockers

Generic (Brand)	Route and Dosage	Uses and Considerations
Phenylalkylamines		
verapamil (Calan SR, Isoptin SR)	A: PO: 40-80 mg t.i.d. A: PO SR: 120-240 mg/day in 2 divided doses; *max*: 480 mg/d	For hypertension (sustained-release form). One of first calcium blockers. Also used for variant angina and cardiac dysrhythmias. Common side effects: dizziness, headache, hypotension, bradycardia, and constipation. *Pregnancy category:* C; PB: 90%; t$^{1/2}$: 3-8 h
Benzothiazepines		
diltiazem HCl (Cardizem, Cardizem CD or SR)	A: PO SR: Initially: 60-120 mg b.i.d.; *max*: 240-360 mg/d	For hypertension (sustained-release form). Also for angina pectoris; IV form for cardiac dysrhythmias (atrial fibrillation). Headache, bradycardia, and hypotension may occur. *Pregnancy category:* C; PB: 70%-80%; t$^{1/2}$: 3.5-9 h
Dihydropyridines		
amlodipine (Norvasc)	A: PO: 5-10 mg/d. Elderly: 2.5-5.0 mg/d	To treat mild and moderate hypertension and angina pectoris. Decreases peripheral vascular resistance (vasodilation). May be used alone or with other antihypertensives. *Pregnancy category:* C; PB: >95%; t$^{1/2}$: 30-50 hours (older adults with hepatic insufficiency: 50-100 hours)
felodipine (Plendil)	A: PO: Initially: 5 mg; *maint*: 5-10 mg/d; *max*: 20 mg/d	Treatment for stage 1 and 2 hypertension, HF, and angina. Potent calcium blocker. Flush, peripheral edema, palpitations, dizziness, and headache may occur. Long duration of action. *Pregnancy category:* C; PB: 99%; t$^{1/2}$: 10-16 h
isradipine (DynaCirc)	*Hypertension*: A: PO: 1.25-10 mg b.i.d.; *max*: 20 mg/d	Management of hypertension, HF, and angina pectoris. For hypertension, drug may be used alone or with a diuretic. *Pregnancy category:* C; PB: 99%; t$^{1/2}$: 5-11 h
nicardipine HCl (Cardene, Cardene SR)	A: PO: 20-40 mg t.i.d. SR: 30-60 mg b.i.d. A: IV: initially: 5 mg/h increase dose PRN; *max*: 15 mg/h C: IV: 1-3 mcg/kg/min	To treat essential hypertension and vasospastic angina. IV therapy for short-term therapy for hypertension. Decreases systemic resistance; heart rate and cardiac output are increased. *Pregnancy category:* C; PB: 95%; t$^{1/2}$: 2-4 h
nifedipine (Procardia)	A: PO: 10-20 mg t.i.d. A: PO SR: 30-90 mg/d; *max*: 180 mg/d	For hypertension and angina pectoris. Potent calcium channel blocker. Common side effects include dizziness, light-headedness, headache, flushing, peripheral edema, and nausea. Drug may be taken alone or with a diuretic. *Pregnancy category:* C; PB: 92%-98%; t$^{1/2}$: 2-5 h
nisoldipine (Sular, Nisocor)	A: PO: 10-20 mg/d in 2 divided doses; *max*: 40 mg/d	To treat hypertension and angina. Can be used alone or combined with another antihypertensive drug. Similar to nifedipine, causing vasodilation, but 10 times more potent than nifedipine. Considered a potent coronary vasodilator. *Pregnancy category:* C; PB: 99%; t$^{1/2}$: 2-14 h

A, Adult; *b.i.d.*, twice a day; *C*, child; *HF*, heart failure; *d*, day; *h*, hour; *IV*, intravenous; *maint*, maintenance; *max*, maximum; *min*, minute; *PB*, protein-binding; *PO*, by mouth; *PRN*, as needed; *SR*, sustained release; *t$^{1/2}$*, half-life; *t.i.d.*, three times a day; *>*, greater than.

amlodipine is longer than other calcium blockers, it is taken once a day.

Pharmacodynamics

Amlodipine may be used alone or with other antihypertensive drugs. Peripheral edema may occur because of its vasodilator effect, so persons with edema may need to take another type of antihypertensive drug. This drug has a long duration of action, so it is prescribed only once a day. Amlodipine may be combined with the ACE inhibitor benazepril, forming Lotrel.

Normally beta-blockers are not prescribed with calcium blockers, because both drugs decrease myocardium contractility. Calcium blockers lower blood pressure better in African Americans than drugs in other categories.

Side Effects and Adverse Reactions

The side effects and adverse reactions of calcium channel blockers include flush, headache, dizziness, ankle edema, bradycardia, and AV block.

Prototype **DRUG CHART 43–4**

AMLODIPINE

Drug Class	**Dosage**
Calcium channel blocker	**A: PO:** 5-10 mg/d
Trade names: Norvasc; Lotrel is a combination of amlodipine with benazepril	**Elderly: PO:** 2.5-5 mg/d
Pregnancy Category: C	
Contraindications	**Drug-Lab-Food Interactions**
Severe hypotension	*Drug:* Increase bradycardia with adenosine.
Caution: Liver disease, HF, aortic stenosis, pregnancy, lactation	*Lab:* May increase amlodipine with grapefruit juice

Pharmacokinetics	**Pharmacodynamics**
Absorption: Gradual; greater than 90% absorbed from GI tract	**PO:** Onset: Gradual
	Peak: 6-9 h
Distribution: PB: greater than 95%	Duration: 24 h
Metabolism: t½: 30-50 hours; elderly, t½: 50-100 h	
Excretion: Urine and feces as inactive metabolites	

Therapeutic Effects/Uses

To treat mild and moderate hypertension and angina pectoris.
Mode of Action: Decreases peripheral vascular resistance (vasodilation), promoting a decrease in blood pressure

Side Effects	**Adverse Reactions**
Peripheral edema, headache, flushing, dizziness, nausea	Reflex tachycardia, marked hypotension

A, Adult; *d,* day; *GI,* gastrointestinal; *h,* hour; *HF,* heart failure; *PB,* protein-binding; *PO,* by mouth; *t½,* half-life.

KEY WEBSITES

Antihypertensive agents: www.nhlbi.nih.gov/hbp/treat/bpd_type.htm
Management of hypertension: www.aafo.org/afp.2003090/853.html
Captopril: www.nlm.nih.gov/medineplus/druginfo/
medmaster/a682823.html

Critical Thinking Case Study

GG, a 72-year-old African American, has heart failure (HF) and diabetes. Her vital signs are: blood pressure 176/94; pulse 92; respirations 30. Her medications include hydrochlorothiazide 50 mg/d, atenolol 50 mg/d, and digoxin 0.25 mg/d.

1. Why was hydrochlorothiazide prescribed for GG? Explain the effects of hydrochlorothiazide on blood pressure. (See Chapter 42.)
2. Abnormal electrolytes and other laboratory test results may occur when taking hydrochlorothiazide. Would the following serum electrolyte and laboratory values be expected to *increase* or *decrease*?
   a. Sodium
   b. Potassium
   c. Calcium
   d. Magnesium
   e. Glucose
   f. Uric acid
3. Why should GG's blood glucose level be monitored while she is taking hydrochlorothiazide?
4. What effect may result when GG takes digoxin and hydrochlorothiazide together? Explain.
5. Atenolol is what type of antihypertensive? Would atenolol be effective in lowering GG's blood pressure if given as the only antihypertensive drug? Explain.
6. How effective is the combination of hydrochlorothiazide and atenolol for controlling GG's blood pressure? Explain.
7. When using a combination drug therapy to correct hypertension, would the dosage for each drug be the same? Explain.

8. When abruptly discontinuing beta-blockers for hypertension without the client taking another antihypertensive, what might occur? Explain how adverse effects can be avoided.

GG's blood glucose is 229. Her drugs for controlling hypertension are changed to prazosin 10 mg t.i.d. Her cholesterol and LDL are elevated. Her serum potassium level was 3.2 mEq/L.

9. Why were GG's hydrochlorothiazide and atenolol discontinued? Explain.
10. What type of antihypertensive is prazosin? Explain the physiologic action of prazosin for lowering the blood pressure.
11. Does prazosin have an effect on the blood glucose level? What effect could prazosin have on GG's abnormal lipid levels? Explain.

GG's ankles have become edematous. Hydrochlorothiazide was prescribed.

12. Why was hydrochlorothiazide again added to the drug regimen?
13. Is the daily prazosin dose within the safe therapeutic prescribed range for GG? Explain. (You may refer to Prototype Drug Chart 43–2.)
14. List the groups of antihypertensive drugs that can cause sodium and water retention.

NCLEX Study Questions

1. GG's blood pressure is 145/90. According to the guidelines for determining hypertension, the stage of her BP is:
   a. normal
   b. prehypertension
   c. stage 1 hypertension
   d. stage 2 hypertension

2. The first-line drug for treating GG's blood pressure might be:
   a. diuretics
   b. alpha blockers
   c. ACE inhibitors
   d. alpha/beta blockers

3. Six months later, GG's blood pressure was 168/86. Her hypertension would be classified as:
   a. stage 1
   b. stage 1 ISH
   c. stage 2
   d. stage 2 ISH

4. The group(s) of antihypertensive drugs that are less effective in African-American clients is/are:
   a. diuretics
   b. calcium-channel blockers and vasodilators
   c. beta blockers and ACE inhibitors
   d. alpha blockers

5. The most frequent diuretic that is combined with an antihypertensive drug is:
   a. chlorthalidone
   b. hydrochlorothiazide
   c. bendroflumethiazide
   d. potassium-sparing diuretic

6. The preferred beta blocker category for treating hypertension is:
   a. beta$_1$ blocker
   b. beta$_2$ blocker
   c. beta$_1$ and beta$_2$ blockers
   d. beta$_2$ and beta$_3$ blockers

7. A common side effect of ACE inhibitors is:
   a. nausea and vomiting
   b. dizziness and headaches
   c. upset stomach
   d. constant, irritated cough

8. Angiotensin II receptor blockers (ARBs) act by:
   a. inhibiting angiotensin-converting enzyme
   b. blocking angiotensin II from AT$_1$ receptors
   c. preventing the release of angiotensin I
   d. promoting the release of aldosterone

Answers: 1. c; 2. a; 3. d; 4. c; 5. b; 6. a; 7. d; 8. b.

44

Anticoagulants, Antiplatelets, and Thrombolytics

ELECTRONIC RESOURCES

evolve

Evolve website (http://evolve.elsevier.com/KeeHayes/pharmacology/):
- *Case Studies*
- *Content Updates*
- *Frequently Asked Questions*
- *Student Review Activities*
- *WebLinks*
- *Additional Reference Material*

Companion CD-ROM:
- *NCLEX Examination Review Questions*
- *Pharmacology Animations*
- *IV Therapy Checklists*
- *Medication Error Checklists*
- *Drug Calculation Problems*
- *Electronic Calculators*
- *Top 200 Drugs with Pronunciations*
- *References from the Textbook*

Outline

Objectives

- Describe the action for anticoagulants, antiplatelets, and thrombolytics.
- Identify the side effects and adverse reactions of anticoagulants, antiplatelets, and thrombolytics.
- Give the nursing processes, including client teaching, for anticoagulants and thrombolytics.

Terms

activated partial thromboplastin time (aPTT), p. 677
acute myocardial infarction (AMI), p. 686
aggregation, p. 676
anticoagulants, p. 677
antiplatelets, p. 683
fibrinolysis, p. 686
international normalized ratio (INR), p. 680
ischemia, p. 686
myocardial infarction, p. 677
necrosis, p. 686
partial thromboplastin time (PTT), p. 677
prothrombin time (PT), p. 680
thromboembolism, p. 686
thrombolytics, p. 686
thrombosis, p. 677

Various drugs are used to maintain or restore circulation. The three major groups of these drugs are (1) anticoagulants, (2) antiplatelets (antithrombotics), and (3) thrombolytics. The *anticoagulants* prevent the formation of clots that inhibit circulation. The *antiplatelets* prevent platelet **aggregation** (clumping together of platelets to form a clot). The *thrombolytics*, popularly called *clot busters*, attack and dissolve blood clots that have already formed. Each of these three drug groups are discussed separately.

Pathophysiology: Thrombus Formation

Thrombosis is the formation of a clot in an arterial or venous vessel. The formation of an arterial thrombus could be caused by blood stasis (because of decreased circulation), platelet aggregation on the blood vessel wall, or blood coagulation. Arterial clots are usually made up of both white and red clots with the white clots *(platelets)* initiating the process, followed by fibrin formation and the trapping of red blood cells in the fibrin mesh. Blood clots found in the veins are from platelet aggregation with fibrin that attaches to red blood cells. Both types of thrombus can be dislodged from the vessel and become an embolus (blood clot moving through the blood stream).

Platelets do not usually stick together unless there is a break in the endothelial lining of a blood vessel. When platelets adhere to the broken surface of an endothelial lining, they synthesize thromboxane A_2, which is a product of prostaglandins and a potent stimulus for platelet aggregation (clumping of platelet cells). The platelet receptor protein that binds fibrinogen, known as *glycoprotein IIb/IIIa,* or GP IIb/IIIa, also promotes platelet aggregation. Thromboxane A_2 and adenosine diphosphate (ADP) increase the activation of this receptor.

As the thrombus inhibits blood flow, fibrin, platelets, and red blood cells (erythrocytes) surround the clot, building the clot's size and structure. As the clot occludes the blood vessel, tissue ischemia occurs.

The venous thrombus usually develops because of slow blood flow. The venous clot can occur rapidly. Small pieces of the venous clot can detach and travel to the pulmonary artery and then to the lung. Inadequate oxygenation and gas exchange in the lungs result.

Oral and parenteral anticoagulants (warfarin and heparin) act primarily to prevent venous thrombosis, whereas antiplatelet drugs act to prevent arterial thrombosis. However, both groups of drugs suppress thrombosis in general.

Anticoagulants

Anticoagulants are used to inhibit clot formation. Unlike thrombolytics, they do *not* dissolve clots that have already formed, but rather act prophylactically to prevent new clots from forming. Anticoagulants are used in clients with venous and arterial vessel disorders that put them at high risk for clot formation. Venous problems include deep vein thrombosis (DVT) and pulmonary embolism, and arterial problems include coronary thrombosis **(myocardial infarction),** presence of artificial heart valves, and cerebrovascular accidents (CVAs, or stroke).

Heparin

Anticoagulants are administered orally or parenterally (subcutaneously [subQ] and intravenously [IV]). Heparin, introduced in 1938, is a natural substance in the liver that prevents clot formation. It was first used in blood transfusions to prevent clotting. Heparin is indicated for rapid anticoagulant effect when a thrombosis occurs because of a deep vein thrombosis (DVT), pulmonary embolism (PE), or an evolving stroke. Heparin is also used in openheart surgery to prevent blood from clotting and in the critically ill client with disseminated intravascular coagulation (DIC). DIC occurs when fibrin clots from within the vascular system, causing excess bleeding. However, the primary use of heparin is to prevent venous thrombosis, which can lead to pulmonary embolism or stroke.

Heparin combines with antithrombin III, which accelerates the anticoagulant cascade of reactions that prevents thrombosis formation. By inhibiting the action of thrombin, conversion of fibrinogen to fibrin does not occur and the formation of a fibrin clot is prevented (Figure 44–1).

Heparin is poorly absorbed through the gastrointestinal (GI) mucosa, and much is destroyed by heparinase, a liver enzyme. Because heparin is poorly absorbed orally, it is given subQ for prophylaxis or IV to treat acute thrombosis. It can be administered as an IV bolus or in IV fluid for continuous infusion. Heparin prolongs clotting time. **Partial thromboplastin time (PTT)** and **activated partial thromboplastin time (aPTT)** are laboratory tests to detect deficiencies of certain clotting factors, and these tests are used to monitor heparin therapy. Heparin can decrease the platelet count, causing thrombocytopenia. If hemorrhage occurs during heparin therapy, the anticoagulant antagonist protamine sulfate is given IV. Protamine can be an anticoagulant, but in the presence of heparin, it is an antagonist to reverse the action of heparin. Before discontinuing heparin, oral therapy with warfarin therapy is begun.

Low-Molecular-Weight Heparins

These derivatives of standard heparin were introduced to prevent venous thromboembolism. Studies have shown that by extracting only the low-molecular-weight fractions of standard heparin through depolymerization, the equivalent of anticoagulation can be achieved with a lower risk of bleeding. Low-molecular-weight heparins (LMWHs) produce more stable responses at recommended doses. As a result, frequent laboratory monitoring of aPTT is not required, because LMWH does not have the standard effect of heparin. Heparin prevents coagulation by combining with Antithrombin III to inactivate factor Xa and thrombin. Low-molecular-weight heparin inactivates the Xa factor, but it is less able to inactivate thrombin.

There are four LMWHs: enoxaparin sodium (Lovenox), dalteparin sodium (Fragmin), danaparoid (Orgaran), and tinzaparin sodium (Innohep). Although danaparoid is considered a LMWH (LMW heparin) drug, it does not have heparin in its structure, so it is referred to as *LMW heparinoid.* The uses for danaparoid are the same as other LMWHs.

The anticoagulant fondaparinux (Arixtra) is a synthetically engineered antithrombotic designed to be effective as a once-daily subcutaneous injection. Categorized as a *selective Factor Xa inhibitor,* fondaparinux is closely related in

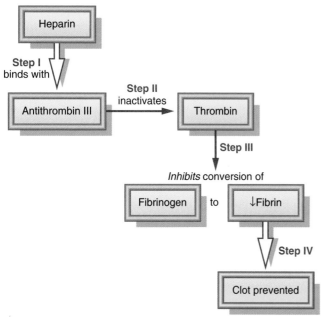

FIGURE 44–1 Action of the parenteral anticoagulant heparin.

structure to heparin and LMW heparins and is used for the same purposes.

These agents are most commonly prescribed to prevent DVT and acute pulmonary embolism after orthopedic or abdominal surgery. Hip- and knee-replacement anticoagulant therapy often includes enoxaparin and danaparoid; abdominal surgery, dalteparin. The drugs can be administered at home, because aPTT monitoring is not necessary, whereas heparin must be given in the hospital. The LMWHs are administered subQ once or twice a day, depending on the drug or drug regimen, and are available in prefilled syringes with attached needles. The client or family member is taught how to administer the subQ injection, which is usually given in the abdomen. The average treatment period lasts 7 to 14 days. The LMWH is usually started in the hospital within 24 hours after surgery (Table 44–1).

The half-life of LMWHs is two to four times longer than that of heparin. Clients should be instructed not to take antiplatelet drugs such as aspirin while taking LMWHs or heparin. Bleeding because of LMWH use is less likely to occur than when heparin is given. LMWH overdose is rare; if bleeding occurs, protamine sulfate is the anticoagulant

Table 44–1

Anticoagulants and Anticoagulant Antagonists

Generic (Brand)	Route and Dosage	Uses and Considerations
Anticoagulants		
Heparins		
heparin sodium (Lipo-Hepin)	A: subQ: 5000-7500 units q6h or 8000-10,000 units q8h A: IV: Bolus: 5000 units, inf: 20,000-40,000 units over 24 h; dose varies according to aPTT level C: IV: units/kg bolus, 50-100 units/kg q4h or 20,000 units/m²/24 h	For thromboembolism as a prophylaxis against clotting. Not given IM because of pain and hematoma. Drugs that inactivate heparin: digitalis, tetracycline, IV penicillin, phenothiazine, and quinidine; aPTT should be monitored. Protamine sulfate is the antidote for bleeding control. Dose is 1-1.5 mg for every 100 units of heparin subQ. *Pregnancy category*: C, PB: 95%; t½: 1-1.5 h
Low-Molecular-Weight Heparins (LMWHs)		
dalteparin sodium (Fragmin)	A: subQ: 2500 international units/d for 5-10 d starting 1-2 h before surgery	For prevention of DVT before surgery and for those at risk of thromboembolism. Similar to enoxaparin. *Pregnancy category*: B; PB: UK; t½: 3-5 h
enoxaparin sodium (Lovenox)	A: subQ: 30 mg b.i.d.	For thromboembolism. Prevents and treats DVT and pulmonary embolism. Bleeding is an adverse reaction. Monitor CBC. *Pregnancy category*: B; PB: UK; t½: 4.5 h
tinzaparin sodium (Innohep)	A: subQ: 175 antiXa international units q24h	To prevent and treat DVT and thromboembolic events. Can be administered in conjunction with warfarin sodium. *Pregnancy category*: UK; PB: UK; t½: 3-4 h
LMW Heparinoids		
danaparoid (Orgaran)	A: subQ: 750 units, q12h	Similar to LMWHs, but does not have heparin structure. Has little effect on thrombin activity and little to no effect on suppressing platelet aggregation. Used to prevent DVT after hip surgery. *Pregnancy category*: B, PB: UK; t½: 24 h

A, Adult; *aPTT*, activated partial thromboplastin time; *b.i.d.*, twice a day; *C*, child; *CBC* complete blood count; *d*, day; *DVT*, deep vein thrombosis; *h*, hour; *HIT*, heparin-induced thrombocytopenia; *IM*, intramuscular; *IV*, intravenous, *inf*, infusion; *INR*, international normalized ratio; *LD*, loading dose; *LMWH*, low-molecular-weight heparin; *maint*, maintenance; *min*, minute; *PB*, protein-binding; *PO*, by mouth; *PT*, prothrombin time; *sec*, second; *subQ*: subcutaneous; *t½*; half-life; *UK*, unknown.

Table 44–1

Anticoagulants and Anticoagulant Antagonists—cont'd

Generic (Brand)	Route and Dosage	Uses and Considerations
Oral Anticoagulants		
Coumarin		
warfarin (Coumadin)	(Prototype Drug Chart 44-1)	
Selective Factor Xa Inhibitors		
fondaparinux (Arixtra)	A: subQ: 2.5 mg/d	Indirectly inhibits thrombin production, and coagulation is suppressed. Closely related to heparin and LMWHs. Used to prevent DVT after hip fracture, hip replacement surgery, and knee-replacement surgery. May cause somewhat more bleeding than LMWHs. Long duration time. *Pregnancy category:* C; PB: UK; $t^{1/2}$: 17-21 h (longer with renal insufficiency)
Direct-Acting Thrombin Inhibitors: Anticoagulants II (Intravenous)		
argatroban (Acova)	A: IV: 2 mcg/kg/min; dose is adjusted to maintain aPTT at 1.5-3 times the baseline	Directly inhibits thrombin (thrombin inhibitor). Same effect as lepirudin. Decreases development of new thrombosis. *Pregnancy category:* B; PB: 54%; $t^{1/2}$: 40-52 min
bivalirudin (Angiomax)	A: IV bolus: 0.75 mg/kg; following 4 h; IV: 1.75 mg/kg/h; following 0.2 mg/kg/h	Bivalirudin binds with and inhibits free-flowing thrombin. Has been effective for use in preventing clot formation in clients with unstable angina who are undergoing cardiac angioplasty. Adverse effect is bleeding. *Pregnancy category:* B; PB: 0%; $t^{1/2}$: 25 min
desirudin (Iprivask)	A: subQ: 15 mg/12 h	Subcutaneous direct thrombin inhibitor; usually given before hip surgery. Given in thigh or abdomen. With renal impairment, dose is decreased. Pregnancy category: B; PB: UK, $t^{1/2}$: 2-3 h
lepirudin (Refludan)	A: IV bolus: 0.4 mg/kg over 15-20 sec; followed by 0.15 mg/kg/h for 2-10 day	Directly inhibits thrombin. Used for prophylaxis and treatment of thrombosis due to HIT. Titrated to aPTT ratio. Liver function should be normal. Adverse effect is bleeding. *Pregnancy category:* B; PB: UK; $t^{1/2}$: 1.3 h
Anticoagulant Antagonists		
protamine sulfate	A: IV: Initially: 1 mg/100 units heparin; administer 10-50 mg in 3-10 min, slow IV push; *max:* 50 mg in any 10 min period	Used to stop bleeding during heparin therapy. Binds and neutralizes heparin. *Pregnancy category:* C; PB: UK; $t^{1/2}$: UK
Vitamin K_1, phytonadione (AquaMEPHYTON, Mephyton, Konakion)	A: PO/IM/IV: 2-10 mg, q12-24h as needed C: subQ/IM: 5-10 mg	For control of bleeding caused by warfarin. If frank bleeding occurs, fresh or frozen plasma or Plasmanate may be needed. Depending on form and route, Vitamin K takes effect in 1 to 24 hours. Hemorrhage is usually controlled in 3 to 6 hours. *Pregnancy category:* C; PB: UK; $t^{1/2}$: UK

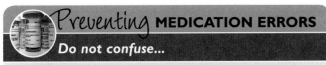

Preventing MEDICATION ERRORS
Do not confuse...

- **Enoxaparin** and **enoxacin**, which are look-alike drugs. Enoxaparin is a low-molecular-weight heparin (LMWH), and enoxacin is a fluoroquinolone antibiotic. Both are generic drugs.

- **Lovenox** and **Lotronex**. Both are trade (brand) name drugs. Lovenox is a trade name for enoxaparin, a LMWH drug. Lotronex is a gastrointestinal (GI) drug.

antagonist used. The dosage for protamine sulfate is 1 mg of protamine for every 1 mg of LMWH given.

Contraindications

The LMWHs are contraindicated for clients with strokes, peptic ulcers, and blood anomalies. These drugs should not be given to clients having eye, brain, or spinal surgery.

Direct Thrombin Inhibitors: Parenteral Anticoagulants II

There are four new parenteral anticoagulants that directly inhibit thrombin from converting fibrinogen to fibrin. These drugs differ from heparin-like anticoagulants. Three of these drugs are given intravenously: argatroban (Acova), bivalirudin (Angiomax), and lepirudin (Refludan). Bivalirudin binds with and inhibits free-flowing thrombin. The fourth drug, desirudin (Iprivask), is administered subcutaneously (see Table 44–1). This group of drugs is more costly than the other anticoagulants.

Oral Anticoagulants

Warfarin (Coumadin), from the coumarin drug family, is the only oral anticoagulant prescribed today. Dicumarol, a coumarin drug, and anisindione from the indanedione group, have been discontinued because of their many side effects. Warfarin is synthesized from dicumarol. Before warfarin was available for human use, it was used in rodenticides to kill rats by causing hemorrhage.

Oral anticoagulants inhibit hepatic synthesis of vita-min K, thus affecting the clotting factors II, VII, IX, and X. Warfarin is used mainly to prevent thromboembolic conditions such as thrombophlebitis, pulmonary embolism, and embolism formation caused by atrial fibrillation, which can lead to a stroke (CVA). Oral anticoagulants prolong clotting time and are monitored by the **prothrombin time (PT),** a laboratory test that measures the time it takes blood to clot in the presence of certain clotting factors which warfarin affects. This laboratory test is usually performed immediately before administering the next drug dose until the therapeutic level has been reached. Today, **international normalized ratio (INR)** is the laboratory test most frequently used to report PT results. It was introduced to account for variabilities in reported PTs from different laboratories. Reagents used in the PT test are compared with an international reference standard and reported as the INR; normal INR is 1.3 to 2. Clients on warfarin therapy are maintained at an INR of 2 to 3. The desired INR for clients who have a mechanical heart valve or recurrent systemic embolism is 2.5 to 3.5, but the desired level could be as high as 4.5.

Monitoring INR at regular intervals is required for the duration of drug therapy. Warfarin (Coumadin) has a long half-life and very long duration. Drug accumulation can occur and lead to external or internal bleeding, so the nurse must observe for petechiae, ecchymosis, tarry stools, and hematemesis and teach the client to do the same at home.

The antidote for warfarin overdose is Vitamin K, but it takes 24 to 48 hours to be effective. Usually a low dose of oral Vitamin K may be recommended for clients with a INR of 5.5. If excessive Vitamin K is given, it make take warfarin 1 to 2 weeks before it can be effective again. For acute bleeding, fresh frozen plasma is indicated.

Parenteral and oral anticoagulants (heparin and warfarin) are presented in Prototype Drug Chart 44–1.

Pharmacokinetics

Heparin is poorly absorbed through the GI mucosa, and much is destroyed by heparinase, a liver enzyme. Heparin is given parenterally, either subcutaneously for prophylactic anticoagulant therapy or IV (bolus or continuous infusion) for an immediate response. Warfarin, an oral anticoagulant, is well absorbed through the GI mucosa; food will delay but not inhibit absorption.

The half-life of heparin is dose-related; high doses prolong the half-life. The half-life of warfarin is 0.5 to 3 days, in contrast to 1 to 2 hours for heparin. Because warfarin has a long half-life and is highly protein-bound, the drug can have cumulative effects. Bleeding can occur, especially if another highly protein-bound drug is administered together with warfarin. Kidney and liver disease prolong the half-life of both heparin and warfarin. Warfarin is metabolized to inactive metabolites that are excreted in urine and bile.

Pharmacodynamics

Heparin, administered for acute thromboembolic disorders, prevents thrombus formation and embolism. It has been effectively used to treat DIC, which causes multiple thrombi in small blood vessels. Warfarin is effective for long-term anticoagulant therapy. The PT level should be 1.5 to 2 times the reference value to be therapeutic, or INR should be 2.0 to 3.0. INR has effectively replaced the use of PT, because PT can vary from laboratory to laboratory and reagent to reagent. Higher INR levels (up to 3.5) are usually required for clients with prosthetic heart valves, cardiac valvular disease, and recurrent emboli. Heparin does not cross the placental barrier, unlike warfarin; warfarin use is not suggested during pregnancy.

Intravenous heparin has a rapid onset; its peak time of action is reached in minutes, and its duration of action is short. After an IV heparin dose, the client's clotting time will return to normal in 2 to 6 hours. SubQ heparin is more slowly absorbed through the blood vessels in fatty tissue. Warfarin (Coumadin) has a long onset of action, peak concentration, and duration of action, so drug accumulation may occur.

Table 44–2 gives the summary comparison between heparin and warfarin, including methods of administration, drug action, uses, contraindications, laboratory tests, side effects, adverse reactions, and antidotes.

Side Effects and Adverse Reactions

Bleeding (hemorrhage) is the major adverse effect of warfarin. Clients should be monitored closely for signs of bleeding (e.g., petechiae, ecchymosis, hematemesis). Laboratory testing of PT or INR should be scheduled at recommended intervals.

Drug Interactions

Because warfarin is highly protein-bound, it is affected by drug interactions. Aspirin, nonsteroidal antiinflammatory drugs (NSAIDs), other types of antiinflammatory drugs, sulfonamides, phenytoin, cimetidine (Tagamet), allopurinol, and oral hypoglycemic drugs for diabetes can displace warfarin from the protein-bound site, causing more free-circulating anticoagulant. Numerous other drugs also increase the action of warfarin, and bleeding is likely to occur. Acetaminophen (Tylenol) should be used instead of aspirin by clients taking warfarin. For frank bleeding resulting from excess free drug, parenteral vitamin K is given as a coagulant to decrease bleeding and promote clotting. However, caution must be used with this approach, because the prothrombin can remain depressed for prolonged periods.

Table 44–1 lists the drug data for the anticoagulants.

Oral Anticoagulant Antagonists

Bleeding occurs in about 10% of clients taking oral anticoagulants. Vitamin K_1 (phytonadione), an antagonist of warfarin, is used for warfarin overdose or uncontrollable bleeding. Usually 1 to 10 mg of vitamin K_1 is given at once, and if it fails to control bleeding, then fresh whole blood or fresh-frozen plasma or platelets are generally given.

Prototype **DRUG CHART 44–1**

HEPARIN AND WARFARIN SODIUM

Drug Class

Anticoagulant
Trade names:
heparin: Lipo-Hepin, Calciparine, ✲Hepalean, Calcilean
Pregnancy Category: C
warfarin: Coumadin, ✲Warfilone
Pregnancy Category: D

Dosage

heparin:
A: subQ: 5000-7500 units q6h or 8000-10,000 units q8h
IV: Bolus: 5000 units; inf: 20,000-40,000 units over 24 h
C: IV: 75 units/kg; then 20 units/kg/h based on aPTT
warfarin:
A: PO: LD: 10 mg/day for 2-3 d; *maint:* 2-10 mg/d
Elderly: PO: 2.5 mg/d
Dose is usually titrated according to INR for adults and the elderly.

Contraindications

heparin/warfarin: Bleeding disorder, peptic ulcer, severe hepatic or renal disease, hemophilia, CVA
warfarin: Blood dyscrasias, eclampsia

Drug-Lab-Food Interactions

Drug: heparin: Increase effect with aspirin, NSAIDs, thrombolytics, probenecid; *decrease* effect with nitroglycerin, protamine
warfarin: Increase effect with amiodarone, aspirin, NSAIDs, sulfonamides, thyroid drugs, allopurinol, histamine$_2$ blockers, oral hypoglycemics, metronidazole, miconazole, methyldopa, diuretics, oral antibiotics, vitamin E; *decrease* effect with barbiturates, laxatives, phenytoin, estrogens, vitamins C and K, oral contraceptives, rifampin
Lab: May increase AST, ALT
Food: Decrease diet rich in vitamin K

Pharmacokinetics

Absorption: *heparin:* subQ or IV; warfarin: PO: Well absorbed
Distribution: PB: *heparin: greater than 80%; warfarin:* 99%
Metabolism: t½: *heparin:* 1-2 h; *warfarin:* 0.5-3 d
Excretion: *heparin:* Slowly in urine and reticulo-endothelial system; *warfarin:* in urine and bile

Pharmacodynamics

heparin:
subQ: Onset: 20-60 min
  Peak: 2 h
  Duration: 8-12 h
IV: Onset: immediate
  Peak: 5-10 min
  Duration: 2-6 h
warfarin:
PO: Onset: greater than 2 d
  Peak: 1-3 d
  Duration: 2.5-5 d

Therapeutic Effects/Uses

heparin/warfarin: To prevent blood clotting
Mode of Action: *heparin:* Inhibits thrombin, which prevents conversion of fibrinogen to fibrin
warfarin: Depression of hepatic synthesis of vitamin K clotting factors (II [prothrombin], VII, IX, and X)

Side Effects

heparin: Itching, burning
warfarin: Anorexia, nausea, vomiting, diarrhea, abdominal cramps, rash, fever

Adverse Reactions

heparin/warfarin: Bleeding, ecchymoses
warfarin: Stomatitis
Life-threatening: heparin/warfarin: hemorrhage

A, Adult; *ALT,* alanine aminotransferase; *aPTT,* activated partial thromboplastin time; *AST,* aspartate aminotransferase; *C,* child; *CVA,* cerebrovascular accident; *d,* day; *h,* hour; *inf,* infusion; *INR,* international normalized ratio; *IV,* intravenous; *LD,* loading dose; *maint,* maintenance; *min,* minute; *NSAIDs,* nonsteroidal antiinflammatory drugs; *PB,* protein-binding; *PO,* by mouth; *subQ,* subcutaneous; *t½,* half-life; ✲, Canadian drug name.

Table 44–2

Comparison of Parenteral and Oral Anticoagulants

Factors to Consider	Heparin	Warfarin (Coumadin)
Methods of administration	Subcutaneously Intravenously	Primarily orally
Drug actions	Binds with antithrombin III, which inactivates thrombin and clotting factors, inhibiting fibrin formation	Inhibits hepatic synthesis of vitamin K, which decreases prothrombin and the clotting factors VII, IX, X
Uses	Treatment of venous thrombosis, pulmonary embolism, thromboembolic complications (e.g., heart surgery, disseminated intravascular coagulation)	Treatment of deep venous thrombosis, pulmonary embolism, transient ischemic attack; prophylactic for cardiac valves
Contraindications/cautions	Hemophilia, peptic ulcer, severe (stage 3 or 4) hypertension, severe liver or renal disease, dissecting aneurysm	Hemophilia, peptic bleeding ulcer, blood dyscrasias, severe liver or kidney disease, acute myocardial infarction, alcoholism
Laboratory tests	Partial thromboplastin time (PTT): 60-70 sec Anticoagulant: 1.5-2 × control in seconds Activated partial thromboplastin time (aPTT): 20-35 sec Anticoagulant: aPTT: up to 40 sec	Prothrombin time (PT): 11-15 sec Anticoagulant: 1.25-2.5 × control in seconds International normalized ratio (INR): 1.3-2 Anticoagulant: INR 2-3 Prosthetic heart valves: INR up to 3.5
Side/adverse effects	Bleeding, hemorrhage, hematoma, severe hypotension	Bleeding, hemorrhage, GI bleeding, ecchymoses, hematuria
Antidote	Protamine sulfate, 1 mg per 100 units of heparin (see Table 44–1)	Vitamin K_1 PO/subQ/IM/IV: 2.5-10 mg, C: subQ/IM: 5-10 mg Infant: 1 mg Vitamin K_4: A: PO/IM/IV: 5-15 mg/day

A, Adult; *C,* child; *d,* day; *GI,* gastrointestinal; *IM,* intramuscular; *IV,* intravenous; *PO,* by mouth; *sec,* second; *subQ,* subcutaneous.

Nursing Process

Anticoagulants: Warfarin (Coumadin) and Heparin

ASSESSMENT

■ Obtain a history of abnormal clotting or health problems that affect clotting, such as severe alcoholism or severe liver or renal disease. Warfarin is contraindicated for clients with blood dyscrasias, peptic ulcer, cerebrovascular accident (CVA), hemophilia, or severe hypertension. Use with caution in client with acute traumatic injury.

■ Obtain a drug and herbal history of current drugs and herbs client takes. Report if a drug-drug or drug-herbal interaction is probable. Warfarin is highly protein-bound and can displace other highly protein-bound drugs, or warfarin could be displaced, which may result in bleeding.

■ Develop a flow chart that lists prothrombin time (PT) or international normalized ratio (INR) and warfarin dosages. A baseline PT or INR should be obtained before warfarin is administered.

NURSING DIAGNOSES

■ Risk for injury (bleeding) related to bleeding because of heparin or warfarin
■ Deficient knowledge related to the side effects of anticoagulants and their action

PLANNING

■ Client's PT will be 1.25 to 2.5 times the control level, or INR will be 2 to 3. For a client receiving heparin, the activated partial thromboplastin time (aPTT) should be checked.
■ Abnormal bleeding will be rapidly addressed while client is taking an anticoagulant. The PT, INR, or aPTT level(s) will be closely monitored.

NURSING INTERVENTIONS

■ Monitor vital signs. An increased pulse rate followed by a decreased systolic pressure can indicate a fluid volume deficit resulting from external or internal bleeding.
■ Monitor PT or INR for warfarin (Coumadin) and aPTT for heparin before administering the anticoagulant. The PT should be 1.25 to 2.5 times the control

level or INR 2 to 3, except for prosthetic heart valves (up to INR 3.5). The platelet count should be monitored, because anticoagulants can decrease platelet count.

■ Check for bleeding from the mouth, nose (epistaxis), urine (hematuria), and skin (petechiae, purpura).

■ Check stools periodically for occult blood.

■ Monitor older adults closely for bleeding. Their skin is thin, and the capillary beds are fragile.

■ Keep anticoagulant antagonists (protamine for heparin and vitamin K for warfarin) available when drug dose is increased or there are indications of frank bleeding. Fresh-frozen plasma may be needed for transfusion.

Client Teaching

General

● Instruct client to inform dentist when taking an anticoagulant. Contacting health care provider may be necessary.

● Advise client to use a soft toothbrush to prevent gums from bleeding.

● Instruct client to shave with an electric razor. Bleeding from shaving cuts may be difficult to control.

● Advise client to have laboratory tests such as PT or INR performed as ordered by health care provider. Warfarin dose is regulated according to the INR derived from the PT.

● Suggest that client carry a medical ID card or wear bracelet (MedicAlert) that lists the person's name, telephone number, and drug taken.

● Encourage client *not* to smoke. Smoking increases drug metabolism, so warfarin dose may need to be increased. If client insists on smoking, notify health care provider.

● Instruct client to check with the health care provider before taking OTC drugs. Aspirin should *not* be taken with warfarin, because aspirin intensifies its action and bleeding is apt to occur. Suggest that client use acetaminophen.

● Inform client that many herbal products (Herbal Alert 44–1) interact with anticoagulants and may increase bleeding. The international normalized ratio (INR) or prothrombin time (PT) should be closely monitored.

● Teach client to control external hemorrhage (bleeding) from accidents or injuries by applying firm, direct pressure for at least 5 to 10 minutes with a clean, dry, absorbent material.

Side Effects

● Advise client to report frank or occult bleeding (petechiae, ecchymosis, purpura, tarry stools, bleeding gums, epistaxis, expectoration of blood).

Diet

● Advise client to avoid large amounts of green, leafy vegetables; broccoli; legumes; soybean oil (rich in vitamin K); coffee, tea, cola (caffeine); excessive alcohol; certain nutritional supplements (coenzyme Q10).

Cultural Considerations ❖

● Have instructions available in the language client speaks/reads most easily. Certain cultural groups may lack understanding of Western approaches to health problems, drug therapy, adverse effects, and follow-up care concerning thrombophlebitis or other conditions that cause thrombus formation.

● Identify conflicts in cultural values and beliefs of client regarding method for treating a vascular problem. Respect traditional practices and incorporate into care plan if harmless. If the method may be harmful, explanations along with a nursing plan should be initiated.

EVALUATION

■ Evaluate the effectiveness of drug therapy. Client's PT or INR values are within the desired range and client is free of significant side effects.

Herbal ALERT 44–1

Anticoagulants

● *Dong quai, feverfew, garlic, ginger, ginkgo,* and *bilberry* may increase bleeding when taken with anticoagulants such as warfarin (Coumadin). Warfarin has an additive effect and increases the international normalized ratio (INR) and prothrombin time (PT).

● Excessive doses of *anise* may interfere with anticoagulants.

● *Ginseng* may decrease the effects of warfarin, thereby decreasing the INR.

● *Alfalfa* may decrease anticoagulant activity.

● *Goldenseal* may decrease the effect of heparin and oral anticoagulants.

● *Black haw* increases the action of anticoagulants.

● *Chamomile* may interfere with the actions of anticoagulants.

● *Valerian* may decrease the effects of warfarin.

Antiplatelet Drugs

Antiplatelets are used to prevent thrombosis in the arteries by suppressing platelet aggregation. Heparin and warfarin prevent thrombosis in the veins.

Antiplatelet drug therapy is mainly for prophylactic use in: (1) prevention of myocardial infarction or stroke for clients with familial history, (2) prevention of a repeat myocardial infarction or stroke, and (3) prevention of a stroke for clients having transient ischemic attacks (TIAs).

Long-term, low-dose aspirin therapy has been found to be both an effective and inexpensive treatment for suppressing platelet aggregation. Aspirin inhibits cyclooxygenase, an enzyme needed by platelets to synthesize thromboxane A_2 (TxA_2). For clients with familial history of stroke or myocardial infarction, the recommended aspirin dose is

Table 44–3

Antiplatelets

Generic (Brand)	Route and Dosage	Uses and Considerations
anagrelide HCl (Agrylin)	A: PO: 1 mg, b.i.d. May be increased by 0.5 mg/wk if necessary. Maintain platelet count: >600,000 mcL	Mild platelet aggregation inhibitor; affects the aggregating agents ADP, cAMP PDE III, and collagen. Adverse reactions include HF, heart block, pulmonary hypertension, cardiomyopathy. Onset: 7-10 d after appropriate dose. *Pregnancy category:* C; PB: UK; t$^{1/2}$: 1.2-1.8 h
aspirin	A: PO: 81-325 mg/d or every other d	For prevention of thrombosis before or after CVA or MI. Client should check with health care provider before taking aspirin for antiplatelet therapy. Aspirin should be avoided with peptic ulcer or liver dysfunction. Enteric-coated preparation decreases GI upset. *Pregnancy category:* D; PB: 76%-90%; t$^{1/2}$: 10-12 h
cilostazol (Pletal)	A: PO: 100 mg, b.i.d. 1 h before or 2 h after AM and PM meals	Inhibits platelet aggregation and is a vasodilator. Also indicated for intermittent claudication. Smoking may decrease serum levels. Adverse reactions include HF, tachycardia, cerebral ischemia, atrial flutter or fibrillation. Pregnancy category: C; PB: 95-98%, t$^{1/2}$: 1-13 h
clopidogrel (Plavix)	(Prototype Drug Chart 44–2)	
dipyridamole (Persantine)	A: PO: 50-100 mg t.i.d.-q.i.d.	For prevention of thromboembolism post-MI and associated with prosthetic devices (heart valves and hip replacement); prevention of TIA. Monitor blood pressure. *Pregnancy category:* B; PB: >91%; t$^{1/2}$: 10-12 h
sulfinpyrazone (Anturane)	A: PO: 200-400 mg b.i.d.; *max:* 800 mg/ day	Used for treating gout. Has antiplatelet function. May be used in AV shunts for hemodialysis to prevent clotting. *Pregnancy category:* C; PB: 95%-99%; t$^{1/2}$: 3 h
ticlopidine (Ticlid)	A: PO: 250 mg b.i.d.	To prevent the risk of strokes and thrombin formation. To treat intermittent claudication and sickle cell disease. Avoid if client has a hematopoietic disorder such as thrombocytopenia or bleeding peptic ulcer. *Pregnancy category:* B; PB: UK: t$^{1/2}$: 24 h-5 d
Combination of Antiplatelet Drugs		
dipyridamole and aspirin (Aggrenox)	*Stroke prevention:* 1 capsule, b.i.d. (aspirin 25 mg and ER-dipyridamole 200 mg)	Combination of aspirin and ER-dipyridamole for stroke prevention with clients who have had TIA
Antiplatelets: Glycoprotein (GP) IIb/IIIa Receptor Antagonists		
abciximab (ReoPro)	A: IV bolus: 0.25 mg/kg given 10-60 min before PTCA. Inject 4.5 ml abciximab into 250 ml of NSS or D$_5$W. Follow with a continuous infusion of 10 mcg/min (17 ml/h) for 12 hours	To prevent acute cardiac ischemia before and following PTCA and for unstable angina. *Pregnancy category:* C; PB: UK; t$^{1/2}$: 30 min
eptifibatide (Integrilin)	A: IV bolus: 180 mcg/kg, then 2 mcg/kg/min for up to 72 h	For acute cardiac syndromes (unstable angina and non-Q-wave MI). Can be used with angioplasty. *Pregnancy category:* B; PB: 25%; t$^{1/2}$: 2.5 h
tirofiban (Aggrastat)	A: IV: 0.4 mcg/kg/min for 30 min, then 0.1 mcg/kg/min for 12-24 h after angioplasty	For acute cardiac syndromes (unstable angina and non-Q-wave MI). May be used with angioplasty. *Pregnancy category:* B; PB: 35% unbound; t$^{1/2}$: UK

ADP, Adenosine diphosphate; *AV,* arteriovenous; *cAMP,* cyclic adenosine monophosphate; *HF,* heart failure; *CVA,* cerebrovascular accident; *d,* day; *ER,* extended release; *GI,* gastrointestinal; *h,* hour; *max,* maximum; *MI,* myocardial infarction; *NSS,* normal saline solution; *PTCA,* percutaneous transluminal coronary angioplasty; *q.i.d.,* four times a day; *t$^{1/2}$,* half-life; *TIA,* transient ischemic attack; *t.i.d.,* three times a day; *UK,* unknown; *wk,* week; *>,* greater than.

81, 162, or 325 mg per day. Because aspirin has prolonged antiplatelet activity, it should be discontinued at least 7 days before surgery.

Other antiplatelet drugs include dipyridamole (Persantine), ticlopidine (Ticlid), clopidogrel (Plavix), anagrelide HCl (Agrylin), abciximab (ReoPro), eptifibatide (Integrilin), and tirofiban (Aggrastat). Clopidogrel, dipyridamole, and ticlopidine have similar effects as aspirin, but they are known as *adenosine diphosphate (ADP) antagonists* affecting platelet aggregation. Cilostazol (Pletal) inhibits platelet aggregation and is a vasodilator that may be used for intermittent claudication. Table 44–3 describes the drugs, dose and route, and uses and considerations for the antiplatelets.

Clopidogrel (Plavix) is an antiplatelet drug frequently used after myocardial infarction or stroke to prevent a second event. It may be prescribed singly or with aspirin. It has been stated that Plavix and aspirin are more effective in inhibiting platelet aggregation if used together than if used as separate antiplatelet therapies. Prototype Drug Chart 44–2 gives the pharmacologic data for clopidogrel (Plavix).

Pharmacokinetics

Clopidogrel (Plavix) is rapidly absorbed and has a high protein-binding power. Studies have not established a relationship between the concentration of the main metabolite and platelet aggregation. The half-life is 8 hours; it is usually prescribed once a day. Excretion of the drug metabolite occurs equally in the urine and feces.

Pharmacodynamics

Clopidogrel (Plavix) prevents platelet aggregation by blocking the binding of adenosine diphosphate (ADP) to the platelet ADP receptor. ADP-mediated activation of the glycoprotein (GP) IIb/IIIa complex inhibits platelet aggregation. Plavix prolongs bleeding time; therefore it should be discontinued for 7 days preceding surgery. The onset of action of Plavix is 1 to 2 hours, and its peak time is 2 to 3 hours. The drug should not be taken if the client has a bleeding peptic ulcer, any active bleeding, or intracranial hemorrhage.

Abciximab, eptifibatide, and tirofiban are used primarily for acute coronary syndromes (unstable angina or non-Q-wave myocardial infarction) and for preventing reocclusion of coronary arteries following percutaneous transluminal coronary angioplasty (PTCA). These drugs are usually given before and after PTCA. The drug of choice for angioplasty is abciximab. Abciximab, eptifibatide, and tirofiban block the binding of fibrinogen to the glycoprotein IIb/IIIa receptor on the platelet surface. They are called *platelet glycoprotein (GP) IIb/IIIa receptor antagonists.* Following IV infusion, the antiplatelet effects for abciximab persist for 24 to 48 hours; for eptifibatide and tirofiban, the antiplatelet effects last for 4 hours.

Herbal products can interact with antiplatelet drugs (Herbal Alert 44–2).

Prototype DRUG CHART 44–2

CLOPIDOGREL BISULFATE

Drug Class

Antiplatelet
Trade name: Plavix
Pregnancy Category: B

Contraindications

Intracranial hemorrhage, peptic ulcer
Caution: Liver disease, GI bleeding, surgery,
    bleeding from trauma

Dosage

A: PO: loading dose: 300 mg and then 75 mg/day

Drug-Lab-Food Interactions

Drug: May *increase* bleeding when taken with NSAIDs;
    interferes with metabolism of phenytoin, warfarin,
    fluvastatin, tamoxifen, tolbutamide, NSAIDs,
    torsemide
Lab: Prolongs bleeding time
Herb: May *increase* bleeding when taken with ginger,
    garlic, ginkgo, feverfew

Pharmacokinetics

Absorption: Rapid
Distribution: PB: 94%-98%
Metabolism: t½: 8 hours
Excretion: 50% urine and 50% feces

Pharmacodynamics

PO: Onset: 1-2 hours
    Peak: 2-3 hours
    Duration: 3 days or longer

Therapeutic Effects/Uses

To prevent recurrence of MI, stroke; prevent vascular death
Mode of Action: Inhibits platelet aggregation. Prevents ADP from binding with the ADP platelet receptor.

Side Effects

Upper RTI, flulike symptoms, dizziness, headaches,
    fatigue, chest pain, diarrhea

Adverse Reactions

None of significance. May cause hypertension,
    bronchitis

A, Adult; *ADP,* adenosine diphosphate; *GI,* gastrointestinal; *PB,* protein-binding; *PO,* by mouth; *MI,* myocardial infarction; *NSAIDs,* nonsteroidal antiinflammatory drugs; *RTI,* respiratory tract infection; *t½,* half-life.

Thrombolytics

Thromboembolism (occlusion of an artery or vein caused by a thrombus or embolus) results in **ischemia** (deficient blood flow) that causes **necrosis** (death) of the tissue distal to the obstructed area. It takes approximately 1 to 2 weeks for the blood clot to disintegrate by natural fibrinolytic mechanisms. If a new thrombus or embolus can be dissolved more quickly, tissue necrosis is minimized, and blood flow to the area is reestablished faster. This is the basis for thrombolytic therapy.

Thrombolytics have been used since the early 1980s to promote the fibrinolytic mechanism (converting plasminogen to plasmin, which destroys the fibrin in the blood clot). The thrombus, or blood clot, disintegrates when a thrombolytic drug is administered within 4 hours after an **acute myocardial infarction (AMI)** (an acute heart attack). Necrosis resulting from the blocked artery is prevented or minimized, and hospitalization time may be decreased. The need for cardiac bypass or coronary angioplasty can be evaluated soon after thrombolytic treatment. A thrombolytic drug should be administered within 3 hours of a thrombolic stroke. These drugs are also used for pulmonary embolism, DVT, noncoronary arterial occlusion from an acute thromboembolism, and thrombolic stroke.

Five commonly used thrombolytics are streptokinase, urokinase, alteplase, reteplase (Retavase), and tenecteplase (TNKase). Streptokinase and urokinase are enzymes that act systemically to promote the conversion of plasminogen to plasmin. Alteplase, also known as *tissue plasminogen activator (tPA)*, is clot-specific and binds to the fibrin surface of a clot, promoting the conversion of plasminogen to plasmin. Plasmin, an enzyme, digests the fibrin in the clot. Plasmin also degrades fibrinogen, prothrombin, and other clotting factors. These five drugs all induce **fibrinolysis** (fibrin breakdown). Prototype Drug Chart 44–3 gives the pharmacologic data for alteplase.

Streptokinase may cause hypotension when first administered. Drug dosage may need to be adjusted. Reteplase (Retavase), a derivative of tPA, is a fairly recent thrombo-

Prototype DRUG CHART 44–3

ALTEPLASE (TISSUE PLASMINOGEN ACTIVATOR [TPA])

Drug Class	Dosage
Thrombolytic agent Trade names: tPA, Activase *Pregnancy Category:* C	**A: IV bolus:** 15 mg, then 50 mg infused over 30 min, then 35 mg infused over 60 min; *max:* 100 mg

Contraindications	Drug-Lab-Food Interactions
Internal bleeding, bleeding disorders, recent CVA, surgery or trauma, bacterial endocarditis, severe liver dysfunction, severe uncontrolled hypertension	*Drug: Increase* bleeding when taken with oral anticoagulants, NSAIDs, cefotetan, plicamycin *Lab: Decrease* in plasminogen, fibrinogen, hematocrit, and hemoglobin

Pharmacokinetics	Pharmacodynamics
Absorption: Direct IV **Distribution:** PB: UK **Metabolism:** t½: 5 min **Excretion:** Urine	**PO:** Onset: Immediate Peak: 5-10 min Duration: 3 hours

Therapeutic Effects/Uses

To dissolve clot following an acute MI, pulmonary embolism, acute ischemic stroke
Mode of Action: Alteplase promotes conversion of plasminogen to plasmin. Plasmin, an enzyme, digests the fibrin matrix of clots. Alteplase initiates fibrinolysis.

Side Effects	Adverse Reactions
Bleeding	*Life-threatening:* intracerebral hemorrhage, stroke, atrial or ventricular dysrhythmias

A, Adult; *CVA,* cerebrovascular accident; *IV,* intravenous; *PB,* protein-binding; *max,* maximum; *min,* minute; *NSAIDs,* nonsteroidal antiinflammatory drugs; *PO,* by mouth; *t½,* half-life; *tPA,* tissue plasminogen activator; *UK,* unknown.

lytic drug. Anticoagulants and antiplatelet drugs increase the risk of hemorrhage; therefore they should be avoided until the thrombolytic effect has passed. The health care provider needs to determine whether the client has taken any of these drugs before seeking treatment.

Pharmacokinetics

The commercial preparation of alteplase (tissue plasminogen activator [tPA]) is identical to natural human tPA, the enzyme that converts plasminogen to plasmin. Alteplase is initially administered as an IV bolus, then infused over 30 minutes, then 60 minutes. A total dose of 100 mg is the recommended maximum; a larger dose could result in the risk of intracranial bleeding. The half-life of alteplase (tPA) is 5 minutes, shorter than the half-life of streptokinase. Alteplase costs about $2750, making it five times more expensive than streptokinase, but about the same as TNKase and reteplase. Allergic reactions to alteplase occur less frequently than to streptokinase, anistreplase, and urokinase.

Pharmacodynamics

Alteplase is similar to natural human tissue plasminogen activator (tPA). It promotes thrombolysis by converting plasminogen to plasmin. Plasmin degrades fibrin, fibrinogen, and factors V, VIII, and XII. Alteplase does not induce hypotension as does streptokinase. Peak action of Alteplase is 5 to 10 minutes. The duration of action is 3 hours.

Side Effects and Adverse Reactions

Allergic reactions can complicate thrombolytic therapy. Anaphylaxis (vascular collapse) occurs more frequently with streptokinase than with the other thrombolytics. If the drugs are administered through an intracoronary catheter after myocardial infarction, reperfusion dysrhythmia or hemorrhagic infarction at the myocardial necrotic area can result. The major complication of thrombolytic drugs is hemorrhage. The antithrombolytic drug aminocaproic acid (Amicar) is used to stop bleeding by inhibiting plasminogen activation, which inhibits thrombolysis.

Table 44–4 lists the drug data for the thrombolytic drugs.

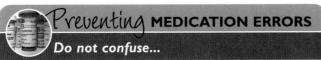

Preventing MEDICATION ERRORS

Do not confuse...

Right Drug

- **Tenecteplase (TNKase)** and **tissue plasminogen activator (tPA)**. These two drugs look alike, and even though they are from the same drug class—thrombolytics—the drugs are different and their administration time is different.

Right Dose and Time

- **TNKase** and **tPA (alteplase)** have different dosages. Their administration time is also different. TNKase is administered as a single dose; tPA (alteplase) is administered in three different doses and times. The first dose is a bolus, and the second and third doses are over 30 minutes and 60 minutes.

Nursing Process

Thrombolytics

ASSESSMENT

- Assess baseline vital signs and compare with future values.
- Check baseline complete blood count (CBC), prothrombin time (PT), or international normalized ratio (INR) values before administration of thrombolytics.
- Obtain a medical and drug history. Contraindications for use of thrombolytics include a recent cerebrovascular accident (CVA), active bleeding, severe hypertension, and anticoagulant therapy. Reported if client takes aspirin or nonsteroidal antiinflammatory drugs (NSAIDs). Thrombolytics are contraindicated for the client with a recent history of traumatic injury, especially head injury.

NURSING DIAGNOSES

- Decreased cardiac output related to acute myocardial infarction (AMI) or coronary artery disease (CAD)
- Anxiety related to severe health problem because of coronary insufficiency or a possible stroke
- Impaired tissue integrity related to coronary insufficiency, heart attack, or stroke
- Risk for injury related to a thrombus or embolus

PLANNING

- The blood clot will be dissolved, and client will be closely monitored for active bleeding.
- Client's vital signs will be monitored for stability during and after thrombolytic therapy.
- Thrombolytic drug should be administered 4 hours after myocardial infarction.

NURSING INTERVENTIONS

- Monitor vital signs. Increased pulse rate followed by decreased blood pressure usually indicates blood loss and impending shock. Record vital signs and report changes.
- Observe for signs and symptoms of active bleeding from the mouth or rectum. Hemorrhage is a serious complication of thrombolytic treatment. Aminocaproic acid can be given as an intervention to stop the bleeding.
- Check for active bleeding for 24 hours after thrombolytic therapy has been discontinued: q15min for the first hour, q30min until the eighth hour, and then hourly.
- Observe for signs of allergic reaction to streptokinase: itching, hives, flush, fever, dyspnea, bronchospasm, hypotension, and/or cardiovascular collapse.
- Avoid administering aspirin or nonsteroidal antiinflammatory drugs (NSAIDs) for pain or discomfort

Table 44-4

Thrombolytics

Generic (Brand)	Route and Dosage	Uses and Considerations
Thrombolytics		
anistreplase (APSAC, Eminase)	A: IV: 30 units over 2-5 min	Treatment following an AMI, causing lysis of thrombi. Decreases infarction size. *Pregnancy category:* C; PB: UK; t$\frac{1}{2}$: 1.5-2 h
reteplase (Retavase)	A: IV bolus: 10 units over 2 min, then repeat 10 units in 30 min (total of 20 units)	To treat coronary thrombosis by causing lysis of thrombi; inhibits fibrin aspect of the thrombus. Derivative of tPA (Alteplase). Considered more effective than tPA with less risk of hemorrhage. *Pregnancy category:* C; PB: UK; t$\frac{1}{2}$: 13-16 min
streptokinase (Streptase, Kabikinase)	*Myocardial infarction:* A: IV: 1,500,000 international units diluted in 45 ml; infuse in 53 ml; infuse over 60 min *Pulmonary embolism:* A: IV: LD: 250,000 international units/h for 24-72 h (24 h for PE; 72 h for DVT)	Dissolves blood clots caused by coronary artery thrombi, DVT, PE; converts plasminogen to plasmin for dissolving fibrin deposits. Should be given after AMI within 4 h. *Pregnancy category:* C; PB: UK; t$\frac{1}{2}$: 20-80 min
tenecteplase (TNKase)	A: IV: *Max:* 50 mg NOTE: Dose is based on body weight.	To reduce mortality associated with AMI. A "clot buster" that can be administered in 5 seconds in one dose. *Pregnancy category:* C; PB: UK; t$\frac{1}{2}$: 11-138 min
alteplase (tissue-type plasminogen activator [tPA], Activase)	(Prototype Drug Chart 44-3)	
urokinase (Abbokinase)	A: IV: LD: 4400 international units/kg diluted and infuse over 10 min, then continuous infusion: 4400 international units/kg over 12 h *Occluded coronary artery:* Dose may be increased.	Same uses as streptokinase. Causes less allergic reaction but is more expensive than streptokinase. Not susceptible to antistreptokinase antibodies. May also be used for peripheral artery occlusion. *Pregnancy category:* B; PB: UK; t$\frac{1}{2}$: 10-20 min
Plasminogen Inactivators		
aminocaproic acid (Amicar)	A: PO/IV: LD: 4-5 g first h Inf: 1-1.25 g/h for 8 h; *max:* 30 g/d	Treatment for excessive bleeding that may result from heart surgery, severe trauma, abruptio placentae, and thrombolytic drugs such as streptokinase, alteplase, and urokinase. Side effects include dizziness, headache, orthostatic, hypotension, and thrombophlebitis. *Pregnancy category:* C; PB: 0%; t$\frac{1}{2}$: 1-2 h

A, Adult; *AMI,* acute myocardial infarction; *d,* day; *DVT,* deep vein thrombosis; *h,* hour; *Inf,* infusion; *IV,* intravenous; *LD,* loading dose; *max,* maximum; *min,* minute; *PB,* protein-binding; *PE,* pulmonary embolism; *t$\frac{1}{2}$,* half-life; *tPA,* tissue plasminogen activator; *UK,* unknown.

when client is receiving a thrombolytic. Acetaminophen can be substituted.
■ Monitor the electrocardiogram (ECG) for the presence of reperfusion dysrhythmias as the blood clot is dissolving; antidysrhythmic therapy may be indicated.
■ Avoid venipuncture/arterial sticks.

Client Teaching

General
• Explain the thrombolytic treatment to client and family. Be supportive.

Side Effects
• Instruct client to report any side effects, such as lightheadedness, dizziness, palpitations, nausea, pruritus, or urticaria.

EVALUATION

■ Determine the effectiveness of drug therapy: clot has dissolved, vital signs are stable, no signs or symptoms of active bleeding, and client is pain free.

KEY WEBSITES

Information on clopidogrel: www.nlm.nih.gov/medicineplus/druginfo/medmaster/a601040.htm
Information on anticoagulation: www.acforum.org
Information on Coumadin: www.cc.nih.gov/ccc/patient_education/drug_nutrient/coumadin1.pdf

Critical Thinking Case Study

TM, age 57, has thrombophlebitis in the right lower leg. IV heparin, 5000 units by bolus, was given. Following the IV bolus, heparin 5000 units given subQ q6h was prescribed. Other therapeutic means to decrease pain and alleviate swelling and redness were also prescribed. An aPTT test was ordered.

1. Was TM's heparin order within the safe daily dosage range?
2. What are the various methods for administering heparin?
3. Why was an aPTT test ordered? How would you determine whether TM is within the desired range? Explain.

After 5 days of heparin therapy, TM was prescribed warfarin (Coumadin) 5 mg PO daily. An INR test was ordered.

4. What is the pharmacologic action of warfarin? Is the warfarin dose within the safe daily dosage range? Explain.

5. What are the half-life and protein-binding for warfarin? If a client takes a drug that is highly protein-bound, would there be a drug interaction? Explain.
6. Why was an INR ordered for TM? What is the desired range?
7. What serious adverse reactions could result with prolonged use or large doses of warfarin?
8. What client teaching interventions should the nurse include? List three.
9. Months later TM had hematemesis. What nursing action should be taken?

NCLEX Study Questions

1. Heparin is effective for treating:
   a. coronary thrombosis
   b. acute myocardial infarction
   c. deep vein thrombosis (DVT)
   d. cerebrovascular accident (CVA—stroke)

2. An antidote for heparin is:
   a. protamine
   b. vitamin K
   c. aminocaproic acid
   d. vitamin C

3. Low-molecular weight heparin (LMWH) has a:
   a. longer half-life than heparin
   b. shorter half-life than heparin
   c. same half-life as heparin
   d. four times shorter half-life than heparin

4. LMWH is usually given to a client in what facility?
   a. Hospital
   b. At home
   c. Clinic
   d. Doctor's office

5. LMWH is administered:
   a. intravenously
   b. intramuscularly
   c. intradermally
   d. subcutaneously

6. The anticoagulant that is administered orally is:
   a. enoxaparin sodium (Lovenox)
   b. warfarin (Coumadin)
   c. bivalirudin (Angiomax)
   d. lepirudin (Refludan)

7. Mrs. TJ is taking warfarin 5 mg daily for atrial fibrillation. Her international normalized ratio (INR) is 3.8. You would consider Mrs. TJ's INR to be:
   a. within normal range
   b. elevated INR range
   c. low INR range
   d. low average INR range

8. The major purpose for antiplatelet drug therapy is to:
   a. dissolve the blood clot
   b. decrease tissue necrosis
   c. inhibit hepatic synthesis of Vitamin K
   d. suppress platelet aggregation

9. The drug used primarily for preventing reocclusion of coronary arteries following a coronary angioplasty is:
   a. clopidogrel (Plavix)
   b. abciximab (ReoPro)
   c. warfarin (Coumadin)
   d. streptokinase

10. The drug category that is given early for the prevention of tissue necrosis following blood clot blockage in a coronary or cerebral artery is:
    a. anticoagulant agent
    b. antiplatelet agent
    c. thrombolytic agent
    d. low-molecular weight heparin (LMWH)

Answers: 1, e; 2, a; 3, a; 4, b; 5, d; 6, b; 7, b; 8, d; 9, b; 10, c.

45

Antilipidemics and Peripheral Vasodilators

ELECTRONIC RESOURCES

evolve

Evolve website (http://evolve.elsevier.com/KeeHayes/pharmacology/):
- *Case Studies*
- *Content Updates*
- *Frequently Asked Questions*
- *Student Review Activities*
- *WebLinks*
- *Additional Reference Material*

Companion CD-ROM:
- *NCLEX Examination Review Questions*
- *Pharmacology Animations*
- *IV Therapy Checklists*
- *Medication Error Checklists*
- *Drug Calculation Problems*
- *Electronic Calculators*
- *Top 200 Drugs with Pronunciations*
- *References from the Textbook*

Outline

Objectives

- Describe the action of the two main drug groups: antilipidemics and peripheral vasodilators.
- Identify the side effects and adverse reactions of antilipidemics and peripheral vasodilators.
- Describe the nursing process, including client teaching, for antilipidemics and peripheral vasodilators.

Terms

antilipidemics, p. 690
apolipoproteins, p. 691
chylomicrons, p. 691
high-density lipoprotein (HDL), p. 691
high sensitivity C-reactive protein (hsCRP), p. 694
homocysteine, p. 694
hyperlipidemia, p. 690
lipoprotein, p. 691
low-density lipoprotein (LDL), p. 691
peripheral vasodilators, p. 690
very low-density lipoproteins (VLDL), p. 691

Various drugs are used to maintain or decrease blood lipid concentrations and promote dilation of vessels. Drugs that lower blood lipids are called *antilipidemics, antihyperlipidemics, antilipemics, and hypolipidemics.* In this chapter, drugs used to lower lipoproteins will be called **antilipidemics**. **Peripheral vasodilators** are drugs that dilate vessels that have been narrowed by vasospasm.

Lipoproteins

Lipids (cholesterol, triglycerides, phospholipids) are bound in the inner shell of protein, which is a carrier that transports lipids in the blood stream. When there is an excess of one or more lipids in the blood, the condition is known as **hyperlipidemia** or *hyperlipoproteinemia.* The four major categories of **lipoprotein** are high-density lipoprotein (HDL), low-density lipoprotein (LDL), very low-density lipoprotein (VLDL), and chylomicrons. **High-density lipoprotein (HDL)**, also known as *friendly* or "good" lipoprotein, is the smallest, most dense lipoprotein, meaning that it contains more protein and less fat than the others. The function of HDL is to remove cholesterol from the blood stream and deliver it to the liver for excretion in bile. **Low-density lipoprotein (LDL)**, the so-called "bad" lipoprotein, contains 50 to 60 percent of cholesterol in the blood stream. With an elevated LDL, there is greater risk for developing atherosclerotic plaques and heart disease. **Very low-density lipoprotein (VLDL)** carries mostly triglycerides and less cholesterol. The **chylomicrons** are large particles that transport fatty acids and cholesterol to the liver. They are composed mostly of triglycerides. Table 45–1 presents the composition of the lipoproteins.

Serum cholesterol and triglyceride measurements are frequently part of a regular physical examination or readmission evaluation and are used as baseline test results. If the levels are high, a 12- to 14-hour fasting lipid profile may be ordered. When cholesterol, triglycerides, and LDL are elevated, the client is at increased risk for coronary artery disease (CAD). Table 45–2 lists the various serum lipids and their reference values (normal serum levels) according to a risk classification.

Apolipoproteins

Apolipoproteins are within the lipoprotein shell and contain apolipoprotein (apo) A-1, apoB, and apoE. The major component of apoA1 is high-density lipoprotein (HDL),

the "friendly" lipoprotein. The major component of apoB is low-density lipoprotein (LDL), which exists in two forms, apoB-100 and apoB-48. ApoB-100 has a very low-density lipoprotein (VLDL) as well as LDL and is a better indicator of risk for coronary artery disease (CAD) than LDL alone.

Nonpharmacologic Methods for Cholesterol Reduction

Before drugs to lower LDL and raise HDL are prescribed, nondrug therapy should be initiated for decreasing blood pressure. Saturated fats and cholesterol in the diet should be reduced. Total fat intake should be 30% or less of caloric intake, and cholesterol intake should be 300 mg daily or less. The client should be advised to read labels on containers and buy appropriate foods. Clients should choose lean meats, especially chicken and fish.

In many cases, diet alone will not lower blood lipid levels. Because 75% to 85% of serum cholesterol is endogenously (internally) derived, dietary modification alone will typically lower total cholesterol levels by only 10% to 30%. This and the fact that adherence to dietary restrictions is often short lived explains why many clients do not respond to diet modification alone.

Exercise is an important aspect of the nonpharmacologic method to reduce cholesterol and increase HDL. For the hypertensive older adult, exercise can be walking and bicycling. If the client is obese, body-weight reduction decreases cholesterol levels and the risk of CAD. Smoking is another risk factor that should be eliminated. Smoking increases LDL cholesterol and decreases the HDL.

Table 45–1

Lipoprotein Groups

Lipoprotein Subgroups	Composition of Lipoproteins			
	Protein (%)	Cholesterol (%)	Triglycerides (%)	Phospholipids (%)
Chylomicrons	1-2	1-3	80-95	3-6
Very low density (VLDL)	6-10	8-20	45-65	15-20
Low density (LDL)	15-20	50-60	4-8	16-20
High density (HDL)	45-55	15-20	2-7	26-32

Modified from Henry J: *Clinical diagnosis and management by laboratory methods*, ed 18, Philadelphia, 1991, Saunders, p. 189.

Table 45–2

Serum Lipid Values

Lipids	Desirable (mg/dl)	Level of Risk for CAD		
		Low Risk (mg/dl)	Moderate Risk (mg/dl)	High Risk (mg/dl)
Cholesterol	150-200	Less than 200	200-240	Greater than 240
Triglycerides	40-150	Values vary with age	Values vary with age	Greater than 190
Lipoproteins				
LDL	Less than 100	100-130	130-159	Greater than 160
HDL	45-60	50-60	35-50	Less than 35

CAD, Coronary artery disease; *HDL*, high-density lipoproteins; *LDL*, low-density lipoproteins.

If nonpharmacologic methods are ineffective for reducing cholesterol, LDL, and VLDL and hyperlipidemia remains, antilipidemic drugs are prescribed to lower blood lipid levels. It must be emphasized to the client that dietary changes need to be made and an exercise program followed even after drug therapy has been initiated. The type of antilipidemics ordered depends on the lipoprotein phenotype (Table 45–3).

Antilipidemics

Drugs that lower lipid levels include bile-acid sequestrants, fibrates (fibric acid), nicotinic acid, cholesterol absorption inhibitor, and hepatic 3-hydroxy-3-methylglutaryl-coenzyme A (HMG-CoA) reductase inhibitors (statins). The statins have fewer adverse effects and are well tolerated.

One of the first antilipidemics was cholestyramine (Questran), introduced in 1959. It is a bile-acid sequestrant that reduces LDL cholesterol (LDL-C) levels by binding with bile acids in the intestine. It is effective against hyperlipidemia type II. This group may be used as an adjunct to the statins. The drug comes in a gritty powder, which is mixed thoroughly in water or juice. Colestipol (Colestid) is another resin antilipidemic similar to cholestyramine. Both are effective in lowering cholesterol. Colesevelam HCl, another bile acid sequestrant similar to cholestyramine and colestipol, is the newer agent and has fewer side effects (less constipation, flatulence, and cramping). Colesevelam also has less effect on the absorption of fat-soluble vitamins than the older agents and is usually the first-choice bile-acid sequestrant drug.

Clofibrate (Atromid-S) and gemfibrozil (Lopid) are fibric acid derivatives that are more effective at reducing triglyceride and VLDL levels than reducing LDL. They are used primarily to reduce hyperlipidemia type IV, but can also be used for type II hyperlipidemia. These drugs are highly protein-bound and should not be taken with anticoagulants, because they compete for protein sites. Anticoagulant dose should be reduced during antilipidemic therapy, and the international normalized ratio (INR) should be closely monitored. Clofibrate, once a popular antilipidemic, is not suggested for long-term use because of its many side effects, such as cardiac dysrhythmias, angina, thromboembolism, and gallstones. Fenofibrate, approved in 1998, has similar actions and some of the same side effects as clofibrate and gemfibrozil. If taken with warfarin, bleeding might occur. It is highly protein-bound.

Nicotinic acid, or niacin (vitamin B_2), reduces VLDL and LDL. Nicotinic acid is actually very effective at lowering cholesterol levels, and its effect on the lipid profile is highly desirable. Because it has numerous side effects and large doses are required, as few as 20% of clients can initially tolerate niacin. However, with proper counseling, careful drug titration, and concomitant use of aspirin, this number can be increased to as high as 60% to 70%.

Ezetimibe (Zetia) is a cholesterol absorption inhibitor that acts on the cells in the small intestine to inhibit cholesterol absorption. It decreases cholesterol from dietary absorption, reducing serum cholesterol, LDL, triglycerides, and apoB levels. Ezetimibe causes only a small increase in HDL. It must be combined with a statin for optimum effect (ezetimibe and simvastatin [Zocor], marketed as Vytorin).

Statins

The statin drugs, first introduced in 1987, inhibit the enzyme HMG CoA reductase in cholesterol biosynthesis; thus the statins are called *HMG CoA reductase inhibitors*. By inhibiting cholesterol synthesis in the liver, this group of antilipidemics decreases the concentration of cholesterol, decreases LDL, and slightly increases HDL cholesterol. Reduction of LDL cholesterol may be seen as early as 2 weeks after initiating therapy. The statin group has been useful in decreasing CAD and reducing mortality rates.

Numerous statins have been approved in the past few years. The present group of statins includes atorvastatin calcium (Lipitor), fluvastatin (Lescol), lovastatin (Mevacor), pravastatin sodium (Pravachol), simvastatin (Zocor), and rosuvastatin calcium (Crestor). Lovastatin was the first statin used to decrease cholesterol. It is effective in lowering LDL (hyperlipidemia type II) within several weeks. Gastrointestinal (GI) disturbances, headaches, muscle cramps, and tiredness are early complaints. With all statins, serum liver enzymes should be monitored, and an annual eye examination is needed, because cataract formation may result. The client should report immediately any muscle aches or weakness which can lead to rhabdomyolysis, a muscle disintegration that can become fatal.

The statins have actions in decreasing serum cholesterol, LDL, VLDL, and triglycerides, and they slightly elevate HDL. Atorvastatin (Lipitor), lovastatin (Mevacor), and simvastatin (Zocor) are more effective at lowering LDL than the other statins. Atorvastatin (Lipitor) is the second most prescribed drug and simvastatin (Zocor) is the fifteenth most prescribed drug out of 200 commonly administered drugs.

Table 45–3
Hyperlipidemia: Lipoprotein Phenotype

Type	Major Lipids
I	Increased chylomicrons and increased triglycerides. Uncommon.
IIA	Increased low-density lipoprotein (LDL) and increased cholesterol. Common.
IIB	Increased very low-density lipoprotein (VLDL), increased LDL, increased cholesterol and triglycerides. Very common.
III	Moderately increased cholesterol and triglycerides. Uncommon.
IV	Increased VLDL and markedly increased triglycerides. Very common.
V	Increased chylomicrons, VLDL, and triglycerides. Uncommon.

Types II and IV are commonly associated with coronary artery disease.

The statin drugs can be combined with other drugs to decrease blood pressure and blood clotting and to enhance the antilipidemic effect. Examples are Advicor (lovastatin and niacin), Caduet (atorvastatin and amlodipine), Pravigard Pac (pravastatin and aspirin), and Vytorin (simvastatin and ezetimibe). These combination drugs, their doses, uses, and effects can be found in Table 45–4.

If antilipidemic therapy is withdrawn, cholesterol and LDL levels return to pretreatment levels. The client taking an antilipidemic should understand that antilipidemic drug therapy is a lifetime commitment for maintaining a decrease in serum lipid levels. Abruptly stopping the statin drug could cause the client to have a threefold rebound effect that may cause death from an AMI.

Table 45–4

Antilipidemics

Generic (Brand)	Route and Dosage	Uses and Considerations
Bile-Acid Sequestrants		
cholestyramine resin (Questran)	A: PO: 4 g t.i.d. a.c. and at bedtime; mix powder in 120-240 ml of fluid; *max:* 24 g/d	First antilipidemic ever produced. For type II hyperlipoproteinemia (LDL). Decrease in LDL apparent in 1 week. Drug powder should be mixed well in fluid. Has no effect on VLDL and HDL, but could increase triglyceride levels. GI upset and constipation can occur. Vitamin A, D, K deficiency may occur because of decreased GI absorption. *Pregnancy category:* C; PB: UK; t$^{1}/_{2}$: UK
colesevelam (Welchol)	A: PO: 3 tablets (625 mg/tablet) b.i.d. (6 tablets daily)	Cholesterol-lowering effect achieved by binding with bile salts in intestines to form insoluble complex with fecal excretions, reducing circulating cholesterol, including LDL. Triglycerides may be slightly increased. Contraindicated with bowel obstruction. May be used in combination with a statin drug. *Pregnancy category:* B; PB: UK; t$^{1}/_{2}$: UK
colestipol HCl (Colestid)	A: PO: 10-30 g/d in divided doses before meals	To reduce cholesterol and LDL levels. Same as cholestyramine. *Pregnancy category:* C; PB: UK; t$^{1}/_{2}$: UK
Fibrates (Fibric Acid)		
clofibrate (Atromid-S)	A: PO: 500 mg q.i.d.	For lowering cholesterol, VLDL, and triglycerides. For types IIB (VLDL), IV, V hyperlipidemia. Drug is more effective for higher cholesterol levels. Therapeutic effect occurs in 2-5 days. Drug should not be taken during pregnancy. Gallstones can occur with long-term use. *Pregnancy category:* C; PB: 90%-95%; t$^{1}/_{2}$: 12-25 h
fenofibrate (Tricor)	A: PO: 67-201 mg/day	Treatment of type IV and V hyperlipidemia, and for hypertriglyceridemia. Specified diet should be part of drug therapy. Monitor serum creatinine levels. *Pregnancy category:* C; PB: 99%; t$^{1}/_{2}$: 21 h
gemfibrozil (Lopid)	A: PO: 600 mg b.i.d. before meals; *max:* 1500 mg/day	For VLDL and elevated triglycerides; LDL may decrease and HDL may increase. For types II (VLDL, LDL), III, IV, V hyperlipidemia. Use in combination with lovastatin contraindicated because of increase in CPK. *Pregnancy category:* B; PB: >90%; t$^{1}/_{2}$: 1.5 h
Nicotinic Acid		
nicotinic acid (Niacin)	A: PO: Initially: 100 mg t.i.d.; maint: 1-3 g/day p.c. in 3 divided doses; *max:* 6 g/day	For VLDL and LDL: types II, III, IV, V hyperlipidemia. Doses are 100 times higher than RDA to lower VLDL. *Pregnancy category:* C; PB: UK; t$^{1}/_{2}$: 45 min
Cholesterol Absorption Inhibitor		
ezetimibe (Zetia)	A: PO: 10 mg daily	Inhibits cholesterol absorption in small intestine. Reduces total cholesterol, LDL, triglycerides. Increases HDL. *Caution* with liver dysfunction and elevated serum transaminase. *Pregnancy category:* C; PB: UK; t$^{1}/_{2}$: UK
Statins (HMG-CoA Reductase Inhibitors)		
atorvastatin calcium (Lipitor)	A: PO: 10 mg/day; *max:* 80 mg/day	To reduce hyperlipidemia (LDL, cholesterol, and triglycerides). May increase digoxin levels. *Caution* in clients with history of liver disease. *Pregnancy category:* X; PB: 98%; t$^{1}/_{2}$, 14 hours

A, Adult; *a.c.*, before meals; *b.i.d.*, twice a day; *CPK*, creatine phosphokinase; *d*, day; *GI*, gastrointestinal; *h*, hour; *HDL*, high-density lipoprotein; *LDL*, low-density lipoprotein; *maint*, maintenance; *max*, maximum; *min*, minute; *PB*, protein-binding; *p.c.*, after meals; *PO*, by mouth; *q.i.d.*, four times a day; *RDA*, recommended daily allowance; *t$^{1}/_{2}$*, half-life; *t.i.d.*, three times a day; *UK*, unknown; *VLDL:* very low-density lipoprotein; *>*, greater than.

Table 45–4

Antilipidemics—cont'd

Generic (Brand)	Route and Dosage	Uses and Considerations
fluvastatin sodium (Lescol)	A: PO: Initially: 20-40 mg at bedtime; maint: 20-80 mg/day	Treatment of types IIA and IIB hyperlipidemia, total cholesterol, and elevated triglycerides. HDL slightly increased. Monitor liver function (liver enzymes). *Pregnancy category:* X; PB: 98%; t$\frac{1}{2}$: 1.2 h
lovastatin (Mevacor)	A: PO: 20-80 mg/day in 1-2 divided doses with meals	Controls cholesterol by inhibiting cholesterol synthesis. Decreases LDL, increases some HDL. Liver enzymes should be monitored. *Pregnancy category:* X; PB: 95%; t$\frac{1}{2}$: 1-2 h
pravastatin sodium (Pravachol)	A: PO: 10-40 mg/day	Decreases serum cholesterol, LDL, VLDL, and triglycerides. HDL slightly increased. Monitor liver enzymes. *Pregnancy category:* X; PB: 55%; t$\frac{1}{2}$: 1.5-2.5 h
rosuvastatin calcium (Crestor)	A: PO: 5 to 40 mg/day; maint: 10 mg/day	Strong statin drug that cuts LDL in half for 52% of recipients. Reduces total cholesterol, LDL, triglycerides. Increases HDL. Serious complication is rhabdomyolysis; muscle pain and weakness should be reported. Liver enzymes should be monitored. *Pregnancy category:* X; PB: 88 %; t$\frac{1}{2}$: 19 h
simvastatin (Zocor)	A: PO: Initially: 5-10 mg/day in evening; maint: 20-80 mg/day in evening; *max:* 80 mg/day	Similar to lovastatin. Monitor liver enzymes. *Pregnancy category:* X; PB: 95%; t$\frac{1}{2}$: UK
Combination Anticholesterol Drugs		
niacin and lovastatin (Advicor)	A: PO: 500 mg niacin/20 mg lovastatin; Also: 750 mg/20 mg; 1000 mg/20 mg; 1000 mg/40 mg	Niacin raises HDL, triglycerides (TGs); lovastatin lowers LDL. Indicated for hypercholesterolemia and mixed dyslipidemia.
amlodipine and atorvastatin (Caduet)	A: PO: 2.5 mg amlodipine/20 mg atorvastatin/day; Also: 2.5 mg/40 mg; 5 mg/10 mg to 5 mg/80 mg; 10 mg/10 mg to 10 mg/80 mg	Combination of calcium channel blocker and statin. Useful in treating hypertension and dyslipidemia. Helpful to clients who take these drugs separately.
Pravigard Pac (aspirin and pravastatin)	A:PO: 81 mg aspirin/20 mg pravastatin/day; also: 81 mg/80 mg; 325 mg/20 mg to 325 mg/80 mg	Used to prevent myocardial infarction and strokes. Increased risk of bleeding, especially with higher aspirin dosages.
ezetimibe/simvastatin (Vytorin)	A: PO: 10/10 mg to 10/80 mg	Combination of ezetimibe (Zetia) and simvastatin (Zocor). Ezetimibe decreases absorption of cholesterol in small intestine; simvastatin interferes with production of cholesterol in liver.

Laboratory Tests

Homocysteine reference values: 4-17 mmol/L (fasting). Homocysteine, an amino acid, is a by-product of protein and is found in eggs, chicken, beef, and cheddar cheese. A high level of homocysteine has been linked to cardiovascular disease, stroke, and the possibility of Alzheimer's disease. It may also promote blood clotting. It has been stated that an increase in serum homocysteine can damage the inner lining of blood vessels and promote a thickening and loss of flexibility in the vessel. Three vitamins that can lower serum homocysteine levels are vitamin B$_6$ (pyridoxine), vitamin B$_{12}$ (cyanocobalamin), and folic acid.

High sensitivity C-reactive protein (hsCRP) reference values: less than 0.175 mg/L; low risk: less than 1 mg/L; moderate risk: 1-3 mg/L; high risk: greater than 3 mg/L. The standard C-Reactive Protein (CP) is a protein that is produced in the liver in response to tissue injury and inflammation. The hsCRP is a highly sensitive test for detecting the inflammatory protein that can be associated with cardiovascular and peripheral vascular disease. It is a test frequently ordered along with cholesterol screen testing. Approximately one third of persons who have had a heart attack have normal cholesterol levels and normal blood pressure. A positive hsCRP test can indicate that the client is at high risk for coronary artery disease (CAD), making it a valuable test for predicting CAD. This test can detect an inflammatory process caused by the build-up of atherosclerotic plaque in the arterial system, particularly the coronary arteries.

Prototype Drug Chart 45–1 lists the data for a frequently prescribed antilipidemic, atorvastatin (Lipitor).

Pharmacokinetics

Atorvastatin (Lipitor) decreases LDL by 25% with lower doses and by 55% with higher doses. It increases HDL, but not to the levels of some of the other statins (pravastatin and simvastatin). It decreases the triglyceride levels by 20% with lower doses and by 50% with higher doses,

Prototype DRUG CHART 45–1

ATORVASTATIN

Drug Class
Antilipidemic, HMG-CoA reductase inhibitor
Trade name: Lipitor
Pregnancy Category: X

Contraindications
Active liver disease, pregnancy
Caution: History of liver disease, increased
  alcohol ingestion, trauma, severe metabolic
  endocrine disorders, uncontrolled seizures

Dosage
A: PO: 10 mg/day; may increase dose up to 80 mg/day
C: Safety is not established

Drug-Lab-Food Interactions
Drug: Decrease effect with antacids, propranolol. May
  increase digoxin level, oral contraceptives. *Increase*
  effects with macrolide antibiotics, antifungals

Pharmacokinetics
Absorption: Rapid
Distribution: PB: 98%
Metabolism: t½: 14 hours; metabolites: 20-30 h
Excretion: Primarily in bile; some in urine

Pharmacodynamics
PO: Onset: 2 wk for decrease in cholesterol
  Peak: 1-2 h; 2-4 wk to be effective
  Duration: 24 h

Therapeutic Effects/Uses
To decrease cholesterol levels and to decrease serum lipids, especially LDL and triglycerides
Mode of Action: Inhibits HMG-CoA reductase, the enzyme necessary for hepatic production of cholesterol.

Side Effects
Rare
Headache, rash/pruritus, constipation/diarrhea,
  sinusitis, pharyngitis

Adverse Reactions
Rhabdomyolysis, myalgia, photosensitivity, cataracts

A, Adult; *C*, child; *h*, hour; *HMG-CoA*, 3-hydroxy-3-methyl-glutaryl coenzyme A; *PO*, by mouth; *PB*: protein-binding; *t½*: half-life; *LDL*, low-density lipoproteins; *wk*, week.

---

a greater reduction than with other statins. Atorvastatin is highly protein-bound, so it is usually prescribed as a once daily dose. It has a half-life of 14 hours, which is moderately long; the half-life for its metabolites is 20 to 30 hours.

Pharmacodynamics

The positive effect of lowering the lipids with atorvastatin is seen in about 2 weeks. The peak time after a dose of atorvastatin is 1 to 2 hours; however, it takes 2 to 4 weeks for therapeutic effect of the drug to be achieved. When the client is taking high doses of atorvastatin or any statins, myopathy and rhabdomyolysis (disintegration of striated muscle fibers) may occur. If client complains of muscle pain or tenderness, it should be reported immediately.

Side Effects and Adverse Reactions

Side effects and adverse reactions of cholestyramine include constipation and peptic ulcer. Constipation can be decreased or alleviated by increasing intake of fluids and foods high in fiber. Early signs of peptic ulcer are nausea and abdominal discomfort, followed later by abdominal pain and distention. To avoid GI discomfort, the drug must be taken with and followed by sufficient fluids.

The many side effects of nicotinic acid (e.g., GI disturbances, flushing of the skin, abnormal liver function [elevated serum liver enzymes], hyperglycemia, hyperuricemia) decrease its usefulness. However, as mentioned, aspirin and careful drug titration can reduce side effects to a manageable level in most clients.

The statin drugs can cause a dose-related increase in liver enzyme levels. Serum liver enzyme levels (alkaline phosphatase, alanine aminotransferase, gamma-glutamyl transferase) should be monitored. Baseline liver enzyme studies should be obtained before initiating statin drug therapy. A slight transient increase in a serum liver enzyme level may be within normal value for the client, but it should be rechecked in a week or so. Clients with acute hepatic disorder should not take a statin drug.

The serious skeletal muscle adverse effect known as *rhabdomyolysis* has been reported with the use of the statin drug class. Clients should be advised to promptly report to the health care provider any unexplained muscle tenderness or weakness, especially if accompanied by fever or malaise.

Table 45–4 lists the drug data for the antilipidemics.

Nursing Process

Antilipidemics (Statins)

ASSESSMENT

■ Assess vital signs and baseline serum chemistry values (cholesterol, triglycerides, aspartate aminotransferase [AST], alanine aminotransferase [ALT], creatine phosphokinase [CPK]).
■ Obtain a medical history. Atorvastatin and statin drugs are contraindicated for clients with a liver disorder. Pregnancy category is X.

NURSING DIAGNOSES

■ Impaired tissue integrity related to atherosclerosis because of hyperlipidemia
■ Anxiety related to elevated cholesterol level because of possible coronary artery disease

PLANNING

■ Client's cholesterol level will be less than 200 mg/dl in 6 to 8 weeks.
■ Client will be taught to choose foods low in fat, cholesterol, and complex sugars.

NURSING INTERVENTIONS

■ Monitor client's blood lipid levels (cholesterol, triglycerides, low-density lipoprotein [LDL], and high-density lipoprotein [HDL]) every 6 to 8 weeks for the first 6 months after any statin therapy, then every 3 to 6 months. For lipid level profile, client should fast for 12 to 14 hours. Desired cholesterol value is less than 200 mg/dl; triglyceride value is less than 150 mg/dl (can vary); LDL is less than 100 mg/dl; and HDL is greater than 60 mg/dl. Cholesterol levels of greater than 240 mg/dl, LDL levels of greater than 160 mg/dl, and HDL levels of less than 35 mg/dl can lead to severe cardiovascular event or cerebrovascular accident (CVA).
■ Monitor laboratory tests for liver function (ALT, ALP, and gamma-glutamyl transferase [GGT]). Antilipidemic drugs may cause liver disorder.
■ Observe for signs and symptoms of GI upset. Taking the drug with sufficient water or with meals may alleviate some of the GI discomfort.

Client Teaching

General

• Advise client that if there is a family history of hyperlipidemia, even children should have a baseline blood lipid level obtained and monitored. Instruct client that children should decrease fatty foods in the diet.

• Emphasize need to comply with drug regimen to lower blood lipids. Side effects should be reported to health care provider.
• Inform client that it may take several weeks before blood lipid levels decline. Explain that laboratory tests for blood lipids (cholesterol, triglycerides, LDL, and HDL) are usually ordered every 3 to 6 months.
• Advise client to have serum liver enzymes monitored as indicated by health care provider. Lovastatin, pravastatin, and simvastatin are contraindicated in acute hepatic disease and pregnancy.
• Instruct client to have an annual eye examination and to report changes in visual acuity.

Clofibrate, Gemfibrozil

• Advise client taking clofibrate that decreased libido and impotence may occur and should be reported. Drug dosage can be changed or another antilipidemic may be ordered.
• Instruct clients with diabetes or those at risk for developing diabetes to monitor blood glucose levels if they take gemfibrozil. Dietary changes or insulin adjustment may be necessary.

Nicotinic Acid

• Instruct client to take the drug with meals to decrease GI discomfort.

Self-Administration

Cholestyramine and Colestipol

• For cholestyramine and colestipol, instruct client to mix the powder well in water or juice.

Side Effects

Cholestyramine, Colestipol, and Nicotinic Acid (Niacin)

• Advise client that constipation may occur with cholestyramine and colestipol. Increasing fluid intake and food bulk should help to alleviate the problem.
• Explain to client that flush is common and should decrease with continued use of the drug. Usually the drug is started at a low dose.
• Advise client that large doses of nicotinic acid can cause vasodilation, producing dizziness and faintness (syncope).

Ezetimibe (Zetia)

• Explain to client that ezetimibe may cause headaches and GI upset. If it continues, notify the health care provider.

Statins

• Explain to client that serum liver enzyme levels are periodically monitored.
• Encourage client to report promptly any unexplained muscle tenderness or weakness that may be caused by rhabdomyolysis.
• Instruct client not to abruptly stop the statin drug, because a serious rebound effect might occur that could lead to an AMI and possible death. Before stop-

ping a statin, client should talk to his or her health care provider.

Diet

- Explain to client that GI discomfort is a common problem with most antilipidemics. Suggest increasing fluid intake when taking the medication.
- Instruct client to maintain a low-fat diet by eating foods that are low in animal fat, cholesterol, and complex sugars. Lovastatin and other antilipidemics are adjuncts to, not substitutes for, a low-fat diet.

Cultural Considerations ❖

- Respect client's belief of how to control his or her cholesterol level.
- Do not criticize folk practices; explanations and modification to plan of care may be necessary if the method client uses is not effective or is unsafe.

EVALUATION

- ▪ Evaluate the effectiveness of the antilipidemic drug. Client's cholesterol level is within desired range.
- ▪ Determine that client is on a low-fat, low-cholesterol diet.

Peripheral Vasodilators

A common problem in older adults is peripheral arterial (vascular) disease (PAD, PVD). It is characterized by numbness and coolness of the extremities, intermittent claudication (pain and weakness of limb when walking but no symptoms at rest), and possible leg ulcers. The primary cause is arteriosclerosis and hyperlipidemia, resulting in atherosclerosis. The arteries become occluded.

Peripheral vasodilators increase blood flow to the extremities. They are used in peripheral vascular disorders of venous and arterial vessels. They are more effective for disorders resulting from vasospasm (Raynaud's disease) than from vessel occlusion or arteriosclerosis (arteriosclerosis obliterans, thromboangiitis obliterans [Buerger's disease]). In Raynaud's disease, cold exposure or emotional upset can trigger vasospasm of the toes and fingers; these clients have benefited from vasodilators. Clients with diabetes mellitus are more likely to have PAD by two to four times the usual rate and are at risk of claudication.

Although the following drugs have different actions, they all promote vasodilation: tolazoline (Priscoline), isoxsuprine (Vasodilan), nicotinyl alcohol, and papaverine (Cerespan, Genabid). Nicotinyl alcohol and papaverine are direct-acting peripheral vasodilators. The alpha-blocker prazosin (Minipress) and the calcium channel blocker nifedipine (Procardia) have also been used as peripheral vasodilators.

Individuals with PAD who are treated with HMG-CoA reductase inhibitors (statins) for dyslipidemia may get improvement for claudication symptoms as well as a decrease in serum lipids. Also, clients with PAD who are hypertensive receive improvement for both conditions when taking the antihypertensive drug ramipril (Altace), an ACE inhibitor. The antiplatelet drugs clopidogrel (Plavix) and aspirin have been used to decrease PAD symptoms. Another antiplatelet drug, cilostazol (Pletal), has been approved by the Food and Drug Administration (FDA) for treating intermittent claudication. It decreases arterial thrombi. The herb ginkgo biloba, taken with an antiplatelet drug, has been used to treat intermittent claudication, because of its vasodilating and antioxidant effects, although this herb has not approved by the FDA. Most of the group of drugs used for treating PAD do not cure the health problem, but can aid in relieving PAD symptoms.

Isoxsuprine hydrochloride, a beta-adrenergic antagonist with slight alpha-adrenergic antagonist effects, is effective for relaxing the arterial walls within skeletal muscles. Prototype Drug Chart 45–2 gives the drug data for isoxsuprine.

Isoxsuprine

Pharmacokinetics

Isoxsuprine is readily absorbed from the GI tract. It has a short half-life of 1.25 to 1.5 hours, and because of this, the drug can be taken three to four times a day.

Pharmacodynamics

Isoxsuprine is a beta$_2$-adrenergic agonist. It causes vasodilation of arteries within the skeletal muscles. Bronchodilation may also occur. This drug has a short onset of action, peak time, and duration of action.

Side Effects and Adverse Reactions

Light-headedness, dizziness, orthostatic hypotension, tachycardia, palpitation, flush, and GI distress may occur.

The effectiveness of peripheral vasodilators in increasing blood flow by vasodilation is questionable in the presence of arteriosclerosis. These drugs may decrease some of the symptoms of cerebrovascular insufficiency. The drug data for the peripheral vasodilators are given in Table 45–5.

Pentoxifylline

Pentoxifylline (Trental), classified as a *hemorrheologic agent*, improves microcirculation and tissue perfusion by decreasing blood viscosity and improving the flexibility of erythrocytes, thus increasing tissue oxygenation. It inhibits aggregation of platelets and red blood cells and helps increase flow through peripheral vessels, because it decreases blood viscosity. It is a derivative of the xanthine group. Pentoxifylline has been approved by the FDA for clients with intermittent claudication and has been prescribed for those with Buerger's disease resulting from arterial occlusions. However, in one research study, pentoxifylline was not determined to be more effective than taking a placebo.

Reactions to an overdose of pentoxifylline include flushing of the skin, faintness, sedation, and GI disturbances. The drug should be taken with food. The client should avoid smoking, because nicotine increases vasoconstriction. Clients taking an antihypertensive drug along with pentoxifylline may need to have the antihypertensive dosage decreased to avoid side effects.

Prototype **DRUG CHART 45–2**

ISOXSUPRINE HCL

Drug Class	**Dosage**
Peripheral vasodilator Trade names: Vasodilan, Vasoprine *Pregnancy Category:* C	**A: PO:** 10-20 mg t.i.d.-q.i.d.
Contraindications	**Drug-Lab-Food Interactions**
Arterial bleeding, severe hypotension, postpartum, tachycardia *Caution:* Bleeding disorders, tachycardia	*Drug:* Decrease blood pressure with antihypertensives
Pharmacokinetics	**Pharmacodynamics**
Absorption: PO: Readily absorbed **Distribution:** PB: UK **Metabolism:** t½: 1.25-1.5 h **Excretion:** In urine	**PO:** Onset: 0.5 h Peak: 1 h Duration: 3 h

Therapeutic Effects/Uses

To increase circulation caused by peripheral vascular disease (Raynaud's disease, arteriosclerosis obliterans) and cerebrovascular insufficiency
Mode of Action: Acts directly on vascular smooth muscle

Side Effects	**Adverse Reactions**
Nausea, vomiting, dizziness, syncope, weakness, tremors, rash, flush, abdominal distention, chest pain	Hypotension, tachycardia, palpitations

A, Adult; *h,* hour; *PB,* protein-binding; *PO,* by mouth; *q.i.d.,* four times a day; *t½,* half-life; *t.i.d.,* three times a day; *UK,* unknown.

Nursing Process

Vasodilators, Isoxsuprine (Vasodilan)

ASSESSMENT

■ Obtain baseline vital signs for future comparison.
■ Assess for signs of inadequate blood flow to the extremities: pallor, coldness of extremity, and pain.

NURSING DIAGNOSES

■ Impaired tissue integrity related to insufficient blood supply
■ Acute pain related to inadequate blood flow to extremity

PLANNING

■ Client's blood flow to the extremities will improve, and client's pain will be controlled.

NURSING INTERVENTIONS

■ Monitor vital signs, especially blood pressure and heart rate. Tachycardia and orthostatic hypotension can be problematic with peripheral vasodilators.

Client Teaching

General
• Inform client that a desired therapeutic response may take 1.5 to 3 months.
• Advise client not to smoke; smoking increases vasospasm.
• Instruct client to use aspirin or aspirin-like compounds only with the health care provider's approval. Salicylates help to prevent platelet aggregation.

Side Effects
• Encourage client to change position slowly but frequently to avoid orthostatic hypotension. Orthostatic hypotension is common when taking high doses of a vasodilator.
• Instruct client to report side effects of isoxsuprine, such as flush, headaches, and dizziness.

Diet
• Suggest that client with gastrointestinal disturbances take isoxsuprine with meals.
• Advise client not to ingest alcohol with a vasodilator, because it may cause a hypotensive reaction.

Table 45–5

Peripheral Vasodilators

Generic (Brand)	Route and Dosage	Uses and Considerations
Alpha-Adrenergic Antagonists		
isoxsuprine HCl (Vasodilan)	(Prototype Drug Chart 45–2)	
tolazoline HCl (Priscoline HCl)	A: subQ/IM/IV: 10-50 mg q.i.d. NB: IV: Initially: 1-2 mg/kg, followed by 1-2 mg/kg/h for 24-48 h; initial dose effect: 30 min	For neonatal pulmonary hypertension. For vascular occlusive diseases in adults. Causes vasodilation and decreases peripheral resistance. Improves circulation in thromboangiitis obliterans, Raynaud's disease, frostbite, and peripheral vasospastic disorders. *Pregnancy category:* C; PB: UK; t½: A: 10 h, NB: 3-10 h
Direct-Acting Peripheral Vasodilators		
ergoloid mesylates (Hydergine)	A: PO/SL: 1 mg t.i.d.; dose may increase to 4-12 mg/d	For cerebrovascular insufficiency. To improve cognitive skills, self-care, and mood, especially in the older adult. SL tablets should be placed under the tongue. May cause GI distress, orthostatic hypotension. *Pregnancy category:* C; PB: UK; t½: 3-12 hours
nicotinyl alcohol (✿Ronigen)	A: PO: 150-300 mg b.i.d.	Acts as vasodilator. Can cause flush and orthostatic hypotension. *Pregnancy category:* UK; PB: UK; t½: UK
papaverine (Pavabid)	A: PO: 100-300 mg q12h or 150 mg q8h SR: 150 mg q12h; *max:* 300 mg q12h IV: 30-120 mg q3h PRN	For arterial spasms. Reduces ischemia of brain, heart, and peripheral vessels. One of the oldest vasodilators. Side effects: flush, GI upset, headaches, increased heart rate and respiration. *Pregnancy category:* C; PB: 90%; t½: 1.5 h
Hemorrheologic		
cilostazol (Pletal)	(See Table 44–3)	
pentoxifylline (Trental)	A: PO: 400 mg t.i.d. with meals	For peripheral vascular disorders. Alleviates intermittent claudication. Improves cerebral function for those with cerebrovascular insufficiency. May decrease stroke incidence for those having recurrent TIAs. *Pregnancy category:* C; PB: UK; t½: 0.5-1 h

A, Adult; *b.i.d.*, twice a day; *d*, day; *GI*, gastrointestinal; *h*, hour; *IM*, intramuscular, *IV*, intravenous; *NB*, newborn; *max*, maximum; *min*, minute; *PB*, protein-binding; *PO*, by mouth; *PRN*, as necessary; *q.i.d.*, four times a day; *subQ*, subcutaneous; *SL*, sublingual; *SR*, sustained-release tablet; *t½*, half-life; *TIA*, transient ischemic attack; *t.i.d.*, three times a day; *UK*, unknown; ✿, Canadian drug.

EVALUATION

- Evaluate the effectiveness of the isoxsuprine therapy; blood flow is increased in the extremities and pain has subsided.
- Client experiences no side effects from the prescribed drug.

KEY WEBSITES

Hyperlipidemia: www.cme.erep.uab.edu/onlineCourses/Hyperlipidemia_TX/ID0346.html
Lipid-lowering treatment: www.nhlbi.nih.gov/health/allhat/
Cholesterol: http://www.nhlbi.nih.gov/health/prof/heart/index.htm#chol

Critical Thinking Case Study

JH had a myocardial infarction (MI) 3 years ago. He was prescribed gemfibrozil (Lopid) 600 mg, twice daily, before meals. His cholesterol remained between 220 and 240 mg/dl and his LDL 140 mg/dl. His anticholesterol drug was changed to simvastatin (Zocor) 20 mg/day in the evening.

1. How does simvastatin differ from gemfibrozil?
2. Why do you think JH's cholesterol drug, gemfibrozil, was changed to simvastatin?
3. While JH is taking simvastatin, which group of serum levels should be monitored?
4. How long after JH took simvastatin should his cholesterol and lipoproteins be checked?
5. What is the maximum dose for simvastatin?
6. JH complains of muscle pain and muscle weakness. What might this indicate?
7. Could JH receive both gemfibrozil and simvastatin? Explain.
8. JH is on vacation and does not have enough simvastatin tablets. What should he do?

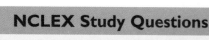

NCLEX Study Questions

1. JR has a serum cholesterol level of 265 mg/dl, triglyceride 235 mg/dl, and LDL 180 mg/dl. These serum levels indicate:
   a. hypolipidemia
   b. normolipidemia
   c. hyperlipidemia
   d. alipidemia

2. The client's cholesterol level should be:
   a. 150 to 200 mg/dl
   b. 200 to 225 mg/dl
   c. 225 to 250 mg/dl
   d. Greater than 250 mg/dl

3. TS's high-density lipoprotein (HDL) is 60 mg/dl. This is:
   a. lower than the desired level of HDL
   b. desired level of HDL
   c. higher than the desired level for HDL
   d. very low HDL level than desired

4. The laboratory tests ordered to determine the presence of the amino acid that can contribute to cardiovascular disease and stroke is:
   a. antidiuretic hormone
   b. homocysteine
   c. ceruloplasmin
   d. cryoglobulin

5. Which serum levels should be monitored when the client is taking a statin drug?
   a. Blood urea nitrogen
   b. Complete blood count
   c. Cardiac enzymes
   d. Liver enzymes

6. What severe skeletal muscle adverse reaction could occur when taking statins?
   a. Myasthenia gravis
   b. Rhabdomyolysis
   c. Dyskinesia
   d. Agranulocytosis

7. A new bile acid sequestrant drug that has fewer side effects than others in the same category is:
   a. clofibrate
   b. cholestyramine
   c. colesevelam
   d. gemfibrozil

8. A client is diagnosed with peripheral arterial disease (PAD). He is prescribed isoxsuprine HCl. The action of isoxsuprine HCl is to:
   a. relax the arterial walls within the skeletal muscles
   b. increase tissue oxygen in the vessels
   c. increase the rigid arteriosclerotic blood vessels
   d. increase intermittent claudication

Answers: 1, c; 2, a; 3, b; 4, b; 5, d; 6, b; 7, c; 8, a.

FIFTEEN

Gastrointestinal Agents

The gastrointestinal (GI) system (tract), comprising the alimentary canal and the digestive tract, begins at the oral cavity of the mouth and ends at the anus. Major structures of the GI system are (1) the oral cavity (mouth, tongue, and pharynx), (2) the esophagus, (3) the stomach, (4) the small intestine (duodenum, jejunum, and ileum), (5) the large intestine (cecum, colon, and rectum), and (6) the anus. The accessory organs and glands that contribute to the digestive process are (1) the salivary glands, (2) the pancreas, (3) the gallbladder, and (4) the liver (Figure XV–1). The main functions of the GI system are digestion of food particles and absorption of the digestive contents (nutrients, electrolytes, minerals, and fluids) into the circulatory system for cellular use. Digestion and absorption take place in the small intestine and to a lesser extent in the stomach. Undigested material passes through the lower intestinal tract with the aid of peristalsis to the rectum and anus, where it is excreted as feces, or stool.

Oral Cavity

The oral cavity, or mouth, starts the digestive process by (1) breaking up food into smaller particles; (2) adding saliva, which contains the enzyme amylase for digesting starch (the beginning of the digestive process); and (3) swallowing, a voluntary movement of food that becomes involuntary (peristalsis) in the esophagus, stomach, and intestines. Swallowing occurs in the pharynx (throat), which connects the mouth and esophagus.

Esophagus

The esophagus, a tube that extends from the pharynx to the stomach, is composed of striated muscle in its upper portion and smooth muscle in its lower portion. The inner lining of the esophagus is a mucous membrane that secretes mucus. The peristaltic process of contraction begins in the esophagus and ends in the lower large intestine. There are two sphincters, the superior esophageal (hyperpharyngeal) sphincter and the lower esophageal sphincter. The lower esophageal sphincter prevents gastric reflux into the esophagus, a condition called *reflux esophagitis*.

Stomach

The stomach is a hollow organ that lies between the esophagus and the intestine. The body of the stomach has lesser and greater curvatures. It can hold 1000 to 2000 ml of gastric contents and empties in 2 to 6 hours (average is 3 to 4 hours), depending on gastric content and motil-

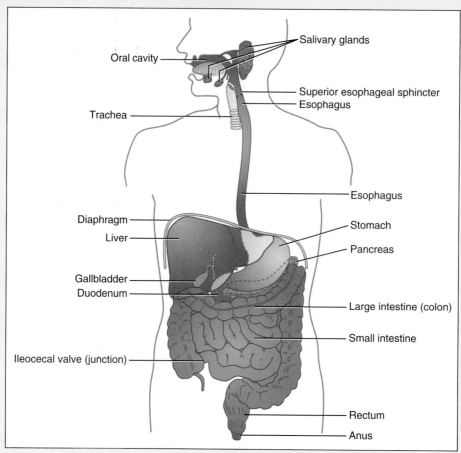

FIGURE XV–I The gastrointestinal system and alimentary canal.

ity. Two sphincters, the *cardiac sphincter*, which lies at the upper opening of the stomach, and the *pyloric sphincter*, located at the lower portion of the stomach or the head of the duodenum, regulate the entrance of food into the stomach.

The interior lining of the stomach has mucosal folds that contain glands that secrete gastric juices. The four types of cells in the stomach mucosa that secrete these juices are (1) *chief cells*, which secrete the proenzyme pepsinogen (pepsin); (2) *parietal cells*, which secrete hydrochloric acid (HCl); (3) *gastrin-producing cells*, which secrete gastrin, a hormone that regulates enzyme release during digestion; and (4) *mucus-producing cells* that release mucus to protect the stomach lining, which extends into the duodenum.

Small Intestine

The small intestine begins at the pyloric sphincter of the stomach and extends to the ileocecal valve at the cecum. Most drug absorption occurs in the duodenum, but lipid-soluble drugs and alcohol are absorbed from the stomach. The lower digestive process begins in the stomach, but most of the digestive contents are absorbed from the small intestine. The duodenum releases the hormone secretin, which suppresses gastric acid secretion, causing the intestinal juices to have a higher pH than the gastric juices. The intestinal cells also release the hormone cholecystokinin, which in turn stimulates the release of pancreatic enzymes and the contrac-

tion of the gallbladder to release bile into the duodenum. Hormones, bile, and pancreatic enzymes (trypsin, chymotrypsin, lipase, and amylase) complete the digestion of carbohydrates, protein, and fat in preparation for absorption.

Large Intestine

The large intestine accepts undigested material from the small intestine, absorbs water, secretes mucus, and with peristaltic contractions moves the remaining intestinal contents to the rectum for elimination. Defecation completes the process.

Drugs for Gastrointestinal Disorders

Vomiting, diarrhea, and constipation are GI problems that frequently require drug intervention. Chapter 46, Drugs for Gastrointestinal Tract Disorders, describes the antiemetics used to control vomiting. This chapter also discusses emetics used to eliminate ingested toxins and drugs, antidiarrheal drugs, and laxatives. The nursing process is considered in relation to each of these drug groups.

Chapter 47, Antiulcer Drugs, discusses drugs used to prevent and treat peptic ulcers (gastric and duodenal). These drugs include tranquilizers, anticholinergics, antacids, histamine₂ blockers, proton pump inhibitors, a pepsin inhibitor, and a prostaglandin analogue antiulcer drug.

46

Drugs for Gastrointestinal Tract Disorders

ELECTRONIC RESOURCES

evolve

Evolve website (http://evolve.elsevier.com/KeeHayes/pharmacology/):
- *Case Studies*
- *Content Updates*
- *Frequently Asked Questions*
- *Student Review Activities*
- *WebLinks*
- *Additional Reference Material*

Companion CD-ROM:
- *NCLEX Examination Review Questions*
- *Pharmacology Animations*
- *IV Therapy Checklists*
- *Medication Error Checklists*
- *Drug Calculation Problems*
- *Electronic Calculators*
- *Top 200 Drugs with Pronunciations*
- *References from the Textbook*

Outline

Objectives

- Compare causes of vomiting, diarrhea, and constipation.
- Explain the actions and side effects of antiemetics, emetics, antidiarrheals, and laxatives.
- Apply the nursing process for the client taking antiemetics, antidiarrheals, and laxatives.
- Describe contraindications to the use of antiemetics, emetics, antidiarrheals, and laxatives.

Terms

Drug groups used to correct or control vomiting, diarrhea, and constipation are antiemetics, emetics, antidiarrheals, and laxatives. Each of these drug groups is discussed separately. Drugs used to treat peptic ulcers are discussed in Chapter 47.

Vomiting

Vomiting (emesis), the expulsion of gastric contents, has a multitude of causes, including motion sickness, viral and bacterial infection, food intolerance, surgery, pregnancy, pain, shock, effects of selected drugs (e.g., antineoplastics), radiation, and disturbances of the middle ear that affect equilibrium. Nausea, a queasy sensation, may or may not precede the expulsion. The cause of the vomiting must be identified. Antiemetics can mask the underlying cause of vomiting and should not be used until the cause has been determined, unless the vomiting is so severe as to cause dehydration and electrolyte imbalance.

Two major cerebral centers—the **chemoreceptor trigger zone (CTZ)**, which lies near the medulla, and the **vomiting center** in the medulla—cause vomiting when stimulated (Figure 46–1). The CTZ receives most of the impulses from drugs, toxins, and the vestibular center in the ear and transmits them to the vomiting center. The neurotransmitter dopamine stimulates the CTZ, which in turn stimulates the vomiting center. Levodopa, a drug with dopamine-like properties, can cause vomiting by stimulating the CTZ. Some sensory impulses, such as odor, smell, taste, and gastric mucosal irritation, are transmitted directly to the vomiting center. The neurotransmitter acetylcholine is also a vomiting stimulant. When the vomiting center is stimulated, the motor neuron responds by causing contraction of the diaphragm, the anterior abdominal muscles, and the stomach. The glottis closes, the abdominal wall moves upward, and vomiting occurs.

Nonpharmacologic measures should be used first when nausea and vomiting occur. If the nonpharmacologic measures are not effective, antiemetics are combined with nonpharmacologic measures. The two major groups of antiemetics are *nonprescription* (antihistamines, bismuth subsalicylate, phosphorated carbohydrate solution) and *prescription* (antihistamines, dopamine antagonists, benzodiazepines, serotonin antagonists, glucocorticoids, cannabinoids, and miscellaneous antiemetics).

Nonpharmacologic Measures

The nonpharmacologic methods of decreasing nausea and vomiting include administration of weak tea, flattened carbonated beverage, gelatin, Gatorade, and Pedialyte (for use in children). Crackers and dry toast may be helpful. When dehydration becomes severe, intravenous (IV) fluids are needed to restore body fluid balance.

Nonprescription Antiemetics

Nonprescription **antiemetics** (antivomiting agents) can be purchased as over-the-counter (OTC) drugs. These drugs are frequently used to prevent motion sickness but have minimal effect on controlling severe vomiting resulting from anticancer agents (antineoplastics), radiation, and toxins. To prevent motion sickness, the antiemetic should be taken 30 minutes before travel. These drugs are not effective in relieving motion sickness if taken after vomiting has occurred.

Selected antihistamine antiemetics such as dimenhydrinate (Dramamine), cyclizine hydrochloride (Marezine), meclizine hydrochloride (Antivert), and diphenhydramine hydrochloride (Benadryl) can be purchased OTC to prevent nausea, vomiting, and dizziness (vertigo) caused by motion. These drugs inhibit vestibular stimulation in the middle ear. Benadryl is also used to prevent or alleviate allergic reactions to drugs, insects, and food by acting as an antagonist to the histamine$_1$ (H$_1$) receptors.

The side effects of antihistamine antiemetics are similar to those of anticholinergics: drowsiness, dryness of the mouth, and constipation. Table 46–1 lists the nonprescription antihistamines used for vomiting caused by motion sickness.

Several nonprescription drugs such as bismuth subsalicylate (Pepto-Bismol) act directly on the gastric mucosa to suppress vomiting. They are marketed in liquid and chewable tablet forms and can be taken for gastric discomfort or diarrhea. Phosphorated carbohydrate solution (Emetrol), a hyperosmolar carbohydrate, decreases nausea and vomiting by changing the gastric pH; it may also decrease smooth-muscle contraction of the stomach. Its effectiveness as an antiemetic has not been verified. Clients with diabetes mellitus should avoid this drug because of its high sugar content.

Antiemetics were once frequently used for the treatment of nausea and vomiting during the first trimester of pregnancy, but they are no longer recommended, because they may cause harm to the fetus. Instead, nonpharmacologic methods should be used to alleviate nausea and vomiting during pregnancy, and OTC antiemetics should be avoided. If vomiting becomes severe and threatens the well-being of the mother and fetus, an antiemetic such as trimethobenzamide (Tigan) can be administered, although this drug is classified as *pregnancy category C*. Other antiemetics may be prescribed cautiously.

Prescription Antiemetics

Common prescription antiemetics are classified into the following groups: (1) antihistamines, (2) anticholinergics, (3) dopamine antagonists, (4) benzodiazepines, (5) serotonin

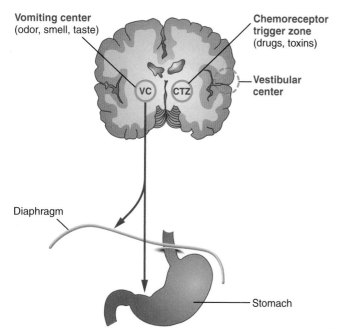

FIGURE 46–1 The chemoreceptor trigger zone and vomiting center.

Labels: Vomiting center (odor, smell, taste); Chemoreceptor trigger zone (drugs, toxins); Vestibular center; VC; CTZ; Diaphragm; Stomach

Table 46–1

Nonprescription Antiemetics: Antihistamine

Generic (Brand)	Route and Dosage	Uses and Considerations
Motion Sickness		
cyclizine HCl (Marezine)	A: PO: 50 mg 0.5 h before travel; may repeat in 4-6 h; *max:* 200 mg/d IM: 50 mg q4-6h PRN C: 6-12 y: PO: 25 mg daily/ t.i.d. *Postoperative vomiting:* A: IM: 50 mg 0.5 h before surgery ends; may repeat q4-6h PRN	Similar to buclizine. Has been used for postoperative nausea and vomiting. *Pregnancy category:* B; PB: UK; $t\frac{1}{2}$: UK
dimenhydrinate (Calm-X, Dimetabs, Dramamine)	A: PO: 50-100 mg q4-6h; *max:* 400 mg/d; IM/IV: 50 mg PRN C: 6-12 y: PO: 25-50 mg PRN; *max:* 150 mg/d C: <2 y: Not recommended	Primarily used to prevent motion sickness. Drowsiness, dizziness, dry mouth, and hypotension may occur. *Pregnancy category:* B; PB: UK; $t\frac{1}{2}$: UK
meclizine HCl (Antivert, Antrizine, Bonine)	A & C >12 y: PO: 25-50 mg 1 h before travel, after meal; may repeat q24h Vertigo: A: PO: 25-100 mg/d in divided doses	Prevention of nausea, vomiting, and dizziness. Drowsiness and dry mouth may occur. *Pregnancy category:* B; PB: UK; $t\frac{1}{2}$: 6 h

A, Adult; *C,* child; *d,* day; *h,* hour; *IM,* intramuscular; *max,* maximum; *PB,* protein-binding; *PO,* by mouth; *PRN,* as needed; *$t\frac{1}{2}$,* half-life; *t.i.d.,* three times a day; *UK,* unknown; *y,* year; *>,* greater than; *<,* less than.

antagonists, (6) glucocorticoids, (7) cannabinoids (for clients with cancer), and (8) miscellaneous. Many of these drugs act as antagonists to dopamine, histamine, serotonin, and acetylcholine, which are associated with vomiting. Antihistamines and anticholinergics act primarily on the vomiting center; they also act by decreasing stimulation of the CTZ and vestibular pathways. The cannabinoids act on the cerebral cortex. Phenothiazines and the miscellaneous antiemetics, such as diphenidol, metoclopramide, and trimethobenzamide, act on the CTZ center. Drug combination therapy is commonly used to manage chemotherapy-induced nausea and vomiting. Lorazepam (Ativan), glucocorticoids, and serotonin (5-HT₃) receptor antagonists are quite effective in combination therapy. Lorazepam, haloperidol, and glucocorticoids are not approved by the Food and Drug Administration (FDA) as antiemetics but are extremely effective when combined for this unlabeled use.

Antihistamines and Anticholinergics

Only a few prescription antihistamines and anticholinergics are used in the treatment of nausea and vomiting. Table 46–2 lists these drugs and their dosages, uses, and considerations.

Side Effects and Adverse Reactions

Side effects include drowsiness, which can be a major problem, dry mouth, blurred vision caused by pupillary dilation, tachycardia (with anticholinergic use), and constipation. These drugs should *not* be used by clients with glaucoma.

Dopamine Antagonists

These agents suppress emesis by blocking dopamine₂ receptors in the CTZ. The categories of dopamine antagonists include phenothiazines, butyrophenones, and metoclo-

pramide. Common side effects of dopamine antagonists are extrapyramidal symptoms (EPS), which are caused by blocking dopamine receptors, and hypotension. See Chapter 26 for a more detailed description of EPS and phenothiazines.

Phenothiazine Antiemetics

Selected piperazine phenothiazines are used to treat nausea and vomiting resulting from surgery, anesthetics, chemotherapy, and radiation sickness. They act by inhibiting the CTZ. When used in clients with cancer, these drugs are commonly given the night before treatment, the day of the treatment, and for 24 hours after treatment. Not all phenothiazines are effective antiemetic agents. When prescribed for vomiting, the drug dosage is usually smaller than when used for psychiatric disorders.

Chlorpromazine (Thorazine) and prochlorperazine edisylate (Compazine) were the first phenothiazines used for both psychosis and vomiting. Promethazine (Phenergan), a phenothiazine introduced as an antihistamine in the 1940s, has a sedative effect and can also be used for motion sickness and management of nausea and vomiting. Promethazine is the most frequently prescribed antiemetic drug. Prototype Drug Chart 46–1 describes the action and effects of promethazine.

Pharmacokinetics

Promethazine is readily absorbed in the gastrointestinal (GI) tract. It has 60% to 90% protein-binding capacity. Promethazine is metabolized by the liver and excreted in urine and feces.

Pharmacodynamics

Promethazine blocks the H₁-receptor sites on effector cells and impedes histamine-mediated responses. The onset of action of oral and intramuscular (IM) administration is 20 minutes, and the duration of action is from 2 to 8 hours. The onset of action of intravenous (IV) promethazine is 5 minutes; the duration of action is the same as the oral preparation.

Table 46–2

Prescription Antiemetics

Generic (Brand)	Route and Dosage	Uses and Considerations
Prescription Antihistamines		
hydroxyzine (Vistaril, Atarax)	A: PO/IM: 25-100 mg t.i.d. or q.i.d. PRN	For postoperative nausea and vomiting, vertigo (dizziness). Given preoperatively with narcotics to decrease nausea. Give hydroxyzine deep IM. Drowsiness and dry mouth usually occur. *Pregnancy category:* C; PB: UK; $t\frac{1}{2}$: 3 h
promethazine (Phenergan)	(Prototype Drug Chart 46–1)	
Anticholinergic		
scopolamine (Transderm-Scop)	A: transdermal patch: 1.5 mg (1 mg dose over 3 days)	For motion sickness. Numerous anticholinergic side effects (dizziness, drowsiness, dry mouth, constipation). Apply patch behind ear at least 4 hours before antiemetic effect is required. Patch is effective for 3 days. Alternate ears if using for longer than 3 days. Wash hands after applying patch disc. Wear no more than one disc/patch at a time. *Pregnancy category:* C; PB: <25%; $t\frac{1}{2}$: 8 h
Dopamine Antagonists		
Phenothiazines		
prochlorperazine maleate (Compazine)	A: PO/IM: 5-10 mg t.i.d.-q.i.d., PRN (give deep IM) SR: 10 mg q12h PR: 5-25 mg PRN C: PO/Rect: 2.5 mg b.i.d.-t.i.d.	Primary use is for severe nausea and vomiting. Secondary use is to reduce anxiety and tension and for psychosis. Drowsiness, dizziness, EPS, and dry mouth may occur. *Pregnancy category:* C; PB: >90%; $t\frac{1}{2}$: 23 h
promethazine (Phenergan)	(Prototype Drug Chart 46–1)	
Butyrophenones		
droperidol (Inapsine)	A: IM/IV: 2.5-10 mg, 0.5-1 h before surgery C: 2-12 y: IM/IV: 0.088-0.165 mg/kg, 0.5-1 h before surgery C: <2 y: Not recommended	Prevention of nausea and vomiting during surgical and diagnostic procedures. May cause hypotension, tachycardia, and EPS. *Pregnancy category:* C; PB: UK; $t\frac{1}{2}$: 2.5 h
Benzodiazepines		
lorazepam (Ativan)	A: PO: 2-6 mg/d in 2-3 divided doses; *max:* 10 mg/d	For prevention of nausea and vomiting resulting from cancer chemotherapy. It is usually administered with an antiemetic such as metoclopramide. *Pregnancy category:* D; PB: 85%; $t\frac{1}{2}$: 10-20 h
Serotonin (5-HT₃) Receptor Antagonists		
dolasetron mesylate (Anzemet)	*Cancer chemotherapy:* A: PO/IV: 100 mg, 1 h before chemotherapy C: >2 y: PO/IV: 1.8 mg/kg 1 h before chemotherapy A & C: PO/IV: *max:* 100 mg	To prevent nausea and vomiting before chemotherapy. Drug can also be used pre- and postoperatively to prevent and treat nausea and vomiting. Acts on serotonin 5-HT₃ receptor in stomach and CTZ. *Pregnancy category:* B; PB: UK; $t\frac{1}{2}$: 10 min to 7 h
granisetron (Kytril)	A: PO: 1 mg b.i.d. (1 h before and 12 h after chemotherapy) A: IV: 10 mcg/kg/30 min before chemotherapy	Prevention of nausea and vomiting caused by cancer chemotherapy. Acts on the CTZ and vomiting center. Headache may occur. *Pregnancy category:* B; PB: 65%; $t\frac{1}{2}$: 4-10 h
ondansetron HCl (Zofran)	A: PO: 8 mg b.i.d. (first dose 30 min before, then 8 h and 16 h after chemotherapy) A: IV: 0.15 mg/kg/30 min before, then 4 and 8 h after chemotherapy (total, 3 doses)	For nausea and vomiting related to cancer chemotherapy, especially treatment with cisplatin. *Pregnancy category:* B; PB: 70%-75%; $t\frac{1}{2}$: 4 h
palonosetron (Aloxi)	A: IV: 0.25 mg over 30 sec, 30 min before chemotherapy	To prevent nausea and vomiting associated with cancer chemotherapy. *Pregnancy category:* B; PB: 62%; $t\frac{1}{2}$: 40 h

A, Adult; *a.c.*, before meals; *AIDS*, acquired immunodeficiency syndrome; *b.i.d.*, two times a day; *C*, child; *CNS*, central nervous system; *CSS*, Controlled Substances Schedule; *CTZ*, chemoreceptor trigger zone; *d*, day; *EPS*, extrapyramidal symptoms; *h*, hour; *IM*, intramuscular; *IV*, intravenous; *max*, maximum; *min*, minute; *PB*, protein-binding; *PO*, by mouth; *PR*, per rectum; *PRN*, as needed; *q.i.d.*, four times a day; *sec*, second; *SR*, sustained release; *t½*, half-life; *t.i.d.*, three times a day; *UK*, unknown; *y*, year; *>*, greater than; *<*, less than.

Table 46-2

Prescription Antiemetics—cont'd

Generic (Brand)	Route and Dosage	Uses and Considerations
Cannabinoids		
dronabinol (Marinol) CSS II	*Chemotherapy-induced nausea:* A: PO: 5 mg/m^2 1-3 h before chemotherapy; then q2-4h after; *max:* 15 mg/m^2/dose	For nausea and vomiting caused by cancer chemotherapy. Taken before and for 24 hours after chemotherapy. Can be an appetite stimulant for clients with AIDS. Common side effects include drowsiness, dizziness, dry mouth, impaired thinking, and euphoria. *Pregnancy category:* B; PB: 98%; t$\frac{1}{2}$: 20-24 h
Miscellaneous		
diphenidol HCl (Vontrol)	*Nausea, vomiting, and vertigo:* A: PO: 25-50 mg q4h PRN; *max:* 300 mg/d C: >6 y: PO: 0.9 mg/kg; *max:* 5.5 mg/kg/d	For nausea, vomiting, and vertigo related to Ménière's disease and middle ear surgery. *Pregnancy category:* C; PB: UK; t$\frac{1}{2}$: 4 h
metoclopramide HCl (Reglan)	A: PO: 10 mg a.c. and at bedtime IV: 1-2 mg/kg 30 min before chemotherapy; then repeat q2h for two doses; then q3h for three doses; infuse diluted solution over not less than 15 min	For nausea and vomiting related to cancer chemotherapy treatment. Increases gastric and intestinal emptying. Avoid alcohol and CNS depressants. EPS may occur. *Pregnancy category:* B; PB: 30%; t$\frac{1}{2}$: 4-7 h
trimethobenzamide HCl (Tigan, Arrestin, Ticon)	A: PO: 250 mg t.i.d.-q.i.d. IM: 200 mg t.i.d.-q.i.d. C: 15-40 kg: PO: 15-20 mg/kg/d divided in three to four doses or 100-200 mg, t.i.d.-q.i.d.	For postoperative nausea and vomiting, motion sickness, and vertigo. Avoid with CNS depressants and if sensitive to benzocaine or similar local anesthetics. *Pregnancy category:* C; PB: UK; t$\frac{1}{2}$: UK
aprepitant (Emend)	A: PO: 125 mg on day 1, 80 mg on days 2 and 3	For nausea and vomiting related to cancer chemotherapy. *Pregnancy category:* B; PB: 95%; t$\frac{1}{2}$: 9-13 h

Drug and Laboratory Interactions

Central nervous system (CNS) depression increases when promethazine is taken with alcohol, narcotics, sedative-hypnotics, and general anesthetics. Anticholinergic effects increase when promethazine is combined with antihistamines, anticholinergics such as atropine, and other phenothiazines. Promethazine may interfere with urinary pregnancy tests, producing false results.

Side Effects and Adverse Reactions

Phenothiazines have antihistamine and anticholinergic properties. The side effects of phenothiazine antiemetics are moderate sedation, hypotension, EPS, CNS effects (restlessness, weakness, dystonic reactions, agitation), and mild anticholinergic symptoms (dry mouth, urinary retention, constipation). Because the dose is lower for vomiting than for psychosis, the side effects are not so severe. Promethazine is relatively free of EPS at antiemetic doses. Table 46-2 lists drug data for phenothiazines and other prescription antiemetics.

Butyrophenones

Haloperidol (Haldol) and droperidol (Inapsine), like phenothiazines, block the dopamine$_2$ receptors in the CTZ. They are used to treat postoperative nausea and the vomiting and emesis associated with toxins, cancer chemotherapy, and radiation therapy. Antiemetic doses of haloperidol are smaller than those required for antipsychotic effects. Like phenothiazines, haloperidol and droperidol are likely to cause EPS if used for an extended time. Hypotension may result; therefore blood pressure should be monitored.

Metoclopramide

Metoclopramide (Reglan) suppresses emesis by blocking the dopamine receptors in the CTZ. It is used in the treatment of postoperative emesis, cancer chemotherapy, and radiation therapy. High doses can cause sedation and diarrhea. With this agent, the occurrence of EPS is more prevalent in children than in adults. Metoclopramide should not be given if the client has GI obstruction, hemorrhage, or perforation.

Benzodiazepines

Selected benzodiazepines indirectly control nausea and vomiting that may occur with cancer chemotherapy. Lorazepam (Ativan) is the drug of choice. Previously diazepam (Valium) was the preferred benzodiazepine. Lorazepam effectively provides emesis control, sedation, anxiety reduction, and amnesia when used in combination with a glucocorticoid and serotonin 5-HT$_3$ receptor antagonist.

Serotonin (5-HT$_3$) Receptor Antagonists

Serotonin antagonists suppress nausea and vomiting by blocking the serotonin receptors (5-HT$_3$) in the CTZ and the afferent vagal nerve terminals in the upper GI tract.

Prototype **DRUG CHART 46–1**

PROMETHAZINE HCl

Drug Class	**Dosage**
Antiemetic: Phenothiazine	**A: PO/PR/IM/IV:** 12.5-25 mg q4-6h PRN
Trade name: Phenergan	**C: PO/PR/IM/IV:** 0.25-0.5 mg/kg q4-6h PRN
Pregnancy Category: C	

Contraindications	**Drug-Lab-Food Interactions**
Hypersensitivity, narrow-angle glaucoma, severe liver disease, intestinal obstruction, blood dyscrasias, bone marrow depression	***Drug:*** Increases CNS depression and anticholinergic effects when taken with alcohol and other CNS depressants
Caution: Cardiovascular disease, liver dysfunction, asthma, respiratory dysfunction, hypertension, elderly and debilitated clients	***Lab:*** False pregnancy test

Pharmacokinetics	**Pharmacodynamics**
Absorption: PO: easily absorbed from GI tract	**PO:** Onset: 20 min
Distribution: PB: 60%-90%	Peak: UK
Metabolism: t½: UK	Duration: 2-8 h
Excretion: In urine and feces	**IM:** Onset: 20 min
	Peak: UK
	Duration: 2-8 h
	IV: Onset: 5 min
	Peak: UK
	Duration: 2-8 h
	PR: Onset: 20 min
	Peak: UK
	Duration: 2-8 h

Therapeutic Effects/Uses

To treat and prevent motion sickness, nausea, and vomiting
Mode of Action: Blocks H_1 receptor sites; inhibits chemoreceptor trigger zone

Side Effects	**Adverse Reactions**
Drowsiness, confusion, anorexia, dry mouth and eyes, constipation, blurred vision, photosensitivity, hypertension, hypotension, transient leukopenia, urinary retention	Extrapyramidal syndrome (tardive dyskinesia, akathisia)
	Life-threatening: Agranulocytosis, respiratory depression

A, Adult; *C*, child; *CNS*, central nervous system; *GI*, gastrointestinal; *h*, hour; *IM*, intramuscular; *IV*, intravenous; *min*, minute; *PB*, protein-binding; *PO*, by mouth; *PR*, per rectum; *PRN*, as needed; *t½*, half-life; *UK*, unknown.

Serotonin antagonists—ondansetron (Zofran), granisetron (Kytril), dolasetron (Anzemet), and palonosetron (Aloxi)—are the most effective of all antiemetics in suppressing nausea and vomiting caused by cancer chemotherapy-induced emesis or emetogenic anticancer drugs. Ondansetron (the first serotonin antagonist), granisetron, and dolasetron do not block the dopamine receptors; therefore, they do not cause EPS as do the phenothiazine antiemetics. These drugs can be administered orally and IV. Ondansetron (Zensana) is a form that is available in an oral spray delivery system. They are also effective in preventing nausea and vomiting before and after surgery. Common side effects include headache, diarrhea, dizziness, and fatigue.

Glucocorticoids (Corticosteroids)

Dexamethasone (Decadron) and methylprednisolone (Solu-Medrol) are two agents that are effective in suppressing emesis associated with cancer chemotherapy. Because these glucocorticoids are administered IV and for only a short while, side effects normally associated with glucocorticoids are minimized. Glucocorticoids are discussed in Chapter 50.

Cannabinoids

Cannabinoids, the active ingredients in marijuana, were approved for clinical use in 1985 to alleviate nausea and vomiting resulting from cancer treatment. These agents may be prescribed for clients receiving chemotherapy who do not respond to or are unable to take other antiemetics. They are contraindicated for clients with psychiatric disorders. Cannabinoids can be used as an appetite stimulant for clients with acquired immunodeficiency syndrome (AIDS). The cannabinoid dronabinol (Marinol) is described in Table 46-2.

Side Effects and Adverse Reactions

Side effects occurring as a result of cannabinoid use include mood changes, euphoria, drowsiness, dizziness, headaches, depersonalization, nightmares, confusion, incoordination, memory lapse, dry mouth, orthostatic hypotension or hypertension, and tachycardia. Less common symptoms are depression, anxiety, and manic psychosis.

Miscellaneous Antiemetics

Diphenidol (Vontrol) and trimethobenzamide (Tigan) are in the class of miscellaneous antiemetics, because they do not act strictly as antihistamines, anticholinergics, or phenothiazines. These drugs suppress impulses to the CTZ. Diphenidol also prevents vertigo by inhibiting impulses to the vestibular area.

Side Effects and Adverse Reactions

The side effects and adverse reactions of the miscellaneous antiemetics are drowsiness and anticholinergic symptoms (dry mouth, increased heart rate, urine retention, constipation, blurred vision). Trimethobenzamide can cause hypotension, diarrhea, and EPS (abnormal involuntary movements, postural disturbances, and alteration in muscle tone).

Table 46-2 lists drug data for the miscellaneous antiemetics along with other prescription antiemetics.

 Nursing Process

Antiemetics

ASSESSMENT

- Determine a history of the onset, frequency, and amount of vomiting and contents of the vomitus. If appropriate, elicit from client possible causative factors such as food (seafood, mayonnaise).
- Obtain a history of present health problems. Clients with glaucoma should avoid many of the antiemetics.
- Record vital signs for abnormalities and for future comparison.
- Assess urinalysis before and during therapy.

NURSING DIAGNOSES

- Imbalanced nutrition: less than body requirements related to inability to ingest food
- Risk for deficient fluid volume related to vomiting

PLANNING

- Client will adhere to nonpharmacologic methods and/or drug regimen to alleviate vomiting
- Client's underlying cause of vomiting will be corrected
- Client will retain small amounts of food

NURSING INTERVENTIONS

- Check vital signs. If vomiting is severe, dehydration may occur, and shocklike symptoms may be present.
- Monitor bowel sounds for hypoactivity or hyperactivity.
- Provide mouth care after vomiting. Encourage client to maintain oral hygiene.

Client Teaching

General

- Instruct client to store drug in airtight, light-resistant container if required.
- Teach client to avoid OTC preparations.
- Direct client not to consume alcohol while taking antiemetics. Alcohol can intensify the sedative effect.
- Advise pregnant women to avoid antiemetics during the first trimester because of possible teratogenic effects on the fetus. Encourage pregnant women to seek medical advice about OTC or prescription antiemetics.

Side Effects

- Tell client to report sore throat, fever, and mouth sores; notify health care provider and have blood drawn for a complete blood count (CBC).
- Alert client to avoid driving a motor vehicle or engaging in dangerous activities, because drowsiness is common with antiemetics. If drowsiness becomes a problem, a decrease in dosage may be indicated.
- Warn client with a hepatic disorder to seek medical advice before taking phenothiazines. Instruct client to report dizziness.
- Suggest to client nonpharmacologic methods of alleviating nausea and vomiting such as flattened carbonated beverages, weak tea, crackers, and dry toast.

Cultural Considerations ❖

- Respect clients' cultural beliefs and alternative methods for treating nausea and vomiting. Discuss with clients the safety of their methods, other nondrug methods, and the purpose of an antiemetic if prescribed.
- An interpreter may be needed to assist non–English-speaking clients to understand the drug schedule for prescribed antiemetics and their side effects.

EVALUATION

- Evaluate the effectiveness of nonpharmacologic methods or antiemetic by noting the absence of vomiting. Identify any side effects that may result from drug.

Emetics

Emetics are drugs used to induce vomiting. When an individual has consumed certain toxic substances, induced vomiting (emesis) may be indicated to expel the substance before absorption occurs. There are many ways to induce vomiting without using drugs, such as putting the finger in the back part of the throat.

Vomiting should not be induced if caustic substances, such as ammonia, chlorine bleach, lye, toilet cleaners, or battery acid, have been ingested. Regurgitating these substances can cause additional injury to the esophagus. To prevent aspiration, vomiting should also be avoided if petroleum distillates are ingested; these include gasoline, kerosene, paint thinners, and lighter fluid. Activated charcoal is given when emesis is contraindicated.

Ipecac

Administration of ipecac has diminished greatly but it is still used when indicated. The American Academy of Clinical Toxicology, the European Association of Poisons Control Centers, and Clinical Toxicologists issued guidelines in 2004 that ipecac syrup should not be administered routinely in the management of poisoned individuals. Ipecac may be appropriate for the client who is alert and if administered within 60 minutes of poisoning.

When the client purchases ipecac, instruct the client to get ipecac *syrup* and *not* ipecac fluid extract, which is more potent and may cause fatalities. When ipecac is kept in the household, it should be kept out of the reach of children. Ipecac syrup induces vomiting by stimulating the CTZ in the medulla and acting directly on the gastric mucosa. Ipecac should be taken with a glass of water (do not give with milk or carbonated beverages). The onset of emesis production following administration of ipecac syrup is usually 15 to 30 minutes. When vomiting is not induced, clients should be treated with an adsorbent, such as activated charcoal, or gastric lavage (Table 46–3). Individuals with bulimia and

anorexia nervosa often abuse ipecac, which may lead to cardiomyopathy, ventricular fibrillation, and death.

Diarrhea

Diarrhea (frequent liquid stool) is a symptom of an intestinal disorder. Causes include (1) foods (spicy, spoiled), (2) fecal impaction, (3) bacteria (*Escherichia coli, Salmonella*) or virus (parvovirus, rotavirus), (4) toxins, (5) drug reaction, (6) laxative abuse, (7) malabsorption syndrome caused by lack of digestive enzymes, (8) stress and anxiety, (9) bowel tumor, and (10) inflammatory bowel disease such as ulcerative colitis or Crohn's disease. Diarrhea can be mild to severe. Antidiarrheals are not to be used for more than 2 days and should not be used if fever is present.

Because intestinal fluids are rich in water, sodium, potassium, and bicarbonate, diarrhea can cause minor or severe dehydration and electrolyte imbalances. The loss of bicarbonate places the client at risk for developing metabolic acidosis. Clients with diarrhea should avoid milk products and foods rich in fat. Diarrhea can develop very quickly and can be life threatening to young clients and older adults, who may not be able to compensate for the fluid and electrolyte losses.

Nonpharmacologic Measures

The cause of diarrhea should be identified. Nonpharmacologic treatment for diarrhea is recommended until the underlying cause can be determined. This includes use of clear liquids and oral solutions (Gatorade; Pedialyte or Rehydralyte [both for use in children]) and IV electrolyte solutions. Antidiarrheal drugs are frequently used in combination with nonpharmacologic treatment.

Traveler's Diarrhea

Traveler's diarrhea, also called *acute diarrhea* and *Montezuma's revenge*, is usually caused by *E. coli*. It ordinarily lasts less than 2 days; however, if it becomes severe, fluoroquinolone anti-

Table 46–3

Emetics and Adsorbent		
Generic (Brand)	**Route and Dosage**	**Uses and Considerations**
Emetics		
ipecac syrup (OTC preparation)	A: PO: 15-30 ml, followed by 200-300 ml tepid water C: >12 y: PO: 15 ml, followed by 200-300 ml tepid water C: <1 y: PO: 5-10 ml, followed by 100-200 ml tepid water	Induces vomiting after poisoning. Should be given within 60 minutes of poisoning to an alert and conscious individual. *Pregnancy category:* C; PB: NA; t½: 2 hr
Adsorbent		
charcoal (CharcoAid, CharcoCaps)	*For poisoning, use CharcoAid:* A: PO: 30-100 g dose in 6-8 oz of water *For flatus, use CharcoCaps:* A: PO: 520 mg, after meals; repeat PRN; *max:* 4 g/d	Promotes absorption of poison/toxic substances. Promotes absorption of intestinal gas. Neither drug is systemically absorbed. *Pregnancy category:* C; PB: NA; t½: NA

A, Adult; *C,* child; *CNS,* central nervous system; *d,* day; *max,* maximum; *NA,* not applicable; *OTC,* over-the-counter; *PB,* protein-binding; *PO,* by mouth; *PRN,* as necessary; *t½,* half-life.

biotics are usually prescribed. Loperamide (Imodium) may be used to slow peristalsis and decrease the frequency of defecation, but it can also slow the exit of the organism from the GI tract. Traveler's diarrhea can be reduced by drinking bottled water, washing fruit, and eating cooked vegetables. Meats should be cooked until well done.

Antidiarrheals

There are various **antidiarrheals** for treating diarrhea and decreasing hypermotility (increased peristalsis). Usually there is an underlying cause of the diarrhea that needs to be corrected as well. The antidiarrheals are classified as (1) opiates and opiate-related agents, (2) somatostatin analogue, (3) adsorbents, and (4) miscellaneous antidiarrheals.

Opiates and Opiate-Related Agents

Opiates decrease intestinal motility, thereby decreasing peristalsis. Constipation is a common side effect of opium preparations. Examples are tincture of opium, paregoric (camphorated opium tincture), and codeine. Opiates are frequently combined with other antidiarrheal agents. Opium antidiarrheals can cause CNS depression when taken with alcohol, sedatives, or tranquilizers. Duration of action of opiates is approximately 2 hours.

Diphenoxylate (Lomotil, Reasec [available in Europe]) is an opiate that has less potential for causing drug dependence than other opiates such as codeine. Difenoxin (Motofen) is an active metabolite of diphenoxylate, but it is more potent than diphenoxylate. Both drugs are combined with atropine to decrease abdominal cramping, intestinal motility, and hypersecretion. Lomotil (diphenoxylate with atropine) is frequently prescribed for "traveler's diarrhea," and Motofen (difenoxin with atropine) is prescribed to treat nonspecific and chronic diarrhea. With prolonged use of these drugs, physical dependence may occur. Diphenoxylate antidiarrheal products are approximately 50% atropine, which will discourage drug abuse. The action and effects of diphenoxylate with atropine (Lomotil) are listed in Prototype Drug Chart 46-2.

Loperamide (Imodium) is structurally related to diphenoxylate but causes less CNS depression than diphenoxylate and difenoxin. It can be purchased as an OTC drug, and it protects against diarrhea, reduces fecal volume, and decreases intestinal fluid and electrolyte losses.

Clients with severe hepatic impairment should not take products containing diphenoxylate, difenoxin, or loperamide. Children and older adults who take diphenoxylate

---

Prototype DRUG CHART 46-2

DIPHENOXYLATE WITH ATROPINE

Drug Class

Antidiarrheal
Trade name: Lomotil
Pregnancy Category: C
CSS V

Contraindications

Severe hepatic or renal disease, glaucoma, severe electrolyte imbalance; children <2 y

Dosage

A: PO: 2.5-5 mg b.i.d.-q.i.d. PRN
C: >2 y: PO: 0.3-0.4 mg/kg/d in 4 divided doses. Use only liquid form (2.5 mg diphenoxylate, 0.025 mg atropine per 5 ml) and product dropper for children <13 y

Drug-Lab-Food Interactions

Drug: Increase CNS depression with alcohol, antihistamines, narcotics, sedative-hypnotics; MAOIs may *enhance* hypertensive crisis
Lab: Increase serum liver enzymes, amylase

Pharmacokinetics

Absorption: PO: Well absorbed
Distribution: PB: UK
Metabolism: t½: 2.5 h
Excretion: In feces and urine

Pharmacodynamics

PO: Onset: 45-60 min
Peak: 2 h
Duration: 3-4 h

Therapeutic Effects/Uses

To treat diarrhea by slowing intestinal motility
Mode of Action: Inhibition of gastric motility

Side Effects

Drowsiness, dizziness, constipation, dry mouth, weakness, flush, rash, blurred vision, mydriasis, urine retention

Adverse Reactions

Angioneurotic edema
Life-threatening: Paralytic ileus, toxic megacolon, severe allergic reaction

A, Adult; *b.i.d.,* twice a day; *C,* child; *CNS,* central nervous system; *CSS,* Controlled Substances Schedule; *d,* day; *h,* hour; *MAOIs,* monoamine oxidase inhibitors; *min,* minute; *PB,* protein-binding; *PO,* by mouth; *PRN,* as necessary; *q.i.d.,* four times a day; *t½,* half-life; *UK,* unknown; *y,* years; >, greater than; <, less than.

are more susceptible to respiratory depression than other age groups.

Pharmacokinetics

Diphenoxylate with atropine is well absorbed from the GI tract. The diphenoxylate is metabolized by the liver mainly as metabolites. There are two half-lives: 2.5 hours for diphenoxylate and 3 to 20 hours for the diphenoxylate metabolites. The drug is excreted in the feces and urine.

Pharmacodynamics

Diphenoxylate with atropine is an opium agonist with anticholinergic properties (atropine); it decreases GI motility (peristalsis). It has a moderate onset of action of 45 to 60 minutes, and the duration of action is 3 to 4 hours. Many side effects are caused by the anticholinergic atropine. Clients with severe glaucoma should take another antidiarrheal that does not have an anticholinergic effect. If this drug is taken with alcohol, narcotics, or sedative-hypnotics, CNS depression can occur.

Somatostatin Analog

Octreotide (Sandostatin) is a somatostatin analogue that is prescribed to inhibit gastric acid, pepsinogen, gastrin, cholecystokinin, and serotonin secretions and intestinal fluid. In addition, it decreases smooth-muscle contractility. It is frequently prescribed for severe diarrhea resulting from metastatic cancer.

Adsorbents

Adsorbents act by coating the wall of the GI tract and adsorbing bacteria or toxins that cause diarrhea. Adsorbent antidiarrheals include kaolin and pectin. These agents are combined in Kaopectate, a mild or moderate antidiarrheal that can be purchased OTC and used in combination with other antidiarrheals. An example is Parepectolin, which contains paregoric (an opiate) and Kaopectate (an adsorbent). Bismuth salts (Pepto-Bismol) are considered adsorbents because they adsorb bacterial toxins. They can also be used as antacids for gastric discomfort. Pepto-Bismol is an OTC drug commonly used to treat traveler's diarrhea. Colestipol and cholestyramine (Questran) are prescription drugs that have been used to treat diarrhea due to excess bile acids in the colon. They are effective, although they have not been approved by the Food and Drug Administration for that purpose. Table 46–4 lists the drug data for antidiarrheal adsorbents.

Miscellaneous Antidiarrheals

Various miscellaneous antidiarrheals are prescribed to control diarrhea. These drugs include furazolidone, lactobacillus, and Parepectolin (paregoric, kaolin, pectin, alcohol). Table 46–4 includes other antidiarrheals.

Antidiarrheals

ASSESSMENT

■ Obtain a history of any viral or bacterial infection, drugs taken, and foods ingested that could be contribut-

ing factors to diarrhea. Many antidiarrheals are contraindicated if client has liver disease, narcotic dependence, ulcerative colitis, or glaucoma.

■ Check vital signs to provide baseline for future comparison and to determine body fluid and electrolyte losses.

■ Determine frequency and consistency of bowel movements.

■ Assess bowel sounds. Hyperactive sounds can indicate increased intestinal motility.

■ Report if client has a narcotic drug history. If opiate or opiate-related antidiarrheals are given, drug misuse or abuse may occur.

NURSING DIAGNOSES

■ Diarrhea related to laxative abuse
■ Imbalanced nutrition: less than body requirements related to misconceptions regarding OTC drugs
■ Risk for imbalanced fluid volume related to diarrhea

PLANNING

■ Client will have bowel movements that are formed.
■ Client's body fluids will be restored.

NURSING INTERVENTIONS

■ Record vital signs. Report tachycardia or systolic blood pressure decrease of 10 to 15 mmHg. Monitor respirations. Opiates and opiate-related drugs can cause central nervous system (CNS) depression.

■ Monitor frequency of bowel movements and bowel sounds. Notify health care provider if intestinal hypoactivity occurs when taking drug.

■ Check for signs and symptoms of dehydration resulting from persistent diarrhea. Fluid replacement may be necessary. With prolonged diarrhea, check serum electrolytes.

■ Administer antidiarrheals cautiously to clients with glaucoma, liver disorders, or ulcerative colitis or to pregnant women.

■ Recognize that drug may need to be withheld if diarrhea continues for more than 48 hours or acute abdominal pain develops.

Client Teaching

General

• Instruct client not to take sedatives, tranquilizers, or other narcotics with drug. CNS depression may occur.
• Inform client to avoid OTC preparations; they may contain alcohol.
• Advise client to take the drug only as prescribed. Drug may be habit-forming; do not exceed recommended dose.
• Encourage client to drink clear liquids.

Table 46–4

Antidiarrheals: Opiates and Opiate-Related, Somatostatin Analogue, Adsorbents, and Miscellaneous

Generic (Brand)	Route and Dosage	Uses and Considerations
Opiates and Opiate-Related		
camphorated opium tincture (paregoric) CSS III	Camphorated: 5-10 ml b.i.d.-q.i.d. C: PO: 0.25-0.5 ml/kg daily-q.i.d.	To decrease incidence of diarrhea. Decreases GI peristalsis. *Pregnancy category:* B (D at term); PB: UK; t¹/₂: 2-3 h
deodorized opium tincture CSS II	A: PO: 0.6 ml or 10 gtt q.i.d. mixed with water; *max:* 6 ml/d C: PO: 0.005-0.01 ml/kg/dose q3-4 h; *max:* 6 doses/d	For acute, nonspecific diarrhea. To treat withdrawal symptoms in neonates of mothers who are addicted to opiates. Not to be used for diarrhea caused by poison. Avoid taking alcohol and CNS depressants. *Pregnancy category:* B (D at term); PB: UK; t¹/₂: 2-3 h
difenoxin and atropine (Motofen) CSS IV	A: PO: Initially: 2 mg; then 1 mg after each loose stool; *max:* 8 mg/d for 2 d C: <2 y: Not recommended	For acute nonspecific and chronic diarrhea. Combination of a synthetic narcotic and atropine. Avoid use in narrow-angle glaucoma. Dry mouth, flush, and tachycardia may occur. *Pregnancy category:* C; PB: UK; t¹/₂: 12-24 h
loperamide HCl (Imodium)	A: PO: Initially: 4 mg; then 2 mg after each loose stool; *max:* 16 mg/d C: 2-5 y: PO: 1 mg t.i.d. C: 6-8 y: PO: 2 mg b.i.d. C: 9-12 y: PO: 2 mg t.i.d.	For diarrhea. Newest OTC drug. Does not affect the CNS. Less than 1% reaches systemic circulation. *Pregnancy category:* B; PB: 98%; t¹/₂: 7-12 h
Somatostatin Analog		
octreotide acetate (Sandostatin)	*Diarrhea related to carcinoid tumors:* A: subQ: Initially 0.05-0.1 mg/d (50-100 mcg/d) in divided doses for 2 wk; then increase according to response; maint: 0.1-0.6 mg/d (100-600 mcg/d) in two to four divided doses; *max:* 0.75 mcg/d (750 mcg/d)	For severe diarrhea resulting from metastatic carcinoid tumors. Suppresses secretion of serotonin, gastrin, and pancreatic peptides. *Pregnancy category:* B; PB: 65%; t¹/₂: 1.5 h
Adsorbents		
bismuth salts (Pepto-Bismol)	*Prevention of traveler's diarrhea:* A: PO: 2 tab q.i.d. a.c. and at bedtime *Treatment:* A: PO: 2 tab or 30 ml q30-60min PRN	For diarrhea, gastric distress. OTC liquid and tablet form. *Pregnancy category:* UK; PB: UK; t¹/₂: UK
kaolin-pectin (Kapectolin, Kaopectate)	A: 60-120 ml after each loose stool C: 6-12 y: 30-60 ml after each loose stool	For diarrhea. Administered after each loose stool. OTC drug. *Pregnancy category:* B; PB: 97%; t¹/₂: 7-14 h
Miscellaneous		
furazolidone (Furoxone)	A: PO: 100 mg q.i.d.; *max:* 400 mg/d C: >1 mo: PO: 5-8 mg/kg/d in four divided doses C: >5 y: 25-50 mg q.i.d.	Management of diarrhea and enteritis caused by bacteria or protozoa. Common side effects include nausea and vomiting. *Pregnancy category:* C; PB: UK; t¹/₂: UK
Parepectolin CSS V	A & C: .12 y: 15-30 ml after each loose stool; *max:* 120 ml/d C: 6-12 y: 5-10 ml after each loose stool; *max:* 40 ml/d	Combination paregoric (an opiate) and Kaopectate. OTC drug, but must be signed for at pharmacy because of opium content. *Pregnancy category:* D; PB: UK; t¹/₂: UK
rifaximin (Xifaxan)	A: PO: 200 mg t.i.d. for 3 days	For treatment of travelers' diarrhea caused by noninvasive strains of *E. coli*. *Pregnancy category:* C; PB: UK; t¹/₂: 5-6 hr

A, Adult; *a.c.*, before meals; *b.i.d.*, twice a day; *C*, child; *CNS*, central nervous system; *CSS*, Controlled Substances Schedule; *d*, day; *GI*, gastrointestinal; *h*, hour; *max*, maximum; *min*, minute; *mo*, month; *OTC*, over-the-counter; *PB*, protein-binding; *PO*, by mouth; *PRN*, as needed; *q.i.d.*, four times a day; *subQ*, subcutaneous; *t¹/₂*, half-life; *tab*, tablet; *t.i.d.*, three times a day; *UK*, unknown; *wk*, week; *y*, year; *>*, greater than; *<*, less than.

- Advise client not to ingest fried foods or milk products until after the diarrhea has stopped.
- Teach client that constipation can result from overuse of antidiarrheal drugs.

Cultural Considerations ❖

- While the more traditional and older individuals in some cultures do not maintain eye contact, the acculturated and more educated usually do maintain eye contact. Do not assume that lack of eye contact means that client is not listening or does not care. It might indicate respect.

EVALUATION

■ Evaluate the effectiveness of the drug; diarrhea has stopped.

■ Monitor long-term use of opiates and opiate-related drugs for possible abuse and physical dependence.

■ Continue to monitor vital signs. Report abnormal changes.

Constipation

Constipation (accumulation of hard fecal material in the large intestine) is a relatively common complaint and a major problem for older adults. Insufficient water intake and poor dietary habits are contributing factors. Other causes include (1) fecal impaction, (2) bowel obstruction, (3) chronic laxative use, (4) neurologic disorders (paraplegia), (5) ignoring the urge to defecate, (6) lack of exercise, and (7) selected drugs, such as anticholinergics, narcotics, and certain antacids.

Nonpharmacologic Measures

Nonpharmacologic management includes diet (high fiber), water, exercise, and routine bowel habits. A "normal" number of bowel movements ranges between one to three a day to three a week. What is normal varies from person to person; the nurse should determine what normal bowel habits are for each client. At times a laxative may be needed, but the client should also use nonpharmacologic measures to prevent constipation.

Laxatives

Laxatives and **cathartics** are used to eliminate fecal matter. Laxatives promote a soft stool, cathartics result in a soft to watery stool with some cramping, and frequently dosage determines whether a drug acts as a laxative or cathartic. Since these terms are often used interchangeably, *laxative* will cover both classes in this chapter. **Purgatives** are "harsh" cathartics that cause a watery stool with abdominal cramping. There are four types of laxatives: (1) osmotics (saline), (2) stimulants (contact or irritants), (3) bulk-forming, and (4) emollients (stool softeners).

Laxatives should be avoided if there is any question that the client may have intestinal obstruction; if abdominal pain is severe; or if symptoms of appendicitis, ulcerative colitis, or diverticulitis are present. Most laxatives stimulate peristalsis. Laxative abuse from chronic use is a common problem, especially in older adults. Laxative dependence can become a problem, so client teaching is an important nursing responsibility.

Osmotic (Saline) Laxatives

Osmotics (hyperosmolar laxatives) include salts or saline products, lactulose, and glycerin. Saline products consist of sodium or magnesium, and a small amount is systemically absorbed. Serum electrolytes should be monitored to avoid electrolyte imbalance. Hyperosmolar salts pull water into the colon and increase water in the feces to increase bulk, which stimulates peristalsis. Saline cathartics cause a semiformed to watery stool according to low or high doses. Good renal function is needed to excrete any excess salts. Saline cathartics are contraindicated for clients with heart failure.

Osmotic laxatives contain three types of electrolyte salts, including (1) sodium salts (sodium phosphate or Phospho-Soda, sodium biphosphate); (2) magnesium salts (magnesium hydroxide [milk of magnesia], magnesium citrate, magnesium sulfate [Epsom salt]); and (3) potassium salts (potassium bitartrate, potassium phosphate). High doses of salt laxatives are used for bowel preparation for diagnostic and surgical procedures. Another laxative used for bowel preparation is polyethylene glycol (PEG) with electrolytes, marketed as *GoLYTELY*. With PEG, however, a large volume of solution, approximately 3 to 4 liters over 3 hours, must be ingested. Clients may be advised to keep GoLYTELY refrigerated to make it more palatable. The positive aspect is that the solution is an isotonic, nonabsorbable osmotic substance that contains sodium salts and potassium chloride; thus it can be used by clients with renal impairment or cardiac disorder.

Lactulose, another saline laxative that is not absorbed, draws water into the intestines to form a soft stool. It decreases the serum ammonia level and is useful in liver diseases, such as cirrhosis. Glycerin acts like lactulose, increasing water in the feces in the large intestine. The bulk that results from the increased water in the feces stimulates peristalsis and defecation.

Side Effects and Adverse Reactions

Adequate renal function is needed to excrete excess magnesium. Clients who have renal insufficiency should avoid magnesium salts. Hypermagnesemia can result from continuous use of magnesium salts, causing symptoms such as drowsiness, weakness, paralysis, complete heart block, hypotension, flush, and respiratory depression.

The side effects of excess lactulose use include flatulence, diarrhea, abdominal cramps, nausea, and vomiting. Clients who have diabetes mellitus should avoid lactulose, because it contains glucose and fructose.

Stimulant (Contact) Laxatives

Stimulant (contact or irritant) laxatives increase peristalsis by irritating sensory nerve endings in the intestinal mucosa. Types include those containing phenolphthalein (Ex-Lax, Feen-A-Mint, Correctol), bisacodyl (Dulcolax), cascara sagrada, senna (Senokot), and castor oil (purgative). Bisacodyl and phenolphthalein are two of the most frequently used and abused laxatives and can be purchased OTC. Results usually occur 6 to 12 hours after ingestion. Bisacodyl and several others of these drugs are used to empty the bowel before diagnostic tests (barium enema). Prototype Drug Chart 46–3 gives the pharmacologic data for the stimulant laxative bisacodyl.

Castor oil is a harsh laxative (purgative) that acts on the small bowel and produces a watery stool. The action is quick, within 2 to 6 hours, so the laxative should not be taken at bedtime. Castor oil is seldom used to correct constipation. It is used mainly for bowel preparation.

Pharmacokinetics

The contact laxative bisacodyl is minimally absorbed from the GI tract. It is excreted in feces, but because of the small amount of bisacodyl absorption, a portion is excreted in urine.

Pharmacodynamics

Bisacodyl promotes defecation. Bisacodyl irritates the colon, causing defecation, and psyllium compounds increase fecal bulk and peristalsis. The onset of action of oral bisacodyl occurs within 6 to 12 hours and with the suppository (rectal administration), within 15 to 60 minutes.

Side Effects and Adverse Reactions

Side effects include nausea, abdominal cramps, weakness, and reddish brown urine caused by excretion of phenolphthalein, senna, or cascara.

With excessive and chronic use of bisacodyl, fluid and electrolyte (especially potassium and calcium) imbalances are likely to occur. Systemic effects occur infrequently, because absorption of bisacodyl is minimal. Mild cramping and diarrhea are side effects of bisacodyl.

Castor oil should not be used in early pregnancy, because it stimulates uterine contraction. Spontaneous abortion may result. Prolonged use of senna can damage nerves, which may result in loss of intestinal muscular tone. Table 46–5 lists the osmotic and stimulant laxatives.

Bulk-Forming Laxatives

Bulk-forming laxatives are natural fibrous substances that promote large, soft stools by absorbing water into the intestine, increasing fecal bulk and peristalsis. These

---

Prototype DRUG CHART 46–3

BISACODYL

Drug Class	**Dosage**
Laxative: Stimulant Trade names: Dulcolax; ✹Apo-Bisacodyl, Bisacolax *Pregnancy Category:* C	**A:** PO: 5-15 mg in AM or PM PRN; max: 30 mg **C:** >6 y: PO: 5-10 mg; 0.3 mg/kg/d **A & C:** >2 y: Rectal supp: 5-10 mg/d **C** <2 y, infants: 5 mg

Contraindications	**Drug-Lab-Food Interactions**
Hypersensitivity, fecal impaction, intestinal/biliary obstruction, appendicitis, abdominal pain, nausea, vomiting, rectal fissures	***Drug:*** *Decrease* effect with antacids, histamine₂ blockers, milk

Pharmacokinetics	**Pharmacodynamics**

Absorption: Minimal (5%-15%)
Distribution: PB: UK
Metabolism: t½: UK
Excretion: In bile and urine
	PO: Onset: 10-15 min
	  Peak: UK
	  Duration: 6-12 h
	PR: Onset: 15-60 min
	  Peak: UK
	  Duration: 6-12 h

Therapeutic Effects/Uses

Short-term treatment for constipation; bowel preparation for diagnostic tests
Mode of Action: Increases peristalsis by direct effect on smooth muscle of intestine

Side Effects	**Adverse Reactions**
Anorexia, nausea, vomiting, cramps, diarrhea	Dependence, hypokalemia ***Life-threatening:*** Tetany

A, Adult; *C,* child; *d,* day; *h,* hour; *max,* maximum; *min,* minute; *PB,* protein-binding; *PO,* by mouth; *PR,* per rectum; PRN, as needed; *supp,* suppository; *t½,* half-life; *UK,* unknown; *y,* year; >, greater than; <, less than; ✹, Canadian drug name.

Table 46–5

Laxatives: Osmotic (Saline) and Stimulant

Generic (Brand)	Route and Dosage	Uses and Considerations
Osmotics: Saline		
glycerin	A: Supp: 3 g C: <6 y: Supp: 1-1.5 g	To relieve constipation. Use with caution for clients with cardiac, renal, or liver disease and for the elderly or dehydrated. *Pregnancy category:* C; PB: UK; $t^{1/2}$: 30-45 min
lactulose (Cephulac, Chronulac, Enulose)	*Chronic constipation:* A: PO: 30-60 ml/d PRN C: PO: 7.5 ml/d after breakfast	For constipation. Also used in liver disease for ammonia elimination. May be used for constipation after barium studies. Poorly absorbed. *Pregnancy category:* C; PB: UK; $t^{1/2}$: UK
magnesium citrate (Citroma, Evac-Q-Mag)	A: PO: 120-240 ml C: PO: 4 ml/kg/dose or half adult dose	For constipation or to complete bowel elimination before diagnostic procedures and surgery. *Pregnancy category:* UK; PB: UK; $t^{1/2}$: UK
magnesium hydroxide (milk of magnesia)	A: PO: 20-60 ml/d C: PO: 0.5 ml/kg/dose	For constipation. Take with a glass of water in morning or evening. With frequent use, good renal function is necessary. *Pregnancy category:* B; PB: UK; $t^{1/2}$: UK
magnesium oxide (Maox, Mag-Ox)	A: PO: 2-4 g at bedtime with 8 oz water Do not use in client with renal failure.	Similar to magnesium hydroxide. *Pregnancy category:* B; PB: UK; $t^{1/2}$: UK
magnesium sulfate (Epsom salt)	A: PO: 10-15 g in 8 oz water C: PO: 5-10 g in water	For complete bowel elimination before surgery. Hypermagnesemia can occur if used frequently. Also used in pregnancy to control seizures with severe toxemia of pregnancy (given IV). Caution for use in renal dysfunction. *Pregnancy category:* B; PB: UK; $t^{1/2}$: UK
sodium biphosphate (Fleet Phospho-Soda)	A: PO: 15-30 ml mixed in water	For constipation or bowel preparation. Contraindicated with HF. *Pregnancy category:* UK; PB: UK; $t^{1/2}$: UK
sodium phosphate with sodium biphosphate (Fleet enema)	*Enema:* A: 60-120 ml C: 30-60 ml	For constipation or bowel preparation for diagnostic procedures. Frequent Fleet enema use may cause fluid imbalance in the elderly. *Pregnancy category:* UK; PB: UK; $t^{1/2}$: UK
Stimulants		
bisacodyl (Dulcolax)	(Prototype Drug Chart 46–4)	
cascara sagrada	A: PO: Tab: 325 mg/d Fluid extract: 1 ml/d Aromatic fluid extract: 5 ml/d	For acute constipation or bowel preparation. Can be mixed with milk of magnesia. Onset: 6-12 h. *Pregnancy category:* C; PB: UK; $t^{1/2}$: UK
castor oil (Neoloid, Purge)	A: PO: 15-60 ml C: 6-12 y: 5-15 ml	For bowel preparation for diagnostic tests. Harsh cathartic or purgative. Not commonly used for constipation. *Pregnancy category:* X; PB: UK; $t^{1/2}$: UK
phenolphthalein (Ex-Lax, Feen-A-Mint, Correctol)	A & C: >12 y: 30-200 mg/d C: 6-12 y: 30-60 mg	For acute constipation. Onset: 6-10 h. Turns urine reddish color. *Pregnancy category:* C; PB: UK; $t^{1/2}$: UK
senna (Senokot)	A: PO: 2 tab or 1-2 tsp (granules) diluted in water; *max:* 4 tab/d	For constipation. Available in granules, syrup, and suppository. Prolonged use may cause fluid and electrolyte imbalances. Flatus and abdominal cramps may occur. *Pregnancy category:* C; PB: UK; $t^{1/2}$: UK
Selective Chloride Channel Activators		
lubiprostone (Amitiza)	A: PO: 24 mcg b.i.d.	For treatment of chronic idiopathic constipation in adults. *Pregnancy category:* C; PB: 94%; $t^{1/2}$: 0.9-1.4 h

A, Adult; *b.i.d.*, twice a day; *C*, child; *HF*, heart failure; *d*, day; *h*, hour; *IV*, intravenous; *max*, maximum; *min*, minute; *PB*, protein-binding; *PO*, by mouth; *PRN*, as needed; *supp*, suppository; $t^{1/2}$, half-life; *tab*, tablet; *tsp*, teaspoon; *UK*, unknown; *y*, year; *>*, greater than; *<*, less than.

agents are nonabsorbable. Defecation usually occurs within 8 to 24 hours; however, it may take up to 3 days after drug therapy is started for the stool to be soft and well formed. Powdered bulk-forming laxatives, which sometimes come in flavored and sugar-free forms, should be mixed in a glass of water or juice, stirred, drunk immediately, and followed by a half to a full glass of water. Insufficient fluid intake can cause the drug to solidify in the GI tract, which can result in intestinal obstruction. This group of laxatives does not cause laxative dependence and may be used by clients with diverticulosis, irritable bowel syndrome, and ileostomy and colostomy (Figure 46–2).

Calcium polycarbophil (FiberCon), methylcellulose (Citrucel), fiber granules (Perdiem), and psyllium hydrophilic mucilloid (Metamucil) are examples of bulk-forming laxatives. Clients with hypercalcemia should avoid calcium polycarbophil because of the calcium in the drug. Prototype Drug Chart 46–4 presents the bulk-forming laxative psyllium (Metamucil).

FIGURE 46–2 Various over-the-counter laxatives are available. The bulk-forming laxatives, such as Metamucil, Perdiem, Citrucel, and FiberCon, do not cause laxative dependence.

Prototype **DRUG CHART 46-4**

PSYLLIUM

Drug Class	**Dosage**
Laxative: Bulk forming Trade names: Metamucil, Naturacil; ✹Karacil *Pregnancy Category:* C	A: PO: 1-2 tsp in 8 oz water/d followed by 8 oz water C: >6 y: PO: 0.5-1 tsp in 4 oz water, followed by ≥4 oz water
Contraindications	**Drug-Lab-Food Interactions**
Hypersensitivity, fecal impaction, intestinal obstruction, abdominal pain	*Drug: Decrease* absorption of oral anticoagulants, aspirin, digoxin, nitrofurantoin
Pharmacokinetics	**Pharmacodynamics**

Absorption: Not absorbed
Distribution: PB: NA
Metabolism: t½: NA
Excretion: In feces
	PO: Onset: 10-24 h
	  Peak: 1-3 d
	  Duration: UK

Therapeutic Effects/Uses

To control chronic constipation
Mode of Action: Acts as bulk-forming laxative by drawing water into intestine

Side Effects	**Adverse Reactions**
Anorexia, nausea, vomiting, cramps, diarrhea	Esophageal or intestinal obstruction if not taken with adequate water *Life-threatening:* Bronchospasm, anaphylaxis

A, Adult; *C,* child; *d,* day; *h,* hour; *NA,* not applicable; *PB,* protein-binding; *PO,* by mouth; *t½,* half-life; *tsp,* teaspoon; *UK,* unknown; >, greater than; ≥, greater than or equal to; ✹, Canadian drug name.

Pharmacokinetics

The bulk-forming laxative Metamucil is a nondigestible and nonabsorbent substance that, when mixed with water, becomes a viscous solution. Because it is not absorbed, there is no protein-binding or half-life for the drug. Metamucil is excreted in the feces.

Pharmacodynamics

The onset of action for Metamucil is 10 to 24 hours. Peak action is 1 to 3 days. The duration of action is unknown.

Side Effects and Adverse Reactions

Bulk-forming laxatives are not systemically absorbed; therefore there is no systemic effect. If bulk-forming laxatives are excessively used, nausea, vomiting, flatus, or diar-

rhea may occur. Abdominal cramps may occur if the drug is used in dry form.

Chloride Channel Activators

Selective chloride channel activators are a new category of laxatives used to treat idiopathic constipation in adults. The first drug in this category is lubiprostone, manufactured by Sucampo Pharmaceuticals. Lubiprostone was approved by the FDA in January 2006. This drug activates chloride channels in the lining of the small intestine, leading to an increase in intestinal fluid secretion and motility. By enhancing the passage of stool lubiprostone relieves constipation, as well as accompanying symptoms of abdominal discomfort, pain, and bloating. Lubiprostone is contraindicated for clients with a history of mechanical GI obstruction, Crohn's disease, diverticulitis, and severe diarrhea. Adverse effects of lubiprostone include nausea, which seems to be dose-dependent, diarrhea, headache, abdominal distention, and flatulence.

Emollients (Stool Softeners)

Emollients are lubricants and stool softeners (surface-acting or wetting drugs) used to prevent constipation. These drugs decrease straining during defecation. Lubricants such as mineral oil increase water retention in the stool. Mineral oil absorbs essential fat-soluble vitamins A, D, E, and K. Some of the minerals can be absorbed into the lymphatic system.

Stool softeners work by lowering surface tension and promoting water accumulation in the intestine and stool. They are frequently prescribed for clients after myocardial infarction or surgery. They are also given before administration of other laxatives in treating fecal impaction. Docusate calcium (Surfak), docusate potassium (Dialose), docusate sodium (Colace), and docusate sodium with casanthranol (Peri-Colace) are examples of stool softeners.

Side Effects and Adverse Reactions

Side effects of mineral oil include nausea, vomiting, diarrhea, and abdominal cramping. This laxative is not indicated for children, older adults, or clients with debilitating diseases, because they might aspirate the mineral oil, resulting in lipid pneumonia.

The docusate group of drugs may cause mild cramping.

Contraindications

Contraindications to the use of laxatives include inflammatory disorders of the GI tract (appendicitis, ulcerative colitis, undiagnosed severe pain that could be caused by inflammation within the intestine [diverticulitis, appendicitis]), pregnancy, spastic colon, or bowel obstruction. Laxatives are contraindicated when any of these conditions is suspected. Table 46–6 presents the drug data for laxatives.

Laxative: Stimulant

ASSESSMENT

- Obtain a history of constipation and possible causes (insufficient water or fluid intake, diet deficient in bulk or fiber, inactivity), frequency and consistency of stools, and general health status.
- Record baseline vital signs for identification of abnormalities and for future comparisons.
- Evaluate renal function.

- Assess electrolyte balance of clients who frequently use laxatives.

NURSING DIAGNOSES

- Constipation related to ignoring urge to defecate
- Risk for deficient fluid volume related to diuretic therapy
- Deficient knowledge related to overuse of laxatives
- Ineffective health maintenance related to lack of ability to make thoughtful judgments

PLANNING

- Client will have a normal bowel elimination pattern.
- Client will exercise, eat foods high in fiber, and have adequate fluid intake to avoid constipation.

NURSING INTERVENTIONS

- Monitor fluid intake and output. Note signs and symptoms of fluid and electrolyte imbalances that may result from watery stools. Habitual use of laxatives can cause fluid volume deficit, electrolyte losses, and loss of urge to defecate.

Client Teaching

General

- Encourage client to increase water intake (if not contraindicated), which will decrease hard, dry stools.
- Advise client to avoid overuse of laxatives, which can lead to fluid and electrolyte imbalances and drug dependence. Suggest exercise to help increase peristalsis.
- Instruct client not to chew tablets but swallow them whole.
- Direct client to store suppositories at less than 86° F (30° C).
- Tell client to take drug only with water to increase absorption.
- Educate client not to take drug within 1 hour of any other drug.
- Remind client that drug is not for long-term use; bowel tone may be lost.
- Warn client to time administration of drug so as not to interfere with activities or sleep.

Side Effects

- Guide client to discontinue use if rectal bleeding, nausea, vomiting, or cramping occurs.

Diet

- Inform client to increase fiber-rich foods such as bran, grains, and fruits.

Cultural Considerations ❖

- Provide explanation and written information as needed related to the use and abuse of stimulant laxa-

Table 46–6

Laxatives: Bulk Forming, Emollients, and Evacuants

Generic (Brand)	Route and Dosage	Uses and Considerations
Bulk Forming		
calcium polycarbophil (FiberCon, Fiberall, Mitrolan)	A: PO: 1 g q.i.d; *max:* 6 g/d C: 6-12 y: PO: 500 mg/d t.i.d.; *max:* 3 g C: 2-5 y: PO: 500 mg/d b.i.d.; *max:* 1.5 g/d	Prevention of constipation. Also used to treat acute nonspecific diarrhea or diarrhea associated with irritable bowel syndrome. For diarrhea, absorbs water and produces formed stool. For constipation, chew tablet and follow with a full glass of water. *Pregnancy category:* C; PB: NA; t½: NA
methylcellulose (Cologel, Citrucel)	A: PO: 5-20 ml t.i.d. in 8-10 oz water C: 5-10 ml b.i.d. with 8 oz water	For constipation. Effects similar to Metamucil. Mix in at least 8 oz of water and take immediately. *Pregnancy category:* UK; PB: NA; t½: NA
psyllium hydrophilic mucilloid (Metamucil)	(Prototype Drug Chart 46–5)	
Emollient: Stool Softeners		
docusate calcium (Surfak)	A: PO: 240 mg/d C: PO: 60-120 mg/d	Prevention of constipation. Stool softener. Acts on small and large intestines; little absorption. When first used may take 1 to 5 days for effect. Available with calcium, potassium, or sodium. Because of sodium content, drug should not be taken if HF is present. *Pregnancy category:* C; PB: NA; t½: NA
docusate potassium (Dialose)	A: PO: 100-300 mg/d	Same as docusate calcium.
docusate sodium (Colace)	A: PO: 50-300 mg/d C: .6 y: 40-120 mg/d	Same as docusate calcium.
docusate sodium with casanthranol (Peri-Colace)	A: PO: 1-2 cap/d C: PO: 1 cap/d	For preventing constipation. Combination drug: docusate sodium 100 mg with casanthranol 30 mg. *Pregnancy category:* C; PB: NA; t½: NA
Emollient: Lubricant		
mineral oil	A: PO: 15-45 ml/at bedtime C: 6-12 y: PO: 5-20 ml	Relief of constipation and fecal impaction. May be useful for those with cardiac disorder and following anorectal surgery. Avoid prolonged use because vitamins A, D, E, and K may be lost. *Pregnancy category:* UK; PB: NA; t½: NA
Evacuant/Bowel Preparation		
polyethylene glycol-electrolyte solution (Colyte, GoLYTELY)	Preparation for GI examination requires 4 h; fasting for 3-4 h A: PO: 240 ml q10-15 min for total of 4 L C: PO: 25-40 ml/kg/h for 4-10 h. Administer via NGT to those unable or unwilling to drink solution (prepared with tap water and refrigerated)	For bowel preparation before GI examination. *Pregnancy category:* C; PB: NA; t½: NA

A, Adult; *b.i.d.,* twice a day; *C,* child; *cap,* capsule; *HF,* heart failure; *d,* day; *h,* hour; *GI,* gastrointestinal; *max,* maximum; *min,* minute; *NA,* not applicable; *NGT,* nasogastric tube; *PB,* protein-binding; *PO,* by mouth; *q.i.d.,* four times a day; *t½,* half-life; *t.i.d.,* three times a day; *UK,* unknown; *y,* year; >, greater than.

tives. Respect values and beliefs of clients from various cultural groups, and incorporate their traditional practices into treatment plan when possible.

EVALUATION

■ Determine the effectiveness of nonpharmacologic methods for alleviating constipation.
■ Evaluate client's use of laxatives in managing constipation. Identify laxative abuse.

Laxative: Bulk Forming

ASSESSMENT

■ Obtain a history of constipation and possible causes (insufficient water or fluid intake, diet deficient in bulk or fiber, inactivity), frequency and consistency of stools, and general health status.

■ Record baseline vital signs for identification of abnormalities and for future comparisons.
■ Assess renal function, urine output, blood urea nitrogen (BUN), and serum creatinine.

NURSING DIAGNOSES

■ Constipation related to inadequate fiber in diet
■ Risk for deficient fluid volume related to overuse of laxatives

PLANNING

■ Client will have a normal bowel elimination pattern.
■ Client will exercise, eat foods high in fiber, and have adequate fluid intake to avoid constipation.

NURSING INTERVENTIONS

■ Check fluid intake and output. Note signs and symptoms of fluid and electrolyte imbalances that may result from watery stools. Habitual use of laxatives can cause fluid volume deficit and electrolyte losses.
■ Monitor bowel sounds.
■ Identify the cause of constipation.
■ Avoid inhalation of psyllium dust.

Client Teaching

General
• Teach client to mix drug with water immediately before use.
• Instruct client *not* to swallow the drug in dry form.
• Direct client to avoid overuse of laxatives, which can lead to fluid and electrolyte imbalances and drug dependence. Suggest exercise to help increase peristalsis.
• Advise client to avoid inhaling psyllium dust; it may cause watery eyes, runny nose, and wheezing.

Side Effects
• Guide client to discontinue use if nausea, vomiting, cramping, or rectal bleeding occurs.

Diet
• Inform client to increase water intake (at least eight 8-oz glasses of fluids per day), which will decrease hard, dry stools.
• Tell client to mix the drug in 8 to 10 oz of water, stir, and drink immediately. At least one glass of extra water should follow. Insufficient water can cause the drug to solidify and lead to fecal impaction.
• Encourage client to increase foods rich in fiber (bran, grains, vegetables, fruits).

Cultural Considerations ❖
• Respect client's cultural beliefs and alternative methods for treating constipation. Suggest nonpharmacologic methods that might be of benefit.

• Provide additional explanation and first-language-appropriate written information as needed about the use and abuse of laxatives.

EVALUATION

■ Determine the effectiveness of nonpharmacologic methods for alleviating constipation.
■ Evaluate client's use of laxatives in managing constipation.
■ Identify laxative abuse.

KEY WEBSITES
Promethazine: http://www.nlm.nih.gov/medlineplus/druginfo/medmaster/a682284.html
Kaolin and Pectin: http://www.nlm.nih.gov/medlineplus/druginfo/medmaster/a601065.html
Activated charcoal: http://www.lifesteps.com/gm/Atoz/ency/charcoal_activated.jsp

 Critical Thinking Case Study

CS, age 34, has been vomiting for 48 hours. In the last 12 hours, CS has had diarrhea. Prochlorperazine (Compazine) 10 mg was administered intramuscularly.

1. What nonpharmacologic measures should the nurse suggest when vomiting occurs?
2. Why was CS given prochlorperazine intramuscularly and not orally or rectally? Prochlorperazine should be given deep intramuscularly. Why?
3. What electrolyte imbalances may occur as a result of vomiting and diarrhea? Explain how they can be replaced.
4. What are the side effects of prochlorperazine? Could these occur to CS? Explain.
5. Could a serotonin antagonist be given to CS instead of prochlorperazine? Explain.

CS was prescribed diphenoxylate with atropine (Lomotil) 2.5 mg t.i.d.

6. Is the Lomotil dosage for CS within the normal prescribed range? Explain.
7. What clinical conditions are contraindicated for the use of Lomotil?
8. What are some of the combination drugs that may be prescribed to control diarrhea? Give their advantages and disadvantages.
9. Explain the similarities of two over-the-counter antidiarrheals. Explain how frequently they should be administered.
10. Do you think CS should receive an adsorbent? Explain.
11. Explain the similarities and differences between ipecac and charcoal.

NCLEX Study Questions

1. A client complains of constipation and requires a laxative. In providing teaching to the client, the nurse reviews the common causes of constipation, which include:
   a. motion sickness
   b. lack of exercise
   c. food intolerance
   d. bacteria *(Escherichia coli)*

2. A client has nausea and is taking ondansetron (Zofran). The nurse explains the action of this drug is to:
   a. stimulate the CTZ
   b. block serotonin receptors in the CTZ
   c. block dopamine receptors in the CTZ
   d. coat the wall of the GI tract and absorb bacteria

3. A client who has constipation is prescribed a bisacodyl suppository. The nurse explains that bisacodyl:
   a. acts on smooth intestinal muscle to gently increase peristalsis
   b. absorbs water into the intestines to increase bulk and peristalsis
   c. lowers surface tension and increases water accumulation in the intestines
   d. pulls hyperosmolar salts into the colon and increases water in the feces to increase bulk

4. A client is using the scopolamine patch (Transderm-Scop) to prevent motion sickness. The nurse teaches the client that common side effects of this drug include:
   a. diarrhea
   b. vomiting
   c. insomnia
   d. dry mouth

5. When metoclopramide (Reglan) is given for nausea, the client is cautioned to avoid:
   a. milk
   b. MAOIs
   c. alcohol
   d. carbonated beverages

Answers: 1, b; 2, b; 3, a; 4, d; 5, c.

47
Antiulcer Drugs

ELECTRONIC RESOURCES

Evolve website (http://evolve.elsevier.com/KeeHayes/pharmacology/):
- *Case Studies*
- *Content Updates*
- *Frequently Asked Questions*
- *Student Review Activities*
- *WebLinks*
- *Additional Reference Material*

Companion CD-ROM:
- *NCLEX Examination Review Questions*
- *Pharmacology Animations*
- *IV Therapy Checklists*
- *Medication Error Checklists*
- *Drug Calculation Problems*
- *Electronic Calculators*
- *Top 200 Drugs with Pronunciations*
- *References from the Textbook*

Outline

Objectives

- Explain the predisposing factors for peptic ulcers.
- Differentiate between peptic ulcer, gastric ulcer, duodenal ulcer, and gastroesophageal reflux disease.
- Describe the actions of seven groups of antiulcer drugs used in the treatment of peptic ulcer: tranquilizers, anticholinergics, antacids, histamine$_2$ blockers, proton pump inhibitors, pepsin inhibitor, and prostaglandin analogue antiulcer.
- Describe client teaching for the following drug groups: anticholinergics, antacids, and histamine$_2$ blockers.
- Differentiate between the side effects of anticholinergics and systemic and nonsystemic antacids.
- Apply the nursing process, including client teaching, to antiulcer drugs.

Terms

Peptic ulcer is a broad term for an ulcer occurring in the esophagus, stomach, or duodenum within the upper gastrointestinal (GI) tract. Ulcers are more specifically named according to the site of involvement: esophageal, gastric, and duodenal ulcers. Duodenal ulcers occur 10 times more frequently than gastric and esophageal ulcers. The release of **hydrochloric acid (HCl)** from the parietal cells of the stomach is influenced by histamine, gastrin, and acetylcholine. Peptic ulcers occur when there is a hypersecretion of hydrochloric acid and pepsin, which erode the GI mucosal lining.

The gastric secretions in the stomach strive to maintain a pH of 2 to 5. **Pepsin**, a digestive enzyme, is activated at a pH of 2, and the acid-pepsin complex of gastric secretions can cause mucosal damage. If the pH of gastric secretions increases to pH 5, the activity of pepsin declines. The **gastric mucosal barrier (GMB)** is a thick, viscous, mucous material that provides a barrier between the mucosal lining and acidic gastric secretions. The GMB maintains the integrity of the gastric mucosal lining and is a defense against corrosive substances. The two sphincter muscles—the *cardiac*, located at the upper portion of the stomach, and the *pyloric*, located at the lower portion of the stomach—act as barriers to prevent reflux of acid into the esophagus and duodenum. Figure 47–1 illustrates common sites of peptic ulcers.

An **esophageal ulcer** results from reflux of acidic gastric secretions into the esophagus as a result of a defective or incompetent cardiac sphincter. A **gastric ulcer** frequently occurs because of a breakdown of the GMB. A **duodenal ulcer** is caused by hypersecretion of acid from the stomach passing into the duodenum because of (1) insufficient buffers to neutralize gastric acid in the stomach, (2) a defective or incompetent pyloric sphincter, or (3) hypermotility of the stomach. **Gastroesophageal reflux disease (GERD)** is inflammation or erosion of the esophageal mucosa caused by a reflux of gastric acid content from the stomach into the esophagus.

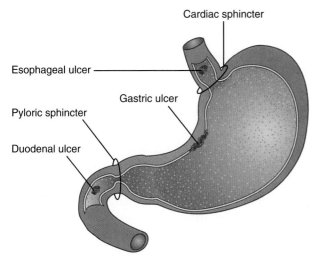

FIGURE 47–1   Common sites of peptic ulcers.

Predisposing Factors in Peptic Ulcer Disease

The nurse needs to assist the client in identifying possible causes of the ulcer and to teach ways to alleviate them. Predisposing factors include mechanical disturbances, genetic influences, bacterial organisms, environmental factors, and certain drugs. Healing of an ulcer takes 4 to 8 weeks. Complications can occur as the result of scar tissue. Table 47–1 lists the predisposing factors for peptic ulcers and their effects.

The classic symptom of peptic ulcers is gnawing, aching pain. With a gastric ulcer, pain occurs 30 minutes to 1.5 hours after eating, and with a duodenal ulcer, 2 to 3 hours after eating. Small, frequent meals of nonirritating foods decrease the pain. With treatment, pain usually subsides in 10 days; however, the healing process may take 1 to 2 months.

A **stress ulcer** usually follows a critical situation such as extensive trauma or major surgery (e.g., burns, cardiac surgery). Prophylactic use of antiulcer drugs decreases the incidence of stress ulcers.

Table 47–1

Predisposing Factors in Peptic Ulcer Disease

Predisposing Factors	Effects
Mechanical disturbances	Hypersecretion of acid and pepsin. Inadequate GMB mucous secretion. Impaired GMB resistance. Hypermotility of the stomach. Incompetent (defective) cardiac or pyloric sphincter.
Genetic influences	Increased number of parietal cells in the stomach. Susceptibility of mucosal lining to acid penetration. Susceptibility to excess acetylcholine and histamine. Excess hydrochloric acid caused by external stimuli.
Environmental influences	Foods and liquids containing caffeine; fatty, fried, and highly spiced foods; alcohol. Nicotine, especially from cigarette smoking. Stressful situations. Pregnancy, massive trauma, major surgery.
Helicobacter pylori	A gram-negative bacterium, *H. pylori* infects gastric mucosa and can cause gastritis, gastric ulcer, and duodenal ulcer. If not eradicated, peptic ulcer may return as frequently as every year. *H. pylori* can lead to atrophic gastritis in some clients. Serology and special breath tests can detect the presence of *H. pylori*.
Drugs	NSAIDs, including aspirin and aspirin compounds, ibuprofen (Motrin, Advil, Nuprin), and indomethacin (Indocin); corticosteroids (cortisone, prednisone); potassium salts; antineoplastic drugs.

GMB, Gastric mucosal barrier; *NSAIDs*, nonsteroidal antiinflammatory drugs.

Helicobacter pylori

Helicobacter pylori, a gram-negative bacillus, is linked with the development of peptic ulcer and known to cause gastritis, gastric ulcer, and duodenal ulcer. When a peptic ulcer recurs after antiulcer therapy, and the ulcer is not caused by nonsteroidal antiinflammatory drugs (NSAIDs) such as aspirin or ibuprofen, the client should be tested for the presence of the bacterium *H. pylori*, which may have infected the gastric mucosa. In the past, endoscopy and a biopsy of the gastric antrum were needed to check for *H. pylori*. Currently a noninvasive breath test, the Meretek UBT, can detect *H. pylori*. This test consists of drinking a liquid containing ^{13}C urea and breathing into a container. If *H. pylori* is present, the bacterial urease hydrolyzes the urea, releasing $^{13}CO_2$, which is detected by a spectrometer. This test is 90% to 95% effective for detecting *H. pylori*. In addition, a serology test may be performed to check for antibodies to *H. pylori*.

There are various protocols for treating *H. pylori* infection, but antibacterial agents are the treatment of choice. The use of only one antibacterial agent is not effective for eradicating *H. pylori*, because the bacterium can readily become resistant to that drug. Treatment to eradicate this bacterial infection includes using a dual-, triple-, or quadruple drug therapy program in a variety of drug combinations, such as amoxicillin (Amoxil), tetracycline (Achromycin V), clarithromycin (Biaxin), omeprazole (Prilosec), lansoprazole (Prevacid), metronidazole (Flagyl), bismuth subsalicylate (Pepto-Bismol), and ranitidine bismuth citrate (Tritec), on a 7- to 14-day treatment plan. The combination of drugs differs for each client according to the client's drug tolerance. A common treatment protocol is the triple therapy of metronidazole (or amoxicillin), omeprazole (or lansoprazole), and clarithromycin (MOC). The drug regimen eradicates more than 90% of peptic ulcer caused by *H. pylori* (Herbal Alert 47–1).

One of the proton pump inhibitors (PPIs) (e.g., omeprazole, lansoprazole) is frequently used as a component of combination drug therapy, because each suppresses acid secretion by inhibiting the enzyme hydrogen or potassium ATPase, which makes gastric acid. These agents block the final steps of acid production. If triple therapy fails to eradicate *H. pylori*, then quadruple therapy using two antibiotics, a PPI, and a bismuth or histamine$_2$ (H$_2$) blocker is recommended. After completion of the treatment regimen, 6 weeks of standard acid suppression, such as H$_2$ blocker therapy, is recommended. Table 47–2 lists various combinations of treatment regimens to eradicate *H. pylori*, and Table 47–3 lists data for the drugs used to treat *H. pylori*.

Gastroesophageal Reflux Disease

Gastroesophageal reflux disease (GERD), also called *reflux esophagitis*, is an inflammation of the esophageal mucosa caused by reflux of gastric acid content into the esophagus. Its main cause is an incompetent lower esophageal sphincter. Smoking and obesity tend to accelerate the disease process. In the United States, 40% to 44% of adults have heartburn, which in many cases is caused by GERD.

Medical treatment for GERD is similar to the treatment for peptic ulcers. This includes the use of the common antiulcer drugs to neutralize gastric contents and reduce gastric acid secretion. Drugs used in treatment include H$_2$ blockers such as ranitidine (Zantac), and PPIs such as omeprazole (Prilosec), lansoprazole (Prevacid), rabeprazole (Aciphex), pantoprazole (Protonix), or esomeprazole (Nexium). A PPI relieves symptoms faster and maintains healing better than an H$_2$ blocker. Once the strictures are relieved by dilation, they are less likely to recur if the client was taking PPIs rather than an H$_2$ blocker.

Effective management of GERD keeps the esophageal mucosa healed and the client free of symptoms, but GERD is a chronic disorder that requires continuous care.

Nonpharmacologic Measures for Managing Peptic Ulcer and Gastroesophageal Reflux Disease

With a GI disorder, nonpharmacologic measures, along with drug therapy, are an important part of treatment. Once the GI problem is resolved, the client should continue to follow nonpharmacologic measures to avoid recurrence of the condition.

Avoiding tobacco and alcohol can decrease gastric secretions. With GERD, nicotine relaxes the lower esophageal sphincter, permitting gastric acid reflux. Obesity enhances the problem of GERD; weight loss is helpful in decreasing symptoms. The client should avoid hot, spicy, and greasy foods, which could aggravate the gastric problem. Certain drugs like NSAIDs, which include aspirin, should be taken with food or in a decreased dosage. Glucocorticoids can cause gastric ulceration and should be taken with food.

To relieve symptoms of GERD, the client should raise the head of the bed, not eat before bedtime, and wear loose-fitting clothing.

Table 47–2

Various Regimens Used to Eradicate Helicobacter pylori

Type of Therapy	Drugs	Treatment Duration	Eradication Rate
Dual therapy	ranitidine bismuth citrate, 400 mg b.i.d. clarithromycin, 500 mg t.i.d.	2-4 wk	82%
	*omeprazole, 40 mg/d clarithromycin, 500 mg t.i.d.	2-4 wk	64%–82%
	*lansoprazole, 30 mg b.i.d. clarithromycin, 400 mg b.i.d.	14 d	72%
Triple therapy	colloidal bismuth subcitrate, 120 mg q.i.d. metronidazole, 250 mg q.i.d.	14 d	96%
	tetracycline, 250 mg q.i.d. OR tetracycline, 500 mg q.i.d.	7 d	83%
	bismuth subsalicylate, 300 mg q.i.d. metronidazole, 500 mg t.i.d. amoxicillin, 500 mg t.i.d. OR	14 d	84%
	bismuth with clarithromycin, 500 mg t.i.d. tetracycline, 500 mg q.i.d.	14 d	93%
	metronidazole, 500 mg b.i.d. OR amoxicillin, 1 g b.i.d. *omeprazole, 20 mg b.i.d. OR lansoprazole, 30 mg b.i.d. clarithromycin, 500 mg b.i.d. *Combinations of:* metronidazole, omeprazole, clarithromycin metronidazole, omeprazole, amoxicillin *lansoprazole, clarithromycin, metronidazole *lansoprazole, amoxicillin, clarithromycin *omeprazole, amoxicillin, clarithromycin	7-14 d	>90%
Quadruple therapy	colloidal bismuth subcitrate, 120 mg q.i.d. tetracycline, 500 mg q.i.d. metronidazole, 500 mg t.i.d. *omeprazole, 20 mg b.i.d. Other combinations may be used	7 d	98%

b.i.d., Twice a day; *d*, days; *q.i.d.*, four times a day; *t.i.d.*, three times a day; *wk*, weeks; >, greater than.
*Other proton pump inhibitors may be substituted for omeprazole and lansoprazole.

Table 47–3

Pharmacologic Agents Used to Treat Helicobacter pylori

Generic (Brand)	Route and Dosage	Uses and Considerations
Antiinfective Agents		
metronidazole HCl (Flagyl, Protostat)	A: PO: 250-500 mg b.i.d., t.i.d., q.i.d.	To treat numerous organisms, including *H. pylori*. Used in combination with other drugs to treat *H. pylori*.
amoxicillin (Amoxil)	A: PO: 500 mg t.i.d.	Used in triple or quadruple therapy for *H. pylori*
clarithromycin (Biaxin)	A: PO: 500 mg b.i.d.-t.i.d.	Used in dual and triple therapy for *H. pylori*
tetracycline	A: PO: 500 mg q.i.d.	Used in triple and quadruple therapy for *H. pylori*
Proton Pump Inhibitors (PPIs)		
omeprazole (Prilosec)	A: PO: 20 mg/d or 40 mg/d	Used in dual, triple, and quadruple therapy for *H. pylori*
lansoprazole (Prevacid)	A: PO: 30 mg b.i.d.	Used in dual and triple therapy for *H. pylori*
esomeprazole (Nexium)	A: PO: 20-40 mg/d	Used in therapy for *H. pylori*
pantoprazole (Protonix)	A: PO: 40-80 mg/d	Used in therapy for *H. pylori*
rabeprazole (Aciphex)	A: PO: 20 mg/d	Used in therapy for *H. pylori*
Antacids		
bismuth subsalicylate	A: PO: 300 mg q.i.d.	Used in combination with other drugs to treat *H. pylori*
colloidal bismuth subcitrate	A: PO: 120 mg q.i.d.	Used in combination with other drugs to treat *H. pylori*
ranitidine bismuth citrate (Tritec)	A: PO: 400 mg b.i.d.	Used in combination with other drugs to treat *H. pylori*

A, Adult; *b.i.d.*, twice a day; *d*, day; *PO*, by mouth; *q.i.d.*, four times a day; *t.i.d.*, three times a day.

Antiulcer Drugs

There are seven groups of antiulcer agents: (1) tranquilizers, which decrease vagal activity; (2) anticholinergics, which decrease acetylcholine by blocking the cholinergic receptors; (3) antacids, which neutralize gastric acid; (4) H_2 blockers, which block the H_2 receptor; (5) PPIs, which inhibit gastric acid secretion, regardless of acetylcholine or histamine release; (6) the pepsin inhibitor sucralfate; and (7) the prostaglandin E_1 analogue misoprostol, which inhibits gastric acid secretion and protects the mucosa. Figure 47–2 illustrates the action of the seven antiulcer drug groups, each of which is discussed separately.

Tranquilizers

Tranquilizers have minimal effect in preventing and treating ulcers; however, they reduce vagal stimulation and decrease anxiety. Librax, a combination of the anxiolytic chlordiazepoxide (Librium) and the anticholinergic clidinium bromide (Quarzan), may be used in the treatment of ulcers.

Anticholinergics

Anticholinergics (antimuscarinics, parasympatholytics) and antacids were the drugs of choice for peptic ulcers for many years. However, with the introduction of H_2 blockers in 1975, anticholinergic use has declined. These drugs relieve pain by decreasing GI motility and secretion. They act by inhibiting acetylcholine and blocking histamine and hydrochloric acid. Anticholinergics delay gastric emptying time, so they are used more frequently for duodenal ulcers than for gastric ulcers. The anticholinergic propantheline bromine (Pro-Banthine) inhibits gastric secretions and is used to treat peptic ulcers.

Anticholinergics should be taken before meals to decrease the acid secretion that occurs with eating. Antacids can slow the absorption of anticholinergics and therefore should be taken 2 hours after anticholinergic administration.

Table 47–4 lists selected anticholinergic drugs used in the treatment of peptic ulcer. Anticholinergics should be used as adjunctive therapy and not as the only antiulcer drug. Anticholinergics are discussed in more detail in Chapter 18.

Side Effects and Adverse Reactions

Anticholinergics have many side effects, including dry mouth, decreased secretions, headache, blurred vision, drowsiness, dizziness, lethargy, palpitations, bradycardia, tachycardia, urinary retention, and constipation. Because anticholinergics decrease GI motility, gastric emptying time is delayed, which can stimulate gastric secretions and aggravate the ulceration.

Antacids

Antacids promote ulcer healing by neutralizing hydrochloric acid and reducing pepsin activity; they do not coat the ulcer. There are two types of antacids: those that have a *systemic* effect and those that have a *nonsystemic* effect.

Sodium bicarbonate, a systemically absorbed antacid, was one of the first antiulcer drugs. Because it has many side effects (sodium excess, causing hypernatremia and water retention; metabolic alkalosis caused by excess bicarbonate; and acid rebound [excess acid secretion]), sodium bicarbonate is seldom used to treat peptic ulcers. Examples of sodium bicarbonate compounds are Bromo-Seltzer and Alka-Seltzer.

Calcium carbonate is most effective in neutralizing acid; however, one third to half of the drug can be systemically absorbed and can cause acid rebound. Hypercalcemia and "milk-alkali syndrome" can result from excessive use of calcium carbonate. Milk-alkali syndrome is intensified if milk products are ingested with calcium carbonate. It is identified by the presence of alkalosis, hypercalcemia, and in severe cases crystalluria and renal failure.

The nonsystemic antacids are composed of alkaline salts such as aluminum (aluminum hydroxide, aluminum carbonate) and magnesium (magnesium hydroxide, magnesium carbonate, magnesium trisilicate, magnesium phosphate). There is a small degree of systemic absorption with these drugs, mainly of aluminum. Magnesium hydroxide has greater neutralizing power than aluminum hydroxide. Magnesium compounds can cause diarrhea, and aluminum and calcium compounds can cause constipation with long-term use. A combination of magnesium and aluminum salts neutralizes gastric acid without causing severe diarrhea or constipation. Simethicone (an antigas agent) is found in many antacids, including Mylanta II, Maalox Plus, and Gelusil II (Figure 47–3). Prototype Drug Chart 47–1 gives the drug data for aluminum hydroxide antacid.

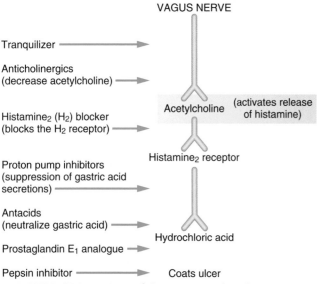

FIGURE 47–2 Actions of the seven antiulcer drug groups.

Table 47–4

Antiulcer: Anticholinergics

Generic (Brand)	Route and Dosage	Uses and Considerations
belladonna tincture	A: PO: 0.6-1 ml t.i.d.-q.i.d. C: PO: 0.1 ml/kg/d in 3-4 divided doses *max*: 3.5 ml/d	For peptic ulcers; decreases gastric secretions. Contraindicated in clients with narrow-angle glaucoma, myasthenia gravis, paralytic ileus, and urinary retention. Dry mouth and constipation can occur. *Pregnancy category*: C; PB: UK; $t^{1/2}$: 18-36 h
clidinium bromide and chlordiazepoxide HCl (Librax)	A: PO: 1-2 cap t.i.d.-q.i.d. a.c., at bedtime	Decreases anxiety and GI distress. Contains a benzodiazepine. *Pregnancy category*: C; PB: UK; $t^{1/2}$: UK
glycopyrrolate (Robinul)	A: PO: 1-2 mg b.i.d.-t.i.d. IM/IV: 0.1-0.2 mg (100-200 mcg) t.i.d.-q.i.d.	For peptic ulcers and gastric disorders caused by hyperacidity. Used as one of the preanesthetic drugs. Same contraindications as belladonna. *Pregnancy category*: B; PB: UK; $t^{1/2}$: UK
propantheline bromine (Pro-Banthine)	A: PO: 15 mg t.i.d. 30 min a.c. and 30 mg at bedtime; *max*: 120 mg/d Elderly: PO: 7.5 mg b.i.d.-t.i.d. a.c. *max*: 90 mg/d	For peptic ulcers; decreases gastric secretions, irritable bowel syndrome, pancreatitis, and urinary bladder spasm. Standard anticholinergic side effects. *Pregnancy category*: C; PB: UK; $t^{1/2}$: 9 h

A, Adult; *a.c.,* before meals; *b.i.d.,* twice a day; *C,* child; *cap,* capsule; *d,* day; *GI,* gastrointestinal; *h,* hour; *IM,* intramuscular; *IV,* intravenous; *max,* maximum; *PB,* protein-binding; *PO,* by mouth; *q.i.d.,* four times a day; $t^{1/2}$, half-life; *t.i.d.,* three times a day; *UK,* unknown.

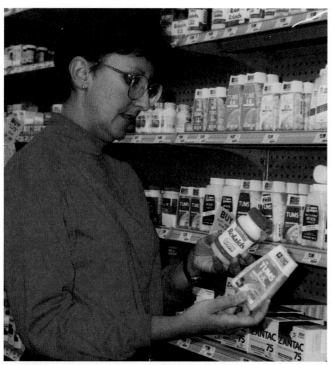

FIGURE 47–3 Numerous over-the-counter antacids are available. This client is deciding which of these antacids would best help relieve her upset stomach.

Pharmacokinetics

Aluminum hydroxide (Amphojel) was one of the first antacids used to neutralize hydrochloric acid. Aluminum products are frequently used to lower high serum phosphate (hyperphosphatemia). Because aluminum hydroxide alone can cause constipation, and magnesium products alone can cause diarrhea, combination drugs such as aluminum hydroxide and magnesium hydroxide (Maalox) have become popular, because they decrease these side effects.

Only a small amount of aluminum hydroxide is absorbed from the GI tract. It is primarily bound to phosphate and excreted in the feces. The small portion that is absorbed is excreted in the urine.

Pharmacodynamics

Aluminum hydroxide neutralizes gastric acid, including hydrochloric acid, and increases the pH of gastric secretions (an elevated pH inactivates pepsin). The onset of action is fairly rapid, but the duration of action varies, depending on whether the antacid is taken with or without food. If the antacid is taken after a meal, the duration of action may be up to 3 hours, because food delays gastric emptying time. Frequent dosing may be necessary if the antacid is given during a fasting state or early in the course of treatment.

The ideal dosing interval for antacids is 1 and 3 hours after meals (maximum acid secretion occurs after eating) and at bedtime. Antacids taken on an empty stomach are effective for 30 to 60 minutes before passing into the duodenum. Chewable tablets should be followed by water. Liquid antacids should also be taken with water (2 to 4 ounces) to ensure that the drug reaches the stomach; however, no more than 4 ounces of water should be taken, because water quickens gastric emptying time.

Antacids containing magnesium salts are contraindicated in clients with impaired renal function because of the risk of hypermagnesemia. Magnesium is primarily excreted by the kidneys; however, hypermagnesemia is usually not a problem unless the client with renal insufficiency is ingesting magnesium. Prolonged use of aluminum hydroxides can cause hypophosphatemia (low serum phosphate). If hyperphosphatemia occurs because of poor renal function, aluminum hydroxide can be given to decrease the phosphate level. In clients with renal insufficiency, aluminum salt ingestion can cause encephalopathy from accumulation of aluminum in the brain. Table 47–5 lists the drug data for antacids.

Prototype DRUG CHART 47–1

ALUMINUM HYDROXIDE

Drug Class

Antiulcer: Antacid
Trade names: Amphojel, AlternaGEL, Alu-Tab
Pregnancy Category: C

Dosage

Antacid:
A: PO: 600 mg 1 h p.c. and at bedtime; chewed, followed by water or milk
Susp: 5-10 ml 1 h p.c. and at bedtime
Hyperphosphatemia:
A: PO: 2 cap or 10-30 ml (regular carbonate suspension) t.i.d.-q.i.d. with meals

Contraindications

Hypersensitivity to aluminum products, hypophosphatemia
Caution: In older adults

Drug-Lab-Food Interactions

Drug: Decrease effects with tetracycline, phenothiazine, isoniazid, phenytoin, digitalis, quinidine, amphetamines. May *increase* effect of benzo-diazepines
Lab: Increase urine pH

Pharmacokinetics

Absorption: PO: Small amount absorbed
Distribution: PB: UK
Metabolism: t½: UK
Excretion: In feces; small amount in urine

Pharmacodynamics

PO: Onset: 15-30 min
Peak: 0.5 h
Duration: 1-3 h

Therapeutic Effects/Uses

To treat hyperacidity, peptic ulcer, and reflux esophagitis; to reduce hyperphosphatemia
Mode of Action: Neutralizes gastric acidity

Side Effects

Constipation

Adverse Reactions

Hypophosphatemia; long-term use can result in GI obstruction

A, Adult; *cap,* capsule; *GI,* gastrointestinal; *h,* hour; *min,* minute; *PB,* protein-binding; *p.c.,* after meals; *PO,* by mouth; *q.i.d.,* four times a day; *Susp,* suspension; *t½,* half-life; *t.i.d.,* three times a day; *UK,* unknown.

 Nursing Process

Antiulcer: Antacids

ASSESSMENT

■ Evaluate client's pain, including type, duration, severity, and frequency.
■ Check client's renal function.
■ Assess for fluid and electrolyte imbalances, especially serum phosphate and calcium levels.
■ Obtain drug history; report probable drug-drug interactions.

NURSING DIAGNOSES

■ Acute pain related to repeated spicy food and alcohol ingestion
■ Ineffective health maintenance related to misuse of antacids
■ Deficient knowledge related to misinterpretation of information

PLANNING

■ Client will be free of abdominal pain after 1 to 2 weeks of antiulcer drug management.

NURSING INTERVENTIONS

■ Avoid administering antacids with other oral drugs, because antacids can delay their absorption. An antacid should definitely not be given with tetracycline, digoxin, or quinidine, because it binds with and inactivates most of the drug. Antacids are given 1 to 2 hours after other medications.
■ Shake suspension well before administering; follow with water.
■ Monitor electrolytes and urinary pH, calcium, and phosphate levels.

Table 47–5

Antiulcer Drugs: Antacids

Generic (Brand)	Route and Dosage	Uses and Considerations
aluminum carbonate (Basaljel)	A: PO: 10-30 ml or 2 tab/cap q2h Extra strength: 5-15 ml	To alleviate gastric hyperacidity related to gastritis, gastric and duodenal ulcers, esophageal reflux, and hiatal hernia. Increases gastric pH and inhibits pepsin activity. Also used to decrease hyperphosphatemia for clients with renal dysfunction. Duration of action is 2 to 3 h when taken 1 h after meals. *Pregnancy category*: C; PB: UK; $t^{1/2}$: UK
aluminum hydroxide (Amphojel, AlternaGEL)	(Prototype Drug Chart 47–1)	
calcium carbonate (Tums, Dicarbosil)	A: PO: 2 tab or 10 ml q2h; *max*: 12 doses/d	To alleviate heartburn, acid indigestion, esophagitis, and hiatal hernia caused by hyperacidity. Also used to treat hyperphosphatemia in clients with renal disorders. OTC drug. One third of drug dose absorbed from GI tract. Constipation can be a problem. *Pregnancy category*: C; PB: UK; $t^{1/2}$: UK
dihydroxyaluminum sodium carbonate (Rolaids Antacid)	A: PO: Chew 1-2 tab PRN	Similar to calcium carbonate, but contains sodium instead of calcium. *Pregnancy category*: C; PB: UK; $t^{1/2}$: UK
magaldrate (Riopan, Lowsium [plus simethicone])	A: PO: 5-15 ml PRN; *max*: 100 ml/d; or 1-2 tab PRN; *max*: 20 tab/d	To alleviate heartburn, gastritis, esophagitis, and peptic ulcers caused by hyperacidity. Contains aluminum and magnesium hydroxide. Low sodium content. Simethicone decreases flatus. Drug is minimally absorbed. *Pregnancy category*: C; PB: UK; $t^{1/2}$: UK
magnesium hydroxide and aluminum hydroxide (Maalox)	A: PO: 2-4 tab PRN; *max*: 16 tab/d or 10-30 ml, 1-3 h p.c. and at bedtime	Same as magaldrate. Caution for clients with renal disorder caused by the magnesium content. OTC drug. *Pregnancy category*: UK; PB: UK; $t^{1/2}$: UK
magnesium hydroxide, aluminum hydroxide, and calcium carbonate (Camalox)	A: PO: 10-20 ml PRN; *max*: 80 ml/d; or 2-4 tab PRN; *max*: 16 tab	Same as magaldrate, but also contains calcium. *Pregnancy category*: UK; PB: UK; $t^{1/2}$: UK
magnesium hydroxide and aluminum hydroxide with simethicone (Aludrox, Mylanta, Mylanta III, Maalox Plus, Gelusil-I, Gelusil-II, Gelusil-M, Di-Gel)	A: PO: 10-20 ml PRN; *max*: 120 ml/d; or 2-4 tab PRN; *max*: 24 tab	Same as magaldrate. Also contains simethicone, which decreases flatus. OTC drug. *Pregnancy category*: UK; PB: UK; $t^{1/2}$: UK
magnesium trisilicate (Gaviscon)	A: PO: 1-2 tab PRN; *max*: 8 tab/d	To relieve gastric disorders caused by hyperacidity. OTC drug. Contains magnesium trisilicate and aluminum hydroxide. *Pregnancy category*: UK; PB: UK; $t^{1/2}$: UK
sodium bicarbonate	A: PO: 0.5 tsp of powder in 8 oz water	Previously used for gastric hyperacidity. Short-acting, potent antacid that is systemically absorbed. Acid-base imbalance could occur. *Pregnancy category*: C; PB: UK; $t^{1/2}$: UK

A, Adult; *cap*, capsule; *d*, day; *GI*, gastrointestinal; *h*, hour; *max*, maximum; *OTC*, over-the-counter; *PB*, protein-binding; *p.c.*, after meals; *PO*, by mouth; *PRN*, as needed; $t^{1/2}$, half-life; *tab*, tablet; *tsp*, teaspoon; *UK*, unknown.

Client Teaching

General
- Instruct client to report pain, coughing, or vomiting of blood.
- Encourage client to drink 2 ounces of water after antacid to ensure that drug reaches the stomach.
- Direct client to take antacid 1 to 3 hours after meals and at bedtime. Do not take antacids at mealtime; they slow gastric emptying time, causing increased GI activity and gastric secretions.
- Advise client to notify health care provider if constipation or diarrhea occurs; the antacid may have to be changed. Self-treatment should be avoided.
- Stress that taking an unlimited amount of the antacid is contraindicated.
- Warn client to avoid taking antacids with milk or foods high in vitamin D.
- Tell client to avoid taking antacids within 1 to 2 hours of other oral medications, because there may be interference with absorption.

- Guide client to check antacid labels for sodium content if on a sodium-restricted diet.
- Alert client to consult with health care provider before taking self-prescribed antacids for longer than 2 weeks.
- Inform client on the use of relaxation techniques.

Self-Administration

- Teach client how to take antacids correctly. Chewable tablets should be thoroughly chewed and followed with water. With liquid antacid, 2 to 4 ounces of water should follow the antacid. Increased amount of water with antacids increases gastric emptying time.

Side Effects

- Direct client to avoid food and beverages that can cause gastric irritation (fatty, spicy meals, caffeine-containing coffee and cola, alcohol).
- Explain to client that stools may become speckled or white.

Cultural Considerations ❖

- Respect client's cultural beliefs and alternative methods for treating GI discomfort. Discuss with client the safety of those methods and the use of drugs prescribed to heal and lessen the symptoms.
- Recognize that clients of various cultural backgrounds may need guidance in understanding the disease process of their GI disturbance. Use of a written plan of care with modification should be considered.

EVALUATION

- Determine the effectiveness of the antiulcer treatment and the presence of side effects. Client should be free of pain, and healing should progress.

Histamine₂ Blockers

The histamine$_2$ (H$_2$) blockers (**histamine$_2$ receptor antagonists**) are popular drugs used in the treatment of gastric and duodenal ulcers. Histamine$_2$ blockers prevent acid reflux in the esophagus (reflux esophagitis). These drugs block the H$_2$ receptors of the parietal cells in the stomach, thus reducing gastric acid secretion and concentration. Antihistamines, used to treat allergic conditions, act against histamine$_1$ (H$_1$); they are not the same as H$_2$ blockers.

The first H$_2$ blocker was cimetidine (Tagamet), introduced in 1975. Cimetidine, which has a short half-life and a short duration of action, blocks about 70% of acid secretion for 4 hours. Good kidney function is necessary, because approximately 50% to 80% of the drug is excreted unchanged in the urine. If renal insufficiency is present, cimetidine's dose and frequency may need to be reduced. Antacids can be given an hour before or after cimetidine as part of the antiulcer drug regimen; however, if they are given at the same time, the effectiveness of the H$_2$ blocker is decreased.

Three H$_2$ blockers, ranitidine (Zantac [1983]), famotidine (Pepcid [1986]), and nizatidine (Axid [1988]), are more potent than cimetidine. In addition to blocking gastric acid secretions, they promote healing of the ulcer by eliminating its cause. Their duration of action is longer, decreasing the frequency of dosing, and they have fewer side effects and fewer drug interactions than cimetidine. Prototype Drug Chart 47–2 gives the pharmacologic data for ranitidine (Zantac), the most frequently prescribed H$_2$ blocker.

Pharmacokinetics

Ranitidine is 5 to 12 times more potent than cimetidine but less potent than famotidine. It is rapidly absorbed and reaches its peak concentration after a single dose in 1 to 3 hours. Ranitidine has a low protein-binding power and a short half-life. With liver disease, the half-life of ranitidine is prolonged. About 50% of the absorbed drug is excreted unchanged in the urine.

Ulcer healing occurs in 4 weeks for 70% of clients and in 8 weeks for 90% of clients taking ranitidine. Large doses of ranitidine are effective for controlling Zollinger-Ellison syndrome, whereas cimetidine is not effective in controlling the symptoms of this disorder.

Pharmacodynamics

Ranitidine inhibits histamine at the H$_2$ receptor site. The drug is effective in treating gastric and duodenal ulcers and can be used prophylactically. It is also useful in relieving symptoms of reflux esophagitis, preventing stress ulcers that can occur following major surgery, and preventing aspiration pneumonitis that can result from aspiration of gastric acid secretions.

Ranitidine has a longer onset of action and duration of action (up to 12 hours) than cimetidine. Because cimetidine has a duration of action of only 4 to 5 hours, it is frequently given three to four times a day.

Famotidine (Pepcid) is 50% to 80% more potent than cimetidine and is five to eight times more potent than ranitidine. It is indicated for short-term use (4 to 8 weeks) for duodenal ulcer and for Zollinger-Ellison syndrome.

Nizatidine (Axid) is the latest H$_2$ blocker. It can relieve nocturnal gastric acid secretion for 12 hours. This drug is similar to famotidine and ranitidine, and none of these agents suppresses the metabolism of other drugs. To prevent recurrence of duodenal ulcers, administer nizatidine 150 mg per day at bedtime or famotidine 20 mg per day at bedtime. Both nizatidine and famotidine have similar protein-binding times and half-lives.

Table 47–6 lists the H$_2$ blockers and their dosages, uses, and considerations.

Side Effects and Adverse Reactions

Side effects and adverse reactions of H$_2$ blockers include headaches, dizziness, constipation, pruritus, skin rash, gynecomastia, decreased libido, and impotence. Ranitidine and famotidine have fewer side effects than cimetidine.

Drug and Laboratory Interactions

Cimetidine interacts with many drugs. By inhibiting hepatic drug metabolism, it enhances the effects of oral anticoagulants, theophylline, caffeine, phenytoin (Dilantin), diazepam (Valium), propranolol (Inderal), phenobarbital, and calcium channel blockers. Cimetidine can cause an increase in blood urea nitrogen (BUN), serum creatinine, and serum alkaline phosphatase. Neither cimetidine nor

Prototype **DRUG CHART 47–2**

RANITIDINE

Drug Class	**Dosage**
Antiulcer: Histamine$_2$ blocker Trade name: Zantac *Pregnancy Category:* B	**A: PO:** 150 mg q12h or 300 mg at bedtime; maint: 150 mg at bedtime **IM:** 50 mg q6-8h **IV:** 50 mg q6-8h diluted **C: PO:** 2-4 mg/kg/d divided q12h **IV:** 1-2 mg/kg/d divided q6-8h
Contraindications	**Drug-Lab-Food Interactions**
Hypersensitivity, severe renal or liver disease *Caution:* Pregnancy, lactation	*Drug: Decrease* absorption with antacids; *decrease* absorption of ketoconazole; *toxicity* with metoprolol *Lab: Increase* serum alkaline phosphatase
Pharmacokinetics	**Pharmacodynamics**
Absorption: PO: well absorbed, 50% **Distribution:** PB: 15% **Metabolism:** t½: 2-3 h **Excretion:** In urine and feces	**PO:** Onset: 15 min Peak: 1-3 h Duration: 8-12 h **IM/IV:** Onset: 10-15 min Peak: 15 min Duration: 8-12 h

Therapeutic Effects/Uses

To prevent and treat peptic ulcers, gastroesophageal reflux, and stress ulcers
Mode of Action: Inhibition of gastric acid secretion by inhibiting histamine at histamine$_2$ receptors in parietal cells

Side Effects	**Adverse Reactions**
Headache, confusion, nausea, vertigo, diarrhea or constipation, depression, rash, blurred vision, malaise	*Life-threatening:* Hepatotoxicity, cardiac dysrhythmias, blood dyscrasias

A, Adult; *C,* child; *d,* day; *h,* hour; *IM,* intramuscular; *IV,* intravenous; *maint,* maintenance; *min,* minute; *PB,* protein-binding; *PO,* by mouth; *t½,* half-life.

Table 47–6

Antiulcer Drugs: Histamine$_2$ Blockers

Generic (Brand)	Route and Dosage	Uses and Considerations
cimetidine (Tagamet)	A: PO: 300 mg q.i.d. with meals and at bedtime or 800 mg at bedtime; maint: 300 mg at bedtime IV: 300 mg q6-8h diluted in 50 ml (administered over 15-30 min) IV: continuous infusion: 37.5 mg/h over 24 h; *max:* 900 mg/d C: PO/IV: 10-40 mg/kg/d divided q6h	For peptic ulcers (gastric and duodenal). First H$_2$ blocker marketed. Many drug interaction and side effects. Duration of action 4-6 h. *Pregnancy category:* B; PB: 20%; t^1/$_2$: 2 h
famotidine (Pepcid)	A: PO: 20 mg q12h or 40 mg at bedtime; maint: 20 mg at bedtime IV: 20 mg q12h diluted C: PO: 0.5-1 mg/kg/d divided q8-12h; *max:* 40 mg/d C: IV: 0.5 mg/kg/d divided q8-12h	For treatment of active duodenal ulcer. Inhibits gastric secretion. More potent than cimeti- dine. *Pregnancy category:* B; PB: 15%-20%; t^1/$_2$: 2.5-4 h
nizatidine (Axid)	A: PO: 150 mg q12h or 300 mg at bedtime; maint: 150 mg at bedtime	Same as famotidine. Also used to treat gastro- esophageal reflux. Give drug after meals or at bedtime. Do not give within 1 h of antacids. *Pregnancy category:* B; PB: 35%; t^1/$_2$: 1-2 h
ranitidine (Zantac)	(Prototype Drug Chart 47–2)	

A, Adult; *C,* child; *d,* day; *h,* hour; *IV,* intravenous; *maint,* maintenance; *max,* maximum; *PB,* protein-binding; *PO,* by mouth; *q.i.d.,* four times a day; *t^1/$_2$,* half-life.

ranitidine should be taken with antacids, because their H₂ blocking action could be decreased. Ranitidine can increase the effect of oral anticoagulants. Table 47–6 lists the drug data for the H₂ blockers.

Nursing Process

Antiulcer: Histamine₂ Blocker

ASSESSMENT

- Determine client's pain, including type, duration, severity, frequency, and location.
- Evaluate GI complaints.
- Check mental status.
- Assess fluid and electrolyte imbalances, including intake and output.
- Monitor gastric pH (>5 is desired), blood urea nitrogen (BUN), and creatinine.
- Determine drug history; report probable drug-drug interactions.

NURSING DIAGNOSES

- Acute pain related to excess gastric secretion

PLANNING

- Client will no longer experience abdominal pain after 1 to 2 weeks of drug therapy.

NURSING INTERVENTIONS

- Do not confuse drug with alprazolam (Xanax).
- Administer drug just before meals to decrease food-induced acid secretion or at bedtime.
- Be alert that reduced doses of drug are needed by older adults, who have less gastric acid. Metabolic acidosis must be prevented.
- Administer IV drug in 20 to 100 ml of solution.

Client Teaching

General

- Instruct client to report pain, coughing, or vomiting of blood.
- Advise client to avoid smoking, because it can hamper effectiveness of drug.
- Remind client that drug must be taken exactly as prescribed to be effective.
- Direct client to separate ranitidine and antacid dosage by at least 1 hour if possible.
- Warn client not to drive a motor vehicle or engage in dangerous activities until stabilized on the drug.
- Tell client that drug-induced impotence and gynecomastia are reversible.
- Educate client in the use of relaxation techniques to decrease anxiety.

Diet

- Teach client to eat foods rich in vitamin B₁₂ to avoid deficiency as a result of drug therapy.
- Alert client to avoid foods and liquids that can cause gastric irritation, such as caffeine-containing beverages, alcohol, and spices.

Cultural Considerations ❖

- Respect client's cultural beliefs and alternative methods for treating GI discomfort. Discuss with client the safety of those methods and the use of drugs prescribed to heal and lessen symptoms.
- Recognize that clients of various cultural backgrounds may need guidance in understanding the disease process of their GI disturbance. Use of a written plan of care with modification should be considered.

EVALUATION

- Determine the effectiveness of the drug therapy and the presence of any side effects or adverse reactions. Client should be free of pain, and healing should progress.

Proton Pump Inhibitors (Gastric Acid Secretion Inhibitors, Gastric Acid Pump Inhibitors)

The PPIs suppress gastric acid secretion by inhibiting the hydrogen/potassium adenosine triphosphatase (ATPase) enzyme system located in the gastric parietal cells. They tend to inhibit gastric acid secretion up to 90% greater than the H₂ blockers (histamine antagonists). These agents block the final step of acid production.

Omeprazole (Prilosec) was the first PPI marketed. Lansoprazole (Prevacid) became available in 1993. In the late 1990s two new PPIs were approved: rabeprazole (Aciphex) and pantoprazole (Protonix). Esomeprazole (Nexium) received Food and Drug Administration (FDA) approval in 2001. These five agents are effective in suppressing gastric acid secretions and are used to treat peptic ulcers and GERD. With lansoprazole, ulcer relief usually occurs in 1 week. Rabeprazole is more effective in treating duodenal ulcers than gastric ulcers, but is most effective for treating GERD and hypersecretory disease (Zollinger-Ellison syndrome). Pantoprazole, the fourth PPI developed, is prescribed to treat short-term erosive GERD. Intravenous pantoprazole is also reported as effective in treating Zollinger-Ellison syndrome. Esomeprazole, the newest PPI, has the highest success rate for healing erosive GERD, more so than omeprazole. Omeprazole promotes irreversible hydrogen or potassium ATPase inhibition until new enzyme is synthesized, which could take days, whereas rabeprazole causes reversible ATPase inhibition. All PPIs in large doses can be combined with antibiotics to treat *H. pylori*. Prototype Drug Chart 47–3 gives the pharmacologic data on lansoprazole.

Prototype DRUG CHART 47–3

LANSOPRAZOLE

Drug Class	**Dosage**
Antiulcer: Proton pump inhibitor Trade name: Prevacid *Pregnancy Category:* C	*Erosive esophagitis:* A: PO: 30 mg daily for 8 wk, then 15 mg daily *GERD* A: PO: 15 mg daily for up to wk C: PO: 1-11 y: 1.5 mg/kg/d *max:* 30 mg/d *Helicobacter pylori:* A: PO: 30 mg b.i.d. for 2 wk in combination therapy *Duodenal ulcer:* A: PO: 15 mg daily for 4 wk
Contraindications	**Drug-Lab-Food Interactions**
Hypersensitivity, pregnancy, lactation	*Drug:* May *decrease* theophylline levels; sucralfate *decreases* lansoprazole bioavailability; may interfere with absorption of ampicillin, ketoconazole, digoxin *Food:* Food *decreases* peak levels
Pharmacokinetics	**Pharmacodynamics**
Absorption: Rapidly absorbed in GI tract **Distribution:** PB: 97% **Metabolism:** t½: 1.5 h **Excretion:** Primarily in urine; also in bile and feces	**PO:** Onset: 2 h Peak: 1.5-3 h Duration: 24 h

Therapeutic Effects/Uses

To treat peptic and duodenal ulcers, GERD, erosive esophagitis, and *H. pylori*
Mode of Action: Suppresses gastric acid secretion by inhibiting hydrogen/potassium ATPase enzyme in gastric parietal cells

Side Effects	**Adverse Reactions**
Headache, dizziness, fatigue, thirst, increased appetite, anorexia, nausea, diarrhea, constipation, rash	Elevated AST, ALT

A, Adult; *ALT,* alanine aminotransferase; *AST,* aspartate aminotransferase; *ATP,* adenosine triphosphate; *b.i.d.,* two times a day; *C,* child; *d,* day; *GERD,* gastroesophageal reflux disease; *GI,* gastrointestinal; *h,* hour; *max,* maximum; *PB,* protein-binding; *PO,* by mouth; *t½,* half-life; *wk,* weeks; *y,* years.

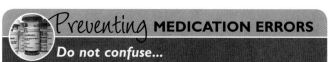

Preventing MEDICATION ERRORS

Do not confuse...

- **Protonix** (a proton pump inhibitor) with **Lotronex** (serotonin 5-HT3 receptor antagonist). These drug names look alike but are from different classes and have different actions. Alosetron (**Lotronex**) is used to treat symptoms of severe irritable bowel syndrome that last longer than 6 months and are unresponsive to traditional therapy.

Pharmacokinetics and Pharmacodynamics

The duration of action for omeprazole is 72 hours and for lansoprazole, 24 hours. These drugs have a short half-life and are highly protein-bound (97%). PPIs should be taken before meals. Caution should be used in clients with hepatic impairment; liver enzymes should be monitored. Possible side effects include headache, dizziness, diarrhea, abdominal pain, and rash. Prolonged use of PPIs may increase the risk of cancer, although this has only been proven in mice, not humans.

Table 47–7 lists the PPIs and their dosages, uses, and considerations.

Drug Interactions

Omeprazole can enhance the action of oral anticoagulants, certain benzodiazepines, and phenytoin, because it interferes with liver metabolism of these drugs. Lansoprazole may decrease theophylline levels. With pantoprazole, no significant drug interactions are reported.

Pepsin Inhibitor (Mucosal Protective Drug)

Sucralfate (Carafate), a complex of sulfated sucrose and aluminum hydroxide, is classified as a pepsin inhibitor, or *mucosal protective drug*. It is nonabsorbable and combines with protein to form a viscous substance that covers the ulcer and protects it from acid and pepsin. This drug does not neutralize acid or decrease acid secretions.

The dosage of sucralfate is 1 gram, usually four times a day before meals and at bedtime. If antacids are added to

Table 47–7

Antiulcer Drugs: Pepsin Inhibitor, Proton Pump Inhibitors, and Prostaglandin Analogue

Generic (Brand)	Route and Dosage	Uses and Considerations
Pepsin Inhibitors		
sucralfate (Carafate)	(Prototype Drug Chart 47–3)	
Proton Pump Inhibitors (Gastric Acid Secretion Inhibitors)		
esomeprazole magnesium (Nexium)	A: PO: 20-40 mg/d	Most effective in treating erosive GERD. Healing usually occurs in 4 to 8 wk. May be combined with amoxicillin or clarithromycin to treat *Helicobacter pylori*. *Pregnancy category*: UK; PB: 97%; t^{1}/$_{2}$: 1-1.5 h.
lansoprazole (Prevacid)	*Duodenal ulcer:* A: PO: 15 mg/d a.c. for 4 wk *Erosive esophagitis:* A: PO: 30 mg/d a.c. for 8 wk	Short-term treatment for duodenal ulcer and erosive esophagitis. Used in drug combination to treat *H. pylori*. Also effective for treating Zollinger-Ellison syndrome. Capsule must be swallowed whole (not chewed or crushed). *Pregnancy category*: B; PB: 97%; t^{1}/$_{2}$: 1.5 h
omeprazole (Prilosec)	*GERD and peptic ulcer:* A: PO: 20 mg/d for 4-8 wk *Hypersecretory:* A: PO: Initially: 60 mg/d; may increase to 120 mg t.i.d.	Treatment of GERD, esophagitis, Zollinger-Ellison syndrome, and *H. pylori*. Poorly absorbed, only 35%-40% in circulation. Antacids can be taken with drug. *Pregnancy category*: C; PB: 95%; t^{1}/$_{2}$: 0.5-1.5 h
pantoprazole (Protonix)	A: PO/IV: 40 mg/d	Treatment of gastric and duodenal ulcers and GERD. Action same as rabeprazole: suppresses gastric acid secretion. *Pregnancy category*: B; PB: UK; t^{1}/$_{2}$: 1-2 h.
rabeprazole (Aciphex)	*Duodenal ulcer/GERD:* A: PO: 20 mg/d *Hypersecretory disease:* A: PO: 60 mg/d or 60 mg b.i.d.	Treatment of duodenal ulcer, GERD, and hypersecretory syndrome (Zollinger-Ellison syndrome). Decreases gastric acid production by inhibiting hydrogen/ potassium ATPase enzyme at gastric parietal cells. *Pregnancy category*: B: PB: UK: t^{1}/$_{2}$: UK
Prostaglandin Analogues		
misoprostol (Cytotec)	A: PO: 100-200 mcg q.i.d. with food C: <18 y: PO: Safety and efficacy not established	Prevention of NSAID-induced gastric ulcer. May be taken during NSAID therapy, including with aspirin. Side effects include diarrhea, abdominal pain, flatulence, nausea, vomiting, constipation, and menstrual spotting. Short duration of action. *Pregnancy category*: X; PB: 85%; t^{1}/$_{2}$: 1.5 h

A, Adult; *a.c.*, before meals; *ATP*, adenosine triphosphate; *b.i.d.*, two times a day; *C*, child; *d*, day; *GERD*, gastroesophageal reflux disease; *h*, hour; *IV*, intravenous; *NSAIDs*, nonsteroidal antiinflammatory drugs; *PB*, protein-binding; *PO*, by mouth; *q.i.d.*, four times a day; *t^{1}/$_{2}$*, half-life; *t.i.d.*, three times a day; *UK*, unknown; *wk*, week; *y*, year; *<*, less than.

decrease pain, they should be given either 30 minutes before or after the administration of sucralfate. Because sucralfate is not systemically absorbed, side effects are few; however, it can cause constipation. If the drug is stored at room temperature in an airtight container, it will remain stable for up to 2 years. Prototype Drug Chart 47–4 shows the action and effects of sucralfate.

Pharmacokinetics

Less than 5% of sucralfate is absorbed by the GI tract. It has a half-life of 6 to 20 hours. Ninety percent of the drug is excreted in feces.

Pharmacodynamics

Sucralfate promotes healing by adhering to the ulcer surface. Onset of action occurs within 30 minutes, and duration of action is short. Sucralfate decreases the absorption of tetracycline, phenytoin, fat-soluble vitamins, and the antibacterial agents ciprofloxacin and norfloxacin. Antacids decrease the effects of sucralfate.

Nursing Process

Antiulcer: Pepsin Inhibitor

ASSESSMENT

■ Evaluate client's pain, including type, duration, severity, and frequency. Ulcer pain usually occurs after meals and during the night.
■ Determine client's renal function. Report urine output of <600 ml/d or <25 ml/h.
■ Assess for fluid and electrolyte imbalances.
■ Measure gastric pH (>5 is desired).

Prototype DRUG CHART 47–4

SUCRALFATE

Drug Class

Antiulcer: Pepsin inhibitor
Trade names: Carafate, ✚Sulcrate
Pregnancy Category: B

Dosage

Active disease:
A: PO: 1 g q.i.d. 1 h a.c. and at bedtime
Maintenance:
A: PO: 1 g b.i.d.

Contraindications

Hypersensitivity
Caution: Renal failure

Drug-Lab-Food Interactions

Drug: Decrease effects with tetracycline, phenytoin,
fat-soluble vitamins, digoxin; *altered absorption* with
ciprofloxacin, norfloxacin, antacids

Pharmacokinetics

Absorption: PO: Minimal absorption (<5%)
Distribution: PB: UK
Metabolism: t½: 6-20 h
Excretion: In urine

Pharmacodynamics

PO: Onset: 30 min
Peak: UK
Duration: 5 h

Therapeutic Effects/Uses

To prevent gastric mucosal injury from drug-induced ulcers (aspirin, NSAIDs); to manage ulcers
Mode of Action: In combination with gastric acid, forms a protective covering on the ulcer surface

Side Effects

Dizziness, nausea, constipation, dry mouth, rash,
pruritus, back pain, sleepiness

Adverse Reactions

None significant

A, Adult; *a.c.*, before meals; *b.i.d.*, twice a day; *h*, hour; *min*, minute; *NSAIDs*, nonsteroidal antiinflammatory drugs; *PB*, protein-binding; *PO*, by mouth; *q.i.d.*, four times a day; *t½*, half-life; *UK*, unknown; ✚, Canadian drug name; <, less than.

NURSING DIAGNOSES

■ Acute pain related to excess gastric secretion

PLANNING

■ Client will be free of abdominal pain after 1 to 2 weeks of antiulcer drug management.

NURSING INTERVENTIONS

■ Administer drug on empty stomach.
■ Administer antacid 30 minutes before or after sucralfate. Allow 1 to 2 hours to elapse between sucralfate and other prescribed drugs; sucralfate binds with certain drugs (e.g., tetracycline, phenytoin), reducing their effect.

Client Teaching

General
• Advise client to take drug exactly as ordered. Therapy usually requires 4 to 8 weeks for optimal ulcer healing. Advise client to continue to take drug even if feeling better.
• Increase fluids, dietary bulk, and exercise to relieve constipation.
• Instruct client in the use of relaxation techniques.
• Monitor for severe, persistent constipation.

• Stress need for follow-up medical care.
• Emphasize cessation of smoking as indicated.

Side Effects
• Direct client to report pain, coughing, or vomiting of blood.

Diet
• Teach client to avoid liquids and foods that can cause gastric irritation: caffeine-containing beverages, alcohol, certain fats, and spices.

Cultural Considerations ❖

• Greet the person by name with the appropriate title: Mr., Mrs., Miss, Ms., or Dr. Wait until client gives permission for you to use the first name.
• Males should not extend the hand in greeting to a female unless she extends her hand first.
• Orthodox Jewish males do not touch females other than their wives, so their failure to take a hand offered in greeting should not be interpreted as a sign of rudeness.

EVALUATION

■ Determine the effectiveness of the antiulcer treatment and the presence of any side effects. Client should be free of pain, and healing should progress.

Prostaglandin Analogue Antiulcer Drug

Misoprostol, a synthetic prostaglandin analogue, is a drug used to prevent and treat peptic ulcer. It appears to suppress gastric acid secretion and increase cytoprotective mucus in the GI tract. It causes a moderate decrease in pepsin secretion. Misoprostol is considered as effective as cimetidine. Clients who complain of gastric distress from NSAIDs such as aspirin or indomethacin prescribed for long-term therapy can benefit from misoprostol. When the client takes high doses of NSAIDs, misoprostol is frequently recommended for the duration of the NSAID therapy. Misoprostol is contraindicated during pregnancy and for women of childbearing age.

Table 47–7 lists the drug data for the pepsin inhibitors, PPIs, and prostaglandin analogue.

KEY WEBSITES

Heartburn, Gastroesophageal Reflux (GER), and Gastroesophageal Reflux Disease (GERD): http://digestive.niddk.nih.gov/ddiseases/pubs/gerd/index.htm

Proton Pump Inhibitors: An Update: http://www.aafp.org/afp/20020715/273.html

Gastritis and Peptic Ulcer Disease: http://www.emedicine.com/emerg/topic820.htm

Critical Thinking Case Study

JH, age 48, complains of a gnawing, aching pain in the abdominal area that usually occurs several hours after eating. He says that Tums help somewhat, but the pain has recently intensified. Diagnostic tests indicate that the client has a duodenal ulcer.

1. Differentiate between peptic ulcer, gastric ulcer, and duodenal ulcer. Explain.
2. What are the predisposing factors related to peptic ulcers? What additional information do you need from JH?
3. What nonpharmacologic measures can you suggest to alleviate symptoms related to peptic ulcer?

The health care provider prescribed Mylanta 2 tsp to be taken 2 hours after meals and ranitidine (Zantac) 150 mg b.i.d. The dose of Mylanta is to be taken either 1 hour before or 1 hour after the ranitidine.

4. JH asks the nurse the purposes for Mylanta and ranitidine. What would be the response?
5. The health care provider may suggest that the client take ranitidine with meals. Why? Why should Mylanta and ranitidine not be taken at the same time?
6. In what ways are ranitidine and cimetidine the same and how do they differ? Explain.
7. As part of client teaching, the nurse discusses side effects of ranitidine with JH. What might be the most effective way to present this information? Develop a plan.

The client states that he drinks beer at lunch and has two gin and tonics in the midafternoon. He states that these drinks help him relax.

8. What nursing intervention should be taken in regard to his alcohol intake?
9. What foods should he avoid?

A week later the client states that he discontinued the prescribed medications because he "felt better." However, the pain recurred and he asked whether he should resume taking the medications.

10. What would be your response? What client teaching should be included?

NCLEX Study Questions

1. A client is diagnosed with peptic ulcer disease. The nurse realizes that predisposing factors for this condition include:
   a. *Helicobacter pylori*
   b. hyposecretion of pepsin
   c. decreased hydrochloric acid
   d. decreased number of parietal cells

2. When a client is given sucralfate (Carafate), the nurse knows that its mode of action is to:
   a. neutralize gastric acidity
   b. inhibit gastric acid secretion by inhibiting histamine at H2 receptors in parietal cells
   c. suppress gastric acid secretion by inhibiting the hydrogen/potassium ATPase enzyme
   d. combine with protein to form a viscous substance that forms a protective covering of ulcer

3. The teaching for a client taking ranitidine includes:
   a. drug-induced impotence is irreversible
   b. administer drug 30 minutes before meals
   c. separate from an antacid by at least one hour
   d. always administer with a magnesium hydroxide

4. When a client complains of pain accompanying a peptic ulcer, an antacid is given, because:
   a. antacids decrease GI motility
   b. antacids decrease gastric acid secretion
   c. aluminum hydroxide is a systemic antacid
   d. antacids neutralize HCl and reduce pepsin activity

5. A client is taking famotidine to inhibit gastric secretions. The side effects of famotidine may include:
   a. diarrhea
   b. dizziness
   c. dry mouth
   d. blurred vision

Answers: 1, a; 2, d; 3, c; 4, d; 5, b.

SIXTEEN

Eye, Ear, and Skin Agents

Many drugs used to treat eye and ear disorders are discussed in other chapters. Antibiotics are covered in Chapters 28, Penicillins and Cephalosporins, 29, Macrolides, Tetracyclines, Aminoglycosides, and Fluoroquinolones, and 30, Sulfonamides. Unit Sixteen discusses in more detail the agents used to treat disorders of the eye, ear, and skin. Chapter 48, Drugs for Disorders of the Eye and Ear, presents medications used to treat eye disorders, particularly glaucoma and ocular infections. Drugs used to treat ear disorders are also covered. Chapter 49, Drugs for Dermatologic Disorders, presents the agents used to treat skin conditions such as acne and psoriasis.

Overview of the Eye

The eyeballs, protected within the orbits of the skull, are controlled by the third, fourth, and sixth cranial nerves and are connected to six extraocular muscles. The eye has three layers: (1) the cornea and sclera; (2) the choroid, iris, and ciliary body; and (3) the retina. Figure XVI–1 illustrates the basic structures of the eye.

The cornea, the anterior covering of the eye, is transparent, enabling light to enter the eye. It has no blood vessels and receives nutrition from the aqueous humor. An abraded cornea is susceptible to infection. Loss of corneal transparency is usually caused by increased intraocular pressure (IOP).

The sclera is the opaque, white fibrous envelope of the eye. Within the sclera are the posterior chamber and the anterior chamber. The posterior chamber has a blind spot, which is not sensitive to light, around the optic nerve. The lens, held in place by ligaments, separates these two chambers. The normally transparent lens focuses light on the retina by changing its shape through a process called *accommodation*.

The anterior chamber, filled with aqueous humor secreted by the ciliary body, lies in front of the lens. The fluid flows into the anterior chamber through a space between the lens and iris. The excess fluid drains into the canal of Schlemm. A rise in intraocular pressure, resulting in glaucoma, occurs with increased production or decreased drainage of aqueous humor.

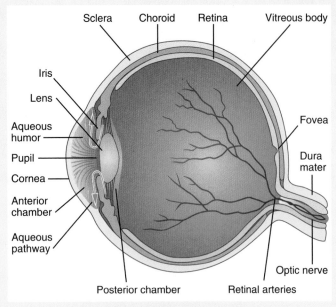

FIGURE XVI–I Basic structures of the eye.

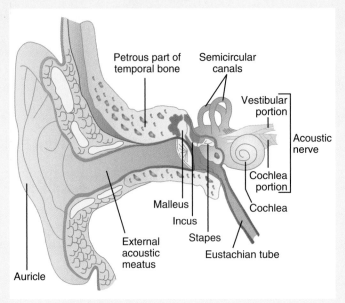

FIGURE XVI–2 Basic structures of the ear.

The choroid, iris, and ciliary body (thickened part of the vascular covering of the eye that provides attachment to ligaments and support to the lens) constitute the second layer. The choroid absorbs light. The iris surrounds the pupil and gives the eye its color. By dilating and constricting, the iris controls the quantity of light reaching the lens.

The retina, the third layer, consists of nerves, rods, and cones that serve as visual sensory receptors. The retina is connected to the brain via the optic nerve.

The eyebrows, eyelashes, eyelids, tears, and corneal and conjunctival reflexes all serve to protect the eye. Bilateral blinking occurs every few seconds during waking hours to keep the eye moist and free of foreign material.

Overview of the Ear

The ear is divided into the external, middle, and inner ear. Figure XVI–2 illustrates the ear's basic structures.

The *external ear* consists of the pinna and the external auditory canal. The external auditory canal transmits sound to the tympanic membrane (eardrum), a transparent partition between the external and middle ear. The eardrum in turn transmits sound to the bones of the middle ear; it also serves a protective function.

The *middle ear*, an air-filled cavity, contains three auditory ossicles (malleus, incus, and stapes) that transmit sound waves to the inner ear. The tip of the malleus is attached to the eardrum; its head is attached to the incus, which is attached to the stapes. The eustachian tube provides a direct connection to the nasopharynx and equalizes air pressure on both sides of the eardrum to prevent it from rupturing. Swallowing, yawning, and chewing gum

help the eustachian tube relieve pressure changes during airplane flights.

The *inner ear*, a series of labyrinths (canals), consists of a bony section and a membranous section. The vestibule, cochlea, and semicircular canals make up the bony labyrinth. The vestibular area is responsible for maintaining equilibrium and balance. The cochlea is the principal hearing organ.

Professional evaluation of ear problems is essential, because hearing loss can result from untreated disorders. Middle ear problems require prescription medications and are not treated with over-the-counter preparations.

Overview of the Skin

Skin, the largest organ of the body, consists of two major layers: the *epidermis* (the outer layer of the skin) and the *dermis* (the layer of skin beneath the epidermis). The functions of the skin include (1) protecting the body from the environment, (2) aiding in body temperature control, and (3) preventing body fluid loss.

The epidermis has four layers: (1) the basal layer (stratum germinativum), the deepest layer lying over the dermis; (2) the spinous layer (stratum spinosum); (3) the granular layer (stratum granulosum); and (4) the cornified layer (stratum corneum), the outer layer of the epidermis. As the epidermal cells migrate to the surface, they die, and their cytoplasm converts to keratin (hard and rough texture), forming keratinocytes. Eventually the keratinocytes slough off as new layers of epidermal cells migrate upward.

The dermis has two layers: (1) the papillary layer, next to the epidermis, and (2) the reticular layer, which is the deeper layer of the dermis. The dermal layers consist of fibroblasts, collagen fibers, and elastic fibers. The collagen and elastic fibers give the skin its strength and elasticity. Within the dermal layer, there are sweat glands, hair follicles, sebaceous glands, blood vessels, and sensory nerve terminals. Figure XVI–3 shows the layers of the skin.

The subcutaneous tissue, primarily fatty tissue, lies under the dermis. Besides fatty cells, subcutaneous tissue contains blood and lymphatic vessels, nerve fibers, and elastic fibers. It supports and protects the dermis.

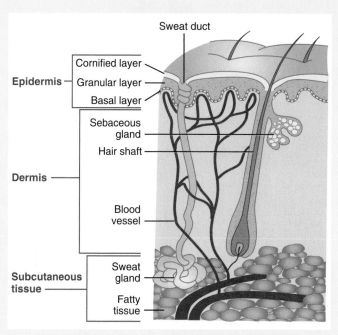

FIGURE XVI–3   Basic structures of the skin.

48

Drugs for Disorders of the Eye and Ear

ELECTRONIC RESOURCES

Evolve website (http://evolve.elsevier.com/KeeHayes/pharmacology/):
- *Case Studies*
- *Content Updates*
- *Frequently Asked Questions*
- *Student Review Activities*
- *WebLinks*
- *Additional Reference Material*

Companion CD-ROM:
- *NCLEX Examination Review Questions*
- *Pharmacology Animations*
- *IV Therapy Checklists*
- *Medication Error Checklists*
- *Drug Calculation Problems*
- *Electronic Calculators*
- *Top 200 Drugs with Pronunciations*
- *References from the Textbook*

Outline

Objectives

- Describe the medication groups commonly used for disorders of the eye and ear.
- Discuss the mechanisms of action, route, side effects and adverse reactions, and contraindications for selected drugs in each group.
- Describe the content of teaching plans for the drug groups presented.
- Describe the nursing process, including client teaching, related to disorders of the eye and ear.

Terms

This chapter describes the most commonly used drugs for eye and ear disorders. Many of these drugs have other uses and are discussed in greater detail in other chapters.

Drugs for Disorders of the Eye

The nurse must be alert to the fact that a variety of systemic diseases have **ophthalmic** (pertaining to the eye) findings that are characteristic. Examples of these systemic disorders are acquired immunodeficiency syndrome (AIDS), coronary vascular disease, muscular and endocrine disorders, and hematologic and neurologic diseases.

Diagnostic Aids

Diagnostic aids are frequently used to locate lesions or foreign objects and to provide local anesthesia to the area. Drugs commonly used as diagnostic aids are presented in Table 48–1.

Topical Anesthetics

Topical anesthetics are used in selected aspects of a comprehensive eye examination and in the removal of foreign bodies from the eye. The two most common topical anesthetics are proparacaine HCl (Ophthaine, Ophthetic) and tetracaine HCl (Pontocaine).

Corneal anesthesia is achieved within 1 minute and generally lasts about 15 minutes. The blink reflex is temporarily lost; therefore the corneal epithelium is not kept moist. To protect the eye, a patch is usually worn over the eye until the effects of the drug are gone. These drugs are *not* to be self-administered by the client. Repeated doses are given only under strict medical supervision.

Antiinfectives and Antiinflammatories

Antiinfectives are frequently used for eye infections. Screen the client for previous allergic reactions. **Conjunctivitis** (inflammation of the delicate membrane covering the eyeball and lining the eyelid) and local skin and eye irritation are possible side effects of topical ophthalmic antiinfective drugs. Examples of frequently occurring ocular conditions treated with antiinfectives include the following:

- Conjunctivitis
- Blepharitis (infection of margins of eyelid)
- Chalazion (infection of meibomian glands of the eyelids that may produce cysts, causing blockage of the ducts)
- Endophthalmitis (inflammation of structures of the inner eye)
- Hordeolum (local infection of eyelash follicles and glands on lid margins)
- Keratitis (corneal inflammation)
- Uveitis (infection of vascular layer of eye [ciliary body, choroid, and iris])

Conjunctivitis is an eye infection that can be bacterial, viral, or allergic in origin. The common ophthalmic antihistamines used to treat allergic conjunctivitis include cromolyn sodium (Crolom), ketotifen fumarate (Zaditor), levocabastine (Livostin), lodoxamide tromethamine (Alomide), olopatadine (Patanol), and pemirolast potassium (Alamast). Burning, headache, and stinging are the most frequent adverse effects.

For more comprehensive information on antiinfectives, see Chapters 28, 29, and 30. The drug data for **optic** (eye) antiinfectives are presented in Table 48–2. Optic antiinflammatories are presented in Table 48–3.

Lubricants

Both healthy and ill persons may need to use eye lubricants. Healthy clients who complain of "dryness of the eyes" use lubricants as artificial tears; lubricants are also used to moisten contact lenses or artificial eyes. Lubricants alleviate discomfort associated with dryness and maintain the integrity of the epithelial surface. They are also used during anesthesia and in acute or chronic central nervous system (CNS) disorders that result in unconsciousness or decreased blinking.

Most lubricants are available over-the-counter (OTC) in both liquid and ointment form. Popular lubricants include Isopto Tears, Tearisol, Ultra Tears, Tears Naturale, Tears Plus, Lens Mate, and Lacri-Lube. Be alert to allergic reactions to preservatives in lubricants.

Antiglaucoma Agents

Pharmacotherapy is the primary approach used to treat glaucoma, which is an increased intraocular pressure (IOP) resulting from excessive production or diminished outflow of aqueous humor. Glaucoma is classified as either (1) *primary* (pathologic change within the eye) or (2) *secondary* (change associated with systemic disease and use of selected drugs). The angle of the anterior chamber also determines the type of glaucoma. The angle can be either *open angle* (diminished outflow of aqueous humor related to degenerative changes in the trabecular meshwork) or *closed angle* (triggered by emotions and drugs that dilate pupils).

Antiglaucoma drugs belong to the following categories: cholinergic and anticholinesterase miotics, beta-adrenergic

Table 48–1
Diagnostic Aids for Eye Disorders

Diagnostic Aid	Purpose
fluorescein sodium	Dye used to demonstrate defects in corneal epithelium. Corneal scratches turn bright green; foreign bodies are surrounded by green ring. Loss of conjunctiva shows orange-yellow. Dye appears in nasal secretions if lacrimal duct patent.
fluorescein sodium and benoxinate HCl (Fluress)	Dye and local anesthetic. Used for short corneal and conjunctival procedures, including removal of foreign bodies.
rose bengal	Preferred dye when superficial conjunctival tissue or corneal pathology or injury suspected.

Table 48–2

Ophthalmic: Antiinfectives

Generic (Brand)	Route and Dosage*	Uses and Considerations
Antibacterials		
chloramphenicol (AK-Chlor, Chloromycetin Ophthalmic)	A & C: Ophthalmic: Instill 1-2 gtt or 0.5-in oint q3-4h for 48 h; increase interval to b.i.d./t.i.d.	Effective against both gram-negative and gram-positive bacteria. For treatment of severe infections or when other antibacterials not effective. Continue treatment for at least 48 h after eye appears normal. *Pregnancy category:* C; PB: NA; t^1/$_2$: NA
ciprofloxacin (Cipro)	A & C >12 y: *Day 1:* 2 gtt q15min for 6 h then 2 gtt q30min for rest of day *Day 2:* 2 gtt qh *Days 3-14:* 2 gtt q4h	Effective against bacterial conjunctivitis. To treat corneal ulceration. Minimal absorption through cornea or conjunctiva. *Pregnancy category:* C; PB: NA; t^1/$_2$: NA
erythromycin (Ilotycin)	A & C >12 y: Oint: 0.5%: 0.5-1 cm daily/ q.i.d.	Most commonly used antibacterial. For superficial ocular infections and prevention of ophthalmia neonatorum. *Pregnancy category:* B; PB: NA; t^1/$_2$: NA
gentamicin sulfate (Garamycin Ophthalmic)	A & C: Sol 0.3%: 1-2 gtt q4h; may increase to 2 gtt qh for severe infections Oint 0.3%: 0.5-in ribbon b.i.d./t.i.d.	For infections of the external eye: *Pregnancy category:* C; PB: NA; t^1/$_2$: NA
norfloxacin (Chibroxin)	A & C >1 y: Sol 3%: instill 1-2 gtt in affected eye(s) q.i.d. for 7 d	For treatment of conjunctivitis. *Pregnancy category:* C; PB: NA; t^1/$_2$: NA
silver nitrate 1% (Dey-Drop)	Neonate: Instill 2 gtt in each eye within 1 h of birth	For prevention and treatment of ophthalmia neonatorum. *Pregnancy category:* C; PB: NA; t^1/$_2$: NA
sulfacetamide (Bleph-10, Sulamyd)	A & C >12 y: Sol: 1 gtt q1-3h while awake; then q3-4h while sleeping	Effectiveness of sulfonamides decreased in the presence of PABA and purulent drainage, hence exudates should be removed before instilling drops. *Pregnancy category:* C; PB: NA; t^1/$_2$: NA
tobramycin (Nebcin, Tobrex)	A & C >12 y: Oint 0.3%: 0.5-in b.i.d./t.i.d Sol 0.3%: 1-2 gtt q4h *For severe infections:* Oint: 0.5-in q3-4h Sol: 2 gtt q30-60 min until improvement, then decrease frequency	For external ocular infections. *Pregnancy category:* D; PB: NA; t^1/$_2$: NA
tetracycline HCl (Achromycin Ophthalmic)	A: Instill 1-2 gtt b.i.d./q.i.d. A: Instill 0.5-in q2-12h	Bacteriostatic action; alternative to silver nitrate for prevention of ophthalmia neonatorum. *Pregnancy category:* D; PB: NA; t^1/$_2$: NA
triple antibiotic ophthalmic ointment (neomycin, polymyxin B Sulfate, bacitracin ophthalmic)	A & C >12 y: 1 cm applied in conjunctival sac q3-4h	Combination dosage form effective against many gram-negative organisms. *Pregnancy category:* C; PB: NA; t^1/$_2$: NA
Antifungal		
natamycin (Natacyn Ophthalmic)	A & C: Sol 5%: 1 gt q2h for 3-4 d; then 1 gt q3h for 14-21 d	May cause transient stinging or temporary blurring of vision. *Pregnancy category:* C; PB: NA; t^1/$_2$: NA
Antiviral		
idoxuridine (IDU, Herplex Liquifilm)	A & C: Sol 1%: Initially: 1 gt q1h during the day and q2h at night; when definite improvement occurs, use 1 gt q2h during the day and q4h at night; continue 3-7 d after healing occurs Oint 0.5%: Place 0.5-in. q4h while awake	To treat cytomegalovirus or herpes simplex keratitis. Store in refrigerator; do not mix with boric acid. If no response in 1 wk, discontinue. *Pregnancy category:* C; PB: NA; t^1/$_2$: NA
trifluridine (Viroptic)	A: Sol 1%: Instill 1 gt into infected eye q2h while awake; *max:* 9 gtt/d until corneal ulcer reepithelialized; then 1 gt q4h for 7 d; *max:* 21 d of treatment	For treatment of herpetic ophthalmic infections and keratoconjunctivitis caused by HSV-1 and HSV-2. *Pregnancy* category: C; PB: NA; t^1/$_2$: NA
vidarabine monohydrate (Vira-A)	A & C: Oint 3%: 0.5-in. 5 × d at 3-h intervals	For treatment of keratoconjunctivitis and herpes simplex keratitis. *Pregnancy category:* C; PB: NA; t^1/$_2$: NA

*To minimize systemic absorption, gently apply pressure on inner canthus.

A, Adult; *b.i.d.,* twice a day; *C,* child; *d,* day; *HSV,* herpes simplex virus; *gt,* drop; *gtt,* drops; *h,* hour; *in,* inch; *max,* maximum; *NA,* not applicable; *oint,* ointment; *PABA,* paraaminobenzoic acid; *PB,* protein-binding; *q.i.d.,* four times a day; *sol,* solution; *t^1/$_2$,* half-life; *t.i.d.,* three times a day; *wk,* week; *y,* year; *>,* greater than.

Table 48–3

Ophthalmic: Antiinflammatories

Generic (Brand)	Route and Dosage*	Uses and Considerations
Nonsteroidals		
*diclofenac sodium (Voltaren)	A: 1 gt to affected eye q.i.d. for 2 wk; start 24 h after cataract surgery	For postoperative inflammation and photophobia. *Pregnancy category:* B; PB: NA; t¹/₂: NA
*flurbiprofen sodium (Ocufen)	A: Instill 1 gt q30min at 2 h before surgery; total dose is 4 gtt	To decrease corneal edema; miosis. *Pregnancy category:* C; PB: NA; t¹/₂: NA
*ketorolac tromethamine (Acular)	A: Sol 0.5%: Instill 1 gt q.i.d.	Efficacy has not been established beyond 1 wk of therapy. Used to relieve itching associated with seasonal allergic conjunctivitis. *Pregnancy category:* C; PB: NA; t¹/₂: NA
*suprofen (Profenal)	*Preoperative:* A: Instill 2 gtt in sac q4h while awake on day preceding surgery; instill 2 gtt in conjunctival sac at 3, 2, and 1 h before surgery	Used to prevent intraoperative miosis. *Pregnancy category:* C; PB: NA; t¹/₂: NA
Corticosteroids		
dexamethasone (AK-Dex Ophthalmic, Decadron, Maxidex)	A & C: Oint: Apply into conjunctival sac t.i.d./q.i.d.; gradually decrease to discontinue. Susp: Instill 2 gtt qh while awake and q2h during night; taper to q3-4h; then t.i.d./q.i.d.	For uveitis, allergic conditions, and inflammation of conjunctiva, cornea, and lids. Should not be used for minor abrasions and wounds. *Pregnancy category:* C; PB: NA; t¹/₂: NA
medrysone (HMS Liquifilm)	A & C: Susp: Initially: Instill 1 gt in conjunctival sac q1-2h (1-2 d); then 1 gt b.i.d./q.i.d.	To treat allergic conditions, burns, inflammation of conjunctiva, cornea, and lids. *Pregnancy category:* C; PB: NA; t¹/₂: NA
prednisolone acetate (Econopred)	A: Initially instill 1-2 gtt in conjunctival sac qh while awake, q2h during night until desired effect; maint: 1 gt q4h. Susp: 0.125% and 1%	To treat uveitis, allergic conditions, burns, and inflammation of conjunctiva, cornea, and lids. *Pregnancy category:* C; PB: NA; t¹/₂: NA
prednisolone sodium phosphate (AK-Pred, Inflamase)	A & Elderly: Sol 0.125% and 1%: 1-2 gtt q1h during day; q2h during night; with response give 1 gt q4h, then 1 gt t.i.d./q.i.d. Oint: thin coat t.i.d./q.i.d.; with response decrease to b.i.d., then daily	To prevent or decrease tissue response to inflammatory process.
Combination: tobramycin 0.3% and dexamethasone 0.1% (TobraDex)	A: 1-2 gtt q2-6h first 24-48h; then q4-6h or less until symptoms decrease; *max:* 20 ml for first treatment. Oint: Apply to conjunctival sac up to t.i.d./q.i.d.; *max:* 8 g for initial treatment. Drops and ointment not recommended for children.	For treatment of fungal, mycobacterial, or viral infection of eye. Combines antiinflammatory power of dexamethasone with antibiotic. Increased tolerability and comfortable pH.

*To minimize systemic absorption, gently apply pressure to inner canthus.
A, Adult; *b.i.d.*, twice a day; *C*, child; *d*, day; *gt*, drop; *gtt*, drops; *h*, hour; *maint*, maintenance; *max*, maximum; *min*, minute; *NA*, not applicable; *oint*, ointment; *PB*, protein-binding; *q.i.d.*, four times a day; *sol*, solution; *susp*, suspension; *t¹/₂*, half-life; *t.i.d.*, three times a day; *wk*, week.

blockers, carbonic anhydrase inhibitors, osmotics, and anticholinergics. Note Herbal Alert 48–1.

Cholinergic Agents (Miotics)

In open-angle glaucoma, **miotics** are used to lower the IOP, thereby increasing blood flow to the retina and decreasing retinal damage and loss of vision. Miotics cause a contraction of the ciliary muscle and widening of trabecular meshwork. The two types of miotics differ in their mechanism of action: (1) *direct-acting cholinergics* (similar to the neurotransmitter acetylcholine), which mediate transmission of nerve impulses at all parasympathetic (cholinergic) nerve sites; and (2) *indirect-acting anticholinesterase* drugs, which inactivate cholinesterase, thereby inhibiting enzymatic destruction of acetylcholine and resulting in pupil constriction and ciliary muscle contraction. Figure 48–1 illustrates increased IOP resulting in glaucoma, and Table 48–4 presents the drug data for commonly prescribed miotics.

Herbal ALERT 48–1

Herbs and Antiglaucoma Agents
- Avoid the use of goldenseal in clients with glaucoma.
- Many herbs alter coagulation; therefore they generally are discontinued before ophthalmic or otic surgery.
- Consult health care provider prior to use of herbs.

Normal flow of aqueous humor

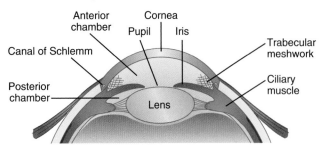

Impeded flow of aqueous humor, resulting in intraocular pressure

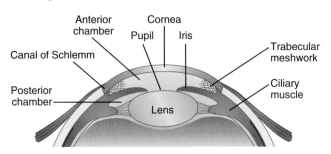

Obstructive flow to canal of Schlemm

FIGURE 48–1 Increased intraocular pressure.

Table 48–4

Miotics: Cholinergics and Beta-Adrenergic Blockers

Generic (Brand)	Route and Dosage	Uses and Considerations
Direct-Acting Cholinergics		
carbachol (Isopto Carbachol)	A: Ophthalmic: 1-2 gtt daily/q.i.d.	To reduce IOP, especially when pilocarpine is ineffective. *Pregnancy category:* C; PB: NA; t¹/₂: NA
pilocarpine HCl (Isopto Carpine)	(Prototype Drug Chart 48–1)	
pilocarpine nitrate (Ocusert Pilo-20, Pilo-40)	(Prototype Drug Chart 48–1)	
echothiophate iodide (Phospholine Iodide)	A: Sol 0.03%-0.25%: 1 gt daily/b.i.d.	Used to treat chronic open-angle glaucoma and glaucoma following cataract surgery. *Pregnancy category:* C; PB: NA; t¹/₂: NA
Indirect-Acting Cholinesterase Inhibitors		
Short Acting		
physostigmine salicylate (Isopto Eserine)	A & C: Oint 0.25%: 0.25 inch 1-3 ×/d Sol 0.25-0.5%: 1-2 gtt up to 4 ×/d	For wide-angle glaucoma. *Pregnancy category:* C; PB: NA; t¹/₂: NA
Long Acting		
demecarium bromide (Humorsol)	A: Sol 0.125-0.25%: 1-2 gtt 2 × wk or 1-2 gtt b.i.d.	Used for open-angle glaucoma when shorter-acting agents have been unsuccessful. Also used for conditions affecting aqueous outflow and accommodative strabismus. *Pregnancy category:* C; PB: NA; t¹/₂: NA
Beta-Adrenergic Blockers		
betaxolol HCl (Betoptic)	A: Susp 0.25% or sol 0.5%: Usual dose 1 gt b.i.d.	Selective beta blocker. Used to decrease elevated IOP in chronic open-angle glaucoma and ocular hypertension. Contraindicated in clients with asthma caused by increased airway resistance from systemic absorption. Use caution in clients receiving oral beta-blockers. *Pregnancy category:* C; PB: NA; t¹/₂: NA
carteolol HCI (Ocupress)	A: Sol 1% sol: 1 gtt b.i.d.	Used for open-angle glaucoma. May potentiate effect of systemic beta-blockers.
levobetaxolol (Betaxon)	A: 1 gt 0.5% susp b.i.d.	Selective beta blocker
levobunolol HCl (Betagan Liquifilm, AKBeta)	A: Sol 0.25%-0.5%: 1-2 gtt daily/b.i.d.	Lowers IOP. *Pregnancy category* C; PB: NA; t¹/₂: NA
timolol maleate (Timoptic)	A: Sol 0.25%-0.5% initially: 1 gt b.i.d.; maint: 1 gt/d once response occurs with initial dosage	Reduces production of aqueous humor. Monitor vital signs during initial therapy. Concurrent use of similar drugs must be individualized. Blurred vision decreases with use. *Pregnancy category:* C; PB: NA; t¹/₂: NA

A, Adult; *b.i.d.*, twice a day; *C*, child; *d*, day; *gt*, drop; *gtt*, drops; *IOP*, intraocular pressure; *maint*, maintenance; *NA*, not applicable; *oint*, ointment; *PB*, protein-binding; *q.i.d.*, four times a day; *sol*, solution; *susp*, suspension; *t¹/₂*, half-life; *t.i.d.*, three times a day; *wk*, week.

Pharmacokinetics

Systemic absorption is possible but not common with the use of miotics. To reduce systemic absorption of eyedrops, the client or nurse should gently apply pressure on the **lacrimal duct** (passage that carries tears into the nose). Pilocarpine, a direct-acting miotic, binds to the ocular tissues; its half-life is unknown. The metabolism and elimination of this drug are also currently unknown.

Pharmacodynamics

Pilocarpine produces **miosis** (contraction of the pupil) and decreases IOP. The onset of action, peak, and duration of action vary with the dose, desired effect, and form. When pilocarpine is administered to produce miosis, its onset of action is 10 to 30 minutes, its time of peak action is unknown, and its duration of action is 4 to 8 hours. When used to reduce IOP, ophthalmic pilocarpine has an unknown onset of action, a peak time of 75 minutes, and duration of action of 4 to 14 hours.

Ocusert is a wafer-thin disk impregnated with time-release pilocarpine. The disk is replaced every 7 days. Clients should check for the presence of the Ocusert disk in the conjunctival sac daily at bedtime and on awakening. With the ocular therapeutic system Ocusert, the onset of action is unknown, the peak is 1.5 to 2 hours, and the duration of action is 7 days.

The drug data for pilocarpine are shown in Prototype Drug Chart 48–1.

Side Effects and Adverse Reactions

Side effects from the use of miotics include headache, eye pain, decreased vision, brow pain, and, less frequently, hyperemia of the conjunctiva. Systemic absorption can cause nausea, vomiting, diarrhea, frequent urination, precipitation of asthmatic attacks, increased salivation, diaphoresis, muscle weakness, and respiratory difficulty. Manifestations of toxicity include vertigo, bradycardia, tremors, hypotension, syncope, cardiac dysrhythmias, and seizures. Atropine sulfate must be available in case of systemic toxicity.

Prototype **DRUG CHART 48–1**

PILOCARPINE

Drug Class

Direct-acting miotic
Trade names: Isopto Carpine, Pilopine HS, Ocusert
   Pilo-20 and –40
Pregnancy Category: C

Dosage

A & C: Sol: 1%-2%, 1-2 gtt, t.i.d./q.i.d.
Gel: Apply 0.5-in ribbon in lower eyelid at bedtime
Ocusert: Replace q7d

Contraindications

Retinal detachment, adhesions between iris and lens,
   acute ocular inflammation; must avoid systemic
   absorption of drug with coronary artery disease,
   obstruction of GI/GU tract, epilepsy, asthma

Drug-Lab-Food Interactions

Drug: Avoid use with carbachol and echothiophate;
   decrease antiglaucoma effects with belladonna
   alkaloids; *decrease* dilation with phenylephrine

Pharmacokinetics

Absorption: PO: Some systemic absorption
Distribution: PB: UK
Metabolism: t½: UK; binds to ocular tissue
Excretion: UK

Pharmacodynamics

Miosis:
Ophthalmic: Onset: 10-30 min
   Peak: 20 min
   Duration: 4-8 h
Reduce IOP:
Ophthalmic: Onset: 45-60 min
   Peak: 75 min
   Duration: 4-14 h
Ocusert: Onset: 1 h
   Peak: 1.5-2 h
   Duration: 7 d
Gel: Onset: 1 h
   Peak: 3-12 h
   Duration: 18-24 h

Therapeutic Effects/Uses

To induce miosis; to decrease IOP in glaucoma
Mode of Action: Stimulation of pupillary and ciliary sphincter muscles

Side Effects

Blurred vision, eye pain, headache, eye irritation,
   brow ache, stinging and burning, nausea, vomiting,
   diarrhea, increased salivation and perspiration,
   muscle tremors, contact allergy
Conjunctival irritation with Ocusert

Adverse Reactions

Dyspnea, hypertension, tachycardia, retinal detachment;
   long term: bronchospasm
Corneal abrasion and visual impairment potential with
   Ocusert

A, Adult; *C,* child; *d,* day; *GI,* gastrointestinal; *gtt,* drops; *GU,* genitourinary; *h,* hour; *in,* inch; *IOP,* intraocular pressure; *min,* minute; *PB,* protein-binding; *PO,* by mouth; *q.i.d.,* four times a day; *sol,* solution; *t½,* half-life; *t.i.d.,* three times a day; *UK,* unknown.

Drug Interactions

Ophthalmic epinephrine, timolol, levobunolol, betaxolol, and systemic carbonic anhydrase inhibitors have the added effect of lowering IOP. Cyclopentolate, ophthalmic belladonna alkaloids, and antidepressants antagonize the therapeutic effects of miotics.

Contraindications

Contraindications to the use of pilocarpine include retinal detachment, adhesions between the iris and lens, and acute ocular infections. Caution is advised for clients with the following conditions: asthma, hypertension, corneal abrasion, hyperthyroidism, coronary vascular disease, urinary tract obstruction, gastrointestinal obstruction, ulcer disease, parkinsonism, and bradycardia.

 Nursing Process

Miotics

ASSESSMENT

■ Obtain medical, herbal, and drug history. Miotics are contraindicated in clients with narrow-angle glaucoma, acute inflammation of the eye, heart block, coronary artery disease, obstruction of the GI or urinary tract, and asthma.
■ Check vital signs. Baseline vital signs can be compared with future findings.
■ Assess client's level of anxiety. The possibility of diminished vision or blindness increases anxiety.
■ Assess client's eye pigment; clients with dark, heavily pigmented irises may benefit from a pilocarpine concentration greater than 4%.

NURSING DIAGNOSES

■ Disturbed sensory perception (visual) related to diagnosis
■ Risk for injury related to impaired vision
■ Anxiety related to possible diminished or loss of vision

PLANNING

■ Client will take miotics as prescribed.
■ Client's intraocular pressure (IOP) will decrease and be within the accepted range.

NURSING INTERVENTIONS

■ Gently apply pressure to the inner canthus to prevent or minimize systemic absorption when administering eyedrops. Some systemic reaction may occur to persons sensitive to drugs of any kind; responses may occur even with small doses.

■ Monitor vital signs. Heart rate and blood pressure may decrease with large doses of cholinergics.
■ Monitor for side effects such as headache, eye pain, and decreased vision.
■ Monitor for postural hypotension. Instruct client to rise slowly from a recumbent position.
■ Check breath sounds for rales and rhonchi; cholinergic drugs can cause bronchospasms and increase bronchial secretions.
■ Maintain oral hygiene if excessive salivation occurs.
■ Keep atropine available as antidote for pilocarpine.

Client Teaching

General

• Instruct client or family on correct administration of eyedrops and ointment; include return demonstration. (Refer to Chapter 3, Figures 3–10 and 3–11.)
• Advise client on need for regular and ongoing medical supervision.
• Inform client not to stop medication suddenly without prior approval of health care provider.
• Advise client to avoid driving or operating machinery while vision is impaired.
• Instruct client on use of relaxation techniques for decreasing anxiety, such as deep breathing, visual imaging, or journaling to express fears, if appropriate.
• Advise client/family of resources available in the community if vision will be diminished or lost.
• Instruct client with glaucoma to avoid atropine-like drugs and goldenseal, which increase IOP. Clients should check labels on OTC drugs or check with a pharmacist.
• Advise client that certain herbal products should be avoided before ophthalmic or otic surgery (see Herbal Alert 48–1).

Self-Administration

• Instruct client/family or both on the correct administration of eyedrops and ointment. Include return demonstration (see Figures 3–10 and 3–11).
• Remove any exudates in eye before applying solution or ointment.
• Allow at least 5 minutes between instillation of another medication.

Ocular Therapeutic Systems (Ocusert)

• Store drug in refrigerator.
• Discard damaged or contaminated disks.
• Explain that the myopia is minimized by inserting the disk in the upper conjunctival sac at bedtime.
• For self-administration, advise clients to follow instructions related to insertion and removal.
• Instruct client to check for presence of disk in conjunctival sac at bedtime and when arising.
• Explain that temporary stinging is expected; notify health care provider if blurred vision or brow pain occurs.

Cholinesterase Inhibitors

- First dose should be administered by health care provider and followed by tonometry reading.
- Instruct client to tightly cap tube, because ointment is inactivated by water.

Cultural Considerations ❖

- Be alert to variations in eye response in African Americans and Filipino clients.
- Depending on client's culture, include the appropriate support person in health teaching and decisions. This need is heightened in conditions with possible loss or diminished vision.
- Use an interpreter as needed.

EVALUATION

■ Evaluate the effectiveness of drug therapy and the presence of side effects. IOP will be within desired range or reduced.

Beta-Adrenergic Blockers

Beta-blockers are first-line drugs in the treatment of glaucoma. Six drugs—betaxolol, carteolol, levobetaxolol, levobunolol, metipranolol, and timolol—are approved for this indication by the Food and Drug Administration (FDA). Beta-adrenergic blockers decrease the production of aqueous humor. The exact mechanism of action is unknown for these agents. Chapter 17 includes a comprehensive discussion of adrenergic blockers. These agents are presented in Table 48–4.

Prostaglandin Analogues

Prostaglandin analogues are currently known to be as effective as beta-blockers in the treatment of glaucoma. Four FDA-approved analogues with fewer side effects than beta-blockers are presented in Table 48–5. When using additional topical ophthalmic agents, allow at least 5 minutes between instillations.

Side Effects and Adverse Reactions

Increased brown pigmentation is most noticeable in individuals with green-brown and yellow-brown irises. When the drug is stopped, the increased pigmentation remains. Systemic reactions are rare. Pigmentation of the eyelid and growth of eyelashes also may occur. Ocular hyperemia is the most common adverse effect; blurred vision, conjunctivitis, dry eye, tearing, and light intolerance were less commonly experienced.

Carbonic Anhydrase Inhibitors

Carbonic anhydrase inhibitors interfere with production of carbonic acid, which leads to decreased aqueous humor formation and decreased IOP. These drugs, initially developed as diuretics, are now also used for the long-term treatment of open-angle glaucoma. Their use is recommended only when pilocarpine, beta-blockers, epinephrine, and cholinesterase inhibitors have not been effective. Table 48–6 presents the drug data for commonly prescribed carbonic anhydrase inhibitors.

Side Effects and Adverse Reactions

Side effects include lethargy, anorexia, drowsiness, paresthesia, depression, polyuria, nausea, vomiting, hypokalemia, and renal calculi. Carbonic anhydrase inhibitors can also cause photosensitivity. Clients frequently discontinue these medications because of their side effects. These drugs are contraindicated during the first trimester of pregnancy and should not be used in persons allergic to sulfonamides.

Carbonic Anhydrase Inhibitors

ASSESSMENT

■ Obtain medical and drug history. Use is contraindicated during first trimester of pregnancy.

Table 48–5		
Prostaglandin Analogues Used to Treat Glaucoma		
Generic (Brand)	**Route and Dosage**	**Uses and Considerations**
latanoprost (Xalatan)	A: 1 gt 0.005% sol daily at bedtime	To lower IOP; generally well tolerated.
bimatoprost (Lumigan)	A: 1 gt 0.03% sol daily at bedtime	Increases outflow of aqueous humor through trabecular meshwork and uveoscleral routes. Onset is 4 h and peak action occurs in 4-12 h.
travoprost (Travatan)	A: 1 gt 0.004% sol daily at bedtime	More effective in African American than non–African Americans. Increases uveoscleral outflow. Onset is 2 h with peak action occurring in 12 h.
unoprostone (Rescula)	A: 1 gt 0.15% sol b.i.d.	Not recommended for children.

A, Adult; *b.i.d.,* twice a day; *gt,* drop; *h,* hour; *IOP,* intraocular pressure; *sol,* solution.

■ Check vital signs. Baseline vital signs can be compared with future readings.
■ Assess level of anxiety. Eye disorders carrying the possibility of blindness may promote high anxiety state in clients.

NURSING DIAGNOSES

■ Disturbed sensory perception (visual) related to diagnosis
■ Risk for injury related to impaired vision
■ Anxiety related to possible diminished or loss of vision

PLANNING

■ Client will take carbonic anhydrase inhibitors as prescribed.
■ Client's intraocular pressure (IOP) will decrease to within the desired range.

NURSING INTERVENTIONS

■ Monitor for side effects such as lethargy, anorexia, drowsiness, polyuria, nausea, and vomiting.
■ Monitor electrolytes, because drug can cause hypokalemia.
■ Increase fluid intake unless contraindicated. Record intake and output; weigh daily.
■ Maintain oral hygiene.

Client Teaching

General
• Encourage use of artificial tears for "dry eyes."

• Encourage client to maintain oral hygiene if mouth is dry; ice chips and sugarless gum are recommended.
• Instruct client not to abruptly discontinue medication. Clients frequently discontinue drug because of side effects.
• Inform client of need for regular and ongoing medical supervision.
• Advise client to avoid driving or operating hazardous machinery while vision is impaired.

Self-Administration
• Instruct client or family on the correct administration of eyedrops and ointment. Include return demonstration. See Figures 3–10 and 3–11.
• Remove any exudate in eye before applying an antiinfective ointment or solution.
• Allow at least 5 minutes between instillation of another medication.

Side Effects
• Advise client to avoid prolonged exposure to sunlight because of the potential for photosensitivity.

Cultural Considerations ❖

• Depending on client's culture, include the appropriate support person in health teaching and decisions. This need is heightened in conditions with possible loss or diminished vision.
• Use interpreter as needed.

EVALUATION

■ Determine effectiveness of drug therapy and presence of side effects. IOP will be within desired range.

Table 48–6

Carbonic Anhydrase Inhibitors

Generic (Brand)	Route and Dosage	Uses and Considerations
acetazolamide (Diamox)	A: PO: 250-1000 mg/d given in divided doses for amounts >250 mg; doses >1000 mg show no increased benefit	To reduce aqueous humor formation, thus lowering IOP. Monitor for dehydration and postural hypotension. Monitor electrolytes. Avoid hazardous activities if drowsy. Most frequently prescribed. *Pregnancy category:* C; PB: UK; t$\frac{1}{2}$ 2-6 h
brinzolamide ophthalmic susp 1% (Azopt)	A: 1 gt t.i.d. C: not recommended	*Topical:* Treatment of elevated IOP in clients with ocular hypertension or open-angle glaucoma by suppressing production of aqueous humor. *Pregnancy category:* UK; PB: UK; t$\frac{1}{2}$: UK
Cosopt (timolol/dorzolamide 0.5%/2%)	1 gt 0.25% in affected eye(s) b.i.d.	Decreases aqueous production. Contraindicated with sulfa allergy. Adverse effects include asthma, bronchospasm, bradycardia, and dyspnea.
dichlorphenamide (Daranide)	A: PO: Initially: 100-200 mg followed by 100 mg q12h until desired response is obtained	Same as brinzolamide. May cause confusion, especially in older adults. *Pregnancy category:* C; PB: UK; t$\frac{1}{2}$: UK
dorzolamide (Trusopt)	A: Sol 2%: 1 gt t.i.d.	Do not use with oral carbonic anhydrase inhibitors. Side effects include burning, stinging, and bitter taste. *Pregnancy category:* UK; PB: UK; t$\frac{1}{2}$: UK

A, Adult; *b.i.d.,* two times a day; *C,* child; *d,* day; *gt,* drop; *h,* hour; *IOP,* intraocular pressure; *PB,* protein-binding; *PO,* by mouth; *t$\frac{1}{2}$,* half-life; *t.i.d.,* three times a day; *UK,* unknown; *>,* greater than.

Table 48–7

Osmotics

Generic (Brand)	Route and Dosage	Uses and Considerations
glycerin	A: PO: 1-1.5 g/kg given 1-1.5 h before surgery	Decreases volume of intraocular fluid to lower ocular tension. Carbohydrate; use with caution in clients with diabetes. *Pregnancy category:* C; PB: UK; t¹/₂: 30-45 min
isosorbide (Ismotic)	A: Sol 45%: 1.5-3 g/kg b.i.d./q.i.d.	Monitor I & O and electrolytes. *Pregnancy category:* C; PB: UK; t¹/₂: 5-9.5 h
mannitol (Osmitrol)	A: IV: Sol 15-20%, 1.5-2 g/kg over 0.5-1 h	Monitor I & O; weigh daily. Contraindicated in severe pulmonary congestion, anuria, and dehydration. Use with caution in clients with HF. *Pregnancy category:* C; PB: UK; t¹/₂: 15-100 min

A, Adult; *b.i.d.*, twice a day; *C*, child; *HF*, heart failure; *h*, hour; *I & O*, intake and output; *IV*, intravenous; *min*, minute; *PB*, protein-binding; *PO*, by mouth; *q.i.d.*, four times a day; *sol*, solution; *t¹/₂*, half-life; *UK*, unknown.

Osmotics

Osmotics are generally used preoperatively and postoperatively to decrease vitreous humor volume, thereby reducing IOP. These drugs are primarily used in the emergency treatment of acute closed-angle glaucoma because of their ability to rapidly reduce IOP. Commonly prescribed osmotic drugs are presented in Table 48–7.

Side Effects and Adverse Reactions

Osmotic medications can cause headache, nausea, vomiting, and diarrhea. Disorientation resulting from electrolyte imbalances can result from use of mannitol and urea, especially in older adults.

Nursing Process

Osmotics

ASSESSMENT

■ Obtain medical and drug history.
■ Check vital signs. Baseline vital signs can be compared with future readings.
■ Assess level of anxiety. Eye disorders carrying the possibility of blindness promote high anxiety state in clients.

NURSING DIAGNOSES

■ Disturbed sensory perception (visual) related to diagnosis
■ Risk for injury related to impaired vision
■ Anxiety related to possible diminished or loss of vision

PLANNING

■ Client's intraocular pressure (IOP) will be lowered.

NURSING INTERVENTIONS

■ Monitor for side effects.
■ Monitor for potassium depletion and electrolyte imbalances.
■ Increase fluid intake unless contraindicated.
■ Record input and output; weigh daily.
■ Monitor changes in level of orientation, especially in older adults.

Client Teaching

General
• Instruct client regarding side effects of drugs.
• Osmotics are usually administered intravenously in a health care setting.

Self-Administration
• Instruct client/family or both on the correct administration of eyedrops and ointment. Include return demonstration. Refer to Figures 3–10 and 3–11.
• Remove any exudates in eye before applying solution or ointment.
• Allow at least 5 minutes between instillation of another medication.

Cultural Considerations ❖
• Depending on client's culture, include the appropriate support person in health teaching and decisions. This need is heightened in conditions with possible loss or diminished vision.
• Use an interpreter as needed.

EVALUATION

■ Determine the effectiveness of drug therapy and presence of side effects. IOP will be within desired range.

Anticholinergic Mydriatics and Cycloplegics

Mydriatics dilate the pupils; **cycloplegics** paralyze the muscles of accommodation. Both are used in diagnostic procedures and ophthalmic surgery. (See the Unit 5 opener for a review of the autonomic nervous system and a comprehensive discussion of anticholinergics.) Anticholinergics actively block acetylcholine, causing both dilation of the pupils and paralysis of the muscles of accommodation by relaxing the ciliary and dilator muscles of the iris. Commonly prescribed anticholinergic mydriatics and cycloplegics are presented in Table 48–8.

Side Effects and Adverse Reactions of Adrenergic Mydriatics

Side effects include headache, brow pain, allergic reaction, and worsening of narrow-angle glaucoma. Adrenergic mydriatics are contraindicated in clients with cardiac dysrhythmias and cerebral atherosclerosis and should be used with caution in older adults and clients with prostatic hypertrophy, diabetes mellitus, or parkinsonism. The health care provider should be notified of blurred vision or loss of sight, difficult breathing, increased perspiration, or flush. The difference in the response of African-American individuals to a mydriatic drug must be taken into consideration. Closely monitor African-American clients for side effects. Filipino eye structure is such that it may be difficult for the health care provider to conduct selected assessments.

Table 48–8

Mydriatics and Cycloplegics

Generic (Brand)	Route and Dosage*	Uses and Considerations
atropine sulfate (Atropisol, Isopto Atropine)	A: Sol 1%: 1-2 gtt up to q.i.d. C: Sol 0.5%: 1-2 gtt up to t.i.d. Oint 1%: Apply in lower eyelid sac up to t.i.d.	Most potent cycloplegic. For refraction, especially in children; for iritis and uveitis. *Not for use with glaucoma or tachycardia.* Wait 5 minutes before using other drugs. *Pregnancy category:* C; PB: NA; t¹/₂: NA
cyclopentolate HCl (AK-Pentolate, Cyclogyl, Pentolair)	A: Sol 0.5%-2%: 1-2 gtt; then 1 gt in 5 min C: 1-2 gtt × 1; may repeat × 1 in 5-10 min with 0.5% or 1% sol	Mydriasis and cycloplegia for eye examination. *Pregnancy category:* C; PB: NA; t¹/₂: NA
dipivefrin HCl (Propine)	A: Sol 0.1%: 1 gt q12h	Control of IOP in chronic open-angle glaucoma. *Pregnancy category:* B; PB: NA; t¹/₂: NA
epinephrine HCl (Epifrin, Glaucon)	A & C: Sol 0.1%-2%: 1-2 gtt d/b.i.d.	For open-angle glaucoma and during eye surgery. Discard brown or precipitate solution. *Pregnancy category:* C; PB: NA; t¹/₂: NA
epinephrine borate (Epinal)	*Surgery:* A: Sol 0.5-1%: Instill 1-2 gtt 3 × *Open-angle glaucoma:* A: Sol 0.5% or 1.0%: Instill 1 gt in eye b.i.d.	For treatment of open-angle glaucoma and during ocular surgery. Contraindicated in narrow-angle glaucoma. Monitor tonometer readings with long-term use. Increased pressor effects. *Pregnancy category:* C; PB: UK; t¹/₂: UK
homatropine hydrobromide (Isopto Homatropine)	A & C: Sol 2% and 5%: 1-2 gtt q3-4h Cy: Use only 2%	Similar to atropine but faster onset and shorter duration. Mydriasis and cycloplegia for eye examination. *Pregnancy category:* C; PB: NA; t¹/₂: NA
phenylephrine HCl (AK-Dilate)	*Mydriasis:* A & C: Sol 2.5% or 10%: Instill 1 gt in eye before examination Mydriasis with vasoconstriction: A & C >12 y: Instill 1 gt in eye; repeat × 1 in 1 h PRN Cy: 2.5% sol: Instill 1 gt in eye; repeat × 1 in 1 h PRN	For eye examination or surgery and treatment of wide-angle glaucoma and uveitis. *Pregnancy category:* C; PB: UK; t¹/₂: UK
scopolamine hydrobromide (Isopto Hyoscine)	A: Sol 0.25%: 1-2 gtt 1 h before examination; 1-2 gtt for treatment up to q.i.d.	Used for clients sensitive to atropine sulfate. More rapid onset and shorter duration than atropine. *Pregnancy category:* C; PB: NA; t¹/₂: NA
tropicamide (Mydriacyl Ophthalmic, Tropicacyl, Opticyl)	*Refraction:* A: 1%: 1-2 gtt; repeat in 5 min Fundus examination: 0.5%: 1-2 gtt 15-20 min before examination	Mydriasis and cycloplegia for eye examination. *Pregnancy category:* C; PB: NA; t¹/₂: NA

*To minimize systemic absorption, apply gentle pressure to lacrimal duct.

A, Adult; *b.i.d.,* twice a day; *C,* child; *Cy,* cycloplegic; *gt,* drop; *gtt,* drops; *h,* hour; *IOP,* intraocular pressure; *min,* minute; *oint,* ointment; *PB,* protein-binding; *PRN,* as needed; *q.i.d.,* four times a day; *sol,* solution; *t¹/₂,* half-life; *t.i.d.,* three times a day; *NA,* not applicable; *UK,* unknown; *y,* year; *>,* greater than.

Side Effects and Adverse Reactions of Cycloplegics

Cycloplegics can cause tachycardia, photophobia, dryness of the mouth, edema, conjunctivitis, and dermatitis. Symptoms of atropine toxicity include dry mouth, blurred vision, photophobia, constipation, fever, tachycardia, confusion, hallucinations, delirium, and coma. Toxicity is treated with physostigmine. Cycloplegics are contraindicated in clients with glaucoma, because they increase IOP.

Refer to Preventing Medication Errors box for examples of eye medications that are commonly confused with other agents.

Drugs for Macular Degeneration

Age-related macular degeneration (ARMD) is a leading cause of vision loss in those 65 and over. The macula is that part of the eye responsible for sharp central vision; damage to the macula blurs central vision in the affected eye. There are two forms of ARMD: "wet," which progresses quite rapidly, and "dry," which slowly destroys vision over a period of years. The wet form is associated with the growth of abnormal blood vessels behind the retina that shift the macula from its normal position. Wet ARMD accounts for 10% to 15% of cases. The vast majority of vision loss from ARMD (85% to 90%) is caused by the dry form, in which the gradual destruction of light-sensitive cells in the macula leads to a blurred or blind spot in the center of vision in one or both eyes. Options for treatment are evolving and include laser treatment, photodynamic therapy, and medications. Pegaptanib (Macugen), an injectable agent, was released in late 2004.

This drug stabilized vision loss in slightly over 50% of clients, but vision improvement was limited to about 10%. A 2006 drug, ranibizumab (Lucentis), stopped vision loss in clinical trials in almost 95% of clients and improved vision in 33% of clients. Ranibizumab is administered as an eye injection every month and is most effective in early phases of wet ARMD.

Administration of Eyedrops and Ointments

Techniques for administering eyedrops and ointments are described in Chapter 3, Boxes 3–3 and 3–4, and illustrated in Figures 3–10 and 3–11. Individuals who wear contact lenses need to be knowledgeable about the products associated with some of the lenses (Figure 48–2).

Clients with Eye Disorders: General Suggestions for Client Teaching

- Eye disorders carrying the possibility of blindness promote a high-anxiety state in clients. Provide time, instructions, and return demonstration in all teaching plans. Use caution with confused or forgetful clients to prevent overdose.
- Instruct client/family that one drop of eye medication is the preferred amount with prescriptions written for 1-2 drops. The eye typically holds the volume of one drop without overflowing. The second drop may cause overflow, greater chance of systemic toxicity, and increased cost of treatment. If a second medication is ordered to be given at the same time, wait at least 5 minutes to instill the second medication.
- Instruct the client or family in the proper administration of eyedrops or ointment. Maintain sterile technique and prevent dropper contamination. Expect some blurriness from ointments. Apply at bedtime, if possible, to avoid safety problems from diminished vision.
- Instruct the client to report changes in vision, blurred vision, vision loss, breathing difficulties, or flush.
- Instruct the client to store the drug in a light-resistant container away from heat.

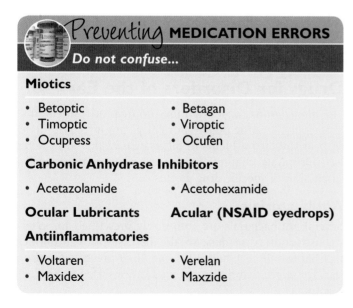

Preventing MEDICATION ERRORS

Do not confuse...

Miotics

- Betoptic
- Timoptic
- Ocupress
- Betagan
- Viroptic
- Ocufen

Carbonic Anhydrase Inhibitors

- Acetazolamide
- Acetohexamide

Ocular Lubricants   Acular (NSAID eyedrops)

Antiinflammatories

- Voltaren
- Maxidex
- Verelan
- Maxzide

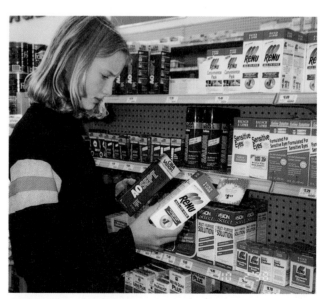

FIGURE 48–2 Clients who wear contact lenses should be knowledgeable about the products associated with some of the lenses.

Table 48–9

Otic: Antiinfectives

Generic (Brand)	Route and Dosage	Uses and Considerations
External		
acetic acid and aluminum acetate (Otic Domeboro)	A & C: Sol 2%: Insert saturated wick, keep moist × 24 h; instill 4-6 gtt q2-3h	Provides an acid medium; has antibacterial activity. Low cost. *Pregnancy category:* UK; PB: NA; t^1/$_2$: NA
boric acid (Ear-Dry), carbamide peroxide (Debrox)	A & C >12 y: Instill 5-10 gtt b.i.d.; tilt head to unaffected side to keep gtt in ear or put cotton plug in outer ear	OTC preparations to dry the ear canal and to loosen and remove impacted wax (cerumen) from the ear canal. Debrox: instill for up to 4 days. If no improvement, call health care provider. *Pregnancy category:* C; PB: NA; t^1/$_2$: NA
chloramphenicol (Chloromycetin Otic)	A & C: Otic sol 0.5%: Instill 2-3 gtt into ear t.i.d.	Topically for infections of ear canal. *Pregnancy category:* C; PB: NA; t^1/$_2$: NA
polymyxin B	A & C: 3-4 gtt t.i.d./q.i.d. for 7-10 days	Usually given in combination with neomycin and hydrocortisone. For disorders of external ear. Discontinue after 10 days to prevent fungal overgrowth. *Pregnancy category:* B; PB: NA; t^1/$_2$: NA
tetracycline (Achromycin)	A & C: 1-2 gtt b.i.d./q.i.d.	Similar to polymyxin B. *Pregnancy category:* D; PB: NA; t^1/$_2$: NA
trolamine polypeptide oleate-condensate (Cerumenex)	A & C: Fill ear canal and insert cotton plug for 15-30 min; flush ear with lukewarm water; repeat × 1 if needed	To loosen and remove impacted wax (cerumen) from ear canal. *Pregnancy category:* C; PB: NA; t^1/$_2$: NA
Internal		
amoxicillin (Amoxil, Augmentin)	A: PO: 250-500 mg q8h C: PO: 20-40 mg/kg/d in 3 divided doses	For treatment of otitis media. Mouth absorbs 80%; food does not prevent absorption. Long duration of action. *Pregnancy category:* B; PB: 20%; t^1/$_2$: 1-1.5 h
ampicillin trihydrate (Polycillin)	A: PO: 250-500 mg q6h IM/IV: 2-8 g/d in divided doses C: PO: 50-200 mg/kg/d in divided doses IM/IV: 50-200 mg/kg/d in divided doses	First broad-spectrum penicillin. GI tract absorbs 50%. Effective against gram-negative and gram-positive bacteria. Individuals allergic to penicillin may also be allergic to ampicillin. *Pregnancy category:* B; PB: 15%-28%; t^1/$_2$: 1-2 h

A, Adult; *b.i.d.*, twice a day; *C*, child; *d*, day; *GI*, gastrointestinal; *gtt*, drops; *h*, hour; *IM*, intramuscular; *IV*, intravenous; *max*, maximum; *min*, minute; *NA*, not applicable; *OTC*, over-the-counter; *PB*, protein-binding; *PO*, by mouth; *q.i.d.*, four times a day; *sol*, solution; *t^1/$_2$*, half-life; *t.i.d.*, three times a day; *UK*, unknown; *y*, year; *>*, greater than.

- Instruct the client not to stop medication suddenly without *prior* approval from the prescribing health care provider.
- Instruct the client to record medications administered. Prepare a chart so the client can record when eye medications are given.
- Instruct the client with glaucoma to avoid atropine-like drugs, which increase IOP. Some drugs for glaucoma are long-acting and require only daily dosing if the client is forgetful or needs another person to administer the medicine.
- Clients should be alerted to check labels on OTC drugs with a pharmacist.
- Instruct the client to carry an identification card or wear a MedicAlert bracelet at all times if allergic to any medications.
- Encourage the client to keep health care appointments.

- Individuals who wear contact lenses need to be knowledgeable about the products associated with care of the lenses.

Drugs for Disorders of the Ear

The medications most often used to treat **otic**, or ear, disorders are the same preparations (e.g., antiinfectives) used to treat similar problems in other areas of the body. Refer to appropriate chapters in the text for a comprehensive discussion of specific drug groups.

Antibacterials

Several antibacterials are commonly prescribed for external use for otic disorders. See the discussions of antibiotics in Chapters 28, 29, and 30. Table 48–9 presents the drug data for selected antibacterial medications used to treat ear disorders.

Table 48–9

Otic: Antiinfectives—cont'd

Generic (Brand)	Route and Dosage	Uses and Considerations
cefaclor (Ceclor)	A: PO: 250-500 mg q8h; *max:* 4 g/d C: PO: 20-40 mg/kg/d in 3 divided doses; *max:* 1 g/d	Second-generation cephalosporin. To treat ampicillin-resistant and gram-negative strains. Third-line drug for otitis media. Not for infants less than 1 month old. Monitor electrolytes in long-term therapy. *Pregnancy* category: B; PB: 25%; t$\frac{1}{2}$: 0.5-1 h
erythromycin (E-Mycin)	A: PO: 250-500 mg q6h IV: 1-4 g/d in 4 divided doses C: PO: 30-50 mg/kg/d in 4 divided doses IV: 20-50 mg/kg/d in 4 divided doses	To treat gram-positive and gram-negative bacterial infections in clients allergic to penicillin. Enteric-coated tablet to prevent gastric acid from destroying drug. *Pregnancy category:* B; PB: 65%; t$\frac{1}{2}$: PO, 1-2 h; IV, 3-5 h
penicillin (Pentids, Pen-V)	*Penicillin G potassium (Pentids):* A: PO: 200,000-500,000 units q6h IM: 500,000-5 million units/d in divided doses IV: 4-20 million units/d in divided doses diluted in IV solution C: PO: 25,000-90,000 units/d in divided doses IV: 50,000-100,000 units/kg/d in divided doses *Penicillin V potassium (Pen-V):* A: PO: 125-500 mg q6h C: PO: 15-50 mg/kg/d in 3-4 divided doses	For otitis media and mastoiditis. Take before or after meals. *Penicillin G:* electrolytes should be monitored; injectable solution is clear. *Penicillin V:* not recommended in renal failure. *Pregnancy category:* B; PB: (G) 60%, (V) 80%; t$\frac{1}{2}$: (G) 0.5-1 h, (V) 0.5 h
sulfonamides (Azulfidine [sulfasalazine], Bactrim [trimethoprim and sulfamethoxazole])	Dose and route vary. See Chapter 29.	Most are highly protein-bound. Increase fluid intake to decrease crystalluria. Side effects include allergic response. Blood disorders may result from long-term use and high doses. Avoid in third trimester of pregnancy. *Pregnancy category:* B, D; PB: 50%-95%; t$\frac{1}{2}$: 4.5-12 h
clarithromycin (Biaxin)	A: PO: 250-500 mg q12h C: PO: 7.5 mg/kg q12h	For otitis media. Cautious use in renal impairment. Efficacy not established in children younger than 12 y. *Pregnancy category:* C; PB: UK; t$\frac{1}{2}$: 3-5 h
amoxicillin and potassium clavulanate (Augmentin)	A: PO: 250 mg q8h C: PO: 40 mg/kg/d divided q8h	For otitis media. Clavulanate inhibits beta lactamase degradation of amoxicillin. *Pregnancy category:* B; PB: UK; t$\frac{1}{2}$: 1-3 h
loracarbef (Lorabid)	A: PO: 200 mg q12h C: PO: 30 mg/kg/d q12h	For otitis media. Second-generation cephalosporin. Use caution in clients with renal impairment and seizures. *Pregnancy category:* B; PB: UK; t$\frac{1}{2}$: 45-60 min

Common conditions requiring antibacterial drugs are acute otitis media (AOM) and acute otitis externa (swimmer's ear). *Streptococcus pneumoniae* is the most common pathogen in children with AOM; no bacteria was found in 20% to 30% of children examined.

Side Effects and Adverse Reactions

Side effects include overgrowth of nonsusceptible organisms. Prior hypersensitivity is a contraindication.

Antiinfectives

ASSESSMENT

■ Obtain a medical and drug history, including any allergies.

■ Check vital signs. Obtain baseline data that can be compared with future findings.

NURSING DIAGNOSES

■ Disturbed sensory perception (auditory) due to diagnosis
■ Pain related to infection

PLANNING

■ Client will be free of ear infection after completion of drug regimen.

NURSING INTERVENTIONS

■ Complete culture and sensitivity before starting drug.
■ Monitor input and output.
■ Report hematuria or oliguria. High doses of antibacterials may be nephrotoxic.
■ Relief of associated pain, if present.
■ Monitor renal function, liver studies, and blood studies (white cell count, red cell count, hemoglobin and hematocrit, bleeding time) as appropriate.
■ Store medication in airtight container.
■ Report dizziness to health care provider.
■ Report fatigue, fever, or sore throat. Any of these symptoms could indicate superimposed infection.

Client Teaching

• Instruct client to complete entire course of medication (usually 10 to 14 days) and *not* to stop medication when the ear(s) "feels better."
• Encourage client to eat yogurt or buttermilk to maintain intestinal flora.
• If client is prone to otitis after swimming or in warm weather, give instruction in how to keep ear canals dry; instillation of drops of alcohol into the ear canal may be helpful. Check with the health care provider.
• Instruct client to wear a MedicAlert bracelet at all times if allergic to medications.

Self-Administration

• Teach client or family about administration of eardrops. Include a return demonstration. Refer to Box 3–5 and Figure 3–12 in Chapter 3.

Cultural Considerations ❖

• Depending on client's culture, include the appropriate support person in health teaching and decisions. This need is heightened in conditions with possible loss or diminished hearing.
• Use interpreter as needed.

EVALUATION

■ Determine the effectiveness of drug therapy and the presence of side effects.

Antihistamine-Decongestants

Antihistamine-decongestants are thought to reduce nasal and middle ear congestion in acute otitis media. (See Chapter 39 for a comprehensive discussion of upper respiratory agents.) Reducing edema around the orifice of the eustachian tube promotes drainage from the middle ear. Numerous OTC antihistamine-decongestant medications are available, including Actifed, Allerest, Dimetapp, Drixoral, Novafed, Ornade, Phenergan, and Triaminic. Common side effects are drowsiness, blurred vision, and dry mucous membranes.

Combination Products

Combination products such as Cortisporin Otic are not held in high regard by most health care providers, who believe that multiple drugs are not necessary if one drug can successfully treat a disorder. These drugs combine local anesthetics or antiinflammatory drugs with antiinfectives.

Ceruminolytics

Cerumen (earwax), produced by glands in the outer half of the ear canal, usually moves to the external os by itself and is washed away. However, **ceruminolytics** are sometimes needed to loosen and remove impacted cerumen from the ear canal. Irrigation with hydrogen peroxide solution (3% diluted to half-strength with water) can flush cerumen deposits out of the ear canal. For chronic impaction, one or two drops of olive oil or mineral oil soften the wax. Cerumenex (prescription) and Debrox (OTC) cost more and are no more effective than the hydrogen peroxide solution.

Administration of Ear Medications

Ear medications are generally contained in a liquid vehicle for ease of administration. Guidelines for the administration of eardrops are given in Box 3–5 and Figure 3–12.

Irrigation

Irrigations of the ear may also be ordered. Irrigation is best accomplished when there is direct visualization of the tympanic membrane (eardrum). It must be done *gently* to avoid damage to the eardrum. Frequently used irrigating solutions include Burow's solution, hydrogen peroxide 3% (with water), hypertonic sodium chloride solution 3%, and acetic acid (vinegar) solution. Contraindications include perforation of the eardrum and prior hypersensitivity.

Clients with Ear Disorders: General Suggestions for Client Teaching

• Instruct the client not to insert any foreign objects into the ear canal.
• Instruct the client to take the drug as prescribed.
• Instruct the client to keep the drug in a light-resistant container.
• Instruct the client about the expected drug effect, dosage, side effects, and when to notify the health care provider.
• Encourage the client to keep follow-up appointments.

Critical Thinking Case Study

MH, age 70, has been on pilocarpine for several days (2% solution, four gtt q.i.d.). She says she must need new glasses because newsprint and the TV picture are a bit "fuzzy."

1. Is any action indicated? If so, what?
2. What additional advice would be appropriate if the client had coronary vascular disease and bradycardia?
3. Are there any expected effects on MH's vital signs? If so, what?
4. What suggestions should MH be given to avoid systemic absorption of the medication?

MZ brings CZ, age 7, to the HMO practice because he has been complaining of pain in his ear for 2 days. Following an assessment the health care provider determines that CZ has an infection in the external right ear canal. Polymyxin B is prescribed to be administered three to four gtt t.i.d. for 14 days.

1. Is the drug regimen appropriate for CZ? What is the nurse's responsibility?
2. What is a consequence of long-term use of this drug?
3. What drug may be used in combination to decrease edema, itching, and redness?

Client teaching is an integral part of the therapeutic drug regimen. Explain the role of the nurse in relation to the following:

4. What position should CZ be in to receive the drugs?
5. What instructions should be given to MZ regarding the administration of eardrops, including the actual positioning of the ear before administering the drops? In what way should these instructions be modified if the child were 2 years old?
6. What advice should you give CZ about putting things in his ear?

NCLEX Study Questions

1. Your client is on mannitol. Contraindications for the use of this drug include:
   a. dehydration
   b. kidney stones
   c. eczema
   d. gout

2. Your client is being prepared for an eye examination. When you take her health history, she tells you she is sensitive to atropine sulfate. What drug might be used instead for the exam?
   a. diclofenac
   b. suprofen
   c. cyclopentolate
   d. betaxolol HCl

3. Your 85-year-old client is taking acetazolamide, a carbonic anhydrase inhibitor. A nursing intervention associated with clients receiving this drug is to monitor:
   a. weight
   b. complete blood count
   c. electrolytes
   d. urine output

4. The prostaglandin analogue more effective in African Americans than non–African Americans is:
   a. latanoprost
   b. bimatoprost
   c. unoprostone
   d. travoprost

5. The primary disadvantage of the use of combination products such as Cortisporin Otic is:
   a. may need only one drug
   b. may not be desired dose
   c. increased cost
   d. less effective

6. What product is recommended to prevent and treat chronic impaction of cerumen?
   a. hydrogen peroxide
   b. rubbing alcohol
   c. charcoal
   d. salt solution

Answers: 1, a; 2, c; 3, c; 4, d; 5, a; 6, a.

49

Drugs for Dermatologic Disorders

ELECTRONIC RESOURCES

evolve

Evolve website (http://evolve.elsevier.com/KeeHayes/pharmacology/):
- *Case Studies*
- *Content Updates*
- *Frequently Asked Questions*

- *Student Review Activities*
- *WebLinks*
- *Additional Reference Material*

Companion CD-ROM:
- *NCLEX Examination Review Questions*
- *Pharmacology Animations*
- *IV Therapy Checklists*
- *Medication Error Checklists*

- *Drug Calculation Problems*
- *Electronic Calculators*
- *Top 200 Drugs with Pronunciations*
- *References from the Textbook*

Outline

Objectives

- Differentiate acne vulgaris, psoriasis, drug-induced dermatitis, and contact dermatitis.
- Describe nonpharmacologic measures used to treat mild acne vulgaris.
- Describe three drugs that can cause drug-induced dermatitis and their characteristic symptoms.
- Compare the topical antibacterial agents used to prevent and treat burn tissue infection.
- Discuss the nursing process, including client teaching, related to commonly used drugs for acne vulgaris, psoriasis, and burns.

Terms

Numerous skin lesions and eruptions require mild to aggressive drug therapy. Some skin disorders include acne vulgaris, psoriasis, eczema dermatitis, contact dermatitis, drug-induced dermatitis, and burn infection. Skin eruptions may result from viral infections (e.g., herpes simplex, herpes zoster), fungal infections (e.g., **tinea pedis** [athlete's foot], **tinea capitis** [ringworm]), and bacterial infections. Please refer to Chapters 28 through 32 for further information on antiinfective agents.

Most treatments for skin eruptions include topical creams, ointments, pastes, gels, lotions, and solutions. Skin lesions may appear as **macules** (flat with varying colors), **papules** (raised, palpable, and less than 1 cm in diameter), **vesicles** (raised, filled with fluid, and less than 1 cm in diameter), or **plaques** (hard, rough, raised, and flat on top). Selected skin disorders and their drug therapy regimens are discussed separately.

Acne Vulgaris

Acne is the most common skin disorder in the United States. **Acne vulgaris** is the formation of papules, nodules, and cysts on the face, neck, shoulders, and back resulting from keratin plugs at the base of the pilosebaceous oil glands near the hair follicles. Of persons with acne, 90% are adolescents. The increase in androgen production that occurs during adolescence increases the production of sebum, an oily skin lubricant. The sebum combines with keratin to form a plug, which results in acne.

Nonpharmacologic Approach

Nonpharmacologic measures should be tried before drug therapy is initiated. A prescribed or suggested cleansing agent is necessary for all types of acne. The skin should be gently cleansed several times a day. Vigorous scrubbing should be avoided. A well-balanced diet is indicated. Megadoses of vitamin A were once used to treat acne. Vitamin A is fat-soluble and retained in tissues, especially the liver, for long periods. Because excessive doses of vitamin A can be highly toxic, megadosing is no longer a valid therapy for treating acne. High doses of vitamin A may also have teratogenic effects on a fetus, producing birth defects. Decreasing emotional stress and increasing emotional support are suggested. If drug therapy is necessary, nonpharmacologic measures should be maintained.

Topical Antiacne Drugs

Mild acne may require gentle cleansing and the use of keratolytics (keratin dissolvers such as benzoyl peroxide, resorcinol, salicylic acid). Benzoyl peroxide is applied as a cream, lotion, or gel once or twice a day. This agent loosens the outer, horny layer of the epidermis.

Tretinoin (Retin-A, Renova), a derivative of vitamin A, is a topical drug for mild to moderate acne that alters keratinization. There are additional antiacne agents, adapalene (Differin), azelaic acid (Azelex), and tazarotene (Tazorac) used to treat mild to moderate acne. Adapalene is similar in action to tretinoin. It has antiinflammatory and comedolytic (eliminates blackheads) properties and tends to be more effective than tretinoin in reducing the number of acne lesions. Adapalene should not be used before or after extended sun exposure or sunburn. It can increase the risk of sunburn and intensify an existing sunburn. Azelaic acid appears as effective as benzoyl peroxide and tretinoin. Adapalene and azelaic acid can cause burning, pruritus, and erythema after several applications; however, this is less common with azelaic acid. Adapalene and tazarotene bind to select retinoid receptors; thus fewer adverse effects are anticipated.

Moderate acne requires a stronger concentration of benzoyl peroxide (10%), and topical antibiotics (e.g., tetracycline, erythromycin, clindamycin, meclocycline) may be added to the treatment regimen. Erythromycin and clindamycin are the most frequently prescribed topical antibiotics and have the fewest side effects.

Systemic Antiacne Drugs

For severe acne, oral antibiotics (e.g., tetracycline [drug of choice] or erythromycin) and topical glucocorticoids may be prescribed. Tetracycline inhibits bacterial protein synthesis. It is used to treat acne with a lower maintenance dose over a period of months. Tetracycline should not be taken with antacids or milk products, because they bind it into an insoluble compound, decreasing its absorption. A major side effect of tetracycline is photosensitivity. Exposure to the sun while taking tetracycline can result in severe sunburn. Pregnant women should not take tetracycline because of possible teratogenic effects on the fetus.

Isotretinoin (Accutane), a derivative of vitamin A, is used for severe cystic acne. It can be administered orally or topically. It decreases sebum formation and secretion, and it has antiinflammatory and antikeratinizing (keratolytic) effects. It can cause adverse reactions such as nosebleeds, pruritus, and inflammation of the eyes and lips. Isotretinoin must not be used during pregnancy because of teratogenic effects. Vitamin A and tetracycline may increase adverse effects. Baseline blood work is required before initiating isotretinoin therapy. Additional cautions associated with isotretinoin include the following: Do NOT: breastfeed, give blood, take other medications or herbal products without first consulting health care provider, drive at night without knowing effect of isotretinoin on night vision, have cosmetic procedures in attempt to smooth skin. Instruct client to contact health care provider and to stop isotretinoin if experiencing muscle weakness, which may be an indication of serious muscle damage. Monitoring of complete blood count (CBC), glucose and lipid levels, and urinalysis on a regular basis is important. Isotretinoin must not be used during pregnancy; its *Pregnancy category* is X. Based on this drug's powerful teratogenicity, a risk-management system to prevent isotretinoin-related teratogenicity was designed by the FDA Dermatologic and Ophthalmic Advisory Committee in 2002. Originally called the *System to Manage Accutane-Related Teratogenicity* (SMART), its purpose was to ensure that no woman be pregnant when treatment was initiated and no woman would become pregnant while taking the drug or for at least one month after completing a therapeutic course of isotretinoin. The iPLEDGE program replaced SMART in December 2005. An Internet-based registry system, iPLEDGE uses a central database to track isotretinoin users and account for all information and access to the drug. Refer to *www.ipledgeprogram.com* for full details. This comprehensive program has rules for the health care provider, client, pharmacist, and wholesaler as follows:

- **Female Client Responsibilities:** Female clients must receive warnings of teratogenicity both orally and in writing. Two negative pregnancy tests are required before starting the drug and one negative test before each monthly refill. Two effective methods of contraception are required 1 month before, throughout the duration, and 1 month after terminating isotretinoin treatment. (Exceptions are total abstinence from intercourse or following hysterectomy.) The client must review iPLEDGE educational materials on a variety of topics, including reasons for contraception when using a drug known to be teratogenic. A signed *Patient Information/Informed Consent* is also required.
- **Health Care Provider Responsibilities:** Registration by the health care provider for the iPLEDGE program is required, and the client must follow up by phone or Internet before treatment, monthly during treatment, and 1 month after treatment is terminated. During these contacts, the client must indicate both birth control methods and respond to questions related to program requirements. After registering and agreeing to follow the iPLEDGE *Program Guide to Best Practices for Isotretinoin*, the health care provider must enter two methods of birth control the client is using and results of monthly pregnancy tests. The initial and all refill prescriptions must also be entered.
- **Pharmacist Responsibilities:** Pharmacists must first be registered with the iPLEDGE program. Isotretinoin must be obtained from a wholesaler also registered with the iPLEDGE program. The pharmacist for each prescription must get authorization from iPLEDGE, confirm with iPLEDGE that prescription date is within 7 days, dispense a 30-day supply (maximum), and indicate the risk-management authorization number on the prescription.
- **Wholesaler Responsibilities:** Wholesaler must be registered with the iPLEDGE program

The iPLEDGE program has recently become less stringent for women of nonchildbearing age and males (refer to website for latest information). Table 49–1 lists the drugs commonly used to control acne vulgaris.

Table 49–1

Drugs for Acne Vulgaris and Psoriasis

Generic (Brand)	Route and Dosage	Uses and Considerations
Acne Vulgaris		
Systemic Preparations		
tetracycline (Sumycin)	A & C >12 y: PO: 250-500 mg b.i.d. *Mild acne:* 250 mg/d or q.o.d.	For moderate to severe acne. Inexpensive. Should not be taken during pregnancy. Should not be taken with milk products or antacids. *Pregnancy category:* D; PB: 65%; t½: 6-12 h
erythromycin (E-Mycin)	A: PO: 250-500 mg b.i.d.	For moderate to severe acne. A substitute for tetracycline. *Pregnancy category:* B; PB: 75%-90%; t½: 1.5-2 h
minocycline HCl (Dynacin)	A: PO: 100 mg b.i.d.	For moderate acne. Should be taken 1h before or 2 h after meals. *Pregnancy category:* D; PB: 90%; t½: 11-24h
Extended release: minocycline HCl (Solodyn)	A: PO: 1 mg/kg once daily	New ER once-daily treatment for nonnodular moderate to severe acne. Effectiveness compared to immediate release formulation; likeliness to cause vertigo is yet to be determined. *Pregnancy category*, D; PB: >90%; t½: UK.
isotretinoin (Accutane, Amnesteem, Claravis, Sotret)	A: PO: 0.5-1mg/kg/d in 2 divided doses. Treat for 15-20 weeks or less if nodule count reduced by >70%; max: 2 mg/kg/d. Take with meals.	For severe acne. Decreases sebum secretion. Used when oral antibiotics have failed. Avoid sunlight, contact lenses and use with tetracycline and vitamin A to reduce toxic effects. Monitor CBC, glucose, and lipid levels. Swallow whole tablet. *Pregnancy category*: X; PB: 99%; t½: 10-20 h
Topical Preparations		
Keratolytic Agents		
azelaic acid (Azelex)	A & C >12 y: Topical: cream 20%; apply b.i.d.	To treat mild to moderate acne. Inhibits hyperactivity of normal melanocytes. Mild pruritus, erythema, dryness, and peeling of skin might result. *Pregnancy category*: B; PB: UK; t½: 12 h

A, Adult; *BSA*, body surface area; *b.i.d.*, twice a day; *b.i.w.*, twice weekly; *C*, child; *d*, day; *DNA*, deoxyribonucleic acid; *FDA*, Food and Drug Administration; *h*, hour; *IV*, intravenous; *max*, maximum; *OC*, oral contraceptive; *PB*, protein-binding; *PO*, by mouth; *q.o.d.*, every other day; *sol*, solution; *subQ*, subcutaneous; *t½*, half-life; *tab*, tablet; *TNF*, tumor necrosis factor; *UK*, unknown; *wk*, week; *y*, year; *>*, greater than.

Table 49–1

Table 49–1

Drugs for Acne Vulgaris and Psoriasis—cont'd

Generic (Brand)	Route and Dosage	Uses and Considerations
benzoyl-peroxide (Benzac, Persa-Gel)	A & C: 2.5%-10% one to four times/d (cream, gel, or lotion)	For mild to moderate acne. Promotes **keratolysis** (removal of horny layer of the epidermis). May cause skin irritation (burning, blistering, swelling).
salicylic acid (Sebulex)	*Antiacne/antiseborrheic:* A & C: 2%-10% cream, gel, shampoo. Use as directed.	For mild to moderate acne; promotes desquamation.
resorcinol (Bicozene)	A & C: 1%-10% cream, ointment, lotion, shampoo	For mild to moderate acne.
resorcinol and sulfur	A & C: 2% resorcinol + 5% sulfur A & C: 2% resorcinol + 8% sulfur Use as directed.	For mild to moderate acne.
Antibiotics		
tetracycline	Ointment: 3% Sol: 2.2 mg/ml	For moderate acne. *Pregnancy category:* B
erythromycin	Ointment: 2% Gel: 1.5%-2%	For moderate acne.
clindamycin (Cleocin)	Gel: $^1/_5$ Lotion: 1% Sol: 1%	For moderate acne.
meclocycline (Meclan)	Ointment, b.i.d.	For moderate acne.
Topical Vitamin A Derivatives		
tretinoin (Retin-A)	Cream: 0.05%-0.1% Gel: 0.025%-0.1% Liquid: 0.05% daily at bedtime	For mild to moderate acne. Vitamin A derivative. May be used with benzoyl peroxide or topical antibiotic. Should not be applied to open wounds. Area should be cleansed first. *Pregnancy category:* B
adapalene (Differin)	A & C >12 y: topical: 0.1% gel; apply daily at bedtime after washing	To treat mild to moderate acne. Do not use before or after extended sun exposure. It intensifies sunburn. Pruritus may occur. *Pregnancy category:* C; PB: UK; t$^1/_2$: UK
Oral Contraceptives		
Estrostep	A: PO: 1 tab daily × 21 d; no tab × 7 d; Take as OC schedule	FDA approved for treatment of acne
Ortho Tri-Cyclen	A: PO: 1 tab daily × 21 d; then no tab × 7 d; take as OC schedule	FDA approved for treatment of acne
Psoriasis		
methoxsalen (Oxsoralen)	A: PO: 10-20 mg 2 h before exposure to therapeutic ultraviolet rays. Topical application before exposure to ultraviolet rays.	For severe psoriasis. Systemic antimetabolite drug. Avoid during pregnancy. Avoid sunlight during drug therapy; sunlight could cause burning and blistering. *Pregnancy category:* C; PB: 80%-90%; t$^1/_2$: >2 h
etretinate (Tegison, Soriatane)	A: PO: 0.5-0.75 mg/kg/d in divided doses, not to exceed 1.5 mg/kg/d	For recalcitrant psoriasis. Related to vitamin A. May take up to 6 months for a response to treatment. *Pregnancy category:* X; PB: 99%; t$^1/_2$: 4-8 d
Topical Preparations		
calcipotriene (Dovonex)	A: Topical: cream, ointment, and scalp sol: 0.005%; apply daily or b.i.d.	To treat mild to moderate plaque psoriasis. Burning, stinging, and erythema may occur. Excess use may increase serum calcium level. *Pregnancy category:* C; PB: UK; t$^1/_2$: UK
calcipotriol/betamethasone dipropionate (Daivobet)	A: Topical: ointment; apply once daily to affected areas	First once-daily topical ointment
coal tar (Estar, PsoriGel)	A: Topical: shampoo, cream, gel, paste, soap, ointment, lotion, solution	For mild to moderate psoriasis. Suppresses DNA synthesis, decreasing mitotic activity. May stain clothing, skin, and hair.
anthralin (Anthra-Derm)	A: Topical: 0.1%-1.0% ointment and cream	For moderate psoriasis. It inhibits DNA synthesis thus suppressing proliferation of the epidermal cells. May stain clothing, skin, and hair.

Continued

Table 49–1

Drugs for Acne Vulgaris and Psoriasis—cont'd

Generic (Brand)	Route and Dosage	Uses and Considerations
tazarotene (Tazorac)	A: Topical: 0.05% and 0.1% gel. Apply in pm to lesions.	Treatment for mild to moderate psoriasis; can also be used for acne. Reduces epidermal inflammation. Photosensitivity can occur.
alefacept (Amevive)	A: IM: 15 mg q wk	For treatment of severe chronic plaque psoriasis. Inhibits T-cell activation. *Pregnancy category:* B; PB: UK; $t^{1/2}$: 270 h
efalizumab (Raptiva)	A: subQ: 1 mg/kg q wk	For treatment of moderate to severe psoriasis. Inhibits T-cell migration & activation of CD 11a. *Pregnancy category:* C PB: UK; $t^{1/2}$: 6 d
etanercept (Enbrel)	A: subQ: 25 mg b.i.w for rheumatoid arthritis; 50 mg b.i.w. for psoriasis	For moderate to severe psoriasis. *Pregnancy category:* B; PB: UK; $t^{1/2}$: 115 h
infliximab (Remicade)	A: IV: 5 mg/kg IV infusion (>120 min) days 0, 2, 6, then q 8 wk for psoriasis	FDA approved in 1999 for treatment of psoriasis *Pregnancy category:* C; PB: UK; $t^{1/2}$: 9.5 d
adalimumab (Humira)	A: subQ: 40 mg q other wk	Human IgG1 monoclonal TNF-alpha antibody. FDA approved in 2002 for rheumatoid arthritis. *Pregnancy category:* B; PB: UK; $t^{1/2}$: 10-20 d
clobetasol propionate (Clobex)	A: Lotion: Apply thin layer twice daily, *max:* 50 g/week Spray: Spray on twice daily, rub in gently & completely. *max:* 50g/wk for 4 consecutive wk Neither product recommended for children under 18 y	Super-high-potency corticosteroid for treatment of moderate to severe plaque psoriasis of up to 20% BSA. Adverse effects include reversible hypothalamic-pituitary-adrenal (HPA) axis suppression & local site burning. Reassess lesions after 2 weeks of treatment. Contraindicated for application to axilla, face, or groin. *Pregnancy category:* D.
Keratolytic Agents salicylic acid, sulfur, resorcinol		See acne vulgaris.

Psoriasis

Psoriasis is a chronic skin disorder that affects 1% to 2% of the U.S. population. It is more common in whites than African Americans. Onset of psoriasis usually appears before the age of 30 years, but it may occur as early as age 10. Psoriasis is characterized by erythematous papules and plaques covered with silvery scales (Figure 49–1). It appears on the scalp, elbows, palms of the hands, knees, and soles of the feet. With psoriasis, epidermal cell growth and epidermal turnover is accelerated to approximately five times the normal expected epidermal growth. Antipsoriatic drug therapy uses preparations such as coal tar products and anthralin to keep the psoriasis in check; however, there are usually periods of remission and exacerbation.

Topical and Systemic Preparations for Psoriasis

Psoriatic scales may be loosened with keratolytics (salicylic acid, sulfur). Topical glucocorticoids are sometimes used for mild psoriasis. Other topical preparations for psoriasis include anthralin (Anthra-Derm, Lasan) and coal tar (Estar, PsoriGel). Applications of 1% anthralin may cause erythema to occur. This agent can stain clothing, skin, and hair. Coal tar products are available in shampoos, lotions, and creams. They have an unpleasant odor and can cause burning and stinging, so they are rarely used. A topical product for mild to moderate psoriasis is calcipotriene (Dovonex), a synthetic vitamin D_3 derivative useful for suppressing cell proliferation. This drug may cause local irritation, but the serious adverse effects are hypercalciuria and hypercalcemia (increased urine and serum calcium levels). A topical antipsoriatic, tazarotene (Tazorac), is used to treat mild to moderate psoriasis. Photosensitivity is a side effect of tazarotene; therefore the client should use sunscreen to avoid severe sunburn.

The anticancer drug methotrexate is a systemic drug that slows high growth fraction. It is prescribed to decrease the acceleration of epidermal cell growth in severe psoriasis. Etretinate (Tegison) is used for severe pustular psoriasis, more so than plaque-type psoriasis. It is used when other agents have failed to control psoriasis. Etretinate has an antiinflammatory effect and inhibits keratinization and proliferation of the epithelial cells. Ultraviolet A (UVA) may be used to suppress mitotic (cell division) activity. Photochemotherapy, a combination of ultraviolet radiation and the psoralen derivative methoxsalen (photosensitive drug), is used to decrease proliferation of epidermal cells. This type of therapy is called *psoralen and ultraviolet A (PUVA)*. PUVA permits lower doses of methoxsalen and ultraviolet A to be given.

FIGURE 49–1 Psoriasis. Typical oval plaque with well-defined borders and silvery scale. (From Habif T: *Clinical dermatology,* St Louis, 2004, Mosby, p. 210.)

High-cost biologic agents are helpful in the management of psoriasis in clients who are refractory to ultraviolet B (UVB) phototherapy and need improved control. Five FDA-approved agents include: alefacept (Amevive), efalizumab (Raptiva); etanercept (Enbrel), infliximab (Remicade), and adalimumab (Humira). These biologic agents are expensive but tend to have fewer side effects with comparable efficacy to other systemic treatments.

Alefacept (Amevive) is a recombinant protein that modifies the inflammatory process and inhibits the activation of memory effector T lymphocytes. No increased rate of opportunistic infections or malignancy has been observed. The drug is administered IM or IV weekly for 12 weeks. Chills are the most common side effect. A second 12-week cycle may be initiated, but with decreased benefits from the first cycle. Weekly monitoring of CBC and T-cell counts is required, and alefacept must be discontinued if the CD4+ T-cell count falls lower than 250 cells per microliter.

Efalizumab (Raptiva) is a humanized therapeutic antibody to treat adults who have severe psoriasis with indication for systemic or phototherapy. Raptiva, a weekly subcutaneous injection, can be self-administered by the client or family. Maintained response is generally seen after 12 weeks of treatment. As an immunosuppressant agent, Raptiva may increase the risk of infection.

Etanercept (Enbrel) is a soluble recombinant human tumor necrosis factor (TNF)-alpha inhibitor. This agent worsens infections, especially tuberculosis (TB). A tuberculin test (PPD) is required prior to initiation of therapy. Etanercept may also worsen heart failure (HF). The drug is administered twice weekly for 12 weeks, then weekly.

Infliximab (Remicade) is a monoclonal antibody that neutralizes TNF-alpha purified protein derivative (PPD). The drug is administered IV at 0, 2, and 6 weeks, then every 8 weeks as tolerated. Opportunistic infection rate is higher than with other agents. A tuberculin test before the start and during treatment is recommended. This drug is associated with demyelinating disease. The major side effect is increased risk of infection. Do not confuse this drug with Reminyl.

Adalimumab is a TNF-alpha inhibitor. The drug is administered subcutaneously every other week.

Table 49–1 lists the drugs used to control psoriasis.

Side Effects and Adverse Reactions: Psoriasis Drugs

- anthralin: Erythema (redness) to normal skin, inflamed eyes, and staining effect.
- coal Tar: Skin irritation, such as burning; photosensitivity; and staining effect.
- etretinate: Anorexia, vomiting, dry skin and nasal mucosa, rash, pruritus, fatigue, bone or joint pain, peeling of skin, and photosensitivity. *Adverse reactions:* Alopecia, cardiac dysrhythmias, hepatitis, and hematuria.
- methoxsalen: Nausea, headache, vertigo, rash, pruritus, and burning and peeling of skin. *Adverse reactions:* Anemia, leukopenia, thrombocytopenia, ulcerative stomatitis, bleeding; alopecia, and cystitis.
- alefacept: Injection site reaction (erythema, itching, pain, swelling), dizziness, throat inflammation, nausea, muscle pain, and chills.
- efalizumab: Headache, chills, fever, nausea, myalgia, and potential of acute infection.
- etanercept: Injection site reaction (erythema, itching, pain, swelling).
- infliximab: Infusion reactions and infections, including reactivation of TB.

Nursing Process

Acne Vulgaris and Psoriasis

ASSESSMENT

- Obtain a history from client of the onset of skin lesions. Note whether there is a familial history of the skin disorder.
- Assess client's skin eruptions. Describe the lesions, location, and drainage, if present.

■ Obtain a culture of a purulent draining skin lesion.
■ Determine baseline vital signs. Report any elevation in temperature.
■ Assess the psychologic effects of skin lesions and changes in body image.

NURSING DIAGNOSES

■ Risk for impaired skin integrity related to side effects of some of the medications
■ Risk for infection due to selected medications
■ Disturbed body image related to skin lesions
■ Risk for situational low self-esteem related to skin lesions

PLANNING

■ Client's skin lesions will be decreased in size or will be absent after drug therapy and skin care.
■ Client will report acceptance of body image.

NURSING INTERVENTIONS

■ Establish rapport, because client may be embarrassed.
■ Apply topical medications to the skin lesions using aseptic technique.
■ Monitor vital signs and report abnormal findings.
■ Check the lesion sites during drug therapy for improvement or adverse reactions to the drug therapy (blistering, swelling, scaling).

Client Teaching

General

• Instruct client not to use harsh cleansers. Tell client to gently clean the skin several times a day.
• Teach client how to apply topical ointments and creams using a clean technique.
• Inform client about the side effects and adverse reactions associated with the drugs taken.
• Tell client to report abnormal findings immediately. Inform client not to take milk or antacids with tetracycline.
• Instruct client to alert the health care provider if pregnant or if there is a possibility of pregnancy. Many agents used to treat acne can cause teratogenic effects on the fetus.
• Advise client to keep health care appointments and have laboratory tests performed as prescribed.

Self-Administration

• Instruct client and family about how to administer biologic agents given via the parenteral route (e.g., preparation and administration of Amevive: diluted solution to be stored in refrigerator and used within 4 hours; do not shake medication; rotate injection sites, leaving at least 1 inch between sites).

Cultural Considerations ❖

• Respect client's cultural beliefs and alternative methods for treating acne vulgaris or psoriasis. Plan may need modification to include pharmacologic treatment for acne or psoriasis.
• Obtain an interpreter when necessary; do not rely on family members, who may not fully disclose because of honor or shame.
• Provide an interpreter with the same background and gender, if possible, especially with sensitive topics.

EVALUATION

■ Evaluate the effectiveness of the drug therapy on the skin lesions. If improvement is not apparent, the drug therapy and skin care regimen may need to be changed.

Verruca Vulgaris (Warts)

The common wart is a hard, horny nodule that may appear anywhere on the body, particularly on the hands and feet. Warts may be benign lesions, or they may be precursors to cancerous lesions, especially those in the genital region. They may be removed by freezing, electrodesiccation, or surgical excision. Drugs used in the treatment of warts include salicylic acid, podophyllum resin, and cantharidin. Salicylic acid promotes desquamation. It can be absorbed through the skin, and salicylism (toxicity) might occur. Podophyllum resin is indicated mainly for venereal warts and is not as effective against the common wart. This drug also can be absorbed through the skin; toxic symptoms such as peripheral neuropathy, blood dyscrasias, and kidney impairment could result if a large area is treated. Podophyllum can cause teratogenic effects and should not be used during pregnancy. Imiquimod (Aldara) and podofilox (Condylox) may be prescribed as alternative agents for podophyllin. Both drugs may be used for topical treatment of external genital and perianal warts.

Cantharidin (Cantharone, Verr-Canth) is used to remove the common wart; however, it can be harmful to normal skin. For treating the common wart, cantharidin is applied to the wart, allowed to dry, and then the wart is covered with a nonporous tape for 24 hours. The procedure can be repeated in 1 to 2 weeks.

Many OTC agents are used to remove warts. The efficacy of some of these is questionable; however, some that contain chemical compounds such as salicylic acid may be effective.

Drug-Induced Dermatitis

An adverse reaction to drug therapy may result in skin lesions that vary from a rash, urticaria, papules, and vesicles to life-threatening skin eruptions such as erythema multiforme (red blisters over a large portion of the body), Stevens-Johnson syndrome (large blisters in the oral and anogenital mucosa, pharynx, eyes, and viscera), and toxic epidermal necrolysis (widespread detachment of the epidermis from underlying skin layers). A hypersensitive reaction to a drug is caused by the formation of sensitizing lymphocytes. If multiple drug therapy is used, the last drug given may be the cause of the hypersensitivity and skin eruptions. The usual skin reactions are a rash that may take several hours or a day to appear and urticaria (hives), which usually take a few minutes to appear. Certain drugs, such as penicillin, are known to cause hypersensitivity.

Other drug-induced dermatitides include discoid lupus erythematosus (DLE) and exfoliative dermatitis. Hydralazine hydrochloride (Apresoline), isoniazid (INH), phenothiazines, anticonvulsants, and antidysrhythmics, such as procainamide (Pronestyl), may cause lupuslike symptoms. If lupus symptoms occur, the drug should be discontinued. Certain antibacterials and anticonvulsants may cause exfoliative dermatitis, resulting in erythema of the skin, itching, scaling, and loss of body hair.

Contact Dermatitis

Contact dermatitis, also called *exogenous dermatitis,* is caused by chemical or plant irritation. A skin rash with itching, swelling, blistering, oozing, or scaling at the affected skin sites characterizes this disorder. The chemical contact may include cosmetics, cleaning products (e.g., soaps, detergents), perfume, clothing, dyes, and topical drugs. Plant contacts include poison ivy, oak, or sumac.

Nonpharmacologic measures include avoiding direct contact with the causative irritant. Protective gloves or clothing may be necessary if the chemical is associated with work. Immediately cleanse the skin area that has been in contact with the irritant. Patch testing may be needed to determine the causal factor.

Treatment may consist of wet dressings containing Burow's solution (aluminum acetate); lotions, such as calamine, that contain zinc oxide; calcium hydroxide solution; and glycerin. Calamine lotion may contain the antihistamine diphenhydramine and is used primarily for plant irritations. If itching persists, antipruritics (systemic diphenhydramine [Benadryl]) may be used. Topical Benadryl is not recommended, as it increases the risk of allergic reaction to systemic Benadryl. Topical antipruritics should not be applied to open wounds or near the eyes or genital area. Other agents used as antipruritics include the following:

- Systemic drugs such as cyproheptadine hydrochloride (Periactin) and trimeprazine tartrate (Temaril)
- Antipruritic baths of oatmeal or Alpha-Keri
- Solutions of potassium permanganate, aluminum subacetate, or normal saline
- Glucocorticoid ointments, creams, or gels

Dexamethasone (Decadron) cream, hydrocortisone ointment or cream, methylprednisolone acetate (Medrol) ointment, triamcinolone acetonide (Aristocort), and flurandrenolide (Cordran) are examples of topical glucocorticoids that aid in alleviating dermatitis. Box 49–1 lists selected topical glucocorticoids according to their potency for relieving the itching and inflammation associated with dermatitis.

A portion of topical glucocorticoids can be systemically absorbed into the circulation. The amount and rate of absorption depend on the vehicle (cream, lotion), drug concentration, drug composition, and skin area to which the glucocorticoid is applied. Absorption is greater where the skin is more permeable—the face, scalp, eyelids, neck, axilla, and genital area. Side effects and adverse reactions may occur with prolonged use of the topical drug or if the drug is continuously covered with a dressing. Prolonged use of topical glucocorticoids can cause thinning of the skin with atrophy of the epidermis and dermis and purpura from small-vessel eruptions; therefore, prolonged use is discouraged.

Hair Loss and Baldness

When the hair shaft is lost and the hair follicle cannot regenerate, male-pattern baldness, or *alopecia,* occurs. Permanent hair loss is associated with a familial history and occurs during the aging process, earlier in some individuals than others. Drugs also known to cause alopecia include the anticancer (antineoplastic) agents, gold salts, sulfonamides, anticonvulsants, aminoglycosides, and some of the nonsteroidal antiinflammatory drugs (NSAIDs) such as indomethacin. Severe febrile illnesses, pregnancy, myxedema (condition resulting from hypothyroidism), and cancer therapies are some of the health conditions contributing to temporary hair loss.

A 2% minoxidil (Rogaine) solution has been approved by the FDA for treating baldness for men and women. A 5% solution is approved for men only. Minoxidil causes vasodilation, increasing cutaneous blood flow. The increased blood flow tends to stimulate hair follicle growth. When the drug is discontinued, however, hair loss occurs within 3 to 4 months. Systemic absorption of minoxidil is minimal, so adverse reactions seldom occur. Occasionally, headaches and a slight decrease in systolic blood pressure occur.

Finasteride (Propecia) is an oral drug used for male baldness. It is available in 1-mg tablets. A 5-mg tablet is prescribed for benign prostatic hyperplasia (BPH). For growing hair, finasteride is effective in 50% of men. It has been reported that it is relatively ineffective in growing hair in older men, even with an increased dose.

Sunscreens

Chemical screens (absorb ultraviolet [UV] radiation) and physical screens (scatter UV radiation) are the two categories of sunscreens. The chemical type accounts for most of the 126 FDA-approved sunscreens. Most absorb UV-UVB, less than one half absorb UVA, and one, avobenzone (Anthelios SX Daily Moisturizing Cream with Sunscreen, PreSun Ultra Screen, Sea & Ski Advanced Sunscreen, Neutro-

Box 49–1

Topical Glucocorticoids

Super High Potency

betamethasone dipropionate, augmented 0.05%, Diprolene (o, g)

clobetasol propionate 0.05%
Clobex (l, sh, s)
Cormax (o, s app)
Olux (f)
Temovate (c, g, o, sc app)
Temovate Emollient (e crm)
fluocinonide 0.1%
Vanos (c)
flurandrenolide 4mcg/sq cm
Cordran (t)
halobetasol propionate 0.05%
Ultravate 0.05% (c, o)

High Potency

amcinonide 0.1%
Cyclocort (c, l, o)
betamethasone dipropionate, augmented 0.05%
Diprolene (c)
Diprolene AF (e crm)
desoximetasone 0.05%
Topicort (g)
desoximetasone 0.25%
Topicort (e crm, o)
diflorasone diacetate 0.05%
Psorcon E (e crm, e oint)
fluocinonide 0.05%
Lidex (c, g, o, so)
Lidex-E (e crm)
halcinonide 0.1%
Halog (c, o, soln)
triamcinolone acetonide 0.5%
Aristocort A (c)
Kenalog (c)

Intermediate Potency

betamethasone valerate 0.12%
Luxiq (f)
clocortolone pivalate 0.1%
Cloderm (c)
desonide 0.5%
DesOwen (c, l, o)
Verdeso (f)

desoximetasone 0.05%
Topicort LP (e crm)
fluocinolone acetonide 0.01%
Derma-Smoothe/FS (oil)
Capex (sh)
fluocinolone acetonide 0.025%
Synalar (c, o)
flurandrenolide 0.025%
Cordran SP (c)
Cordran (o)
flurandrenolide 0.05%
Cordran (l, o)
Cordran-SP (c)
fluticasone propionate 0.005%
Cutivate (o)
fluticasone propionate 0.05%
Cutivate (c, l)
hydrocortisone probutate 0.1%
Pandel (c)
hydrocortisone butyrate 0.1%
Locoid (c, o, soln)
hydrocortisone valerate 0.2%
Westcort (c, o)
mometasone furoate 0.1%
Elocon (c, l, o)
prednicarbate 0.1%
Dermatop (e crm, o)
triamcinolone acetonide 0.1%
Aristocort A (c, o)
Kenalog (c, l)
triamcinolone acetonide 0.2%
Kenalog (a)

Low Potency

Alclometasone dipropionate 0.05%
Aclovate (c, o)
Fluocinolone acetonide 0.01%
Synalar (soln)
Hydrocortisone base or acetate 0.5%
Cortisporin (c)
Hydrocortisone base or acetate 1%
Cortisporin (o)*
Hytone (c, o)
U-cort (c)
Vytone (c)*

C, Cream; *e crm,* emollient cream; *e oint,* emollient ointment; *f,* foam; *g,* gel; *l,* lotion; *o,* ointment; *sh,* shampoo; *s,* spray; *s app,* scalp application; *soln,* solution; *t,* tape.
*Denotes that product has more than one active ingredient.
Data from *Nurse Practitioners' Prescribing Reference,* 14:119, Spring 2007.

gena Ultra Sheer Dry-Touch Sunblock), protects against UVA and B. Physical screens prevent skin penetration of UV. Examples of these products are titanium dioxide and zinc oxide, generally applied to limited areas of the body such as nose and ears.

Ultraviolet radiation causes many problems, including premature aging of the skin, burns, and skin cancer. Sunscreens protect against sunburn photosensitivity to selected drugs but do not guard against melanoma and basal cell carcinoma. Sun protection factor (SPF) is a rating on sunscreen products of protection against UVB radiation. The highest rating approved by FDA is SPF 30+; however, SPF 15 is not one half the protection of SPF 30. A higher protection rating is not proportional to the amount of UVB radiation blocked. For example, SPF 15 blocks 93% of UVB and SPF 30 blocks 96.7%. Sunscreens (SPF greater than 15) are recommended for children over 6 months of age and all adults.

Using common sense is the best way to protect the skin. Ultraviolet radiation is most intense between 10:00 AM and 3:00 PM. Apply an appropriate sunscreen for the circumstances at least 30 minutes (sunscreens with PABA or padimate allow 2 hours) before going out into the sun. Sunscreen will protect for about 2 hours when applied properly and not exposed to moisture (through swimming or sweating). Wearing protective clothing (a wide-brimmed hat, sunglasses, and long-sleeve shirt) is a good idea. When using DEET (insect repellent) together with sunscreens, apply DEET first to avoid decreased effectiveness of the sunscreen.

Burns and Burn Preparations

Burns from heat (thermal burns), electricity (electrical burns), and chemical agents (chemical burns) can cause skin lesions. Burns are classified according to degree and tissue depth of burns and are described in Table 49–2.

A moderately severe sunburn is an example of a *first-degree burn*. A severe sunburn can result in a *second-degree burn*. A burn needs immediate attention, regardless of the degree and tissue depth of the burn.

For first-degree and minor burns, a cold wet compress should be applied to the burned area to constrict blood vessels and decrease swelling. This treatment also decreases the amount of pain. The quicker the burn area is cooled, the less tissue damage occurs. No greasy ointment, butter, or greasy dressing should be applied, because they can inhibit heat loss from the burn and increase the damage to the tissues. A nonprescription antibiotic, such as bacitracin with polymyxin B (Polysporin), may be used for minor burns. Used separately, polymyxin B and neomycin are not drugs of choice, because they do not have a broad-spectrum effect. With chemical burns, the clothing should be removed immediately and the skin thoroughly flushed with water.

Persons with second- and third-degree burns that involve the dermis and subcutaneous tissue should undergo treatment in a burn center or other hospital setting. Intravenous therapy is started immediately, and a nonnarcotic or narcotic analgesic is given for pain. Burn areas are cleansed with sterile saline solution and an antiseptic such as povidone-iodine (Betadine). If a povidone-iodine solution is used, it should be determined that the client is not allergic to iodine or seafood. Broad-spectrum topical antibacterials, usually effective against many gram-positive and gram-negative organisms and yeast infections, are applied to burn areas to prevent infection. Examples of these antibacterials include mafenide acetate (Sulfamylon), silver sulfadiazine (Silvadene), silver nitrate 0.5% solution, and nitrofurazone (Furacin). Prototype Drug Chart 49–1 lists the drug data for the antibacterial agent mafenide acetate (Sulfamylon).

Mafenide Acetate

Pharmacokinetics

Mafenide acetate is absorbed through the skin and metabolized by the liver to a metabolite. The drug is excreted in the urine. The drug and its metabolite are strong carbonic anhydrase inhibitors, which may lead to acid-base imbalances (e.g., metabolic acidosis and respiratory alkalosis) and fluid loss from the mild diuretic effect. If respiration becomes rapid, labored, or shallow, the cream should be discontinued for a few days until the acid-base balance is restored.

Pharmacodynamics

Mafenide, a sulfonamide derivative, interferes with bacterial cell-wall synthesis and metabolism and is bacteriostatic. It is used as a topical water-soluble antibacterial agent to prevent or combat a burn infection. After the burn is cleansed and debrided, $\frac{1}{16}$ inch of mafenide cream is applied to the affected area one to two times daily and is covered lightly with a dressing. The client may complain of a burning sensation when the drug is applied.

Table 49–3 lists selected topical medications for burns and their strengths, uses, and considerations.

Silver Sulfadiazine

Silver sulfadiazine (Silvadene, SSD) is commonly used to prevent and treat sepsis in second- and third-degree burns. It acts on the cell membrane and cell wall to produce bactericidal effects. Unlike mafenide, it is *not* a carbonic anhydrase inhibitor. It is contraindicated at or near term pregnancy.

One percent or less of the silver is absorbed, and up to 10% of sulfadiazine is absorbed. Side effects and adverse reactions may include skin discoloration, burning sensation, rashes, erythema multiforme, skin necrosis, and possible leukopenia.

Table 49–2

Degree and Tissue Depth of Burns

Type	Degree	Depth	Characteristics
Superficial epidermal	First	Epidermis	Erythema (redness), painful
Partial thickness superficial	First-second	Epidermis, upper dermis	Blistering, very painful
Deep thickness	Second	Epidermis, lower dermis	Mottled, blistering, intense pain
Full thickness	Third	Epidermis, dermis, nerve ending involvement, subcutaneous tissue	Pearly white skin, charred, no pain

Prototype DRUG CHART 49–1

MAFENIDE ACETATE

Drug Class	**Dosage**
Topical antiinfective Trade names: Sulfamylon Cream *Pregnancy Category:* C	**A & C: Topical:** Apply $\frac{1}{16}$-in. layer evenly to affected area daily/b.i.d.; reapply as necessary
Contraindications	**Drug-Lab-Food Interactions**
Hypersensitivity, inhalation injury *Caution:* Renal failure	None known

Pharmacokinetics	**Pharmacodynamics**
Absorption: Some absorbed **Distribution:** PB: UK **Metabolism:** t½: UK **Excretion:** In urine	**Topical: Onset:** On contact Peak: 2-4 h Duration: As long as applied

Therapeutic Effects/Uses

To treat second- and third-degree burns; to prevent organism invasion of burned tissue areas; to treat burn infections
Mode of Action: Inhibits bacterial cell wall synthesis

Side Effects	**Adverse Reactions**
Rash, burning sensation, urticaria, pruritus, swelling	Metabolic acidosis, respiratory alkalosis, blistering, superinfection ***Life-threatening:*** Bone marrow suppression, fatal hemolytic anemia

A, Adult; *b.i.d.,* two times a day; *C,* child; *h,* hour; *in,* inch; *PB,* protein-binding; *t½,* half-life; *UK,* unknown.

Table 49–3

Topical Antiinfectives: Burns

Generic (Brand)	Route and Dosage	Uses and Considerations
nitrofurazone (Furacin)	0.2% Cream, ointment, sol *Adjunctive therapy:* Apply directly or to dressing daily for second- to third-degree burns; q4-5d for second-degree burns with scant exudates	For second- and third-degree burns. Can cause photosensitivity; avoid sunlight. May cause contact dermatitis. *Pregnancy category:* C; PB: NA; t½: NA
mafenide acetate (Sulfamylon) silver nitrate	(Prototype Drug Chart 49–1) 0.5 sol; 10%, 25% sticks; apply only to affected area 2-3 ×/wk for 2-3 wk	For second- and third-degree burns. Dressings are soaked in 0.5% silver nitrate solution and then removed before they dry. Effective against some gram-negative organisms. May cause electrolyte imbalance (hypokalemia) if used extensively. *Pregnancy category:* C; PB: NA; t½: NA
silver sulfadiazine (Silvadene, SSD)	1% Cream, apply daily-b.i.d. in $\frac{1}{16}$-in. layer	Prevent and treat infection of second- and third-degree burns. Ten percent of the drug is absorbed. Excessive use or extensive application area may cause sulfa crystals (crystalluria). *Pregnancy category:* C; PB: NA; t½: NA

b.i.d., Twice a day; *d,* day; *NA,* not applicable; *PB,* protein-binding; *t½,* half-life; *in,* inch; *sol,* solution; *wk,* week.

Nursing Process

Topical Antiinfectives: Burns

ASSESSMENT

■ Assess burned tissue for infection. Culture an oozing wound.
■ Check client's vital signs. Report abnormal findings, such as elevated temperature.
■ Determine fluid status. Report signs and symptoms of hypovolemia or hypervolemia.

NURSING DIAGNOSES

■ Risk for infection related to loss of skin integrity
■ Pain related to thermal injury
■ Disturbed body image related to loss of skin integrity

PLANNING

■ Aseptic technique will be enforced when caring for burned tissue, and tissue will be free from infection.

NURSING INTERVENTIONS

■ Administer prescribed analgesia before application, if needed.
■ Cleanse burned tissue sites using aseptic technique.
■ Apply topical antibacterial drug and dressing with sterile technique.
■ Monitor client's fluid balance and renal function.
■ Monitor client for side effects and adverse reactions to topical drug.
■ Monitor client's vital signs and be alert for signs of infection. Use with caution in client with acute renal failure.
■ Closely monitor client's acid-base balance, especially in the presence of pulmonary or renal dysfunction.
■ Store drug in dry place at room temperature.

Client Teaching

General

● Instruct client and family about changes in respiratory status.

Self-Administration

● Explain to client and family the care given to the burned tissue areas, using aseptic technique.
● Instruct client and family how to apply topical agent and dressings to the burned areas.
● Instruct client and family on signs and symptoms of infection and to report them promptly to the health care provider.

Cultural Considerations ❖

● In many cultures the extended family structure is important for health teaching and providing support.
● Do not assume that a positive response means a definite "yes" or understanding (it may be simply a show of politeness).

EVALUATION

■ Evaluate effectiveness of treatment interventions to burned tissue areas by determining whether healing is proceeding and sites are free from infection.

Critical Thinking Case Study

MG, age 15, complains about numerous blackheads and large raised pimples on her face. She seeks help from a health care provider.

1. To assist in identifying her skin problem, what should the health history and assessment include?
2. Which nonpharmacologic measures might you discuss with MG in caring for her facial skin condition?

MG's skin disorder does not improve. Her health care provider says she has acne vulgaris and has prescribed benzoyl peroxide and oral tetracycline.

3. MG asks the nurse how to use benzoyl peroxide. What should the explanation of the method and frequency for the use of benzoyl peroxide include?
4. What should be included in the client teaching related to the use of oral tetracycline?
5. What other agents for acne might MG use? Explain their uses and side effects.
6. MG asks whether she will have to remain on benzoyl peroxide and oral tetracycline for the rest of her life. What is the answer or course of action? Explain.

NCLEX Study Questions

1. The purpose of keratolytic agents is to remove:
   a. a horny layer of dermis
   b. a horny layer of epidermis
   c. erythematous lesions
   d. hair follicles

2. Nursing implications for health teaching with clients taking isotretinoin include which of the following? (Select all that apply.)
   a. Avoid sunlight
   b. Monitor weight
   c. Monitor CBC, glucose, lipids
   d. Do not breast feed or give blood

3. Nursing implications of the new biologic agents for the management of psoriasis include:
   a. daily weight
   b. monitor electrolytes
   c. assess lesions
   d. monitor CBC and T-cell count

4. The drug used to treat male-pattern baldness is which of the following:
   a. dexamethasone
   b. PABA
   c. minoxidil
   d. finasteride

5. BR has second- and third-degree burns over 25% of his body. Mafenide acetate has been ordered. What acid-base imbalance can result from its use? (Select all that apply.)
   a. Metabolic acidosis
   b. Metabolic alkalosis
   c. Respiratory alkalosis
   d. Respiratory acidosis

6. Based on your client's prolonged use of glucocorticoids, your assessment includes:
   a. obesity
   b. thinning of the skin
   c. erythematous lesions
   d. purpura

Answers: 1, b; 2, a, c, d; 3, c; 4, d; 5, a, c; 6, b, d.

SEVENTEEN

Endocrine Agents

$\mathcal{T}$he endocrine system consists of ductless glands that secrete hormones into the bloodstream. *Hormones* are chemical substances synthesized from amino acids and cholesterol that act on body tissues and organs and affect cellular activity. Hormones can be divided into two categories: (1) proteins or small peptides and (2) steroids. Hormones from the adrenal glands and the gonads are steroid hormones; the others are protein hormones. The *endocrine glands* include the pituitary (hypophysis), thyroid, parathyroid, adrenal, gonads, and pancreas. Figure XVII–1 illustrates the location and functions of these glands. This unit discusses the hormonal activity of the endocrine glands.

Pituitary Gland

The pituitary gland, or hypophysis, is located at the base of the brain and has two lobes, the anterior pituitary (adenohypophysis) and the posterior pituitary (neurohypophysis). The anterior pituitary gland is called the *master gland,* because it secretes hormones that stimulate the release of other hormones from target glands, including the thyroid, parathyroids, adrenals, and gonads. The posterior pituitary gland secretes two neurohormones—antidiuretic hormone (ADH), or vasopressin, and oxytocin. Figure XVII–2 shows the anterior and posterior pituitary glands and the types of hormones secreted.

Anterior Pituitary Gland

The anterior pituitary hormones are (1) thyroid-stimulating hormone (TSH), (2) adrenocorticotropic hormone (ACTH), and (3) the gonadotropins (follicle-stimulating hormone [FSH] and luteinizing hormone [LH]). They control the synthesis and release of hormones from the thyroid, adrenals, and ovaries. Other hormones secreted from the anterior pituitary include growth hormone (GH), prolactin (PL), and melanocyte-stimulating hormone (MSH). The amount of each hormone secreted from the anterior pituitary is regulated by a negative feedback

system. If excess hormone is secreted from the target gland, hormonal release from the anterior pituitary is suppressed. If there is a lack of hormone secretion from the target gland, there will be an increase in that particular anterior pituitary hormone.

FIGURE XVII–I   The endocrine glands.

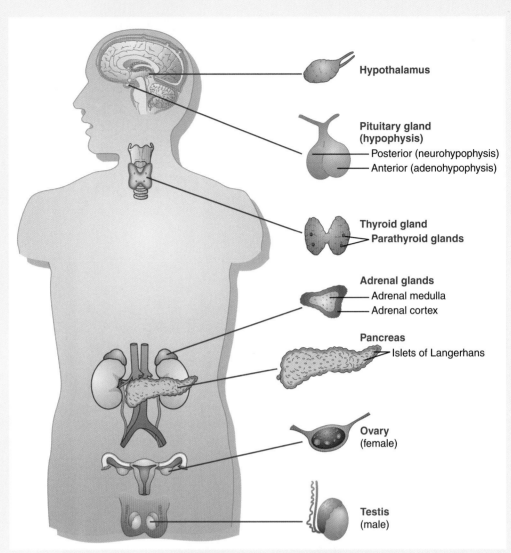

Hypothalamus

Pituitary gland (hypophysis)
— Posterior (neurohypophysis)
— Anterior (adenohypophysis)

Thyroid gland
— Parathyroid glands

Adrenal glands
— Adrenal medulla
— Adrenal cortex

Pancreas
— Islets of Langerhans

Ovary (female)

Testis (male)

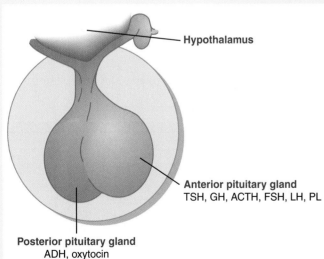

Hypothalamus

Anterior pituitary gland
TSH, GH, ACTH, FSH, LH, PL

Posterior pituitary gland
ADH, oxytocin

FIGURE XVII–2   The anterior and posterior pituitary glands. *ACTH,* Adrenocorticotropic hormone; *ADH,* antidiuretic hormone; *FSH,* follicle-stimulating hormone; *GH,* growth hormone; *LH,* luteinizing hormone; *PL,* prolactin; *TSH,* thyroid-stimulating hormone.

Thyroid-Stimulating Hormone

The anterior pituitary gland secretes TSH in response to thyroid-releasing hormone (TRH) from the hypothalamus. TSH, or thyrotropic hormone, stimulates the release of thyroxine (T_4) and triiodothyronine (T_3) from the thyroid gland. Hypersecretion of TSH can cause hyperthyroidism and thyroid enlargement, and hyposecretion can cause hypothyroidism. Serum TSH levels should be checked to determine whether there is a TSH deficit or excess. TSH and T_4 levels are frequently measured to differentiate pituitary from thyroid dysfunction. A decreased T_4 level and a normal or elevated TSH level can indicate a thyroid disorder.

Adrenocorticotropic Hormone

Secretion of ACTH occurs in response to corticotropin-releasing factor (CRF) from the hypothalamus. ACTH from the anterior pituitary stimulates the release of glucocorticoids (cortisol), mineralocorticoids (aldosterone), and androgen from the adrenal cortex (adrenal glands). Elevated serum cortisol from the adrenal cortex inhibits ACTH and CRF release. When the cortisol level is low, ACTH secretion is stimulated, which in turn stimulates the adrenal cortex to release more cortisol. More ACTH is secreted in the morning than in the evening.

Gonadotropic Hormones

The gonadotropic hormones regulate hormone secretion from the ovaries and testes (the gonads). The anterior pituitary gland secretes the gonadotropic hormones FSH, LH, and prolactin. FSH promotes the maturation of follicles in the ovaries and initiates sperm production in the testes. LH combines with FSH in follicle maturation and estrogen production and promotes secretion of androgens from the testes. Prolactin stimulates milk formation in the glandular breast tissue after childbirth. Estrogen, progesterone, and testosterone are discussed in Chapters 55, Drugs for Women's Health and Reproductive Disorders, and 56, Drugs for Men's Health and Reproductive Disorders, respectively.

Growth Hormone

GH, or somatotropic hormone (STH), acts on all body tissues, particularly the bones and skeletal muscles. The amount of GH secreted is regulated by growth hormone-releasing hormone (GH-RH) and growth hormone-inhibiting hormone (GH-IH, or somatostatin) from the hypothalamus. Sympathomimetics, serotonin, and glucocorticoids can inhibit the secretion of GH.

Posterior Pituitary Gland

The posterior pituitary gland (neurohypophysis) secretes ADH (vasopressin) and oxytocin. Interconnecting nerve fibers between the hypothalamus and the posterior pituitary gland allow ADH and oxytocin to be synthesized in the hypothalamus and stored in the posterior pituitary gland. ADH increases the reabsorption of water from the renal tubules, returning it to the systemic circulation. Secretion of ADH is regulated by the serum osmolality (concentration of the vascular fluid). An increase in serum osmolality increases the release of ADH from the posterior pituitary; more water is then absorbed from the renal tubules to dilute the vascular fluid. Excess ADH can overload the vascular system. A decrease in serum osmolality decreases the release of ADH, promoting more water excretion from the renal tubules. Oxytocin stimulates contraction of the smooth muscles of the uterus; it is discussed in Chapter 53, Female Reproductive Cycle II: Labor, Delivery, and Preterm Neonatal Drugs.

Thyroid Gland

Located anterior to the trachea, the thyroid gland has two lobes that are connected by a bridge of thyroid tissue. The thyroid gland secretes two hormones, thyroxine (T_4) and triiodothyronine (T_3 liothyronine). These hormones affect nearly every tissue and organ by controlling their metabolic rate and activity. Stimulation by the thyroid hormones results in an increase in cardiac output, oxygen consumption, carbohydrate use, protein synthesis, and breakdown of fat (lipolysis). Thyroid hormones also affect body heat regulation and the menstrual cycle. Thyroid hormone levels in the blood are regulated by negative feedback. The anterior pituitary gland secretes TSH, which stimulates the thyroid gland to produce T_4 and T_3. An increased amount of circulating thyroid hormones suppresses the release of TSH, and a decreased amount increases the release of TSH by the adenohypophysis.

Parathyroid Glands

There are four parathyroid glands (two pairs) that lie on the dorsal surface of the thyroid gland. The parathyroid gland secretes parathormone, or parathyroid hormone (PTH), which regulates calcium levels in the blood. A decrease in serum calcium stimulates the release of PTH. PTH increases calcium levels by (1) mobilizing calcium from the bone, (2) promoting calcium absorption from the intestine, and (3) promoting calcium reabsorption from the renal tubules. Calcitonin, a hormone produced primarily by the thyroid gland and to a lesser extent by the parathyroid and thymus glands, inhibits calcium reabsorption by bone and increases renal excretion of calcium. Calcitonin counteracts the action of PTH.

Adrenal Glands

The adrenal glands, located at the top of each kidney, consist of two separate sections—the adrenal medulla (the inner section) and the adrenal cortex (the section surrounding the adrenal medulla). The adrenal medulla releases the catecholamines epinephrine and norepinephrine and is linked with the sympathetic nervous system. The adrenal cortex produces two major types of hormones (corticosteroids)—glucocorticoids and mineralocorticoids. The principal glucocorticoid is cortisol, and the principal mineralocorticoid is aldosterone. The adrenal cortex also produces small amounts of androgen, estrogen, and progestin. Glucocorticoids have a profound influence on electrolytes and the metabolism of carbohydrates, protein, and fat, and glucocorticoid deficiencies can result in serious illness and even death.

Pancreas

The pancreas, located to the left of and behind the stomach, is both an exocrine and an endocrine gland. The exocrine section of the pancreas secretes digestive enzymes into the duodenum; these enzymes are discussed in Unit Fifteen, Gastrointestinal Agents. The endocrine section has cell clusters called *islets of Langerhans*. The alpha islet cells produce glucagon, which breaks glycogen down to glucose in the liver, and the beta cells secrete insulin, which regulates glucose metabolism. Insulin, an antidiabetic agent, is used to control diabetes mellitus. Antidiabetic agents are discussed in Chapter 51.

Drugs For Endocrine Disorders

Chapters 50, Endocrine Drugs: Pituitary, Thyroid, Parathyroid, and Adrenal Disorders, and 51, Antidiabetics, discuss the drugs used to diagnose and treat endocrine disorders. Chapter 50 discusses the agents for disorders involving the pituitary gland, thyroid gland, parathyroid gland, adrenal gland, and ADH. The parenteral and oral antidiabetic drugs (hypoglycemic drugs) are described in Chapter 51.

50

Endocrine Drugs: Pituitary, Thyroid, Parathyroid, and Adrenal Disorders

ELECTRONIC RESOURCES

Evolve website (http://evolve.elsevier.com/KeeHayes/pharmacology/):
- *Case Studies*
- *Content Updates*
- *Frequently Asked Questions*
- *Student Review Activities*
- *WebLinks*
- *Additional Reference Material*

Companion CD-ROM:
- *NCLEX Examination Review Questions*
- *Pharmacology Animations*
- *IV Therapy Checklists*
- *Medication Error Checklists*
- *Drug Calculation Problems*
- *Electronic Calculators*
- *Top 200 Drugs with Pronunciations*
- *References from the Textbook*

Outline

Objectives

- Compare the hormones secreted from the adenohypophysis and the neurohypophysis.

- Differentiate the actions and uses of the pituitary hormones, thyroxine (T_4), triiodothyronine (T_3), parathyroid hormone (PTH), and glucocorticoids.

- Describe the side effects of thyroxine (T_4) and triiodothyronine (T_3).

- Compare the nursing process, including client teaching, of drug therapy related to hormonal replacement or hormonal inhibition for the pituitary, thyroid, parathyroid, and adrenal glands.

Terms

This chapter describes drugs used for hormonal replacement and for inhibition of hormonal secretion from the pituitary, thyroid, parathyroid, and adrenal glands. The gonadal, or sex, hormones are discussed in Chapters 55 and 56. Before reading Chapters 50 and 51 the student or nurse should review the introduction to Unit XVII (Endocrine Agents), which describes the locations of the endocrine glands and the hormones they secrete. Knowledge of the various **endocrine** (ductless glands that produce internal secretions that flow to all parts of the body) hormones and their functions facilitates an understanding of the drugs that act on the endocrine glands.

Pituitary Gland

Anterior Lobe

The pituitary gland (**hypophysis**) has an anterior and a posterior lobe. The anterior pituitary gland, called the **adenohypophysis**, secretes the following hormones that target glands and tissues:

- Growth hormone (GH), which stimulates growth in tissue and bone
- Thyroid-stimulating hormone (TSH), which acts on the thyroid gland
- Adrenocorticotropic hormone (ACTH), which stimulates the adrenal gland
- Gonadotropins (follicle-stimulating hormone [FSH] and luteinizing hormone [LH]), which affect the ovaries. (FSH and LH are discussed in more detail in Chapter 55.)

Drugs with adenohypophyseal properties used to stimulate or inhibit glandular activity are discussed according to their therapeutic use. The negative feedback system that controls the amount of hormonal secretion from the pituitary gland and the target gland is discussed in the introduction to Unit XVII.

Growth Hormone

Two hypothalamic hormones regulate GH: (1) growth hormone-releasing hormone (GH-RH) and (2) growth hormone-inhibiting hormone (GH-IH; somatostatin). Growth hormone does not have a specific target gland. It affects body tissues and bone; GH replacement stimulates linear growth when there is a GH deficiency. Growth hormone drugs cannot be given orally, because they are inactivated by gastrointestinal enzymes. Subcutaneous (subQ) or intramuscular (IM) administration of GH is necessary

If a child's height is well below the standard for a specified age, GH deficiency may be diagnosed, and dwarfism can result. Growth hormone replacement is very expensive (approximately $20,000 for 1 year), so various tests are performed to determine whether this therapy is essential. Because GH acts on newly forming bone, it must be administered before the epiphyses are fused. Administration of GH over several years can increase height by a foot. Prolonged GH therapy can antagonize insulin secretion and eventually cause diabetes mellitus. Athletes should be advised not to take GH to build muscle and physique because of its effects on blood sugar and other side effects.

Drug Therapy: Growth Hormone Deficiency

Somatrem (Protropin) and somatropin (Humatrope) are two growth hormones used to treat growth failure in children because of pituitary GH deficiency. Somatropin is a product that has the identical amino acid sequence as human growth hormone. Somatrem also has the identical sequence of pituitary GH plus an additional amino acid. Development of antibodies to somatrem has occurred in 30% to 40% of clients during the first 3 to 6 months of therapy, but in 95% of these clients, this has not decreased the effectiveness of the somatrem treatment. Somatropin is contraindicated in pediatric clients who have growth deficiency due to Prader-Willi syndrome and are severely obese or who have severe respiratory impairment, because fatalities associated with these risk factors have been reported.

Drug Therapy: Growth Hormone Excess

Gigantism (excessive growth during childhood) and **acromegaly** (excessive growth after puberty) can occur with GH hypersecretion and are frequently caused by a pituitary tumor. If the tumor cannot be destroyed by radiation, the prolactin-release inhibitor bromocriptine can inhibit the release of GH from the pituitary.

Octreotide (Sandostatin) is a potent synthetic somatostatin used to suppress GH release. It can be used alone or with surgery or radiation. This drug is expensive. GI side effects are common. This drug can also be used for severe diarrhea resulting from carcinoid tumors.

Table 50–1 lists the drugs used to replace or inhibit GH.

Thyroid-Stimulating Hormone

The adenohypophysis secretes **thyroid-stimulating hormone (TSH)** in response to thyroid-releasing hormone (TRH) from the hypothalamus, and TSH stimulates the thyroid gland to release thyroxine (T_4) and triiodothyronine (T_3, or liothyronine). Excess TSH secretion can cause hyperthyroidism, and a TSH deficit can cause hypothyroidism. Hypothyroidism may be caused by a thyroid gland disorder (primary cause) or a decrease in TSH secretion (secondary cause). Thyrotropin (Thytropar), a purified extract of TSH, is used as a diagnostic agent to differentiate between primary and secondary hypothyroidism (see Table 50–1).

Adrenocorticotropic Hormone

The hypothalamus releases corticotropin-releasing factor (CRF), which stimulates the pituitary corticotrophs to secrete **adrenocorticotropic hormone (ACTH)**. ACTH secretion stimulates the release of glucocorticoids (cortisol), mineralocorticoids (aldosterone), and androgen from the adrenal cortex. Usually ACTH and cortisol secretions follow a diurnal rhythm in which the ACTH and cortisol secretion is higher in the early morning and then decreases through the day. Stresses such as surgery, sepsis, and

Table 50–I

Anterior and Posterior Pituitary Hormones

Generic (Brand)	Route and Dosage	Uses and Considerations
Anterior Lobe		
Growth Hormone (GH)		
sermorelin acetate (Geref)	*Diagnostic:* A & C: IV: 0.3-1 mcg/kg	Diagnostic test to determine if pituitary gland is secreting GH.
somatrem (Protropin)	*Growth hormone deficiency:* C: subQ/IM: 100 mcg/kg (0.1 mg/kg) × 3 wk or 0.2 units/kg 3 × wk; 48-h interval is recommended between doses	For growth hormone replacement to treat dwarfism. Affects growth of most body tissues and promotes bone growth at epiphyseal plates of long bones. *Pregnancy category:* C; PB: 20%-25%; $t^{1/2}$: 20-30 min
somatropin (Humatrope, Nutropin, Genotropin)	C: subQ/IM: 60 mcg/kg (0.06 mg/kg) 3 × wk or 0.16 international units/kg 3 × wk; 48-h interval is recommended between doses	For treating growth hormone deficiency. Promotes bone growth at epiphyseal plates of long bones. *Pregnancy category:* D; PB: UK; $t^{1/2}$: 15-60 min
Growth Hormone Suppressant Drugs		
bromocriptine mesylate (Parlodel)	A: PO: 1.25-2.5 mg daily × 3 d; range: 10-30 mg/d; *max:* 100 mg/d	To treat acromegaly. Also used with pituitary radiation or surgery to decrease GH levels. Will decrease lactation and prolactinoma. *Pregnancy category:* C; PB: 93%; $t^{1/2}$: 4.5 h (first phase), 45 h (last phase), average: 15 h
octreotide acetate (Sandostatin)	A: subQ: 50-100 mcg t.i.d.	To treat acromegaly. To treat severe diarrhea associated with metastatic carcinoid and other tumors. *Pregnancy category:* B; PB: 65%; $t^{1/2}$: 2.5 h
lanreotide acetate (Somatuline Depot)	A: subQ: Initially 90 mg q4 wk for 4 months; then 60-120 mg q4wk for 4 months	To suppress GH. Monitor glucose levels. *Pregnancy category:* C; PB: 69-78%; $t^{1/2}$: 23-30 d
Thyroid-Stimulating Hormone (TSH)		
thyrotropin (Thyrogen, Thytropar)	*Hypothyroidism and treatment of thyroid cancer:* A: subQ/IM: 10 international units/d for 1-3 d; cancer treatment: 3-8 d	For diagnosing cause of hypothyroidism (pituitary or thyroid). Radioiodine study follows last injection. *Pregnancy category:* C; PB: UK; $t^{1/2}$: 35 min with normal thyroid
Adrenocorticotropic Hormone (ACTH)		
corticotropin (Acthar); corticotropin, repository (H.P. Acthar gel)	(Prototype Drug Chart 50–1)	
cosyntropin (Cortrosyn)	A & C >2 y: IM/IV: 0.25 mg over 2 min C: <2 y: IM: 0.125 mg IV: 0.125 mg at 0.04 mg/h over 6 h	For diagnostic testing to differentiate between pituitary and adrenal cause of adrenal insufficiency. Obtain plasma cortisol level before and 30 min after cosyntropin administration. *Pregnancy category:* C; PB: UK; $t^{1/2}$: 15 min
Posterior Lobe		
Antidiuretic Hormone (ADH)		
desmopressin acetate (DDAVP)	*Diabetes insipidus (DI):* A: Intranasal: 0.1-0.4 ml/d in divided doses C: <12 y: Intranasal: 0.05-0.3 ml/d in divided doses	For treating DI, hemophilia A, von Willebrand disease. Can have a long duration of action (5 to 21 h). *Pregnancy category:* B; PB: UK; $t^{1/2}$: 1.25 h
desmopressin (Stimate)	A: subQ/IV: 2-4 mcg in 2 divided doses C: <12 y: Inf: 0.3 mcg/kg diluted in 10 ml of NSS over 15-30 min	Same as for desmopressin acetate.
lypressin (Diapid)	*Diabetes insipidus:* A & C: Intranasal: 1-2 sprays per nostril q.i.d.	Prevention or control of DI caused by insufficient ADH. To decrease polydipsia, polyuria, and dehydration. Duration of action is 3 to 8 hours. *Pregnancy category:* B; PB: UK; $t^{1/2}$: 15 min
vasopressin (aqueous) (Pitressin)	*Diabetes insipidus:* A: subQ/IM: 5-10 units, b.i.d.-q.i.d. C: subQ/IM: 2.5-10 units, b.i.d.-q.i.d.	For treating DI. For relief of intestinal distention. Decreases GI bleeding from esophageal varices. Can also be given intranasally. Promotes reabsorption of water from renal tubules. Duration of action 2 to 8 h. *Pregnancy category:* X; PB: UK; $t^{1/2}$: 15 min
vasopressin tannate/oil (Pitressin Tannate)	A: IM: 1.5-5.0 units, q2-3d C: IM: 1.25-2.5 units, q2-3d	Same as for vasopressin. Action is longer because of the oil.

A, Adult; *ADH,* antidiuretic hormone; *b.i.d.,* twice a day; *C,* child; *d,* day; *DI,* diabetes insipidus; *GI,* gastrointestinal; *h,* hour; *IM,* intramuscular; *inf,* infusion; *IV,* intravenous; *min,* minute; *NSS,* normal saline solution; *PB,* protein-binding; *PO,* by mouth; *q.i.d.,* four times a day; *subQ,* subcutaneous; $t^{1/2}$, half-life; *t.i.d.,* three times a day; *UK,* unknown; *wk,* week; *y,* year; >, greater than; <, less than.

trauma override the diurnal rhythm, causing an increase in secretions of ACTH and cortisol.

The ACTH drug corticotropin (Acthar) is used to diagnose adrenal gland disorders, to treat adrenal gland insufficiency, and as an anti-inflammatory drug in the treatment of allergic response. Administration of ACTH intravenously (IV) should increase the serum cortisol level in 30 to 60 minutes if the adrenal gland is functioning. If steroid deficiency is caused by pituitary insufficiency, ACTH should eventually stimulate cortisol production. ACTH decreases the symptoms of multiple sclerosis during its exacerbation phase. Prototype Drug Chart 50–1 lists the actions and effects of corticotropin (Acthar).

Pharmacokinetics

Corticotropin stimulates the adrenal gland to secrete corticosteroids. The aqueous and gel preparations are well absorbed into the circulation. Zinc is added to some formulations to slow the absorption rate. A portion of the drug is bound to protein; however, the percentage is un-

known. The half-life of the drug is 15 to 20 minutes. It is excreted in the urine.

Pharmacodynamics

Corticotropin suppresses the inflammatory and immune responses. It is also prescribed to treat adrenal insufficiency secondary to inadequate corticotropin secretion. The drug is administered intramuscularly (IM) and IV. Its onset of action, peak concentration time, and duration of action are prolonged when it is injected IM. The IV preparation is in an aqueous form; therefore its actions are faster than those of the gel and zinc-additive preparations.

Drug Interactions

Corticotropin has numerous drug interactions. Diuretics and anti-*Pseudomonas* penicillins such as piperacillin can decrease the serum potassium level (hypokalemia). If the client is taking a digitalis preparation and hypokalemia is present, digitalis toxicity can result. Phenytoin, rifampin, and barbiturates increase the metabolic rate, which can

---

Prototype DRUG CHART 50–1

CORTICOTROPIN, REPOSITORY CORTICOTROPIN, CORTICOTROPIN-ZINC HYDROXIDE

Drug Class

Pituitary adrenocorticotropic hormone
Trade names:
corticotropin: Acthar, ACTH
corticotropin, repository: H.P. Acthar Gel
corticotrophin–zinc hydroxide: Cortrophin zinc
Pregnancy Category: C

Dosage

Diagnostic testing:
A: IV: 10-25 units in 500 ml D_5W q8h
subQ/IM: 20 units, q.i.d.
Repository injection:
A: subQ/IM: 40-80 units, q24-72h
Acute multiple sclerosis:
A: subQ/IM: 80-120 units/d for 2-3 wk

Contraindications

Severe fungal infection, HF, peptic ulcer
Caution: Hepatic disease, psychiatric disorders, myasthenia gravis

Drug-Lab-Food Interactions

Drug: Increase ulcer formation with aspirin; may *increase* effect of potassium-wasting diuretics; *decrease* effects of oral antidiabetics (hypoglycemics) or insulin

Pharmacokinetics

Absorption: IM: Well absorbed
Distribution: PB: UK
Metabolism: t½: 15-20 minutes
Excretion: In urine

Pharmacodynamics

IM: Onset: <6 h
  Peak: 6-18 h
  Duration: 12-24 h
IV: Onset: UK
  Peak: 1 h
  Duration: UK

Therapeutic Effects/Uses

To diagnose adrenocortical disorders; acts as an antiinflammatory agent; to treat acute MS
Mode of Action: Stimulates adrenal cortex to secrete cortisol

Side Effects

Nausea, vomiting, increased appetite, mood swing (euphoria to depression), petechiae, water and sodium retention, hypokalemia, hypocalcemia

Adverse Reactions

Edema, ecchymosis, osteoporosis, muscle atrophy, growth retardation, decreased wound healing, cataracts, glaucoma, menstrual irregularities
Life-threatening: Ulcer perforation, pancreatitis

A, Adult; *HF,* heart failure; *d,* day; *h,* hour; *IM,* intramuscular; *IV,* intravenous; *MS,* multiple sclerosis; *q.i.d.,* four times a day; *subQ,* subcutaneous; *PB,* protein-binding; *t½,* half life; *UK,* unknown; *wk,* week; *<,* less than.

decrease the effect of the ACTH drug. Persons with diabetes may need increased insulin and oral antidiabetic (hypoglycemic) drugs because ACTH stimulates cortisol secretion, which increases the blood sugar level.

Posterior Lobe

The posterior pituitary gland, known as the **neurohypophysis**, secretes **antidiuretic hormone (ADH)** (vasopressin) and oxytocin. (Oxytocin is discussed in Chapter 53.)

ADH promotes water reabsorption from the renal tubules to maintain water balance in the body fluids. When there is a deficiency of ADH, large amounts of water are excreted by the kidneys. This condition, **diabetes insipidus (DI)**, can lead to severe fluid volume deficit and electrolyte imbalances. Head injury and brain tumors resulting in trauma to the hypothalamus and pituitary gland can also cause DI. Fluid and electrolyte balance must be closely monitored in these clients, and ADH replacement may be needed. The ADH preparations vasopressin (Pitressin) and desmopressin acetate (DDAVP) can be administered intranasally or by injection.

Table 50–1 lists the drugs used for pituitary disorders and their dosages, uses, and considerations.

Nursing Process

Pituitary Hormones

ASSESSMENT

- Obtain baseline vital signs for future comparison. Report abnormal results.
- Determine client's urinary output and weight.
- Assess client for an infectious process. Corticotropin can suppress signs and symptoms of infection.
- Note client's physical growth. Compare child's growth with reported standards. Report findings.

NURSING DIAGNOSES

- Ineffective health maintenance related to lack of ability to maintain drug regimen
- Delayed growth and development related to deficient stimulation of growth hormone

PLANNING

- Client will be free of pituitary disorder with appropriate drug regimen.

NURSING INTERVENTIONS

Antidiuretic Hormone (ADH)

- Monitor vital signs. Increased heart rate and decreased systolic pressure can indicate fluid volume loss resulting from decreased ADH production. With less ADH secretion, more water is excreted, decreasing vascular fluid (hypovolemia).

- Record urinary output. Increased output can indicate fluid loss caused by a decrease in ADH.

Adrenocorticotropic Hormone (ACTH), Corticotropin

- Avoid administering corticotropin to clients with adrenocortical hyperfunction. Corticotropin stimulates the release of cortisol from the adrenal glands.
- Monitor the growth and development of a child receiving corticotropin.
- Observe client's weight. If a weight gain occurs, check for edema. A side effect of corticotropin (ACTH) is sodium and water retention.
- Watch carefully for adverse effects when corticotropin is discontinued. Dose should be tapered and not stopped abruptly, because adrenal hypofunction may result.
- Check laboratory findings, especially electrolyte levels. Electrolyte replacement may be necessary.

Growth Hormone (GH)

- Monitor blood sugar and electrolyte levels in clients receiving GH. Hyperglycemia can occur with high doses.

Client Teaching

Adrenocorticotropic Hormone (ACTH)

- Advise client to adhere to the drug regimen. Discontinuation of certain drugs, such as corticotropin, can cause hypofunction of the gland being stimulated.
- Direct client to decrease salt intake to decrease or avoid edema. Potassium supplement may be needed.
- Instruct client to report side effects such as muscle weakness, edema, petechiae, ecchymosis, decrease in growth, decreased wound healing, and menstrual irregularities.

Growth Hormone (GH)

- Advise athletes not to take GH because of its side effects. GH can be effective for children whose height is markedly below the expected norm for their age. Because GH acts on newly forming bone, it should be administered before the epiphyses are fused.
- Inform client with diabetes to closely monitor blood sugar levels. Insulin regulation may be necessary.
- Suggest that client or family monitor client's growth rate.

Cultural Considerations ❖

- There is sometimes a lack of understanding in some cultural groups in regard to the purpose and use of GH. The health care provider needs to emphasize that these are not drugs for building muscles and that they can cause many serious side effects, such as diabetes mellitus, when abused.

EVALUATION

- Evaluate the effectiveness of the drug therapy.

Thyroid Gland

Thyroxine (T_4) and **triiodothyronine** (T_3) are secreted by the thyroid gland. The functions of T_4 and T_3 are to regulate protein synthesis and enzyme activity and to stimulate mitochondrial oxidation. Approximately 20% of circulating T_3 is secreted from the thyroid gland, and 80% of T_3 comes from the degradation of about 40% of T_4, which occurs in the periphery. T_4 and T_3 are carried in the blood by thyroxine-binding globulin (TBG) and albumin, which protect the hormones from being degraded. T_3 is more potent than T_4, and only unbound free T_3 and T_4 are active and produce a hormonal response.

Feedback mechanisms regulate T_4 and T_3 secretion from the thyroid gland. The hypothalamus releases thyrotropin-releasing hormone (TRH), which stimulates the release of TSH from the pituitary gland. TSH stimulates the synthesis and release of T_4 and T_3 from the thyroid gland. Excess free T_4 and T_3 inhibit the hypothalamus-pituitary-thyroid (HPT) axis, which results in decreased TRH and TSH secretion. Likewise, too low an amount of T_4 and T_3 increases the function of the HPT axis.

For thyroid deficiency (hypothyroidism), synthetic T_4 and T_3 may be prescribed, either alone or in combination. When the thyroid gland secretes an overabundance of thyroid hormones (hyperthyroidism), antithyroid drugs are usually indicated.

Hypothyroidism

Hypothyroidism, a decrease in thyroid hormone secretion, can have either a primary cause (thyroid gland disorder) or a secondary cause (lack of TSH secretion). Primary hypothyroidism occurs more frequently. Decreased T_4 and elevated TSH levels indicate primary hypothyroidism, the causes of which are acute or chronic inflammation of the thyroid gland, radioiodine therapy, excess intake of antithyroid drugs, and surgery. **Myxedema** is severe hypothyroidism in the adult; symptoms include lethargy, apathy, memory impairment, emotional changes, slow speech, deep coarse voice, edema of the eyelids and face, thick dry skin, cold intolerance, slow pulse, constipation, weight gain, and abnormal menses. In children, hypothyroidism can have a congenital (**cretinism**) or prepubertal (juvenile hypothyroidism) onset. Drugs containing T_4 and T_3, alone or in combination, are used to treat hypothyroidism.

Drug Therapy: Hypothyroidism

Levothyroxine sodium (Levothroid, Synthroid) is the drug of choice for replacement therapy for the treatment of hypothyroidism. It increases the levels of T_3 and T_4. Levothyroxine is also used to treat simple goiter and chronic lymphocytic (Hashimoto) thyroiditis.

Liothyronine (Cytomel) is a synthetic T_3 that has a short half-life and duration of action; it is not recommended for maintenance therapy. Liothyronine is better absorbed from the GI tract than levothyroxine, and because of its rapid onset of action and short half-life, it is frequently used as initial therapy for treating myxedema.

Liotrix (Euthroid, Thyrolar) is a mixture of levothyroxine sodium and liothyronine sodium in a 4:1 ratio. For treating hypothyroidism, there is no significant advantage to using liotrix over levothyroxine sodium alone, because levothyroxine converts T_4 to T_3 in the peripheral tissues.

The drug thyroid is seldom used. Some clients with hypothyroidism may benefit from this agent.

Prototype Drug Chart 50–2 presents the drug data for the synthetic thyroid drug levothyroxine.

Pharmacokinetics

Levothyroxine (T_4) is a synthetic thyroid hormone preparation. The GI mucosa absorbs 50% to 75% of levothyroxine. It is highly protein-bound, and when administered with other highly protein-bound drugs like oral anticoagulants, side effects can result. The half-life of levothyroxine is longer than that of liothyronine. Levothyroxine is excreted in the bile and feces.

Pharmacodynamics

Levothyroxine increases metabolic rate, cardiac output, protein synthesis, and glycogen use. The peak concentration time and duration of action are much longer with levothyroxine than with liothyronine. Liotrix is a combination of T_4 and T_3 with a greater concentration of T_4.

Drug Interactions

Many drug interactions are associated with T_4 and T_3 drugs. Thyroid preparations increase the effect of oral anticoagulants because of drug displacement from the protein-binding sites. When either of these drugs is taken with an adrenergic agent (e.g., decongestant or vasopressor), the cardiac and central nervous system (CNS) actions are increased. Levothyroxine and liothyronine can decrease the effectiveness of digitalis preparations. Estrogen can increase the effect of liothyronine. Insulin and oral antidiabetic drug dosages may need to be increased.

Table 50–2 lists the drug data for natural and synthetic thyroid preparations.

Hyperthyroidism

Hyperthyroidism is an increase in circulating T_4 and T_3 levels, which results from an overactive thyroid gland or excessive output of thyroid hormones from one or more thyroid nodules. Hyperthyroidism may be mild with few symptoms or severe, as in thyroid storm in which death may occur from vascular collapse. **Graves disease**, or **thyrotoxicosis**, is the most common type of hyperthyroidism caused by hyperfunction of the thyroid gland. It is characterized by a rapid pulse (*tachycardia*), palpitations, excessive perspiration, heat intolerance, nervousness, irritability, exophthalmos (bulging eyes), and weight loss.

Hyperthyroidism can be treated by surgical removal of a portion of the thyroid gland (subtotal thyroidectomy), radioactive iodine therapy, or antithyroid drugs, which inhibit either synthesis or release of thyroid hormone. Any of these treatments can cause hypothyroidism. Propranolol (Inderal) can control cardiac symptoms like palpitations

Prototype DRUG CHART 50–2

LEVOTHYROXINE SODIUM

Drug Class
 	
Thyroid hormone
Trade names: T_4, Synthroid, Levothroid; ✚Eltroxin
Pregnancy Category: A
	Dosage
	
	A: PO: Initially: 25-50 mcg/d (0.025-0.05 mg/d); maint:
	    50-200 mcg/d (0.05-0.2 mg/d)
	IV: 0.2-0.5 mg initial dose; 0.1-0.2 mg/d until stable and
	    then PO
	C: >3 y: PO: 5-6 mcg/kg/d or 50-100 mcg/d (0.05-0.1
	    mg/d)

Contraindications
 	
Thyrotoxicosis, myocardial infarction (MI),
    severe renal disease
Caution: Cardiovascular disease, hypertension,
    angina pectoris
	Drug-Lab-Food Interactions
	
	Drug: Increase cardiac insufficiency with epinephrine;
	increase effects of anticoagulants, tricyclic antide-
	pressants, vasopressors, decongestants; *decrease*
	effects of antidiabetics (oral and insulin), digitalis
	products; *decrease* absorption with cholestyramine,
	colestipol

Pharmacokinetics
 	
Absorption: PO: 50%-75%
Distribution: PB: 99%
Metabolism: t½: 6-7 days
Excretion: In bile and feces
	Pharmacodynamics
	
	PO: Onset: UK
	    Peak: 24 h-1 wk
	    Duration: 1-3 wk
	IV: Onset: 6-8 h
	    Peak: 24-48 h
	    Duration: UK

Therapeutic Effects/Uses

To treat hypothyroidism, myxedema, and cretinism
Mode of Action: Increase metabolic rate, oxygen consumption, and body growth

Side Effects	**Adverse Reactions**

Nausea, vomiting, diarrhea, cramps, tremors,
    nervousness, insomnia, headache, weight loss
	Tachycardia, hypertension, palpitations
	Life-threatening: Thyroid crisis, angina pectoris, cardiac
	    dysrhythmias, cardiovascular collapse

A, Adult; *C,* child; *d,* day; *h,* hour; *IV,* intravenous; *maint,* maintenance; *PB,* protein-binding; *PO,* by mouth; *t½,* half life; *UK,* unknown; *wk,* week; *y,* year; ✚, Canadian drug name; >, greater than.

---

and tachycardia that result from hyperthyroidism. It does not lower T_4 and T_3.

Drug Therapy: Hyperthyroidism

The purpose of antithyroid drugs is to reduce the excessive secretion of thyroid hormones (T_4 and T_3) by inhibiting thyroid secretion. The use of surgery (subtotal thyroidectomy) and radioiodine therapy frequently leads to hypothyroidism. Thiourea derivatives (thioamides) are the drugs of choice used to decrease thyroid hormone production. This drug group interferes with synthesis of thyroid hormone. Thiourea derivatives do not destroy thyroid tissue, but rather block thyroid hormone action.

Propylthiouracil (PTU) and methimazole (Tapazole) are effective thioamide antithyroid drugs. They are useful for treating thyrotoxic crisis and in preparation for subtotal thyroidectomy. Methimazole does not inhibit peripheral conversion of T_4 to T_3 as does PTU; however, it is 10 times more potent and it has a longer half-life than PTU. Pro-

longed use of thioamides may cause a goiter because of the increased TSH secretion and inhibited T_4 and T_3 synthesis. Minimal doses of thioamides should be given when indicated to avoid goiter formation.

Strong iodide preparations such as Lugol's solution have been used to suppress thyroid function for clients who have undergone subtotal thyroidectomy as a result of Graves disease. Sodium iodide administered IV is useful for the management of thyrotoxic crisis. Table 50–2 gives the drug data for antithyroid drugs used to treat hyperthyroidism.

Drug Interactions

Thyroid drugs interact with many other drugs. When used with oral anticoagulants (e.g., warfarin [Coumadin]), they can cause an increase in the anticoagulation effect. In addition, thyroid drugs decrease the effect of insulin and oral antidiabetics; digoxin and lithium increase the action of thyroid drugs; and phenytoin (Dilantin) increases serum T_3 level.

Table 50–2

Thyroid Hormone: Replacements and Antithyroid Drugs

Generic (Brand)	Route and Dosage	Uses and Considerations
Thyroid Replacements: Hypothyroidism		
levothyroxine sodium (Synthroid)	(Prototype Drug Chart 50–2)	
liothyronine sodium (Cytomel)	A: PO: Initially: 5-25 mcg/d; *maint:* 25-75 mcg/d C: PO: Initially: 5 mcg/d, >3 y: 25-75 mcg/d	For hypothyroidism. Synthetic T_3 drug. Faster acting than other thyroid drugs. Effects seen in 24 to 72 h. Cardiac side effects. *Pregnancy category:* A; PB: 99%; $t^{1/2}$: 1-1.5 h
liotrix (Euthroid, Thyrolar)	A: PO: Initially: 15-30 mcg/d, increased q2-3wk; *maint:* 60-120 mcg/d C: PO: Initially: same as adult	For hypothyroidism. Synthetic T_4 and T_3 drug; 4:1 ratio. Onset of action immediate. Duration of action 72 h. Common side effects include irritability, nervousness, insomnia, tachycardia, weight loss. *Pregnancy category:* A; PB: 99%; $t^{1/2}$: <7 d
thyroid (Armour Thyroid, Thyrar)	A: PO: Initially: 15-60 mg/d, increased monthly as needed; *maint:* 60-180 mg/d C: PO: 15 mg/d, increased q2wk as needed	For hypothyroidism to reduce goiter size. Natural form obtained from animals. T_4 and T_3: 4:1 ratio. Onset of action is slow; long duration of action (weeks). Common side effects include irritability, nervousness, insomnia, tachycardia, and weight loss. *Pregnancy category:* A; PB: 99%; $t^{1/2}$: <7 d (T_3: 1-2 h; T_4: 6-7 h)
Antithyroid Drugs: Hyperthyroidism		
Thioamides		
methimazole (Tapazole)	A: PO: Initially: 15-60 mg/d in 3 divided doses; *maint:* 5-15 mg q8h C: PO: Initially: 0.4 mg/kg/d in divided doses; *maint:* 0.2 mg/kg/d in 3 divided doses	For treating hyperthyroidism. Inhibits thyroid hormone synthesis. Onset of action: 1 wk for effect. Rash, urticaria, headache, and GI upset may occur. *Pregnancy category:* D; PB: 0%; $t^{1/2}$: 5-13 h
propylthiouracil (PTU)	A: PO: Initially: 300-450 mg/d in divided doses; *maint:* 150-300 mg/d C: 6-10 y: PO: 50-150 mg/d in divided doses C: >10 y: PO: Same as adult or 150 mg/m²/d	For treating hyperthyroidism, Graves disease. Inhibits conversion of T_4 and T_3. May be used before surgery or radioactive iodine treatment, palliative control of toxic goiter. *Pregnancy category:* D; PB: 75%-80%; $t^{1/2}$: 1-2 h
Iodine		
Strong iodine solution (Lugol's solution, potassium iodide solution)	A & C: PO: 0.1-0.3 ml (3-5 gtt) t.i.d. *Thyroid crisis:* A & C: PO: 1 ml in water p.c. t.i.d.	For hyperthyroidism. To reduce size and vascularity of thyroid gland. Dilute drug and administer after meals; sip through straw to avoid discoloration of teeth. Maximum effect after 10 to 15 days. *Pregnancy category:* D; PB: UK; $t^{1/2}$: UK

A, Adult; *C,* child; *d,* day; *GI,* gastrointestinal; *gtt,* drops; *h,* hour; *maint,* maintenance; *PB,* protein-binding; *p.c.,* after meals; *PO,* by mouth; *$t^{1/2}$,* half-life; T_4, thyroxine; $T3$, triiodothyronine; *t.i.d.,* three times a day; *UK,* unknown; *wk,* week; *y,* year; >, greater than; <, less than.

 Nursing Process

Thyroid Hormone: Replacement and Antithyroid Drugs

ASSESSMENT

■ Determine baseline vital signs to compare with future data. Report abnormal results.
■ Check serum T_3, T_4, and thyroid-stimulating hormone (TSH) levels. Report abnormal results.

Thyroid Replacement

• Obtain a history of drugs client currently takes. Be aware that thyroid drugs enhance the action of oral anticoagulants, sympathomimetics, and antidepressants and decrease the action of insulin, oral hypoglycemics, and digitalis preparation. Phenytoin and aspirin can enhance the action of thyroid hormone.

Antithyroid Drugs

- Assess for signs and symptoms of a thyroid crisis (thyroid storm), including tachycardia, cardiac dysrhythmias, fever, heart failure, flushed skin, apathy, confusion, behavioral changes, and later hypotension and vascular collapse. Thyroid crisis can result from a thyroidectomy (excess thyroid hormones released), abrupt withdrawal of antithyroid drug, excess ingestion of thyroid hormone, or failure to give antithyroid medication before thyroid surgery.

NURSING DIAGNOSES

- Ineffective health maintenance related to inability to maintain drug regimen
- Ineffective tissue perfusion related to hyposecretion of thyroid hormone
- Activity intolerance related to generalized weakness

PLANNING

- Client's signs and symptoms of hypothyroidism will be alleviated within 2 to 4 weeks with prescribed thyroid drug replacement, and the client will not experience side effects.
- Client's signs and symptoms of hyperthyroidism will be alleviated in 1 to 3 weeks with the prescribed antithyroid drug.

NURSING INTERVENTIONS

- Record vital signs. With hypothyroidism, the temperature, heart rate, and blood pressure are usually decreased. With hyperthyroidism, tachycardia and palpitations usually occur.
- Monitor client's weight. Weight gain commonly occurs in clients with hypothyroidism.

Client Teaching

Thyroid Drug Replacement for Hypothyroidism
- Encourage client to take drug at the same time each day, preferably before breakfast. Food will hamper absorption rate.
- Teach client to check warnings on OTC drug labels. Avoid OTC drugs that caution against use by persons with heart or thyroid disease.
- Direct client to report symptoms of hyperthyroidism (tachycardia, chest pain, palpitations, excess sweating) caused by drug accumulation or overdosing.
- Suggest that client carry a MedicAlert card, tag, or bracelet with the health condition and thyroid drug used.

Diet: Hypothyroidism
- Caution client to avoid foods that can inhibit thyroid secretion (strawberries, peaches, pears, cabbage, turnips, spinach, kale, Brussels sprouts, cauliflower, radishes, and peas).

Antithyroid Drugs for Hyperthyroidism
- Instruct client to take the drug with meals to decrease gastrointestinal symptoms.
- Advise client about the effects of iodine and its presence in iodized salt, shellfish, and OTC cough medicines.
- Emphasize the importance of drug compliance; abruptly stopping the antithyroid drug could bring on thyroid crisis.
- Teach client the signs and symptoms of hypothyroidism: lethargy, puffy eyelids and face, thick tongue, slow speech with hoarseness, lack of perspiration, and slow pulse. Hypothyroidism can result from treatment of hyperthyroidism.
- Advise client to avoid antithyroid drugs if pregnant or breastfeeding. Antithyroid drugs taken during pregnancy can cause hypothyroidism in the fetus or infant.

Self-Administration
- Demonstrate to client how to take a pulse rate. Instruct client to monitor the pulse rate and report increases or marked decreases in pulse rate.

Side Effects
- Teach client the side effects of antithyroid drugs: skin rash, hives, nausea, alopecia, loss of hair pigment, petechiae or ecchymoses, and weakness.
- Advise client to contact the health care provider if a sore throat and fever occur while taking antithyroid drugs. A serious adverse reaction of antithyroid drugs is agranulocytosis (loss of white blood cells). A complete blood count should be monitored for leukopenia.

Cultural Considerations ❖

- Recognize that various cultural groups may need guidance in understanding the disease process of hypothyroidism or hyperthyroidism. Support client and family member who may be dismayed about the symptoms of either of these health problems and lack knowledge of the prescribed drug therapy for management of the thyroid condition. Additional time in explanations and a written plan of care may be necessary for non–English-speaking persons.

EVALUATION

Thyroid Replacement

- Evaluate the effectiveness of the thyroid drug and drug compliance.
- Continue monitoring for side effects from drug accumulation or overdosing.

Antithyroid Drugs

- Evaluate the effectiveness of the antithyroid drug in decreasing signs and symptoms of hyperthyroidism. If signs and symptoms persist after 2 to 3 weeks of therapy, other methods for correcting hyperthyroidism may be necessary.

Prototype **DRUG CHART 50–3**

CALCITRIOL

Drug Class

Vitamin D analogue
Trade name: Rocaltrol
Pregnancy Category: C

Dosage

A: PO: 0.25 mcg/d

Contraindications

Hypersensitivity, hypercalcemia, hyperphosphatemia,
   hypervitaminosis D, malabsorption syndrome
Caution: Cardiovascular disease, renal calculi

Drug-Lab-Food Interactions

Drug: Increase cardiac dysrhythmias with digoxin,
   verapamil; *decrease* calcitriol absorption with
   cholestyramine
Lab: Increase serum calcium with thiazide diuretics,
   calcium supplements

Pharmacokinetics

Absorption: PO: Well absorbed
Distribution: PB: UK; crosses the placenta
Metabolism: t½: 3-8 h
Excretion: Mostly in feces

Pharmacodynamics

PO: Onset: 2-6 h
   Peak: 10-12 h
   Duration: 3-5 d

Therapeutic Effects/Uses

To treat hypoparathyroidism and manage hypocalcemia in chronic renal failure
Mode of Action: Enhancement of calcium deposits in bones

Side Effects

Anorexia, nausea, vomiting, diarrhea, cramps,
   drowsiness, headache, dizziness, lethargy,
   photophobia

Adverse Reactions

Hypercalciuria, hyperphosphatemia, hematuria

A, Adult; *d*, day; *h*, hour; *PB*, protein binding; *PO*, by mouth; *t½*, half life; *UK*, unknown.

Parathyroid Glands

The parathyroid glands secrete **parathyroid hormone (PTH)**, which regulates calcium levels in the blood. A decrease in serum calcium stimulates the release of PTH. Calcitonin decreases serum calcium levels by promoting renal excretion of calcium. The functions of PTH and calcitonin are discussed in the introduction to Unit XVII.

Parathyroid hormone agents treat hypoparathyroidism, and synthetic calcitonin treats hyperparathyroidism. Hypocalcemia (serum calcium deficit) can be caused by PTH deficiency, vitamin D deficiency, renal impairment, or diuretic therapy, and PTH replacement helps correct the calcium deficit. The action of PTH is to promote calcium absorption from the GI tract, promote reabsorption of calcium from the renal tubules, and activate vitamin D.

Calcitriol

Calcitriol is a vitamin D analogue that promotes calcium absorption from the GI tract and secretion of calcium from bone to the bloodstream. Prototype Drug Chart 50–3 describes the drug data related to calcitriol.

Pharmacokinetics

Calcitriol is readily absorbed from the GI tract. Its half-life is moderate (3 to 8 hours). Most of the drug is excreted in feces.

Pharmacodynamics

Calcitriol is given for the management of hypocalcemia. It increases serum calcium levels by promoting calcium absorption from the intestines and renal tubules. Calcitriol has a long onset of action, peak action, and duration of action.

Hyperparathyroidism can be caused by malignancies of the parathyroid glands or ectopic PTH hormone secretion from lung cancer, hyperthyroidism, or prolonged immobility, during which calcium is lost from bone. Table 50–3 lists the drugs used to treat hypoparathyroidism and hyperparathyroidism.

Nursing Process

Parathyroid Hormone Insufficiencies

ASSESSMENT

■ Note serum calcium level. Report abnormal results.
■ Assess for symptoms of tetany in hypocalcemia: twitching of mouth, tingling and numbness of fingers, carpopedal spasm, spasmodic contractions, and laryngeal spasm.

Table 50-3

Drug Therapies for Parathyroid Disorders

Generic (Brand)	Route and Dosage	Uses and Considerations
Treatment for Hypoparathyroidism and Hypocalcemia: Vitamin D Analogues		
calcifediol (Calderol)	A: PO: Initially: 300-350 mcg/wk PO: 50-100 mcg/d or 100-200 mcg every other day	For bone disease and hypocalcemia associated with chronic renal disease and dialysis. *Pregnancy category:* C; PB: UK; t^{1}/$_2$: 12-22 d
calcitriol (Rocaltrol)	(Prototype Drug Chart 50-3)	
dihydrotachysterol (Hytakerol)	A: PO: 0.75-2.5 mg/d for 4 d, then 0.2-1 mg/d C: PO: 1-5 mg/d for 4 d, then 0.5-1.5 mg/d	For treatment of hypoparathyroidism associated with hypocalcemia and for pseudohypoparathyroidism. Serum calcium levels should be monitored weekly during early therapy. Clients should avoid taking thiazide diuretics to prevent causing possible hypercalcemia. *Pregnancy category:* A; PB: UK; t^{1}/$_2$: UK
ergocalciferol (Drisdol)	A & C: PO/IM: 50,000-200,000 international units/d or 1.25-5.0 mg/d	For hypoparathyroidism and rickets. Larger dose may be required in vitamin D-resistant rickets. Enhances calcium and phosphorus absorption. Long duration of action. *Pregnancy category:* C; PB: UK; t^{1}/$_2$: 12-24 h
Treatment for Hyperparathyroidism and Hypercalcemia		
calcitonin-human (Cibacalcin); calcitonin-salmon (Miacalcin)	*Human:* A: subQ: Initially: 0.5 mg/d; maint: 0.25 mg/d-0.5 mg b.i.d. *Salmon:* A: subQ/IM: Initially: 4 international units/kg/d; *maint:* 4-8 international units/kg q12h	For treating Paget disease (osteitis deformans), hyperparathyroidism, and hypercalcemia. Calcitonin-salmon is more potent than calcitonin-human. Calcitonin decreases serum calcium by binding at receptor sites on osteoclast. *Pregnancy category:* C; PB: UK; t^{1}/$_2$: 1-1.5 h
etidronate (Didronel)	A: PO: 5-10 mg/kg/d; *max:* 20 mg/kg/d	For Paget disease; for hypercalcemia caused by antineoplastic therapy. *Pregnancy category:* B; PB: UK; t^{1}/$_2$: 6 h
cinacalcet (Sensipar)	A: PO: 30 mg b.i.d. initially; titrate individualized dose q2-4wk	For treatment of hyperparathyroidism and hypercalcemia. *Pregnancy category:* C; PB: 93-97; t^{1}/$_2$: 30-40 h

A, Adult; *b.i.d.*, two times a day; *C*, child; *d*, day; *h*, hour; *IM*, intramuscular; *maint*, maintenance; *max*, maximum; *PB*, protein-binding; *PO*, by mouth; *subQ*, subcutaneous; *t^{1}/$_2$*, half-life; *UK*, unknown; *wk*, week.

NURSING DIAGNOSES

- Diarrhea related to adverse effects of calcitriol
- Deficient fluid volume related to fluid loss from vomiting and polyuria

PLANNING

- Client's serum calcium level will be within the normal range.

NURSING INTERVENTIONS

- Monitor serum calcium level. Normal reference value is 8.5 to 10.5 mg/dl, or 4.5 to 5.5 mEq/L. Serum calcium <8.5 mg/dl, or <4.5 mEq/L, indicates hypocalcemia. Serum calcium >10.5 mg/dl, or >5.5 mEq/L, indicates hypercalcemia. Serum ionized calcium levels are usually used, because much of the calcium is protein-bound and is nonionized and nonactive.

Client Teaching

Hypoparathyroidism
- Direct client to report symptoms of tetany (see Assessment).

Hyperparathyroidism
- Instruct client to report signs and symptoms of hypercalcemia: bone pain, anorexia, nausea, vomiting, thirst, constipation, lethargy, bradycardia, and polyuria.
- Advise women to inform health care provider about pregnancy status before taking calcitonin preparation.
- Encourage client to check OTC drugs for possible calcium content, especially if client has an elevated serum calcium level. Some vitamins and antacids contain calcium. Tell client to contact health care provider before taking drugs with calcium.

EVALUATION

- Monitor the effectiveness of drug therapy.
- Continue monitoring for signs and symptoms of hypocalcemia (tetany) when commercially prepared calcitonin has been given.

Adrenal Glands

The paired **adrenal glands** consist of the adrenal medulla and adrenal cortex. The adrenal cortex produces two types of hormones, or corticosteroids: glucocorticoids (cortisol) and mineralocorticoids (aldosterone). Cortisol is secreted by the adrenal glands in response to the hypothalamus-pituitary-adrenal (HPA) axis as a result of the feedback mechanism. A decrease in serum cortisol levels increases CRF and ACTH secretions, which stimulate the adrenal glands to secrete and release cortisol. An increased serum cortisol level exerts the negative feedback mechanism, which inhibits the HPA axis, resulting in less cortisol being released. Additional physiologic functions related to the hormones secreted from the adrenal medulla and adrenal cortex are described in the introduction to Unit XVII.

Corticosteroids promote sodium retention and potassium excretion. A sodium ion is reabsorbed from the renal tubule in exchange for a potassium ion; the potassium ion is then excreted. Because of their influence on electrolytes and carbohydrate, protein, and fat metabolism, a deficiency of corticosteroids can result in serious illness or death. A decrease in corticosteroid secretion is called *adrenal hyposecretion* (adrenal insufficiency, or **Addison disease**) and an increase in corticosteroid secretion is called *adrenal hypersecretion* (**Cushing syndrome**).

Glucocorticoids

Glucocorticoids are influenced by ACTH, which is released from the anterior pituitary gland. They affect carbohydrate, protein, and fat metabolism and muscle and blood cell activity. Because of their many mineralocorticoid effects, glucocorticoids can cause sodium absorption from the kidney, resulting in water retention, potassium loss, and increased blood pressure. Cortisol, the main glucocorticoid, has antiinflammatory, antiallergic, and antistress effects. Indications for glucocorticoid therapy include trauma, surgery, infections, emotional upsets, and anxiety. Table 50–4 lists the physiologic aspects of adrenal hyposecretion (Addison disease) and hypersecretion (Cushing syndrome).

Most of the wide variety of glucocorticoid drugs, frequently called *cortisone drugs*, are synthetically produced. These drugs have several routes of administration: oral, parenteral (IM or IV), topical (creams, ointments, lotions), and aerosol (inhaler). The IM route, although seldom used, should be administered deep in the muscle. The subQ route is not recommended. Chapter 39 has more on glucocorticoids for respiratory use, and topical glucocorticoids are discussed in Chapter 49.

Glucocorticoids are used to treat many diseases and health problems, including inflammatory, allergic, and debilitating conditions. Among the inflammatory conditions that may require glucocorticoids are autoimmune disorders (e.g., multiple sclerosis, rheumatoid arthritis, myasthenia gravis); ulcerative colitis; glomerulonephritis; shock; ocular

Table 50–4

Physiologic Data: Adrenal Hyposecretion and Hypersecretion

Body System	Adrenal Hyposecretion	Adrenal Hypersecretion
Metabolism		
Glucose	Hypoglycemia	Hyperglycemia
Protein	Muscle weakness	Muscle wasting; thinning of skin; poor wound healing; osteoporosis; fat accumulation in face, neck, and trunk (protruding abdomen, "buffalo hump"); hyperlipidemia; high cholesterol
Fat		
Central nervous system	Apathy, depression, fatigue	Increased neural activity; mood elevation; irritability; seizures
Gastrointestinal	Nausea, vomiting, abdominal pain	Peptic ulcers
Cardiovascular	Tachycardia, hypotension, cardiovascular collapse	Hypertension; edema; heart failure
Eyes	None	Cataract formation
Fluids and electrolytes	Hypovolemia; hyponatremia; hyperkalemia	Hypervolemia; hypernatremia; hypokalemia
Blood cells	Anemia	Increased red blood cell count and neutrophils; impaired clotting

and vascular inflammations; head trauma with cerebral edema; polyarteritis nodosa; and hepatitis. Allergic conditions include asthma, drug reactions, contact dermatitis, and anaphylaxis. Debilitating conditions are mainly caused by malignancies. Organ transplant recipients may require glucocorticoids to prevent organ rejection.

There are many glucocorticoids, some more potent than others. Dexamethasone (Decadron) has been used to treat severe inflammatory response resulting from head trauma or allergic reactions. An inexpensive glucocorticoid frequently prescribed is prednisone. Prototype Drug Chart 50–4 describes the pharmacologic data for prednisone.

Pharmacokinetics

Prednisone is readily absorbed from the GI tract. It has a short half-life of 3 to 4 hours, and it has a moderately high protein-binding power. Prednisone is excreted primarily in the urine.

Pharmacodynamics

The major actions of prednisone are to suppress an acute inflammatory process and for immunosuppression. It prevents cell-mediated immune reactions. Peak action occurs in 1 to 2 hours, and its duration of action is long (1 to 1.5 days).

Commonly used glucocorticoid drugs are listed in Table 50–5. Most of the glucocorticoids are pregnancy category C drugs. Agents used for adrenocortical insufficiency contain both glucocorticoids and mineralocorticoids, whereas drugs for antiinflammatory or immunosuppressive use contain mostly glucocorticoids.

Side Effects and Adverse Reactions

The side effects and adverse reactions of glucocorticoids that result from high doses or prolonged use include increased blood sugar, abnormal fat deposits in the face and trunk (so-called *moon face* and *buffalo hump*), decreased extremity size, muscle wasting, edema, sodium and water retention, hypertension, euphoria or psychosis, thinned skin with purpura, increased intraocular pressure (glaucoma), peptic ulcers, and growth retardation. Long-term use of glucocorticoid drugs can cause adrenal atrophy (loss of adrenal gland function). When drug therapy is discontinued, the dose should be tapered to allow the adrenal cortex to produce cortisol and other corticosteroids. Abrupt withdrawal of the drug can result in severe adrenocortical insufficiency.

Drug Interactions

Glucocorticoids increase the potency of drugs taken concurrently, including aspirin and nonsteroidal antiinflammatory drugs (NSAIDs), thus increasing the risk of

---

Prototype DRUG CHART 50–4

PREDNISONE

Drug Class

Adrenal hormone: glucocorticoid
Trade names: Deltasone, Meticorten, Orasone, Panasol-S, ✣Apo-Prednisone, Winpred
Pregnancy Category: C

Contraindications

Hypersensitivity, psychosis, fungal infection
Caution: Diabetes mellitus

Dosage

A: PO: 5-60 mg/d in divided doses
C: PO: 0.1-0.15 mg/kg/d in 2-4 divided doses or 4-5 mg/m^2/d in 2 doses

Drug-Lab-Food Interactions

Drug: Increase effect with barbiturates, phenytoin, rifampin, ephedrine, theophylline; *decrease* effects of aspirin, anticonvulsants, isoniazid (INH), antidiabetics, vaccines

Pharmacokinetics

Absorption: PO: Well absorbed
Distribution: PB: 65%-91%; crosses the placenta
Metabolism: t½: 3-4 h
Excretion: In urine

Pharmacodynamics

PO: Onset: UK
Peak: 1-2 h
Duration: 24-36 d

Therapeutic Effects/Uses

To decrease inflammatory occurrence; as an immunosuppressant; to treat dermatologic disorders
Mode of Action: Suppression of inflammation and adrenal function

Side Effects

Nausea, diarrhea, abdominal distention, increased appetite, sweating, headache, depression, flush, mood changes

Adverse Reactions

Petechiae, ecchymosis, hypertension, tachycardia, osteoporosis, muscle wasting
Life-threatening: GI hemorrhage, pancreatitis, circulatory collapse, thrombophlebitis, embolism

A, Adult; *C*, child; *d*, day; *GI*, gastrointestinal; *h*, hour; *PB*, protein-binding; *PO*, by mouth; *t½*, half-life; *UK*, unknown; ✣, Canadian drug name.

Table 50–5

Adrenal Hormones: Glucocorticoids, Mineralocorticoid, and Glucocorticoid Inhibitors

Generic (Brand)	Route and Dosage	Uses and Considerations
Glucocorticoids		
Short Acting		
cortisone acetate (Cortone Acetate)	A: PO/IM: 20-300 mg/d; decrease dose periodically	For adrenocortical insufficiency. Contains glucocorticoid and mineralocorticoid. Decreases inflammatory process. Oral dose rapidly absorbed from the GI tract. Administer deep IM. Give oral dose with food. *Pregnancy category:* C; PB: UK; t$\frac{1}{2}$: 0.5-12 h
hydrocortisone (Cortef, Hydrocortone)	A: PO: 20-240 mg/d in 3-4 divided doses IV: 15-240 mg (phosphate) q12h Rectal supp: 10-25 mg	For adrenocortical insufficiency and inflammation. Parenteral form: hydrocortisone sodium phosphate. Acetate form of drug may be injected into joints. Available in cream, ointment, lotion, and spray. *Pregnancy category:* C; PB: 79%; t$\frac{1}{2}$: 2-12 h
Intermediate Acting		
methylprednisolone (Medrol, Solu-Medrol [sodium succinate], Depo-Medrol [acetate])	A: PO: 4-48 mg/d in one or more divided doses IM/IV: Succinate: 10-40 mg q4h-q6h IM: Acetate: 40-80 mg/wk	For treating inflammatory conditions such as arthritis, bronchial asthma, allergic reactions, and cerebral edema. *Pregnancy category:* C; PB: UK; t$\frac{1}{2}$: 3.5 h
prednisolone (Hydeltrasol [sodium phosphate])	A: PO: 2.5-15 mg b.i.d.-q.i.d. IV: Phosphate: 2-30 mg q12h C: PO: 0.14-2 mg/kg/d in a single or divided doses	For antiinflammatory or immunosuppressive effect. For parenteral use. Can be injected into joints and soft tissue. Potent steroid. *Pregnancy category:* C; PB: 80%-90%; t$\frac{1}{2}$: 3.5 h (tissue: 18-36 h)
prednisone	(Prototype Drug Chart 50–4)	For antiinflammatory or immunosuppressive effect. *Pregnancy category:* C; PB: UK; t$\frac{1}{2}$: 2-5 h
triamcinolone (Aristocort, Kenacort, Azmacort, Kenalog)	A: PO: 4-48 mg/d in 2-4 divided doses Topical preparations: cream, ointment	
Long Acting		
beclomethasone dipropionate (Vancenase AQ, Beconase AQ)	A: Inhal: 2 puffs t.i.d.-q.i.d.	Inhalation for treating bronchial asthma and bronchial inflammation. Also to treat seasonal rhinitis. Like all glucocorticoid inhalants, for prophylactic use. NOT for acute asthmatic attack. *Pregnancy category:* C; PB: 87%; t$\frac{1}{2}$: 5-15 h
betamethasone (Celestone)	A: PO: 0.6-7.2 mg/d in single or divided doses IM/IV: 1-9 mg/d; *max:* IM: 12 mg/d	Potent antiinflammatory steroid drug. May be injected into joints. Also effective for treating bronchial asthma, arthritis, severe allergic reactions, and cerebral edema. Should be taken with food. *Pregnancy category:* C; PB: 64%-90%; t$\frac{1}{2}$: 3-5 h
dexamethasone (Decadron)	*Inflammation:* A: PO: 0.25-4 mg b.i.d.-q.i.d. IM: 4-16 mg q1-3wk C: PO: 0.2 mg/kg/d in divided doses *Shock:* A: IV: 1-6 mg/kg as a single dose (IV push in IV fluids)	Potent antiinflammatory drug. For acute allergic disorders, asthma attack, cerebral edema, and unresponsive shock. For diagnosis of Cushing syndrome and depression. Can be administered IV push or in IV fluids. Give oral dose with food. *Pregnancy category:* C; PB: 80%-90%; t$\frac{1}{2}$: 3-4 h
parumethasone acetate (Haldrone)	A: PO: 0.5-6 mg t.i.d-q.i.d. C: PO: 58-200 mcg/kg/d in 3-4 divided doses	For treating inflammatory conditions and allergic reactions. Similar to prednisone. Give with food. With long-term therapy do not abruptly stop dosing. *Pregnancy category:* C; PB: 95%; t$\frac{1}{2}$: 3-45 h
Mineralocorticoids		
fludrocortisone acetate (Florinef Acetate)	A & C: PO: 0.1-0.2 mg/d	For treating adrenocortical insufficiency, Addison disease. Also for salt-losing adrenogenital syndrome. Used only for its mineralocorticoid effects. *Pregnancy category:* C; PB: 92%; t$\frac{1}{2}$: 3.5 h

A, Adult; *ACTH*, adrenocorticotropic hormone; *b.i.d.*, twice a day; *C*, child; *d*, day; *GI*, gastrointestinal; *h*, hour; *IM*, intramuscular; *inhal*, inhalation; *IV*, intravenous; *PB*, protein-binding; *PO*, by mouth; *q.i.d.*, four times a day; t$\frac{1}{2}$, half-life; *t.i.d.*, three times a day; *UK*, unknown; *wk*, week.

Continued

Table 50–5

Adrenal Hormones: Glucocorticoids, Mineralocorticoid, and Glucocorticoid Inhibitors—cont'd

Generic (Brand)	Route and Dosage	Uses and Considerations
Glucocorticoid Inhibitors		
aminoglutethimide (Cytadren)	*Cushing syndrome:* A: PO: 250 mg q6h; *max:* 2 g/d	Hormone antagonist: adrenal steroid inhibitor. May be used to treat Cushing syndrome associated with adrenal adenoma or carcinoma and ACTH-secreting tumors. Blocks first step in steroid synthesis. *Pregnancy category:* D; PB: UK; t^1/$_2$: 13 h
ketoconazole (Nizoral)	A: PO: 200-400 mg/d	Usually used in conjunction with surgery or radiation to inhibit glucocorticoid synthesis. Needs higher dose to suppress steroid synthesis than to treat fungal infection. *Pregnancy category:* C; PB: UK; t^1/$_2$: 8 h
Mitotane and Diagnosis for Adrenal Gland Dysfunction		
mitotane (Lysodren)	A: PO: 2-6 g/d, q6-8h. Dose may be increased; *max:* 16 g/d	Antineoplastic agent that suppresses action of adrenal gland. Used to treat Cushing syndrome. *Pregnancy category:* C; PB: UK; t^1/$_2$: 18-160 d
Diagnosis for Adrenal Gland Dysfunction		
metyrapone (Metopirone)	A: PO: 30 mg/kg at midnight or 750 mg q4h × 6 doses, 4 days before ACTH administration C: PO: 15 mg/kg q4h × 6 doses	For diagnosing secondary adrenal insufficiency. Blocks cortisol synthesis in adrenals. Caution: may cause acute adrenal insufficiency. *Pregnancy category:* UK; PB: UK; t^1/$_2$: 1-2.5 h
corticotropin (Acthar)	Diagnostic test for adrenal and pituitary function	(Prototype Drug Chart 50–1)
cosyntropin (Cortrosyn)	Diagnostic test for adrenal and pituitary function	(Table 50–1)

GI bleeding and ulceration. Use of potassium-wasting diuretics (e.g., HydroDIURIL, Lasix) with glucocorticoids increases potassium loss, resulting in hypokalemia. Glucocorticoids can decrease the effect of oral anticoagulants (e.g., warfarin [Coumadin]).

Barbiturates, phenytoin, and rifampin decrease the effect of prednisone. Prolonged use of prednisone can cause severe muscle weakness.

Dexamethasone, a potent glucocorticoid, interacts with many drugs. Phenytoin, theophylline, rifampin, barbiturates, and antacids decrease the action of dexamethasone, whereas NSAIDs, including aspirin, and estrogen increase its action. Dexamethasone decreases the effects of oral anticoagulants and oral antidiabetics. When the drug is given with diuretics or anti-*Pseudomonas* penicillin preparations, the serum potassium level may decrease markedly. Glucocorticoids can increase blood sugar levels, so insulin or oral antidiabetic drug dosage may need to be increased.

Glucocorticoid Inhibitors

The antifungal drug ketoconazole (Nizoral) and the antineoplastic hormone antagonists mitotane (Lysodren) and aminoglutethimide (Cytadren) inhibit glucocorticoid synthesis. Ketoconazole is effective in treating clients with Cushing syndrome and is useful as an adjunct to surgery or radiation. High doses should be avoided, because this drug can induce fatal ventricular dysrhythmias. Aminoglutethi-

mide is frequently prescribed for temporary treatment of selected clients with Cushing syndrome, especially clients with adrenal adenoma or carcinoma, ectopic ACTH-producing tumors, or adrenal hyperplasia.

Mineralocorticoids

Mineralocorticoids, the second type of corticosteroid, secrete aldosterone. Aldosterone is controlled by the renin-angiotensin system, not by ACTH. These hormones maintain fluid balance by promoting the reabsorption of sodium from the renal tubules. Sodium attracts water, resulting in water retention. When *hypovolemia* (decrease in circulating fluid) occurs, more aldosterone is secreted to increase sodium and water retention and restore fluid balance. With sodium reabsorption, potassium is lost and hypokalemia (potassium deficit) can occur. Some glucocorticoid drugs also contain mineralocorticoids; these include cortisone and hydrocortisone. A severe decrease in the mineralocorticoid aldosterone leads to hypotension and vascular collapse, as seen in Addison disease. Mineralocorticoid deficiency usually occurs with glucocorticoid deficiency, frequently called *corticosteroid deficiency.*

Fludrocortisone (Florinef) is an oral mineralocorticoid that can be given with a glucocorticoid. It can cause a negative nitrogen balance; therefore a high-protein diet is usually indicated. Because potassium excretion occurs with the use of mineralocorticoids and glucocorticoids, the serum potassium level should be monitored.

Nursing Process

Adrenal Hormone: Glucocorticoids

ASSESSMENT

- Note baseline vital signs for future comparison.
- Assess laboratory test results, especially serum electrolytes and blood sugar. Serum potassium level usually decreases and blood sugar level increases when a glucocorticoid such as prednisone is taken over an extensive period.
- Obtain client's weight and urine output to use for future comparison.
- Assess client's medical and herbal history. Report if client has glaucoma, cataracts, peptic ulcer, psychiatric problems, or diabetes mellitus. Glucocorticoids can intensify these health problems.

NURSING DIAGNOSES

- Deficient knowledge of drug discontinuation related to lack of recall
- Excess fluid volume related to fluid retention
- Risk for impaired tissue integrity related to side effect of a rash

PLANNING

- The client's side effects of glucocorticoid therapy will be minimal.
- The client's inflammatory process will abate.

NURSING INTERVENTIONS

- Determine vital signs. Glucocorticoids such as prednisone can increase blood pressure and sodium and water retention.
- Administer glucocorticoids only as ordered. Routes of administration include oral, intramuscular (not in the deltoid muscle), intravenous, aerosol, and topical. Topical glucocorticoid drugs should be applied in thin layers. Rashes, infection, and purpura should be noted and reported.
- Record weight. Report weight gain of 5 lbs in several days; this would most likely be caused by water retention.
- Monitor laboratory values, especially serum electrolytes and blood sugar. Serum potassium level could decrease to <3.5 mEq/L, and blood sugar level would probably increase.
- Watch carefully for signs and symptoms of hypokalemia: nausea, vomiting, muscular weakness, abdominal distention, paralytic ileus, and irregular heart rate.
- Assess for side effects from glucocorticoid drugs when therapy has lasted more than 10 days and the drug is taken in high dosages. The cortisone preparation should not be abruptly stopped, because adrenal crisis can result.
- Monitor older adults for signs and symptoms of increased osteoporosis. Glucocorticoids promote calcium loss from bone.
- Report changes in muscle strength. High doses of glucocorticoids promote loss of muscle tone.

Client Teaching

General

- Advise client to take drug as prescribed. Caution client *not* to abruptly stop the drug. When drug is discontinued, dose is tapered over 1 to 2 weeks.
- For short-term use (<10 days) of glucocorticoids such as prednisone or other cortisone preparations, the drug dose still needs to be tapered. Prepare a schedule for client to decrease the dose over 4 to 5 days. For example, take one tab q.i.d.; next day, take one tab t.i.d.; next day, take one tab b.i.d.; and then take one tab daily.
- Direct client not to take cortisone preparations (oral or topical) during pregnancy unless necessary and prescribed by the health care provider. These drugs may be harmful to the fetus.
- Inform client that certain herbal laxatives and diuretics may interact with a glucocorticoid drug and may increase the severity of hypokalemia (Herbal Alert 50–1).
- Instruct client to avoid persons with respiratory infections, because these drugs suppress the immune system. This is especially important if client is receiving a high dose of glucocorticoids.
- Teach client receiving glucocorticoids to inform other health care providers of all drugs taken, especially before surgery.
- Encourage client to have a MedicAlert card, tag, or bracelet stating the glucocorticoid drug taken.

Self-Administration

- Instruct client how to use an aerosol nebulizer. Warn client against overuse of the aerosol to avoid possible rebound effect.

Herbal ALERT 50–1

Herbs and Corticosteroids

- Herbal laxatives (*cascara, senna*) and herbal diuretics (*celery seed, juniper*) can decrease serum potassium levels. When these herbs are taken with corticosteroids, hypokalemia can become more severe.
- *Ginseng* taken with corticosteroids may cause central nervous system stimulation and insomnia.
- *Echinacea* may counteract the effects of corticosteroids.
- *Licorice* potentiates the effect of corticosteroids and may cause a substantial decrease in serum potassium level.

Side Effects

• Teach client to report signs and symptoms of drug overdose or Cushing syndrome: moon face, puffy eyelids, edema in the feet, increased bruising, dizziness, bleeding, and menstrual irregularity.

Diet

• Instruct client to take cortisone preparations at mealtime or with food. Glucocorticoid drugs can irritate gastric mucosa and cause peptic ulcer.
• Advise client to eat foods rich in potassium, such as fresh and dried fruits, vegetables, meats, and nuts. Prednisone promotes potassium loss and hypokalemia.

Cultural Considerations ❖

• Recognize that various cultural groups need guidance in understanding the disease process of Cushing syndrome. Explain to the family that their family member is not "dumb or disinterested," but has an adrenal problem. Explain that the symptoms do not "go away" and may be progressive if prescribed therapy is not followed.

EVALUATION

■ Evaluate the effectiveness of glucocorticoid drug therapy. If the inflammation has not improved, a change in drug therapy may be necessary.
■ Continue monitoring for side effects, especially when client is receiving high doses of glucocorticoids.

KEY WEBSITES

Levothyroxine: http://www.nlm.nih.gov/medlineplus/druginfo/medmaster/a682461.html

Myxedema Coma: Diagnosis and Treatment: http://www.aafp.org/afp/20001201/2485.html

Vasopressin (Pitressin): http://www.med.umich.edu/ccmu/vasopressin.htm

Critical Thinking Case Study

MP, age 68, had a severe allergic reaction to shellfish. She was taken to the emergency room. A single dose of dexamethasone 100 mg IV (direct IV over 30 seconds) was ordered. MP weighs 65 kg.

1. Why is MP receiving dexamethasone IV? Is the dosage of dexamethasone within safe therapeutic range? Explain.
2. Describe the various ways for administering dexamethasone IV. By what other routes can dexamethasone be administered?
3. What additional health information and assessment may aid the health care provider in treating MP's serious health problem?

Twenty-one tablets of prednisone, 5 mg each, were prescribed to be taken over 5 days, with tapering daily doses. The first day would be 10 mg q.i.d.; the second day, 10 mg t.i.d.; the third day, 10 mg b.i.d.; the fourth day, 10 mg once daily; and the fifth day, 5 mg once daily.

4. Why was prednisone ordered and not oral dexamethasone? Explain.
5. What is the purpose for tapering prednisone doses? Explain.
6. Is the drug dose within safe therapeutic range? Explain.
7. Should MP have side effects such as peripheral edema caused by water and sodium retention as a result of tapered prednisone doses? Explain.
8. What is the difference between prednisone and prednisolone?
9. What are the adverse reactions from prolonged use of prednisone?
10. What are the nursing interventions and client teaching for MP and clients who take prednisone?

NCLEX Study Questions

1. A client is receiving the growth hormone drug somatrem (Protropin) to stimulate growth in tissue and bone for the treatment of dwarfism. The nurse understands that this drug simulates a hormone from the:
   a. adrenal gland
   b. thyroid gland
   c. anterior pituitary gland
   d. posterior pituitary gland

2. A client is given desmopressin acetate. The nurse knows that this drug is to treat:
   a. gigantism
   b. diabetes mellitus
   c. diabetes insipidus
   d. adrenal insufficiency

3. A client is taking levothyroxine (Synthroid). For which of the following adverse effects would the nurse monitor the client?

   a. Tachycardia
   b. Drowsiness
   c. Constipation
   d. Weight gain

4. The nurse is administering dihydrotachysterol (Hytakerol) to a client. The nurse realizes that the action of this drug is to treat:
   a. inflammation
   b. Paget's disease
   c. hypercalcemia
   d. hypoparathyroidism

5. A client is given corticotropin (Acthar). The nurse knows to monitor the client for:
   a. weight gain
   b. hyperkalemia
   c. hypoglycemia
   d. hypercalcemia

51

Antidiabetics

ELECTRONIC RESOURCES

Evolve website (http://evolve.elsevier.com/KeeHayes/pharmacology/):
- Case Studies
- Content Updates
- Frequently Asked Questions
- Student Review Activities
- WebLinks
- Additional Reference Material

Companion CD-ROM:
- NCLEX Examination Review Questions
- Pharmacology Animations
- IV Therapy Checklists
- Medication Error Checklists
- Drug Calculation Problems
- Electronic Calculators
- Top 200 Drugs with Pronunciations
- References from the Textbook

Outline

Objectives

Terms

Diabetes Mellitus
Insulin
Nursing Process: Antidiabetics: Insulin

Oral Antidiabetic Drugs (Oral Hypoglycemic Drugs)
Nursing Process: Oral Antidiabetics
Other Antidiabetic Agents
Hyperglycemic Drugs

Key Websites

Critical Thinking Case Study

NCLEX Study Questions

Objectives

- Compare type 1 and type 2 diabetes mellitus.
- Describe the symptoms of diabetes mellitus.
- Explain a hypoglycemic reaction and describe the symptoms.
- Differentiate among rapid-acting, intermediate-acting, and long-acting insulins and combination mix.
- Determine the peak concentration time for four types of insulin action and when a hypoglycemic reaction is most likely to occur.
- Explain the action of oral antidiabetic drugs and their side effects.
- Differentiate between the action of insulin, oral antidiabetic agents, and glucagon.
- Apply the nursing process to the client taking insulin and oral antidiabetic agents.

Terms

About 18.5 million persons in the United States have diabetes mellitus, approximately 6 million of whom are adults unaware that they have this disease. Complications from uncontrolled diabetes are the third leading cause of death. In the sixteenth century, diabetes was traced to Egyptian writings about "honeyed urine." Insulin, the protein hormone used to control diabetes, was not available for client use until 1921. In the 45 to 65 age group, Native Americans, Hispanics, and African Americans have a two to three times higher incidence of diabetes mellitus than whites.

Antidiabetic drugs are used primarily to control diabetes mellitus, a chronic disease that affects carbohydrate metabolism. There are two groups of antidiabetic agents: (1) insulin and (2) oral hypoglycemic (antidiabetic) drugs. **Insulin**, a protein secreted from the beta cells of the pancreas, is necessary for carbohydrate metabolism and plays an important role in protein and fat metabolism. The beta cells make up 75% of the pancreas, and the alpha cells that secrete glucagon, a hyperglycemic substance, occupy approximately 20% of the pancreas. **Oral hypoglycemic drugs**, also known as **oral antidiabetic drugs** (to avoid confusion with the term *hypoglycemic reaction*), are synthetic preparations that stimulate insulin release or otherwise alter the metabolic response to hyperglycemia.

Diabetes Mellitus

Diabetes mellitus, a chronic disease resulting from deficient glucose metabolism, is caused by insufficient insulin secretion from the beta cells. This results in high blood sugar *(hyperglycemia)*. Diabetes mellitus is characterized by the three *p*'s: **polyuria** (increased urine output), **polydipsia** (increased thirst), and **polyphagia** (increased hunger). Diabetes *mellitus* is a disorder of the pancreas, whereas diabetes *insipidus* is a disorder of the posterior pituitary gland, discussed in detail in Chapter 50.

The four types of diabetes are presented in Table 51–1. Viral infections, environmental conditions, and genetic factors contribute to the onset of **type 1 diabetes mellitus**. **Type 2 diabetes mellitus** is the most common type of diabetes. Some sources suggest that heredity and obesity are the major factors that cause type 2 diabetes. With type 2 diabetes, there is some beta-cell function with varying amounts of insulin secretion. Hyperglycemia may be controlled for some type 2 diabetes with oral antidiabetic *(hypoglycemic)* drugs and a diet prescribed by the American Diabetic Association; however, about one third of clients with type 2 diabetes need insulin. Clients with type 2 diabetes who use one or two oral antidiabetic drugs may become insulin-dependent years later.

Certain drugs increase blood sugar and can cause hyperglycemia in prediabetic persons. These include glucocorticoids (cortisone, prednisone), thiazide diuretics (hydrochlorothiazide [HydroDIURIL]), and epinephrine. Usually the blood sugar level returns to normal after the drug is discontinued.

During the second and third trimesters of pregnancy, the levels of the hormones progesterone, cortisol, and human placental lactogen (hPL) increase. These increased hormone levels can inhibit insulin usage. This is a contributing factor for the occurrence of gestational diabetes mellitus (GDM) during pregnancy. Glucose is then mobilized from the tissue and lipid storage sites. After pregnancy, the blood glucose level may decrease; however, some clients may develop diabetes, whereas others may develop type 2 diabetes mellitus in later years.

Insulin

Insulin is released from the beta cells of the islets of Langerhans in response to an increase in blood glucose. Oral glucose load is more effective in raising the serum insulin level than an intravenous (IV) glucose load. Insulin promotes the uptake of glucose, amino acids, and fatty acids and converts them to substances that are stored in body cells. Glucose is converted to glycogen for future glucose needs in the liver and muscle, thereby lowering the blood glucose level. The normal range for blood glucose is 60 to 100 mg/dl and 70 to 110 mg/dl for serum glucose. When the blood glucose level is greater than 180 mg/dl, *glycosuria* (sugar in the urine) can occur. Increased blood sugar acts as an osmotic diuretic, causing polyuria. When blood sugar remains elevated (>200 mg/dl), diabetes mellitus occurs.

Table 51–1

Types and Occurrences of Diabetes Mellitus

Types of Diabetes Mellitus	Additional Names	Percentage of Occurrences
Type 1	Insulin-dependent diabetes mellitus (IDDM); also called *juvenile-onset diabetes*	10%-12%
Type 2	Non-insulin-dependent diabetes mellitus (NIDDM); also called *maturity-onset or adult-onset diabetes*	85%-90%
Secondary diabetes (medications, hormonal changes)		2%-3%
Gestational diabetes mellitus (GDM)		<1% (2% to 5% of all pregnancies)

< Less than.

Beta Cell Secretion of Insulin

The beta cells in the pancreas secrete approximately 0.2 to 0.5 units/kg/daily. A client weighing 70 kg (154 pounds) secretes 14 to 35 units of insulin a day. More insulin secretion may occur if the person consumes a greater caloric intake. A client with diabetes mellitus may require 0.2 to 1 units/kg/daily. The higher range may be because of obesity, stress, or tissue insulin resistance.

Commercially Prepared Insulin

Parenteral (injectable) insulin is obtained from pork and beef pancreas when the animals are slaughtered. Pork insulin is closely related to human insulin, having only one different amino acid; beef insulin has four different amino acids. Human insulin (Humulin) was introduced in 1983 and is produced by two separate methods: (1) changing the different amino acid of pork insulin or (2) using deoxyribonucleic acid (DNA) technology. Pork insulin is a weaker allergen than beef insulin, and the use of human insulin has a low incidence of allergic effects and insulin resistance. Insulin is made more pure than previously, especially the Humulin produced by DNA technology, which results in fewer side effects. Human insulins administered subcutaneously (subQ) are absorbed faster and have a shorter duration than animal insulins. Newly diagnosed clients with insulin-dependent diabetes are usually prescribed human insulin. In addition, clients in whom hyperglycemia develops during pregnancy or who already have diabetes and become pregnant are usually prescribed human insulin. If a client has been taking animal (pork or beef) insulin without experiencing any untoward effects, it is not necessary to change to human insulin.

The concentration of insulin is 100 units/ml or 500 units/ml (U100/ml, U500/ml), and the insulin is packaged in a 10-ml vial (see the figures on insulin in Chapter 4D). Insulin 500 units is only available in short-acting regular insulin (Humulin R, Novolin R). Insulin 500 units is seldom used except in emergencies and for clients with serious insulin resistance (>200 units/daily). Insulin 40 units is no longer used in the United States, although it is still used in other countries. Insulin syringes are marked in units of 100 units per 1 ml for insulin U100. Insulin syringes must be used for accurate dosing. To prevent dosage errors, the nurse must be certain that there is a match of the insulin concentration with the calibration of units on the insulin syringe. Before use, the client or nurse must roll, not shake, cloudy insulin bottles to ensure that the insulin and its ingredients are well mixed. Shaking a bottle of insulin can cause bubbles and an inaccurate dose. Insulin requirements vary; usually less insulin is needed with increased exercise, and more insulin is needed with infections and high fever.

Administration of Insulin

Insulin is a protein and *cannot* be administered orally because gastrointestinal (GI) secretions destroy the insulin structure. It is administered subQ, at a 45- to 90-degree angle. The 90-degree angle is made by raising the skin and fatty tissue; the insulin is injected into the pocket between the fat and the muscle. In a thin person with little fatty tissue, the 45- to 60-degree angle is used. Regular insulin is the *only* type that can be administered IV.

The site and depth of insulin injection affect absorption. Insulin absorption is greater when given in the deltoid and abdominal areas than when given in the thigh and buttock areas. Insulin administered subQ has a slower absorption rate than if it is administered IM. Heat and massage could increase subQ absorption. Cooling the subQ area can decrease absorption.

Insulin is usually given in the morning before breakfast. It can be given several times a day. Insulin injection sites should be rotated to prevent **lipodystrophy** (tissue atrophy or hypertrophy), which can interfere with insulin absorption. *Lipoatrophy* (tissue atrophy) is a depression under the skin surface that primarily occurs in females and children. A frequent cause of an atrophied area is the use of animal insulins (beef and pork). *Lipohypertrophy* (tissue hypertrophy) is a raised lump or knot on the skin surface that is more common in males. It is frequently caused by repeated injections into the same subQ site. The client needs to develop a "site rotation pattern" to avoid lipodystrophy and to promote insulin absorption. There are various insulin rotation programs, such as an 8-day rotation schedule (insulin is given at a different site each day). The American Diabetic Association suggests that insulin be injected daily at a chosen site for 1 week. Injections should be 1.5 inches apart (a knuckle length) at a site area each day. When a client requires two insulin injections a day (morning and evening), one site should be chosen on the right side (morning) and one site chosen on the left side (evening). Figure 51–1 illustrates sites for insulin injections. A record of injection area sites and dates administered should be kept.

Illness and stress increase the need for insulin. Insulin doses should *not* be withheld during illness, including infections and stress. Hyperglycemia and ketoacidosis may result from withholding insulin.

Types of Insulin

There are several standard types of insulin: rapid acting, short acting, intermediate acting, long acting, and combinations. Rapid and short-acting insulins are in clear solution without any added substance to prolong the insulin action. Intermediate-acting insulins are cloudy and may contain protamine, a protein that prolongs the action of insulin, or zinc, which also slows the onset of action and prolongs the duration of activity.

Rapid-acting insulins include insulin lispro (human analog [Humalog]), human insulin aspart [rDNA origin] (NovoLog), and for oral inhalation human insulin [rDNA origin] (Exubera). Lispro insulin is formed by reversing two amino acids in human regular insulin (Humulin). Insulin aspart [rDNA origin] (NovoLog) is another human insulin analog in which a single amino acid (proline) has

FIGURE 51–1 Sites for insulin injection.

been substituted with aspartic acid to help prevent the molecules from clumping together to allow quicker entry into blood circulation. Lispro and insulin aspart act faster than regular insulin, so they MUST NOT be administered more than 5 minutes before mealtime. Clients who are insulin-dependent and who take rapid-acting insulin usually require intermediate-acting insulin as well.

Insulin human [rDNA origin] (Exubera) powder was the first orally inhaled insulin treatment option approved by the FDA (January 2006) to control hyperglycemia. Exubera was dispensed in 1 or 3 mg dose "blisters," which are small, foil dose packets. The action of rapid-acting insulin begins in 5 to 15 minutes, and the duration of action is 2 to 4 hours. This method was used primarily to provide mealtime insulin supplements and not to meet basal insulin needs. Intermediate-acting insulin was still needed. Exubera was not recommended in clients with lung disease, such as asthma or COPD due to variation of lung function. Also, Exubera was contraindicated in clients who have smoked within the last 6 months. The systemic insulin exposure is expected to be 2 to 5 times greater than in non-smokers. The smoker would be at risk for hypoglycemia.

Despite remaining safe and effective, insulin human [rDNA origin] (Exubera) was removed from the market by Pfizer on January 16, 2008 due to such a small number of clients taking Exubera. Inhaled insulin is expensive. Nektar Therapeutics, who originally developed Exubera may partner with another pharmaceutical company to market this type of insulin in the future.

Short-acting insulin has an onset of action in 30 minutes to 1 hour. The peak action occurs in 2 to 4 hours, and the duration of action is 6 to 8 hours. Regular (unmodified, crystalline) insulin is short-acting insulin that can be administered IV and subQ. Regular insulin is generally given 30 minutes before meals.

Intermediate-acting insulins include neutral-protamine-Hagedorn (NPH), Lente, Humulin N, and Humulin L. Isophane insulins like NPH and Humulin N contain protamine, a protein that prolongs the action of insulin. Lente and Humulin L contain zinc, which also prolongs the insulin action time. The onset of intermediate-acting insulin is 1 to 2 hours, peak action occurs in 6 to 12 hours, and the duration of action is 18 to 24 hours.

Insulin glargine (Lantus) is long-acting insulin with an onset of one hour. It is evenly distributed over a 24-hour duration of action; thus it is administered once a day, usually at bedtime. Incidence of nocturnal hypoglycemia is not as common as with other insulins because of its continuous sustained release. Insulin detmir (Levemir) is another long-acting insulin that peaks in 6 to 8 hours and lasts for 12 to 24 hours. These two insulins are analogues of human insulin. Approved by the FDA in 2000, Glargine was the first long-acting recombinant DNA (rDNA origin) human insulin for clients with types 1 and 2 diabetes. Glargine and detmir are available in prefilled 3-ml cartridge for the "OptiPen One" insulin pen device. Some clients complain of more pain at the injection site with the administration of glargine than with NPH insulin.

Combination insulins are commercially premixed. These include Humulin 70/30, Novolin 70/30, Humulin 50/50, and Humalog Mix 75/25. These combinations are widely used. The Humulin 70/30 vials or prefilled disposable pens contain 70% of human insulin isophane (intermediate-acting insulin, NPH) and 30% regular (fast-acting) insulin. The exterior of an insulin pen resembles a fountain pen. The Humulin 50/50 vial or pen contains 50% isophane (NPH) insulin and 50% regular insulin. The Humalog 75/25 mix is available in vials or prefilled disposable pens and contains 75% lispro protamine insulin and 25% lispro "rapid" insulin. Humalog 75/25 helps prevent hypoglycemia, which could occur with the 70/30 or 50/50 combination insulins, and helps control hyperglycemia more effectively. The 75/25 pen contains 300 units of insulin and does not require refrigeration after first use. It can be stored at room temperature for up to 10 days. With these combinations of insulin, the client does not have to mix regular and NPH insulins as long as one of these combinations is effective. However, some clients need less than 25% or 30% regular insulin and more intermediate-acting insulin. Such a client needs to mix the two insulins in the prescribed proportions.

Regular insulin can be mixed with protamine or zinc insulin in the same syringe. Mixing insulin can alter the absorption rate. When regular insulin is mixed with Lente insulin, a portion of the effect of regular insulin is lost. Less regular insulin effect is lost when mixed with NPH than when mixed with Lente, but Lente insulin causes less allergic response than NPH.

Insulin Resistance

Antibodies develop over time in persons taking animal insulin. This can slow the onset of insulin action and extend its duration of action. Antibody development can cause insulin resistance and insulin allergy. Obesity can also be a causative factor for insulin resistance. Skin tests with different insulin preparations may be performed to determine whether there is an allergic effect. Human and regular insulins produce fewer allergens.

Storage of Insulin

Unopened insulin vials are refrigerated until needed. Once an insulin vial has been opened, it may be kept (1) at room temperature for 1 month or (2) in the refrigerator for 3 months. Insulin is less irritating to the tissues when injected at room temperature. Insulin vials should not be put in the freezer. In addition, insulin vials should not be placed in direct sunlight or in a high-temperature area. Prefilled syringes should be stored in the refrigerator and should be used within 1 to 2 weeks. Opened insulin vials lose their strength after approximately 3 months.

Prototype Drug Chart 51–1 compares regular insulin with NPH insulin.

Prototype DRUG CHART 51–1

INSULINS

Drug Class

Antidiabetic: Insulin
Humalog (Lispro)—rapid acting
Regular Humulin R—short acting
Humulin N—intermediate acting
Glargine (Lantus)—long acting
Pregnancy Category: B

Dosage

Varies according to client's blood sugar

Contraindications

Hypersensitivity to beef, pork, zinc, protamine insulins
Caution: Hypersensitivity

Drug-Lab-Food Interactions

Drug: Increased hypoglycemic effect with aspirin, oral anticoagulant, alcohol, oral hypoglycemics, beta-blockers, tricyclic antidepressants, MAOIs, tetracycline; *decreased* hypoglycemic effect with thiazides, glucocorticoids, oral contraceptives, thyroid drugs, smoking

Pharmacokinetics

Absorption: Lispro and Humulin R rapidly absorbed from subQ injection site. Humulin N is absorbed at a slower rate. Glargine is absorbed at a slow evenly distributed rate.
Distribution: PB: UK
Metabolism: t½: varies with type of insulin
Excretion: Mostly in urine

Pharmacodynamics

Lispro (Humalog):
subQ: Onset: 5-15 min
 Peak: 30-60 min
 Duration: 3-4 h
Regular Humulin R:
subQ: Onset: 30-60 min
 Peak: 2-3 h
 Duration: 4-8 h
Humulin N:
subQ: Onset: 1-2 h
 Peak: 4-12 h
 Duration: 18-24 h
Glargine (Lantus):
subQ: Onset: 1 h
 Peak: None
 Duration: 24 h

Therapeutic Effects/Uses

To control diabetes mellitus; to lower blood sugar
Mode of Action: Insulin promotes use of glucose by body cells

Side Effects

Confusion, agitation, tremors, headache, flushing, hunger, weakness, lethargy, fatigue, urticaria; redness, irritation or swelling at insulin injection site

Adverse Reactions

Tachycardia, palpitations, hypoglycemic reaction, rebound hyperglycemia (Somogyi effect), lipodystrophy
Life-threatening: Shock; anaphylaxis

h, Hour; *MAOI,* monoamine oxidase inhibitor; *min,* minute; *PB,* protein-binding; *subQ,* subcutaneous; *t½,* half-life; *UK,* unknown.

Pharmacokinetics

All insulins can be administered subQ, but only regular insulin can be given IV. The half-life varies. Insulin is metabolized by the liver and muscle and excreted in the urine.

Pharmacodynamics

Insulin lowers blood sugar by promoting use of glucose by the body's cells. Insulin is also active in the storage of glucose as glycogen in muscles. The onset of action of rapid-acting insulin given subQ is 5 to 15 minutes. The onset of action of regular insulin given subQ is 30 minutes to 1 hour and 10 to 30 minutes given IV. The onset of action of intermediate-acting insulin is 1 to 2 hours. The peak action of insulins is important because of the possibility of hypoglycemic reaction (insulin shock) occurring during that time. The peak time for regular insulin is 2 to 4 hours and for intermediate-acting insulin, 6 to 12 hours. The nurse needs to assess for signs and symptoms of hypoglycemic reaction: nervousness, tremors, confusion, sweating, and increased pulse rate. Orange juice, sugar-sweetened beverages, or hard candy should be kept available and given if a reaction occurs.

Regular insulin can be given several times a day, especially during the regulation of insulin dosage. Intermediate- and long-acting insulins are usually administered once a day. Regular insulin (3 to 15 units) can be mixed with intermediate-acting insulin (Humulin N), especially if rapid onset of action is needed. When switching from pork to human insulin, the client may require an adjustment of insulin dose, because human insulin has a shorter duration of action.

Sliding-Scale Insulin Coverage

Insulin may be administered in adjusted doses that depend on individual blood glucose test results. When the diabetic client has extreme variances in insulin requirements (e.g., stress from hospitalization, surgery, illness, infection), adjusted dosing or sliding scale insulin coverage provides a more constant blood glucose level. Blood glucose testing is performed several times a day at specified intervals (usually before meals). A preset scale usually involves directions for the administration of rapid- or short-acting insulin.

Drug Interactions

Drugs such as thiazide diuretics, glucocorticoids (cortisone preparations), thyroid agents, and estrogen increase the blood sugar; therefore insulin dosage may need adjustment. Drugs that decrease insulin needs are tricyclic antidepressants, monoamine oxidase (MAO) inhibitors, aspirin products, and oral anticoagulants.

Table 51–2 lists the drug data for the rapid-acting, intermediate-acting, and long-acting insulins.

Side Effects and Adverse Reactions: Hypoglycemic Reactions and Ketoacidosis

When more insulin is administered than needed for glucose metabolism, a **hypoglycemic reaction**, or **insulin shock**, occurs. The person may exhibit nervousness, trembling, and lack of coordination, have cold and clammy skin, and complain of a headache. Some clients become combative and incoherent. Giving sugar orally or IV in-

creases the use of insulin, and the symptoms disappear immediately.

In response to an excessive dose of insulin, diabetic clients may develop the Somogyi effect. This hypoglycemic condition usually occurs in the predawn hours of 2:00 to 4:00 AM. A rapid decrease in blood glucose during the night-time hours stimulates a release of hormones (e.g., cortisol, glucagon, epinephrine) to increase blood glucose by lipolysis, gluconeogenesis, and glycogenolysis creating the Somogyi effect. Management of the Somogyi effect involves monitoring blood glucose between 2:00 AM and 4:00 AM and reducing the bedtime insulin dosage.

Hyperglycemia on awakening is known as the *dawn phenomenon*. The client usually awakens with a headache and reports night sweats and nightmares. Management of the dawn phenomenon involves increasing the bedtime dose of insulin.

With an inadequate amount of insulin, sugar cannot be metabolized, and fat catabolism occurs. The use of fatty acids (ketones) for energy causes **ketoacidosis** (diabetic acidosis or diabetic coma). Table 51–3 gives the signs and symptoms of hypoglycemic reaction and ketoacidosis.

Insulin Pen Injectors

An insulin pen resembles a fountain pen. The pen contains a disposable needle and a disposable insulin-filled cartridge. Insulin pens come in two types: prefilled and reusable. These insulin-filled pens are considered to deliver an insulin dose more accurate than the traditional 100 unit syringe and vial.

To operate the insulin pen, the insulin dose is obtained by turning the dial to the number of insulin units needed. The capacity of these prefilled and reusable insulin pens is 151 to 300 units, or 1.5 to 3 ml. Some insulin pens can measure the insulin dose to as low as 0.5 to 2 units. Insulin pens available on the market include Novolog FlexPen (Novo Nordisk), Humalog-Pen (Lilly), Apidra OptiClik injection pen (Sanofi-aventis), Lantus SoloSTAR (Sanofi), and Levemir FlexPen (Novo Nordisk). Insulin pens tend to be more expensive delivery systems, but their advantages may outweigh the extra cost.

The use of insulin pens increases the client's compliance with the insulin regimen. The convenience of the pen is most appealing. The client may choose to use the insulin pen for its portability (e.g., at work or while traveling). The traditional method for administering insulin may be used at other times. The cost of insulin in vials is somewhat less than the prefilled insulin pens, but most clients state that less injection pain is associated with the insulin pens than with the traditional insulin syringe.

Insulin Pumps

There are two types of insulin pumps: implantable and portable. The implantable insulin pump is surgically implanted in the abdomen. It delivers basal insulin infusion and bolus doses with meals, administered either intraperitoneally or IV. With the use of implantable insulin pumps, fewer hypogly-

Table 51–2

Antidiabetics: Insulins

Generic (Brand)	Route and Dosage	Pregnancy Category	Half-Life	Onset	Peak	Dura-tion
Rapid acting						
insulin lispro (Humalog) insulin aspart [rDNA origin] (NovoLog) insulin glulisine (Apidra)	A: 0.5-1.0 unit/kg/day, dose individualized	*Humalog:* B *NovoLog, Apidra:* C	26-81 min	5-15 min	*Humalog, Apidra:* 30-90 min *NovoLog:* 1-3 h	*Humalog:* 2-5 h *NovoLog:* 3-5 h *Apidra:* 1-2.5 h
Short acting						
insulin regular (Humulin R, Novolin R, regular insulin)	A & C: subQ/IV: 100 units/ml; dose individualized	B	10 min-1 h	30 min	2-4 h	6-8 h
Intermediate acting						
insulin isophane NPH (Humulin N, Novolin N)	(Prototype Drug Chart 51–1)	B	13 h	1-2 h	6-12 h	18-24 h
insulin zinc suspension Lente (Humulin L, Novolin L)	A & C: subQ: 100 units/ml; dose individualized	B	13 h	1-2 h	8-12 h	18-24 h
Long acting						
Ultralente insulin	Same as Lente	B	13 h	5-8 h	14-20 h	30-36 h
insulin glargine (Lantus)	Dose individualized	C	UK	1 h	None	24 h
Combinations*						
Humulin 70/30 (isophane NPH 70%, regular 30%)	Dose individualized	B	13 h	0.5 h	4-8 h	22-24 h
insulin isophane NPH 50/50 (Humulin (NPH 50%, regular 50%)	Dose individualized	B	13 h	0.5 h	4-8 h	24 h
Humalog 75/25 (lispro prot-amine 75%, lispro 25%)	Dose individualized	B	<13 h	5-15 min	0.5-6 h	20-24 h

A, Adult; *C*, child; *h*, hour; *IV*, intravenous; *min*, minute; *NPH*, neutral-protamine-Hagedorn; *subQ*, subcutaneous; *UK*, unknown; <, less than.
*Protamine and zinc suspensions are added to regular insulin.

cemic reactions occur and the blood glucose levels are controlled. Long-term effectiveness of the pump is under study.

Portable or external insulin pumps, also called *continuous subQ insulin infusion (CSII)*, have been available since 1983. The external insulin pump keeps blood glucose levels as close to normal as possible. The insulin pump is a battery-operated device that uses regular insulin, which is stored in a reservoir syringe placed inside the device. The unit is the size of a cell phone and weighs about 3.5 ounces. It delivers both basal insulin infusion (continuous release of a small amount of insulin) and bolus doses with meals. Infusions are programmed by the client. About three basal rates are programmed a day; however the client can adjust the rate according to changes in activity. The insulin can be delivered by bolus (the client pushes a button to deliver a bolus dose at meals).

Insulin is delivered from the device through a plastic tube with a metal or plastic needle placed subQ by the client. The needle can be inserted into the abdomen, upper thigh, or upper arm. Only regular insulin is used. Modified insulins (NPH and Lente) are not used because of unpredictable control of blood sugars. The pump delivers exactly as much regular insulin as the client programs.

The ongoing insulin delivery therapy helps to decrease the risk of severe hypoglycemic reaction and maintains glucose (glycemic) control. Glucose levels should be monitored at least daily with or without an insulin pump.

Most insulin pumps have a memory of the last 24 boluses (time and day). An alarm is sounded when insulin is not delivered. The pump can be disconnected from the insertion site for bathing, swimming, and other activities; however, it is recommended that it not be discontinued for longer than 1 to 2 hours.

Success of insulin pump therapy depends on the individual's knowledge and compliance related to insulin use and the diabetic state. The person with type 1 diabetes mellitus may benefit most from the use of insulin pump therapy. This insulin delivery method is considered more

Table 51–3

Hypoglycemic Reaction and Diabetic Ketoacidosis

Reaction	Signs and Symptoms
Hypoglycemic reaction (insulin shock)	Headache, light-headedness Nervousness, apprehension Tremor Excess perspiration; cold, clammy skin Tachycardia Slurred speech Memory lapse, confusion, seizures Blood sugar level <60 mg/dl
Diabetic ketoacidosis (hyperglycemic reaction)	Extreme thirst Polyuria Fruity breath odor Kussmaul breathing (deep, rapid, labored, distressed, dyspnea) Rapid, thready pulse Dry mucous membranes, poor skin turgor Blood sugar level 251 mg/dl

>, Greater than; < less than.

effective than the use of multiple injections of regular and modified types of insulins and lessens the long-term diabetic complications.

Insulin Jet Injectors

Insulin jet injectors shoot insulin, without a needle, directly through the skin into the fatty tissue. Because the insulin is delivered under high pressure, stinging, pain, burning, and bruising may occur. This method of insulin insertion is not indicated for children or older adults. This type of device is also expensive, costing approximately 2 to 10 times as much as the subQ dose.

Nursing Process

Antidiabetics: Insulin

ASSESSMENT

■ Identify the drugs client currently takes. Certain drugs such as alcohol, aspirin, oral anticoagulants, oral antidiabetics, beta-blockers, tricyclic antidepressants, monoamine oxidase inhibitors (MAOIs), and tetracycline increase the hypoglycemic effect when taken with insulin. Note that thiazides, glucocorticoids, oral contraceptives, thyroid drugs, and smoking can increase blood sugar.

■ Assess the type of insulin and dosage. Note whether it is given once or multiple times a day.

■ Note vital signs and blood sugar levels. Report abnormal findings.

■ Determine client's knowledge of diabetes mellitus and the use of insulins.

■ Check for signs and symptoms of a hypoglycemic reaction (insulin shock) and hyperglycemia or ketoacidosis.

NURSING DIAGNOSES

■ Risk for impaired tissue integrity related to failure to rotate insulin injection sites
■ Imbalanced nutrition: more than body requirements related to excessive intake in relationship to metabolic need
■ Risk for injury related to confusion from a hypoglycemic reaction

PLANNING

■ Client's blood sugar will be within normal values (70 to 110 mg/dl).

NURSING INTERVENTIONS

■ Monitor vital signs. Tachycardia can occur during an insulin reaction.
■ Determine blood glucose levels and report changes. The reference value is 60 to 100 mg/dl for blood glucose and 70 to 110 mg/dl for serum glucose.
■ Prepare a teaching plan based on client's knowledge of health problem, diet, and drug therapy.

Client Teaching

General

• Instruct client to immediately report symptoms of hypoglycemic (insulin) reaction: headache, nervousness, sweating, tremors, rapid pulse; and symptoms of a hyperglycemic reaction (diabetic acidosis): thirst, increased urine output, sweet fruity breath odor.

• Advise client that hypoglycemic reactions are more likely to occur during the peak action time. Most diabetics know whether they are having a hypoglycemic reaction, but some have a higher tolerance to low blood sugar and can have a severe hypoglycemic reaction without realizing it.

• Explain that orange juice, sugar-containing drinks, and hard candy may be used when a hypoglycemic reaction begins.

• Teach family members to administer glucagon by injection if client has a hypoglycemic reaction and cannot drink sugar-containing fluid.

• Inform client that certain herbs may interact with insulin and oral antidiabetic drugs. A hypoglycemic or hyperglycemic effect might occur (Herbal Alert 51–1).

• Instruct client about the necessity for compliance with prescribed insulin therapy and diet.

• Advise client to obtain a MedicAlert card, tag, or bracelet indicating the health problem and insulin dosage.

Self-Administration

• Direct client how to check blood sugar with a glucometer (Sure Touch, One Step, Accu-Chek). Figure 51–2 illustrates use of a glucometer.

- Instruct client in care of insulin container and syringes. Inform client taking NPH or Lente insulin with regular insulin that the regular insulin should be drawn up before the NPH or Lente insulin.

Diet

- Advise client taking insulin to eat the prescribed diet on a consistent schedule. Diet information may be obtained from the American Diabetes Association or a nutritionist.

Cultural Considerations ❖

- Provide additional instructions about insulin action, administration, reactions, and possible complications in the language client speaks/reads most easily.
- Follow-up by a community health nurse may be needed to assist client's compliance with insulin use, diet, and exercise regimens.
- Identify conflicts in values and beliefs and explain the composition of insulin, because client may prefer to avoid pork insulins for religious reasons.

FIGURE 51–2 A 10-year-old child uses a glucometer to check her blood sugar level.

Herbal ALERT 51–1

Antidiabetic Agents

- *Chromium* may decrease insulin requirements.
- *Black cohosh* may potentiate the hypoglycemic effects of insulin and oral antidiabetic drugs.
- *Garlic, bitter melon, aloe,* and *gymnema* can increase insulin levels and therefore may cause hypoglycemia when used with insulin or oral antidiabetic drugs. They can have a direct hypoglycemic effect.
- *Ginseng* can lower blood glucose levels. When taken with insulin or an oral antidiabetic (hypoglycemic) drug, hypoglycemic effects or reaction may occur.
- *Bilberry* may increase hypoglycemia when taken with insulin or oral antidiabetics.
- *Cocoa, rosemary,* and *stinging nettle* decrease therapeutic effect of insulin and oral antidiabetic drugs (have a hyperglycemic effect).

EVALUATION

- Evaluate effectiveness of insulin therapy by noting whether blood sugar level is within the accepted range.
- Determine client's knowledge of the signs and symptoms of hypoglycemic or hyperglycemic reaction.

Oral Antidiabetic Drugs (Oral Hypoglycemic Drugs)

First- and Second-Generation Sulfonylureas

Oral antidiabetic drugs, also called *oral hypoglycemics,* were discovered in the early 1940s in France. Persons with type 2 diabetes use these drugs; persons with type 1 diabetes should *not* use them. Clients with type 2 diabetes have some degree of insulin secretion by the pancreas. The sulfonylureas, a group of antidiabetics chemically related to sulfonamides but lacking antibacterial activity, stimulate pancreatic beta cells to secrete more insulin. This increases the insulin cell receptors, increasing the ability of the cells to bind insulin for glucose metabolism.

The sulfonylureas are classified as first- and second-generation. The first-generation sulfonylureas are divided into short-acting, intermediate-acting, and long-acting antidiabetics. Tolbutamide (Orinase) is a first-generation short-acting sulfonylurea. Acetohexamide (Dymelor) and tolazamide (Tolinase) are first-generation intermediate-acting sulfonylureas. Chlorpropamide (Diabinese) is a first-generation long-acting sulfonylurea.

The second-generation sulfonylureas were first used in Europe; in 1984 they were approved by the FDA for use in the United States. The newer sulfonylureas increase the tissue response to insulin and decrease glucose production by the liver. They have greater hypoglycemic potency than the first-generation sulfonylureas. Effective doses for the second-generation drugs are lower than first generation dosages. They have a longer duration and cause fewer side effects. The second-generation drugs have less displacement potential from protein-binding sites by other highly protein-bound drugs, such as salicylates and warfarin (Coumadin), than first-generation drugs. Second-generation sulfonylureas should not be used when liver or kidney dysfunction is present. A hypoglycemic reaction is more likely to occur in older adults.

Second-generation sulfonylureas include glimepiride (Amaryl) and glipizide (Glucotrol, Glucotrol XL), which directly stimulate the beta cells to secrete insulin, thus decreasing the blood glucose level. Glimepiride improves postprandial glucose levels. It may be used in combination with insulin in persons with type 2 diabetes. Side effects include GI disturbances such as nausea, vomiting, diarrhea, and abdominal pain.

Table 51–4 lists drug data for the sulfonylureas. Prototype Drug Chart 51–2 lists the actions and effects of the second-generation sulfonylurea glipizide.

Table 51–4

Oral Antidiabetics

Generic (Brand)	Route and Dosage	Uses and Considerations
First-Generation: Short Acting		
tolbutamide (Orinase)	A: PO: 510-3000 mg/d in 2-3 divided doses	For managing type 2 diabetes. Chemically related to sulfonamides but no antiinfective effect. Hypoglycemic reaction may occur if overdosed. *Pregnancy category:* C; PB: >90%; t½: 4-7 h
First-Generation: Intermediate Acting		
acetohexamide	A: PO: 251 mg/d before breakfast; *max:* 1.5 g/d	For managing mild to moderately severe type 2 diabetes mellitus. *Pregnancy category:* C; PB: UK; t½: 5-6 h
tolazamide (Tolinase)	A: PO: 100-251 mg/d in 1-2 divided doses; *max:* 1 g/d	Same as acetohexamide. Diet and exercise should be part of diabetic therapy. Duration of action 10 to 20 hours. *Pregnancy category:* C; PB: 90%; t½: 7 h
First-Generation: Long Acting		
chlorpropamide (Diabinese)	A: PO: Initially: 100-251 mg/d; maint: 100-510 mg/d in 1-2 divided doses; *max:* 751 mg/d	For managing type 2 diabetes. May be given to selected type 1 clients for reducing insulin doses. Diet and exercise should be a part of diabetic therapy. Duration of action 24 h. May cause water and sodium retention. *Pregnancy category:* C; PB: 95%; t½: 36 h
Second Generation		
glipizide (Glucotrol)	(Prototype Drug Chart 51–2)	
glyburide nonmicronized (DiaBeta, Micronase)	A: PO: Initially: 1.25-5 mg/d; maint: 1.25-20 mg q.i.d./ b.i.d.; *max:* 20 mg/d	Same as chlorpropamide. Potent drug. Duration of action 10 to 24 h. *Pregnancy category:* B; PB: 90%-95%; t½: 10 h
glyburide micronized (Glynase)	A: PO: 1.5-3 mg/d in AM; maint: 3-4.5 mg/d; *max:* 12 mg/d in 1 or 2 divided doses	For type 2 diabetes. Same as glyburide nonmicronized.
glimepiride (Amaryl)	A: PO: Initially: 1-2 mg a.c.; maint: 1-4 mg/d a.c.; *max:* 8 mg/d a.c.	To treat clients with type 2 diabetes. May be used in combination with insulin. Can lower the 2-hour postprandial glucose levels significantly. GI disturbances may occur. *Pregnancy category:* C; PB: 99.5%; t½: 5-9 h
Nonsulfonylureas		
Biguanides		
metformin (Glucophage)	(Prototype Drug Chart 51–3)	
Alpha-Glucosidase Inhibitors		
acarbose (Precose)	A: PO: Initially 25 mg 1-3 × 3 daily with meals; *max:* 150 mg/d <60 kg, 300 mg/d if >60 kg	For managing hyperglycemia in type 2 diabetes mellitus. Used as monotherapy or in combination with a sulfonylurea. *Pregnancy category:* B; PB: UK; t½: 2 h
miglitol (Glyset)	A: PO: 25-100 mg t.i.d. with meals	For managing type 2 diabetes. May be taken with a sulfonylurea or as monotherapy with diet and exercise. GI disturbances may occur. *Pregnancy category:* B; PB: ,4%; t½: 2 h
Thiazolidinediones (Insulin-Enhancing Agents)		
pioglitazone HCl (Actos)	A: PO: 15-45 mg/d	Management of type 2 diabetes. It improves glycemic control and decreases insulin resistance. It inhibits gluconeogenesis and increases sensitivity to insulin in muscle and fatty tissues. For monotherapy; can be combined with sulfonylurea or insulin. Liver enzymes should be monitored. *Pregnancy category:* C; PB: 99%; t½: 3-7 h
rosiglitazone maleate (Avandia)	A: PO: 4-8 mg/d; or 2-4 mg b.i.d.	Management for type 2 diabetes. Improves blood glucose control and increases insulin sensitivity. Can increase resumption of ovulation in premenopausal women. For monotherapy use; maybe combined with metformin. Diet, exercise, and monitoring liver enzymes are suggested. Replaced troglitazone (Rezulin), which was removed from the market because it caused severe liver problems. *Pregnancy category:* C; PB: 99.8%; t½: 3-4 h

A, Adult; *a.c.,* before meals; *b.i.d.,* twice a day; *d,* day; *GI,* gastrointestinal; *h,* hour; *maint,* maintenance; *max,* maximum; *PB,* protein-binding; *PO,* by mouth; *q.i.d.,* four times a day; *t½,* half-life; *t.i.d.,* three times a day; *UK,* unknown; >, greater than; <, less than.

Table 51–4

Oral Antidiabetics—cont'd

Generic (Brand)	Route and Dosage	Uses and Considerations
Meglitinides		
repaglinide (Prandin)	A: PO: 0.5-4 mg a.c. b.i.d., t.i.d., q.i.d.; *max*: 16 mg/d	To manage type 2 diabetes. May be taken alone or in combination with metformin. Similar in action to sulfonylureas but not in structure. Increases beta-cell secretion of insulin. *Pregnancy category*: C; PB: 98%; t½: 1 h
nateglinide (Starlix)	A: PO: 60-120 mg a.c. t.i.d.; *max*: 540 mg/d	To treat type 2 diabetes. Increases release of insulin from beta cells. May be used alone or in combination with metformin. *Pregnancy category*: UK; PB: 98%; t½: 1.5 h
Incretin Modifiers		
sitagliptin phosphate (combination form: sitagliptin phosphate + metformin [Januvia])	A: PO: 100 mg/d	For managing type 2 diabetes mellitus. Used in combination with exercise and diet. *Pregnancy category*: B; PB: 38%; t½: 12 h
Fixed Combination Oral Antidiabetic Drugs		
glyburide/metformin (Glucovance)	A: PO: Initially: 1.25/251 mg (glyburide/metformin) daily or b.i.d. with meals. Increase dose at 2-wk intervals; maint: 2.5/510 mg or 5/510 mg/d or b.i.d. with meals; *max*: 20/2000 mg/d	For managing type 2 diabetes mellitus. May be used when glucose is not controlled with either drug alone. Contraindicated for clients with renal insufficiency because of risk of developing lactic acidosis. *Pregnancy category*: B-D; PB: UK; t½: UK

Pharmacokinetics

Glipizide is well absorbed from the GI tract and highly protein-bound. Glipizide is metabolized by the liver. The primary metabolites are inactive and excreted mainly in urine.

Pharmacodynamics

Glipizide (Glucotrol, Glucotrol XL) is the most common sulfonylurea drug prescribed for type 2 diabetes mellitus. It lowers blood sugar by stimulating pancreatic beta cells to secrete insulin. The onset of action of acetohexamide usually occurs within 15 to 30 minutes, and the peak action time is between 1 and 2 hours. Glipizide is normally given once a day in the morning because of its long duration of action of 24 hours.

Side Effects, Adverse Reactions, and Contraindications

The side effects of most oral antidiabetic drugs are similar to those of insulin. Taking antidiabetic drugs without adequate food can lead to an insulin reaction with signs and symptoms such as nervousness, tremors, and confusion. Adverse reactions include hematologic disorders, such as aplastic anemia, leukopenia, and thrombocytopenia. Seizures and coma may also occur. Sulfonylureas are contraindicated in type 1 diabetes (no functioning beta cells), diabetic ketoacidosis, pregnancy, and lactation and during stress, surgery, or severe infection.

The major side effect of sulfonylureas is hypoglycemia. Acarbose, which is often used in combination with sulfonylureas does not cause hypoglycemia unless it is taken with a sulfonylurea or insulin. It can cause increased flatulence (gas), diarrhea, and abdominal distention.

Drug Interactions

Aspirin, oral anticoagulants, MAO inhibitors, sulfonamides, and some NSAIDs can increase the action of sulfonylureas, especially first generation, by binding to plasma proteins and displacing sulfonylureas. Because this causes increased free sulfonylurea, an insulin reaction can result. The action of sulfonylureas is decreased by concurrent administration of thiazide diuretics, isoniazid, phenytoin, and corticosteroids. Clients should be alerted not to drink alcohol while taking sulfonylureas, because alcohol increases the half-life, and a hypoglycemic reaction can result.

Nonsulfonylureas

Expanding knowledge of glucose metabolism has revealed new mechanisms for the management of type 2 diabetes. The drugs metformin and acarbose use different methods to control serum glucose levels following a meal. Unlike the sulfonylureas, which enhance insulin release and receptor interaction, these drugs affect the hepatic and GI production of glucose.

Biguanides: Metformin (Glucophage)

Metformin is a biguanide compound that acts by decreasing hepatic production of glucose from stored glycogen. This diminishes the increase in serum glucose following a meal and blunts the degree of postprandial hyperglycemia. Metformin also decreases the absorption of glucose from the small intestine, and there is evidence that it increases

Prototype DRUG CHART 51–2

GLIPIZIDE

Drug Class Glipizide: Sulfonylurea, first-generation Trade names: Glucotrol, Glucotrol XL *Pregnancy Category:* C	**Dosage** A: PO: Initially 2.5-5 mg before meals daily; maintenance: 10-15 mg daily before meals; (dose should be divided if >15 mg); *max:* 40 mg/d A: PO: ER: 5-10 mg/d
Contraindications Diabetic ketoacidosis *Caution:* Hepatic or renal dysfunction, elderly, debilitated or malnourished, adrenal or pituitary insufficiency	**Drug-Lab-Food Interactions** *Drug:* Alcohol may produce a disulfiram-like reaction (flushing, headache, sweating, nausea, violent vomiting, weakness); Hypoglycemia may be potentiated by oral anticoagulants, MAO inhibitors, salicylates, probenecid, sulfonamides, cimetidine, clofibrate, phenylbutazone *Lab:* Altered liver function tests *Food:* None known
Pharmacokinetics **Absorption:** Rapidly absorbed from GI **Distribution:** PB: 90%-95% **Excretion:** Primarily in urine	**Pharmacodynamics** PO: Onset: 15-30 min Peak: 1-2 h Duration: 24 h

Therapeutic Effects/Uses

To control hyperglycemia in type 2 diabetes mellitus
Mode of Action: Directly stimulates beta cells in pancreas to secrete insulin, indirectly alters sensitivity of peripheral
insulin receptors, allowing increased insulin binding

Side Effects Drowsiness, headache, confusion, visual disturbances, anxiety, hunger, anorexia, nausea, constipation, diarrhea	**Adverse Reactions** Hypoglycemia, tachycardia *Life-threatening:* Seizures, coma, respiratory depression

A, Adult; *d,* day; *GI,* gastrointestinal; *h,* hour; *MAO,* monoamine oxidase; *max,* maximum; *min,* minute; *PB,* protein-binding; *PO,* by
mouth; *ER,* extended release; *t½,* half-life; >greater than.

---

insulin receptor sensitivity as well as peripheral glucose uptake at the cellular level. Unlike sulfonylureas, metformin does not produce hypoglycemia or hyperglycemia. It can cause GI disturbances.

Metformin is 51% to 60% bioavailable and is absorbed primarily from the small intestine. It does not undergo hepatic metabolism and is eliminated unchanged in the urine. It is not recommended for clients with renal impairment. Monotherapy with metformin is effective; however, when combined with a sulfonylurea, the drug is useful in cases resistant to oral antidiabetics (oral hypoglycemics). Metformin therapy should be withheld for 48 hours before and after the client undergoes IV contrast dye, because lactic acidosis or acute renal failure may develop.

Alpha-Glucosidase Inhibitors: Acarbose (Precose) and Miglitol (Glyset)

Acarbose acts by inhibiting the digestive enzyme in the small intestine responsible for the release of glucose from complex carbohydrates (CHO) in the diet. By inhibiting alpha glucosidase, the CHO cannot be absorbed and therefore pass into the large intestine. Acarbose has no demonstrated systemic effects and is not absorbed into the body in significant amounts. It does not cause a hypoglycemic reaction. Acarbose is intended for use in clients who do not achieve results with diet alone. Miglitol (Glyset), like acarbose, inhibits alpha glucosides. Miglitol is absorbed from the GI tract. This drug will not cause hypoglycemia, but if taken with a sulfonylurea or insulin, hypoglycemia could occur.

Thiazolidinediones

Troglitazone (Rezulin) was the first drug in this group, approved by the FDA in 1997. Because of severe liver problems and deaths associated with this drug, it was removed from the market in early 2000. Pioglitazone (Actos) and rosiglitazone (Avandia) were considered safer thiazolidinedione drugs, but in 2007 a warning was added to the Avandia packaging after the FDA issued a statement that Avandia users may be at greater risk for heart attack and possibly death (Prototype Drug Chart 51–3). These two drugs can be prescribed for monotherapy or combined with other oral antidiabetic drugs. Pioglitazone can be taken in combination

Prototype **DRUG CHART 51–3**

METFORMIN

Drug Class

Metformin: Biguanide
Trade names: Glucophage, Glucophage XL
Pregnancy Category: B

Dosage

A: PO: Initial: 510 mg/d-t.i.d. with meals; increase dose
  gradually; *max:* 2510 mg/d
A: PO: ER: 510 mg/day with evening meal; *max:*
  2000 mg/d

Contraindications

Hypersensitivity, concurrent infection, hepatic
  or renal dysfunction, cardiopulmonary
  insufficiency, alcoholism
Caution: Pregnancy, lactation

Drug-Lab-Food Interactions

Drug: Hypoglycemia may be potentiated by captopril,
  nifedipine, procainamide, quinidine, digoxin,
  furosemide, triamterene, cimetidine, ranitidine, azole
  antifungals, trimethoprim, vancomycin, quinine; Io-
  dinated contrast dyes may lead to lactic acidosis or
  acute kidney failure
Lab: Altered liver function tests
Food: None known

Pharmacokinetics

Absorption: 51-60% absorbed
Distribution: PB: 0%
Metabolism: t½: 6.2-17.6 h
Excretion: Primarily in urine

Pharmacodynamics

PO: Onset: UK
  Peak: 1-3 h
  Duration: UK

Therapeutic Effects/Uses

To control hyperglycemia in type 2 diabetes mellitus
Mode of Action: Increases binding of insulin to receptors, improves tissue sensitivity to insulin, increases glucose
  transport into skeletal muscles and fatty tissues, decreases glucose production in the liver by reducing gluconeogenesis, and reduces glucose absorption from the intestines

Side Effects

Dizziness, fatigue, headache, agitation, bitter
  or metallic taste, anorexia, nausea, vomiting,
  diarrhea

Adverse Reactions

Lactic acidosis; malabsorption of amino acids, vitamin
  B_{12}, and folic acid
Life-threatening: Lactic acidosis

A, Adult; *d,* day; *h,* hour; *max,* maximum; *PB,* protein-binding; *PO,* by mouth; *ER,* extended release; *t½,* half-life; *t.i.d.,* three times
a day; *UK,* unknown.

---

with sulfonylurea or insulin, and rosiglitazone may be combined with metformin. These drugs do not induce hypoglycemic reactions if taken alone. They decrease insulin resistance and improve blood glucose control.

Meglitinides

Repaglinide (Prandin) and nateglinide (Starlix) are classified as meglitinide oral antidiabetic agents. They stimulate the beta cells to release insulin. The action of repaglinide and nateglinide is similar to that of sulfonylureas. These agents can be used alone or in combination with metformin for clients with type 2 diabetes mellitus. They are short-acting antidiabetic drugs. They should not be prescribed for clients with liver dysfunction because of a possible decreased liver metabolism rate. More of the drug could remain in the body, which may cause a hypoglycemic reaction.

Incretin Modifier

The oral antidiabetic sitagliptin phosphate (Januvia) is classified as an incretin modifier (dipeptidyl peptidase-4

[DPP-4] inhibitor) for treatment of type 2 diabetes mellitus. The action of sitagliptin is to increase the level of incretin hormones, increase insulin secretion, and decrease glucagon secretion to reduce glucose production. This incretin modifier is used as adjunct treatment with exercise and diet to reduce both fasting and postprandial plasma glucose levels.

Guidelines for Oral Antidiabetic (Hypoglycemic) Therapy for Type 2 Diabetes

The following are criteria for the use of oral antidiabetic drugs:

- Onset of diabetes mellitus at age 40 years or older
- Diagnosis of diabetes for less than 5 years
- Normal weight or overweight
- Fasting blood glucose equal to or less than 200 mg/dl
- Less than 40 units of insulin required per day
- Normal renal and hepatic function

Oral Antidiabetics

ASSESSMENT

■ Identify the drugs client currently takes. Aspirin, alcohol, sulfonamides, oral contraceptives, and monoamine oxidase inhibitors (MAOIs) increase the hypoglycemic effect; a decrease in oral antidiabetic drug may be needed. Glucocorticoids (cortisone), thiazide diuretics, and estrogen increase blood sugar.

■ Note vital signs and blood sugar levels. Report abnormal findings.

■ Determine client's knowledge of diabetes mellitus and the use of oral antidiabetics.

NURSING DIAGNOSES

■ Risk for injury related to side effect of visual disturbances

■ Imbalanced nutrition: more than body requirements related to excessive intake of food

■ Deficient knowledge related to lack of exposure to teaching about taking adequate food with oral antidiabetics

PLANNING

■ Client's blood sugar will be within normal serum levels (70 to 110 mg/dl).

■ Client will adhere to prescribed diet, blood testing, and drug.

NURSING INTERVENTIONS

■ Determine vital signs. Oral antidiabetics increase cardiac function and oxygen consumption, which can lead to cardiac dysrhythmias.

■ Administer oral antidiabetics with food to minimize gastric upset.

■ Monitor blood glucose levels and report changes. The reference value is 60 to 100 mg/dl for blood glucose and 70 to 110 mg/dl for serum glucose.

■ Prepare a teaching plan based on client's knowledge of health problems, diet, and drug therapy.

Client Teaching

General

• Advise client that hypoglycemic (insulin) reaction can occur when taking an oral hypoglycemic drug, especially the sulfonylureas. This drug stimulates the release of insulin from the beta cells of the pancreas. Oral antidiabetics are *not* insulin. Normally, clients with diabetes mellitus type 1 do not have functioning beta cells and should *not* take oral antidiabetics, only

insulin. Sulfonylureas are prescribed for clients with diabetes mellitus type 2.

• Teach client to recognize symptoms of hypoglycemic reaction (headache, nervousness, sweating, tremors, rapid pulse) and symptoms of hyperglycemic reaction (thirst, increased urine output, sweet fruity breath odor).

• Explain that insulin might be needed instead of an oral antidiabetic drug during stress, surgery, or serious infection. Blood sugar levels are usually elevated during stressful times.

• Instruct client about the necessity for compliance to diet and drug.

• Advise client to obtain a MedicAlert card, tag, or bracelet indicating the health problem and antidiabetic dosage.

Self-Administration

• Direct client how to check blood sugar level with a glucometer. Client should record and report abnormal results.

Side Effects

• Advise client to report side effects such as vomiting, diarrhea, and rash.

Diet

• Instruct client not to ingest alcohol with antidiabetic drugs to avoid a hypoglycemic reaction. Food taken with oral antidiabetics will decrease gastric irritation.

• Advise client taking oral antidiabetics to eat the prescribed diet on schedule. Delaying or missing a meal can cause hypoglycemia.

• Explain the use of orange juice, sugar-containing drinks, or hard candy when a hypoglycemic reaction begins. Explain importance of reporting such problems to the health care provider.

• Direct client to take oral antidiabetics with food to decrease gastric irritation.

Cultural Considerations ❖

• Respect client's cultural beliefs and alternative method for treating "sugar in the urine" and elevated blood sugar levels. Discuss with client (the use of an interpreter may be necessary) the safety of the methods and the use of oral antidiabetic drugs to correct the problem. If client takes an oral antidiabetic drug to decrease the blood glucose level, emphasize the importance of checking the blood sugar levels daily or as indicated. Hypoglycemic reaction can result from increased doses of oral antidiabetic agents and insufficient dietary intake.

EVALUATION

■ Evaluate the effectiveness of drug therapy by noting whether blood sugar levels are within the accepted range.

Other Antidiabetic Agents

Exenatide (Byetta) is an antidiabetic agent from Amylin Pharmaceuticals and Eli Lilly and Company that was approved by the FDA in April 2005. This agent has been placed in a new classification of drugs known as *incretin mimetics* that improve beta-cell responsiveness, which improves glucose control in people with type 2 diabetes mellitus. The actions of exenatide are to enhance insulin secretion, increase beta-cell responsiveness, suppress glucagon secretion, slow gastric emptying, and reduce food intake. Exenatide is not a substitute for insulin and should not be administered to patients with type 1 diabetes mellitus, diabetic ketoacidosis, severe renal dysfunction, or severe GI disease. Common adverse effects that occur with exenatide include headache, dizziness, jitteriness, nausea, vomiting, and diarrhea. Exenatide is administered by injectable prefilled pens in twice-a-day dosing and has significantly improved A1C levels and weight loss in many individuals.

Pramlintide acetate (Symlin) is another antidiabetic agent from Amylin Pharmaceuticals, approved by the FDA in March 2005 for adults with type 1 and type 2 diabetes mellitus. The primary purpose of pramlintide is to improve postprandial glucose control in diabetic patients who are using insulin but are unable to achieve and maintain glucose control. The actions of pramlintide are to suppress glucagon secretion, slow gastric emptying, and modulate appetite by inducing satiety. Suppression of glucagon secretion reduces postprandial hepatic glucose for approximately 3 hours. By slowing gastric emptying, the absorption rate of glucose is reduced. Satiety promotes reduced food intake. Common adverse effects include dizziness, anorexia, nausea, vomiting, and fatigue. Pramlintide is administered by subcutaneous injection before meals in the abdomen or thigh; it is never given in the arm.

Hyperglycemic Drugs

Glucagon

Glucagon is a hyperglycemic hormone secreted by the alpha cells of the islets of Langerhans in the pancreas. Glucagon increases blood sugar by stimulating glycogenolysis (glycogen breakdown) in the liver. It protects the body cells, especially those in the brain and retina, by providing the nutrients and energy needed to maintain body function.

Glucagon is available for parenteral use (subQ, IM, and IV). It is used to treat insulin-induced hypoglycemia when other methods of providing glucose are not available. For example, the client may be semiconscious or unconscious and unable to ingest sugar-containing products. Clients with diabetes who are prone to severe hypoglycemic reactions (insulin shock) should keep glucagon in the home, and family members should be taught how to administer subQ or IM injections during an emergency hypoglycemic reaction. The blood glucose level begins to increase within 5 to 20 minutes after administration. Recently IV glucagon has been used in the acute treatment of beta-blocker overdose and profound shock.

Diazoxide

Oral diazoxide (Proglycem), which is chemically related to thiazide diuretics, increases blood sugar by inhibiting insulin release from the beta cells and stimulating release of epinephrine (Adrenalin) from the adrenal medulla. This drug is not indicated for hypoglycemic reaction; rather, it is used to treat chronic hypoglycemia caused by hyperinsulinism due to islet cell cancer or hyperplasia. The parenteral form of diazoxide (Hyperstat) is prescribed for malignant hypertension. Hypotension does not usually occur with oral diazoxide.

Diazoxide has a long half-life and is highly protein-bound. Its onset of action is 1 hour, and the duration of action is 8 hours. Most of the drug is excreted unchanged in urine.

Critical Thinking Case Study

TC, age 32, was diagnosed with diabetes mellitus after the birth of her first child; her blood sugar level was 180 mg/dl. Her serum glucose level has been maintained within the normal range with acetohexamide 251 mg/daily.

1. Why was TC, at her age, taking an oral antidiabetic drug instead of insulin?
2. Acetohexamide is indicated for what type of diabetes mellitus? When should acetohexamide not be taken?
3. Should acetohexamide be taken with sulfonamides, aspirin, NSAIDs, cimetidine, alcohol, or insulin? Why or why not?
4. Why should TC monitor her blood sugar using a home glucometer?

Two years later, TC became pregnant again. Acetohexamide was discontinued, and Humulin N insulin 25 units was prescribed. Since the birth of her second child, she has remained on Humulin N 25 U daily.

5. Give a possible reason why the health care provider changed the antidiabetic drug to insulin when TC became pregnant.
6. Humulin N is similar to what other type of insulin? How do these two types differ?
7. Give the onset, peak, and duration of action for Humulin N insulin. When is an insulin reaction most likely to occur with Humulin N?
8. What are the pros and cons for TC to receive Humulin 70/30 insulin?
9. What are the signs and symptoms of a hypoglycemic reaction?
10. What should be included in client teaching?

TC asks the nurse if she can take acetohexamide again instead of insulin, because she is eating the "right foods."

11. What should the response be?

NCLEX Study Questions

1. A client is diagnosed with type 2 diabetes mellitus. The nurse is aware that which of the following is true?
   a. Client is most likely a teenager
   b. Client is most likely a child under 10
   c. Heredity and obesity are major causative factors
   d. Viral infections contribute most to disease development

2. Antidiabetic drugs are designed to control signs and symptoms of diabetes mellitus. The nurse primarily expects a decrease in:
   a. blood glucose
   b. fat metabolism
   c. glycogen storage
   d. protein mobilization

3. A client is to receive insulin prior to breakfast, and breakfast tray delivery is variable. The nurse knows that _____ insulin should not be administered until the breakfast tray has arrived and the client is ready to eat.
   a. Humulin N
   b. Humalog (Lispro)
   c. glargine (Lantus)
   d. regular Humulin R

4. A client is receiving a daily dose of Humulin N insulin at 7:30 AM. The nurse expects the peak effect of this drug to occur at:
   a. 8:15 AM
   b. 10:30 AM
   c. 5:00 PM
   d. 11:00 PM

5. When the client is prescribed glipizide (Glucotrol), the nurse knows that side effects/adverse effects include:
   a. tachypnea
   b. tachycardia
   c. increased alertness
   d. increased weight gain

EIGHTEEN

Reproductive and Gender-Related Agents

This unit comprises seven chapters that focus on reproductive and gender-related drugs. Chapters 52, 53, 54, and 55 address agents specifically associated with female health and disorders. Drugs used throughout the female reproductive cycle, including pregnancy and preterm labor, are comprehensively discussed in Chapter 52, Female Reproductive Cycle I: Pregnancy and Preterm Labor Drugs. Chapter 53, Female Reproductive Cycle II: Labor, Delivery, and Preterm Neonatal Drugs, covers labor and delivery. Chapter 54, Postpartum and Newborn Drugs, focuses on the pharmacology of the postpartum and neonatal period. Chapter 55, Drugs for Women's Health and Reproductive Disorders, details the variety of oral contraceptive products and the drugs used to treat uterine dysfunction, including premenstrual syndrome, endometriosis, and menopausal discomforts. Chapter 56, Drugs for Men's Health and Reproductive Disorders, describes androgens and anabolic steroids, antiandrogens, and other drugs related to male reproductive health and disorders. Chapter 57, Drugs for Infertility and Sexually Transmitted Diseases, concludes this unit with a discussion of drugs used for these specific reproductive health issues.

Female Reproductive Processes

The uterus is a pear-shaped, hollow, very muscular organ located in the pelvic cavity between the rectum and the bladder; it is connected to the vagina by the cervix (Figure XVIII–1). Three distinct layers compose the uterine wall: the outer layer (perimetrium); the muscular middle layer (myometrium); and the inner mucosal layer (endometrium).

The myometrium is a network of involuntary (smooth) muscles divided into three layers, with the muscles of each layer configured in different patterns. For example, the outer muscles are arranged longitudinally to assist with cervical effacement (thinning and shortening) and to expel the fetus at the time of delivery. Muscles in the middle layer are arranged in a figure-8 design. These muscles are extremely important in the control of bleeding (hemostasis). Blood vessels are threaded throughout these muscles, and when a contraction occurs, the vessels are

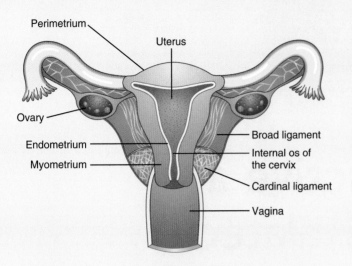

FIGURE XVIII–1 Anatomy of the female reproductive system.

compressed, creating a hemostatic effect. Circular muscle fibers are found in the area of the internal os and help control its sphincter. These circular muscles keep the fetus contained in the uterus for the normal gestational period. It is these muscles that stretch (dilate) the cervix to a diameter of 10 cm during labor. When all three muscle layers work together during labor, contractions cause cervical dilation and descent and delivery of the infant.

The Menstrual Cycle

The reproductive cycle is hormonally controlled by interactions between the endocrine and reproductive systems. The hypothalamus secretes gonadotropin-releasing hormone (Gn-RH), which stimulates the anterior pituitary to synthesize and release follicle-stimulating hormone (FSH) and luteinizing hormone (LH). These gonadotropins stimulate the ovaries to produce estrogen and progesterone, respectively.

In most women the menstrual cycle lasts 28 days (range of 22 to 34 days). The ovarian hormones estrogen and progesterone regulate the cycle, which has three ovarian phases: follicular, ovulatory, and luteal. Endometrial phases occur simultaneously with these ovarian phases.

The *follicular phase* occurs during days 1 to 14 of the cycle. Days 1 to 6 of this period constitute the menstrual phase and days 7 to 14, the proliferative phase. During the total 14-day period, FSH increases and follicles begin to mature within the ovary. One graafian follicle from the group matures and swells by days 10 to 13, ruptures on day 14, and releases the ovum to the fallopian tube. The *ovulatory phase* occurs on day 14 when the ovum is released. The *luteal phase* occurs from days 15 to 28 and includes the secretory phase of the endometrial cycle. During this period, estrogen and progesterone are produced by the ovarian corpus luteum (the ruptured graafian follicle), reaching peak levels 8 days into the phase. Changes occur in the endometrium for optimal implantation of a fertilized ovum. FSH and LH levels decrease, mediated by dopa-

mine, norepinephrine, and serotonin. Estrogen and progesterone are withdrawn immediately before menstruation, and the endometrial prostaglandin level increases. The cycle begins anew with the follicular phase. In cycles that are nonovulatory, hormonal secretion of estrogen, FSH, and LH is erratic; there is also an alteration in the usual amount of progesterone. These physiologic alterations become the basis for planning and implementing pharmacologic interventions.

Male Reproductive Processes

There are three male reproductive processes: *spermatogenesis*, or sperm production; regulation of male sexual functioning; and sexual intercourse.

Male Reproductive Anatomy and Physiology

The anatomy of the male sexual organs is depicted in Figure XVIII–2. The external reproductive organs include the penis, the scrotum, and the testes. The penis consists of three cylindrical bodies of erectile tissue: two corpora cavernosa and the corpus spongiosum. With sexual excitement, the vascular spaces fill with blood to produce an erection (Figure XVIII–3).

The scrotum has two compartments, each of which holds a testis, epididymis, and spermatic cord. The spermatic cord supports the testis and includes the vas deferens, blood vessels, nerves, and muscle fibers.

Each testis contains seminiferous tubules in which spermatogenesis occurs. The sperm then move into the epididymis. This leads into the vas deferens, the source of about 20% of ejaculate, or semen. On either side of the prostate gland, a seminal vesicle empties seminal fluid into the ampulla. Seminal fluid contains fructose to provide energy for the sperm, prostaglandins, fibrinogen, and a sperm-activating factor.

The contents of the ampulla and the seminal vesicles empty into an ejaculatory duct that leads through the body of the prostate to empty into the urethra. Prostatic fluid, which constitutes about 20% of semen, empties from the prostate gland into the ejaculatory duct. The urethra carries semen to its distal end. The urethral glands along the length of the urethra and the bulbourethral glands near the prostatic end of the urethra supply the urethra with mucus. The bulbourethral glands secrete alkaline preejaculatory fluid to protect sperm from the acidity of the urethra.

Hormonal Regulation of Male Reproductive Functioning and Spermatogenesis

Gn-RH from the hypothalamus stimulates the anterior pituitary gland to secrete two major gonadotropins, LH and FSH, in both men and women. LH stimulates the interstitial Leydig cells of the testes to mature and produce testosterone. There is a direct relationship between the amount

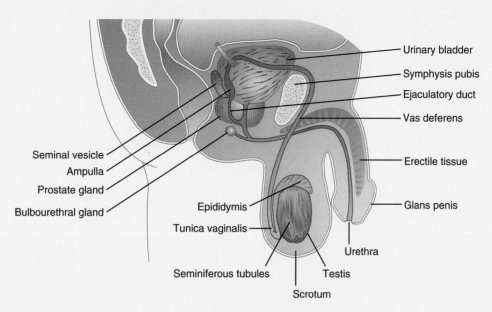

FIGURE XVIII–2 Anatomy of the male reproductive system.

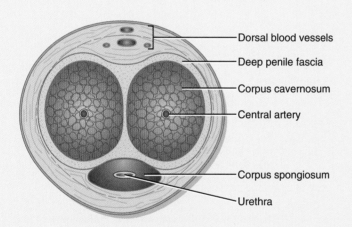

FIGURE XVIII–3 Erectile tissue of the penis.

of circulating LH and the amount of testosterone produced. Testosterone is also produced to a lesser extent in the adrenal cortex and in the ovaries of women.

In men, FSH stimulates the Sertoli cells to begin conversion of spermatids into mature sperm. In addition, the Sertoli cells are stimulated to secrete estrogens, which may promote spermatogenesis. For spermatogenesis to be complete, testosterone must be secreted simultaneously by the Leydig cells and diffused into the seminiferous tubules.

Testosterone is the precursor of two classes of sex steroids: 5-alpha-reduced androgens and estrogens. The net effect of endogenous androgens is the sum of the effects of the 5-alpha-reduced metabolite *dihydrotestosterone* and its estrogen derivative, *estradiol*. Most testosterone is loosely bound by plasma protein and circulates for 15 to 30 minutes before it is fixed to target tissues or metabolized. Most testosterone fixed to target cells is then converted to its active form, dihydrotestosterone.

The rate of testosterone production is controlled by a negative feedback loop. With increased testosterone, the hypothalamus decreases production of Gn-RH (Figure XVIII–4). With sperm production, the Sertoli cells release a hormone called *inhibin*, which suppresses FSH production by the anterior pituitary, maintaining a constant rate of spermatogenesis. It is not known how, before puberty, the brain stimulates the hypothalamus to begin Gn-RH secretion, but if the brain is not intact, this may not occur.

Sexual Function

The human sexual response cycle consists of five phases: desire, excitement, plateau, orgasm, and resolution. Sexual desire is the stimulus that causes an individual to initiate or be receptive to sexual activity. During the excitement phase, the man experiences penile erection. Men are incapable of engaging in sexual intercourse without this arousal. The plateau phase is characterized by genital enlargement, mucous secretion, generalized muscle tension, hyperventilation, tachycardia, and increased blood pressure. During the orgasmic phase, the vas deferens, seminal vesicles, ejaculatory duct, and penile urethra contract three or four times over a few seconds causing the man to ejaculate. During resolution, there is a refractory period in which pelvic vasocongestion declines and generalized muscle relaxation takes place.

Process of Fertilization

Fertilization, or *conception*, occurs when a sperm penetrates an ovum, usually in the distal third of the fallopian tube.

In a single ejaculation, between 200 and 400 million spermatozoa are deposited in the vagina. Sperm move up the female reproductive tract using the flagellar motion of their tails. It takes an average of 4 to 6 hours for the sperm to reach the distal fallopian tube. Semen contains prosta-

FIGURE XVIII–4 Hypothalamic-pituitary-gonadal feedback loops. (From Fogel CI, Lauver D: *Sexual health promotion*, Philadelphia, 1990, Saunders, p. 339.)

glandins that may enhance uterine motility to facilitate sperm migration. The ciliary action of the fallopian tubes enhances migration of the ovum to the uterus and of sperm toward the ovary.

Uterine enzymes capacitate the sperm by altering their glycoprotein coat. In an acrosomal reaction, the sperm release the enzyme hyaluronidase, which breaks through the outer layer of the ovum. The moment one sperm penetrates the ovum, a chemical reaction occurs that blocks other sperm from entering. Cellular division begins immediately in what is now called the *zygote*, or fertilized egg.

After 3 days, the zygote enters the uterus. It has now differentiated into an inner solid mass of cells, the *blastocyst,* and an outer layer, the *trophoblast.* Progesterone secreted by the corpus luteum of the ovary maintains a favorable uter-

ine environment to nourish the blastocyst until *implantation* in the uterine lining occurs. The blastocyst develops into the embryo and the amniotic membrane, whereas the trophoblast develops into the chorionic membrane and the fetal side of the placenta. The maternal portion of the placenta develops under the site of the blastocyst's implantation. The *placenta* is the structure through which oxygen, nutrients, and metabolic wastes pass between the maternal and fetal circulations for the duration of pregnancy. The placenta begins to function by the fourth week of pregnancy. Within the first 8 weeks of pregnancy, organ systems are differentiated, and it is during this period that the fetus is most vulnerable to teratogens. Growth of the fetus throughout pregnancy depends on adequate oxygenation and nutrition, the metabolic environment, freedom from infection, and integrity of the mother's reproductive tract.

52

Female Reproductive Cycle I: Pregnancy and Preterm Labor Drugs

Robin Webb Corbett and Laura K. Williford Owens

ELECTRONIC RESOURCES

Evolve website (http://evolve.elsevier.com/KeeHayes/pharmacology/):
- *Case Studies*
- *Content Updates*
- *Frequently Asked Questions*
- *Student Review Activities*
- *WebLinks*
- *Additional Reference Material*

Companion CD-ROM:
- *NCLEX Examination Review Questions*
- *Pharmacology Animations*
- *IV Therapy Checklists*
- *Medication Error Checklists*
- *Drug Calculation Problems*
- *Electronic Calculators*
- *Top 200 Drugs with Pronunciations*
- *References from the Textbook*

Objectives

- Explain potential health-promoting and detrimental effects of substances ingested by the woman during the prenatal period.
- Describe the drugs that alter uterine muscle contractility.
- Describe drug therapy used during preterm labor to decrease the incidence or severity of neonatal respiratory dysfunction.
- Describe systemic and regional medications for pain control during labor.
- Describe the drugs used in gestational hypertension.
- Describe the nursing process, including client teaching, associated with the drugs used during pregnancy and preterm labor.

Terms. . . . .

. . . .

This chapter focuses on the pharmacologic aspects of pregnancy in cycle I and labor and delivery in cycle II. Topics include prenatal health promotion and drugs used for uterine dysfunction during labor and delivery, pain control during labor, and gestational hypertension.

Physiology of Pregnancy

Because pregnancy is a change in the normal physiology of the body, the normal and expected pharmacokinetics and pharmacodynamics of medications also change. Some of the changes in drug action during pregnancy include (1) the effect of circulating steroid hormones on the liver's metabolism of drugs, (2) a woman's reduced gastrointestinal motility and increased gastric pH, (3) increased glomerular filtration rate and increased renal perfusion, resulting in more rapid renal excretion of drugs, (4) expanded maternal circulating blood volume, resulting in dilution of drugs, and (5) alteration in the clearance of drugs in later pregnancy, resulting in a decrease in serum and tissue concentrations of drugs. Because of the alteration in the normal physiology of the body, medications should not be ordered in lower doses with longer intervals between doses because of the possibility of subtherapeutic serum and tissue concentrations.

In addition to the aforementioned effects on medication during pregnancy, other factors, such as late pregnancy and labor, can alter the half-lives of some medications. Antibiotics and barbiturates are examples of medications that have shorter half-lives during pregnancy. In contrast to later pregnancy, labor can actually increase the half-life of some medications—analgesics, hypnotics, and antibiotics, for example. Labor affects half-life, because it is believed that drug clearance decreases as a result of transient reduced blood flow associated with uterine contractions when the mother is in a supine position. In certain disease states during pregnancy, concern arises as to the effects of these conditions on medication. Disorders such as diabetes and gestational hypertension may result in decreased renal perfusion and subsequent drug accumulation.

The placenta plays an important role in drug use and metabolism. It was thought for some time that the placenta played a barrier role, but it is now known that the placenta plays a major role as the organ of exchange for numerous substances, including medications. It allows some substances to transfer quickly or slowly between mother and fetus, depending on variables such as (1) maternal and fetal blood flow, (2) the molecular weight of the substance (low-molecular-weight substances cross more readily than do higher-molecular-weight substances, and most medications fall into the low-molecular-weight class, which means they would readily cross the placenta), (3) the degree of ionization of the drug molecule (the more ionized the molecule, the less readily it crosses the placenta), (4) the degree of protein-binding (highly bound drugs do not cross readily), (5) the metabolic activity of the placenta (the metabolic activity can biotransform molecules into active metabolites that can affect the fetus), and (6) maternal dose.

Guidelines for medication administration during pregnancy must include determination that the benefits of prescribing a drug outweigh potential short- or long-term risks to the maternal-fetal system. Careful selection and monitoring for the minimum effective dose for the shortest interval in the therapeutic range are required. Consideration must be given to alterations related to the physiologic changes of pregnancy.

Liver metabolism of medications is much slower in the fetus as a result of the immaturity of the liver. Therefore drug metabolism is slower in the fetus, which can cause more evident or longer drug effects than on the mother. The degree of fetal exposure to a drug and its breakdown products are more important to fetal outcome than the rate at which the drug is transported to the fetus.

The mechanisms by which drugs cross the placenta are analogous to the way in which drugs infiltrate breast tissue. Lactation results in increased blood flow to the breasts, and drugs accumulate in adipose breast tissue through simple diffusion. Long-term effects on infants from drugs in breast milk are unknown, but medications that do accumulate in breast milk are known, and the breastfeeding mother should be alerted to the potential accumulation.

Despite prenatal education, public service announcements, and information conveyed through the media, use of legal and illicit drugs by pregnant women continues. Additionally, health care providers may prescribe drugs for maternal disorders that indirectly affect the fetus. However, it is important to note that most drugs required by pregnant women can be used safely. It is estimated that half the medications taken by pregnant women are over-the-counter (OTC) drugs. The drugs most commonly ingested during pregnancy (other than illicit drugs) are iron supplements and vitamins, antiemetics, antacids, stool softeners, nasal decongestants, mild analgesics, and antibiotics. Pregnant women who use or have questions regarding the use of OTC medications should be discouraged from using such medications until they consult with their health care provider or their pharmacist.

Drugs conclusively determined to be safe for the embryo are limited in number. Clinical trials can be resources for reliable drug information; however, it is unethical to test for the safety and efficacy of medications in pregnant women. Animal studies are required during drug testing, but the information obtained from such studies is difficult to extrapolate to humans. Case reports used for such information can be of limited value because they usually present isolated occurrences. A commonly used source of information about drug safety in pregnancy is the Food and Drug Administration's (FDA) category system. The categories were created to assist with safe prescribing and informed counseling of the pregnant patient requiring medication.

There are many known **teratogens** (substances that cause developmental abnormalities). Timing, dose, and duration of exposure are of crucial importance in determining the teratogenicity of a given drug. In humans the teratogenic period begins 2 weeks after conception. During the first 2 weeks, the embryo is not susceptible to teratogenesis. At this time of development, exposure to teratogens may result in either death of the embryo or minor cellular damage without congenital birth defects. From 2 gestational weeks through the next 10 weeks is the period of organogenesis (development of major structures and organs). Examples of adverse effects of selected illicit substances commonly used during pregnancy are presented in Table 52–1.

Therapeutic Drug and Herbal Use in Pregnancy

The most common indications for use of medications during pregnancy are nutritional supplementation with iron, vitamins, and minerals and treatment of nausea and vomiting, gastric acidity, and mild discomforts, but caution must be exercised (Herbal Alert 52–1).

Herbal ALERT 52–1

Pregnancy

Just as prescription and over-the-counter (OTC) medications are not generally recommended during pregnancy, herbal preparations are also to be avoided. The following herbs in particular should be avoided:
- *Sage:* stimulates uterus
- *Kava kava:* decreases platelets
- *Garlic* and *gingko biloba:* increase bleeding when used with anticoagulants
- *Ginseng:* may decrease action of anticoagulants
- *St. Johns wort:* mutagenic risk to cells of developing embryo and fetus

Use of these herbal products may be especially deleterious during pregnancy.

Iron

During pregnancy, approximately twice the normal amount of iron is needed to meet fetal and maternal daily requirements: 27 mg daily during pregnancy compared with 18 mg daily for nonpregnant women 19 to 30 years of age. Supplementation with iron is not generally necessary until the second trimester, when the fetus begins to store iron; the goal is to prevent *maternal* iron deficiency anemia, not to supply the fetus. The fetus is adequately supplied through the placenta, although the mother is deficient. The time of greatest iron demand is during the third trimester: 22.4 mg daily compared with 6.4 mg daily and 18.8 mg daily for the first and second trimesters (National Academy of Sciences, 2000, p. 347).

Although a normal diet generally provides the 18-mg recommended daily allowance (RDA) of iron for nonpregnant clients, nonanemic pregnant women are usually instructed to supplement using a dosage that provides 60 mg of elemental iron; anemic clients should receive 120 mg of elemental iron. The elemental iron content of the most common iron salts includes ferrous sulfate 20% (300 mg of ferrous sulfate is equivalent to 60 mg elemental iron), exsiccated ferrous sulfate 30%, ferrous gluconate 12%, and ferrous fumarate 33%. The estimated net iron cost of pregnancy is approximately 800-1000 mg. This iron cost is calculated as 250 mg basal losses + 320 mg deposition in fetal and placental tissue + 500 mg increased hemoglobin mass + 350 mg iron loss in blood associated with delivery (National Academy of Sciences, 2000, pp. 345-346). Clients are advised to continue supplements for 6 weeks postpartum.

Pregnant women generally have a decreased hematocrit early in the third trimester. Those with levels less than 30% will have their supplemental iron dosages increased and complete blood counts with platelet and ferritin measured. In those found to have true iron-deficiency anemia, response to iron supplementation is usually noted in 5 to 7 days, with a modest reticulocytosis and a rise in the hemoglobin in 3 weeks. No teratogenic effects have been reported with physiologic doses. Numerous OTC and prescription iron products are available in varying dosages, which differ in the amount of elemental iron contained in the form of iron salts. Examples are listed in Table 52–2.

Adverse Reactions

Common side effects of iron supplements include nausea, constipation, black tarry stools, gastrointestinal irritation, epigastric pain, vomiting, and diarrhea.

Nursing Implications

Liquid forms can cause temporary discoloration of the teeth and therefore should be diluted and administered through a plastic straw. Iron supplements are best absorbed on an empty stomach and when administered with water or juice (concurrent administration of 200 mg ascorbic acid/vitamin C per 30 mg of elemental iron increases

Table 52-1

General Adverse Effects of Selected Substances Commonly Abused during Pregnancy

Substance	Maternal Effects	Fetal Effects*
Alcohol (high risk: 6 oz or more/d)	1 oz (2 drinks) absolute alcohol 2 ×/wk: increased risk of spontaneous abortion (2-4 times)	Fetal alcohol syndrome (FAS): mild to moderate mental retardation, altered facial features, growth retardation, low birth weight, small head circumference, hypotonia, and poor motor coordination. Full FAS seen only in some children; others display only fetal alcohol effect (FAE)
Caffeine	2 cups increase epinephrine concentrations after 30 min and decrease intervillous blood flow with potential for spontaneous abortion (dosage and gestational period related)	Excess consumption (>6-8 cups/d) likely toxic to embryo. No evidence of teratogenicity
Cocaine	48-h clearance via urine. Increased incidence of spontaneous abortion in first trimester. Continued use or sporadic use related to premature delivery and abruptio placentae secondary to placental vasoconstriction and hyperextension	4-5 d clearance time via urine of newborn because of liver immaturity and lack of cholinesterase. Intrauterine growth retardation, decreased head circumference, intrauterine cerebral infarction. No true withdrawal syndrome, but increased irritability, hyperreflexia, and tremulousness. Deficient organization and interactive abilities. By month 4, still exhibits hypertonicity, tremulousness, and impaired motor development. By month 6, effects may appear to be self-limited, but long-term research needed
Heroin	First trimester spontaneous abortion, premature delivery, inadequate maternal calorie and protein intake	Neonatal meconium aspiration syndrome; decreased weight and length through postnatal month 9 (weight and length catch up by month 12); smaller head circumference (with no catch up); impaired interactive abilities (hard to console and engage); inconsistent behavioral responses; increased tremulousness and irritability
Marijuana	Heavy use (5 or more marijuana cigarettes per week): shortened gestation (<37 wk); may hasten delivery through uterine stimulation	No higher incidence of serious birth defects caused solely by marijuana. Higher incidence of meconium passage during labor
Tobacco/nicotine	Degenerative placental lesions with areas of poor oxygen exchange; higher incidence of abruptio placentae; placenta previa, vaginal bleeding during pregnancy; possible PROM; possible amnionitis; less likely to choose to breastfeed	Short stature, smaller head and arm circumferences; no increase in mortality rate or congenital anomalies (some evidence of increased oral clefts); increased respiratory infections beyond the perinatal period; possible shorter attention span beyond perinatal period
Methadone	If taken before pregnancy, will need to slow detoxification during pregnancy and decrease dose 5 mg every 2 wk. Do not detoxify before week 14 of gestation because of increased risk of spontaneous abortion	Smaller weight and length through postnatal month 9 (catch up on weight and length by month 12); smaller head circumference (no catch up); withdrawal-induced fetal distress if mother detoxifies after week 32 of gestation
Barbiturates	CNS depression; lethargy; sleepiness; subtle mood alterations and impaired judgment/fine motor skills for 24 h No known inhibitory effect on uterine tone or contractility. Selective anticonvulsant activity without anesthesia effects may warrant use in pregnancy for seizure disorders Active labor with imminent delivery is a contraindication, because no antagonist drug is available	Rapidly cross placenta; with excessive use/high doses cause CNS depression, leading to respiratory depression, hyperactivity, and decreased sucking reflex
Tranquilizers	Dose-dependent; toxic reactions include ataxia, syncope, vertigo, and drowsiness; control of acute eclamptic seizures during labor	Benzodiazepine (diazepam [Valium]) use in first trimester not associated with oral clefts or other anomalies. Chronic third trimester or labor exposure in high doses associated with hypotonia, hypothermia, hyperbilirubinemia, and poor sucking reflex. Effects may be enhanced if systemic analgesics also given to mother. Fetal effects are prolonged

*Inner city children with prenatal drug exposure scored significantly lower on measures of language, school readiness skills, impulse control and visual attention span/sequencing at 5 years of age when compared to nondrug exposed children from a comparable environment (Pulsifer, Butz, Forzn & Belcher, 2008).

CNS, Central nervous system; d, day; h, hour; min, minute; PROM, premature rupture of fetal membranes; wk, week; <, less than; >, greater than.

Table 52–2

Iron Products

Generic (Brand)	Route and Dosage	Uses and Considerations
Ferrous sulfate (Fer-In-Sol, Feosol, Fero-Gradumet, Mol-Iron, Fer-Iron)	A: PO: 300-600 mg/d in divided doses 325 mg/d sufficient to meet needs of non-iron-deficient pregnant client; with iron deficiency, should receive 325 mg 2-3 ×/d	Hematinic; for iron deficiency anemia; prophylaxis for iron deficiency in pregnancy. Replaces iron stores needed for RBC development Absorption PO is 5%-30% in intestines; therefore GI side effects. Toxic reactions include pallor, hematemesis, shock, cardiovascular collapse, and metabolic acidosis. Contraindicated in hypersensitivity and peptic ulcer. Decreased absorption of tetracycline, penicillamine, and antacids; increased absorption with ascorbic acid; decreased absorption with eggs, milk, coffee, and tea. Can reduce availability of zinc from the diet *Nursing implications:* Taking iron at bedtime helps avoid GI upset. Absorption of iron is promoted when taken with orange juice or other vitamin C source. Use straw (elixir); swallow tablet/capsule whole; take with water on empty stomach. Sit upright 30 min after dose to decrease reflux. Increase fluids, activity, and dietary bulk. Keep away from children Peak reticulocytosis: 5-10 d; hemoglobin values increase: 2-4 wk *Pregnancy category:* A; PB: UK; t½: UK; onset: 3-10 d; duration: 3-4 mo
Ferrous gluconate (Fergon) Ferrous fumarate (Fumasorb, Femiron, Feostat, Fumerin)	A: PO: 200-600 mg t.i.d. A: PO: 200 mg t.i.d. or q.i.d.	Same as above Same as above

A, Adult; *d*, day; *GI*, gastrointestinal; *min*, minute; *mo*, month; *PB*, protein-binding; *PO*, by mouth; *q.i.d.*, four times a day; *RBC*, red blood cell; *t½*, half-life; *t.i.d.*, three times a day; *UK*, unknown; *wk*, week.

the absorption of iron). However, if gastric irritation does occur, administer with food. Iron supplementation may inhibit the absorption of several medications, and appropriate separation of the doses should be followed. For example, iron supplementation should be administered 2 hours before or 4 hours after antacids. Additional examples of medications that may require separation in dose include levodopa, levothyroxine, methyldopa, penicillamine, quinolones, and tetracyclines. For the same reasons, do not administer iron with milk, cereals, tea, coffee, or eggs.

Folic Acid

Folic acid supplementation as part of pre-conception planning improves the outcome of pregnancy. During pregnancy, folic acid (vitamin B$_9$, folate) is needed in increased amounts. Folic acid deficiency early in pregnancy can result in spontaneous abortion or birth defects, especially neural tube defects (failure of the embryonic neural tube to close properly, leading to spina bifida or skull and brain malformations). Deficiency of folic acid may also contribute to premature birth, low birth weight, and premature separation of the placenta *(abruptio placentae)*. In the United States, approximately 4000 pregnancies a year are affected by neural tube defects. Controlled clinical trials have demonstrated that folic acid supplementation can reduce this incidence by as much as 50%.

The RDA for folic acid in the nonpregnant client is 180 mcg, but the American College of Obstetricians and Gynecologists (ACOG) recommends that all women of childbearing age ingest 400 mcg of folic acid daily for birth defect prevention. (During pregnancy the RDA rises to 600 mcg.) The reason behind ACOG's recommendation is the high incidence of unplanned and unrecognized pregnancies. The neural tube closes within the first 4 weeks of pregnancy (18-26 days after conception); therefore it is important that women consume the recommended amounts of folic acid per day. For women who have had a pregnancy that was affected by a neural tube defect, higher doses of folic acid are recommended: 4 mg starting 1 to 3 months before conception.

The recommended amount should be ingested from folate-enriched foods and supplementation, because the amount of naturally occurring folic acid ingested in foods will vary from day to day, and the folic acid from these sources is not well absorbed. Examples of folate-enriched foods include bread, rolls, flour, cornmeal, rice, pasta, and cereals.

Adverse Reactions

Side effects of folic acid supplementation are not common but include allergic bronchospasm, rash, pruritus, erythema, and general malaise. Clients should be aware that folic acid supplementation may cause urine to turn more intensely yellow.

Multiple Vitamins

Prenatal vitamin preparations are routinely recommended for pregnant women. These preparations generally supply vitamins A, D, E, C, B complex (B_1, B_2, B_3, B_5, B_6), B_{12}, iron, calcium, and other minerals. The role of prenatal vitamins in preventing congenital defects (e.g., cleft lip or palate, limb defects) remains undetermined.

Poor food habits cannot be rectified through supplements alone; vitamins are used most effectively by the body when taken with meals. Calories and protein are not supplied by supplements.

Megadoses of vitamins and minerals during pregnancy will not improve health and may cause harm to the fetus, the pregnant client, or both. Large doses of vitamin A can be teratogenic, and excessive ingestion of vitamins D, E, and K may also be toxic.

Practitioners should consider cultural food practices and beliefs in regard to the use of prenatal vitamins. For example, in Mexico some people view vitamins as a *hot* food that should not be ingested during pregnancy (Darby 2007). Cultural sensitivity is important in assessment and teaching regarding herbs, foods, and nonprescription and prescription drugs.

Drugs for Minor Discomforts of Pregnancy

The average prenatal client uses three drugs during pregnancy, two of which are vitamin and mineral supplements. Drug ingestion is most likely during the first and the third trimesters, when the minor discomforts of pregnancy tend to be most bothersome. Many of the complaints associated with pregnancy will be related to the gastrointestinal (GI) tract (nausea and vomiting, heartburn, constipation). The etiology of nausea and vomiting is unclear. Physiologically, nausea is purported to be related to increased human chorionic gonadotropin (hCG) levels of pregnancy. The increased progesterone of pregnancy, which relaxes smooth muscle, contributes to the discomforts of heartburn and constipation. The physiologic reason is that elevated female sex hormones during pregnancy change the motility of the GI tract. Additionally, the enlarging uterus displaces the bowel.

Nausea and Vomiting

Nausea and vomiting (morning sickness) during early pregnancy are major complaints for most (about 88%) pregnant women, but *hyperemesis gravidarum* (severe nausea and vomiting which may require hospitalization for hydration and nutrition) occurs with much lower incidence (1% to 3%). Nausea and vomiting are common, possibly because of increased levels of hCG, estrogens, and progesterone, and changes in the metabolism of carbohydrates. Nonpharmacologic measures to decrease nausea and vomiting include (1) eating crackers, dry toast, bread, dry cereal, or other complex carbohydrates before rising; (2) avoiding fatty or highly seasoned foods; (3) eating small, frequent meals; (4) drinking fluids between rather than with meals; (5) drinking apple juice or flat carbonated beverages between meals; (6) eating a high-protein bedtime snack; (7) stopping or cutting down on smoking; and (8) taking an iron supplement at bedtime. These measures work well for most women, but if vomiting is severe, fluid replacement and pharmacologic measures may be necessary.

The Food and Drug Administration (FDA) has *not* approved any drug for morning sickness, nor is there consensus among health care providers who do prescribe drug therapy as to the best agents. Antiemetic drug studies often find that affected women rate even placebo agents as helpful. Examples of commonly used antiemetics include phenothiazines (promethazine), antihistamines (doxylamine), anticholinergics (scopolamine), prokinetic agents (metoclopramide), and ginger. Table 52–3 presents examples of the most commonly used drugs for management of nausea and vomiting during pregnancy.

Many women may choose to use ginger to help treat nausea and vomiting associated with pregnancy, but there is insufficient evidence to determine the safety and efficacy of its use during pregnancy. Recent studies suggest that ginger can be safely used, but as with all medications and herbal supplements, encourage the pregnant client to discuss the use of ginger with her health care provider.

Women who experience nausea and vomiting may experience gastric distress if they are also taking supplemental iron; taking the iron supplement with food, at bedtime, or temporary suspension of therapy may help. It is suggested that prenatal vitamins be taken at the time of day the client is least likely to experience emesis, because there is a high incidence of nausea and vomiting associated with prenatal vitamins. For clients with continued iron-induced gastric distress, many health care providers recommend taking two Flintstones vitamins with iron. Salting food to taste may help to replace vomited chloride; foods rich in potassium and magnesium may also help replace lost nutrients.

Clients whose symptoms persist and who experience weight loss and dehydration may require intravenous (IV) rehydration, including replacement of electrolytes and vitamins. Antiemetic therapy (probably with phenothiazines) may be used.

Heartburn

Heartburn *(pyrosis)* is a burning sensation in the epigastric and sternal regions that occurs with reflux of acidic stomach contents. The incidence of heartburn during pregnancy is common, up to 80%. Pregnant clients experience decreased motility in the GI tract as a result of the normal increase in the hormone **progesterone**. Progesterone also relaxes the cardiac sphincter (the sphincter leading into the stomach from the esophagus, also called the *lower esophageal sphincter*), making reflux activity *(reverse peristalsis)*

Table 52–3

Drugs for Management of Nausea and Vomiting during Pregnancy (Recommendation not Implied)

Generic (Brand)	Route and Dosage	Uses and Considerations
Antihistamines meclizine (Antivert)	PO: 20-50 mg/d	*Mechanism of action:* Considered mild; available as OTC drug. Sites of action: labyrinth and CNS. Blocks CTZ, which acts on vomiting center *Side effects:* Dizziness, drowsiness, dry mouth and nose, blurred vision, diplopia, urinary retention, urticaria, rash, and headache. Cardiovascular effects can include hypotension, palpitations, and tachycardia *Contraindications:* Hypersensitivity to drug or any component *Warnings/precautions:* Use with closed-angle glaucoma. Increased effect of alcohol, tranquilizers, and narcotics *Pregnancy category:* B; metabolized in liver and excreted unchanged in feces and as metabolites in urine. t½: 6 h; onset: 1-2 h; duration: 8-24 h
Phenothiazines promethazine (Phenergan)	PO, IV, IM, PR: 12.5-25 mg q4-6h prn	*Mechanism of action:* Blocks postsynaptic mesolimbic dopaminergic receptors in the brain; exhibits a strong alpha-adrenergic blocking effect and depresses the release of hypothalamic and hypophyseal hormones; competes with histamine for the H_1 receptor *Adverse reactions:* Dizziness, drowsiness, excitation, fatigue, insomnia, photosensitivity reactions, nausea, vomiting, and constipation *Contraindications:* Hypersensitivity to drug or any component of the formulation; CNS depression or coma *Warnings/precautions:* Use caution in cardiovascular disease, not for subQ or intraarterial administration; injection may contain sulfites which may cause allergic reactions in some clients *Pregnancy category:* C, t½: 9-16 h; onset IM 20 min, IV 3-5 min, duration 2-6 h
Anticholinergics scopolamine (Scopace)	PO, IM, IV, subQ: 0.3-0.65 mg q4-6h	*Mechanism of action:* Antagonizes histamine and serotonin *Adverse reactions:* Confusion, drowsiness, headache, fatigue, dry skin, constipation, vomiting, bloated feeling. Cardiovascular side effects include orthostatic hypotension, ventricular fibrillation, tachycardia, palpitations *Contraindications:* Hypersensitivity to the active ingredient or any component of the formulation. Narrow-angle glaucoma, acute hemorrhage, GI or GU obstruction, tachycardia secondary to cardiac insufficiency, and myasthenia gravis *Warnings/precautions:* Use with caution in hepatic or renal impairment *Pregnancy category:* C; onset IM 0.5-1 h, duration 4-6 h
Prokinetic Agents metoclopramide (Reglan)	PO: 10-15 mg QID 30 min a.c.	*Mechanism of action:* Blocks dopamine receptors in chemoreceptor trigger zone of the CNS, causes enhanced motility and accelerated gastric emptying without stimulating secretions *Adverse reactions:* Restlessness, drowsiness, diarrhea, weakness, insomnia *Contraindications:* Hypersensitivity to metoclopramide or any component of the formulation. GI obstruction, perforation or hemorrhage; pheochromocytoma; history of seizure disorder *Pregnancy category:* B; t½ 4-7 h; onset 0.5-1 h, duration 1-2 h
Other trimethobenzamide (Tigan, T-Gen)	200 mg rectally q6-8h	*Mechanism of action:* Obscure action; may be mediated through CTZ. Does not inhibit direct impulse to vomiting center. Chemically classified as an ethanolamine derivative. Precautions include use in client with cardiac dysrhythmias, narrow-angle glaucoma, asthma, and pyloroduodenal obstruction. Rectal doses of the drug are more unpredictable *Side effects:* Drowsiness, headache, blurred vision, diarrhea, depression, hypotension, muscle cramps, allergic reactions, and extrapyramidal symptoms; blood dyscrasias *Contraindications:* Benzocaine, hypersensitivity to drug. Use suppository form in neonates or preterm infants *Warning/precaution:* Avoid use in acute emesis to avoid masking of symptoms *Drug interactions:* Phenothiazines/barbiturates, belladonna *Pregnancy category:* C; t½: UK; onset: PO/PR: 10-40 min; IM: 15-35 min; duration: 3-4 h

a.c., Before meals; *CNS,* central nervous system; *CTZ,* chemoreceptor trigger zone; *d,* day; *GI,* gastrointestinal; *GU,* genitourinary; H_1, histamine$_1$; *h,* hour; *IM,* intramuscular; *IV,* intravenous; *min,* minute; *OTC,* over-the-counter; *PO,* by mouth; *PR,* by rectum; *PRN,* as needed; *subQ,* subcutaneous; *t½,* half-life; *UK,* unknown.

more likely. Digestion and gastric emptying are slower than in the nonpregnant state. Heartburn is common when a pregnant client sits or lies down soon after eating a normal meal, only to have her gravid uterus exert upward pressure on her stomach, causing increased reflux activity and the perception of hyperacidity. Heartburn is a disorder of the second and third trimesters of pregnancy.

Nonpharmacologic measures are preferred in the management of heartburn. These include (1) limiting the size of meals; (2) avoiding highly seasoned, fried, or greasy foods; (3) avoiding gas-forming foods (e.g., cabbage, beans, onions); (4) eating slowly and chewing thoroughly; (5) avoiding citrus juices; (6) drinking adequate fluids, but not with meals; and (7) avoiding reclining immediately after eating.

Antacids should be considered first-line therapy if the client does not respond to nonpharmacologic therapy. The antacids of choice for the pregnant client include nonsystemic low-sodium products (those considered dietetically sodium-free) containing aluminum and magnesium (in the form of hydroxide) in combination. These two ingredients can be found in the combined form of magaldrate (also called *hydroxymagnesium aluminate*). Discourage the long-term use or large doses of magnesium antacids, because fetal renal, respiratory, cardiovascular, and muscle problems may result. Some products also include simethicone (Mylicon), an antiflatulent used to decrease the surface tension of GI gas bubbles, burst the bubbles, and promote rapid gas expulsion. Additionally, sucralfate is likely safe during pregnancy, because the drug is not systemically absorbed. Calcium carbonate antacid preparations may be avoided in pregnancy because of the rebound effect following acid neutralization. Tums are frequently taken by pregnant women for heartburn, but because Tums are calcium-based, excessive use may contribute to the constipation of pregnancy.

Most clients do not realize that remedies commonly used by nonpregnant women (e.g., baking soda [sodium bicarbonate], antacids such as Alka-Seltzer, Bromo-Seltzer, Rolaids) can be harmful during pregnancy. Selection of the wrong antacid can result in diarrhea, constipation, or electrolyte imbalance. The combination of nonpharmacologic measures plus minimal use of safe antacids should effectively meet the pregnant client's needs.

Liquid antacids are the preparations most commonly used in pregnancy because of their uniform dissolution, rapid action, and greater activity. Tablets are also acceptable, particularly for convenience, provided these are thoroughly chewed and the client maintains an adequate fluid intake.

Histamine$_2$ receptor antagonists (H$_2$RAs) can be used during pregnancy, but only if the client has failed initial treatment with antacids, and their use is recommended by a health care provider. The teratogenicity of these medications is unknown; however, cimetidine, ranitidine, famotidine, and nizatidine have received the FDA's pregnancy category B rating. H$_2$RAs work by competitively and revers-

ibly binding to the histamine receptors of the parietal cells, causing a reduction in gastric acid secretion. The onset of action is generally in 1 hour and can persist for 6 to 12 hours.

There is even less experience with the use of proton pump inhibitors. These medications work to suppress gastric acid secretion by inhibiting the proton pump on the surface of the parietal cells. With the recent release of Prilosec OTC (omeprazole), pregnant clients may be inquisitive about its use for heartburn during pregnancy. Encourage clients to discuss the options with their provider. Currently the use of omeprazole is limited to cases in which the benefits of therapy far outweigh the risks.

Table 52–4 presents medications for heartburn commonly used during pregnancy.

Constipation

Constipation is a frequent occurrence during pregnancy. Its cause may be related to hormonal changes, specifically progesterone, which decreases GI motility. Like heartburn, nonpharmacologic treatments for constipation should be tried first. These include (1) increasing fluid intake, (2) increasing dietary fiber intake, and (3) moderate physical exercise.

If the aforementioned methods do not work, treatment is indicated, and the safest agents are considered the bulk-forming preparations containing fiber (for example, Metamucil), because these agents are not systemically absorbed. Also, docusate sodium, a stool softener, would be appropriate as first-line treatment during pregnancy. Agents that should be reserved for occasional use include milk of magnesia, magnesium citrate, lactulose, sorbitol, bisacodyl, and senna.

Castor oil should be avoided during pregnancy, because it can stimulate uterine contractions. Mineral oil should also be avoided, because it can reduce the absorption of fat-soluble vitamins such as vitamin K. Low levels of vitamin K in the neonate can result in hemorrhage.

Pain

Up through week 26 of pregnancy, headaches resulting from hormonally induced body changes, sinus congestion, or eye strain are quite common. It is not unusual for the pregnant client to experience backaches, joint pains, round ligament pain (resulting in mild abdominal aches and twinges), and pain from minor injuries. Nonpharmacologic pain relief measures should be tried initially. These include rest, a calming environment, relaxation exercises, alteration in routine, mental imagery, ice packs, warm moist heat, postural changes, correct body mechanics, and changes in the height and style of footwear.

Acetaminophen

Acetaminophen (Tylenol), a para-aminophenol analgesic, is a pregnancy category B drug. It is the most commonly ingested nonprescription drug during pregnancy. Acetaminophen may be used during all trimesters of pregnancy

Table 52–4

Over-the-Counter Antacids Commonly Used in Pregnancy

Generic (Brand)	Route and Dosage	Uses and Considerations
aluminum hydroxide (Amphojel)	A: PO: As directed*	Contains aluminum hydroxide gel (320 mg) per 300 mg tablet or per 5 ml; ANC 8; contains saccharin and sorbitol. OTC preparation. *Use:* For heartburn secondary to reflux *Action:* Neutralization of gastric acidity *Side effects:* Constipation *Adverse reactions:* Dehydration, hypophosphatemia (long-term use), GI obstruction *Drug interactions:* Decreased effects with tetracycline, phenothiazine, benzodiazepines, isoniazid, digoxin; follow dose with water *Pregnancy category:* C; PB: UK; t½: UK; onset: 15-30 min; peak: 0.5 h; duration: 1-3 h
magnesium hydroxide and aluminum hydroxide with simethicone (Mylanta Extra Strength Liquid, Almacone)	40 to 125 mg PO q.i.d. after meals and at bedtime; up to 500 mg/d	*Mylanta Extra Strength Liquid:* Each 5 mL contains aluminum hydroxide (400 mg), magnesium hydroxide (400 mg), simethicone (40 mg), parabens, saccharin, sorbitol and sodium (2 mg) OTC *Almacone Tablets:* Each tablet contains aluminum hydroxide (200 mg), magnesium hydroxide (200 mg), simethicone (20 mg) OTC. Tablets must be thoroughly chewed. *Use:* Same as above with addition of antiflatulence action. *Action:* Neutralization of gastric acidity and antiflatulence. *Adverse effects:* Acid rebound may occur. Aluminum based antacids may cause constipation while magnesium based antacids have a laxative effect. Aluminum and magnesium based combination antacids are given to balance the constipation and laxative effects. Do not administer magnesium based antacids in women with renal disease. *Drug interactions:* Concurrent administration with digoxin, indomethacin, or iron salts may decrease absorption of these drugs. Concurrent administration with chlordiazepoxide decreases rate of chlordiazepoxide absorption. Pharmacologic effect decreased with benzodiazepines, captopril, corticosteroids, fluoroquinolones, histamine H₂ antagonists, hydantoins, ketoconazole, penicillamine, phenothiazines, salicylates, and ticlopidine with antacids. Pharmacologic effect increased with levodopa, sulfonylureas, and valporic acid. *Pregnancy category:* C; PB: UK; t½: UK.
magaldrate with simethicone (Riopan Plus tablets, Riopan Plus suspension)	As directed*	*Riopan Plus Tablets:* Each contains magaldrate (480 mg) and simethicone (20 mg); ANC 13.5; chewable; contains sorbitol. *Riopan Plus Suspension:* Each 5 ml contains magaldrate (540 mg) and simethicone (20 mg); ANC 15; contains saccharin. *Use:* Same as above. *Action:* Same as above. *Side effects:* Same as above. *Adverse reactions:* Same as above. *Drug interactions:* Decreased absorption of phenothiazines, isoniazid, fluoroquinolones, tetracyclines *Pregnancy category:* C; t½: UK; PB: UK; onset: immediate; peak: UK; duration: prolonged.

*Dosage recommendations for antacid preparations should be clarified by the health care provider; however, as a general rule, no more than 12 tablets or 12 tsp should be taken in a 24-hour period, depending on the strength of the product. Major side effects are a change in bowel habits (diarrhea or constipation), nausea, vomiting, alkalosis, and hypermagnesemia. Owing to their action on gastric pH (increased) and their propensity to bind with other drugs to form poorly absorbed complexes, antacids figure in numerous drug interactions. Antacids should not be given within 2 hours of iron, digitalis products, tetracycline, or phenothiazine.

A, Adult; *ANC,* acid-neutralizing capacity (per tablet or 5 ml); *d,* day; *GI,* gastrointestinal; *h,* hour; *min,* minute; *OTC,* over-the-counter; *PB,* protein-binding; *PO,* by mouth; *q.i.d.,* four times a day; *t½,* half-life; *tsp,* teaspoon; *UK,* unknown.

in therapeutic doses on a short-term basis for its analgesic and antipyretic effects. The drug is a weak prostaglandin inhibitor and does not have significant antiinflammatory effects. Refer to Prototype Drug Chart 25–1 in Chapter 25 for the actions, effects, and safe use of acetaminophen.

Pharmacokinetics

The rate of absorption is dependent on the rate of gastric emptying. Acetaminophen is 20% to 50% protein-bound and crosses the placenta during pregnancy; it is also found in low concentrations in breast milk. Acetaminophen is partially hepatically metabolized into inactive metabolites; however, a highly active metabolite (N-acetyl-p-benzoquinone) produced when the drug is taken in large doses can have potential liver and kidney toxicity. The half-life is 2 to 3 hours. To date there is no concrete evidence of fetal anomalies associated with the use of acetaminophen, and no adverse effects have been noted in breastfed infants of mothers who used the drug while pregnant or breastfeeding.

Pharmacodynamics

Use of acetaminophen during pregnancy should not exceed 12 tablets per 24 hours of a 325-mg formulation (regular strength) or 8 tablets per 24 hours of a 500-mg (extra strength) formulation (because of the potential for kidney and liver toxicity). The drug should be taken at 4- to 6-hour intervals. Onset of effects following oral ingestion is within 10 to 30 minutes; peak action occurs at 1 to 2 hours; duration lasts from 3 to 5 hours.

Adverse Reactions

Most clients without preexisting renal or hepatic disease tolerate acetaminophen well. Clients with hypersensitivity to the compound should not use it. Acetaminophen should be used cautiously in clients at risk for infection because of the possibility of masking signs and symptoms. The most frequent adverse reactions are skin eruptions, urticaria, unusual bruising, erythema, hypoglycemia, jaundice, hemolytic anemia, neutropenia, leukopenia, pancytopenia, and thrombocytopenia.

Aspirin

Aspirin (ASA, Bayer, Ecotrin, Halfprin), a salicylate, is classified as a mild analgesic. Aspirin is a pregnancy category C drug (which changes to category D if full-dose aspirin is used in the third trimester). Aspirin is discussed in detail in Chapter 25.

Aspirin is a prostaglandin synthetase inhibitor with antipyretic, analgesic, and antiinflammatory properties. Teratogenic effects have not been shown conclusively, but the risk of anomalies is perceived to be small.

Aspirin can inhibit the initiation of labor and actually prolong labor through its effects on uterine contractility, therefore its use is not recommended during pregnancy. In addition, aspirin use late in pregnancy is associated with greater maternal blood loss at delivery. There may be increased risk of anemia in pregnancy and of antepartum hemorrhage as well. Hemostasis is affected in the newborn whose mother ingested aspirin during the last 2 months of pregnancy (even without use during the actual week of delivery). The platelets are unable to aggregate to form clots, and it appears that this is not a reversible effect after delivery; the infant has to wait for its own bone marrow to produce new platelets.

Nursing Process

Antepartum Drugs

ASSESSMENT

- Gather comprehensive medical, drug (illicit, nonpharmacologic and pharmacologic), and herbal history.

- Obtain baseline vital signs.
- Identify clients at risk for substance abuse, and collaborate with other professionals to plan strategies to minimize risks.
- Assess drug history to determine whether antacid use will interfere with absorption.
- Review history of aspirin use when admitting a client in labor. If aspirin has been used, alert the staff and monitor for increased bleeding.
- Ascertain any medical history of alcoholism, liver disease, viral infection, and renal deficiencies. Acetaminophen should be used cautiously in these clients.

NURSING DIAGNOSES

- Deficient knowledge related to health maintenance needs during pregnancy
- Deficient knowledge related to potential fetal outcomes from exposure to teratogens

PLANNING

- Client will use and avoid various drugs during pregnancy as advised.
- Client will discuss drugs (illicit, OTC, prescribed), and herbal use with health care provider or pharmacist prior to use.

NURSING INTERVENTIONS

General

- Be cognizant that drug use may be part of multiple substance abuse and may also involve maternal-neonatal infections.
- Stress the importance of prenatal care, and discuss fears client may have about health care professionals and concerns about legal action in the event of substance abuse.

Specific

- Instruct on nonpharmacologic and pharmacologic measures to relieve common pregnancy discomforts.
- Refer to tobacco, alcohol, or drug treatment program if appropriate.
- Instruct on nutritional and therapeutic supplements needed during pregnancy.
- Monitor hemoglobin/hematocrit of prenatal clients per agency protocol.

Iron

- Question client about nausea, constipation, and bowel habit changes if taking iron preparations.
- Give diluted liquid iron preparation through a plastic straw to prevent discoloration of teeth.
- Store iron in a light-resistant container.
- Be cognizant that client may have false-positive result of occult blood in stool if taking iron.

Client Teaching

General

- Advise pregnant woman that tobacco, alcohol, and heavy caffeine use may have adverse effects on the fetus.
- Instruct client that before taking drugs (illicit, OTC, prescribed) to discuss with health care provider secondary to teratogenic potential.
- Advise client planning to breastfeed to discuss drugs (illicit, OTC, prescribed) with health care provider.

Aspirin/Acetaminophen

- Advise client to take acetaminophen rather than aspirin during pregnancy; aspirin is particularly contraindicated during the third trimester.

Antepartum Drugs

- Instruct client not to take nonsteroidal antiinflammatory drugs (NSAIDs) with acetaminophen.

Caffeine/Alcohol/Nicotine

- Advise client to limit coffee and caffeine ingestion from none to 1 to 2 cups per day and to limit other sources of caffeine (tea, cola, soft drinks, chocolate, certain drugs).
- If caffeine is allowed by the health care provider, teach client to space limited caffeine intake evenly throughout the day, because caffeine passes readily to the fetus, who cannot metabolize it. Caffeine can decrease intervillous placental blood flow.
- Advise client to use decaffeinated products or dilute caffeinated products.
- Suggest that client use herbal products carefully because of occasionally harmful ingredients (see Herbal Alert 52–1).
- If client plans to breastfeed, tell her that 1% of the caffeine she consumes will appear in her breast milk within 15 minutes. Therefore, although a cup of coffee is not a problem, it is not wise to drink several cups of coffee in succession; excess caffeine will accumulate in the infant's tissues. The infant lacks enzymes to adequately clear the caffeine for 7 to 9 months after birth.
- Instruct client not to drink alcohol if she is pregnant, because no safe level of alcohol has been determined, and even minimal exposure has resulted in fetal alcohol effect and moderate/excess exposure has resulted in fetal alcohol syndrome.
- Advise client that smoking can cause the loss of nutrients such as vitamins A and C, folic acid, cobalamin, and calcium. Tobacco use may contribute to a shortened gestation and low-birth-weight infants.

Antacids

- Advise that antacids should not be taken within 1 hour of taking an enteric-coated tablet, because the acid-resistant coating may dissolve in the increased alkaline condition of the stomach, and the medica-

tion will not be released in the intestine as intended. Stomach upset may result.
- Advise client to store antacid liquid suspension at room temperature (or place under refrigeration to improve palatability), not to let it freeze, and to shake the bottle well before pouring.

Iron

- Instruct client about dietary sources of iron, which include organ meats (liver), red meat, nuts and seeds, wheat germ, spinach, broccoli, prunes, and iron-fortified cereals.
- Explain to client that if supplemental iron is taken between meals, increased absorption (and also increased side effects) may result. Taking iron 1 hour before meals is suggested. Give with juice or water, but not with milk or antacids.

Self-Administration for Iron and Antacids

- Advise client to swallow the iron tablets whole, not to crush them. Liquid iron preparations should be taken with a plastic straw to avoid staining the teeth.
- Caution client not to take antacids with iron, because antacids impair absorption and are generally discouraged during pregnancy. Iron and antacids should be taken 2 hours apart if both are prescribed.

Side Effects for Iron and Antacids

- Advise client to keep iron tablets away from children. Iron tablets look like candy, and death has been reported in small children who have ingested 2 g or less of ferrous sulfate. Iron is a leading cause of fatal poisoning in children.
- Advise client that there may be a change in bowel habits when taking antacids. Aluminum and calcium carbonate products can cause constipation, whereas magnesium products can cause diarrhea. Many antacids contain a combination of ingredients to reduce adverse effects.

EVALUATION

- ■ Evaluate the effectiveness of the prescribed drug therapy. Report side effects.
- ■ Evaluate client's understanding of possible effects on the fetus with maternal use of drugs (prescribed, OTC, and illicit) and the use of tobacco and alcohol.

Drugs that Decrease Uterine Muscle Contractility

Preterm Labor

Preterm labor (PTL) is labor that occurs between 20 and 37 weeks of pregnancy, involving a fetus with an estimated weight between 500 and 2499 g. Regular contractions occur at less than 10-minute intervals over 30 to 60 minutes and are strong enough to result in 2-cm cervical dilation and 80% effacement. Preterm labor occurs in approximately

8% to 10% of all pregnancies. Preterm infants who survive very early delivery have significant physiologic challenges to overcome, so PTL that progresses to preterm delivery accounts for most perinatal morbidity and mortality (excluding fetuses with anomalies) in the United States.

Although PTL has no single known cause, certain risk factors have been identified: maternal age younger than 18 or older than 40 years, low socioeconomic status, previous history of preterm delivery (17% to 37% chance of recurrence), intrauterine infections (e.g., bacterial vaginosis), polyhydramnios, multiple gestation, uterine anomalies, antepartum hemorrhage, smoking, drug use, urinary tract infections, and incompetent cervix. Attempts to arrest PTL are contraindicated in: (1) pregnancy of less than 20 weeks' gestation (confirmed by ultrasound), (2) bulging or premature rupture of membranes (PROM), (3) confirmed fetal death or anomalies incompatible with life, (4) maternal hemorrhage and evidence of severe fetal compromise, and (5) chorioamnionitis.

Nonpharmacologic treatment measures for PTL include bed rest, hydration (ingestion of six to eight glasses of fluids daily or more, IV fluid bolus), pelvic rest (no sexual intercourse or douching), and screening for intrauterine and urinary tract infections. Client assessment will include uterine activity (frequency, duration, and intensity), vaginal bleeding or discharge, and fetal monitoring.

Tocolytic Therapy

When clients in true PTL (with cervical change) have no contraindications, they become candidates for **tocolytic therapy** (drug therapy to decrease uterine muscle contractions) using beta$_2$-adrenergic receptor agonists (e.g., terbutaline [Brethine]) or the calcium antagonist magnesium sulfate. The goals in tocolytic therapy are to: (1) interrupt or inhibit uterine contractions to create additional time for fetal maturation in utero, (2) delay delivery so antenatal corticosteroids can be delivered to facilitate fetal lung maturation, and (3) allow safe transport of the mother to an appropriate facility if required.

Table 52–5 lists the most commonly used drugs to decrease preterm uterine contractions.

Beta-Sympathomimetic Drugs

Beta-sympathomimetic drugs act by stimulating beta$_2$-receptors on uterine smooth muscle. The frequency and intensity of uterine contractions decrease as the muscle re-

Table 52–5

Drugs Used to Decrease Uterine Contractility

Generic (Brand)	Route and Dosage	Uses and Considerations
Beta-Adrenergic Agents		
terbutaline (Brethine)	Follow agency protocols for specific directives plus individual health care provider's order; may be given subQ; usually therapy is 0.25 mg subQ to 0.5 mg subQ every 3 to 4 h	Sympathomimetic beta$_2$-adrenergic agonist. Partially metabolized in the liver; excreted by the kidneys. 40%-50% rate of tocolytic breakthrough and recurrence of preterm labor 3 wk after start of PO therapy may require repeat therapy (may be due to desensitization of beta receptors over time)
		Current research focused on use of low-dose continuous subQ pumps that are portable and can deliver intermittent bolus doses based on data reflecting peak need periods. Pumps are cost-effective with high client satisfaction. Increases in maternal pulse and FHR. Rapidly crosses placenta; breastfeeding not contraindicated because of short half-life
		Drug interactions: Additive effect with CNS depressants (narcotics, sedative-hypnotics) and neuromuscular blocking agents
		Pregnancy category: B; t½: 11-16 h; onset: 15 min IV/subQ and 30-45 min PO; duration: 4-8 h PO and 1.5-4 h subQ; peak serum levels: 0.5-1 h IV/subQ and 1-2 h PO
Calcium Antagonists		
magnesium sulfate	Follow agency protocols for specific directives plus individual physician orders for concentration and ml/h IV. Usual LD: 4-6 g in 100 ml over 15-20 min; *maint:* 40 g in 1 L of IVF at 2-4 g/h. Dose based on serum magnesium levels, deep tendon reflex assessment, and uterine response	Calcium antagonist and CNS depressant. Relaxes uterine smooth muscle through calcium displacement. Must be given by infusion pump for accurate dosage. Freely crosses placenta. Few contraindications allow for use in clients who exhibit life-threatening complications. Maternal magnesium levels monitored through serum analyses, DTR, respiratory rate, and urinary output
		Elevated levels may be evident in newborn for 7 d; observe newborn for 24-48 h for signs of toxicity if mother treated close to delivery; breastfeeding not contraindicated
		Antidote: calcium gluconate 1 g given IV over 3 min
		Pregnancy category: B; onset: immediate by IV; duration: 30 min

CNS, Central nervous system; *d,* day; *DTR,* deep tendon reflex; *FHR,* fetal heart rate; *h,* hour; *IV,* intravenous; *IVF,* intravenous fluid; *LD,* loading dose; *maint,* maintenance; *min,* minute; *PO,* by mouth; *subQ,* subcutaneous; *t½,* half-life; *wk,* week.

laxes. Terbutaline (Brethine) is commonly used. It is approved for medicinal use but not specifically as a tocolytic. Terbutaline can effectively decrease uterine contractions; however, the literature indicates that knowledge about the long-term effects of this drug is still lacking.

Pharmacokinetics

Clients with mild contractions may be initially given subcutaneous terbutaline (Brethine) followed by a series of subcutaneous (subQ) injections of the drug. Clients are monitored to determine whether and when contractions diminish or cease. Terbutaline is minimally protein-bound (25%) and metabolized via the liver to inactive metabolites. Its half-life is 11 to 16 hours. Oral therapy or subcutaneous pump therapy with terbutaline may be prescribed for longer-term maintenance.

Pharmacodynamics

Oral terbutaline has an onset of action of 30 to 45 minutes, a peak plasma/serum concentration of 1 to 2 hours, and a duration of action of 4 to 8 hours. IV and subcutaneous terbutaline have an onset of action within 15 minutes, a peak serum concentration level in 30 to 60 minutes, and a duration of action of 1.5 to 4 hours subQ.

Adverse Reactions

Maternal side effects include tremors, malaise, weakness, dyspnea, tachycardia, increased systolic blood pressure, decreased diastolic blood pressure, chest pain, nausea, vomiting, diarrhea, constipation, erythema, sweating, hyperglycemia, and hypokalemia. Many of these effects are associated with terbutaline's cross-reactivity with $beta_1$-adrenergic receptors. More serious adverse reactions include pulmonary edema, dysrhythmias, ketoacidosis, and anaphylactic shock.

Fetal side effects include tachycardia and potential hypoglycemia resulting from fetal hyperinsulinemia caused by maternal hyperglycemia.

Drug Interactions

The increased effects of general anesthetics can produce additive hypotension. Pulmonary edema can occur with concurrent use of corticosteroids. Cardiovascular effects may be additive with other sympathomimetic drugs, such as epinephrine, albuterol, and isoproterenol. Beta-adrenergic blocking agents, such as propranolol HCl, nadolol, pindolol, timolol maleate, and metoprolol tartrate, antagonize beta-sympathomimetics.

Magnesium Sulfate

Magnesium sulfate, a calcium antagonist and central nervous system depressant, relaxes the smooth muscle of the uterus through calcium displacement. Administered IV, the drug has a direct depressant effect on uterine muscle contractility. The drug increases uterine perfusion, which has a therapeutic effect on the fetus. This drug, which is also less expensive, may be safer to use than the beta-sympathomimetics, because it has fewer adverse effects. It can also be used when beta-sympathomimetics are contraindicated (e.g., in women with diabetes and cardiovascular disease). The drug is excreted by the kidneys and crosses the placenta. The maintenance dose must be titrated to keep uterine contractions under control, and magnesium levels are drawn based on the clinical response of the client. Magnesium sulfate therapy is contraindicated in clients who have myasthenia gravis; impaired kidney function and recent myocardial infarction are relative contraindications. Clients with renal impairment may require adjusted dosages.

Adverse Reactions

Dosage-related side effects in the maternal client include flushing, feelings of increased warmth, perspiration, dizziness, nausea, headache, lethargy, slurred speech, sluggishness, nasal congestion, heavy eyelids, blurred vision, decreased GI action, increased pulse rate, and hypotension. Increased severity is evidenced by depressed reflexes, confusion, and magnesium toxicity (respiratory depression and arrest, circulatory collapse, cardiac arrest). Side effects in the fetus are decreased fetal heart rate variability, and in the neonate, slight hypotonia with diminished reflexes and lethargy for 24 to 48 hours.

If maternal neurologic, respiratory, or cardiac depression is evidenced, the antidote is calcium gluconate (10 mg IV push over 3 minutes).

Nursing Interventions during Tocolytic Therapy

- Monitor vital signs, FHR, fetal activity, and uterine activity as ordered. Report respirations fewer than 12 per minute, which may indicate magnesium sulfate toxicity.
- Monitor I & O. Report urinary output less than 30 ml/h.
- Assess breath and bowel sounds as ordered, or at least every 4 hours.
- Assess deep tendon reflexes (DTR) and clonus before initiation of therapy and as ordered. Notify health care provider of changes in DTR (areflexia or hyporeflexia) and clonus.
- Weigh daily.
- Monitor serum magnesium levels as ordered (therapeutic level is 4 to 7 mg/dl).
- Have calcium gluconate (1 g given IV over 3 minutes) available as an antidote.
- Observe newborn for 24 to 48 hours for magnesium effects if drug was given to mother before the delivery.

Nursing Process

Beta₂-Adrenergic Agonists: Brethine (Terbutaline)

ASSESSMENT

■ Identify risks for preterm labor (PTL) early in pregnancy.

■ When a client has preterm uterine contractions, obtain a history, complete physical assessment, vital signs, fetal heart rate (FHR), and urine specimen for screening for intrauterine infection and urinary tract infection.

NURSING DIAGNOSES

■ Risk for activity intolerance related to nonpharmacologic and pharmacologic interventions for PTL

■ Ineffective health maintenance related to nonpharmacologic and pharmacologic interventions for PTL and the long-term implications for the woman and her fetus/infant

■ Deficient knowledge related to etiology and nonpharmacologic and pharmacologic interventions for PTL

■ Fear related to potential for early labor and birth

PLANNING

■ Client's preterm uterine contractions will cease by resting in left side-lying position, increasing fluid intake, assuming pelvic rest, and following tocolytic therapy as directed.

■ Client has no progressive cervical change.

NURSING INTERVENTIONS

■ Monitor and assess uterine activity and FHR.

■ Maintain client in left lateral position as much as possible to facilitate uteroplacental perfusion.

■ Monitor vital signs per unit protocol, specifically maternal pulse. Report maternal heart rate greater than 110 beats/min.

■ Report auscultated cardiac dysrhythmias. An electrocardiogram (ECG) may be ordered.

■ Auscultate breath sounds every 4 hours. Notify health care provider if respirations are more than 30 per minute or if there is a change in quality (wheezes, rales, coughing).

■ Monitor daily weight to assess fluid overload; strict intake and output (I & O) measurement.

■ Report baseline FHR over 180 beats/min or any significant increase in uterine contractions from pretreatment baseline.

■ Report persistence of uterine contractions despite tocolytic therapy.

■ Report leaking of amniotic fluid, any vaginal bleeding or discharge, or complaints of rectal pressure.

■ Be alert to presence of maternal hyperglycemia and hypokalemia and hypoglycemia in the newborn delivered within 5 hours of discontinued beta-sympathomimetic drugs.

■ Assist clients on bed rest and home tocolytic therapy to plan for assistance with self-care and family responsibilities.

Client Teaching
General

• Inform client of the signs and symptoms of PTL (menstrual-type cramps, sensation of pelvic pressure, low backache, increased vaginal discharge, and any abdominal discomfort).

• Instruct client that if she experiences PTL contractions, initial action should be to void, recline on her left side to increase uterine blood flow, and drink extra fluids. Emphasize that she should notify her health care provider if uterine contractions do not cease or if they increase in frequency.

• Explain side effects of beta-sympathomimetic drugs. Report heart palpitations or dizziness to health care provider.

• Instruct client to take drugs regularly and as prescribed.

• Advise client to contact the health care provider before taking any other drugs while on tocolytic drug therapy.

Cultural Considerations ❖

• Provide an interpreter with the same ethnic background and gender if possible, especially with sensitive topics and stress situations.

EVALUATION

■ Evaluate the effectiveness of the tocolytic drug by noting six or fewer uterine contractions in 1 hour or per provider order.

■ Evaluate client's understanding of nonpharmacologic measures for decreasing preterm contractions: bed rest, increasing oral fluid intake, pelvic rest, and lying on her left side.

■ Continue monitoring client's vital signs, FHR, and uterine activity. Report any change immediately.

Corticosteroid Therapy in Preterm Labor

The desired outcome of tocolytic therapy is prevention or cessation of PTL. Clients at risk for preterm delivery (24 to 34 weeks' gestation) should receive antenatal corticosteroid therapy with betamethasone (Celestone) or dexamethasone. Administration of corticosteroids accelerates

Table 52–6

Prenatal Therapy for Surfactant Development

Generic (Brand)	Route and Dosage	Uses and Considerations
betamethasone (Celestone)	IM: 12 mg IM q24h × 2 doses	Corticosteroid. Given to prevent RDS in preterm infants by injecting mother before delivery to stimulate surfactant production in the fetal lung. Not effective in treating preterm infant after delivery. Most effective if given at least 24 h (preferably 48-72 h) but less than 7 d before delivery in week 33 or before. Contraindicated in severe gestational hypertension and in systemic fungal infection. Simultaneous use with terbutaline may enhance risk of pulmonary edema. Drug can mask signs of chorioamnionitis; therefore drug not usually given with ruptured membranes. Metabolized in the liver and excreted by the kidneys; crosses the placenta; enters breast milk. Therapy less effective with multifetal birth and with male infants. No data available related to breastfeeding. *Pregnancy category:* C; PB: 64%; t½: 6.5 h; onset: 1-3 h; peak: 10-36 min IV; duration: 7-14 d
Dexamethasone (Decadron)	IM: 6 mg q12h × 4 doses	Same as betamethasone

d, Day; *h,* hour; *IM,* intramuscular; *IV,* intravenous; *min,* minute; *PB,* protein-binding; *RDS,* respiratory distress syndrome; *t½,* half-life.

lung maturation and lung surfactant development in the fetus in utero, thereby decreasing the incidence and severity of respiratory distress syndrome (RDS) and increasing survival of preterm infants. Antenatal therapy decreases infant mortality, RDS, and intraventricular bleeds in neonates born between 24 to 34 gestational weeks (Chan, Johnson 2006). The effects and benefits of corticosteroid administration are believed to begin 24 hours after administration and last for up to 1 week.

Surfactant is made up of two major phospholipids: sphingomyelin and lecithin. Sphingomyelin initially develops in greater quantity (from about the 24th week) than lecithin. However, by the 33rd to 35th weeks of gestation, lecithin production peaks, making the ratio of the two substances about 2:1 in favor of lecithin. This is called the **L/S (lecithin/sphingomyelin) ratio**, measured in the amniotic fluid. The L/S ratio is a predictor of fetal lung maturity and risk for neonatal RDS.

Clients with gestational hypertension, PROM, placental insufficiency, some types of diabetes, or narcotic abuse may have amniotic fluid with higher than expected L/S ratios for the gestational date because of a stress-induced increase in endogenous corticosteroid production.

Betamethasone (Celestone)

When PTL occurs before the 33rd week of gestation, corticosteroid therapy with betamethasone may be prescribed. The usual dose is 12 mg intramuscularly (IM) every 24 hours for two doses.

Adverse Reactions

Side effects of betamethasone are rare but include seizures, headache, vertigo, edema, hypertension, increased sweating, petechiae, ecchymoses, and facial erythema.

Dexamethasone

In clinical controlled trials, there is insufficient evidence to recommend betamethasone over dexamethasone, because the two have not been compared. Dexamethasone has a rapid onset of action and a shorter duration of action; therefore, it must be prescribed in a shorter frequency compared with betamethasone. The recommended antepartum regimen for dexamethasone is 6 mg IM every 12 hours for four doses. *Do not confuse dexamethasone with desoximetasone.*

Adverse Reactions

The potential adverse reactions associated with dexamethasone therapy include insomnia, nervousness, increased appetite, headache, hypersensitivity reactions, and arthralgias. Table 52–6 provides information for the reviewed corticosteroids.

Nursing Process

Betamethasone (Celestone)

ASSESSMENT

- Assess for history of hypersensitivity.
- Assess vital signs; report abnormal findings.
- Assess fetal heart rate (FHR).

NURSING DIAGNOSES

- Fear related to potential for preterm labor and birth with uncertain fetal outcome secondary to fetal immaturity
- Risk for infection

PLANNING

■ Client will not deliver within 24 hours of receiving betamethasone (Celestone).

NURSING INTERVENTIONS

■ Shake the suspension well. Avoid exposing to excessive heat or light.

■ Inject into large muscle, but *not* the deltoid, to avoid local atrophy.

■ Monitor maternal vital signs.

■ Maintain accurate intake and output.

■ Check blood glucose if used for client with diabetes.

Cultural Considerations ❖

• Provide an interpreter with the same ethnic background and gender if possible, especially when dealing with sensitive topics and stress situations.

EVALUATION

■ Continue monitoring client's vital signs. Report changes.

■ Continue monitoring FHR. Report changes.

■ Monitor neonate for hypoglycemia and presence of neonatal sepsis.

Drugs for Gestational Hypertension

Gestational hypertension (elevated blood pressure without proteinuria after 20 gestational weeks in clients normotensive prior to pregnancy), the most common serious complication of pregnancy, can have devastating maternal and fetal effects (ACOG 2002). Gestational hypertension has replaced the term *pregnancy-induced hypertension (PIH)*, still commonly used in clinical discussions, albeit no longer correct. With proper management of gestational hypertension, the prognosis for both mother and infant is good. Hypertensive disorders are reported in 12% to 22% of all pregnant clients, with 5% to 8% of all pregnancies reflecting incidence of **preeclampsia** (gestational hypertension with proteinuria) (Chan, Johnson 2006). The condition is most often observed after 20 weeks' gestation, intrapartum, and during the first 72 hours postpartum. The cause of preeclampsia remains unknown, although numerous hypotheses exist. The pathophysiology of preeclampsia and **eclampsia** (new-onset grand mal seizures in a client with preeclampsia) is believed to be related to decreased levels of vasodilating prostaglandins with resulting vasospasm (ACOG, 2002). The major predisposing risk factors for the development of preeclampsia are listed in Box 52–1.

Box 52–1

Predisposing Factors in Preeclampsia

• African American
• Primigravida (first pregnancy)
• History of preeclampsia
• Younger than 20 or older than 35 years of age (especially as primigravida)
• Multifetal gestation
• Family history of preeclampsia
• Gestational trophoblastic disease
• Pregestational diabetes mellitus
• Preexisting hypertensive, vascular, or renal disease
• Overweight
• Antiphospholipid antibody syndrome

The two categories of gestational hypertension—preeclampsia and eclampsia—are based on clinical manifestations. Preeclampsia is the presence of hypertension (systolic blood pressure >140 mmHg or diastolic blood pressure >90 mmHg) and proteinuria ($\geq$300 mg in 24-hour urine collection) in a normotensive prepregnant client after the 20th week of gestation. Preeclampsia is subdivided into *mild* preeclampsia and *severe* preeclampsia (Table 52–7 for comparison).

About 5% of preeclamptic clients, notably those without adequate prenatal care, progress to eclampsia, in which seizure activity occurs and the perinatal mortality rate is about 20%. Early diagnosis of preeclampsia with appropriate treatment keeps most preeclamptic clients from progressing to this stage. About 25% of eclampsia occurs postpartum.

A severe sequela of preeclampsia is known as **HELLP syndrome** (defined by *H*emolysis, *E*levated *L*iver enzymes, and *L*ow *P*latelet count), which occurs in about 2% to 12% of clients with gestational hypertension. Clients who manifest severe preeclampsia are most likely to also have HELLP syndrome.

Two primary treatment goals in preeclampsia, in addition to delivery of an uncompromised fetus and psychologic support for the client and her family, are reduction of vasospasm and prevention of seizures.

Delivery of the infant and placenta (products of conception) is the only known cure for preeclampsia. Vaginal delivery is preferred so that anesthesia or surgical risks will not be added. Labor induction via cervical ripening may be initiated to facilitate labor. For a vaginal delivery, epidural or combined epidural and spinal anesthesia are frequently performed for pain management while promoting uteroplacental circulation. Maternal hypotension is a significant concern for hypertensive clients who have epidurals. In contrast, parturients with worsening preeclampsia or fetal distress may be delivered via cesarean section. Clients with HELLP syndrome may have their labor induced for a vaginal delivery at 32 or more weeks' gestation. For clients with HELLP syndrome who are at less than 32 weeks' gestation, cesarean delivery may be considered.

Table 52–7

Comparison of Mild and Severe Preeclampsia and Eclampsia

Mild Preeclampsia	Severe Preeclampsia	Eclampsia
Blood pressure increase to >140 and/or >90 diastolic but <160 systolic	Blood pressure increase of >160/110 on two occasions at least 6 h apart (client on bed rest)	Signs and symptoms of mild or severe preeclampsia and 1 grand mal seizure
Proteinuria >300 mg in 24 h or +1 ± 2 on dipstick; edema not generalized; noted in hands, feet	Proteinuria >5 gm in 24 h or 3+ or greater in two random samples 4 hours apart; edema generalized; found in face (periorbital, coarse features), hands, lower extremities (ankles), abdomen, and dependent areas	
Weight gain >1 lb/wk before 32 wk or >2.5 lb/wk after 34 wk	Weight gain up to 10 lb in 1 wk	
Deep tendon reflexes in arms and legs only slightly increased (0: no response; 1+: sluggish/low; 2+: normal active; 3+: brisk)	Deep tendon reflexes in arms and legs hyperactive (4+: hyperactive/transient clonus; 5+: brisk; clonus sustained)	
Adequate urinary output (1 ml/kg/h)	Oliguria present (<400 ml per 24 h)	
No major cerebral or visual symptoms	Cerebral or visual symptoms, particularly blurred vision, spots, flashing lights, and/or persistent and severe headache in frontal area	
May have mild frontal headache		
No epigastric pain	Epigastric pain may be present; pulmonary edema, cyanosis	

h, Hour; *wk*, week; >, greater than; <, less than.

If a client's disease progresses to the point of eclampsia (maternal seizure), delivery is generally postponed for 1 to 3 hours if fetal status allows. The labor induction or cesarean delivery is an additional stressor for the client who exhibits acidosis and hypoxia resulting from seizure. Ideally once vital signs are stabilized with improved urinary output and decreased acidosis/hypoxia, delivery is pursued.

Nonpharmacologic treatments for preeclampsia might potentially include activity reduction, lying on the left side, increased dietary protein (supplemental 90 g/day), psychosocial therapy, and biofeedback, but the aforementioned recommendations have been studied and shown not to have clinically beneficial effects. Therefore, drug therapy is commonly used for treatment.

Methyldopa (Aldomet), hydralazine (Apresoline), and Labetalol (Trandate) are considered first-line therapy for preeclampsia, because they have been most widely used in pregnant women and their safety and efficacy for mother and fetus have been established. Additional alternatives include beta-blockers, prazosin, nifedipine, and clonidine. Beta-blockers are generally considered safe, but there is a potential for impairment of fetal growth if used early in pregnancy. Nifedipine, a calcium channel blocker, has been used with no major problems. Diuretics should be avoided because of the potential alteration in plasma volume. Angiotensin-converting enzyme inhibitors should be avoided in the second and third trimesters because of the potential for fetal renal toxicity.

Table 52–8 presents the drug data for the two most commonly used drugs for treating preeclampsia, magnesium sulfate and hydralazine.

Adverse Reactions of Methyldopa (Aldomet)

Observe the client for peripheral edema, anxiety, nightmares, drowsiness, headache, dry mouth, drug fever, and mental depression. These are the most common potential adverse reactions.

Adverse Reactions of Hydralazine (Apresoline)

Observe the client for headache, nausea, vomiting, nasal congestion, dizziness, tachycardia, palpitations, and angina pectoris. Avoid a sudden decrease in maternal blood pressure, which may cause fetal hypoxia. Hydralazine has no known direct adverse effects on the fetus.

Adverse Reactions of Magnesium Sulfate

Early signs of increased magnesium levels include lethargy, flushing, feelings of increased warmth, perspiration, thirst, sedation, heavy eyelids, slurred speech, hypotension, depressed deep tendon reflexes (DTR), and decreased muscle tone. Adverse reactions generally occur with serum magnesium sulfate levels greater than 10 mEq/L. Therapeutic levels are 4 to 7mEq/L. Loss of patellar reflexes is often the first sign of magnesium toxicity and may be seen at 8-10 mEq/L. Respiratory depression may manifest at levels greater than 10-15 mEq/L and cardiac arrest at levels greater than 20-25 mEq/L.

Table 52–8

Drugs Used in Severe Preeclampsia

Generic (Brand)	Route and Dosage	Uses and Considerations
magnesium sulfate	LD: 6 g in 20 min IV; piggyback via infusion pump; maint: 2/h IV via infusion pump	Prevention and treatment of seizures related to preeclampsia. Acts as CNS depressant. Decreases acetylcholine from motor nerves, which blocks neuromuscular transmission and decreases incidence of seizures. Secondary effect is reduction in blood pressure as magnesium sulfate relaxes smooth muscle
		Secondarily affects peripheral vascular system with increased uterine blood flow caused by vasodilation and some transient BP decrease during first hour; also inhibits uterine contractions. Depresses DTRs and respiration; maintenance dose depends on reflexes, respiratory rate, urinary output, and magnesium level. Production of abnormally high serum magnesium level is main risk
		Therapeutic levels range from 4-7 mEq/L; effective in preventing seizures. Client is at risk if respiratory rate <12/min, urinary output <30 ml/h, DTR is absent or hyporeflexic. Patellar reflexes disappear with serum magnesium levels of 8-10 mEq/L. Maternal respiratory depression may occur with levels greater than 10-15 mEq/; cardiac arrest with levels >20-25 mEq/L. Notify health care provider of any of the above
		Can be given IV or IM (infrequent). Should not be given parenterally to clients with heart block, or myocardial damage. Use with caution in clients with renal impairment
		Absorbed magnesium is excreted by kidneys; excreted in breast milk, but not a contraindication to breastfeeding
		Contraindications: myasthenia gravis. Relative contraindications: myocardial damage or heart block
		Antidote: calcium gluconate 1 g slow IV push over 3 min
		Pregnancy category: B; PB: UK; t½: UK; onset: IV immediate, IM 1 h; duration: IV 30 min, IM 3-4 h; infusion usually stopped 24 h postpartum
hydralazine hydrochloride (Apresoline)	IV push: 5-10 mg doses IV every 20 min to maximum cumulative total of 20 mg or until blood pressure is controlled	Antihypertensive agent. Acts by causing arteriolar vasodilation. Usually lowers diastolic BP more than systolic BP. Objective of treatment is to maintain diastolic BP between 90 and 110 mmHg. Usually not given to pregnant preeclamptic client with diastolic BP >105 mmHg because of risk of reduced intervillous blood flow. Clients with impaired renal function may require lower doses
	IM & PO routes not usually used	*Parenteral: onset:* 5-20 min; peak: 10-80 min; duration: 2-6 h; well tolerated; maternal tachycardia and increased cardiac output and oxygen consumption may occur
		Oral: onset: 20-30 min; peak: 1-2 h; duration: 2-4 h
methyldopa (Aldomet, ♣Apo-Methyldopa	IV: 250-1000 mg every 6-8 h, *max:* 1 gm every 6 h	*Mechanism of action:* Stimulates central alpha-adrenergic receptors, resulting in decreased sympathetic outflow to heart, kidneys, and peripheral vasculature
	PO: 250 mg b.i.d., *max:* 4 gm/d	*Contraindications:* Hypersensitivity to methyldopa or any component of formulation. Active hepatic disease, liver disorders previously associated with use of methyldopa, concurrent use with MAOIs
		Warnings/precautions: Sedation is usually transient during initial treatment and dosage increases
labetalol (Trandate)	IV: 20 mg IV, followed by 40 mg, then 80 mg, then 80 mg every 10 min until blood pressure is controlled or maximum cumulative dose of 220 mg is given	*Pregnancy category:* B; t½: 75-80 min, onset 3-6 h; duration 12-24 h

b.i.d., Two times a day; *BP*, blood pressure; *CNS*, central nervous system; *d*, day; *DTR*, deep tendon reflex; *h*, hour; *IM*, intramuscular; *IV*, intravenous; *LD*, loading dose; *maint*, maintenance; *MAOIs*, monoamine oxidase inhibitors; *min*, minute; *PB*, protein-binding; *PO*, by mouth; *t½*, half-life; *UK*, unknown; >, greater than; <, less than, ♣, Canadian drug.

Decreased variability is commonly seen on the fetal heart rate tracing. If the client received magnesium sulfate close to the time of delivery, the neonate may exhibit low Apgar scores, hypotonia, lethargy, weakness, and potential respiratory distress. The fetal level of magnesium generally reaches more than 90% of maternal levels within 3 hours of administration. There is no evidence linking congenital defects and maternal hypocalcemia or hypermagnesemia. The greater risk to the fetus is from maternal preeclampsia with resulting decreased placental blood flow and intrauterine growth retardation.

Gestational Hypertension

ASSESSMENT

■ Review baseline vital signs from early pregnancy and BP readings during prenatal visits.
■ Identify client history that may predispose client to preeclampsia.

NURSING DIAGNOSES

■ Deficient fluid volume related to shift of intravascular fluid to extravascular space as outcome of vasospasm with subsequent elevated arterial hypertension
■ Deficient knowledge related to preeclampsia, diagnosis, treatment modalities, common outcomes for mother and infant
■ Risk for inadequate tissue perfusion and risk to fetal well-being secondary to vasospasm
■ Risk for maternal injury related to seizure activity and magnesium toxicity
■ Anxiety related to possible preterm hospitalization and delivery with possible adverse fetal or maternal outcomes

PLANNING

■ Client's blood pressure will be maintained within acceptable ranges.
■ Client will verbalize understanding of preeclampsia, etiology, signs and symptoms and nonpharmacologic and pharmacologic treatment measures.
■ Client will comply with planned preeclampsia treatment regimen.
■ Fetus will tolerate impaired uteroplacental perfusion and subsequent delivery without injury.
■ Therapeutic magnesium levels will be maintained.
■ Plan for magnesium sulfate infusion for at least 24 hours postpartum.

Client Teaching

General
• Teach client about preeclampsia and implications for mother, fetus, and newborn.
• Provide client with information about nonpharmacologic and pharmacologic treatment measures for preeclampsia.

Safety
• Instruct client to lie in the left lateral recumbent position, and explain the rationale.
• Teach client signs and symptoms of progressive preeclampsia and when to seek medical assistance.
• Explain to client that fetal well-being will be assessed through biophysical profile (BPP), nonstress test (NST), or contraction stress test at frequent intervals, depending on the health care provider and preeclampsia severity (e.g., NST and/or BPP 1-2 ×/week).
• Educate family regarding possibility of seizures and appropriate actions to take if seizures occur.

Diet
• Provide nutritional counseling in regard to need for additional protein intake (90 g) to make up for urinary protein losses, normal sodium diet, and importance of adequate fluid intake.
• Explain to client the rationale for daily weights.

Magnesium Sulfate
• Explain to client why she will have a Foley catheter, infusion pump, continuous fetal monitoring, and assessment of deep tendon reflex (DTR) and clonus. Explain that therapy will extend into the postpartum period 24 to 48 hours, depending on the agency and health care provider.
• Explain to client about visitor restrictions and that she will be in a low-stimulation environment.
• Tell client that she will likely experience flush, warm sensation, and possibly nausea and vomiting during the initial loading dose.
• Tell client that evidence of magnesium levels that are within therapeutic range include decreased appetite, some speech slurring, double vision, and weakness.

Hydralazine
• Explain to client that nurses will be monitoring pulse and BP almost constantly until they become stable after administration, then every 15 minutes thereafter. Explain that an electronic BP monitor may be used to obtain constant readings. Some providers will request manual BP measurements.
• Explain to client the need for careful measuring of I & O.
• Tell client she may experience headache as a side effect of the drug.

NURSING INTERVENTIONS

Magnesium Sulfate

■ Continuous electronic fetal monitoring.
■ Monitor for maternal toxicity. Lethargy and weakness result from blocking of neuromuscular transmission. Diaphoresis, flushing, feeling of warmth, and nasal congestion are results of vasodilation from relaxation of smooth muscle.
■ Have airway suction, resuscitation equipment and emergency drugs available.
■ Have antidote available. Calcium gluconate (1 g) IV is given over 3 minutes.
■ Maintain client in left lateral recumbent position in low-stimulation environment. Provide close observation.
■ For IM administration, use Z-track technique and rotate sites (drug is painful and irritating).

■ Monitor BP, pulse, and respiratory rate per agency protocol; monitor DTR, clonus, and I & O (with urimeter) every hour. Some providers will request manual BP measurements.

■ Monitor temperature, breath sounds, and bowel sounds every 4 hours.

■ Check urine for protein every hour.

■ Assess for epigastric pain, headache, visual symptoms (blurred vision and scotoma), sensory changes, edema, level of consciousness, and seizure activity on ongoing basis.

■ Monitor serum magnesium levels according to agency protocol for range between 4 to 7mEq/L.

■ Notify physician if following are observed:

• Respirations less than 12/min

• Absence of DTR

• Urinary output less than 30 ml/h

• Systolic BP greater than or equal to 160 mm Hg, unless ordered otherwise

• Magnesium level greater than 7 mEq/L

• Absent bowel sounds or altered breath sounds

• Epigastric pain or right upper quadrant pain (associated with hepatic edema causing stretching of the liver capsule), headache, visual symptoms (blurred vision and scotoma), sensory changes, change in affect or level of consciousness, seizure activity

■ Monitor laboratory reports for low platelet count, elevated liver enzymes (AST, LDH), bilirubin levels. Observe for evidence of excessive bleeding.

■ Monitor fetal status. FHR baseline should remain 110 to 160 beats per minute (bpm).

■ Monitor 24-hour urinary protein lab results if ordered (≥300 mg/24 h is abnormal).

■ Monitor client for magnesium toxicity.

■ Monitor newborn for effects of placental exposure to excess magnesium sulfate. Although infrequent, newborn side effects include lethargy, neurologic or respiratory depression, and muscle hypotonia.

Hydralazine

■ Take pulse and BP every 5 minutes when drug is administered or monitor with an electronic BP device until stabilized, then every 15 minutes. Some providers will request manual BP measurements.

■ Observe for maintenance of diastolic BP between 90 and 110 mm Hg or as ordered.

■ Observe for change in level of consciousness and headache.

■ Monitor I & O to avoid hypotensive episodes or overload.

■ Monitor fetal heart rate (FHR).

Cultural Considerations ❖

• Provide an interpreter with the same ethnic background and gender if possible, especially with sensitive topics and stress situations.

Client Teaching

General

• Instruct client to avoid exposure to infection.

• Remind client with diabetes to check her glucose level as ordered.

Side Effects

• Instruct client to report immediately any breathing difficulty, weakness, or dizziness.

• Instruct client to report changes in stool, easy bruising, bleeding, blurred vision, unusual weight gain, and emotional changes.

EVALUATION

■ Evaluate the effectiveness of therapy to reduce BP (hydralazine).

■ Continue monitoring vital signs. Report changes.

■ Document the effect of teaching and learning opportunities on client's knowledge deficit about preeclampsia treatment modalities and outcomes.

■ Note fetal well-being secondary to treatment with drugs as evidenced by fetal monitoring and fetal movement assessment.

■ Monitor maternal physiologic changes in relation to magnesium sulfate levels.

■ Continue monitoring FHR. Report changes.

KEY WEBSITES

American College of Obstetricians and Gynecologists: http://www.acog.org

ePregnancy: http://www.epregnancy.com

Pregnancy and Drugs: http://www.fda.gov

Critical Thinking Case Study

TA (gravida 3, para 0) has a history of spontaneous abortion at 10 weeks' gestation and a preterm delivery and demise of a neonate at 21 weeks' gestation. At her 28-week prenatal visit, she reports increased clear vaginal discharge and feelings of pelvic pressure. Examination of her cervix reveals 2-cm dilation and a presenting fetal part low in the pelvis. TA is admitted to the hospital and uterine activity is documented. Terbutaline therapy is ordered for treatment of preterm labor. The nurse prepares for terbutaline administration by the subQ route.

1. How will terbutaline therapy be initiated? What intervals and dosages should be anticipated?
2. What maternal and fetal side effects should the nurse expect to observe?
3. What should TA be told about the drug effects she will experience?

4. How should the nurse respond to TA's questions about the risks of preterm delivery?

After 24 hours of terbutaline subQ therapy, uterine contractions have been reduced to two to three per hour. TA is to be discharged home after oral terbutaline therapy is initiated. The nurse is preparing TA's discharge teaching.

5. What dose and administration schedule would the nurse expect to be ordered?
6. What should TA be advised to do if she forgets or misses an oral dose of terbutaline?
7. What instructions should be given to TA about her activity and diet?
8. TA asks whether the side effects of terbutaline will continue. What is an appropriate nursing response?
9. What signs and symptoms should TA be advised to report?

NCLEX Study Questions

1. A serum alpha fetal protein (AFP) is done to detect:
   a. gestational diabetes   c. neural tube defects
   b. preeclampsia   d. group B strep

2. Ms. James is Rh negative. Following her amniocentesis the nurse would administer:
   a. RhoGAM   c. hepatitis B
   b. rubella   d. Motrin

3. A nurse is teaching a prenatal client how best to decrease the gastrointestinal distress she experiences with her prenatal vitamins. The nurse tells the client to:
   a. take the prenatal vitamin between meals
   b. take the prenatal vitamin with food
   c. take the prenatal vitamin with orange juice
   d. take the prenatal vitamin with milk

4. A nurse employed in an infertility clinic is working with a pre-conceptual couple. The nurse advises the woman to take _____ for at least 3 months prior to becoming pregnant to prevent fetal neural tube defects.
   a. iron   c. folic acid
   b. ginger   d. pyridoxine

5. A nurse in the prenatal clinic is reviewing telephone messages she needs to return that afternoon. Of the following, which one should the nurse call first?
   a. A primigravida, 10 gestational weeks, with nausea and vomiting and requesting information about ginger
   b. A gravida 2, 35 gestational weeks, with Braxton Hicks contractions and requesting information about caffeine
   c. A gravida 2, 32 gestational weeks, gestational diabetic with a blood sugar of 132 and requesting information about her insulin
   d. A primigravida, 28 gestational weeks, with pre-eclampsia and requesting information about taking Motrin for a headache

6. The therapeutic level for magnesium sulfate is:
   a. 4-7 mEq/L   c. 10-15 mEq/L
   b. 7-10 mEq/L   d. 15-20 mEq/L

7. The first sign of magnesium toxicity is:
   a. lethargy
   b. respirations less than 12/minute
   c. loss of patellar reflexes
   d. positive clonus

8. Camella has been receiving magnesium sulphate IV for 24 hours to treat her severe preeclampsia. On assessment you find the following: temperature 37.3° C, pulse 88, respirations 14, BP 138/76, 21 patellar reflexes and negative ankle clonus. Your priority nursing intervention is:
   a. obtain a stat magnesium sulfate level
   b. discontinue magnesium sulfate
   c. contact the physician
   d. continue to monitor

9. Patrice, an 19-year-old primigravida, 8 gestational weeks, is in the prenatal clinic for her first exam. She complains of nausea and vomiting "every morning." Which comment made by Patrice would indicate the need for further instruction?
   a. "My friend gave me gingersnap cookies to eat."
   b. "I have been eating dry crackers before I get up."
   c. "I have tried to avoid foods with strong smells."
   d. "I have been drinking chamomile tea to help the nausea and vomiting."

53

Female Reproductive Cycle II: Labor, Delivery, and Preterm Neonatal Drugs
Robin Webb Corbett and Laura K. Williford Owens

Outline

Objectives

Terms

Drugs for Pain Control during Labor
Analgesia/Sedation
Nursing Process: Pain Control Drugs
Anesthesia
Nursing Process: Regional Anesthetics

Drugs that Enhance Uterine Muscle Contractility
Oxytocin
Nursing Process: Enhancement of Uterine Contractility: Oxytocins
Ergot Alkaloids
Nursing Process: Other Oxytocics: Ergonovine and Methylergonovine

Surfactant Therapy in Preterm Birth
Synthetic Surfactant
Nursing Process: Beractant (Survanta), Calfactant (Infasurf), and Poractant Alfa (Curosurf)

Key Websites

Critical Thinking Case Study

NCLEX Study Questions

Objectives

- Critique systemic and regional medications for pain control during labor, their action, side effects, and nursing implications.
- Describe the nursing process, including client teaching, associated with the drugs used during labor and delivery.
- Compare drugs used to enhance uterine contractility during labor and following placental expulsion, their action, side effects, and nursing implications.
- Describe the nursing process associated with the administration of surfactant therapy for preterm neonates.

Terms

Drugs for Pain Control during Labor

Labor and delivery are divided into four stages, the first three specific to labor and delivery. During the first stage, the dilating stage, cervical effacement and dilation occur; the cervix thins and becomes fully dilated at 10 cm. The first stage consists of three phases categorized by cervical dilatation. These three phases are the latent phase (0 to 4 cm), the active phase (4 to 7 cm), and the transition phase (8 to 10 cm). The second stage of labor, the pelvic stage, begins with complete cervical dilatation and ends with delivery of the newborn (Figure 53–1). During the third stage of labor, the placenta separates from the uterine wall and is delivered. The fourth stage of labor, or the first 1 to 4 hours postpartum, is a period of physiologic stabilization for the mother and initiation of familial attachment.

During the first stage of labor, uterine contractions produce progressive cervical effacement and dilatation. As the first stage of labor progresses, uterine contractions become stronger, longer, and more frequent, and discomfort increases. Pain and discomfort in labor are caused by uterine contraction, cervical dilatation and effacement, hypoxia of the contracting myometrium, and perineal pressure from the presenting part. Pain perception is influenced by physiologic, psychologic, social, and cultural factors, in particular, the woman's past experience with pain, anticipation of pain, fear and anxiety, knowledge deficit of the labor and delivery process, and involvement of support persons.

Before administering pharmacologic treatment, nonpharmacologic measures should be initiated. Nonpharma-

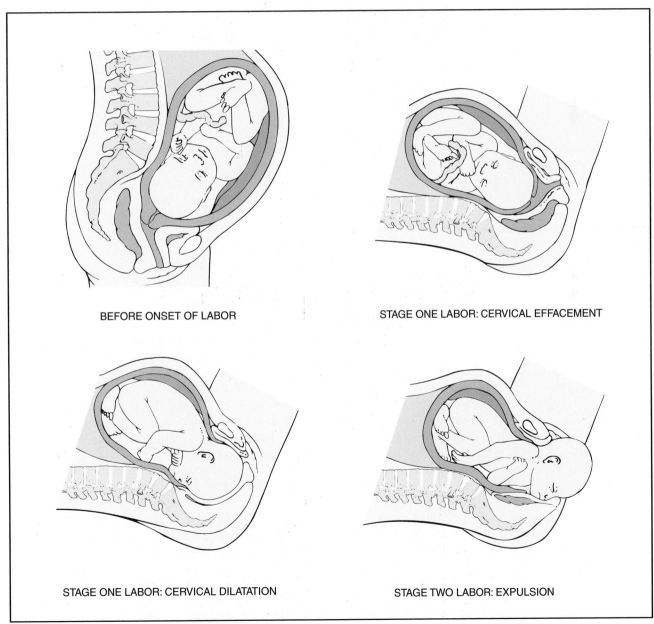

BEFORE ONSET OF LABOR

STAGE ONE LABOR: CERVICAL EFFACEMENT

STAGE ONE LABOR: CERVICAL DILATATION

STAGE TWO LABOR: EXPULSION

FIGURE 53–1 First and second stages of labor. (From Nichols F, Zwelling E: *Maternal-newborn nursing: theory and practice*, Philadelphia, 1997, WB Saunders.)

cologic measures for pain relief during labor include (1) ambulating, (2) supportive positioning of the gravid uterus and promoting uterine perfusion, (3) using touch and massage, (4) using hygiene and comfort measures, (5) involving support persons, (6) using breathing and relaxation techniques, (7) transcutaneous electrical nerve stimulation, (8) hypnosis, (9) acupuncture, and (10) using hydrotherapy (warm water tubs and showers).

Other nonpharmacologic measures include alternative and complementary medicine. Of particular concern is the use of herbal supplements by the pregnant client later in pregnancy to stimulate labor. For example, some women ingest pregnancy toner tea, which includes the components raspberry, nettles, dandelion, alfalfa, and peppermint leaf. Other herbal supplements used include blue cohosh, castor oil, red raspberry leaf, and evening primrose oil. Pregnant women may self-administer, or the practice may be part of their traditional beliefs and framework of health. Concerns with herbal supplements are related to the often numerous physiologic active components of the herbs, adulterants, inconsistent dosing, and lack of proven efficacy. Herbs taken in later pregnancy may contribute to preterm labor or increased bleeding at delivery. Nurses must be culturally sensitive to the use of herbal supplements and health practices during pregnancy, specifically in the later gestational weeks.

When pharmacologic intervention is needed for pain relief, drugs are used as an adjunct to nonpharmacologic measures. Drugs should be selected to not only decrease the client's pain but also minimize side effects for the fetus or newborn and mother. Pain relief in labor can be obtained with systemic analgesics and regional anesthesia. Analgesics alter the client's perception and sensation of pain without producing unconsciousness.

Analgesia/Sedation

Systemic medications used during labor include sedative-tranquilizers, narcotics agonists, and mixed narcotic agonist-antagonists; these may be administered orally (sedative-hypnotic drugs), intravenously (IV), or intramuscularly (IM) (Table 53–1). Because of the variable response and blood levels with intramuscular administration, these drugs are more commonly administered intravenously. These medications should be administered at the onset of the uterine contraction, because parenteral administration at the onset of the contraction decreases neonatal drug exposure as blood flow is decreased to the uterus and fetus.

The sedative-tranquilizer drugs are most commonly given for false labor, latent labor, or with ruptured membranes without true labor. These drugs may also be administered to minimize maternal anxiety and fear. These drugs promote rest and relaxation and decrease fear and anxiety, but they do not provide pain relief. The sedative drugs most commonly used are barbiturates or hypnotics—generally secobarbital sodium (Seconal) and pentobarbital sodium (Nembutal). Other drugs, such as phenothi-

azine derivatives and hydroxyzine, can be given alone during early labor or in combination with narcotic agonists when the client is in active labor. In addition to decreasing anxiety and apprehension, these drugs potentiate the analgesic action of the opioids and minimize emesis. These drugs include promethazine (Phenergan), a phenothiazine, and hydroxyzine hydrochloride (Vistaril), a sedative-hypnotic.

The second group of drugs given for active labor are narcotic agonists. These drugs may be administered parenterally or via regional blocks. When administered with neuraxial anesthesia, a lower dose of anesthetic is required for effective pain relief, thereby minimizing side effects. These drugs interfere with pain impulses at the subcortical level of the brain. To effect pain relief, opioids interact with mu and kappa receptors. For example, morphine sulfate activates both mu and kappa receptors.

Meperidine (Demerol) is the most commonly prescribed synthetic opioid for pain control during labor. A second narcotic agonist used for pain relief during labor is fentanyl (Sublimaze). Fentanyl is a short-acting synthetic opioid that is best administered IV because of its short duration of action. Morphine sulfate may also be used for pain control in active labor, but it is less frequently used. High doses of opioids are required for effective labor analgesia when administered parenterally.

The third group of systemic medications used for pain relief in labor are opioids with mixed narcotic agonist-antagonist effects. These drugs exert their effects at more than one site—often an agonist at one site and an antagonist at another. The two most commonly used narcotic-agonist-antagonist drugs are butorphanol tartrate (Stadol) and nalbuphine (Nubain). A primary advantage of these drugs is their *dose ceiling effect*. This means additional doses do not increase the degree of respiratory depression, maternal and/or neonatal, so there is less respiratory depression with these drugs than with opioids. The respiratory depression ceiling effect is believed to result from activation of kappa agonists and weak mu antagonists.

Adverse Reactions

Adverse effects of sedative-hypnotic drugs (secobarbital, pentobarbital) include paradoxically increased pain and excitability, lethargy, subdued mood, decreased sensory perception, and hypotension. Fetal and neonatal side effects include a decreased fetal heart rate (FHR) variability and neonatal respiratory depression, sleepiness, hypotonia, and delayed breastfeeding with a poor sucking response for up to 4 days.

The side effects of phenothiazine derivatives and antiemetics/antihistamines (promethazine, hydroxyzine) include confusion, disorientation, excess sedation, dizziness, hypotension, tachycardia, blurred vision, headache, restlessness, weakness, and urinary retention with *promethazine*; drowsiness, dry mouth, dizziness, headache, blurred vision, dysuria, urinary retention, and constipation with *hydroxyzine*. Decreased FHR variability occurs, and the neo-

Table 53–1

Common Systemic Medications Used for Pain Relief in Labor

Generic (Brand)	Route and Dosage	Uses and Considerations
Sedative-Hypnotics		
secobarbital (Seconal)	IM: 50-100 mg PO: 100-200 mg	Used to decrease anxiety during latent phase of labor. Onset: 15-30 min; peak: 15-30 min; duration: 1-4 h. No effects on uterine tone or contractility; rapidly crosses placenta; can cause decreased variability in FHR because of decreased CNS control over heart rate. No antagonist for barbiturates, so secobarbital administered only if delivery not expected for 24-48 h. May have prolonged depressant effects on neonate. Excreted in breast milk. Compatible with breastfeeding. May increase CNS depression with alcohol, narcotics, antihistamines, tranquilizers, and MAOIs. Avoid valerian, St. John's wort, kava kava, gotu kola. *Pregnancy category:* D; PB: 45%-60%; t½: 15-40 h
pentobarbital (Nembutal)	IV: Initial: 100-200 mg	Short-acting barbiturate. Sedative. *Pregnancy category:* D. See Prototype Drug Chart 17–1
Promethazine (Phenergan)	IM/IV: 12.5-50 mg q3-4h or IM: 25-50 mg with 25-75 mg meperidine or IV: 15-25 mg with 25-75 mg meperidine; repeat if needed; *max:* 100 mg in 24 h	A phenothiazine antihistamine; used as adjunct to narcotic analgesics during first stage of labor; antiemetic properties. Onset: IM: 20 min; IV: 3-5 min. Do not give subcutaneously. To prevent or minimize tissue damage during IV administration, dilute, administer via running IV line at port furthest from patient's vein and administer through a large bore vein if possible. Instruct patient to report signs of pain and burning with administration. Used alone to promote rest and sleep; potentiates action of narcotic agonists, reducing narcotic doses. May cause decreased variability in FHR; contraindicated during lactation. At term, rapidly crosses placenta; fetal and maternal blood concentrations in equilibrium in 15 min, with infant levels persisting for 4 h. Transient hypotonia, lethargy, and electroencephalographic changes for 3 d in newborn. May cause maternal tachycardia; may impair newborn platelet aggregation. If given with meperidine, give slowly at beginning of contraction over several minutes to decrease amount of drug perfused immediately to the fetus via placenta. *Adverse reactions:* dizziness, dry mouth, excessive sedation, weakness, blurred vision, and restlessness. *Pregnancy category:* C; PB: 35%-55%; t½: 22h
promethazine HCl (Phenergan)	IV:12.5-25 mg IM: 25-50 mg q4-6 h; repeat if needed	Antianxiety agent; antihistamine; antiemetic; sedative-hypnotic. Used alone early in labor or later to potentiate action of narcotic agonists. Onset: IV: 3-5 min; IM: 20 min; peak: IV/IM: UK; duration: 2-6 h. IV is not the preferred route for administration but is the frequent route for obstetrical clients. Solution for IV may be diluted in 25-100 ml NS or D₅W and infused over 15-30 m at a rate <25 mg/m Use Z-track injection for IM to reduce pain. Intraarterial or subQ administration not recommended (thrombus and digital gangrene can occur). Extravasation can result in sterile abscesses and marked tissue induration. Use with caution in clients with chronic obstructive pulmonary disease and asthma. Crosses placenta. Possible respiratory depression if drug administered near delivery. Can cause decreased variability in FHR. Breastfeeding not recommended. No effect on labor or neonatal Apgar scores. *Adverse reactions:* hypotension, drowsiness, dizziness, ataxia; may cause CNS depression with alcohol, analgesics, barbiturates, narcotics; may decrease effects of epinephrine. *Pregnancy category:* C; PB: 93%; t½: 3 h
hydroxyzine pamoate (Vistaril)	*Anxiety:* PO: 25-100 mg *Preoperative sedation:* 50-100 mg IM: 25-100 mg	Anxiolytic; antiemetic; antihistamine. Used for anxiety and preoperative and postoperative adjunctive for sedation. Onset: 15-30 min; peak: 2 h; duration: 4-6 hours. Administer deep in large muscle. Do not give IV or subQ. Additive effects may be noted with use of ethanol, St. John's wort, kava kava, anticholinergics and CNS depressants. *Pregnancy category:* C; PB: UK; t½: 3-7 h
Narcotic Agonists		
fentanyl citrate (Sublimaze)	IM/IV: 25-50 mcg or IM: 50-100 mcg	IV onset: 1-2 min; peak: 3-5 min; duration: 30-60 min; IM onset: 7-15 min; peak: 20 -30 min; duration: 1-2 h. Is 50-100 times as potent as morphine. Muscle rigidity may occur with too rapid IV administration. Inject over 3-5 min. Crosses placenta and excreted in breast milk. Watch for respiratory depression in neonates of mothers who receive this drug in labor. May see withdrawal symptoms in neonate if mother was regular opioid user during pregnancy. Be alert to risk of overdose in clients using CNS depressants, phenothiazines, ethanol and tricyclic antidepressants. Herbal interactions include increased CNS depression with the use of St John's wort, kava kava and gotu kola. Contraindicated in clients with severe asthma. *Pregnancy category:* C; PB: UK; t½: 2-4 h

CNS, Central nervous system; *d,* day; *FHR,* fetal heart rate; *h,* hour; *IM,* intramuscular; *IV,* intravenous; *MAOI,* monoamine oxidase inhibitor; *max,* maximum; *min,* minute; *PB,* protein-binding; *PO,* by mouth; *PRN,* as needed; *subQ,* subcutaneous; *t½,* half-life; *UK,* unknown; *<,* less than, *>,* greater than.

Continued

Table 53–1

Common Systemic Medications Used for Pain Relief in Labor—cont'd

Generic (Brand)	Route and Dosage	Uses and Considerations
morphine sulfate	IM/IV: 5-10 mg or IV 2-5 mg q4h	Opioid; binds to CNS opiate receptors and inhibits ascending pain pathways. Used for relief of moderate to severe pain, for preoperative medication, and as supplement to anesthesia. Onset: IM: 20-30 min; IV: 3-10 min. Peak: IM: 0.5-1 h; IV: 20 min. Duration: IM: 3-4 h; IV: 3-5 h. Have naloxone available as antidote. If naloxone is necessary for maternal and fetal respiratory depression, give to mother and infant. CNS depressants and tricyclic antidepressants may potentiate effects of morphine. Cautious use with MAO inhibitors and meperidine. Use of selective serotonin reuptake inhibitors (SSRIs) or meperidine may precipitate serotonin syndrome. Use with caution in patients with biliary tract disease and seizure disorders. May see withdrawal symptoms in narcotic-dependent clients. May see withdrawal symptoms in neonates of narcotic dependent clients. May cause drowsiness and respiratory depression, sedation, euphoria, hallucinations, headache, palpitations. Do not give if respirations <12/min. Morphine crosses the placenta. Use with caution in clients delivering preterm infant, because fetus may exhibit decreased beat-to-beat variability on FHR monitor. Newborn may have moderate CNS depression, hypotonia at birth, and mild behavioral depression. When giving IV, dilute in 4-5 ml of sterile water and administer slowly (15mg over 3-5 min). Herbal interactions include increased CNS depression with valerian, St John's wort, kava kava, gotu kola. Enters breast milk, compatible with breastfeeding for single doses of morphine. Chronic morphine use may have adverse neonatal effects and is not recommended. *Pregnancy category:* C (D, if prolonged use or high at-term dose); PB: 30%-35%; t½: 2-4 h
Mixed Narcotic Agonist-Antagonists		
butorphanol tartrate (Stadol)	IV: 0.5-1 mg q1.5-2h or 1-2 mg q4h	Mixed opioid agonist/antagonist. IV onset: 5-10 min; peak: 4-5 min; duration: 3-4 h. Herbal interactions include increased CNS depression with the use of valerian, St John's wort, kava kava, and gotu kola. Avoid use in opiate-dependent clients who have not been detoxified; may cause withdrawal syndrome. Cautious use in clients with renal or hepatic dysfunction. For use in pregnancies >37 gestational weeks and no fetal distress. Alternative analgesic should be used if delivery anticipated in 4 h or less. If breastfeeding, take dose immediately after breastfeeding or 3-4 hours prior to next feeding. *Pregnancy category:* C/D; PB: 80%; t½: 2.5-4 h
nalbuphine (Nubain)	IV: 5-10 mg q2-3h	Mixed opioid agonist/antagonist. Narcotic. Onset: 2-3 m; peak: 2-3 min; duration: 3-6 h. Limited respiratory depression. Less analgesic effect than morphine. About 10%-15% of laboring women experience hallucinations with nalbuphine. Cautious use in clients with renal or hepatic dysfunction. Avoid use in opiate-dependent clients, may cause withdrawal syndrome. Monitor for fetal bradycardia. Monitor newborn for respiratory depression or bradycardia. Inject slowly over at least 2-3 min. If breastfeeding, take immediately after breastfeeding or 3-4 h prior to next feeding. Herbal interactions include increased CNS depression with valerian, St John's wort, kava kava, gotu kola. Toxicity can be reversed with naloxone. *Pregnancy category:* B; PB: UK; t½: 5 h

nate can experience moderate central nervous system (CNS) depression, hypotonia, lethargy, poor feeding, and hypothermia.

The adverse effects of opioids depend on the responses activated by the mu and kappa receptors. Activation of mu receptors result in analgesia, decreased gastrointestinal (GI) motility, euphoria, respiratory depression, sedation, and physiologic dependence. In contrast, activation of kappa receptors results in analgesia, decreased gastrointestinal motility, miosis, and sedation. When parenterally administered, the side effects of opioids include nausea, vomiting, sedation, orthostatic hypotension, pruritus, and maternal and neonatal respiratory depression. The associated nausea and vomiting result from stimulation of the chemoreceptor trigger zone in the medulla. Motor block is another concern. Mothers may not walk after delivery until they are able to maintain a straight leg raise against downward pressure as applied by the practitioner. Fetal and neonatal effects include a diminished FHR variability and depression of neonatal respirations and Apgar scores. Depression of neonatal neurobehavior is evidenced by lowered Apgar scores. For example, with meperidine, neonatal respiration occurs within 2 to 3 hours after administration. Neonatal respiratory depression may require reversal by administration of naloxone (Narcan). Through inhibition of both mu and kappa receptors, naloxone (Narcan) may reverse the effects of opioids. NOTE: With maternal administration of naloxone (Narcan) there will be a subsequent increase in pain. See Chapter 18 for a discussion of neonatal naloxone dosing and administration.

Narcotic agonist drugs (morphine, fentanyl) can cause orthostatic hypotension, nausea, vomiting, headache, sedation, hypotension, and confusion. Decreased FHR variability and neonatal CNS depression can occur with meperidine.

Mixed narcotic agonist-antagonist drugs (Stadol, Nubain) can cause nausea, clamminess, sweating, sedation, respiratory depression, vertigo, lethargy, headache, and flush. Side effects in the fetus and neonate include decreased FHR variability, moderate CNS depression, hypotonia at birth, and mild behavioral depression.

Pain Control Drugs

ASSESSMENT

- Assess client's level of pain using agency pain scale.
- Assess client's cultural framework to determine the use of complementary and alternative medicine in later pregnancy and beliefs regarding laboring.
- Assess the laboring client's behavior for relaxation and progress of labor in relation to expected norms.
- Assess client's verbal and nonverbal behavior for data supportive or nonsupportive of coping with labor.
- To determine effectiveness of pain management, obtain baseline vital signs, BP, breath sounds, quality of uterine contractions, degree of effacement and dilation, and fetal heart rate (FHR) before administering analgesic.
- Question client regarding use of complementary and alternative medicine (to include herbal supplements) during pregnancy.
- Screen for drug history to ascertain potential for drug-drug interactions.
- Assess cultural expectations related to pain experiences.

NURSING DIAGNOSES

- Acute pain related to progressive labor
- Fear of pain related to labor
- Anxiety related to uncertainty about labor experience and personal coping ability

PLANNING

- Client will verbalize a level of pain she is comfortable with during the labor and delivery process.
- Client will demonstrate minimal to no side effects of pain-control drugs during labor.

- Client will verbalize a decrease in pain on a scale of 1 to 10 or per agency pain scale.

NURSING INTERVENTIONS

- Incorporate client's cultural beliefs and framework of health in plan of care.
- Offer appropriate analgesia for stage and phase of labor and anticipated method of delivery. Encourage client and her support persons to participate in decision making about analgesia.
- Document administration of drug per agency protocol.
- Provide appropriate safety measures after administration of drugs.
- Check compatibility chart for any mixing of drugs.
- Verify that correct antidote drugs are available.
- Within agency protocols, safe obstetric practice, and client preferences, administer drugs before maximum intensity of pain and anxiety.
- Assess client's level of pain using agency-appropriate pain scale within 30 to 60 minutes after analgesic administration.

Sedative-Hypnotics: Barbiturates

- Do not give if active labor is imminent.
- Monitor FHR; expect decreased variability.

Phenothiazine Derivatives

Promethazine (Phenergan)
- If administered by IV route, give at onset of the uterine contraction. Administer at a rate not to exceed 25 mg/min.
- Monitor amount of promethazine client receives in 24 hours; monitor maternal heart rate following administration.

Hydroxyzine (Vistaril)
- Administer IM (Z-track technique) only. Do not give subQ or IV.

Narcotic Agonists and Mixed Narcotic Agonist-Antagonists

- Assess client parity, obstetrical delivery history and anticipated time until delivery.
- Because of risk of neonatal respiratory depression, do not administer when delivery is likely within the next 2 hours.
- Monitor urine output.
- Monitor FHR, assessing for fetal well-being before and during drug administration.

Fentanyl (Sublimaze)

- Generally not given before active labor. Have Naloxone (Narcan) available as antidote if needed.
- If drug is administered IV, administer slowly at beginning of a contraction over several minutes to decrease

the amount of drug perfused to the fetus via the placenta.

- Assess respirations. Must be >12 before administration.
- Provide restful environment as adjunctive therapy.
- Keep bed rails up when client is nonambulatory and have client solicit assistance with ambulation.
- Monitor FHR, assessing for fetal well-being before and during drug administration.
- Have neonatal naloxone (Narcan) available.

Butorphanol Tartrate (Stadol)

- Monitor for signs of narcotic withdrawal in narcotic-dependent clients.
- Monitor for maternal and/or neonatal respiratory depression.
- Assess respirations. Must be greater than 12 before administration.
- IM: inject deep into muscle. If given IV, give slowly at onset contraction. Do not administer subQ.
- Provide restful environment as adjunctive therapy.
- Monitor FHR tracing, assessing for fetal well-being before and during drug administration.
- Keep bed rails up when client is nonambulatory, and have client solicit assistance with ambulation.
- Have naloxone (Narcan) available.

Client Teaching

General

- Instruct client concerning the following: (1) drugs ordered, (2) route of administration and reason, (3) expected effects of drug on labor, and (4) potential drug effects on client and fetus or newborn.
- Tell client that most drugs used for pain relief in labor and delivery are not given by mouth, because the gastrointestinal tract functions more slowly during labor, and drug absorption is decreased, making the oral route ineffective.

Safety

- Instruct client about safety precautions that will be used while receiving the drug, including the following: (1) positioning in bed, (2) side rails, (3) assistance with ambulation.

Cultural Considerations ❖

- Acknowledge and incorporate client's cultural belief framework into nursing care.
- Assess client's use of complementary and alternative medicine (to include herbal supplements) during pregnancy and labor.
- Recognize cultural influences on client's perception of and expression of discomfort and pain.
- Provide an interpreter as appropriate.

EVALUATION

- Evaluate effectiveness of the drug in alleviating the pain.
- Evaluate fear and anxiety in regard to pain and ability to cope with the labor experience.
- Monitor maternal respirations, heart rate, BP, uterine contractions, dilatation and effacement, and FHR for alterations from baseline. Report deviations beyond those expected with a normally progressing labor.
- Document findings, using agency protocols and obstetric nursing standards of care.

Anesthesia

Anesthesia in labor and delivery represents the loss of painful sensations with or without loss of consciousness. There are two types of pain experienced in childbirth. *Visceral pain* from the cervix and uterus is carried by sympathetic fibers and enters the neuraxis at the thoracic 10, 11, 12, and lumbar 1 spinal levels. Early labor pain is transmitted to T11 to T12 with later progression to T10 and L1. *Somatic pain* is caused by pressure of the presenting part and stretching of the perineum and vagina. This pain is the pain of the transition phase and the second stage of labor and is transmitted to the sacral 2, 3, and 4 areas by the pudendal nerve.

Regional Anesthesia

Regional anesthesia achieves pain relief during labor and delivery without loss of consciousness. Injected local anesthetic agents temporarily block conduction of painful impulses along sensory nerve pathways to the brain (Table 53–2). Regional anesthesia allows the client to experience labor and childbirth with relief from discomfort in the blocked area. There are primarily two types of anesthesia: (1) local anesthetic agents for local infiltration (e.g., episiotomy) and (2) regional blocks (e.g., epidural [Table 53–3]). The most common peridural anesthesias include spinal, epidural, and combined spinal-epidural and pudendal (Figure 53–2). Other less commonly administered regional blocks include caudal and paracervical blocks. The anesthesiologist or nurse anesthetist is responsible for administering regional anesthesia. Nurses may assist with administration of anesthesia and monitor the client for drug effectiveness and side effects during and after administration.

Women receiving parenteral analgesic for labor and delivery may require more focused anesthesia for episiotomies and for repair of perineal lacerations. Local anesthetic agents may be administered alone, and the anesthetic agent primarily administered is lidocaine. Burning at the site of injection is the most common side effect.

Spinal anesthesia, also known as a *saddle block*, is injected in the subarachnoid space at the T10 to S5 dermatome (Figure 53–3). This anesthesia may be a single dose or administered as a combined spinal epidural. Spinal anesthesia is administered immediately before delivery or

Table 53–2

Anesthetic Agents Used in Obstetrics

Anesthetic Agent	Usual Concentration	Usual Dose (mg)	Onset	Average Duration (minutes)	Clinical Use
chloroprocaine	1-2	400-600	Rapid	15-30	Local or pudendal
	2-3	300-750		30-60	Epidural
tetracaine	0.2	4	Slow	70-150	Low spinal block
	0.5	7-10	Fast	75-150	Spinal for cesarean
lidocaine	1	200-300	Rapid	30-60	Local or pudendal block
	2	300-450		60-90	Epidural for cesarean
	5	50-75		45-60	Spinal for cesarean, PP tubal ligation, and vaginal delivery
bupivacaine	0.5	75-100	Slow-moderate	90-150	Epidural for cesarean
	0.25	20-25	Moderate	60-90	Epidural for labor
	0.75	7.5-11		60-120	Spinal for cesarean
ropivacaine	0.5	75-100	Slow-moderate	90-150	Epidural for cesarean
	0.25	20-25	Slow-moderate	60-90	Epidural for labor

PP, Postpartum.

Table 53–3

Regional Anesthesia for Labor and Delivery

Type of Anesthesia	Administered When	For	Administered Where	Area Blocked	Key Points
Perineal infiltration (local)	Immediately before delivery or late 2nd stage	Episiotomies Repair of episiotomies, tears	Perineum	Perineum	Rapid onset No maternal CNS depression Does not affect pain, uterine contraction
Paracervical	1st stage of labor	Vaginal delivery	Around cervix	Nerves of uterus T10-L1	Rarely done Fetal bradycardia most common complication Maternal seizures from intravascular injections Contraindicated in clients with uteroplacental insufficiency or preexisting fetal distress
Pudendal	2nd stage of labor	Vaginal delivery, outlet forceps delivery	Pudendal nerve, S2-S4, transvaginally	Perineum and lower vagina	Maternal complications uncommon Fetal complications rare High failure rate with this block Inadequate anesthesia for mid-forceps delivery, postpartum repair of cervix & manual exploration of uterine cavity Blind sticks by provider increases risk of exposure to HIV or other virus Infrequently used
Caudal	After labor is well established	Vaginal delivery	Caudal canal 3-5 cm above the coccyx	Perineum	Mother may feel contractions, have ability to push & have effective perineal analgesia Rarely used
Spinal	Immediately before delivery or late 2nd stage	Vaginal delivery with forceps / vacuum C-section	*Saddle block:* sacral anesthesia *More commonly:* subarachnoid space at T10 to S5 dermatome	*Vaginal delivery:* umbilicus to toes *C-section:* below xiphoid process to toes	Postdural puncture headache (PDPH) May be used with high risk obstetric & obese Client may feel visceral discomfort with C-section It is advised that clients receiving low molecular weight heparin (LMWH) wait 10-12 hours after LMWH before epidural or spinal administration; MD must evaluate Side effects with intrathecal opioids include pruritus and nausea and vomiting. Complications with intrathecal opioids include fetal bradycardia and maternal respiratory depression.

Continued

Table 53–3

Regional Anesthesia for Labor and Delivery—cont'd

Type of Anesthesia	Administered When	For	Administered Where	Area Blocked	Key Points
Epidural 　Single dose 　Intermittent epidural bolus 　Continuous epidural infusion 　Patient Controlled Epidural Analgesia (PCEA) 　Combined spinal-epidural (CSE)	Generally at 4-5 cm dilation, but refer to agency policy	Vaginal delivery with forceps/vacuum C-section	Lumbar epidural space L3-L4 or L4-L5 Single bolus injected in subarachnoid space & epidural catheter in lumbar epidural space	*Vaginal delivery:* T10-S5 dermatome, umbilicus to toes *C-section:* T4/T8-S5 dermatome, nipple/xyphoid process to toes (would be large single bolus epidural)	Need for frequent injections unless receiving continuous epidural infusion Need for increased doses of anesthetics in comparison to spinal Maternal hypotension: monitor blood pressure Assess for unilateral block Need for bolus (500-1000 ml) of crystalloid (LR) solution prior to administration May prolong 2nd stage of labor Increased incidence of instrumental deliveries (forceps/vacuum) It is advised that clients receiving low molecular weight heparin (LMWH) wait 10-12 hours after LMWH before epidural or spinal administration; MD must evaluate Side effects with epidural/intrathecal opioids include pruritus and nausea and vomiting. Complications with epidural/intrathecal opioids include fetal bradycardia and maternal respiratory depression
General anesthesia	Prior to delivery	C-sections Urgent situations, medical issues require general anesthesia, epidural/spinal contraindicated	IV agents with rapid sequence inhalation anesthesia induction	Loss of consciousness	Unable to witness/participate in birth Antacid given preoperatively to prevent complications of gastric acid aspiration

late in the second stage when the fetal head is on the perineal floor. Drugs frequently administered either alone or in combination with the local anesthetic for a vaginal delivery include lidocaine (20 to 40 mg), bupivacaine (1.25 to 2.5 mg) with sufentanil (10 mcg), or fentanyl (25 mcg). Dosages vary depending on administration of the anesthetic agent plain or with epinephrine. Spinal anesthesia has a rapid onset, requires less local anesthetic, and may be used with high-risk obstetric and obese clients. Postdural puncture headache is a primary concern, occurring 6 to 48 hours after dural puncture; it may also occur after accidental dura puncture with epidural anesthesia. Treatment for postdural headache includes analgesics, increased fluids, and bed rest. With resistant headaches, 500 mg of caffeine in 500 ml normal saline may be given over 2 hours. Autologous blood patching (10 to 20 ml) is the most effective means to treat post dural headache.

Lumbar epidurals may be administered as a single injection, intermittent injections, continuous patient-controlled epidural anesthesia (PCEA), and as a combined spinal-epidural (Figure 53–3). Epidurals may be administered as a single anesthetic agent or with opioids or epinephrine. Single-dose epidural anesthesia is infrequently used as analgesia and is limited to the single dosing action. Intermittent epidural bolus dosing was once commonly used for pain relief. Doses of the local anesthetic were injected intermittently via an epidural catheter. Limitations of this method included the need for frequent injections and decreased pain control because of the dosing schedule. Most frequently clients now receive a continuous epidural infusion, which provides more consistent drug levels and more effective pain relief. Rescue doses are given as necessary to achieve pain relief.

Opioids are administered with the local anesthetic to more effectively control the somatic pain of transition and second-stage labor pain. The opioids most frequently used in combination with the local anesthetic (e.g., 0.125% bupivacaine or 0.2% ropivacaine) are fentanyl or sufentanil. Fentanyl or sufentanil are lipophilic opioids commonly

FIGURE 53–2 A, Membranes and spaces of spinal cord and levels of sacral, lumbar, and thoracic nerves. B, Cross-section of vertebra and spinal cord. (From Lowdermilk D, Perry S: *Maternity and women's health care*, ed 9, St Louis, 2007, Mosby.)

used with continuous or PCEA epidural. These opioids offer rapid analgesia and fewer side effects than hydrophilic opioids. In contrast, morphine sulfate and hydromorphone are hydrophilic opioids. They have a slower onset of action, variable duration, and increased side effects, specifically respiratory depression (Table 53–4).

Another additive to the local anesthetic is epinephrine. Epinephrine increases the duration of the local anesthetic and decreases its uptake and clearance from the cerebrospinal fluid (CSF), while enhancing the intensity of the neural blockade. Single and intermittent injections have

wide variations in drug levels and less effectively controlled pain. A continuous lumbar epidural allows a more evenly spaced drug level; less anesthetic is required to provide more effective pain control. Continuous-infusion PCEA gives the client control of her anesthesia at a basal infusion rate of 6 ml/h, a 5-ml bolus dose, and a 10-minute lockout. Frequently single, intermittent, and PCEA will require rescue doses to improve analgesia.

Lastly, combined spinal-epidural (CSE) analgesia couples the rapid analgesia and specificity of catheter placement of spinal anesthesia with continuous infusion via

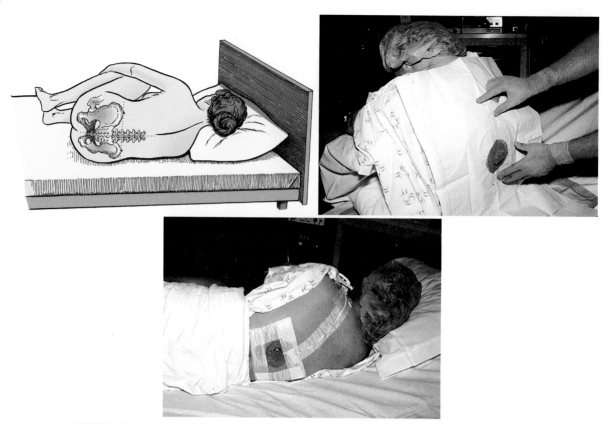

FIGURE 53–3 Positions for epidural blocks. (Photos courtesy of Michael S. Clement, MD, Mesa, Arizona. From Lowdermilk D, Perry S: *Maternity and women's health care*, ed 9, St Louis, 2007, Mosby.)

catheter of epidural anesthesia, providing pain relief for later labor.

Controversy exists regarding the effect of regional analgesia, specifically epidurals, on the progress of labor. Some studies indicate no significant effect on labor, whereas other research has demonstrated a decreased maternal urge to push and increased length of labor.

Anesthesia for cesarean deliveries may be general, spinal, or epidural. General anesthesia may be necessary for emergency deliveries, when spinal or epidural anesthesias are contraindicated. It allows for rapid anesthesia induction and control of the airway. Before the administration of general anesthesia, Bicitra 30 ml is orally administered to decrease gastric acidity. Antacids are administered to decrease complications from gastric acid aspiration. Other medications that may be used in place of Bicitra are cimetidine 300 mg, ranitidine 50 mg, or metoclopramide 10 mg.

Table 53–4

Parenteral Opioids for Labor and Delivery

Opioid	Dosage	Analgesic Effect Begins	Peak Analgesic Effect	Duration of Action
meperidine (Demerol)	IM 50-100 mg	IM 10-45 min	IM 40-50 min	IM & IV 3-4 h
	IV 25-50 mg	IV 5 min	IV 5-10 min	IM 1-2 h
fentanyl (Sublimaze)	IM 50-100 mcg	IM 7-8 min	IM 30 min	IV 30-60 min
	IV 25-50 mcg	IV almost immediately	IV 3-5 min	IM & IV 4-6 h
morphine sulfate	IM 5-10 mg	IM 15-60 min	IM 1-2 h	IM & IV 3-6 h
	IV 2-5 mg	IV 5-10 min	IV 20 min	IM & IV 3-4 h
nalbuphine (Nubain)	IM 10-20 mg	IM <15 min	IM 60 min	
	IV 10 mg	IV 12-30 min	IV 30 min	
butorphanol (Stadol)	IM 1-4 mg	IM 5-10 min	IM 30-60 min	
	IV 2 mg	IV 10 min	IV 30-60 min	

h, Hour; *IM*, intramuscular; *IV*, intravenous; *min*, minute; <, less than.

More commonly epidural or spinal anesthesia is administered for cesarean births. Spinal anesthesia is the more common choice for cesareans because of rapid onset, increased reliability, and improvement in spinal needle design (smaller gauge and shape [Sprotte needle]) with subsequent reduction in postdural headaches. For epidural inductions the test dose is given, followed by administration of the local anesthetics: lidocaine 1.5% to 2%, bupivacaine 0.5%, or chloroprocaine 3%. Epinephrine may be added, as may opioids (fentanyl 50 to 100 mcg, sufentanil 10 to 20 mcg, or Duramorph 3 to 5 mg), which are administered after clamping of the cord. Epidural provides pain relief for 18 to 24 hours. With spinal anesthesia, the local anesthetics most commonly administered are lidocaine 5% (60 to 75 mg), bupivacaine 0.75% (8 to 15 mg), or tetracaine 1% (7 to 10 mg). Epinephrine 0.2 mg and the opioids fentanyl 10-25 mg or sufentanil 10 mcg or Duramorph 0.10 to 0.25 mg may also be administered. With the additives, spinal anesthesia also provides 18 to 24 hours of pain relief.

Contraindications to peridural anesthesia are clients with skin infection at the injection site, coagulopathies, active neurologic disease, severe aortic or mitral stenosis, prior sensitivity to anesthetic agent, and hypovolemia. Of particular importance is client understanding of the procedure and informed consent.

Adverse effects from local anesthetic agents depend on their chemical properties, but primarily the CNS and cardiovascular systems are affected. CNS generally precede cardiovascular effects, with the exception of bupivacaine, in which adverse effects occur at the same drug level. Maternal systemic hypotension is the most frequent complication of regional anesthesia. Adverse CNS effects include dizziness, confusion, headache, slurred speech, metallic taste, nausea, vomiting, seizures, and coma. Cardiovascular symptoms include hypertension and tachycardia initially, followed by hypotension, cardiac arrhythmias and cardiac arrest. Fetal distress occurs secondary to maternal hypotension and subsequent reduced uteroplacental perfusion.

Adverse effects from regional anesthetics vary, depending on the agent and mode of delivery. With spinal and epidural anesthesia, a primary concern is maternal hypotension. Hypotension is defined as a decrease in systolic blood pressure greater than 20% to 30% of the baseline blood pressure or below 100 mmHg. To decrease maternal hypotension before epidural placement, an IV bolus of 500 to 1000 ml of crystalloids is given. Women with hypotension are positioned on their left side to facilitate placental perfusion then administered a rapid bolus dose of crystalloid IV solution. If the maternal hypotension does not improve with the fluid bolus, then ephedrine 5 to 15 mg is administered IV. Maternal block is a primary consideration and is decreased with administration of lower concentrations of the regional local anesthetics. Women receiving Duramorph frequently complain of pruritus, which may be effectively relieved with diphenhydramine (Benadryl) administration.

Nursing Process

Regional Anesthetics

ASSESSMENT

- Check history for drug sensitivity to local anesthetic agents.
- Assess client's "labor plan" with expectations for coping with labor and beliefs about use of analgesia and anesthesia.
- Assess knowledge about regional anesthesia.
- Assess cervical dilation and effacement and labor progress.
- Monitor fetal status.
- Review history for presence of any contraindications to regional anesthesia; notify anesthesia provider.

NURSING DIAGNOSES

- Acute pain related to progressive labor with diminished coping ability
- Deficient knowledge related to inexperience with regional anesthesia/analgesia
- Risk for impaired fetal gas exchange due to maternal hypotension secondary to epidural block
- Impaired physical mobility secondary to regional anesthesia
- Risk for urinary retention secondary to regional anesthesia

PLANNING

- Client will verbalize desired amount of pain relief during labor.
- Client will remain normotensive and maintain a normal pulse rate; fetal heart rate (FHR) will remain within normal parameters.
- Client will not experience bladder distention.
- Client will be able to discuss use of regional anesthesia for labor and delivery pain control.

NURSING INTERVENTIONS

General
- Assess hydration status before regional anesthesia is given; monitor for anesthetic hypotensive effects. Provide bolus IV fluids as ordered, usually 500-1000 ml prior to regional anesthesia administration.
- Insert Foley catheter prior to administration to monitor maternal fluid status.
- Position and support client on her left side or as instructed by anesthesia provider.
- Monitor progress of labor for any decrease in frequency or intensity of uterine contractions.
- Monitor maternal vital signs and FHR.

- Have emergency drugs and ephedrine, antihistamines, oxygen, and resuscitation equipment available.
- Be aware of how to place client in Trendelenburg position if necessary.
- Monitor for postdural puncture headache; notify anesthesia provider.

Spinal

- Assess uterine contractions; anesthetic agent must be given immediately after a contraction.
- Monitor BP for hypotensive effects per agency protocol. Have oxygen with positive pressure ventilation equipment readily available.
- Assess level of analgesia following administration and sensory and motor status following delivery.
- Document procedure per agency protocol.

Epidural

- Ensure that client has 500 to 1000 ml IV bolus of an isotonic solution before the procedure to increase circulatory volume and prevent maternal hypotension.
- Monitor FHR and progress of labor and keep in mind that anesthetic can inhibit fetal descent.
- Monitor BP for hypotensive effects per agency protocol.
- Assess level of analgesia following administration.
- If maternal hypotension occurs, maintain client on left side and increase rate of IV fluids. Notify health care provider.
- Assess for bladder distention. If voiding cues are unsuccessful (e.g., placement in semi-Fowler position, privacy, running water over the perineum, running water over the hand), then catheterize.
- Before allowing client to ambulate after delivery, assess sensory and motor status.
- Conduct ongoing pain assessment. If nature of pain changes, contact the anesthesia provider to evaluate anesthesia needs.
- Document procedure per agency protocol.

Caudal

- Place client in position requested by anesthesia provider for administration.

Paracervical Block

- Maintain continuous FHR monitoring for fetal bradycardia after administration.
- Monitor maternal BP.

Client Teaching

- Discuss technique, potential benefits, and side effects of client's particular method of anesthesia.

Side Effects

- Instruct client that regional anesthetics may slow labor and some clients may need a drug to enhance uterine contractions.
- Assess client for postdural puncture headache after spinal anesthesia or after accidental dura puncture with epidural. Instruct client that bed rest, oral analgesics, caffeine, or a autologous blood patch may be used for headache pain relief.

Skill

- Instruct client how to curl into position for epidural administration. Instruct client that forceps or vacuum extraction may be needed for delivery (because of the reduction of the "urge to push" sensation).
- Instruct client how to assume the left lateral or other position as requested by anesthesia provider for caudal anesthesia.

Safety

- Instruct client receiving epidural anesthesia that she will have an IV and close monitoring of FHR and uterine contractions secondary to anesthesia.

EVALUATION

- Evaluate BP compared with preprocedure baseline; also evaluate FHR for alterations in variability and for decelerations.
- Evaluate effectiveness of anesthetic in relieving discomfort. Also evaluate for uniformity of anesthesia; if lateralization or if "patchy," notify anesthesia provider.
- Assess for bladder distention. If voiding cues are unsuccessful (e.g., placement in semi-Fowler position, privacy, running water over the perineum, running water over the hand), then catheterize.
- Before allowing client to ambulate after delivery, assess sensory and motor status.
- Evaluate uterine fundus for firmness.

Spinal Block (Subarachnoid Block)
Adverse Reactions

Client: Hypotension; paresthesia or nerve injury, high/spinal block (respiratory muscles are impaired by block), postdural puncture headache, neuritis, block failure. NOTE: Headache is less common because of the small size (25 gauge) of needle used. Client may have nausea, vomiting, backache, urinary retention, apnea with total spinal, or infection. *Fetus or neonate:* None, unless secondary to maternal hypotension, then FHR late decelerations.

Normal Dose

Vaginal delivery: bupivacaine 1.25-2.5 mg (with sufentanil 10 mcg or fentanyl 25 mcg) or 5% lidocaine 20-40 mg injected intrathecally. *Cesarean delivery:* lidocaine 5% (60-75 mg), bupivacaine 0.75% (8-15 mg), tetracaine 1%

(7-10 mg) with epinephrine 0.2 mg and/or fentanyl 10-25 mcg or sufentanil 10 mcg or Duramorph 0.10-0.25 mg.

Nursing Implications

Client needs to be well hydrated; administer bolus of 500-1000 ml crystalloid solution as ordered. Cervix should be fully dilated before administration. Anesthetic should be given immediately after a contraction to avoid impairing neonate's respiratory efforts. Client is generally placed sitting or in curled side-lying position for administration. Monitor blood pressure every 1 to 2 minutes for the first 10 minutes. After administration, monitor BP every 5 to 10 minutes. Assess level of analgesia. Treat maternal hypotension due to uterine displacement by placing a wedge under hip.

Contraindications

Infection at puncture site, increased intracranial pressure, allergy to local anesthetics, coagulopathies, severe hypovolemia, severe aortic or mitral stenosis, or lack of client consent.

Indication

Need for high degree of pain relief for delivery. Used primarily for cesarean delivery, forceps delivery, or in the postpartum period for repair of traumatic lacerations of the perineum or removal of retained placenta; infrequently used for labor. *When given:* Immediately before delivery; late in second stage when fetal head is on the perineum (for vaginal delivery). *Area blocked:* Umbilicus to toes with vaginal delivery. Immediately below xyphoid process to toes with cesarean delivery. *Injection site:* With client in sitting or side-lying position, anesthetic injected into subarachnoid space at L4-L5.

Lumbar Epidural Block (Single Dose)
Adverse Reactions

Client: Hypotension, paresthesia or nerve injury, neuritis, postdural headache with accidental puncture of dura, epidural hematoma, and high/total block (respiratory muscles are impaired by block). NOTE: Headache is less common because of the small size (25 gauge) of needle used. Client may have nausea, vomiting, backache, urinary retention, infection, catheter complications, intravascular injection, direct spinal cord injury and bloody tap. *Fetus or neonate:* Few, unless secondary to maternal hypotension, then FHR late decelerations.

Normal Dose

Vaginal delivery: bupivacaine 0.125%-0.25%, lidocaine 1%, or chloroprocaine 2% (8-15 ml), or sufentanil 10-15 mcg or 100-200 mcg fentanyl in 10 ml of saline, or bupivacaine 0.0625% plus fentanyl 50 mcg or sufentanil 10 mcg. *Cesarean delivery:* lidocaine 1.5%-2% or bupivacaine 0.5% or chloroprocaine 3% with epinephrine or sodium bicarbonate 1 ml/10 ml local anesthetic and/or fentanyl 50-100 mcg

or sufentanil 10-20 mcg or Duramorph 3-5 mg given after the umbilical cord is clamped.

Nursing Implications

Before epidural, client is well hydrated with 500-1000 ml of dextrose-free intravenous fluids. A test dose (3 ml of lidocaine & 1.5% epinephrine) is administered by the anesthesiologist or nurse anesthetist and used to confirm correct placement of catheter; if local anesthetic is injected into vein, client may experience dizziness, ringing in ears, numb mouth, metallic taste, or toxic response. Loss or reduction of bearing-down reflex means low forceps or vacuum extraction may be needed for delivery. May slow progress of labor. Maternal lateral positioning is done to prevent aortocaval compression. Maternal diastolic blood pressure should be less than 110 mmHg before initiating the epidural. When maternal hypotension occurs, place the client on her left side, infuse IV fluids rapidly, and administer ephedrine 5-15 mg IV. Monitor BP every 1 to 2 minutes for the first 10 minutes, then every 10-30 minutes until the block wears off. Assess level of analgesia. After delivery, assess motor strength prior to ambulation. Of particular importance is the assessment of bilateral analgesia for pain relief during labor. If unilateral analgesia occurs, client is turned to opposite side and more anesthetic is injected.

Contraindications

Infection at site, increased intracranial pressure, allergy to local anesthetics, coagulopathies, severe hypovolemia, severe aortic or mitral stenosis, or lack of client consent.

Indication

Pain relief in first and second stages of labor. *When given:* Active labor, 5-6 cm dilated in a primipara, 3-4 cm in a multipara. *Area blocked:* T12-S5 (entire pelvis) in area of dorsal root ganglion, with varying degrees of motor and sensory loss depending on dosage and agent injected. *Injection site:* Epidural space (potential space between the dura mater and vertebral canal from cranium to sacrum) between L2-L3 or L3-L5 or L4-L5; *not* in the dura. Never injected above L1, where the spinal cord ends. Nerves run off and down the spinal canal, where they free-float and are easily moved aside by the epidural needle. The goal is to bathe the nerves with dispersed local anesthetic.

Continuous Lumbar Epidural Block Using Indwelling Catheter in Epidural Space
Adverse Reactions

Client: Hypotension, paresthesia or nerve injury, postdural headache with accidental puncture of dura. NOTE: Headache is less common because of the small size (25 gauge) of needle used. Client may have nausea, vomiting, backache, urinary retention, infection, catheter complications, intravascular injection, direct spinal cord injury and bloody tap. *Fetus or neonate:* Few, unless secondary to maternal hypotension, then FHR late decelerations.

Normal Dose

Continuous infusion options (rate is 8-15 ml/hr): bupivacaine 0.04%-0.125% plus fentanyl 1-2 mcg/ml or sufentanil 0.1-0.3 mcg/ml or bupivacaine 0.125% without opiate.

Nursing Implications

Before epidural, client is well hydrated with 500-1000 ml of dextrose-free IV fluids. Test dose (3 ml of lidocaine & 1.5% epinephrine) is administered by the anesthesiologist or nurse anesthetist and used to confirm correct placement of catheter; if local anesthetic is injected into vein, client may experience dizziness, ringing in ears, numb mouth, metallic taste, or toxic response. Loss or reduction of bearing-down reflex means low forceps or vacuum extraction may be needed for delivery. May slow progress of labor. Maternal lateral positioning is done to prevent aortocaval compression. Maternal diastolic blood pressure should be less than 110 mmHg before initiating the epidural. When maternal hypotension occurs, place the client on her left side, infuse IV fluids rapidly, and administer ephedrine 5-15 mg IV. Monitor BP every 1-2 minutes for the first 10 minutes and then every 10-30 minutes until the block wears off. Assess level of analgesia. After administration of the anesthetic, assess motor strength prior to ambulation. Breakthrough pain is treated by increased infusion rate of rescue dose of anesthetic.

Indication

Pain relief during first and second stages. This is the most widely used anesthesia method for labor pain management. Useful for prolonged labor. *When given:* Progressive active labor, 5-6 cm dilated in a primipara, 3-4 cm in a multipara. *Area blocked:* Same as for lumbar epidural block. *Injection site:* Same as for lumbar epidural block.

Advantages

Provides continuous anesthesia from stage 1 through delivery and perineal repair. Client can feel movement and pressure but no pain. Can be used for vaginal delivery or cesarean birth. Sensory level can be altered and density of the block can be manipulated. Can be used to deliver epidural morphine PF (Duramorph) or fentanyl (Sublimaze) into epidural space for regional analgesia (highly effective). Clients may experience pruritus, which may be effectively relieved with diphenhydramine (Benadryl) or naloxone (Narcan) infusions.

Considerations

Loss or reduction of bearing-down reflex means that forceps or a vacuum extraction may be needed for delivery. Requires an increased amount of local anesthetic agent. Bupivacaine is used in low concentration (as low as 1/16%) and may be combined with fentanyl (Sublimaze).

Complications

Same as for lumbar epidural block.

Side Effects

Pruritus (in 2 to 3 hours when drug reaches upper thoracic segments), urinary retention, and nausea and vomiting related to ineffective hydration to prevent hypotension during labor.

PCEA (Patient Controlled Epidural Administration)
Adverse Reactions

Client: Hypotension, paresthesia or nerve injury, postdural headache with accidental puncture of dura. Note: Headache is less common because of the small size (25 gauge) of needle used. Client may have nausea, vomiting, backache, urinary retention, infection, catheter complications, intravascular injection, direct spinal cord injury and bloody tap. *Fetus or neonate:* Few, unless secondary to maternal hypotension, then FHR late decelerations.

Nursing Implications

Before epidural, client should be well hydrated with 500-1000 ml of dextrose-free IV fluids. Test dose (3 ml of lidocaine & 1.5% epinephrine) is used to confirm correct placement of catheter; if local anesthetic is injected into vein, client may experience dizziness, ringing in ears, numb mouth, metallic taste, or toxic response. Loss or reduction of bearing-down reflex means low forceps or vacuum extraction may be needed for delivery. May slow progress of labor. Maternal lateral positioning is done to prevent aortocaval compression. Maternal diastolic blood pressure should be less than 110 mmHg before initiating the epidural. When maternal hypotension occurs, place the client on her left side, infuse IV fluids rapidly, and administer ephedrine 5-15 mg IV. Monitor BP every 1 to 2 minutes for the first 10 minutes and then every 10-30 minutes until the block wears off. Assess level of analgesia. After delivery, assess motor strength prior to ambulation. Breakthrough pain is treated by increased infusion rate of rescue dose of anesthetic.

Indication

Pain relief during first and second stages. Useful for prolonged labor. *When given:* Progressive active labor, 5-6 cm dilated in a primipara, 3-4 cm in a multipara. *Area blocked:* Same as for lumbar epidural block. *Injection site:* Same as for lumbar epidural block.

Advantages

Provides continuous anesthesia from stage 1 through delivery and perineal repair. Client can feel movement and pressure but no pain. Client is in control, and dose may be self-titrated according to her perception of pain. Sensory level can be altered and density of the block can be manipulated. Can be used to deliver epidural morphine PF (Duramorph) or fentanyl (Sublimaze) into epidural space for regional analgesia (highly effective). Clients may experience pruritus, which may be effectively relieved with diphenhydramine (Benadryl) or naloxone (Narcan) infusions.

Considerations

Loss or reduction of bearing-down reflex means that forceps or a vacuum extraction may be needed for delivery. Requires an increased amount of local anesthetic agent. Bupivacaine is used in low concentration (as low as 1/16%) and may be combined with fentanyl (Sublimaze).

Complications

Same as for lumbar epidural block.

Side Effects

Pruritus (in 2 to 3 hours when drug reaches upper thoracic segments), urinary retention, and nausea and vomiting related to ineffective hydration to prevent hypotension during labor.

Combined Spinal-Epidural
Adverse Reactions

Client: Hypotension, paresthesia or nerve injury, post-dural headache. NOTE: Headache is less common because of the small size (25 gauge) of needle used. Client may have nausea, vomiting, backache, urinary retention, infection, catheter complications, intravascular injection, direct spinal cord injury, and bloody tap. Proper catheter placement is not assured; this becomes a problem if an epidural catheter is needed for emergency analgesic administration. *Fetus or neonate:* Few, unless secondary to maternal hypotension, then FHR late decelerations.

Normal Dose

Spinal: 25 mcg fentanyl or 10 mcg sufentanil in 1 ml PF saline; epidural is initiated with bupivacaine 0.04%-0.125% plus fentanyl 1-2 mcg/ml or sufentanil 0.1-0.3 mcg/ml or bupivacaine 0.125% without opiate.

Nursing Implications

Before epidural, client is well hydrated with 500-1000 ml of dextrose-free IV fluids. Test dose (3 ml of lidocaine & 1.5% epinephrine) is used to confirm correct placement of catheter; if local anesthetic is injected into vein, client may experience dizziness, ringing in ears, numb mouth, metallic taste, or toxic response. Loss or reduction of bearing-down reflex means low forceps or vacuum extraction may be needed for delivery. May slow progress of labor. Maternal lateral positioning is done to prevent aortocaval compression. Maternal diastolic blood pressure should be less than 110 mmHg before initiating the epidural. When maternal hypotension occurs, place the client on her left side, infuse IV fluids rapidly, and administer ephedrine 5-15 mg IV. Monitor BP every 1 to 2 minutes for the first 10 minutes and then every 10-30 minutes until the block wears off. Assess level of analgesia. After delivery, assess motor strength prior to ambulation. Breakthrough pain is treated by increased infusion rate of rescue dose of anesthetic.

Indication

Pain relief during first and second stages. Spinal can help with early labor pain and epidural with pain management during active labor. *When given:* Progressive active labor. *Area blocked:* Same as for spinal and lumbar epidural block. *Injection site:* Same as for spinal and lumbar epidural block.

Advantages

Provides continuous anesthesia from stage 1 through delivery and perineal repair. Client can feel movement and pressure but no pain. Sensory level can be altered and density of the block can be manipulated. Can be used to deliver epidural morphine PF (Duramorph) or fentanyl (Sublimaze) into epidural space for regional analgesia (highly effective). Clients may experience pruritus, which may be effectively relieved with diphenhydramine (Benadryl) or naloxone (Narcan). Administration of a combination of local anesthetic and opioid more effectively blocks the somatic pain of transition and second-stage labor.

Considerations

Loss or reduction of bearing-down reflex means that forceps or a vacuum extraction may be needed for delivery. Requires an increased amount of local anesthetic agent. Bupivacaine is used in low concentration (as low as $^1/_{16}$%) and may be combined with fentanyl (Sublimaze).

Complications

Same as for lumbar epidural block.

Side Effects

Pruritus (in 2 to 3 hours when drug reaches upper thoracic segments), urinary retention, and nausea and vomiting related to ineffective hydration to prevent hypotension during labor.

Caudal (a Type of Epidural Anesthesia)
Indication

Pain in first and second stages of labor. *When given:* Active labor. *Area blocked:* Perineum; masks uterine contractions. *Injection site:* Epidural space through sacral hiatus (S4).

Advantages

Useful for women with metabolic, lung, and heart disease. Very rapid perineal anesthesia and muscle relaxation. Can be used continuously.

Considerations

Increased need to use forceps or vacuum extraction because there is a loss of urge to push. Risk of systemic toxic reactions. Level of anesthesia is more difficult to obtain.

Paracervical Block
Indication

Pain during first stage. Due to high incidence of fetal bradycardia, paracervical block is infrequently administered. *When given:* Active phase of first stage; may be repeated periodically until 8-cm dilated. *Area blocked:* Uterus, cervix, and vagina; masks uterine contractions. *Injection site:* Submucosa of the fornix of the vagina lateral to the cervix.

Advantages

Rapid onset. Lasts 60 to 90 minutes. Relieves pain of cervical dilation and contractions. Does not block lower vagina or perineum.

Considerations

Rapid absorption (because injected into a very vascular area). Does not provide anesthesia for delivery or episiotomy repair. Has variable effects on labor progress.

Side Effects

Client: Hematomas in tissue around injection site. *Fetus:* Mild to severe bradycardia or prolonged FHR deceleration with decreased variability are common.

Pudendal Block
Indication

For low forceps deliveries, episiotomy, and laceration repair. *When given:* Immediately before birth. *Area blocked:* Perineum; pudendal nerves. *Injection site:* Transvaginally, behind each sacrospinous ligament to block pudendal nerves.

Considerations

None. Not useful for pain management in first stage of labor.

Side Effects

None.

Local Infiltration
Indication

For episiotomy and perineal laceration repair. *When given:* Just before delivery or repair. *Area blocked:* Local area adjacent to injection. *Injection site:* Perineal subcutaneous tissue.

Advantage

No effect on FHR or client's vital signs.

Considerations

May not obtain complete relief of pain and may need additional injections; requires large amount of local anesthetic agent.

Side Effects

Client: Mild discomfort and/or burning during injection. *Fetus or neonate:* None.

Relative Contraindications to Regional Anesthesia

The following are relative contraindications to regional anesthesia:

- Morbid obesity
- Severe gestational hypertension (increased risk of profound hypotension associated with underlying disease state)
- Coagulation disorders and risk of bleeding secondary to decreased platelets (client should have a normal partial thromboplastin time and platelet count)
- Generalized sepsis or local infection at needle insertion site

Drugs that Enhance Uterine Muscle Contractility

Uterotropic drugs enhance uterine contractility by stimulating the smooth muscle of the uterus. Oxytocin, the ergot alkaloids, and some prostaglandins constitute the uterotropics.

Oxytocin is synthesized in the hypothalamus and is transported to nerve endings in the posterior pituitary. The hormone is released by the nerve endings under appropriate stimulation; capillaries absorb the substance and carry it into the general circulation, where it facilitates uterine smooth muscle contraction.

In the presence of adequate estrogen levels (those normally achieved by the third trimester), IV oxytocin stimulates uterine contraction. Oxytocin, prepared in synthetic form and marketed as Pitocin, is approved by the Food and Drug Administration (FDA) for labor induction and labor augmentation. Box 53–1 presents common medical reasons for induction.

Before **labor induction** (process of causing or initiating labor) begins, risks and benefits and the status of mother and fetus must be assessed. Informed consent for induction must be obtained. The gestational age of the fetus must be considered, together with position of the fetus (head down and deep in the pelvis) and size of the fetus in relation to the client's pelvis. The client's **cervical ripening** (softening of the cervix) is also assessed; the cervix is ripe, and thus ready for induction, when it is soft and progressing in effacement and partial dilation. An objective scoring system called the **Bishop score** (scoring system to assist in

---

Box 53-1

Indications for Labor Induction

- Pregnancy-induced hypertension
- Chronic hypertension
- Membrane rupture >24 hours
- Chorioamnionitis
- Postdates (>42 weeks' gestation)
- Intrauterine growth retardation (IUGR)
- Positive contraction stress test (CST)
- Maternal diabetes mellitus (classes B-F)
- Maternal renal disease
- Isoimmunization
- Intrauterine fetal death

predicting whether labor induction may be successful) is used to assess readiness for induction. Elements assessed in the modified Bishop Scoring System are dilation, effacement, station, cervical consistency, and cervical position. Modified Bishop scores of 8 or greater are associated with a successful labor induction.

Some clients are not suitable candidates for labor induction, because the risks of the procedure outweigh the potential benefits. Box 53–2 presents some major contraindications to labor induction.

Two approaches of labor induction are used to ripen, efface, and begin cervical dilation in pregnant women at term (or near term) with a medical or obstetric indication for labor induction: *mechanical methods* and *prostaglandins*.

One mechanical method involves insertion of a Foley catheter through an undilated cervix and internal os with subsequent inflation of the bulb. The Foley catheter bulb provides a mechanical stimulation similar to "stripping of the membranes." When the Foley "falls out," the client is started on IV oxytocin. A second mechanical method is insertion of an extraamniotic saline infusion with a balloon catheter to induce labor. A third mechanical method is membrane "stripping." With membrane stripping, there is release of prostaglandin F_2 from the decidua or prostaglandin E_2 from the cervix. Spontaneous labor has been induced within 72 hours of membrane stripping with no increase in infection rates. Amniotomy, artificial rupture of the membranes, is commonly performed in women with a partially dilated and effaced cervix. When done at 5 cm, dilated spontaneous labor is shortened by 1 to 4 hours without an increase in maternal or fetal complications. Chorioamnionitis and cord compression have been reported.

The second approach to labor induction uses administration of dinoprostone, the naturally occurring form of prostaglandin E_2 (PGE_2). It is thought that intracervically or intravaginally administered PGE_2 acts to create cervical effacement and softening through a combination of contraction-inducing and cervical-ripening properties, possibly secondary to an increased submucosal water content and collagen degradation resulting from collagenase secretion in response to PGE_2. One approach uses prefilled syringes of commercially prepared dinoprostone cervical gel 0.5 mg. (Prepidil gel); the gel is introduced just inside the cervical os. A second approach is the placement in the posterior vaginal fornix of a vaginal insert (Cervidil) containing 10 mg of controlled-release dinoprostone at 0.3 mg/h.

Prostaglandin E_1 is also effective in stimulating cervical ripening, although administration is an off-label use. Cytotec or misoprostol (prostaglandin E_1) may be administered intravaginally or orally. Dosing ranges from 25 to 50 mcg every 3 to 4 hours.

Side effects associated with the use of prostaglandins include uterine hyperstimulation, which may be treated with terbutaline sulfate. Uncommonly some patients may experience chills, fever, vomiting and diarrhea. Contraindications to the use of prostaglandins include active vaginal bleeding and known allergies to prostaglandins. With hepatic or renal disease, cautious use of prostaglandin E_2 is recommended; its use is contraindicated in patients with glaucoma. Contraindications for prostaglandin E_1 include a previous cesarean delivery or hysterotomy.

Table 53–5 presents the dosage, uses, and considerations for administration of dinoprostone for cervical ripening.

Oxytocin

In addition to labor induction, IV oxytocin can also be used for labor augmentation. It facilitates smooth-muscle contraction in the uterus of a client already in labor but experiencing inadequate **uterine contractility** (tightening and shortening of uterine muscles). The client with **uterine inertia** (uterine inactivity or hypotonic contractions) may be more responsive to oxytocin than the client who has not begun labor; therefore a lower starting dose will be needed.

In both labor induction and **labor augmentation** (stimulation of effective uterine contractions once labor has begun), oxytocin is infused at a prescribed individualized dosage rate, and this rate is increased, decreased, or maintained at fixed intervals based on uterine and fetal response. The objective is to establish an adequate contraction pattern that promotes labor progress, generally represented by contractions every 2 to 3 minutes that last for 50 to 60 seconds with moderate intensity. It is important that the client receiving oxytocin not experience uterine hyperstimulation, which causes markedly increased pain and compromised FHR patterns secondary to impaired placental perfusion. Continuous nursing observation during labor induction or augmentation is critical. The need for an accurate infusion rate requires the use of an infusion pump with oxytocin as an IV piggyback line. Once cervical dilation has reached 5 to 6 cm, and an ade-

---

Box 53–2

Contraindications to Labor Induction

- Disproportion between fetal head and maternal pelvis (cephalopelvic disproportion)
- Unfavorable fetal presentation (transverse or breech)
- Documented fetal intolerance of uterine contractions
- Prematurity
- Placenta previa or suspected abruptio placentae
- Severe pregnancy-induced hypertension
- Multiparity (6 or more)
- Multifetal gestation
- History of uterine trauma
- Previous major surgery in the area of the cervix or uterus
- Prior classical uterine incision
- Active genital herpes infection
- Umbilical cord prolapse
- Excessive amniotic fluid causing overdistended uterus

Table 53–5

Dinoprostone for Cervical Ripening

Generic (Brand)	Route and Dosage	Uses and Considerations
dinoprostone cervical gel, 0.5 mg (Prepidil gel)	Intracervical: Prepidil contains 0.5 mg of dinoprostone in 2.5 ml of gel for intracervical use. Repeat in 6-12 h if negative cervical or uterine response. The maximum 24 h dose is 1.5 mg, supplied in 3 doses. Before beginning oxytocin after the Prepidil administration there should be a 6- to 12-h delay	A naturally occurring form of prostaglandin E_2 (PGE_2). Used to ripen unfavorable cervix at or near term in pregnant women needing labor induction. Metabolized in lung, liver, and kidney; eliminated by kidney. Must be administered in a hospital. Clients may have a reactive nonstress test before first dose. Monitor uterine activity and FHR; suggest a 20-min FHR strip before doses. Gel must be at room temperature before administration and is administered by sterile technique. Gel must not be placed above level of cervical os. Client is to remain recumbent 15-30 min following administration of gel and 2 h after insert administration. Drug may augment other oxytocic agents; therefore no concomitant use; sequential use 6-12 h after gel is recommended. Insert may be inserted with minimal amount of water-soluble lubricant. Wear sterile gloves when administering gel or insert. Contraindicated in clients with prostaglandin hypersensitivity, cephalopelvic disproportion (CPD), ruptured membranes, and unexplained vaginal bleeding. Use gel with caution in clients with asthma, seizures, glaucoma, increased intraocular pressure, cardiovascular, renal, or hepatic disease. Not recommended for clients in whom oxytocic drugs are contraindicated or with prolonged uterine contractions; not recommended in clients with placenta previa or active genital herpes (vaginal delivery not indicated). *Adverse reactions:* uterine hyperstimulation, nausea, vomiting, diarrhea, back pain, warm feeling in vagina, and dinoprostone-induced fever, fetal distress. Treat dinoprostone-induced fever, which occurs in about 50% of clients, with tepid baths and increased fluids. Fever is not to be treated with aspirin. Assess vaginal discharge frequently during use. *Pregnancy category:* C; PB: UK; t½: UK; onset: 10-60 min; peak: UK; duration: 12 h
dinoprostone (Cervidil vaginal inserts)	Vaginal: Cervidil contains 10 mg of dinoprostone in a timed release insert, releasing 0.3 mg/h. Insert is left in place for 12 h. Oxytocin may be started 30-60 min after removal of the insert. In contrast to the gel, the insert may be removed with FHR decelerations or uterine hyperstimulation Ripening unfavorable cervix: Intravaginal: 10 mg over 12 h; remove 12 h after insertion or at onset of active labor	Remove insert and have oxygen or beta-adrenergic drugs to treat uterine hyperstimulation. Use insert at room temperature. Provider should wear sterile gloves to decrease risk of absorption as inserted high into the vagina. Assess cervical dilatation and effacement at the time of insertion. After administration, client remains in lying position for 30 min-2 h. Monitor FHR and uterine stimulation during use. Have medication available for frequent gastrointestinal side effects of abdominal cramping, diarrhea, nausea, and vomiting. Contraindicated in clients with prostaglandin hypersensitivity, cephalopelvic disproportion (CPD), ruptured membranes, and unexplained vaginal bleeding. Use insert with caution in clients with asthma, seizures, glaucoma, increased intraocular pressure, cardiovascular, renal, or hepatic disease. Not recommended for clients in whom oxytocic drugs are contraindicated or with prolonged uterine contractions; not recommended in clients with placenta previa or active genital herpes (vaginal delivery not indicated). *Adverse reactions:* uterine hyperstimulation, nausea, vomiting, diarrhea, back pain, warm feeling in vagina, and dinoprostone-induced fever, fetal distress. Treat dinoprostone-induced fever, which occurs in about 50% of clients, with tepid baths and increased fluids. Fever is not to be treated with aspirin. Assess vaginal discharge frequently during use. Onset: UK; peak: UK; duration: up to 2-3 h. *Pregnancy category:* C; PB: UK; t½: UK

FHR, Fetal heart rate; *h,* hour; *min,* minute; *PB,* protein-binding; *t½,* half-life; *UK,* unknown.

quate contraction pattern is evident, the rate of oxytocin infusion can often be slowed or stopped.

Following delivery, oxytocin 10 to 20 mg is usually added to an existing IV solution to help the uterus stay contracted and thus close the uterine sinuses at the placental site. The drug can also be given IM after delivery of the placenta.

Prototype Drug Chart 53–1 shows the actions and effects of oxytocin.

Oxytocin (Pitocin, Syntocinon) is well absorbed from the nasal mucosa when administered intranasally for milk letdown. The protein-binding percent is low, and the half-life is 1 to 9 minutes. It is rapidly metabolized and excreted by the liver.

The onset of action of oxytocin administered IM is in 3 to 5 minutes, the peak concentration time is unknown, and the duration of action is 2 to 3 hours. The onset of action of oxytocin administered by IV is immediate, the peak con-

Prototype DRUG CHART 53–1

OXYTOCIN

Drug Class

Oxytocic
Trade names: Pitocin, Syntocinon
Pregnancy Category: X

Dosage

For induction or augmentation of labor:
A: IV: 10 units (1 amp) diluted in 1000 ml lactated
  Ringer's to 10 milliunits/ml. (Resulting concentration is
  10 milliunits oxytocin per 1 ml of IV fluid.) Connect to
  primary IV line close to needle site as a piggyback
  line. Low-dose oxytocin regimen: start oxytocin at
  0.5-1 or 1-2 milliunits/min with an incremental dose
  of 1-2 milliunits/min; *max:* 20 milliunits/min. High-
  dose oxytocin regimen: begin oxytocin at 6 milliunits/
  min IV with an increase in dose by 6 milliunits/min every 15 min; *max:* 40 milliunits/min.
Postdelivery:
A: IV: 10-20 units added to 1000 ml electrolyte or
  dextrose solution; infuse at rate to prevent uterine
  atony IM: 10 units after delivery of the placenta
Nasal spray: One spray into one or both nostrils 2-3 min
  before nursing or pumping; not for use during
  pregnancy

Contraindications

Proven cephalopelvic disproportion, fetal intolerance
  of labor, hypersensitivity, anticipated nonvaginal
  delivery, pregnancy (intranasal spray)

Drug-Lab-Food Interactions

Drug: Hypertension with vasopressors, cyclopropane
  anesthetics

Pharmacokinetics

Absorption: PO: Not well absorbed, intranasal
  and IM very rapidly
Distribution: PB: Low; widely distributed in extracellular
  fluid; minute amounts in fetal circulation
Metabolism: t½: 1-9 min; rapidly metabolized by liver
Excretion: In urine

Pharmacodynamics

IM: Onset: 3-5 min
  Peak: 40 min
  Duration: 2-3 h
IV: Onset: Within 1 min
  Peak: UK
  Duration: 1 h
Intranasal: Onset: Few minutes
  Peak: UK
  Duration: UK

Therapeutic Effects/Uses

To induce or augment labor contractions; to treat uterine atony; to stimulate milk letdown (intranasal spray)
Mechanism of Action: Promotes uterine contractions by increasing intracellular concentrations of calcium in uterine
  myometrial tissue, thereby increasing the activity of the calcium-dependent phosphorylating enzyme myosin light-
  chain kinase. The nasal spray works by forcing milk into larger ducts and sinuses. This occurs because oxytocin
  promotes milk ejection by causing contraction of the smooth-muscle fibers surrounding the breast alveoli and lac-
  tiferous ducts.

Side Effects

Maternal effects with undiluted IV use only:
  hypertension, dysrhythmias, tachysystole, and uterine
  hyperstimulation. Tachysystole is 6 or more uterine
  contractions in a 20-min window. (Hyperstimulation
  is defined as uterine contractions lasting at least
  2 min or 5 or more contractions in a 10-min window.)

Adverse Reactions

Seizures, water intoxication if given in electrolyte-free
  solution or at a rate greater than 20 milliunits/min.
  (Water intoxication is manifested by nausea,
  vomiting, hypotension, tachycardia, and cardiac
  arrhythmias.)
Life-threatening: *Client:* Intracranial hemorrhage,
  cardiac dysrhythmias, asphyxia
  Fetus: jaundice, hypoxia

A, Adult; *amp*, ampule; *h*, hour; *IM*, intramuscular; *IV*, intravenous; *min*, minute; *PB*, protein-binding; *PO*, by mouth; *t½*, half-life;
UK, unknown.

centration time is unknown, and the duration of action is 1 hour. The onset of action of intranasally administered oxytocin is a few minutes, the peak concentration time is unknown, and the duration of action is 20 minutes.

The medication is diluted and administered IV piggyback for induction or augmentation of labor. Pitocin is diluted in a variety of ways and administered via infusion pump in ml/min dosing with the volume determined by the dilution. IV administration of undiluted oxytocin is not recommended because of the risk of a sudden, acute hypotensive response.

Concurrent use of vasopressors can result in severe hypertension. Hypotension can occur with concurrent use of cyclopropane anesthesia and with undiluted IV push administration.

Nursing Process

Enhancement of Uterine Contractility: Oxytocins

ASSESSMENT

■ Obtain client informed consent prior to induction or augmentation.
■ Confirm term gestation before inducing or augmenting labor.
■ Collect accurate baseline data before beginning infusion, including maternal pulse and blood pressure (BP), uterine history, uterine activity, and fetal heart rate (FHR) pattern.
■ Interview client and review history to ascertain that there are no contraindications.

NURSING DIAGNOSES

■ Deficient knowledge related to drugs used to promote uterine contractility

PLANNING

■ Oxytocin will enhance uterine contractions without adverse maternal or fetal effects.
■ Client's vital signs will be within acceptable ranges throughout labor, delivery, and postpartum period.
■ FHR will demonstrate normal rate, pattern, and variability throughout labor and delivery.

NURSING INTERVENTIONS

■ Have tocolytic agents and oxygen readily available.
■ Monitor intake and output.
■ Monitor maternal pulse and BP, uterine activity, and FHR during oxytocin infusion.
■ Maintain client in sitting or lateral recumbent position to promote placental infusion.

■ Monitor for signs of uterine rupture, which include FHR decelerations, sudden increased pain, loss of uterine contractions, hemorrhage, and rapidly developing hypovolemic shock.

Client Teaching

• Inform client that drug is given IV and dosage adjusted in response to uterine contraction pattern.
• For milk letdown, teach client timing and method of nasal administration.

EVALUATION

• Evaluate for effective labor progress.
• Monitor maternal vital signs and FHR. Report changes in vital signs and FHR, specifically late decelerations and any vaginal bleeding.

Ergot Alkaloids

The **ergot alkaloids** (one of a large group of alkaloids derived from a fungus) act by direct smooth-muscle-cell receptor stimulation. These drugs are not used during labor, because they can cause sustained uterine contractions (tetanic contractions), which would result in fetal hypoxia and possibly rupture of the uterus. The uterus becomes more sensitive to these drugs too. After delivery, however, sustained contractions are effective in the prevention or control of postpartum hemorrhage and the promotion of uterine involution.

The two most commonly used ergot derivatives are ergonovine maleate (Ergotrate Maleate tablets) and methylergonovine maleate (Methergine). Methylergonovine maleate can be given by mouth. IV administration is not recommended and is given only in emergency situations. If Methergine is given IV, administer 0.2 mg over 1 minute. Transient significant elevations in BP can occur, particularly after IV infusion. Clients with gestational hypertension or peripheral vascular diseases should not receive ergot derivatives. Table 53–6 presents the most commonly used uterotonic drugs.

Side Effects and Adverse Reactions

Side effects of ergot alkaloids include uterine cramping, nausea and vomiting, dizziness, hypertension with IV administration, sweating, tinnitus, chest pain, dyspnea, itching, and sudden severe headache. Signs of ergot toxicity (**ergotism**) include pain in arms, legs, and lower back; numbness; cold hands and feet; muscular weakness; diarrhea; hallucinations; seizures; and blood hypercoagulability.

Table 53–6

Uterotonic Drugs Commonly Used to Enhance Uterine Contractility

Generic (Brand)	Route and Dosage	Uses and Considerations
oxytocin (Pitocin, Syntocinon)	(Prototype Drug Chart 53–1)	
ergonovine maleate (Ergotrate)	PO: 0.2-0.4 mg (1-2 tablets) q6-12h over 48 h	Oxytocic; ergot alkaloid. Direct stimulation of vascular smooth muscle, producing vasoconstriction of peripheral and cerebral vessels; used to prevent and treat postpartum or postabortion hemorrhage caused by uterine atony or subinvolution. *PO* onset: 6-15 min; duration: 3 h. Metabolized in liver; excreted in urine. Do not use in clients with coronary artery disease, hypertension, gestational hypertension. Contraindicated before delivery of placenta. Use with caution in clients with sepsis or hepatic or renal impairment. *Adverse reactions:* diaphoresis, palpitations, transient chest pain, thrombophlebitis, seizures, cerebrovascular accidents, dizziness, headache, nausea, vomiting, tinnitus, dyspnea. *Pregnancy category:* X; PB: UK; t½: 2 h
methylergonovine maleate (Methergine)	PO: 0.2-0.4 mg, q6-12h; *max:* 1 wk IM: 0.2 mg after delivery of anterior shoulder (if full obstetric supervision), after delivery of placenta, or postpartum; repeat q2-4h; oral doses may follow parenteral IV: Same as for IM; but slowly over 1 min with careful monitoring of BP (IV route for acute emergencies only [e.g., bleeding])	Prevention and treatment of postpartum hemorrhage, subinvolution, and postabortion hemorrhage. Exhibits similar smooth-muscle action to ergotamine, but primarily affects smooth muscle, producing sustained contractions and shortening third stage of labor. *IV* onset: immediate; duration: 45 min. *IM* onset: 2-5 min; duration: 3 h. *PO* onset: 5-25 min; duration: 3 h. Metabolized in liver; eliminated in urine. Not routinely administered IV because of possible sudden hypertensive and cerebrovascular accidents; limit use with clients with hypertension (especially IV). Contraindicated with maternal sepsis, labor induction, threatened spontaneous abortion; do not use with vasodepressors, other ergot alkaloids, or vasoconstrictors. Appears in breast milk, but interference with breastfeeding is less than with ergonovine. *Adverse reactions:* transient hypertension, diaphoresis, palpitations, dizziness, headache, nausea, vomiting, tinnitus, transient chest pain, dyspnea. *Pregnancy category:* C; PB: UK; t½: biphasic: initial: 1-5 min; terminal: 30 min-2 h

BP, Blood pressure; *h*, hour; *IM*, intramuscular; *IV*, intravenous; *max*, maximum; *min*, minute; *PB*, protein-binding; *PO*, by mouth; *t½*, half-life; *UK*, unknown; *wk*, week.

 Nursing Process

Other Oxytocics: Ergonovine and Methylergonovine

ASSESSMENT

■ Assess lochia and uterine tone before giving ergonovine or methylergonovine.
■ Assess effectiveness of uterine massage and oxytocin administration on local flow and uterine tone.
■ Recognize that these two drugs have a vasoconstrictive effect, which may cause hypertension. Ergonovine is more vasoconstrictive than methylergonovine.
■ Obtain baseline BP before administration.

NURSING INTERVENTIONS

■ Monitor client's BP per agency protocol.
■ Protect drugs from exposure to light.
■ Monitor for side effects or symptoms of ergot toxicity (ergotism). Notify physician if systolic BP increases by 25 mmHg or diastolic BP by 20 mmHg over baseline.

Client Teaching

• Instruct client that she will feel more intense uterine cramps after receiving the drug but may receive analgesics for pain.

Safety

• Instruct client to avoid smoking. Nicotine increases the vasoconstrictive properties of these drugs.

Side Effects

• If client is breastfeeding, explain that the drug lowers serum prolactin levels with the potential to inhibit postpartum lactation. Ergonovine has greater potential to inhibit lactation than methylergonovine.

Cultural Considerations ❖

• Recognize cultural influence on client's expression or lack of expression of discomfort and/or pain.
• Provide an interpreter as appropriate.

EVALUATION

■ Evaluate effectiveness of drug by assessment of lochia and uterine tone. Count and weigh perineal pads as appropriate.

■ Continue monitoring maternal vital signs, specifically pulse and BP. Report changes in maternal vital signs, continued excessive vaginal bleeding, or uterine atony.

Surfactant Therapy in Preterm Birth

Synthetic Surfactant

One approach to respiratory difficulties in the preterm infant is surfactant replacement therapy. This is used to prevent the development of **respiratory distress syndrome (RDS)** (respiratory disease of the newborn with absence, deficiency or alteration in surfactant production). **Surfactant** (a lipoprotein in the alveoli which reduces surface tension of pulmonary fluids and keeps alveoli open during expiration) replacement therapy is also used to decrease the severity of RDS following diagnosis. Supplementing the amount of endogenous surfactant available to maintain distention of the alveolar sacs is the focus of this therapy.

Currently the FDA has approved the use of beractant (Survanta), calfactant (Infasurf), and poractant alfa (Curosurf). Beractant (Survanta) lowers alveolar surface tension during respiration and stabilizes alveoli. Beractant (Survanta) intratracheal suspension, a natural bovine-lung extract, contains phospholipids, neutral lipids, fatty acids, and surfactant-associated proteins to which colfosceril palmitate (DPPC), palmitic acid, and tripalmitin are added. Beractant (Survanta) does not require reconstitution. Calfactant (Infasurf) is a calf-lung surfactant that can be used pre-ventilatory for prevention of RDS or post-ventilatory for treatment. Poractant alfa (Curosurf) is porcine-lung surfactant and is indicated for rescue treatment. All three of these products define *prophylactic* and *rescue* use differently (Table 53–7) and have different dosing and administration requirements for each use.

All products require a patent endotracheal (ET) tube for administration and specified alterations in positioning the infant throughout the procedure to ensure even drug dispersion. These precise position changes allow gravity to assist in the distribution of the product in the lungs, particularly at the alveolar surface.

Rales and moist breath sounds may be a transient finding following administration of these products, particularly with beractant (Survanta). Additionally, transient oxygen desaturation has occurred with poractant alfa (Curosurf), and airway obstruction has occurred in 39% of infants in clinical studies with calfactant (Infasurf). Unless obvious signs of airway obstruction are noted, suctioning should not be performed for 2 hours after administration.

Surfactant replacement therapy has been found effective in reducing the severity of RDS; rapid improvements in lung compliance and oxygenation may require immediate decreases in ventilator settings to prevent lung overdistention and pulmonary air leak.

Preventing MEDICATION ERRORS

Do not confuse...

- **Methylergonovine** (Methergine) with **terbutaline** sulfate (Brethine). These drugs have opposite actions! Be alert to packaging, which is very similar. Both are amber ampules with colored neck bands wrapped in foil and amber plastic packaging. Do not store these drugs together.

- **Fentanyl citrate** (Sublimaze) with **Sufentanil** (Sufenta). Fentanyl citrate and Sufentanil are both phenylpiperidines and opioid analgesics for moderate to severe pain, working as mu receptor agonists. The parenteral dose of fentanyl is 0.1 mg and its equivalent dose of sufentanil is 10 mcg. Fentanyl and sufentanil may be administered as analgesic adjuncts or primary anesthetic agents during general or epidural anesthesia.

- **Promethazine hydrochloride** (Phenergan) with **promazine hydralazine** (Sparine). Promethazine hydrochloride is a phenothiazine antihistamine and antiemetic. Sparine is categorized as an antipsychotic drug.

Adverse Reactions

Side effects during administration have included incidents of reflux of product up the ET tube with decreases in oxygenation. Dosing is slowed or halted if the infant (1) becomes dusky colored, (2) becomes agitated, (3) experiences transient bradycardia, (4) has oxygen saturation increases of more than 95%, (5) experiences improved chest expansion, or (6) has arterial or transcutaneous CO_2 levels less than 30 mm Hg. Pulmonary hemorrhage has been seen in infants treated with Exosurf. Suctioning before dosing decreases the chance for ET tube blockage during dosing. No long-term complications or sequelae of synthetic surfactant therapy have been reported.

Nursing Process

Beractant (Survanta), Calfactant (Infasurf), and Poractant Alfa (Curosurf)

ASSESSMENT

■ Assess for informed consent. Separate consents are needed for multifetal birth.
■ Assess infant's vital signs.

NURSING DIAGNOSES

■ Impaired gas exchange related to inadequate lung surfactant

PLANNING

■ Infant's oxygen requirement and respiratory effort will decrease.
■ Infant's need for mechanical ventilation will be quickly reduced.
■ Infant will experience no respiratory distress within 1 hour of surfactant administration.

NURSING INTERVENTIONS

Beractant (Survanta) Intratracheal Suspension
• Prepare drug in adequate time for drug to warm to room temperature for 20 minutes or in hand for at least 8 minutes. Do not artificially warm drug.
• Do not shake drug.

Table 53–7

Postnatal Surfactant Therapy for Prevention and Treatment of Respiratory Distress Syndrome

Generic (Brand)	Route and Dosage	Uses and Considerations
beractant (Survanta) intratracheal suspension	4 ml/kg per dose ET (divide into 4 quarter doses and give each quarter dose with infant in different position) in one of two modes: *Prophylaxis:* 1 dose within 15 min of birth if possible; repeat in 6 h if respiratory distress continues; maximum 4 doses in 24 h (6 h apart). *Rescue:* 4 ml/kg intratracheally (also divide into 4 quarter doses and give each quarter dose with different infant positioning). Give dose as soon as RDS is diagnosed, preferably within 8 h of birth. Repeat in 6 h, giving a maximum of 4 doses in 24 h	beractant (Survanta) contains phospholipids, neutral lipids, fatty acids, and surfactant-associated proteins to which colfosceril palmitate (DPPC), palmitic acid, and tripalmitin are added. Each 1 ml contains 2.5 mg phospholipids. Must be given by health care personnel experienced with ventilators as prevention or rescue in treatment of RDS. Administered through a 5 French end-hole catheter as a dosing catheter inserted into ET tube. Following administration of each quarter dose, catheter removed from ET tube and infant ventilated for 30 sec until stable. *Prophylaxis* defined as use in infants less than 1250 g at high risk for RDS or larger infants with evidence of pulmonary immaturity. *Rescue* defined as treatment of infants with moderate to severe RDS. Biophysical effects occur at the alveolar surface; lowers surface tension on alveolar surfaces during respiration and stabilizes alveoli against collapse at resting pressures. Infants should be frequently monitored with arterial or transcutaneous measurement of systemic oxygen or carbon dioxide. Does not require reconstitution. Drug should appear off-white to light brown. Swirl vial gently; DO NOT SHAKE. Some foaming is normal. Store at 36°-46° F (2°-8° C); warm 20 min at room temperature or in hand for at least 8 min. Do not artificially warm. For prevention dose, begin preparation before infant's birth. Do not warm or return drug to refrigerator more than once. Protect from light. No known contraindications. *Adverse reactions:* transient bradycardia, oxygen desaturation (associated with dosing procedure); ET tube reflux; ET blockage, pallor, vasoconstriction, hypotension, hypocarbia, hypercarbia, and apnea. All reactions resolve with symptomatic treatment
calfactant (Infasurf)	3 ml/kg of birth weight as soon as possible after birth. Give as 2 doses of 1.5 ml/kg each every 12 h for total of 3 doses	Must be given by health care personnel experienced with ventilators and RDS. Stabilization of the premature infant with hypoxemia should occur before administration of calfactant therapy. Give preferably within 30 min after birth. Give through an ET tube. Draw dose with 20-G needle; avoid foaming. Does not require reconstitution. Do not dilute or shake. Gently agitate for dispersion of drug. Drug does not have to be warmed before administration. Refrigerate at 36°-46° F (2°-8° C) and protect from light. No known contraindications. *Adverse reactions:* bradycardia, airway obstruction, apnea, hypoventilation, cyanosis, ET tube reflux, ET blockage
poractant alfa (Curosurf)	2.5 ml/kg of birth weight. Up to 2 additional doses of 1.25 ml/kg birth weight can be every 12 h; maximum dose 5 ml/kg	Administered via 5 French catheter inserted into ET tube. With infant positioned either right or left side dependent, administer one half dose into each main bronchus. Must be given by health care personnel experienced with ventilators and RDS. Do not suction airways for 1 h after surfactant instillation unless airway obstruction occurs. Multiple-dose regimen has evidenced efficacy. Ventilator inspiratory pressures should be reduced immediately if chest expansion improves substantially after dosing. Contraindications are previous hypersensitivity to any component of poractant alfa formulations. *Adverse reactions:* increased incidence of patent ductus arteriosus, hypotension, transient oxygen desaturation, apnea, and flushing

ET, Endotracheal; *h,* hour; *min,* minute; *RDS,* respiratory distress syndrome; *sec,* second.

- Provide only off-white to light brown product for use in procedure.
- Assist with positioning of infant after each quarter dose as detailed in protocol.

Calfactant (Infasurf)

- Avoid excessive foaming.
- Draw up dose using 20-gauge or larger needle.
- Administer through side port of endotracheal (ET) tube.
- Administer medication with infant on one-for-one dose, and turn to opposite side for subsequent dose.
- Administer while ventilation is continued over 20 to 30 breaths for each dose, with small bursts during inspiratory cycles.

Beractant (Survanta) Intratracheal Suspension and Calfactant (Infasurf)

- Monitor infant carefully for chest expansion, color, arterial blood gases, oxygen saturation, heart rate, facial expression, ET tube patency, BP, and electrocardiogram.
- Monitor ventilator pressure readings and breath sounds.
- Expect the infant's lungs to sound wet after administration; do not suction through the endotracheal tube for 2 hours.

Poractant Alfa (Curosurf)

- Draw up doses using 20-gauge or larger needle.
- Suction before dosing.
- Mucous plugging of the ET tube can occur during or after dosing.
- Do not suction airways for 1 hour after surfactant instillation unless signs of airway obstruction are present.
- Monitor ventilator inspiratory pressures, which should be reduced immediately if chest expansion improves after dosing administration.

Client Teaching

General

- Explain to parents what respiratory distress syndrome is and how surfactant helps the infant.
- Explain to parents the purpose of multiple monitoring devices to reduce unrealistic fears about the neonate's condition.
- Ensure informed consent for usage.

Side Effects

- Encourage parents to verbalize understanding about risks associated with use of the drug.

EVALUATION

- Evaluate preadministration breath sounds and ventilator pressure readings to compare with postadministration findings

 Critical Thinking Case Study

TA (gravida 3, para 0) is at 42 weeks' gestation. At her prenatal visit, her health care provider notes signs and symptoms of pregnancy-induced hypertension and advises TA of the plan to induce labor after administration of prostaglandin gel. TA asks the nurse, "Can you help me understand all this?"

1. What objective tool (scoring system) can be used to predict the extent to which TA's cervix is "ripe" and therefore favorable for successful induction?

TA's health care provider orders Prepidil gel for use in the cervix.

2. What will be accomplished with the use of the gel?
3. Who will administer the gel?
4. How often can the gel be administered?
5. How long after the last dose of gel can the IV oxytocic medication be started to induce labor?
6. Why is there a waiting period before starting the oxytocin?
7. Further questioning reveals that TA has been ingesting a pregnancy tonic that includes herbal supplements since she was 36 weeks' gestation. List three concerns specific to pregnancy.

It is now 16 hours since TA first had the gel inserted. Upon responding to TA's call light, the nurse finds her in the bathroom upset that she feels nauseous, occasionally vomiting a little stomach fluid, and complaining that her stool is "really watery." "Is something wrong?" TA asks.

8. Analysis of the data about TA's symptoms support what conclusion?
9. What nursing actions might be taken to support TA?
10. When TA returns to bed and the external fetal monitor is reapplied, what data should the nurse collect, record, and report to the obstetric provider?

It is now 24 hours since TA had her first gel instillation and 6 hours since her last insertion. A vaginal examination reveals that TA's cervix is soft, 50% effaced, 3 cm dilated, and the presenting part is at 2 station. Contractions are 5 minutes apart and mild. The health care provider elects to begin an oxytocin infusion.

11. TA asks how a medicine "running into my arm is able to make my uterus contract." How would one explain the mode of action of oxytocin to TA?
12. Why is the oxytocin infusion run through a secondary line attached as a "piggyback" to the primary line? At which port along the primary line is the piggyback inserted and why?

Critical Thinking Case Study

13. Why is oxytocin administered via an infusion pump? What is the measurement for dosing?
14. What actions in regard to the IV equipment setup should be taken as safety measures before starting the oxytocin?
15. What drugs should be nearby in the event of an emergency with the oxytocin?
16. What information should be recorded during the infusion?
17. While setting up the oxytocin infusion, a nurse in training asks what criteria to use to know when to slow the rate or stop the infusion. You correctly respond that

contractions would be _____ minutes apart with _____ intensity and the cervix would be dilated at least _____ cm.

18. If uterine hyperstimulation occurs, explain how to handle the situation. Address the following:
Position TA; rationale: _____
IV fluids; rationale: _____
Oxygen; rationale: _____
19. TA asks what side effects can occur if she receives a continuous lumbar epidural. What is the appropriate response?

NCLEX Study Questions

1. LW is to receive 10 mg Nubain slow IV push for pain relief during labor. Nubain is administered:
   a. during the uterine contraction
   b. at the end of the uterine contraction
   c. between uterine contractions
   d. at any time during the contractions

2. MB is to have a lumbar epidural anesthesia. Prior to the anesthesiologist administering the epidural, the priority nursing intervention is to administer:
   a. an antacid, Bicitra
   b. an antiemetic, Phenergan
   c. a bolus of 500-1000 cc of a crystalloid IV solution
   d. a RhoGAM injection

3. AE is a 33-year-old in active labor and experiencing "back labor" with intense pain in her lower back. An effective nursing intervention is:
   a. counterpressure against the sacrum
   b. pant-blow breathing techniques
   c. effleurage
   d. conscious relaxation or guided imagery

4. TM has an epidural for pain control during her labor. In your assessment you note a drop in her blood pressure. The priority nursing intervention is to:
   a. administer low-flow oxygen
   b. turn her on her left side
   c. assess her urinary output
   d. monitor her vaginal bleeding

5. JP is to have a stat cesarean section. Prior to her surgery the nurse administers Bicitra. The purpose of administering an antacid is to:
   a. prevent infection
   b. neutralize gastric contents
   c. reduce the need to use postoperative pain medication
   d. prevent postoperative vomiting

6. Spinal anesthesia with Duramorph is administered to a client for pain relief during a cesarean section. The client complains of itching. The nurse prepares to administer which prn medication?
   a. diphenhydramine (Benadryl)
   b. fentanyl (Sublimaze)
   c. butorphanol tartrate (Stadol)
   d. lidocaine

7. A nurse administered beractant (Survanta) to a premature infant to prevent respiratory distress syndrome (RDS). In assessing the infant's lungs the nurse auscultated rales and moist breath sounds. The priority nursing intervention is:
   a. notify the provider
   b. suction immediately to remove the beractant (Survanta)
   c. turn the infant "back to sleep"
   d. document; this is a normal transient finding

8. LS is a 28 y/o G2P1001 at 40 weeks on Pitocin for augmentation of her labor. She is having increasing pain and asking for her PRN pain meds. External fetal monitoring shows her contraction frequency to be 30 seconds, her contraction duration between 90 to 120 seconds, and intensity 95 mmHg. The fetal heart rate is 135-145 and reactive. What is your priority nursing intervention?
   a. Give pain medication and continue to monitor
   b. Increase Pitocin to change labor pattern
   c. Stop Pitocin and call her health care provider
   d. Prepare for cesarean section

Answers: 1. a; 2. c; 3. a; 4. b; 5. b; 6. a; 7. d; 8. c.

54

Postpartum and Newborn Drugs

Robin Webb Corbett and Laura K. Williford Owens

ELECTRONIC RESOURCES

Evolve website (http://evolve.elsevier.com/KeeHayes/pharmacology/):
- Case Studies
- Content Updates
- Frequently Asked Questions
- Student Review Activities
- WebLinks
- Additional Reference Material

Companion CD-ROM:
- NCLEX Examination Review Questions
- Pharmacology Animations
- IV Therapy Checklists
- Medication Error Checklists
- Drug Calculation Problems
- Electronic Calculators
- Top 200 Drugs with Pronunciations
- References from the Textbook

Outline

Objectives

- Discuss the purpose, action, side effects, and nursing implications of the drugs commonly administered during the postpartum period.
- Discuss the purpose, action, side effects, and nursing implications of the drugs administered to the newborn.
- Describe the nursing process, including client teaching, related to drugs used during the postpartum period and drugs administered to the newborn immediately after delivery.

Terms

This chapter focuses on pharmacologic considerations for mothers and infants after delivery. Nonpharmacologic measures and pharmacologic agents related to the relief of common maternal discomforts during the postpartum period are also described. In addition, drugs commonly administered to newborns immediately after delivery are included. It is important to note that for some cultures, pregnancy is perceived as a cold state, so warm foods and activities are encouraged to balance the body. Failure to do so, it is believed, may contribute to later poor health. For example, women of Mexican American ethnicity need to avoid chilling and exposure to drafts. Therefore perineal cold compresses may not be accepted by these women. Japanese women may prefer to take their postpartal medications with warm water rather than cold water. Cultural values also influence infant care. It is important for nurses to be culturally sensitive to the pregnant client's cultural belief framework and try to include this framework in provision of care and establishing rapport with the client.

Drugs Used during the Postpartum Period

During the **puerperium** (the period from delivery until 6 weeks postpartum), the maternal body physically recovers from antepartal and intrapartal stressors and returns to its prepregnant state.

Pharmacologic and nonpharmacologic measures commonly used during the postpartum period have five primary purposes: (1) to prevent uterine atony and postpartum hemorrhage (see Chapter 52); (2) to relieve pain from uterine contractions, perineal wounds, and hemorrhoids; (3) to enhance or suppress **lactation** (production and release of milk by mammary glands); (4) to promote bowel function; and (5) to enhance immunity (Box 54–1).

Whenever possible, nonpharmacologic measures are preferred to the use of drugs or are used in conjunction with drugs (Herbal Alert 54–1 addresses the use of herbs during the postpartum period.) Postpartum nursing care ideally occurs as a partnership between the nurse and the new family. To enhance health and wellness, the nurse collaborates with the mother and family to strengthen the new mother's self-confidence and ability to handle her own health challenges. The nurse's role in this system is threefold:

- To assess and discuss postpartal physical changes and pain management with the client and determine both healing progress within a standard and effectiveness of medications
- To teach the client and administer postpartal medications
- To teach the client and administer narcotic analgesics (as prescribed) when pain control by nonnarcotic products is ineffective.

Box 54–1

Routine Postpartum Medication Orders

Vaginal Delivery Postpartum Medications

Standing Orders

oxytocin (Pitocin) 20 units in 1 L D$_5$LR or 10 units IM
ferrous sulfate (FeSO$_4$) 325 mg PO b.i.d.-t.i.d.
Prenatal vitamin 1 tab PO daily
Motrin 800 mg t.i.d.

PRN Orders

docusate sodium (Colace) 100 mg PO b.i.d. PRN for constipation OR
Dulcolax suppository PR PRN for constipation
A & D cream or Lanolin PRN if breastfeeding
Rubella vaccine if not immunized

Cesarean Birth Postpartum Medications

Standing Orders

cefazolin (Ancef) 1 g IVPB X 1 dose at time of cesarean section
oxytocin (Pitocin) 20 units in 1 L D5LR or 10 units IM
POD 1
ferrous sulfate (FeSO$_4$) 325 mg PO b.i.d.-t.i.d.
Prenatal vitamin 1 tab PO daily
Motrin 800 mg t.i.d.

PRN Orders

POD 1
nalbuphine (Nubain) 5-10 mg subQ or IV q2-3h OR
meperidine (Demerol) 50-75 mg IM q3-4h PRN pain
acetaminophen/codeine (Tylenol No. 3) 1-2 tab PO q3-4h PRN for pain OR
oxycodone/acetaminophen (Percocet) 1 tab PO q6h PRN for pain
hydroxyzine (Vistaril) 25-50 mg IM q3-4h PRN nausea
prochlorperazine (Compazine) 10 mg IV q4-6h PRN nausea OR
promethazine (Phenergan) 25-50 mg IV q3-4 h PRN nausea
A & D cream or Lanolin PRN if breastfeeding
POD 2
bisacodyl (Dulcolax) suppository PR PRN for constipation OR
magnesium hydroxide (milk of magnesia) 30 ml PO q6h PRN
simethicone (Gas-X) 80 mg PO q.i.d. PRN for bloating and/or gas
Rubella vaccine (Meruvax II) subQ if not immunized

b.i.d., Twice a day; *h,* hour; *IM,* intramuscular; *IVPB,* intravenous piggyback; *PO,* by mouth; *PRN,* as needed; *q.i.d.,* four times a day; *subQ,* subcutaneous; *tab,* tablet; *t.i.d.,* three times a day.
Data from Chan PD, Johnson SM: *Gynecology and obstetrics,* Laguna Hills, Calif, 2006, Current Clinical Strategies Publishing.

Pain Relief for Uterine Contractions

"Afterbirth pains" may occur during the first few days postpartum when uterine tissue experiences ischemia during contractions, particularly in multiparous women and when breastfeeding. Nonsteroidal agents may be used to control postpartal discomfort and pain, with narcotic agents reserved for more severe pain such as that experienced by the

Herbal ALERT 54–1

Use of Herbs during Lactation

Herbal supplements are not generally recommended during lactation. The herbal supplements listed below are contraindicated for breastfeeding women:

aloe
pennyroyal (Hedeoma pulegeoides)
belladonna
black tea (Camellia sinensis)
blessed thistle (Cnicus benedictus)
bromelain
buckthorn bark
burdock (Arctium lappa)
cascara sagrada bark
cat's claw (Uncaria tomentosa; U. guianensis)
chondroitin
coltsfoot leaf
comfrey
danshen (Salvia miltiorrhiza)
DHEA
echinacea (E. angustifolia; E. pallida; E. purpurea)
ephedra (Ephedra spp.)/ma-huang
eucalyptus oil (Eucalyptus globulus)
flaxseed & flaxseed oil
goldenseal (Hydrastis canadensis)
hops (Humulus lupulus)
kava kava
lavender
licorice (Glycyrrhiza glabra) and DGL (deglycyrrhizinated licorice)
milk thistle
oleander (Nerium indicum; N. oleander)
red clover (Trifolium pratense)
red yeast
saw palmetto
senna leaf, peppermint oil, and caraway oil
shark cartilage
tea tree oil (Melaleuca alternifolia); do not apply to breast or nipple
yohimbe bark (Corynanthe johimbe; Pausinystalia johimbe)

Data from Brener T, Doyle R: Nursing 2007 drug handbook, New York, 2007, Lippincott Williams & Wilkins: Nursing herbal medicine handbook, New York, 2006, Lippincott Williams & Wilkins; 2006 Mosby's drug consult, St Louis, 2006, Elsevier.

Box 54–2

Commonly Used Postpartum Systemic Analgesics

acetaminophen (Tylenol)
acetaminophen/codeine (Tylenol No. 3)
acetaminophen & propoxyphene (Darvocet-N 50, Darvocet-N 100)
ibuprofen (Motrin)
codeine sulfate
ketorolac tromethamine (Toradol)
meperidine (Demerol)
morphine sulfate
nalbuphine (Nubain)
oxycodone acetaminophen (Percocet)

are not ambulatory, all factors that contribute to decreased bowel activity. In addition, respiratory assessment is important for clients receiving opioids, because respiratory depression may occur. Frequently nonsteroidal agents like ibuprofen (Advil, Motrin) and ketorolac tromethamine (Toradol) are used to control postpartum discomfort and pain. Nonsteroidal antiinflammatory drugs (NSAIDs) inhibit the enzyme cyclooxygenase (COX), of which there are two isoenzymes, COX-1 or COX-2; both decrease prostaglandin synthesis. These drugs are effective in relieving mild to moderate pain, including postpartum uterine contractions, episiotomy, hemorrhoids, and perineal wounds. NSAIDs commonly cause gastrointestinal (GI) irritation, and it is recommended that clients take them with a full glass or water or with food to minimize GI distress. With administration of NSAIDs, a lower narcotic dosage may control pain as a result of the additive analgesic effect. The use of NSAIDs requires ongoing assessment for GI bleeding. These drugs inhibit platelet synthesis and may prolong bleeding time. Client teaching with this category of drugs is important, because some NSAIDs may be purchased over the counter (OTC). Client teaching includes avoidance of these drugs while pregnant; symptoms of GI bleeding (dark, tarry stools, blood in urine, and coffee-ground emesis); and avoidance of the concurrent use of alcohol, aspirin, and corticosteroids, which may increase the risk of GI toxicity.

Pain Relief for Perineal Wounds and Hemorrhoids

Pregnancy and the delivery process increase the pressure on perineal soft tissue. The tissue may become ecchymotic or edematous. Increased edema, ecchymosis, and pain may occur if an **episiotomy** (incision made to enlarge the vaginal opening to facilitate newborn delivery) or perineal laceration is present. Perineal assessment may be facilitated by the acronym, REEDA. The perineum is assessed for redness (R), ecchymosis (E), edema (E), discharge (D), and approximation (A). In addition, hemorrhoids that developed during pregnancy may be exacerbated by the pushing during labor. Comfort measures (ice packs imme-

client after cesarean delivery, tubal ligation, or extensive perineal laceration. Box 54–2 presents a list of systemic analgesics commonly used during the postpartum period.

Because some systemic analgesics (e.g., codeine, meperidine, oxycodone) can cause decreased alertness, it is important for the nurse to observe the client as she cares for her newborn to ensure safety. Clients who receive opioids, such as morphine sulfate or codeine sulfate, should be assessed for bowel function and respirations. With continued opioid use, client assessment of bowel history is necessary, because these drugs can exacerbate the constipation of pregnancy. During the intrapartum period, women are NPO (nothing by mouth) or ingest limited liquids and

Table 54-1

Drugs Used to Relieve Pain from Perineal Wounds and Hemorrhoids

Generic (Brand)	Route and Dosage	Uses and Considerations
Perineal Wounds (Episiotomy or Laceration)		
benzocaine (Americaine, Dermoplast)	Spray liberally t.i.d. or q.i.d. 6-12 in from perineum following perineal cleansing Supplied as aerosol benzocaine 20%	Local anesthetic; inhibits impulses from sensory nerves by decreasing permeability of cell membrane to sodium ions. Apply 6-12 in from affected area. Peak: 1 min; duration: 30-60 min. Hydrolyzed in the plasma and liver (to lesser extent) by cholinesterase; eliminated as metabolites in urine. Well absorbed from mucous membranes and traumatized skin. Contraindicated in secondary bacterial infection of tissue and known hypersensitivity
witch hazel pads (Tucks [50% witch hazel with glycerin, water, and methylparaben]) (may also be used for hemorrhoids)	Apply premoistened pads t.i.d. or q.i.d. to wound site	Precipitates protein, causing tissue to contract. May be chilled/refrigerated in original container for additional comfort. If liquid, pour over ice and dip absorbent pads into solution; change when diluted. Medical intervention should be sought if rectal bleeding is present. *Side effect:* local irritation (discontinue use)
Hemorrhoids		
hydrocortisone acetate 10 mg (Anusol-HC, Tucks Ointment [pramoxine HCl 1%, mineral oil 46.7%, zinc oxide 12.5%])	1 suppository b.i.d. for 3-6 d	Relieves pain and itching from irritated anorectal tissue. Anusol-HC contains hydrocortisone acetate, acts as an antiinflammatory agent. Available without hydrocortisone. Wear gloves. Onset: UK; peak: UK; duration: UK. Contraindicated with hypersensitivity. If second infection in tissue, discontinue. If anorectal symptoms do not improve in 7 d or if bleeding, protrusion, or seepage occurs, inform health care provider. Not to be used if fourth-degree perineal laceration. Not known if excreted in breast milk; use cautiously. *Pregnancy category:* C
hydrocortisone acetate 1% and pramoxine HCl 1% topical aerosol (Proctofoam-HC)	1 applicator transferred to a 2 × 2 in pad and placed against rectum inside peripad b.i.d. or t.i.d. and after bowel movements	Topical corticosteroid aerosol foam with same action and considerations as above. Also available in nonsteroidal preparation. Shake foam aerosol before use. Onset: UK; peak: UK; duration: UK. Extent of percutaneous absorption of topical corticosteroids is determined by vehicle integrity, epidermal barrier, and use of occlusive dressings. Not known if any quantity detectable in breast milk. *Side effects:* burning, itching, irritation; dryness, infrequent folliculitis reactions
dibucaine ointment, USP 1% (Nupercaine)	Apply as above t.i.d. or q.i.d., using no more than 1 tube in 24 h	Local anesthetic ointment containing dibucaine 1%. Action same as benzocaine. Onset: within 15 min; peak: UK; duration: 2-4 h. Do not use if rectal bleeding is present. Do not use near eyes or over denuded surfaces or blistered areas. Do not use if known hypersensitivity to amide-type anesthetics. *Side effects:* burning, tenderness, irritation, inflammation, contact dermatitis, urticaria, cutaneous lesions, edema. *Pregnancy category:* C

b.i.d., Two times a day; *d,* day; *h,* hour; *in,* inch; *min,* minute; *q.i.d.,* four times a day; *t.i.d.,* three times a day; *UK,* unknown.

diately after birth, tightening of the buttocks before sitting, use of peribottles and cool and warm sitz baths) and selected topical agents (witch hazel and Nupercainal ointment) may relieve pain and minimize discomfort (Table 54–1). Note that rectal suppositories should not be used by women with fourth-degree perineal lacerations.

Side Effects and Adverse Reactions

The most commonly reported side effects of topical or local agents (e.g., witch hazel) include burning, stinging, tenderness, edema, rash, tissue irritation, sloughing, and tissue **necrosis** (death of tissue caused by disease or injury). The most commonly reported side effects of hydrocortisone local or topical drugs include burning, pruritus, irritation, dryness, **folliculitis** (skin inflammation resulting from contact with an irritating substance or allergen),

allergic contact dermatitis, and secondary infection. These side effects are more likely to occur when **occlusive** (i.e., obstructive) dressings are used.

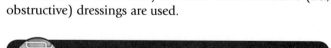

ASSESSMENT

■ Assess client's cultural framework for health.
■ Assess client's pain using agency pain scale. Assess the perineal area for wounds and hemorrhoids (size, color,

location, pain scale, REEDA (*r*edness, *e*cchymosis, *e*dema, *d*ischarge, *a*pproximation).
■ Check the expiration dates on topical spray cans, bottles, and ointment tubes.
■ Assess for presence of infection in perineal site; avoid use of benzocaine on infected perineal tissue.

NURSING DIAGNOSES

■ Acute pain related to episiotomy, perineal laceration, or hemorrhoids
■ Deficient knowledge of causes of pain and discomfort; inexperience with treatment measures, nonpharmacologic and pharmacologic

PLANNING

■ Client's perineal discomfort will be alleviated by use of topical sprays, compresses, sitz baths, and ointment.

NURSING INTERVENTIONS

■ Incorporate client's cultural framework of help in nursing plan of care.
■ Instruct client in use of the peribottle. Use warm water and direct water on the perineum from front to back (clean to dirty).
■ Do not use benzocaine spray when perineal infection is present.
■ Shake benzocaine spray can. Administer 6 to 12 inches from perineum with client lying on her side with top leg up and forward to provide maximum exposure. This can also be done with one foot on the toilet seat.
■ Use witch hazel compresses (Tucks or witch hazel solution) with an ice pack and a peri-pad to apply cold to the affected area in addition to the active agent.
■ Store Anusol HC suppositories below 86° F (30° C), but protect from freezing. Use gloves for administration. If client is breastfeeding, assess to determine whether client is ready to switch to preparation without hydrocortisone (goal is to discontinue use of suppositories as quickly as possible).
■ Check lot numbers and expiration dates.
■ Use of Proctofoam-HC needs to be explained carefully to client, because directions instruct the client to place the agent inside the anus, which is not generally done with obstetric clients (they may have perineal wounds that extend into the anus). Rectal suppositories should not be used by the client with a fourth-degree perineal laceration.

Client Teaching: Perineal Wounds: Topical Spray Containing Benzocaine

General
• Describe the process of perineal wound healing.
• Explain expected action and side effects.

• Instruct client that the drug is not for prolonged use (no more than 7 days) or for application to a large area.
• Instruct client with bleeding hemorrhoids to use the drug carefully and to keep her health care provider informed if condition exacerbates or does not improve within 7 days.

Self-Administration
• Apply three to four times daily or as directed.
• Apply without touching sensitive area.
• Hold can 6 to 12 inches from affected area. Administer the spray by either lying on the side in bed while spraying the treatment from behind or by standing with one foot on a chair or toilet seat.

Safety
• Assess use of complementary and alternative medicines, including herbal supplements.
• Avoid contact of the medication with eyes.
• Instruct client not to use a perineal heat lamp following application, because this could cause tissue burns.
• If condition exacerbates or symptoms recur within a few days, notify the health care provider and discontinue use until directed.
• Keep medication out of the reach of children in postpartum unit and later at home. If ingested, contact poison control center immediately.
• Store below 120° F (49° C). Dispose of empty can without puncturing or incinerating.

Client Teaching: Witch Hazel Compresses

General
• Explain expected action and side effects of product. Cooling, soothing sensation may provide relief of itching, burning, and irritation at episiotomy site or from hemorrhoids.
• Notify health care provider if condition exacerbates or does not improve within 7 days.

Self-Administration
• Pour liquid witch hazel over chipped ice; place soft, clean, absorbent squares in solution; squeeze square to eliminate excess moisture; fold and place moist square against episiotomy site or hemorrhoids.
• If using commercial medicated pads, entire container may be placed in the refrigerator.
• Avoid touching the surface of the pad placed next to the perineal wound.
• Instruct client when to change the compress and show how to place ice bag and peri-pad over the compress.

Safety
• Do not insert medicated pads into the rectum.
• Keep product away from children.
• Do not use if rectal bleeding is present.

Side Effects
- Discontinue use if local irritation occurs.

Client Teaching: Hemorrhoids: Tucks Ointment and Tucks Suppositories

General
- Explain expected effects of product use: relief of burning, itching, and discomfort from irritated anorectal tissues by soothing, lubricating, and coating mucous membranes.
- Explain that topical analgesia lasts for several hours after use.
- Tell client to store below 86° F (30° C) so suppositories do not melt but do not freeze.

Self-Administration
- Apply *ointment* externally in postpartum period.
- Place *suppository* in lower portion of anal canal. *Caution:* products usually are not inserted rectally if fourth-degree lacerations are present.
- Apply small quantity of *ointment* onto 2 × 2-inch gauze square; place inside peripad against swollen anorectal tissue approximately 5 times per day.
- If *suppository* is ordered, tell client to keep refrigerated but not frozen. Remove wrapper before inserting in rectum (hold suppository upright and peel evenly down sides). Do not hold suppository for prolonged period, because it will melt. If suppository softens before use, hold in foil wrapper under cold water for 2 to 3 minutes.

Safety
- Ascertain client hypersensitivity to any of the components of the ointment (e.g., pramoxine HCl 1%, mineral oil 46.7%, zinc oxide 12.5%).
- Avoid contact of the medication with eyes.

Side Effects
- Ointment may occasionally cause burning sensation in some clients, especially if anal tissue is not intact.
- If erythema, irritation, edema, or pain develops or increases, discontinue use and consult health care provider.
- Notify health care provider if bleeding occurs.

Client Teaching: Hydrocortisone & Pramoxine (Proctofoam-HC) and Pramoxine HCl (Procto-Foam NS)

General
- Explain expected action and side effects of product. Explain that pramoxine HCl is not chemically related to "-caine"-type local anesthetics, and there is decreased chance of cross-sensitivity reactions in clients allergic to other local anesthetics.

Self-Administration
- Tell client that product is for anal or perianal use only and is not to be inserted into rectum.

- Shake can vigorously before use.
- Fully extend applicator plunger; hold can upright to fill applicator.
- Express contents of applicator onto a 2 × 2-inch gauze pad and place inside peripad against rectum.
- Use two to three times daily and after bowel movements.
- Take the applicator apart after each use and wash with warm water.

Safety
- Keep aerosol container away from children in postpartum unit and later at home.
- Store below 120° F (49° C).
- Dispose of aerosol container without puncturing or incinerating.
- Avoid contact of the medication with eyes.

Side Effects
- Tell client it is unknown whether topical administration of corticosteroids could result in sufficient systemic absorption to produce detectable quantities in breast milk. Burning, itching, irritation, dryness, and folliculitis occasionally occur, especially if occlusive dressings are used.

Client Teaching: Dibucaine Ointment 1% (Nupercainal Ointment)

General
- The ointment is poorly absorbed through intact skin, but it is well absorbed through mucous membranes and excoriated skin.
- Effects should be perceived within 15 minutes and last for 2 to 4 hours.

Self-Administration
- Express ointment from the applicator on a tissue or 2 × 2-inch gauze pad and place against the anus. Do not insert applicator into the rectum.

Safety
- Do not use product near the eyes, over denuded surface or blistered areas, or if there is rectal bleeding.
- Do not use more than one tube (30-g size) in 24 hours.
- Keep medication out of the reach of children.

Side Effects
- Ask client if there is any known hypersensitivity to amide-type anesthetics; if so, product is contraindicated.
- Local effects may include burning, tenderness, irritation, inflammation, and contact dermatitis; inform health care provider if these occur.
- Other side effects may include edema, cutaneous lesions, and urticaria.

- Provide an interpreter with the same ethnic background and gender if possible, especially with sensitive topics.

EVALUATION

■ Reevaluate client's perception of pain following use of nonpharmacologic and pharmacologic measures. Identify need for additional client teaching.

■ Reassess perineal and anal tissues for integrity, healing, and any side effects.

Lactation Suppression

In the past, lactation was commonly controlled through drug therapy with one of three agents: chlorotrianisene (Tace), Deladumone OB (combination of estrogen plus androgen in the form of estradiol valerate and testosterone enanthate), or bromocriptine mesylate (Parlodel). Estrogenic substances are much less popular than in the past because of the increased incidence of thrombophlebitis associated with the high dosage needed to suppress lactation and concerns about potential carcinogenic effects. Although these drugs are not used now, your clients and their families may ask about these medications, which were given in the past for lactation suppression. Presently nonpharmacologic measures (wearing a supportive bra 24 h/day for 10 to 14 days, breast binding, and axillary ice packs) are recommended for lactation suppression (Table 54–2).

Promotion of Bowel Function

Constipation is common during the postpartum period. The residual effects of progesterone on smooth muscle decreases peristalsis, and this added to decreased

Table 54–2

Nonpharmacologic Measures for Common Postpartum Needs

Indication	Intervention
Uterine contractions	Client positioned on abdomen with pillow under abdomen × 20-30 min for 3-4 d
	Distraction, breathing techniques, therapeutic touch, relaxation, guided imagery, ambulation
	No heat to abdomen because of risk of uterine relaxation and increased bleeding
Perineal wound resulting from episiotomy or laceration	Ice packs/glove (covered in thin, absorbent material to protect tissue) for 6-8 h after delivery
	Client positioned on side as much as possible with pillow between legs
	Early and frequent ambulation
	Perineal exercises (Kegel exercises)
	Cool sitz bath 2-3 h after delivery
	Warm sitz bath 12-24 h after delivery 3-4 × per d
	Area cleansed front to back using perispray squeeze bottle, cleansing shower, or Surgi-Gator
	Client tightens buttocks or squeezes buttocks together before sitting and sits tall and flat, not rolled back onto coccyx
	No tampons, douche, or feminine hygiene sprays
	No intercourse until after lochia has ceased or as advised by health care provider
Hemorrhoids	As above but particularly:
	Ice
	Sims position to help increase venous return
	Warm, moist heat; sitz bath
	Witch hazel pads (e.g., Tucks)
Lactation suppression	Tight bra or binder worn continuously for 10-14 d
	Normal fluid intake
	No manipulation or stimulation of breasts
Engorgement	As above, plus ice to axillary area of breasts if client is bottle feeding the newborn, or apply warm compresses if client is breastfeeding
	Express a small amount of colostrum or milk (if breastfeeding) by hand expression before putting infant to breast to facilitate latching on
Sore or cracked nipples	Absorbent breast pads worn to keep moisture away from nipples
	No soap on nipples
	Air-dry nipples after nursing
	Express a small amount of breast milk on nipples to be used as a protective lubricant
	Apply hypoallergenic purified lanolin (Lansinoh, PureLan) or similar cream or ointment to the nipples, which may be used as a protective lubricant and promote healing
	For cracked nipples do not use Lansinoh as it may trap bacteria contributing to yeast infections.
	For cracked nipples use comfort gel pads
	No nipple shields because they can promote chafing
	Do not limit infant's nursing time at breast; otherwise milk ducts will not be emptied, and increased pressure may occur
	Proper positioning for feeding; nursing be initiated on the less sore nipple
	Suction broken with little finger after feeding to prevent pulling on nipple

d, Day; *h,* hour; *min,* minute.

liquid intake during labor, decreased activity, and relaxation of the abdominal muscles amplifies the problem. Clients who deliver by cesarean section are even more likely to experience constipation and **flatus** (intestinal gas). Nonpharmacologic measures (e.g., high-fiber foods, early ambulation, drinking at least 64 ounces of fluids a day, and promptly responding to the defecation urge) are generally instituted after delivery.

Pharmacologic measures include the use of stool softeners, laxative stimulants, and for the postcesarean client, **antiflatulents** (used to treat excessive gas in the stomach and intestines) (Table 54–3). (See Chapter 46 for additional information).

Table 54–3

Drugs Used to Promote Postpartum Bowel Function

Generic (Brand)	Route and Dosage	Uses and Considerations
docusate sodium (Colace) 550 mg with 3 mg sodium, 100-mg capsule with 5 mg sodium (Dulcolax Stool Softener) 100 mg with 5 mg sodium docusate calcium (Surfak) 240-mg capsule	100 mg PO b.i.d. 50-400 mg PO daily in 1-4 divided doses; usual dosage is 50-360 mg daily	Reduces surface tension of the oil-water interface of the stool, resulting in enhanced incorporation of water and fat and subsequent stool softening. Onset: 12-72 h. Docusate salts are interchangeable (amount of Na, Ca, or K per dosage is clinically insignificant). Do not use concomitantly with mineral oil. Contraindicated if intestinal obstruction, acute abdominal pain, nausea, or vomiting is present. Do not use >1 wk. Prolonged, frequent, or excessive use may cause bowel dependence or electrolyte imbalance. Compatible with breastfeeding. *Side effects:* rash. *Pregnancy category:* C; PB: NA; t½: NA
sennosides with docusate sodium (Peri-Colace, Senokot); docusate sodium 50 mg; sennosides, 8.6 mg	1-2 tablets PO usually at bedtime	Mild stimulant laxative. Should be taken with full glass of water. Onset: 8-12 h, but may require up to 24 h. Do not use if abdominal pain, nausea, or vomiting present. Compatible with breastfeeding. *Adverse reactions:* rash, abdominal cramping, diarrhea, nausea. *Pregnancy category:* C; PB: NA; t½: NA
bisacodyl USP (Dulcolax) (suppository 10 mg or tablet 5 mg)	2-3 tablets PO or 1 suppository, 5-15 mg daily given as a single dose	Stimulant laxative. Irritates smooth muscle of the intestine, possibly the colon and intramural plexus; alters water and electrolyte secretion, increasing intestinal fluid and producing laxative effect. Onset PO: 6-10 h; rectally: 15 min-1 h. Absorption: 5% absorbed systemically following oral or rectal form. Metabolized in the liver to conjugated metabolites; excreted in breast milk, bile, and urine. Do not crush tablets (enteric coated). Do not administer within 1 h of milk or antacid, because enteric coating may dissolve, resulting in abdominal cramping and vomiting. *Side effects:* abdominal cramps, nausea, vomiting, rectal burning, electrolyte and fluid acidosis or alkalosis, hypocalcemia. *Pregnancy category:* C
magnesium hydroxide (milk of magnesia)	30 ml PO PRN daily or in divided doses	Laxative. Acts by increasing and retaining water in intestinal lumen, causing distention that stimulates peristalsis and bowel elimination. Onset: 4-8 h. Excreted by kidneys (absorbed portion); unabsorbed portion excreted in feces. Poses risk to client with renal failure, because 15%-30% of magnesium is systemically absorbed. Use with caution in clients with impaired renal function, because hypermagnesemia and toxicity may occur as a result of decreased renal clearance of absorbed magnesium. Contraindicated in clients with colostomy, ileostomy, abdominal pain, nausea, vomiting, fecal impaction, and renal failure. Drug interactions may occur with tetracyclines, digoxin, indomethacin, or iron salts, isoniazid. Milk of magnesia concentrate is 3× as potent as regular-strength product. *Side effects:* abdominal cramps, nausea. *Adverse reactions:* hypotension, hypermagnesemia, muscle weakness, and respiratory depression. *Pregnancy category:* B
magnesium hydroxide with mineral oil (Phillips MO)	30-60 ml PO daily	Mild saline laxative. Acts by drawing water into gut, increasing intraluminal pressure and intestinal motility. Onset: 0.5-6 h. *Pregnancy category:* B. Equivalent to magnesium hydroxide
mineral oil	15-45 ml PO daily or in divided doses	Lubricant laxative eases passage of stool by decreasing water absorption and lubricating the intestine. Onset: 6-8 h; peak: UK; duration: UK. May impair absorption of fat-soluble vitamins (A, D, E, K), oral contraceptives, coumarin, and sulfonamides. Avoid bedtime doses because of risk of aspiration (lipid pneumonitis). Do not give with food or meals because of risk of aspiration and decreased fat-soluble vitamin absorption. Contraindicated in clients with ileostomy, colostomy, appendicitis, ulcerative colitis, and diverticulitis. Best administered on an empty stomach. *Side effects:* nausea, vomiting, diarrhea, and abdominal cramps. *Pregnancy category:* C; PB: NA; t½: NA

b.i.d., Twice a day; *d,* day; *h,* hour; *min,* minute; *NA,* not applicable; *PB,* protein-binding; *p.c.,* after meals; *PO,* by mouth; *q.i.d.,* four times a day; *t½,* half-life; *t.i.d.,* three times a day; *UK,* unknown; >, greater than.

Continued

Table 54–3

Drugs Used to Promote Postpartum Bowel Function—cont'd

Generic (Brand)	Route and Dosage	Uses and Considerations
senna (Senokot)	10-15 ml syrup at bedtime.; 2-4 tablets PO b.i.d.	Stimulant laxative. Acts by local irritant effect on colon to promote peristalsis and bowel evacuation. Also increases moisture content of stool by accumulating fluids in intestine. Onset: 6-24 h. Metabolized in liver; eliminated in feces (viable) and urine. Drug interactions may occur with monoamine oxidase inhibitors (MAOIs), disulfiram, metronidazole, and procarbazine. May discolor urine or feces. Liquid syrups contain 7% alcohol. May create laxative dependence and loss of bowel function with prolonged use. Contraindicated in clients with fluid and electrolyte disturbances, abdominal pain, and nausea and vomiting. Excreted in breast milk. *Pregnancy category:* C; t½: NA
simethicone (Gas-X chewable tablets, 80 mg; Extra Strength Gas-X chewable tablet, 125 mg; Gas-X Extra Strength softgel, 125 mg, Phazyme tablet, 90 mg, capsule, 125, 180 mg; Mylanta Gas Relief chewable tablet, 80 mg; Mylanta Gas Relief Maximum Strength chewable tablet, 125 mg)	1 tablet or softgel four times a day after meals and at bedtime; *max:* 6 tablets or 4 softgels/24 h	Antiflatulent. Acts by dispersing and preventing formation of mucus-surrounded gas pockets in GI tract; changes surface tension of gas bubbles and allows them to coalesce, making them easier to eliminate as belching and rectal flatus. Must be chewed thoroughly before swallowing; suggest client drink a full glass of water after tablets are chewed. Onset: UK. Excreted unchanged in the feces. May interfere with results of guaiac tests of gastric aspirates. Double doses should not be taken to make up for missed doses. Store below 104° F (40° C) in well-closed container. No known side effects. *Pregnancy category:* C; t½: UK

Side Effects and Adverse Reactions

The following side effects have been reported:

- docusate sodium (Colace): Bitter taste, throat irritation, rash
- sennosides and docusate sodium (Peri-Colace): Nausea, abdominal cramping, diarrhea, and rash
- bisacodyl suppositories (Dulcolax): Proctitis and inflammation
- magnesium hydroxide (milk of magnesia): Abdominal cramps and nausea
- senna (Senokot): Nausea, vomiting, diarrhea, abdominal cramps; can also cause diarrhea in breastfed infants
- mineral oil: Nausea, vomiting, diarrhea, abdominal cramps; if aspirated, lipid pneumonitis may occur

Nursing Process

Laxatives

ASSESSMENT

- Note time of delivery, predelivery food and fluid intake, ambulation and activity, and predelivery bowel habits. Obtain history of bowel problems.

- Assess client's bowel sounds in all four quadrants (particularly postcesarean delivery) and note abdominal distention.
- Assess the perineal area for wounds, hemorrhoids, and episiotomy (REEDA).

NURSING DIAGNOSES

- Risk for constipation related to perineal discomfort, decreased peristalsis, and use of opioids
- Risk for discomfort related to first postdelivery bowel movement (especially if episiotomy, hemorrhoids, or perineal wounds are present)

PLANNING

- Client will have a bowel movement by 2 to 4 days postpartum.
- Client will resume normal prepregnancy bowel elimination pattern within 4 to 6 weeks.

NURSING INTERVENTIONS

Docusate Sodium (Colace) and Sennosides with Docusate Sodium (Peri-Colace)

- Store at room temperature.
- If a liquid preparation is ordered, give with milk or fruit juice to mask bitter taste.
- Take with a full glass of water.
- Assess client for any history of laxative dependence.

- Drug interaction may occur with mineral oil, phenolphthalein, or aspirin.

Bisacodyl USP (Dulcolax)

- Store tablets and suppositories below 77° F (25° C) and avoid excess humidity.
- Do not crush tablets.
- Do not administer within 1 to 2 hours of milk or antacid, because enteric coating may dissolve, resulting in abdominal cramping and vomiting.
- Take with a full glass of water.

Mineral Oil

- Do not give with or immediately after meals.
- Give with fruit juice or carbonated drinks to disguise taste.

Magnesium Hydroxide (Milk of Magnesia)

- Shake container well.
- Do not give 1 to 2 hours before or after oral drugs because of effects on absorption.
- Take with a full glass of water.
- Note that milk of magnesia concentrate is three times as potent as regular-strength product.
- Give laxative 1 hour before or 1 hour after any oral antibiotic.

Senna (Senokot)

- Protect from light and heat.

Simethicone (Gas-X)

- Administer after meals and at bedtime.
- If chewable simethicone tablets ordered, instruct client to chew tablets thoroughly before swallowing and follow with a full glass of water.

Client Teaching: General

- Instruct client that stool softeners are given to enable a bowel movement without straining.
- Instruct clients that continued laxative use may result in laxative dependence.
- Instruct client that measures to prevent and treat constipation include drinking 6-8 glasses of fluid/ day, ingesting foods high in fiber (bran, fruits, vegetables), and increasing daily ambulation and activity. Instruct clients to avoid/minimize ingestion of gas-forming foods (beans, cabbage, onions) and to increase ambulation/activity.
- Instruct clients regarding temperature and storage requirements for particular drugs.

Client Teaching: Docusate Sodium (Colace) and Sennosides with Docusate Sodium (Peri-Colace)

- Drink at least six 8-oz glasses of liquid daily. Drink one glass of fluid with each dose.

- Take liquid forms with milk or fruit juice to mask bitter taste.
- Explain that many laxatives contain sodium. Tell client to check with health care provider or pharmacist before using laxative if on a low-sodium diet.
- Do not take drug if already taking mineral oil or having acute abdominal pain, nausea, vomiting, or signs of intestinal obstruction.
- Do not use products for longer than 1 week. Advise that prolonged, frequent, or excessive use may result in dependence on drug or electrolyte imbalance.
- Report to health care provider if skin rash occurs or if stomach or intestinal cramping occurs and does not diminish.

Client Teaching: Senna (Senokot)

- Instruct client that drug may discolor urine or feces to yellow-green.
- Instruct client to discontinue the drug if abdominal pain, nausea, or vomiting occurs.
- Instruct client that syrup form is 7% alcohol.

Client Teaching: Mineral Oil

- Instruct client not to take other laxatives (e.g., docusate products) if she is already taking mineral oil.
- Instruct client to take mineral oil on an empty stomach; do not take with food or meals because of risk of aspiration and decreased fat-soluble vitamin absorption.
- Avoid bedtime doses because of risk of aspiration.
- Instruct client to report nausea, vomiting, diarrhea, or abdominal cramping.

Client Teaching: Magnesium Hydroxide (Milk of Magnesia)

- Laxative action generally occurs in 4 to 8 hours.
- Take with a full glass of water.
- Note whether dose is regular strength or concentrated form of drug, because concentrate is three times as potent as regular strength.
- Drug may interact with tetracyclines, digoxin, indomethacin, iron salts, isoniazid; notify health care provider if any of these drugs are used.
- Instruct client to report any muscular weakness, diarrhea, or abdominal cramps.

Client Teaching: Simethicone (Gas-X)

- Drug will help relieve flatus and associated pain. Take after meals. If chewable tablets are ordered, instruct client to chew tablets thoroughly, drink a full glass of water.
- If a dose is missed, take it as soon as possible; however, if the time is close to the next scheduled dose, skip the missed dose and take the scheduled dose. Do not take double doses.

Cultural Considerations ❖

- Provide an interpreter with the same ethnic background and gender if possible, especially with sensitive topics.
- Be culturally cognizant that different cultures discuss elimination in different ways. Be aware of cultural beliefs and practices.

EVALUATION

- Evaluate for return of prepregnancy regular bowel function.

Immunizations

Rh$_O$(D) Immune Globulin

An Rh-negative client who lacks the Rh factor in her own blood may carry a fetus who is either Rh-negative or Rh-positive. During pregnancy, minimal amounts of fetal blood may cross the placenta. Also, an abortion (spontaneous, therapeutic, or induced), amniocentesis, ectopic pregnancy, previa, and abruption result in some mixing of maternal and fetal blood. Subsequently anti-D antibodies develop in an Rh-negative mother with an Rh-positive fetus; with the development of these antibodies, the mother becomes sensitized (Figure 54–1). If mother and fetus are both Rh-negative, no incompatibility exists to trigger the maternal antibody response, but if the fetus is Rh-positive, the Rh-negative mother is at risk for **Rh sensitization** (i.e., the development of protective antibodies against incompatible Rh-positive blood). The immunoglobulin IgM is formed and cannot cross the placenta. Later IgD antibodies develop, which may cross the placenta with isoimmunization to the D antigen and subsequent hemolysis of fetal red blood cells. Prenatal D isoimmunization occurs in approximately 1% to 2% of Rh-negative women. In later exposure, as with subsequent pregnancies, there is a more rapid IgG (secondary) immune response and increased potential for fetal hemolysis in an Rh-positive fetus. The protective antibodies, once formed, remain throughout life and may result in hemolytic difficulties for fetuses in subsequent pregnancies. Maternal blood is assessed for the D antibody at the initial prenatal laboratory evaluation and at 28 to 29 gestational weeks. Human D immunoglobulin (RhoGAM, Rh$_O$[D] immune globulin) is rou-

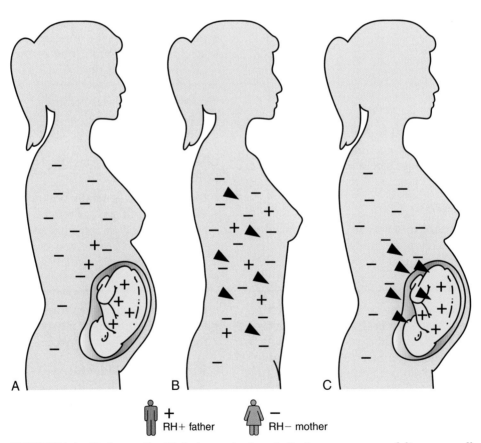

+ RH+ father

– RH– mother

FIGURE 54–1 Understanding Rh isoimmunization. A, During pregnancy or delivery, a small amount of fetal blood may enter the mother's circulation. B, When the mother is Rh-negative and is pregnant with an Rh-positive fetus, the mother's immune system responds by producing anti-Rh$_O$(D) antibodies. C, In subsequent pregnancies, these antibodies cross the placenta and enter the fetal circulation; when the fetus is Rh-positive, the anti-Rh$_O$(D) antibodies will attack the fetal red blood cells and cause hemolysis. (From Nichols F, Zwelling E: *Maternal-newborn nursing: theory and practice*, Philadelphia, 1997, Saunders.)

Table 54–4

Rh$_O$(D) Immune Globulin (RhoGAM)

Route and Dosage	Uses and Considerations
IM in deltoid	A sterile concentrated solution of gamma globulin prepared from human serum containing antibodies to the Rh factor (D antigen), also expressed as anti-Rh$_O$(D). Administered to unsensitized Rh-negative clients. Action is to suppress active antibody response and formation of anti-Rh$_O$(D) in Rh-negative clients exposed to fetal Rh-positive blood. Promotes destruction of Rh-positive fetal cells in maternal serum before mother can make antibodies that would cause hemolysis of fetal RBCs in Rh-positive fetuses and newborns in subsequent pregnancies. Use with *caution* in clients with thrombocytopenia, bleeding disorders, and IgA deficiency. Contraindicated in clients with known hypersensitivity to immune globulins or thimerosal, transfusion of Rh$_O$(D)-positive blood in previous 3 mo or previous sensitization to Rh$_O$(D). 1 vial (300 mcg) prevents maternal sensitization if fetal RBC volume that entered maternal circulation is <15 ml. If the estimated fetal blood and maternal mixing is 30 ml, then an additional 300 mcg is administered. When 15 ml maternal-fetal blood mixing has occurred, a fetal RBC should be performed to determine the appropriate dose. Appears in breast milk (not absorbed by infant). *Adverse reactions:* lethargy, splenomegaly, elevated bilirubin, myalgia, temperature elevation; most commonly (rare) fever and pain at injection site. *Pregnancy category:* C; t½: 23-26 d
300 mcg (1 vial) (standard dose)	Given at 28 wk gestation as prophylaxis and again after normal delivery (within 72 h) with negative direct and indirect Coombs test. Also 300 mcg (standard dose) given after amniocentesis. Larger than standard dose may be given if the Kleihauer-Betke analysis shows large fetal-maternal blood transfusion has occurred
50 mcg (1 vial) (microdose)	Given after abortion or ectopic pregnancy before 13 gestational wk. Because it is a blood product, some clients may refuse because of religious beliefs

d, Day; *IgA*, immunoglobulin A; *IM*, intramuscular; *mo*, month; *RBC*, red blood cell; *t½*, half-life; *wk*, week; >, greater than; <, less than.

tinely administered to women with maternal/fetal blood mixing, such as following an abortion, ectopic pregnancy, or amniocentesis. Dosage depends on gestation: 50 mcg (a microdose) of D immunoglobulin is administered before 13 gestational weeks and 300 mcg is given thereafter. During the postpartum period, D immune globulin should be administered within 72 hours. For women with abruption, previa, cesarean births, or manual placental removal, a Kleihauer-Betke analysis (serum test) should be done, because greater than 30 ml of fetal-maternal bleeding may have occurred, necessitating an increased dose of D immunoglobulin. In this case, 300 mcg of D immunoglobulin is given for each 30 ml of "estimated fetal whole blood" in the maternal circulation. Therefore one full dose (300 mcg) provides enough antibody to prevent Rh sensitization if the volume of red blood cells entering the circulation is 15 ml or less. When 15 ml or more is suspected, a fetal red cell count should be performed to determine the appropriate dose.

The Rh sensitization process can be prevented through the administration of **Rh$_O$(D) immune globulin (Rho-GAM)** to unsensitized Rh-negative clients after each actual or potential exposure to Rh-positive blood (Table 54–4).

Adverse Reactions

Adverse reactions include hypotension, chills, dizziness, fever, headache, pruritus, rash, abdominal pain, diarrhea, and injection site reactions (discomfort, mild pain, redness, and swelling).

Nursing Process

Rh$_O$(D) Immune Globulin

ASSESSMENT

■ Determine blood type and Rh status of all prenatal clients.

■ Assess client for her understanding of both her own and her partner's Rh status.

■ Ask client about previous pregnancies and their outcome; ask whether she has ever received Rh$_O$(D) immune globulin.

■ Follow agency protocols for Rh blood testing for client and infant at time of delivery.

■ Assess client's religious beliefs, because some clients may refuse Rh$_O$(D) immune globulin, considering it to be a blood product. Postpartum, assess data about newborn's Rh type. If infant is Rh-negative, no need for drug. If infant is Rh-positive *and* Rh-negative mother is not sensitized (negative indirect Coombs test) *and* infant has a negative direct Coombs test, mother is a candidate to receive the injection to prevent antibody production or "sensitization".

■ Obtain client's written consent before administration. A refusal form is required in some agencies if the drug is declined.

■ Assess for history of allergy to immune globulin products.

NURSING DIAGNOSES

■ Deficient knowledge related to Rh incompatibility and sensitization
■ Deficient knowledge related to $Rh_O(D)$ immunoglobulin (RhoGAM) purpose, action, and side effects

PLANNING

■ Client will receive $Rh_O(D)$ immune globulin (Rho-GAM) as indicated within 72 hours after delivery or abortion.
■ Client will be able to discuss Rh sensitization and actions indicated during subsequent pregnancies.

NURSING INTERVENTIONS

■ Document Rh workup and eligibility of client to receive drug. Convey information in verbal report and in client record using agency protocol.
■ Check lot numbers on vial and laboratory slip for agreement before administration; check expiration date. Check identification band and laboratory slip for matching number. Return required slips to laboratory or blood bank.
■ Administer $Rh_O(D)$ immune globulin: dose (microdose/standard dose) according to gestational weeks and exposure and route according to provider orders and agency. Administer intramuscularly. Normally administered in deltoid muscle within 72 hours after delivery, but if more than 72 hours, administer as soon as possible up to 28 days.
■ Intravenous administration of $Rh_O(D)$ immune globulin is possible though infrequent. Check provider orders and dose. If IV administration, then reconstitute with normal saline. Store at 36° F to 46° F (2° C to 8° C).
■ Have epinephrine available to treat anaphylaxis.

Client Teaching

General
• Explain the action, purpose, and side effects of the drug.
• Instruct client to avoid live virus vaccines for 3 months following administration.
• Provide written documentation of date of administration for client's personal health record.

Cultural Considerations ❖
• Provide an interpreter with the same ethnic background and gender if possible, especially with sensitive topics.

EVALUATION

■ Evaluate client's understanding of the need for $Rh_O(D)$ immune globulin.

Rubella Vaccine

Maternal rubella, also called *German measles*, is a potentially devastating infection for the fetus, depending on gestational age. If an unimmunized woman (rubella titer <1:10 or negative titer) contracts the virus during the first trimester, a high rate of abortion and neurologic and developmental sequelae associated with **congenital rubella syndrome** (transmission of the rubella virus to the fetus via the placenta) may result. Cataracts, glaucoma, deafness, heart defects, and mental retardation are seen with this syndrome. When infection occurs after the first trimester, there is less risk of fetal damage because of the developmental stage of the fetus. There is no treatment for maternal or congenital rubella infection. The goals are immunization and prevention of rubella in women of childbearing age (Table 54–5).

Table 54–5

Rubella Virus Vaccine, Live, MSD (Meruvax II) (Ra27/3 Strain)

Route and Dosage	Uses and Considerations
Given subQ: 0.5 ml into outer upper arm	Live virus vaccine for immunization against rubella (German measles). Dose is same for all persons, using either single dose or multidose vials. Do not give immune serum globulin (ISG) concurrent with vaccine. Contraindicated in pregnant women and clients with anaphylactoid reactions to neomycin and/or gelatin, febrile respiratory illness or other febrile infection, active untreated tuberculosis, or immune deficiency conditions. Vaccinated persons can shed but not transmit the virus. Defer vaccination for 3 mo after blood or plasma transfusions and also after human serum immune globulin. Postpartum clients who received blood products may be vaccinated if repeat titer is drawn 6-8 wk later to ensure that seroconversion occurred. Excreted in breast milk; use caution. Important for client to use contraceptive method for 4 weeks following administration, because rubella is teratogenic. Rubella titer may be reassessed 3 mo after administration. *Side effects:* burning, stinging at injection site; malaise; fever; headache; slight rash 2-4 wk after injection; joint pain 1-3 d within 1-10 wk of injection. *Pregnancy category:* C

d, Day; *mo,* month; *subQ,* subcutaneous; *wk,* week.

Adverse Reactions

Side effects are generally mild and temporary. Burning or stinging at the injection site is caused by the acidic pH of the vaccine. Regional lymphadenopathy, **urticaria** (i.e., skin rash caused by an allergic reaction), rash, malaise, sore throat, fever, headache, polyneuritis, arthralgia, and moderate fever are occasionally seen.

Nursing Process

Rubella Vaccine

ASSESSMENT

■ Review history and laboratory results to determine need for rubella vaccine.

■ A rubella titer of less than 1:8/1:10 (agency lab), negative, or not immunized indicates need for rubella vaccine administration.

■ Rubella vaccine is contraindicated if client verbalizes (or if chart review indicates) any of the following. Document presence of any of these factors:

  ■ Pregnant

  ■ Receipt of whole blood transfusions, plasma transfusion, or human immune serum globulin within the past 3 months

  ■ History of anaphylactic or anaphylactoid reactions to neomycin (dose contains 25 g of neomycin)

  ■ History of anaphylactic or anaphylactoid reactions to gelatin or gelatin-containing products

  ■ Received other virus vaccines within 1 month (Do not give less than 1 month before or after other virus vaccines.)

  ■ Immunosuppressed, radiation therapy, untreated active tuberculosis (TB), AIDS or symptomatic HIV

  ■ Blood dyscrasias, leukemia, lymphomas of any type, or other malignant neoplasms affecting bone marrow or lymphatic system

  ■ Any febrile or respiratory illness or other acute illness

■ Determine whether client is also a candidate to receive $Rh_O(D)$ immune globulin (RhoGAM). Administration of both drugs may result in suppression of rubella antibodies with need to recheck rubella titer in approximately 3 months.

NURSING DIAGNOSES

■ Deficient knowledge related to risk of rubella infection and benefit of prevention

■ Risk for injury related to rubella infection in subsequent pregnancy secondary to lack of immunity

PLANNING

■ Client will receive rubella vaccine to protect against rubella (German measles).

■ Client will plan to prevent pregnancy for 3 months following subQ injection.

NURSING INTERVENTIONS

■ Protect vaccine from light and store at 35.6° F to 46.4° F (2° C to 8° C) before reconstitution.

■ Reconstitute with diluent provided and administer within 8 hours. Administer 0.5 ml vaccine subQ in upper outer arm. Do not administer IV.

■ If tuberculin skin test is to be done, administer it before or simultaneously with rubella vaccine (may have temporary depression in tuberculin skin sensitivity). If MMR has been given prior to tuberculin skin test, postpone tuberculin skin test until 4-6 week after MMR administration. If giving both simultaneously, use the Mantoux test.

Skill: Reconstitution

• Single-dose vial: withdraw entire amount of diluent into syringe.

• Inject total volume into vial of lyophilized vaccine and agitate to mix thoroughly.

• Withdraw entire contents into syringe and inject total volume of restored vaccine.

• Have epinephrine readily available in case of anaphylactic reaction.

• Clearly convey in verbal report and documentation that vaccination has occurred.

• Record date of administration, lot number, manufacturer, name, and title to comply with agency policy.

Client Teaching

General

• Discuss with client the importance of immunity to rubella, and help her understand the need to obtain titers to determine immune status.

• Discuss the importance for use of effective contraception for 4 weeks after vaccine injection. Identify contraceptive method of choice and document instruction.

• Reassure client that there is no risk to her from being near small children who received the injection, even if she is pregnant and not immune.

• Instruct parents regarding the drug action, purpose, and side effects.

Safety

• Recommend that client have titer rechecked in 3 months if she also received RhoGAM.

Side Effects

• The most common side effect is burning or stinging at injection site; some also experience malaise, fever, headache, and slight rash about 2 to 4 weeks after injection. About 1 to 10 weeks after injection, some may experience joint pain that lasts 1 to 3 days.

Cultural Considerations ❖

• Provide an interpreter as appropriate.

EVALUATION

■ Evaluate the need for rubella vaccine and administration to women with titer less than 1:8/1:10 (agency lab), not immunized, or negative titer.

Drugs Administered to the Newborn Immediately after Delivery

Drugs administered to the newborn in the immediate period after birth are (1) erythromycin ophthalmic ointment to provide prophylaxis against eye infections (required by U.S. public health law and all states) and (2) vitamin K to prevent hemorrhagic disease of the newborn (Table 54–6). Anti-infective agents may be applied to the cord stump (e.g., alcohol or Triple Dye) during the first few hours after birth; however, current literature supports "dry cord care" with no agents applied.

Side Effects and Adverse Reactions

Erythromycin Ophthalmic Ointment. Side effects include chemical conjunctivitis in about 20% of newborns, which manifests as edema and inflammation lasting about 24 to 48 hours. This may interfere slightly with eye-to-eye contact between parents and the newborn.

Phytonadione Vitamin K_1, (Aqua-MEPHYTON). Side effects include pain and edema at the injection site. Some allergic reactions, manifested by urticaria and rash, have been reported. Newborns who receive larger doses may exhibit hyperbilirubinemia and jaundice resulting from competition for binding sites.

Nursing Process

Drugs Administered to the Newborn after Delivery

ASSESSMENT

Erythromycin Ophthalmic Ointment (Ilotycin Ophthalmic)

■ Assess newborn for signs of hypersensitivity.

Phytonadione (Vitamin K_1, Mephyton, Aqua-MEPHYTON)

■ Assess newborn for bleeding from umbilical cord, circumcision site, nose, and gastrointestinal tract, and for generalized ecchymoses.

NURSING DIAGNOSES

■ Risk for injury related to infectious process (congenital) or transient low prothrombin levels in the newborn

---

Table 54–6

Drugs Administered to the Newborn Immediately after Delivery

Generic (Brand)	Route and Dosage	Uses and Considerations
erythromycin ophthalmic ointment (Ilotycin Ophthalmic)	Half-inch ribbon of ointment placed in lower conjunctival sac of each eye (beginning at inner canthus) within 1 h of delivery	Prevention of gonococcal conjunctivitis and chlamydial conjunctivitis (**ophthalmia neonatorum**), which can cause blindness. Source of infection is birth canal. Contains antibiotic (erythromycin) in sterile base of mineral oil and white petrolatum. Has bactericidal or bacteriostatic action based on concentration per gram and target organisms present. Mandatory administration in the U.S. *Side effects:* Chemical conjunctivitis (swelling, inflammation 24-48 h)
phytonadione (Vitamin K_1, Mephyton, Aqua-MEPHYTON)	0.5-1 mg IM in vastus lateralis (preferably) or rectus femoris within 1 h after birth (Check health care provider or agency standing orders for dosage)	Prevention of hemorrhagic disease of the newborn. Anticoagulant antagonist. An aqueous colloidal solution of vitamin K_1. Newborn does not receive adequate vitamin K transplacentally and is unable to synthesize vitamin initially because of limited intestinal flora; therefore production of clotting factors in liver is hindered and low prothrombin levels are evidenced. Phytonadione facilitates production of clotting factors equal to natural vitamin K. Newborns of mothers who received oral anticoagulants, anticonvulsants, antituberculosis drugs or recent antibiotics during pregnancy may need higher dosage 6-8 h after the first injection. *Side effects:* Pain and edema at injection site; possible allergic reactions include urticaria and rash; those who receive larger doses may exhibit hyperbilirubinemia and jaundice.

h, Hour; *IM*, intramuscular; *in*, inch.

PLANNING

■ Newborn will experience minimal or no side effects from drugs routinely administered after delivery.

NURSING INTERVENTIONS

Erythromycin Ophthalmic Ointment

■ See Chapter 3 for procedure for administration of eye ointment.

■ Promote bonding by facilitating eye contact between parents and infant during this period, but delay instillation no longer than 1 hour after delivery.

■ Wear gloves for administration of eye ointment. Do not place tube of ointment under radiant warmer with infant before administration.

■ Administer erythromycin ophthalmic ointment prior to administration of phytonadione and hepatitis B (with maternal consent only) injections. Infant may cry following injections, making administration of ophthalmic ointment more difficult.

■ Administer erythromycin ophthalmic ointment (ribbon of ointment about 1 cm long) from inner canthus to outer canthus in lower conjunctival sac of each eye. Do not touch eye with applicator.

■ Following administration, close eyes to more evenly distribute ointment. After 1 minute, may blot eye with gauze to remove excess ointment. Do not irrigate eyes following instillation.

Phytonadione (Vitamin K$_1$, Mephyton, Aqua-MEPHYTON)

■ Protect drug from light because of photosensitivity of the preparation.

■ Cleanse anterolateral site before injecting drug; if alcohol is used, allow to dry prior to drug administration.

■ Wear gloves when administering phytonadione (vitamin K)

■ If phytonadione (vitamin K) is in a glass vial, withdraw medication with a filter needle. Change needles and use a 25 gauge, $^5/_8$-inch needle to administer in either the vastus lateralis (preferred) or the rectus femoris muscle.

■ Stabilize infant's leg prior to administration of phytonadione (vitamin K).

■ Observe injection site for edema and inflammation (Figure 54–2). Refer to Chapter 3 for a complete discussion of safe pediatric drug injection sites.

■ Administer phytonadione prior to circumcision.

Client Teaching: Erythromycin Ophthalmic Ointment (Ilotycin Ophthalmic)

• Instruct parents regarding the drug action, purpose, and side effects. Instructing parents about drug administration is mandatory in the United States.

• Tell parents that any edema around eyes usually disappears within 24 to 48 hours.

• Explain that administration of eye prophylaxis is federally and state mandated and that there is no risk to vision from the ointment.

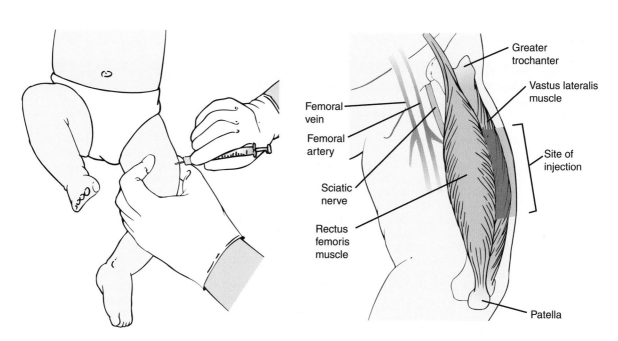

FIGURE 54–2 Site for giving an intramuscular injection to a newborn shortly after birth. (From Nichols F, Zwelling E: *Maternal-newborn nursing: theory and practice,* Philadelphia, 1997, Saunders.)

Client Teaching: Phytonadione (Vitamin K1, Mephyton, Aqua-MEPHYTON)

- Instruct parents regarding the drug action, purpose and side effects.

EVALUATION

- Evaluate for newborn bleeding, specifically days 2 and 3 after administration of phytonadione (Vitamin K, Mephyton, Aqua-MEPHYTON).
- Evaluate for drug hypersensitivity or side effects.
- Evaluate parents' understanding about medications administered to their newborns.

Immunization during the Newborn Period before Discharge

The American Academy of Pediatrics and the Centers for Disease Control and Prevention (CDC) have recommended that immunization against hepatitis B virus (HBV) begin in the newborn period. The HBV infection may result in serious long-term liver disease, cancer, and death in adulthood. The goal of immunization is to reduce the number of chronic carriers of the virus in the population, thus preventing HBV infection.

In pregnancy, HBV transmission occurs vertically, primarily at the time of delivery. The recombinant hepatitis B (Engerix-B, Recombivax HB) provides passive immunization for the newborn (Table 54–7). The current recommendation is that newborns receive recombinant hepatitis B and if appropriate, hepatitis B immunoglobulin (HBIG) injections intramuscularly (IM) in the anterolateral thigh (vastus lateralis [preferred] or rectus femoris muscles) following a protocol based on the mother's HBsAg-positive or -negative status. These injections require signed maternal consent prior to administration. Infants born to HBsAg-negative mothers will receive only recombinant hepatitis B (Engerix-B, Recombivax HB). Infants born to HBsAg-positive mothers will receive concurrent injections of both HBIG and hepatitis B vaccine (Engerix-B, Recombivax HB) in separate sites, because it is believed that infection can be prevented in 90% of newborns.

Hepatitis B Vaccine

ASSESSMENT

- Review prenatal record laboratory data for maternal HBsAg status. Validate whether infant is to receive hepatitis B vaccine singly or in concert with hepatitis B immune globulin (HBIG).
- Assess parental knowledge of immunizations, purpose, and childhood immunization schedule.
- Assess for hypersensitivity to yeast (recombinant HB).
- Assess for written maternal consent for newborn vaccine before administration.

NURSING DIAGNOSES

- Risk for injury related to hepatitis B infection
- Deficient knowledge related to hepatitis B, maternal prophylaxis, and pediatric immunization schedule

Table 54–7

Hepatitis B Immunization in the Newborn Period

Generic (Brand)	Route and Dosage	Uses and Considerations
hepatitis B vaccine (Engerix-B, Recombivax HB)	For newborns of HBsAg negative, HBsAg-positive mothers and unknown hepatitis B status: *Engerix-B:* 0.5 ml (10 mcg) IM within 12 h after birth (first dose); second dose at 1-2 mo and final dose at age ≥24 weeks (6 mo). *Recombivax HB:* 0.5 ml (5 mcg) IM within 12 h after birth (first dose), repeated at 1 mo and 6 mo.	Hepatitis B vaccine is a recombinant vaccine that provides passive immunization against all subtypes of HBV. Given to all infants regardless of HBsAg status of mother. Unvaccinated infants *younger than* 12 mo with a mother or primary care giver with acute hepatitis B should be given HBIG because of risk of becoming an HBV carrier following infection (also start HBV vaccine series). Must be injected IM into vastus lateralis (preferably) or rectus femoris; never inject IV. Following three doses, >90% of infants and children will seroconvert 95%-99%. Protection in those who seroconvert will last 3-7 y with a single booster. Contraindicated if hypersensitivity to any component of vaccine or yeast. *Neonatal side effects:* soreness at injection site with edema, warmth, erythema, and induration. *Pregnancy category:* C
		Newborns of HBsAg-positive mothers should also receive HBIG 0.5 ml IM within 12 h of birth. May be given concurrently with first dose of hepatitis B vaccine in separate site (opposite thigh). Newborns of mothers with HBsAg-unknown status whose maternal results are positive within 7 days of birth should receive HBIG (0.5 ml) IM in thigh not used for vaccine.

h, Hour; *HBIG,* hepatitis B immune globulin; *HBsAg,* hepatitis B surface antigen; *HBV,* hepatitis B virus; *IM,* intramuscular; *IV,* intravenous; *mo,* month; *y,* year; *>,* greater than.

PLANNING

■ The newborn will receive correct dosage of hepatitis B vaccine before discharge, including HBIG if indicated.

■ The newborn's caregiver will keep scheduled appointments with primary health care provider and verbalizes plans to continue childhood immunizations as recommended by the current immunization schedule.

NURSING INTERVENTIONS

Skill
- Shake vial well before withdrawal of medication.
- Discard if other than slightly opaque white suspension.
- Cleanse anterolateral site before injecting drug. If alcohol is used, allow to dry prior to drug administration.
- Inject complete contents of vial; do not dilute.
- Have epinephrine available for allergic reaction.
- If mother refuses hepatitis B vaccine (Engerix-B, Recombivax HB) or HBIG, note in maternal and newborn chart. Assess agency protocol, because some agencies document medication refusal. Monitor newborn's temperature post injection per agency protocol.

Safety
- Give IM in vastus lateralis (preferably) or rectus femoris.
- Document administration and site in chart.
- Record lot number, expiration date, name, and title in chart.
- Store product at 35.6° F to 46.4° F (2° C to 8° C).
- Do not freeze (because freezing destroys potency).

- Do not confuse hepatitis B vaccine (Engerix-B, Recombivax) and HBIG or Haemophilus B (Hib) vaccine, because these drugs have different dosages.

Client Teaching

General
- Inform mother of implications of her hepatitis B surface antigen (HBsAg)-positive or HBsAg-negative status for her newborn, and recommend interventions.
- Have mother read literature and sign consent for vaccine administration. Place original/copy in newborn's chart as per agency protocol. Instruct parents regarding childhood immunizations as recommended by the current immunization schedule. Inform mother when repeat doses need to be given. Give mother written information regarding the immunization schedule and infant immunization record. Document administration of hepatitis B on infant immunization record.

EVALUATION

■ Evaluate mother's understanding of the need for hepatitis B vaccine for her newborn.

Critical Thinking Case Study

TA, age 17, gravida 4, para 1, came to the hospital for labor induction/augmentation at 42 weeks' gestation because of her prolonged pregnancy and signs and symptoms of pregnancy-induced hypertension. TA's mother arrived at the hospital when TA was 8 cm dilated in time for the latter stages of TA's labor. Her mother remained as TA's support person throughout the delivery, which occurred at 6:00 AM by vacuum extraction. TA had a continuous epidural for her labor and delivery. An episiotomy was done at the time of delivery, and a fourth-degree laceration occurred. A cluster of hemorrhoids was evident. Baby JA, weighing 8 lbs 7 oz, had Apgar scores of 7 and 9. The infant is alert and active. TA lives with her mother and has been going to high school while working part time in an automotive parts store. TA wants to keep her infant and to breastfeed "for at least 3 months." She plans to finish school and return to work in 6 weeks.

Immediately after the delivery, you conduct an assessment of TA, analyze the data, and determine and prioritize her nursing care needs. The same is done for the newborn.

1. Based on the data supplied about her delivery, what is the priority nursing diagnosis for TA?
2. What is an outcome-based goal for the diagnosis given?
3. How should the nurse intervene in regard to the episiotomy during the early postpartum period, integrating both pharmacologic and nonpharmacologic measures? Orders include benzocaine spray, witch hazel pads, Proctofoam-HC, and ibuprofen tablets (200 mg) at the bedside.
4. TA verbalizes that her grandmother wants her to eat warm soup that she will bring to the hospital. She also told TA not to take a shower for 4 weeks. What further assessment is necessary?

Baby JA's newborn medications must be administered within the first hour following delivery. Bonding for TA and JA should also be promoted at this time.

Critical Thinking Case Study

5. Within the standard, how should bonding be promoted, including eye contact between mother and infant, while eye prophylaxis is also administered?

6. What steps should be followed to instill the ointment into the infant's eyes, including safety aspects for the nurse administering the ointment?

7. What should TA be taught about the side effects of eye prophylaxis?

8. How should the reason for the vitamin K_1 injection for the infant be explained to TA in terms she can understand?

9. What steps should be followed to prepare and give the vitamin K_1 injection, including safety aspects for the nurse administering the injection?

TA is Rh negative. The blood type of the infant's father is unknown. A cord blood was drawn on the infant at the time of delivery. Based on TA's historical data, answer the following:

10. What is a concern in terms of defining TA as a likely or unlikely $Rh_O(D)$ immune globulin candidate? What information about the mother and infant is needed to aid in the decision?

Assuming TA is a $Rh_O(D)$ immune globulin candidate, answer the following:

11. What is a nursing diagnosis for TA?

12. What is an outcome-based goal for the diagnosis given?

13. What is the timeframe in which $Rh_O(D)$ immune globulin should be administered? Explain the rationale for this timeframe.

14. What are appropriate verbal and written documentation in regard to $Rh_O(D)$ immune globulin administration, both before and after administration?

15. TA's chart reveals that her rubella titer is 1:6. What orders should be expected in regard to rubella vaccine?

16. Neomycin is listed as a known allergy in TA's medication administration record. Considering TA's titer, the standing health care provider's order, and knowledge

about this vaccine, how should this situation be handled?

17. In a situation in which a mother is both a rubella and $Rh_O(D)$ immune globulin candidate, with both products being administered, what is the focus of client teaching for TA in regard to the rubella titer?

Because of her episiotomy, TA is concerned about her first postdelivery bowel movement. It is explained to her that the docusate with sennosides product in her self-administered medication packet will help.

18. TA says that she does not want to take the docusate because she plans to breastfeed. What is the appropriate nursing diagnosis based on TA's communication?

19. How should TA's concerns be addressed, based on knowledge of the product and breastfeeding?

TA asks what can be done about her hemorrhoids. The mode of action of the ordered pharmacologic products is explained to her. She then states, "So I just have to insert this syringe-type applicator into my rectum once I fill it from the big can?"

20. Analyze TA's statement. What is correct and incorrect concerning the knowledge?

21. What nursing diagnosis is appropriate for TA based on the information supplied?

22. What client teaching is needed for TA?

Baby JA is ordered to receive hepatitis B vaccine before discharge. TA is HBsAg-negative.

23. Which newborns are eligible to receive hepatitis B vaccine?

24. How many doses constitute the total series, and what is the duration for these?

25. Why is this vaccine given to newborns? Why is this important in today's society?

26. TA asks how long the infant's immunity should last. How should she be answered?

27. Where would one expect to find the vaccine stored?

28. What is the written documentation required with administration of this vaccine?

NCLEX Study Questions

1. Client AB asks the nurse why her baby is receiving a vitamin K injection. The nurse's best response is based upon the knowledge that:
   a. vitamin K causes an increase in newborn platelets
   b. a newborn's liver is too immature to produce vitamin K
   c. the newborn cannot synthesize vitamin K without intestinal flora
   d. vitamin K is not produced in bone marrow until an infant is 8 days old

2. In assessing the postpartum client the nurse notes saturation of two peripads in less than 1½ hours. The priority intervention is:
   a. palpate the fundus and massage if boggy
   b. prepare to administer pitocin IV
   c. prepare to administer Methergine
   d. assess maternal blood pressure and pulse for hypovolemic shock

3. Two hours after delivery LW complains of pain from her episiotomy. The most effective nursing intervention is a(n):
   a. sitz bath for 20 minutes
   b. application of cold compresses to the perineum
   d. temperature 100.1° F
   c. blood pressure 148/92

4. MW is being discharged from the hospital. In reviewing her chart the nurse notes she is Rubella-negative. Your teaching will include using an effective contraceptive to prevent pregnancy, because she is at increased risk of congenital anomalies for the next:
   a. 1 week
   b. 4 weeks
   c. 3 months
   d. 6 months

5. Prior to administering the newborn medication _____, it is mandatory to have maternal signed consent.
   a. erythromycin
   b. vitamin K
   c. hepatitis B
   d. betamethasone

6. Prior to administering MMR vaccine to DS at discharge, you ask about allergies. If she says she has an allergy to _____, you would withhold the vaccine and notify her provider.
   a. baker's yeast
   b. eggs
   c. duck meat or duck feathers
   d. gelatin

7. The nurse is mentoring a new graduate preparing to administer the vitamin K injection to a newborn. Which muscle site selected by the new graduate would indicate the need for further teaching?
   a. Anterolateral thigh
   b. Vastus lateralis
   c. Rectus femoris
   d. Gluteus maximus

8. Methergine is prescribed for a client with postpartum hemorrhage. What finding would contraindicate administering Methergine to this client?
   a. Respirations 12
   b. Pulse 62
   c. Blood pressure 148/92
   d. Temperature 100.1° F

Answers: 1, c; 2, a; 3, b; 4, b; 5, c; 6, d; 7, d; 8, c.

55

Drugs for Women's Health and Reproductive Disorders

Sandra Elliott

ELECTRONIC RESOURCES

evolve

Evolve website (http://evolve.elsevier.com/KeeHayes/pharmacology/):
- *Case Studies*
- *Content Updates*
- *Frequently Asked Questions*
- *Student Review Activities*
- *WebLinks*
- *Additional Reference Material*

Companion CD-ROM:
- *NCLEX Examination Review Questions*
- *Pharmacology Animations*
- *IV Therapy Checklists*
- *Medication Error Checklists*
- *Drug Calculation Problems*
- *Electronic Calculators*
- *Top 200 Drugs with Pronunciations*
- *References from the Textbook*

Objectives

- Describe the types, expected actions, and side effects of oral contraceptive products.
- Recognize new hormonal/pharmacologic products related to conception control.
- Explain the expected effects of medications used to treat dysfunctional uterine bleeding, premenstrual syndrome, endometriosis, menopausal symptoms, and osteoporosis.
- Describe the nursing process, including client teaching, associated with drugs used for women's health and disorders.

Terms

Oral contraceptive products and medications used for uterine dysfunction and menopause are described in this chapter. Nursing interventions and client teaching are emphasized.

Oral Contraceptive Products

Among the various methods of contraception available, **oral contraceptives** (known as *the pill*), enjoy wide popularity because of their ease of use and high degree of effectiveness with relative safety for most women. With chemicals similar to the hormones estrogen and progesterone, oral contraceptives act by preventing ovulation. The effectiveness of oral contraceptives can be compromised by concurrent use of some medications (e.g., antibiotics) or herbal products (Herbal Alert 55–1). When these steroidal agents were first approved for use by the Food and Drug Administration (FDA) in 1960, little was known about the best combinations of drugs to use, or their optimum doses. Adverse side effects, particularly circulatory disorders, were frequent. Subsequent research has resulted in lower-dose drugs. Research continues to focus on actual and potential short- and long-term benefits and risks associated with use of low-dose oral contraceptives, particularly in the areas of circulatory risks and carcinogenesis. New administration forms (e.g., long-acting progestin-releasing subcutaneous implants) and immunologic methods of contraception are other areas of current research.

There are two main types of oral contraceptives: estrogen-progestin combination products (OCPs), and progestin-only products (POPs), sometimes called *the minipill*. Combination products have the lowest pregnancy rate.

Estrogen-Progestin Combination Products

Combined estrogen-progestin oral contraceptive products prevent pregnancy by suppressing pituitary release of follicle-stimulating hormone (FSH) and luteinizing hormone (LH), which are needed to mature a graafian follicle in the ovary, thereby inhibiting ovulation. These agents also create changes in the endometrium that make it less favorable for implantation of a fertilized ovum. In addition, the quantity and viscosity of the cervical mucus is changed by progestins, making it hostile to sperm. Alterations in motility within the fallopian tube may also impede the movement of the ova.

The most commonly prescribed oral contraceptive products are the estrogen-progestin combinations. These formulations are differentiated based on the strength of the individual components and whether estrogen or progesterone effects predominate. The amount of estrogen varies among the available products. Low-dose combination products have 35 mcg or less of ethinyl estradiol or 50 mcg or less of mestranol. The synthetic progesterone **progestin** incorporated in the combination products reduces the effects of estrogen. The goal of therapy is to identify the product that offers the best contraceptive protection throughout the menstrual cycle while producing the fewest unwanted side effects as a result of either the estrogen or the progestin component.

There are three types of combination products: monophasic, biphasic, and triphasic. The *monophasics*, the most common, provide a fixed ratio of estrogen to progestin throughout the menstrual cycle. In *biphasics*, the amount of estrogen is fixed throughout the cycle, but the amount of progesterone varies (reduced in the first half and increased in the second half) to provide for proliferation of the endometrium and secretory development similar to the physiologic process. Ortho-Novum 10/11 is an example of a biphasic (Phase 1, 10 days; Phase 2, 11 days.) The *triphasics*, the newest combination products, deliver low doses of both hormones with minimal side effects, including breakthrough bleeding. With triphasics, the amount of either estrogen or progesterone varies throughout the cycle in different ratios during three phases (e.g., Phase 1, 5 days; Phase 2, 7 days; Phase 3, 9 days). Ortho Tri-Cyclen is an example of a triphasic pill that varies the dosage of progestin. Estrostep is an example of a triphasic pill that varies the dosage of estrogen. Both have FDA indications for the treatment of acne.

Seasonale was the first FDA-approved extended-cycle birth control pill. The 91-day regimen (84 active pills/ 7 placebo pills) of Seasonale reduces a woman's periods from 13 to just 4 per year. Women who may benefit from an extended cycle regimen include those with menstrual disorders such as endometriosis, dysmenorrhea, PMS, and ovarian cysts. Seasonale is now available as generic Quasense.

Seasonique is another extended-cycle birth control pill that gives women four periods per year instead of 12. With Seasonique, women get a low dose of estrogen (0.1 mg of ethinyl estradiol) *during* their period, which may provide benefits including less breakthrough bleeding. Users of extended-cycle birth control pills may be more likely to experience bleeding or spotting between periods; such bleeding and spotting tends to decrease during later cycles as women keep taking the drug. **Extended-cycle regimen pills always have a Sunday start**.

Lybrel is the first *continuous*-dose oral contraceptive pill to be FDA approved. It is also seeking FDA approval for the treatment of PMDD. Lybrel comes in a 28-day pill pack and contains 90 micrograms of levonorgestrel and 20 micrograms of ethinyl estradiol.

Loestrin 24 Fe is a 24-day active hormonal regimen of 1 milligram of norethindrone acetate and 20 micrograms of ethinyl estradiol tablets, plus 4 ferrous fumarate tablets.

Herbal ALERT 55–1

St. John's Wort

St. John's wort (*Hypericum perforatum*) may reduce the effectiveness of contraceptive steroids. This may also result in breakthrough bleeding.

It is the first birth-control pill approved in the United States that provides 24 days of active hormonal therapy and 4 days of iron supplement pills. Its advertising promises to give women "shorter, lighter periods".

Yasmin with drospirenone (drsp) is a combination pill (ethinyl estradiol 30 mcg; drospirenone 3 mg). While the progestins in other combination oral contraceptives are derived from testosterone, drospirenone is the only progestin derived from spironolactone, not testosterone. Drospirenone may increase serum potassium. Women should not take Yasmin if they have kidney, liver, or adrenal disease, because this could cause serious heart and health problems. Other drugs may also increase potassium. Women should have a blood test to check their potassium level if they have a chronic condition requiring daily long-term treatment with any of the following medications: NSAIDs (such as ibuprofen, naproxen), taken long-term and daily for arthritis or other diseases or conditions; potassium-sparing diuretics (spironolactone and others); potassium supplementation; ACE inhibitors (Capoten, Vasotec, Zestril, and others); angiotensin-II receptor antagonists (Cozaar, Diovan, Avapro, and others); and heparin.

Yaz, is a new monophasic oral contraceptive and the first pill to combine 20 mcg of ethinyl estradiol with the progestin drospirenone (drsp). The 24-day active hormone pill regimen of Yaz results in less hormonal fluctuation than traditional oral contraceptive pills that provide 21 days of active pills. As with Yasmin, Yaz contains the progestin drospirenone, a spironolactone analogue with antimineralocorticoid properties. The 24-day active hormone pill regimen of Yaz combined with the 30-hour half life of drospirenone results in less hormonal fluctuation between cycles, compared to traditional oral contraceptives with 21 days of active pills and seven days of placebos. Preclinical studies indicate that drospirenone also provides an antiandrogenic effect, which means that it counteracts the effects of male hormones in the body. Yaz is FDA approved for the treatment of premenstrual dysphoric disorder (PMDD) as well as acne. It has the same precautions as Yasmin.

Femcon Fe is the first chewable birth control pill. Femcon Fe spearmint-flavored pills can be swallowed or chewed.

Progestin-Only Products

The progestin-only oral contraceptive, called the mini-pill, acts primarily by altering the cervical mucus and secondarily by altering the endometrium to inhibit implantation. Ovulation is also inhibited in some clients through blockage of LH release. These products were designed to further decrease circulatory side effects. There is, however, a lower pregnancy prevention rate, which increases further if a client misses a pill, because these drugs do not suppress activity of the hypothalamus and pituitary to the same degree as the combination products. **If the minipill is taken more than 3 hours late, a back-up contraceptive method should be used for 48 hours.** There are no placebo pills

in a pack of progestin-only pills. All 28 pills contain active hormones. An increase in the amount of breakthrough bleeding is also noted. Examples of progestin-only products include Ovrette, Ortho Micronor, and Nor-QD. Table 55–1 presents selected examples of the various oral contraceptive formulations.

Pharmacokinetics

Combination Products. Ethinyl estradiol is rapidly absorbed orally. It undergoes significant first-pass metabolism and elimination via the liver. Mestranol is converted in the liver to ethinyl estradiol, which is 97% to 98% bound to plasma proteins. The half-life varies from 6 to 20 hours. Excretion is via bile and urine in a conjugated form. There is some enterohepatic recirculation.

Progestin-Only Products. Progestins are also well absorbed orally. Peak plasma levels occur from 0.5 to 4 hours after ingestion, depending on the particular compound. Norethynodrel and ethynodiol diacetate are converted to norethindrone. Levonorgestrel is bioavailable and does not undergo first-pass liver metabolism; norethindrone undergoes first-pass metabolism and is 65% available. The progestins are bound to plasma proteins and to sex hormone-binding globulin. The half-life of norethindrone varies from 5 to 14 hours; the half-life of levonorgestrel is 11 to 45 hours.

Dosage Schedule

Combination Products. Most monophasic products are available in 21- and 28-tablet packages. The 28-tablet packages include seven placebo tablets called *counters* (or some formulations contain an iron supplement), so that the client continues to take one tablet each day rather than having to remember starting and stopping dates. Clients are instructed to take one tablet every day at approximately the same time each day. Many products require the client to start the tablets on the Sunday following the first day of menstruation. If menstruation actually starts on Sunday, the client starts her tablets that day. Other products instruct the client to start her tablets on day 5 of the menstrual cycle (day 1 is the day she begins menstruation). If the client is on a 21-day regimen, she restarts her next cycle following a 7-day break whether her bleeding has stopped or not. If a Sunday start is used, a backup method (such as condoms or a diaphragm) needs to be used for a minimum of 7 days. Other products instruct the client to start her tablets on day 1 of the menstrual cycle (which is the day she begins menstruation). A backup method is not needed with this method.

With the "Quick Start" method the pill can be started on any day of the week regardless of where a woman is in her cycle, as long as pregnancy has been ruled out. There is no medical reason for a woman to wait until Sunday or for her menses. Many providers recommend that a woman should start her pills as soon as possible and to use a backup method for contraception for one week. After one week on the combination products the woman is protected from pregnancy.

The biphasic and triphasic products are taken in phases and are color-coded to assist the client. They too are available in 21- and 28-day regimens and are started within the

Table 55–1

Oral Contraceptives

Product	Amount of Estrogen (mcg)	Amount of Progestin (mg)
Combination Products: Listed by Decreasing Estrogen Content		
Monophasic Products		
Norinyl 1 + 50 (21 days)	50 mestranol	1 norethindrone
Genora 1/50	50 mestranol	1 norethindrone
Demulen 1/50	50 ethinyl estradiol	1 ethynodiol diacetate
Ortho-Novum 1/35	35 ethinyl estradiol	1 norethindrone
Norinyl 1 + 35	35 ethinyl estradiol	1 norethindrone
Modicon	35 ethinyl estradiol	0.5 norethindrone
Brevicon	35 ethinyl estradiol	0.5 norethindrone
Ovcon 35	35 ethinyl estradiol	0.4 norethindrone
Demulen 1/35	35 ethinyl estradiol	1 ethynodiol diacetate
Desogen	30 ethinyl estradiol	0.15 desogestrel
Loestrin Fe 21 1.5/30	30 ethinyl estradiol	1.5 norethindrone acetate
Lo/Ovral	30 ethinyl estradiol	0.3 norgestrel
Levlen	30 ethinyl estradiol	0.15 levonorgestrel
Levlite	20 ethinyl estradiol	0.10 levonorgestrel
Loestrin 21 1/20	20 ethinyl estradiol	1 norethindrone acetate
Biphasic Products		
Ortho-Novum 10/11	Same formulation as above but different colors for tablets	
Triphasic Products		
Tri-Norinyl	*Phase I (7 days):* 35 ethinyl estradiol	0.5 norethindrone
	Phase II (9 days): 35 ethinyl estradiol	1 norethindrone
	Phase III (5 days): 35 ethinyl estradiol	0.5 norethindrone
Ortho Tri-Cyclen	*Phase I (7 days):* 35 ethinyl estradiol	0.18 norgestimate
	Phase II (7 days): 35 ethinyl estradiol	0.215 norgestimate
	Phase III (7 days): 35 ethinyl estradiol	0.25 norgestimate
Ortho-Novum 7/7/7	*Phase I (7 days):* 35 ethinyl estradiol	0.5 norethindrone
	Phase II (7 days): 35 ethinyl estradiol	0.075 norethindrone
	Phase III (7 days): 35 ethinyl estradiol	1 norethindrone
Tri-Levlen	*Phase I (6 days):* 30 ethinyl estradiol	0.05 levonorgestrel
	Phase II (5 days): 40 ethinyl estradiol	0.075 levonorgestrel
	Phase III (10 days): 30 ethinyl estradiol	0.125 levonorgestrel
Triphasil	Same as above	
Progestin-Only Products: Listed by Decreasing Progestin Content		
Ortho Micronor		0.35 norethindrone
Nor-QD		0.35 norethindrone
Ovrette		0.075 norgestrel

guidelines previously presented. For example, the biphasic Ortho-Novum 10/11 requires 10 white tablets for 10 days, followed by 11 peach tablets for 11 days. With a 21-day regimen, the client stops for 7 days; with a 28-day regimen, the client takes seven green inert tablets during this period before beginning the next cycle. The triphasic Ortho-Novum 7/7/7 works similarly. White tablets are taken for 7 days, light peach for 7 days, darker peach for 7 days, followed by 7 days off or 7 green inert tablets. Exceptions to these guidelines include the triphasics Triphasil 21 and Tri-

Levlen 21, which are started on the first day of the menstrual cycle with the designated color code followed for 6 days, 5 days, and 10 days, respectively. These too are available in 21- and 28-day packaging.

Yasmin (drospirenone/ethinyl estradiol), is the first oral contraceptive with progestin to reduce water retention. The dosage is drospirenone/ethinyl estradiol, 3 mg/0.03 mg daily for 21 days; then one inert tablet daily (white tablet) for 7 days. It is contraindicated in women with renal, hepatic, or adrenal insufficiency. Monitor potassium level during the first cycle if there is risk of hyperkalemia (taking drugs that increase potassium, such as angiotensin-converting enzyme [ACE] inhibitors, angiotension receptor blockers, nonsteroidal antiinflammatory drugs [NSAIDs], potassium-sparing diuretics). Potential adverse effects include headache, menstrual disorder, and breast pain.

Progestin-Only Products. The progestin-only products are taken one tablet at the same time daily without interruption. The tablets should begin being taken on the first day of menstruation.

Missed Doses

Clients occasionally miss a tablet. If only one tablet is missed, it is unlikely that ovulation will occur. However, the risk increases with each additional missed dose. Table 55–2 presents guidelines for missed doses of oral contraceptives.

Contraindications

Not every client is a candidate for use of oral contraceptives. Box 55–1 lists contraindications to their use.

Drug Interactions

The effectiveness of some drugs is impaired by oral contraceptives; other drugs impair the effectiveness of oral contraceptives. Box 55–2 lists examples of drugs for which the nurse should maintain a high index of suspicion for interactive effects with oral contraceptives. Clients receiving low-dose formulations of oral contraceptives need to be particularly cautious about potential interactions.

Side Effects and Adverse Reactions

The risk of death from the use of oral contraceptives is less than the risk from pregnancy, especially if the client does not exhibit contraindications listed in Box 55–1. Most side effects are related to differences in the estrogen-progestin ratio of the products and the client's response.

Side effects primarily caused by an excess of estrogen include nausea, vomiting, dizziness, fluid retention, edema, bloating, breast enlargement, breast tenderness, chloasma (slightly more in dark-skinned clients exposed to sunlight on higher dose tablets), leg cramps, decreased tearing, corneal curvature alteration, visual changes, vascular headache, and hypertension (in about 1% to 5% of previously normotensive clients within the first few months).

Side effects primarily caused by estrogen deficiency include vaginal bleeding (breakthrough bleeding, especially in the first few cycles after starting therapy) that lasts several days (usually during days 1 to 14), oligomenorrhea (especially after long-term use), nervousness, and **dyspareunia** (painful sexual intercourse) secondary to atrophic vaginitis.

Table 55–2	
Guidelines for Missed Doses of Oral Contraceptives	

Missed Dose	Recommendations
Combination Products	
One tablet	Take tablet as soon as realized OR Take two tablets the next day OR Take one tablet, discard missed tablet, continue schedule, but use secondary form of contraception until menses begin.
Two tablets	Take two tablets as soon as realized with next tablet at the usual time OR Take two tablets daily for the next 2 days and resume regular schedule PLUS use a secondary form of contraception for the rest of the cycle.
Three tablets	Start a new package of tablets 7 days after the last tablet was taken. Use another form of contraception until tablets have been taken for 7 consecutive days.
Progestin-Only Products	
One or more tablets	Take tablet as soon as realized and follow with next tablet at regular time PLUS use back-up method of contraception for 48 h

h, Hour.

Box 55–1

Contraindications for Oral Contraceptives

Absolute Contraindications

Pregnancy (known or suspected)
Breastfeeding <6 weeks postpartum
Hypertension 160/100 or with vascular disease
Heavy smokers (>15 cig/day) over the age of 35 y
Migraine with aura
Diabetic nephropathy/retinopathy/neuropathy, or diabetes of >20 y duration
Vascular disease
Past or current history of deep venous thrombosis (DVT)/ pulmonary embolism (PE)
Past or current history of stroke
Major surgery with prolonged immobilization or any surgery on the legs
Current history of ischemic heart disease, valvular heart disease
Multiple risk factors for cardiovascular disease (e.g., older age, smoking, diabetes, hypertension)
Active viral hepatitis
Cirrhosis
Benign or malignant liver tumors
Breast cancer of <5 y duration
Known or suspected endometrial cancer

Cautious Use

Undiagnosed genital bleeding
Postpartum <21 d
Over the age of 35 and smokes <15 cig/d
Under the age of 35 and smokes >15 cig/d
Gallbladder disease
Past history of breast cancer >5 y ago
Use of drugs that affect liver enzymes (e.g., anticonvulsants, rifampin, griseofulvin)
Mild hypertension without other risk factors for cardiovascular disease
Hyperlipidemia
Non-insulin dependent diabetes
Known hyperlipidemias

cig, Cigarettes; *d,* day; *y,* year; > greater than; < less than.

Box 55–2

Drug Interactions with Oral Contraceptives

Enzyme-Inducing Drugs

(Use Higher Dose Pill or Alternative Form of Contraception)

rifampin
rifabutin
griseofulvin
dilantin
phenobarbital
topiramate
Tegretol

Non-Enzyme-Inducing Drugs

(Use Back-up Method for Duration of Treatment Plus 7 Days)

ampicillin
doxycycline
tetracycline

condoms unless they are confident that both partners are free of human immunodeficiency virus (HIV) and other sexually transmitted infections.

Adverse reactions of a more severe nature include increased risk of superficial and deep venous thrombosis, pulmonary embolism, cerebrovascular accident (thrombotic stroke), myocardial infarction, and acceleration of preexisting but undiagnosed breast tumors.

 Nursing Process

Oral Contraceptives

ASSESSMENT

■ Obtain a record of client's drug and herbal use.
■ Obtain baseline BP and weight. Report abnormal findings. Determine pregnancy status.
■ Assess for history of smoking, hypertension, and all contraindications listed in Box 55–1.
■ Recognize the need for periodic reassessment of baseline data and side effects. Most clients should be seen in 1 to 3 months after beginning regimen.

NURSING DIAGNOSES

■ Deficient knowledge related to fertility pattern
■ Deficient knowledge related to contraceptive method(s)
■ Noncompliance related to contraceptive method selected
■ Risk for impaired liver function related to contraceptive methods containing estrogen

Side effects primarily caused by an excess of progestin include increased appetite, weight gain, oily skin and scalp, acne, depression, vaginitis from yeast *(Candida),* excess hair growth, decreased breast size, and amenorrhea after cessation of use (1% to 2% of clients).

Side effects primarily caused by progestin deficiency include dysmenorrhea, bleeding late in the cycle (days 15 to 21), heavy menstrual flow with clots, or amenorrhea. There may also be changes in laboratory values, including thyroid and liver function, blood glucose, and triglycerides.

The combined oral contraceptive pill may increase the vascularity of the cervical epithelium, extend the area of cervical ectopy, and alter certain immune parameters. Advise pill users to use male or female latex or polyurethane

■ Nausea related to contraceptive methods containing estrogen

PLANNING

■ Client will choose a contraceptive method suitable for her lifestyle and risk factors.
■ Client will take oral contraceptives as prescribed and will report side effects that occur.

NURSING INTERVENTIONS

■ Separate personal views from those of client regarding contraception and use of specific products.
■ Recognize that many clients on oral contraceptives abandon the method within a year; therefore plan to provide client with alternatives.
■ Non-nursing mothers can begin combination oral contraceptives 3 to 4 weeks postpartum, regardless of whether menstruation has spontaneously occurred.

Client Teaching

General

• Remind client that these drugs should be used only under a health care provider's direction.
• Inform client that concurrent use of some drugs and herbal products decreases the effectiveness of oral contraceptives. Client should use a second form of contraception during these times (see Herbal Alert 55-1).
• Review with client the following aspects of oral contraceptives:

Advantages

• Easy to use and has low failure rate
• Minimal risks for women who do not smoke
• Contraception is not linked to the sexual act
• Decreased pregnancy fears may increase sexual responsiveness
• Suppressed pain at ovulation
• Decreased dysmenorrhea
• Regular, predictable menses
• Lighter, shorter menstrual flow
• Decreased iron-deficiency anemia resulting from decreased menstrual flow
• 80% to 90% reduced risk of functional ovarian cysts
• May provide protection against benign breast lesions and uterine and ovarian cancers
• Reduced risk of pelvic inflammatory disease
• Lower risk of ectopic pregnancy
• Decreased menstrual migraine-type headache
• No evidence that breast cancer is caused or increased by use of oral contraceptives
• Decreased chance of endometrial cancer (possibly because of progestin) in younger women not past menopause; protection may last up to 10 years after pills have been stopped if a client has used them long-term

• Thromboembolism risk does not appear related to duration of oral contraceptive use, but rather to the dose of estrogen (lower-dose products less risky).

Disadvantages

• If not monogamous, increased risk of acquiring sexually transmitted diseases (STDs), because no barrier is involved
• Bothersome side effects
• Requires medical follow-up after first 3 to 6 months, which may, in addition to cost of pills, be perceived as expensive in terms of time and money
• Requires daily administration
• Expense (generally $35 to $45/ month)
• Need for a prescription, which limits access
• Most prescription companies only allow one to three months to be dispensed at a time

Safety

• Counsel client not to smoke tobacco because of the increased cardiovascular risks.
• Advise client to use barrier method of contraception during the first month of oral contraceptive use and for 3 months after discontinuing use and before trying to conceive.
• Provide instructions about dealing with missed pills (see Table 55-2).
• Tell client to report any effects from the pill to a health professional so that the therapy can be adjusted to suit her own particular needs. Encourage her not to give up and discontinue use of the pills.
• Tell client to report breakthrough bleeding or spotting, because she may need a change in dose of oral contraceptive.
• Tell client to always report that she takes oral contraceptives when seeing a health care provider because of possible synergistic or antagonistic responses to other therapies.
• Nursing mothers should delay use of combined oral contraceptives until after breastfeeding is completed; another method should be selected.

Side Effects

• Acquaint client with the rare but possible side effects that are considered serious, including thrombophlebitis, pulmonary embolus, myocardial infarction, cerebral vascular accident, and retinal vein thrombosis.
• As an outcome of discussion about serious side effects, teach client the acronym ACHES for dangerous side effects that must be reported to a health care provider:
A = Abdominal pain (severe)
C = Chest pain or shortness of breath
H = Headaches that are severe; dizziness, weakness, numbness, speech difficulties
E = Eye disorders including blurring or loss of vision
S = Severe leg pain or swelling in the calf or thigh

More Common Side Effects
- Inform client that her menstrual flow may be less in amount and duration because of thinning of the endometrial lining.
- Determine whether client wears contact lenses and discuss how to handle dry eyes caused by decreased tearing and alterations in the shape of the cornea.
- Tell client who experiences post-pill amenorrhea that 95% of women have regular periods within 12 to 18 months. In addition, tell her that those who participate in endurance fitness activities may have increased post-pill amenorrhea.
- Inform client of a possible decrease in libido caused by alteration in vaginal secretions and decreased levels of testosterone.

Skill
- Teach client to do a monthly breast self-examination.

Diet
- Counsel client to moderate caffeine intake because elimination of caffeine may be decreased because of oral contraceptives.
- Tell client to take her pill with a snack at night or after meals to help eliminate nausea and also to take the pill at the same time each day.

Cultural Considerations ❖
- Be aware of different cultures' contraception practices.
- Consider the role of each partner in the specific culture regarding decision making about contraception method.

EVALUATION

- Evaluate client's compliance with the oral contraceptive regimen.

Other Methods of Contraception

Alternative methods of contraception are suited to clients who select not to take a pill on a daily basis or who are unable to comply with the daily dosing. If a woman is unable to take the pill because of contraindications, then *all* methods that contain estrogen, such as the patch and the ring, are contraindicated.

Implanon

The newest implant, Implanon, was FDA approved in July 2006. It is a single implant containing the progestin etonogestrel. It is effective for 3 years. Amenorrhea may occur in about 20% of clients. The single implant is easier and faster to insert and remove. Its advantages include decreased menstrual and ovulatory cramping or pain. Implanon has less bleeding than with Norplant. Organon, the manufacturer, has provided training for all providers who intend to insert or remove this device. This is intended to remove some of the problems that Norplant had with inadequate training of the providers, which made the device difficult to remove.

Depo-Provera

Long-acting injectable progestin, known as *medroxyprogesterone acetate (Depo-Provera)*, requires only one injection every 3 months. The injection acts by suppressing ovulation and changing the pH of the vaginal mucosa to an environment less hospitable to sperm. The injection (150 mg, best absorbed when it is administered Z-track in the ventrogluteal site) is relatively inexpensive. The site of the injection is documented, so that injection sites are rotated. The client is given a personalized calendar for subsequent doses. Like oral contraceptives, there is no protection against sexually transmitted diseases (STDs). The method is safe for postpartum clients to receive before discharge following delivery; clients may also breastfeed while using this contraceptive. The most common side effects reported include initially irregular menstruation and spotting (menstruation may cease in about 1 year). Women who smoke may complain of headaches (usually relieved by acetaminophen). In addition, other side effects include weight gain, bloating, decreased libido, hair loss, and depression. In rare instances, serious side effects may occur, including chest pain, hemoptysis, abdominal pain, shortness of breath, and numbness in the extremities. The drug is contraindicated in cases of undiagnosed vaginal bleeding or known or suspected pregnancy. When injections are discontinued, some clients may experience delayed resumption of fertility for a year or more.

Depo-subQ Provera 104 is now also available. The medroxyprogesterone acetate injectable suspension is now in a subQ form administered at 104 mg/0.65 ml to women every 3 months (12 to 14 weeks). Depo-subQ Provera 104 is indicated for the prevention of pregnancy in women of childbearing potential. Women who use either Depo-subQ Provera 104 or IM Depo-Provera long-term should be counseled about the loss of bone mineral density (BMD). The new black box warning further notes that bone loss is greater with increased duration of use, may not be completely reversible, and that Depo-Provera should be used as a long-term birth control method (e.g., longer than 2 years) only if other birth control methods are "inadequate." If abnormal bleeding associated with Depo-subQ Provera 104 is severe, appropriate investigation and treatment should be instituted.

The Patch

Ortho Evra is the first weekly form of birth control. The patch consists of a norelgestromin/ethinyl estradiol transdermal system. It is a thin plastic patch placed on the skin of the buttocks, stomach, upper outer arm, or upper torso once a week for 3 weeks in a row. A new patch is used each week for 3 weeks. The fourth week is patch-free to allow for menses. The patch releases combined estrogen and progesterone that protect against pregnancy for 1 month.

The patch prevents ovulation, thickens cervical mucus to prevent fertilization, and prevents a fertilized egg from implanting in the uterus. It is up to 99.7% effective, but it is not effective against STDs. Advantages include having no pill to take daily; the ability to become pregnant returns quickly when use is stopped; there is less menstrual flow and cramping, acne, iron deficiency anemia, excess body hair, premenstrual symptoms, and vaginal dryness; it reduces the risk of ovarian and endometrial cancers, pelvic inflammatory disease, breast cysts, ovarian cysts, and **osteoporosis** (loss of bone mass predisposing client to fractures); and there are fewer occurrences of ectopic pregnancy.

Disadvantages of the patch include skin reaction at the site of application, menstrual cramps, a change in vision or the inability to wear contact lenses, and it may not be as effective for women who weigh more than 198 pounds. Serious side effects are similar to the pill, including blood clots, heart attack, and stroke; women who are over 35 and smoke are at a greater risk. Other side effects include temporary irregular bleeding, weight gain or loss, breast tenderness, and nausea.

NuvaRing

NuvaRing is a 2-inch-diameter indwelling ring inserted into the vagina to release estrogen and progestin in quantities comparable to oral contraceptives. Effectiveness is reported at 98%, reflecting a rate similar to other leading contraceptives. The client inserts the ring during the first 5 days of the menstrual cycle. She then removes the ring after 3 weeks, remains "ring-free" for 1 week, and then inserts a new ring. Backup contraception is recommended during the first 7 days after the *first* ring is placed. During this time, the hormones reach an appropriate protective level. Then contraception is expected to be continuous, provided the ring is correctly inserted. If the ring slips out and remains out for more than 3 hours, additional contraception is required until the ring has been in place for 7 days. Possible side effects include vaginal discharge, irritation, or infection. There is some risk of blood clots or heart attack, which is increased in clients who smoke (similar to that associated with other hormonal contraceptives). NuvaRing does not protect against STDs or HIV infection. Its price is reported to be comparable with name-brand oral contraceptives.

Nonoxynol 9

Nonoxynol-9-based spermicide products are no longer advised for sexually-transmitted infection (STI) protection. The spermicide can cause vulvovaginal abrasions and altered vaginal flora, which could increase the susceptibility to HIV. Nonoxynol-9 products are available as vaginal foam, suppositories, film or sponges.

The Today Sponge is a polyurethane sponge impregnated with nonoxynol 9. This contraceptive product was discontinued in 1995 because of manufacturing problems, but is now again available over-the-counter in stores.

Other Barrier Methods

Both male and female condoms are available over the counter without a prescription. The female condom is a polyurethane (plastic) pouch with flexible rings at each end. It is inserted deep into the vagina like a diaphragm. The ring at the closed end holds the pouch in the vagina. The ring at the open end stays outside. Male condoms are available in latex, lambskin, and polyurethane. Latex condoms offer very good protection against HIV. Other barrier methods include the FemCap, cervical cap, and diaphragm, which require a medical visit for proper fitting.

Intrauterine Devices

Other alternatives to oral contraceptives are intrauterine devices (IUDs). The IUD is a safe method of contraception with a high client satisfaction rare and high efficacy. IUDs are safe for use in women who are at low risk for acquiring STDs. There are higher expulsion rates in nulliparous women. Currently there two IUDs are on the market.

The ParaGard T 380A releases copper, which interferes with sperm motility and fertilization as a result of inflammation of the endometrium. The ParaGard may increase the average monthly blood loss during menses by about 35%; NSAIDs may diminish this effect. It may also increase dysmenorrhea. ParaGard can remain in place for up to 10 years.

The Mirena levonorgestrel-releasing intrauterine system (LNG-IUS) causes cervical mucus to become thicker so sperm cannot enter the upper reproductive tract or reach the ovum. Changes in uterotubal fluid also impair sperm migration. Alteration of endometrium prevents implantation of the fertilized ovum. The Mirena has some anovulatory effect. Menorrhagia improves by 90%. There is an improvement in dysmenorrhea. There is a 20% chance of amenorrhea by 1 year and 60% by 5 years. The Mirena is as effective as female sterilization, it may decrease a woman's risk of pelvic inflammatory disease (PID) by 60%, and it has a decreased risk of ectopic pregnancy. The Mirena is effective for 5 years.

Medical Abortion

Medical abortion is a way to end a pregnancy that is less than 63 days from the first day of the last period (LMP). Methotrexate stops the pregnancy in the uterus. It may also be used to treat an *early* ectopic pregnancy. Mifepristone (RU486) blocks the hormone progesterone. Without progesterone, the lining of the uterus breaks down, ending the pregnancy. Misoprostol is then given to cause the uterus to contract and empty.

Emergency Contraception

Emergency contraception (EC) has been available for more than 25 years. Also called *postcoital contraception,* EC can prevent pregnancy after unprotected intercourse. It may be

Preventing MEDICATION ERRORS
Do not confuse...

- **Mifepristone** (RU486) with **Misoprostol** (Cytotec) or **Methotrexate**. Mifepristone is used for early pregnancy termination by blocking progesterone. Lack of progesterone causes the uterine lining to shed and ends the pregnancy. Misoprostol causes the uterus to contract and is used for early pregnancy termination or for cervical ripening at any gestational age. It can also be used to control postpartum hemorrhage. Methotrexate is a folate antagonist used to treat ectopic pregnancy.

Table 55–3

Emergency Contraception: The Yuzpe Regimen

Pill Brand	Manufacturer	Pills per Dose (Every 12 h for 2 Doses)
Alesse	Wyeth-Ayerst	5 pink pills
Aviane	Duramed	5 orange pills
Cryselle	Barr	4 white pills
Enpresse	Barr	4 orange pills
Lessina	Barr	5 pink pills
Levlen	Berlex	4 light orange pills
Levlite	Berlex	5 pink pills
Levora	Watson	4 white pills
Lo/Ovral	Wyeth-Ayerst	4 white pills
Low-Ogestrel	Watson	4 white pills
Nordette	Wyeth-Ayerst	4 light orange pills
Portia	Barr	4 pink pills
Seasonale	Barr	4 pink pills
Tri-Levlen	Berlex	4 yellow pills
Triphasil	Wyeth-Ayerst	4 yellow pills
Trivora	Watson	4 pink pills
Progestin-Only Pills		
Ovrette	Wyeth-Ayerst	20 yellow pills *or* 40 yellow pills in one dose
Plan B	Barr	1 white pill *or* 2 white pills in one dose

h, Hour.

prescribed in two ways: using hormonal contraceptive pills or inserting a copper-releasing IUD (ParaGard). The pills contain hormones that reduce the risk of pregnancy when started within 120 hours (5 days) of unprotected intercourse. This treatment is more effective the sooner it begins. The only documented contraindication to EC is an established pregnancy, because EC is ineffective in this case.

The Yuzpe regimen, named after Canadian professor Albert Yuzpe, consists of 0.1 mg dl-norgestrel (or its equivalent) followed by a second dose 12 hours later. The Yuzpe regimen prevents about 60% to 75% of expected pregnancies. About 50% of users experience nausea and 20% report vomiting, which can reduce client adherence.

The EC pills delay or prevent ovulation; interfere with tubal transport of the embryo, egg, or sperm; and change the hormones necessary for the preparation of the uterine lining. They decrease the risk of pregnancy by 75% for each act of unprotected sexual intercourse; birth control pills have a much higher rate of effectiveness—almost 100%. The major side effect is nausea; an over-the-counter (OTC) antinausea medicine (e.g., diphenhydramine 25 to 50 mg) may be helpful if taken 1 hour before the EC. Irregular menstrual bleeding is another side effect. If a woman does not begin menstruation within a few days of the expected time, she should take a pregnancy test. Clients who are unable to take estrogen should not take the usual EC pill dosage. See Table 55–3 for combined oral contraceptives used for EC.

If pregnancy is already established or if implantation occurred since the unprotected sexual intercourse, the pregnancy is not disrupted. EC pills do not result in an abortion, and there are no reports of harm to the fetus. EC can be used when needed. EC is not as effective as taking oral contraceptives or using condoms as directed (i.e., consistently and correctly).

Plan B

In 1999 the FDA approved the first progestin-only Emergency Contraceptive Pill available in the U.S., known as *Plan B*. In August 2006 the FDA approved Plan B without

a prescription for women age 18 or older, but a prescription is needed for women 17 and younger. Plan B should be taken within 3 days (72 hours) after unprotected sex, but may still be effective 120 hours (5 days) after intercourse. If taken within 24 hours of unprotected intercourse, it was found to reduce the risk of pregnancy by 95%. The two 0.75-mg doses of levonorgestrel may be combined into a single more-convenient 1.5-mg dose with no effect on efficacy or side effects. Plan B cause less nausea than estrogen-containing emergency contraceptive methods.

A copper IUD may be inserted within 5 days of unprotected intercourse and removed after the woman's next menstrual period, or it may remain in place as a method of birth control for up to 10 years.

The hotline for EC information is 1-888-NOT-2-LATE, and the website is: *http://ec.princeton.edu*.

The following contraceptives are no longer on the market in the United States.

Lunelle

Lunelle (a combination of medroxyprogesterone acetate and estradiol cypionate) was a contraceptive that inhibited secretion of gonadotropin, thereby preventing follicular maturation and ovulation. An IM injection of medroxyprogesterone acetate 25 mg and estradiol cypionate 5 mg per 0.5 ml suspension was administered every 28 to 30 days, not to exceed 33 days. Lunelle was taken off the market in 2001 because of manufacturing problems.

Norplant

Norplant (approved in December 1990), used low-dose levonorgestrel in six matchstick-shaped Silastic implants placed under the skin of the upper arm. Norplant was considered effective for 5 years. Norplant is no longer available because of manufacturing problems.

Preven

The Preven Emergency Contraceptive Kit contained the Yuzpe regimen of emergency contraceptive pills (two pills per dose, taken 12 hours apart), a pregnancy test, and instructions for use. It was approved by the FDA and was the first product specifically labeled and marketed for emergency contraception. It caused more nausea than Plan B, which is currently available. Preven has been taken off the market and is no longer available.

Drugs Used to Treat Hormone Dysfunction

Uterine dysfunction is common in premenstrual syndrome, endometriosis, and menopause. This section describes these entities and presents current pharmacologic approaches to management. The menstrual cycle is described in this unit's introduction.

Premenstrual Syndrome

Premenstrual syndrome (PMS), first formally described and named in 1931, comprises a collection of varied physical, emotional, and behavioral symptoms. Box 55–3 lists some commonly reported symptoms of PMS; more than 150 have been recorded in the literature.

Box 55–3

Symptoms of Premenstrual Syndrome

- Bloating in lower abdomen
- Weight gain
- Headache (migraine)
- Increased appetite
- Cravings for foods high in sugar or salt
- Breast soreness
- Fatigue
- Sleep disorders
- Backaches
- Acne flare-ups
- Joint pain
- Constipation
- Feelings of being out of control
- Emotional lability
- Tension
- Anxiety
- Difficulty with concentration
- Irritability
- Agitation
- Depression
- Suicidal thoughts
- Rage

PMS can result in decreased work effectiveness and impaired interpersonal relationships. PMS affects 40% of all adult women (four to five million in the United States) to some degree, with about 5% exhibiting debilitating symptoms. There is a family history associated with the syndrome, but it is not hereditary. The syndrome is seen most commonly in women in their thirties and early forties, but it also affects adolescents. PMS occurs in a repetitive regular pattern during the **luteal phase** (days 15 to 28) of the menstrual cycle; it decreases during the **follicular phase** (days 1 to 14).

Nursing Process

Premenstrual Syndrome

ASSESSMENT

- Obtain history of premenstrual syndrome (PMS) symptoms, such as bloating, weight gain, headache, and increased appetite (see Box 55–3).

NURSING DIAGNOSES

- Deficient knowledge related to the menstrual cycle and etiology of related alterations in mood and comfort
- Ineffective coping related to signs and symptoms
- Interrupted family processes related to diagnosis

PLANNING

- Client will verbalize relief from PMS from nonpharmacologic and pharmacologic measures.

NURSING INTERVENTIONS

- Provide quality client and family education in a supportive manner that encourages family communication.

Client Teaching

General

- Express that symptoms are real and that "crazy feelings" do not mean client is crazy.
- Explain menstrual cycle and current knowledge about PMS verbally, in writing, and graphically.
- Share current research findings regarding PMS and known treatment modalities with client, her family, and community groups.
- Encourage client to include aerobic exercise in her regular activity pattern three to five times each week.
- Describe and discuss stress-reduction activities.
- Encourage family communication regarding PMS symptoms experienced by client so that the family understands client's behavior.

- Suggest sources for, and potential value of, support groups.

Self-Administration
- Have client keep a log of symptoms experienced during her menstrual cycle to better link events with symptoms.
- If alprazolam (Xanax) is ordered, discuss issues of dependency and withdrawal.
- If danazol is ordered, refer to the guidelines for use of this drug in the Nursing Process box on endometriosis and Table 55–4.

Diet
- Encourage client to take therapeutic doses of vitamin and mineral supplements with meals.
- Encourage a low-fat, low-salt, high-carbohydrate diet. Suggest four to six small meals and portable snacks (bagels, rice cakes).
- Decrease caffeine intake and increase water consumption.
- Limit alcoholic beverages; these may precipitate headaches.

EVALUATION

■ Evaluate the effectiveness of the nonpharmacologic and pharmacologic measures for relief of PMS.

There is no universal agreement about the definition, etiology, symptoms, or treatment of PMS. The most widely held theory is that PMS is linked to estrogen and progesterone levels and the relationship of these hormones to other brain chemicals. The symptoms are observed during the luteal phase when levels are high and decrease when drugs that inhibit gonadotropin-releasing hormone (Gn-RH) and ovulation are used. Other hypotheses center on the release of endogenous opiates (beta-endorphins), disruptions in central nervous system neurotransmitters (resulting in mood swings), and the role of prolactin secretion.

Diagnosis of PMS is made when the client's symptoms are documented as consistently occurring at about the same time and in the same way during a defined number of menstrual periods. Other endocrine abnormalities need to be ruled out. One difficulty with diagnosis is that PMS is not consistent, because every cycle is not the same; therefore measurement is problematic, particularly because every symptom that occurs associated with a menstrual cycle is not PMS.

Treatment of PMS includes nonpharmacologic and pharmacologic measures. There is not one curative therapy or a way to know what therapy may be best for a particular client other than trial and error.

Nonpharmacologic treatment includes expression of empathy, support from family and others, correction of knowledge deficits about PMS and the menstrual cycle, exercise, and dietary changes (e.g., limiting salty foods, alcohol, caffeine, chocolate, concentrated sweets; eating four

to six small high-carbohydrate, low-fat meals, which help stabilize blood sugar levels and enhance mood). Stress reduction is helpful, as is aerobic exercise, which is believed to have a regulatory effect on estrogen and progesterone secondary to hypothalamic stimulation. These measures may help the client feel proactive regarding her situation, give her a sense of overall well being, and improve her general health. In addition, endorphin levels are heightened, which is found to be helpful.

Pharmacologic treatment remains largely empirical, because research has not consistently been done under double-blind, placebo-controlled conditions. Some clients experience improvement with selected symptoms through use of vitamin B_6 (popular with self-help groups but not found superior to placebo) or vaginal or rectal progesterone suppositories (200 to 400 mg twice daily), which are commonly used but not documented as effective and have some long-term effects. In addition, individuals who exhibit depressive symptoms tend to get worse with progesterone use because of its depressant effects. Other pharmacologic trials include diuretics (not recommended) and prostaglandin inhibitors; bromocriptine (Parlodel) (2.5 mg twice daily started on day 10 of cycle and taken until menstruation begins) for breast soreness; and alprazolam (Xanax) (0.25 mg three times daily from day 20 of cycle to day 2 of menses, followed by one tablet per day) for treatment of anxiety, irritability, and depression. Reducing dietary caffeine decreases breast tenderness more than by pharmacologic intervention. One theory under study is that stronger antiprostaglandins (e.g., NSAIDs) will prove useful when taken in conjunction with vitamin therapy that contains magnesium, calcium, pyridoxine, vitamin E, and zinc. This drug regimen should begin when PMS symptoms start and continue through the beginning of the menstrual period. Oral contraceptives, such as Yaz and Lybrel, have recently been approved by the FDA for treatment of PMDD.

Sarafem (fluoxetine hydrochloride) is an FDA-approved prescription treatment that relieves the mood and physical symptoms of premenstrual dysphoric disorder (PMDD), a severe form of PMS. It is a selective serotonin reuptake inhibitor (SSRI). Symptom relief includes a decrease in irritability, mood swings, fatigue, tension, and breast tenderness. SSRIs block the uptake of serotonin into human platelets and regulate serotonin use by the brain.

Two other forms of experimental (not approved by the FDA) hormonal anovulatory treatment are danazol and Gn-RH agonists. These formulations, which are also approved for treatment of endometriosis, are presented in Table 55–4.

Endometriosis

Endometriosis is the abnormal location of endometrial tissue outside the uterus in the pelvic cavity; it has no single, clearly identifiable cause. Possible etiologies are retrograde menstruation (backward movement of endometrial cells through the fallopian tubes out into the abdomen) or

Table 55–4

Drug Therapy for Endometriosis

Generic (Brand)	Route and Dosage	Uses and Considerations
danazol	PO: 400 mg b.i.d. for 4-6 mo; can extend to 9 mo; can restart if symptoms return	Pituitary gonadotropin inhibitory agent. No estrogenic or progestational action. Suppresses and atrophies intra- and extrauterine tissue. Menses cease during therapy, and no ovulation occurs; pain is relieved. Ovulation/menses usually recur within 90 d after treatment Therapy started during menstruation or after pregnancy. If therapy is for fibrocystic breast disease, breast carcinoma must be ruled out before treatment. Commonly used for women with infertility associated with endometriosis. Used for PMS on investigational basis *Contraindications:* pregnancy; breastfeeding; abnormal genital bleeding; impaired heart, liver, or kidney function; severe hypertension Can alter some laboratory values (e.g., decreased HDL, increased LDL). Can increase insulin requirements and, if given with warfarin, cause a prolonged PT. *Adverse effects:* depression, headache, hot flashes, weight gain, androgenic effects, hemorrhagic cystitis, hematuria, hepatotoxicity, cholestatic hepatitis, acne, rashes, oily skin, hirsutism, bloating, muscle cramps, voice deepening (irreversible), hearing loss, mood swings, anxiety, fatigue, nausea, vomiting, diarrhea, constipation. Also produces atherogenic lipid profile. Many clients cannot tolerate side effects and discontinue drug Alternate doses may be used for clients with hereditary angioedema and fibrocystic breast disease. *Pharmacokinetics:* Therapeutic effects occur within 3 wk of daily therapy. Absorbed well orally; peak action: 2-4 h. Biotransformed by the liver; excreted in the urine. *Pregnancy category:* X; t½: 4.5 h
Gonadotropin-Releasing Hormone (Gn-RH) Agonists		
leuprolide acetate for depot suspension (Lupron Depot 3.75)	IM: 3.75 mg q mo for up to 6 mo	As an agonist, initially stimulates FSH and LH, but over time creates prolonged suppression, which causes decreased ovarian secretion of estrogen/progesterone, resulting in a hypoestrogenic state. Lack of hormonal stimulation causes regression of displaced endometrial tissue. Contains no androgen. Found as effective as danazol in reducing extent of endometriosis Initial dose best given during day 1-3 of menstrual cycle to avoid affecting a pregnancy. Barrier contraceptives should be used during treatment, because pregnancy is possible Minimal changes produced in lipid profile. Normal function returns in 4 to 12 wk after treatment discontinued Retreatment not recommended, because safety data beyond 6 mo are not available. *Contraindications:* actual or potential pregnancy, undiagnosed vaginal bleeding, breastfeeding (because it is unknown if drug is excreted in breast milk). *Side effects:* hot flashes, headaches, decreased libido, vaginal dryness, night sweats, mood changes, mild bone loss (usually regained within 6 mo of finishing treatment) FDA classification 3B* *Pharmacokinetics:* Therapeutic levels detected for at least 4 wk after injection; 85%-100% released within 4 wk with no accumulation. *Pregnancy category:* X; PB: 46%; t½: 3-4.2 h
nafarelin acetate (Synarel Nasal Solution)	400 mcg daily, administered as one spray (200 mcg) into one nostril in morning and one spray (200 mcg) into other nostril in evening for up to 6 mo	Contains no androgen. Controlled studies comparing nafarelin (400 mg) and danazol (600 or 800 mcg/d) found higher hypoestrogenic (therapeutic state), but less androgenic side effects. Found comparable in reducing extent of endometriosis and in effect on associated client symptoms. Maintains LDL/HDL ratio. Return of normal function in 4-12 wk after treatment discontinued *Contraindications:* clients sensitive to Gn-RH, Gn-RH analogs, or inert substances included in product; actual or potential pregnancy; undiagnosed vaginal bleeding; breastfeeding. Clients with rhinitis should have a topical decongestant prescribed by health care provider and use at least 30 min after nafarelin *Side effects:* effects seen in a natural menopause caused by a hypoestrogenic state, notably hot flashes, vaginal dryness, decreased libido, headaches, and emotional lability. FDA classification 1B† *Pharmacokinetics:* peak action: 10-40 min. Drug elimination after intranasal administration has not been studied. PB: 80%; t½: approximately 30 h (range 0.8-10 h)

*A new formulation of a compound already on the market that offers a modest therapeutic gain over currently available agents.
†A new chemical entity that offers a modest therapeutic gain over currently available agents.
b.i.d., Twice a day; *d,* day; *FDA,* Food and Drug Administration; *FSH,* follicle-stimulating hormone; *Gn-RH,* gonadotropin-releasing hormone; *h,* hour; *HDL,* high-density lipoproteins; *IM,* intramuscular; *LDL,* low-density lipoproteins; *LH,* luteinizing hormone; *min,* minute; *mo,* month; *PB,* protein-binding; *PMS,* premenstrual syndrome; *PO,* by mouth; *PT,* prothrombin time; *t½,* half-life; *wk,* week.

spread through the lymphatic or vascular systems. Regardless of cause, the displaced endometrial tissue is found affixed to the ovaries, the posterior surface of the uterus, the uterosacral ligaments, the broad ligaments, or the bowel. The displaced tissue responds to hormonal control, particularly estrogen from the ovaries, in the same way as the tissue inside the uterus. Thus, when menstruation occurs, this extrauterine tissue also bleeds. As the number of menstrual cycles increases, inflammation, scar tissue formation, and adhesions result.

Clients with endometriosis may be symptomatic (about 75%) or asymptomatic (those diagnosed during infertility work-ups). The diagnosis is based on symptoms and laparoscopic evidence of endometrial tissue. Symptoms include severe low-back and pelvic pain that increases with menstruation. Painful, sometimes bloody, bowel movements during menstruation have been reported, as has painful sexual intercourse (dyspareunia). Irregular bleeding (spotting) before and after menses is common. Long term, there is an association with primary or secondary infertility; about 25% to 40% of infertile women exhibit the condition. Endometriosis may obstruct or affect the motility of the fallopian tubes. There is also a risk that nearby organs (e.g., urinary and gastrointestinal tracts) may become obstructed by invasion of endometrial tissue.

Endometriosis is found most often in women who have delayed childbearing until their thirties, although it may occur during adolescence. There is an increased prevalence rate of 7% for siblings and daughters of affected women. Approximately five million women in the United States have endometriosis. Affected women may exhibit increased ectopic pregnancy rates and difficult pregnancies and labors.

Some success for the treatment of endometriosis has been seen with the use of a laser during laparoscopy to remove or destroy endometrial growths.

Three drugs are approved for use in endometriosis: danazol and two Gn-RH agonists, leuprolide acetate (Lupron Depot) and nafarelin acetate (Synarel). Danazol has been the drug of choice, but use of the Gn-RH agonists is increasing. Danazol suppresses the release of FSH and LH. These drugs are presented in Table 55–4.

In long-term and highly painful endometriosis that has not been controlled with drug therapy or laparoscopy, hysterectomy (including ovary removal) may be elected.

Endometriosis

ASSESSMENT

■ Obtain a complete client history, including menstrual history.

■ Identify client's fertility plans.
■ Review chart for baseline liver function studies and pregnancy test.

Leuprolide Acetate
• Review client's history for risk factors associated with major bone loss; the drug may pose an additional risk.

NURSING DIAGNOSES

■ Pain (acute and chronic) related to hormonally controlled displaced endometrial tissue
■ Activity intolerance related to painful menstrual cycles
■ Deficient knowledge related to menstrual cycle, displaced endometrial tissue, etiology of pain, and treatment options

PLANNING

■ Client will be free of pain/discomfort resulting from endometriosis with the use of danazol, leuprolide acetate, or nafarelin acetate.

NURSING INTERVENTIONS

Danazol
■ Assess client for signs of anxiety about delaying fertility and the time involved in treatment.
■ Recall that the drug must be started during client's menstrual period.

Leuprolide Acetate
■ Store product and diluent at room temperature.
■ Must be reconstituted and used immediately (no preservatives). Reconstituted product must be shaken to create a milky suspension.

Client Teaching: Danazol
General
• Discuss the purpose, action, and side effects of the drug with client. Explain that this medication suppresses FSH and LH. Explain that the medication is expensive. Explain length of treatment.
• Plan with client for the use of a back-up nonhormonal form of birth control.
• Tell client that menses will usually return in 2 to 3 months after treatment.
• Tell client to have one menstrual cycle after treatment is completed before trying to conceive.

Side Effects
• Suggest that client wear minipads for spotting during the first month of therapy and to report any bleeding to her health care provider.
• Discuss removal of unwanted hair and skin care for acne prevention. If acne occurs, consult a dermatologist.

- Suggest that client wash her face and hair more often because of oily scalp and skin and to use oil-free makeup and shampoo.
- If muscle cramps occur, advise client to do warm-up exercises before active workout and to gradually increase exertion.

Diet
- Ask client to keep a food history. Suggest increased exercise to help offset weight gain that is experienced by 75% (average 4 kg); suggest caloric control plan based on history.
- Increase water consumption.
- Consider use of calcium supplements

Skill
- Review breast self-examination with client.

Client Teaching: Leuprolide Acetate

General
- Explain to client that the drug causes a temporary state of menopause.
- Explain that the treatment process requires one injection each month.
- Explain that the drug is palliative and temporarily effective in reducing symptoms. It does not create a change in basic physiology, metabolism, or hormone production. When treatment is complete, whatever is normal for client will return over time.
- Advise client that initially there may be an increase in clinical signs and symptoms of endometriosis, but these will disappear.
- Explain that 6 months is the accepted duration of therapy for gonadotropin-releasing hormone (GnRH) agonists. Safety data are available only for 6-month use. Retreatment is not recommended.

Self-Administration
- Remind client that she must use a nonhormonal contraceptive method during treatment.

Side Effects
- If client is concerned about potential bone loss, state that one 6-month course of treatment has been found to cause only a small loss. However, clients who are at higher risk for bone loss caused by chronic alcoholism, tobacco use, strong family history of osteoporosis, or chronic use of anticonvulsants or corticosteroids should carefully discuss the decision for or against therapy with this drug. Suggest client add weight-bearing exercise and walking or low-impact aerobics to offset bone loss.
- Stress that client must be consistent in receiving her doses of the drug; otherwise breakthrough bleeding or ovulation can occur.
- Tell client to inform the health care provider if menstruation persists while being treated.

- Discuss mood changes secondary to hormonal changes with drug and possible emotional lability; suggest support network and resource groups.
- If vaginal dryness occurs, suggest client use water-based lubricants and try alternate sexual positions for intercourse.
- If night sweats occur, suggest cotton bedclothes and change of clothes; resist chills by gradually exposing body from under bed covers to room air. Contact health care provider if sleep disturbances persist.

Diet
- Suggest increased calcium-based food products.

Client Teaching: Nafarelin Acetate

General
- Explain that precise guidelines must be followed by client if the treatment is to be effective.
- Ask client if she is allergic to any component of the drug, including nafarelin base, benzalkonium chloride, acetic acid, sodium hydroxide, hydrochloride, or sorbitol.
- Tell client that the action of the drug, guidelines for birth control use, hypoestrogenic effects, and return of normal function are the same as for leuprolide acetate.
- Advise client that the medication is expensive, is provided as a 30-day supply, and needs to be continued for 6 months of therapy without interruption.

Self-Administration
- Stress that client must use the drug twice a day (every 12 hours) for the full duration of treatment.
- Tell client to start the drug between days 2 and 4 of the menstrual period.
- Client must be told of the need to prime the spray pump only before the first use. The sprayer is designed to deliver the exact dose each time. A fine spray will occur after 7 to 10 pushes on the pump. If a thin stream occurs, she should call her pharmacist immediately.
- Tell client to store the bottle upright, below 86° F (30° C), and out of light. Because she must use it every 12 hours, it is suggested she put it near her toothbrush or other regularly used product (morning and night).
- Tell client to record each dose on the supplied chart and to refill prescription so as not to miss any doses.
- Tell client it is permissible to use a nasal decongestant spray (with health care provider's knowledge) while on nafarelin. Use the nafarelin spray first and allow 30 minutes to elapse before using the decongestant spray.
- Instruct client to blow her nose to clear both nostrils before using the drug. She should bend forward and place the spray tip in one nostril aimed at the back and outer side of her nose. She should close the other

nostril with her finger and then spray one time while sniffing gently, then tilt her head back to spread the drug over the back of the nose. She must be told *not* to spray in the second nostril unless told to do so by her doctor. Alternate nostrils are used for each dose.

Side Effects
- Advise client that she may note irregular vaginal spotting or bleeding, which should decrease and stop unless doses are missed.
- Similar to leuprolide.

Diet
- Suggest increased calcium-based food products.

EVALUATION

- Evaluate the effectiveness of the drug regimen. If pain or discomfort persists, notify the health care provider. Drug dose adjustment may be necessary.

Menopause

The transitional process experienced by women as they move from the reproductive into the nonreproductive stage of life is called the *female climacteric*, a natural event. Women perceive the "change of life" experience in an individualized way on a continuum from no difficulty to severe difficulty. This phase of life occurs for most women somewhere between their late thirties to late fifties. The climacteric has three stages—premenopause, menopause, and postmenopause—during which certain physiologic events occur.

The premenopausal period may last for more than 5 years before true menopause occurs. During this period, menstrual variations become evident. For example, menstrual periods may occur as usual, be lighter in flow, or last a shorter time. They may begin, stop, and then start again or be of longer duration with a heavier flow that may contain blood clots. Sudden episodes of vasodilation (hot flashes) also begin to occur in some women. Others experience vaginal dryness. These unpredictable changes may last for several years and are probably caused by alterations in the hypothalamic-pituitary-ovarian feedback system.

Menopause is defined as the permanent end of menstruation caused by decreased ovarian function. This natural event is documented as having occurred once a woman has had no menstrual periods for 1 year. The triggering event for the onset of natural menopause is not known. The average age at menopause is about 50 years (range 45 to 55 years). Women who experience menopause before age 40 are said to have had *premature menopause*. Menopause can also occur abruptly as a secondary effect of surgical removal of the ovaries (oophorectomy), radiologic procedures in which ovarian function is destroyed, severe infection, ovarian tumors, or as a temporarily induced state for treatment of conditions such as endometriosis.

Postmenopause is the stage when the body adapts to a new hormonal environment. Although the production of estrogen and progesterone from the ovaries decreases during the late premenopausal and early postmenopausal periods, the ovary is able to secrete androgens (testosterone) in varying amounts as a result of the influence of increased LH levels. During postmenopause, androstenedione (the main androgen secreted by the ovaries and adrenal cortex, which is present in reduced amounts postmenopause) is converted into estrone, a naturally occurring estrogen formed in extraglandular tissue of the brain, liver, kidney, and adipose tissue. This represents the main source of available estrogen once the ovaries lose the ability to produce estradiol. Table 55–5 presents common physical effects associated with the climacteric.

Hormone and Estrogen Replacement Therapy

Hormone replacement therapy (HRT) is the most prevalent treatment for the relief of vasomotor symptoms and vaginal dryness. Oral estrogen, most commonly in the form of conjugated estrogens, is taken by the client together with the synthetic hormone progestin in one of several treatment regimens. The progestin is added to minimize the risk of endometrial hyperplasia and endometrial cancer from the use of estrogen alone. The progestin, however, has potential negative effects, including potential PMS-type symptoms, breast pathology, and alterations in lipid metabolism. Thus progestin partially blunts the beneficial effects of estrogen. The client has much to consider when deciding on a course of action.

The Women's Health Initiative (WHI) was a randomized, controlled, primary prevention trial that recruited 16,608 women between 1993 and 1998. The WHI focused on risk-and-benefit strategies that could reduce the incidence of heart disease, breast and colorectal cancer, and fractures in postmenopausal women. Results of the first arm of the WHI were released in May 2002. The results concluded that HRT should *not* be prescribed for long-term prevention of chronic diseases. HRT is associated with increased risk of breast cancer, thromboembolism, coronary heart disease, and stroke. HRT should *only* be used for the treatment of menopausal symptoms, at the lowest dose possible, for the shortest duration possible, usually less than 5 years.

Hormone therapy is no longer recommended *solely* for the purpose of preventing osteoporosis, although the study demonstrated a reduction in hip and vertebral fractures by one third using HRT. Other medications can help prevent osteoporosis and fractures, and these agents appear to carry lower risks for conditions such as breast cancer or heart disease. Other drug therapies include bisphosphonates, which can reduce the breakdown of bone. Another class of drug, selective estrogen receptor modulators, or SERMs, are a new class of synthetic estrogens that act like estrogens in certain parts of the body (such as the

Table 55-5

Common Physical Effects Associated with the Female Climacteric

Hypoestrogenic State	Effects
Irregular menstruation	Variable frequency, duration, flow
Vasodilation	Hot flashes with transient sensations of intense heat in upper chest, neck, and head; visible flushing; sweating; chills; tachycardia; sleep disruption
Vaginal alterations	Dryness; decreased lubrication during sexual stimulation; thinning. Decreased acidity and increased irritation response to stressors such as intercourse can cause increased vaginitis (itching, burning, discharge). Increased incidence of prolapse/cystocele
Decreased bone mass (osteoporosis)	Backache, reduced height, and sudden fracture, particularly in thin, fair, small-boned women and those with a family history, no pregnancies, sedentary lifestyle, inadequate diet, smoking, alcohol use, or use of drugs that increase calcium loss (anticonvulsants, corticosteroids). Most rapid decrease in mass (particularly in hips, spine, and torso) occurs in first 3-5 y postmenopause and slows after age 65 years
Additional Effects Caused by Menopause Combined with Natural Aging	
Urethral disorders	Loss of urethral tone, painful urination, frequency, and stress incontinence
Decreased breast size	
Decreased skin elasticity	Facial, neck, and hand wrinkling; variations in quantity and distribution of body hair
Lower HDL levels	Increased risk (3×) for cardiovascular disease as LDL levels increase
Abdominal fat development	Greater degree of central android abdominal fat accumulates because of altered peripheral resistance to insulin and increase in type II diabetes as aging progresses (lower incidence in estrogen users)
Hyperinsulinemia	Signs and symptoms of low blood sugar
Short-term memory loss	

HDL, High-density lipoproteins; *LDL,* low-density lipoproteins; *y,* year.

bones) while leaving other parts unaffected. Evista is an example of a SERM used to treat osteoporosis.

For all women, lifestyle recommendations for healthy bones include a diet high in calcium (postmenopausal women should be taking 1200 to 1500 mg of calcium per day), a multivitamin containing vitamin D, and regular weight-bearing exercise such as walking.

In the United States the typical approach to HRT is to take oral estrogen in the lowest dose to control symptoms for days 1 to 25 of the month, with the addition of progesterone (Provera) 10 mg from days 16 to 25 or estrogen and progesterone to be taken together every day without any days off.

Currently there is no absolutely correct HRT management regimen. Health care providers may prescribe either cyclic or continuous estrogen with progestin or a combined continuous approach. Other regimens are also used.

Dosage forms for the various types of HRT include oral, transdermal, vaginal cream or suppositories, injections, pellets, or vaginal rings. The natural or biologic estrogens are composed of estrones (including conjugated equine estrogens, esterified estrogens, and piperazine estrone sulfate) and estradiols (including micronized estradiol and estradiol valerate or 17 β-estradiol). These are preferred for use in postmenopausal clients rather than the synthetic estrogens (ethinyl estradiol, mestranol) used for oral contraception. Synthetic estrogens are believed to be more taxing to the renal and hepatic systems than are biologic estrogens. Conjugated estrogens, mixtures of natural estrogens isolated from the urine of pregnant mares, are the most commonly used preparations for **estrogen replace-**

ment therapy (ERT) (hormones for treating symptoms of menopause and decreasing the risks of cardiovascular disease and osteoporosis in postmenopausal women). Premarin, the most frequently used conjugated estrogen product, is presented in Prototype Drug Chart 55-1.

The newest form of hormone therapy (HT) is Angeliq (0.5 mg drospirenone and 1 mg estradiol). It is the only HT with the unique progestin drospirenone (found in Yasmin and Yaz) and carries the same precautions as those drugs.

Dosage Forms

The oral route is most commonly used; it is well tolerated by most clients and relatively easy to use, but it does require daily dosing. Some clients experience gastrointestinal (GI) upsets, particularly nausea and vomiting. A client with GI disorders such as colitis, irritable bowel syndrome, peptic ulcer, or malabsorption may receive inconsistent doses with oral administration, necessitating the use of another dosage form. Oral estrogens have a particularly

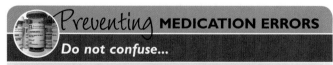

Preventing MEDICATION ERRORS

Do not confuse...

• **Premarin** with **Prempro** or **Premphase.** Premarin is estrogen *only* for hormone replacement therapy. Both Prempro and Premphase have combined estrogen and progesterone for use by women with an intact uterus to prevent uterine hyperplasia when estrogen is used.

Prototype **DRUG CHART 55–1**

CONJUGATED ESTROGENS

Drug Class

Estrogen replacement
Trade names: Premarin, Premphase, Prempro
Pregnancy Category: X

Contraindications

Breast or reproductive cancer, undiagnosed genital
  bleeding, pregnancy, lactation, thromboembolitic
  disorders, smoking
Caution: Cardiovascular disease, severe renal or
  hepatic disease, smoking, diabetes mellitus

Dosage

A: PO: 0.3-1.25 mg/d cyclically (with or without
  progestins); most often 0.625 mg/d

Drug-Lab-Food Interactions

Drug: Increase effects with corticosteroids; *decrease*
  effects of anticoagulants, oral hypoglycemics;
  decrease effects with rifampin, anticonvulsants,
  barbiturates; *toxicity* with tricyclic antidepressants

Pharmacokinetics

Absorption: PO: Well absorbed
Distribution: PB: Widely distributed; crosses placenta
  and enters breast milk
Metabolism: t½: UK
Excretion: In urine and bile

Pharmacodynamics

PO/IV: Onset: Rapid
  Peak: UK
  Duration: UK
IM: Onset: Delayed

Therapeutic Effects/Uses

To relieve vasodilation, hot flashes, and vaginal dryness
Mode of Action: Development and maintenance of female genital system, breast, and secondary sex characteristics;
  increased synthesis of protein

Side Effects

Nausea, vomiting, fluid retention, breast tenderness,
  leg cramps, breakthrough bleeding, chloasma

Adverse Reactions

Jaundice, thromboembolic disorders, depression,
  hypercalcemia, gallbladder disease
Life-threatening: Thromboembolism, cerebrovascular
  accident, pulmonary embolism, myocardial infarction,
  endometrial cancer

A, Adult; *d*, day; *IM*, intramuscular; *IV*, intravenous; *PB*, protein-binding; *PO*, by mouth; *t½*, half-life; *UK*, unknown.

---

beneficial effect on lipids by increasing high-density lipo-proteins. Although the oral route does result in complete absorption from the GI tract, there is greater impact upon liver proteins.

Medroxyprogesterone acetate (Provera), the progestin most often administered in combination with the estrogen, is taken orally. Examples of progestin products are given in Table 55–6.

The transdermal skin patch (the Estraderm Transdermal System) is a convenient method, because it does not require daily dosing. The patch is applied to intact skin in the prescribed dosage. Generally the lower abdomen is used, but other sites (except for the breasts) may be used. The patch is applied twice a week for 3 weeks, rotating sites, followed by 1 week without use of the patch to allow for normal withdrawal bleeding. The transdermal patch allows for absorption of the estrogen (17 β-estradiol) directly into the bloodstream through a membrane that limits the absorption rate. The advantage is that the GI tract and liver are bypassed initially, which results in less nausea and vomiting and less impact on liver proteins.

ClimaraPro is a thin translucent patch containing 0.015 mg/day of levonorgestrel and 0.045 mg/day of estradiol. It is the first once-a-week combined hormone therapy approved to treat menopausal symptoms such as hot flashes. The transdermal patch allows for continuous delivery of hormones at much lower doses than in oral HRT.

Vaginal cream preparations are used in the treatment of vaginal atrophy, which causes painful intercourse and urinary difficulties. These preparations contain conjugated estrogens and are rapidly absorbed into the bloodstream via the mucous membranes that lines the vagina. Vaginal creams may be used in conjunction with another method, such as tablets or the transdermal patch.

Estring is an elastomer ring containing 2 mg of 17 beta-estradiol, the major naturally occurring estrogen produced in the ovaries of fertile women. The Estring ring is inserted into the upper portion of the vagina, where it releases 50% to 60% of the estradiol, providing a consistent low dose of estrogen for 3 months. Estring is used to treat local symptoms of urogenital atrophy, which affects 20% to 40% of postmenopausal women.

Table 55–6

Estrogens and Progestins

Generic (Brand)	Route and Dosage	Pregnancy Category
Conjugated Estrogens		
Premarin	(Prototype Drug Chart 55–1)	X
Steroidal Estrogens		
estradiol (Estrace, Estraderm)	*Menopausal/hypogonadism:* PO: 1-2 mg/d for 21 d, then 7-10 d off cycle; may repeat cycle. *Patch:* 10-20 cm² system 2×/wk, in above cycle. *Breast cancer:* 10 mg t.i.d. *Prostate cancer:* 1-2 mg t.i.d. *Atrophic vaginitis:* Cream: 2-4 g/d for 1-2 wk; maint: 1 g 2×/wk	X
estradiol cypionate (Depo-Estradiol Cypionate)	*Menopausal symptoms:* IM: 1-4 mg q3-4wk. *Hypogonadism:* IM: 1.5-2 mg q mo	X
esterified estrogens (Menest)	*Menopausal symptoms:* PO: 0.3-1.25 mg/d for 3 wk, then 7-10 d off cycle. *Breast cancer:* PO: 10 mg t.i.d. *Prostate cancer:* 1.25-2.5 mg t.i.d.	X
estrone (Theelin)	*Hypogonadism:* 0.1-2 mg/wk. *Prostate cancer:* 2-4 mg 3×/wk	X
estropipate (Ogen)	*Hypogonadism:* 1.25-7.5 mg/d for 3 wk, then 7-10 d off cycle	X
Progesterone	*Menopausal/hypogonadism:* 100 mcg daily for 7 d, then 7 d off cycle; *maint:* q wk *DUB:* IM: 5-10 mg/d for 7 d. *Amenorrhea:* IM: 5-10 mg/d for 6-8 d	X
Medroxyprogesterone acetate (Provera, Depo-Provera)	*DUB/amenorrhea:* 5-10 mg/d for 5-10 d. *Endometriosis:* IM: 150 mg q3mo	X
megestrol acetate (Megace)	*Breast cancer:* PO: 40 mg q.i.d. *Endometrial cancer:* 40-320 mg/d in divided doses	X
Norethindrone	*DUB/amenorrhea:* 5-20 mg/d on days 5-25 of menstrual cycle	X

Consult a health care provider on the latest research.
b.i.d., Twice a day; *d,* day; *DUB,* **dysfunctional uterine bleeding** (excessive menstrual flow or too frequent menstruation); *IM,* intramuscular; *maint,* maintenance; *mo,* month; *PO,* by mouth; *q.i.d.,* four times a day; *t.i.d.,* three times a day; *wk,* week.

Femring is the first and only vaginal ERT to treat moderate to severe hot flashes, night sweats, and vaginal dryness in menopause. Femring contains estradiol acetate, an estrogen, contained in a soft, flexible silicone ring. It is inserted into the upper vagina for 3 months. It may be left in place during intercourse and treatment for vaginal infections.

Estrogel 0.06% is a synthetic plant-based transdermal estradiol gel applied once daily for the treatment of moderate to severe vasomotor symptoms. A thin film is applied to one arm from the shoulder to wrist. The gel dries in 2 to 5 minutes. Estrogel is packaged in a non-aerosol, metered dose pump that is designed to deliver 1.25 g of gel per compression. A progestin should be used with an intact uterus.

Estrasorb is the first prescription topical emulsion for estrogen therapy. Estrasorb delivers consistent levels of estradiol into the bloodstream in a lotion-like emulsion, applied daily to the skin on the legs for the relief of moderate to severe vasomotor symptoms. Estrasorb should be applied in a comfortable sitting position to clean, dry skin on both legs each morning. A progestin should be used with an intact uterus.

Contraindications

Contraindications to ERT include pregnancy, history of endometrial or breast cancer within the last 5 years, history of thromboembolic disorders, acute liver disease or chronic impaired liver function, gallbladder or pancreatic disease, poorly controlled hypertension, undiagnosed genital bleeding, and endometriosis. Lifestyle factors such as smoking, known to enhance the risk of thromboembolism, should be considered in the treatment decision. The client with a history of fibroid tumors is not started on ERT for a full year after the last menstruation, because estrogen would likely result in tumor growth. The hypoestrogenic state associated with natural menopause usually causes existing fibroids to shrink. The presence of fibrocystic breast disease, diabetes, or obesity may require extra caution.

Contraindications to HRT in conjunction with estrogen are the same as those for ERT. It is important to rule out the presence of known or suspected breast cancer before progestins are used.

Pharmacokinetics

The natural estrogens are completely and rapidly absorbed from the GI tract and rapidly metabolized by the liver, necessitating daily doses when oral products that are nonesterified (a process that delays metabolism and lengthens action) are used. About 80% of estradiol is bound to sex hormone-binding globulin, with 2% unbound and the rest bound to albumin. Estradiol is converted to estrone in the enterohepatic circulation and is conjugated and excreted via the urine. Progestin (Provera) is rapidly absorbed and metabolized primarily in the liver with excretion via the kidney; distribution of the agent is not well described.

Osteoporosis

Over half of U.S. women over the age of 50 have osteoporosis or osteopenia, placing them at risk for a bone fracture. The most serious fracture site is the hip. Hip fracture is the second most common reason for older women being placed in nursing homes, exceeded only by Alzheimer's disease.

Nursing Interventions

Prevention of osteoporosis includes 1200 mg of calcium daily if not taking estrogen; those taking hormones need only 1000 mg. Vitamin D supplementation (400 international units/day) is needed for women who do not receive daily doses of sunlight. Smoking cessation should be encouraged, because smoking interferes with vitamin D absorption. Daily weight-bearing exercise strengthens the bones, increases muscle strength, and enhances balance. To prevent falls, loose rugs should be removed, adequate lighting provided, and handrails installed where appropriate. Caution should be used in clients who are prescribed medications that cause hypotension or dizziness.

Medications

Estrogen is *no longer* recommended for the sole treatment and prevention of osteoporosis, because other medications are available that have a lower risk of cardiac disease, breast cancer, and blood clots.

Menostar (estradiol transdermal system) is 14 mcg of estrogen in a transdermal, once-a-week patch for prevention of postmenopausal osteoporosis. This estrogen patch is the lowest transdermal dose available. It is available for women who are unable to tolerate alternative therapies. For women with an intact uterus, a progestin is only recommended every 6 to 12 months.

Alendronate (Fosamax) is a bisphosphonate used to treat osteopenia and osteoporosis. It is available in a daily or weekly dose. It must be taken with 8 oz of water, 30 minutes before ingesting any food, liquids, or medication, and the client must remain upright for 30 minutes. Once-a-week dosing has made this a first-line therapy. Common side effects include abdominal pain and acid reflux.

Ibandronate sodium (Boniva) is a once-a-month bisphosphonate indicated for the treatment and prevention of osteoporosis in postmenopausal women. It has the same directions for use and side effects as the other bisphosphonates.

Risedronate (Actonel) is also available in a daily or weekly dose. It has similar directions for use and side effects as the bisphosphonates.

Raloxifene (Evista) is a selective estrogen receptor modulator (SERM) that increases bone mineral density, decreases bone turnover, and reduces vertebral fractures. A secondary analysis of women with breast cancer in osteoporotic women treated with raloxifene showed a decrease in the risk of breast cancer. Side effects include hot flashes and increased risk of DVT.

Teriparatide (Fortéo) is for the treatment of postmenopausal osteoporosis. It is administered 20 micrograms subQ on a daily basis. It can be used by both men and women who have had a fracture related to osteoporosis, or who have multiple risk factors for fracture and who cannot use other osteoporosis treatments.

Calcitonin and parathyroid hormone are used only for the treatment, not prevention, of osteoporosis.

Nursing Process

Estrogen Replacements

ASSESSMENT

- Assess the following baseline data:
  - Height and weight
  - Usual physical activity

Diet
- Family history and personal risk factors regarding osteoporosis and cardiovascular disease
- Client's menstrual history
- Nature of the family members' climacteric experience
- Current experience with the climacteric and the drugs client uses
- Assess client's perception of menopause.
- Assess client's attitude toward resumption of menstrual periods.

NURSING DIAGNOSES

- Sexual dysfunction related to signs and symptoms of diagnosis
- Disturbed body image related to changes in body related to menopause
- Health-seeking behaviors related to seeking relief of symptoms

PLANNING

- Client will verbalize menopausal symptoms and the nonpharmacologic and pharmacologic measures that may aid in alleviating symptoms.

NURSING INTERVENTIONS

- Educate women about the nature of the climacteric, its potential effects, and nonpharmacologic as well as pharmacologic treatment. Place current educational materials in health and community sites.
- Indicate on the laboratory slip or specimen that client takes hormone replacement therapy (HRT).
- Administer at bedtime to decrease adverse effects.

Client Teaching

General
- Review the risk-to-benefit ratio for use of estrogen replacement therapy (ERT).
- Review the contraindications to HRT.
- Advise client to have a breast examination, pelvic examination, and Pap test, before starting HRT.

- Tell client that warm weather and stress exacerbate vasodilation/hot flashes.
- Advise client to use a fan, drink cool liquids, wear layered cotton clothes, decrease intake of caffeine and spicy foods, and talk with her health care provider about the use of vitamin E to cope more comfortably with vasodilation. Individuals with diabetes, hypertension, or rheumatic heart disease should use vitamin E in low doses with the health care provider's approval.
- Encourage client on HRT to have medical follow-up every 6 to 12 months, including a blood pressure check and breast and pelvic examinations.
- Suggest that client carry sanitary pads or tampons for breakthrough bleeding or irregular menstruation.
- Stress the need to use nonhormonal birth control, because irregular menstruation may create anxiety about pregnancy. Tell client to plan to use birth control for 2 years. If she has progesterone-induced bleeding, the only way to determine whether she is truly menopausal is by hormone assay.
- Suggest to client that she use a water-soluble vaginal lubricant to reduce painful intercourse (dyspareunia) and prevent trauma.
- Advise client to decrease use of antihistamines and decongestants if she experiences vaginal dryness.
- Advise client to wear cotton underwear and pantyhose with a cotton liner and to avoid douches and feminine hygiene products.
- Suggest that client take Premarin with progestin after meals to avoid nausea and vomiting.
- Tell client to report any heavy bleeding (flooding) and to have her hematocrit and hemoglobin evaluated.
- Tell client to report bleeding that occurs between menstruation or return of bleeding after cessation of menstruation.
- Advise client starting on HRT that the withdrawal bleeding that occurs from days 25 to 30 is normal and not the same as cyclic menstrual periods. Tell her that this bleeding will usually last only 2 to 3 days and that she will not experience the same degree of premenstrual symptoms she may have had with regular menstruation.
- Advise client to report if bleeding occurs other than on days 25 to 30 once she has started on HRT.
- Tell client that the withdrawal bleeding does not signify that she can become pregnant.
- Advise client that after HRT is discontinued, there may be a recurrence of menopausal signs and symptoms such as hot flashes.

Self-Administration
- Teach client to perform regular breast self-examination.
- If client uses vaginal cream, review the application procedure and suggest that she wear minipads.
- If client uses the transdermal patch, tell her to open the package and apply it immediately, holding it in place for about 10 seconds; to check the edges to ensure adequate contact; to use the abdomen (except waistline) for the patch; to rotate the sites with at least 1 week before reuse of a site; to not use the breast as a site; to not put the patch on an irritated or oily area; to reapply the patch if it loosens or apply a new one; and to follow the same cycle schedule.

Diet
- Discuss the use of yogurt containing *Acidophilus* or *Lactobacillus* as a way of maintaining normal bacterial flora in the vagina.
- Tell client that she may experience an occasional hot flash on days 25 to 30 when she goes through withdrawal bleeding. Instruct client to stop treatment and contact a health care provider if she has headache, visual disturbances, signs of thrombophlebitis, heaviness in legs, chest pain, or breast lumps.
- Tell client that if she wants to stop HRT, she should do so with the guidance of her health care provider.
- Suggest that client at risk for osteoporosis (1) exercise consistently (e.g., walking or bicycling), (2) eat a well-balanced diet (low in red meat and sugar) with 1200 mg calcium/d if premenopausal or 1200 to 1500 mg/d if menopausal, and (3) avoid smoking and alcohol.

EVALUATION

- Evaluate the effectiveness of the nonpharmacologic or pharmacologic measures for premenopausal symptoms.
- Determine whether side effects occur. Plan with the client alternative measures to control menopausal symptoms.

KEY WEBSITES

Planned Parenthood: www.plannedparenthood.org
The Contraceptive Report: www.contraceptiononline.org/
Managing Contraception: www.managingcontraception.com

Critical Thinking Case Study

TA (gravida 3, para 1) is ready to leave the hospital following her delivery of baby JA. Pregnancy-induced hypertension had developed during the pregnancy, but she had no prior history of hypertension. She plans to breastfeed for 3 months. She desires contraception and asks questions about hormonally controlled birth control methods.

1. TA asks whether she can take combination birth control pills while breastfeeding. What is a nursing diagnosis for TA based on her communication?

2. The nurse tells her she may breastfeed and start using combination pills in about 6 weeks, once the milk flow is established. Is this information correct or incorrect? Why?

3. TA asks if there are any advantages to using oral contraceptives rather than a diaphragm. What are four advantages and four disadvantages the nurse could include in her discussion?

4. TA tells you she smokes three fourths of a pack of cigarettes a day. How does this information affect the decision for or against oral contraceptive use?

5. TA starts to use combination birth control pills and calls the clinic, upset that she has forgotten to take one pill. What would the clinic nurse correctly tell TA to do? How might the nurse in the postpartum unit have better prepared TA for this situation?

6. Because milk flow needs to be established before starting on combination birth control pills, what should be recommended to TA about contraception upon leaving the hospital? Consider that TA had a fourth-degree episiotomy and hemorrhoids.

7. TA states that when she has "bad allergies," she sometimes takes OTC antihistamines. How should TA be advised?

8. How should TA be advised to take her birth control pills?

9. Injectable progestin (Depo-Provera) is recommended as an alternative method for contraception. What advantage might this product have for TA over the oral products?

10. What should TA be advised about regarding the use of Depo-Provera while breastfeeding?

11. What implication does TA's smoking have in regard to known side effects with Depo-Provera?

12. Why should the site in which a Depo-Provera injection is given be documented?

13. How should the way Depo-Provera works be explained to TA?

14. TA asks how long it will take to regain her fertility once she stops using the Depo-Provera injection. What is the correct response to her question?

NCLEX Study Questions

1. Key factors the nurse should address in a teaching plan for oral contraceptive use include all but:
   a. explanations of ACHES
   b. all herbal supplements are considered safe with birth control pills
   c. will not protect from STDs
   d. important to take pills at the same time every day

2. Advantages of Depo-Provera include all but:
   a. predictable menstrual cycles
   b. safe while breastfeeding
   c. discrete: no pills to carry or visible patches
   d. relatively inexpensive

3. Which are not common symptoms associated with PMS?
   a. Fatigue
   b. Headache
   c. Acne
   d. Hair loss

4. Effective treatment modalities for the symptoms of PMS include all but:
   a. limitation of alcoholic beverages
   b. high fat, low carbohydrate diet
   c. decreased caffeine intake
   d. increased water intake

5. Indications for hormone therapy include all but:
   a. relief of hot flashes
   b. relief of vaginal atrophy
   c. prevention of cardiovascular disease
   d. relief of night sweats

6. Routes of administration of hormone replacement therapy include all but:
   a. shampoo
   b. oral tablets
   c. vaginal ring
   d. transdermal patch

Answers: 1, b; 2, a; 3, d; 4, b; 5, c; 6, a.

56

Drugs for Men's Health and Reproductive Disorders

Kathleen J. Jones

ELECTRONIC RESOURCES

Evolve website (http://evolve.elsevier.com/KeeHayes/pharmacology/):
- Case Studies
- Content Updates
- Frequently Asked Questions
- Student Review Activities
- WebLinks
- Additional Reference Material

Companion CD-ROM:
- NCLEX Examination Review Questions
- Pharmacology Animations
- IV Therapy Checklists
- Medication Error Checklists
- Drug Calculation Problems
- Electronic Calculators
- Top 200 Drugs with Pronunciations
- References from the Textbook

Outline

Objectives

- Describe the feedback loop comprising hypothalamic, anterior pituitary, and gonadal hormones.
- Describe the role of testosterone in development of primary and secondary male sex characteristics and in spermatogenesis.
- Differentiate common conditions for which androgen therapy and antiandrogen therapy are indicated.
- Describe clients for whom androgen therapy is particularly risky.
- Assess clients for therapeutic and adverse effects of androgen therapy.
- Compare and contrast commonly prescribed medications that can impair male sexual function.
- Explain the nursing process, including client teaching, related to drugs used to treat male reproductive disorders.

Terms

This chapter discusses drug regimens for various altera-tions in male reproductive health other than the sexu-ally transmitted diseases (STDs), which are addressed in Chapter 57 because of their association with infertility, particularly among women.

Reproductive health requires the production of ade-quate quantities of various hypothalamic, pituitary, and gonadal hormones as well as the appropriate hormone receptors. It requires normal development and patency of the reproductive tract. In addition, reproductive health implies that men and women at developmentally appro-priate life stages are fertile (i.e., able to produce gametes [sperm or eggs]). Finally, reproductive health entails the ability to engage in sexual intercourse with ejaculation by the male.

Alterations in reproductive health reflect a wide range of developmental, endocrine, infectious, inflammatory, hy-pertrophic, malignant, and psychoemotional processes. To gain a better understanding of ways in which reproductive health is affected, reproductive processes are reviewed.

The male reproductive processes, including anatomy and physiology, sperm production, regulation of male sexual functioning, and sexual intercourse, are discussed in the introduction to Unit XVI.

The drug family most clearly associated with male re-productive processes is the androgens. Because anabolic steroids and antiandrogens impact male reproduction, they are also discussed.

Substances Related to Male Reproductive Disorders

Androgens

Androgens, or male sex hormones, affect sexual processes, accessory sexual organs, cellular metabolism, and bone and muscle growth. The actions and effects of natural an-drogens are listed in Prototype Drug Chart 56–1. **Testos-terone**, the main androgen, is synthesized primarily in the testes and to a lesser extent in the adrenal cortex. In women the ovaries synthesize small amounts of testosterone. In men, normal plasma concentrations of testosterone are 250 to 1000 mg/dl, with circadian fluctuations.

Pharmacokinetics

In men, about 98% of circulating testosterone is bound to protein. It is the unbound fraction that is biologically active. Estrogen elevates the production of sex hormone-binding globulin; therefore more circulating testosterone is bound in women.

The half-life of endogenous free testosterone in the blood is 10 to 20 minutes. Exogenous testosterone is absorbed orally, but because as much as 50% is metabolized on its first pass through hepatic circulation, high doses are needed to achieve effective plasma levels. Synthetic androgens have longer half-lives. Testosterone can be combined with esters to form esterified testosterone, in an oil base, to achieve a dura-tion of action of up to 4 weeks.

Testosterone is excreted mainly in the urine as the metabolites an-drosterone and etiocholanolone. About 6% of the hormone is excreted unaltered in the feces. Synthetic androgens may be excreted as unal-tered hormone or as metabolites. In some tissues the action of testos-terone depends on its reduction to 5-alpha-dihydrotestosterone, whereas in other tissues testosterone itself is the active hormone. In the central nervous system, the metabolite estradiol affects hormonal action.

Pharmacodynamics

Testosterone is responsible for the development of male characteristics. These include the fetal development and maturation of the male repro-ductive system and the development of secondary sex characteristics such as pubic hair growth, beard and body hair growth, baldness, deep-ening of the male voice, thickening of the skin, sebaceous gland activity, increased musculature, bone development, and red blood cell formation.

The mechanism for these effects may be increased protein formation in the target cells. Dihydrotestosterone with its receptor acts at binding sites on the chromosomes. Increased ribonucleic acid (RNA) poly-merase activity and increased synthesis of specific RNA and proteins result, accounting for the anabolic effects of testosterone.

The testes produce testosterone in utero. After birth until just before puberty, production is negligible. During puberty testosterone produc-tion increases rapidly and continues until later adulthood. As men age the number of Leydig cells decreases, sperm production declines, and luteinizing hormone (LH) and follicle-stimulating hormone (FSH) levels rise. Levels of unbound testosterone are reduced in older men to one third to one fifth the peak value. "Andropause" is beginning to receive attention as a health issue affecting older men, particularly those older than 70 years. If men experience osteoporosis and anemia, and if their testosterone levels are less than or equal to 300ng/dl, testosterone re-placement therapy should be considered.

Indications for Androgen Therapy

Various androgens and their uses are identified in Table 56–1.

Hypogonadism. The clearest indication for androgen therapy is **hypogonadism**. Hypogonadism occurs when there is insufficient testosterone production by the testes. Hypogonadism can be primary, reflecting testicular abnor-mality, or secondary, reflecting hypothalamic or pituitary failure. Severely affected boys do not experience puberty. Lack of libido, impotence, decreased bone density, or the onset of vasomotor flushing also can occur. The timing and extent of treatment depend on the clinical manifestations.

Artificial induction of puberty is undertaken after boys reach 15 to 17 years of age. Hypothalamic and pituitary function is assessed. A 4- to 6-month trial of androgen therapy is implemented, followed by a like period of rest for reevaluation. If prolonged therapy is required, testos-terone cypionate or testosterone enanthate is given, start-ing with 100 mg given intramuscularly (IM) every 2 weeks for 6 to 12 months, with a gradual increase to 200 mg ev-ery 2 weeks. It takes 3 or 4 years for sexual development to occur. Plasma testosterone levels should be monitored and dosages adjusted as needed to maintain normal levels.

Another form of treatment is transdermal testosterone skin patches that are applied daily to the scrotum or other sites. The patches eliminate the need for injections and provide circadian fluctuations in dosage.

Constitutional Growth Delay. A height of two or more standard deviations below the mean for age and sex occurs in 2.5% of normal children. This tends to be of greater concern for boys. Delay in bone growth seems to be of little consequence by the time boys reach the age of

Prototype DRUG CHART 56–1

TESTOSTERONE

Drug Class	**Dosage**

Androgen
Trade names: Andro-Cyp 100, Depandro 100,
   Depotest-100, Duratest-100, Depo-Testosterone,
   Testred Cypionate 200, Virilon, depAndrogyn, Everone
Pregnancy Category: X
CSS III
	Androgen replacement:
	PO: 10-40 mg/d
	Buccal: 5-20 mg/d
	subQ: 150-450 mg q3-6 mo
	IM: 10-30 mg 2-3 times/wk
	Metastatic carcinoma of the breast:
	PO: 200 mg/d
	Buccal: 200 mg/d
	IM: 100 mg 3 times/wk

Contraindications	**Drug-Lab-Food Interactions**

Pregnancy, nephrosis, hypercalcemia, pituitary
   insufficiency, hepatic dysfunction, benign
   prostatic hypertrophy, prostatic cancer, history of
   myocardial infarction, prepubertal status, non–
   estrogen-dependent breast cancer
Caution: Hypertension, hypercholesterolemia,
   coronary artery disease, gynecomastia, renal disease,
   seizure disorders; prepubescent clients, older adults
	Drug: Increases effects of anticoagulants; *decreases*
	   effect with barbiturates, phenytoin, phenylbutazone;
	   antagonizes calcitonin, parathyroid; corticosteroids
	   exacerbate edema
	Lab: Decreases blood glucose in diabetics; *increases*
	   serum cholesterol, thyroid, liver function, hematocrit

Pharmacokinetics	**Pharmacodynamics**

Absorption: IM: Well absorbed
Distribution: PB: 98%
Metabolism: t½: 10-100 min
Excretion: In urine and bile
	IM: Onset: UK
	   Peak: UK
	   Duration: cypionate enanthate: 2-4 wk; base,
	      propionate: 1-3 d

Therapeutic Effects/Uses

To achieve normal androgen levels; to slow progress of estrogen-dependent breast cancers
Mode of Action: Development and maintenance of male sex organs and secondary sex characteristics

Side Effects	**Adverse Reactions**

Abdominal pain, nausea, diarrhea, constipation,
   hives, irritation at injection site, increased salivation,
   mouth soreness, increased or decreased libido,
   insomnia, aggressive behavior, weakness, dizziness,
   pruritus
	Acne, masculinization, irregular menses, urinary
	   urgency, gynecomastia, priapism, red skin, jaundice,
	   sodium and water retention, allergic reaction,
	   depression, habituation
	Life-threatening: Hepatic necrosis, hepatitis, hepatic
	   tumors, respiratory distress

CSS, Controlled Substances Schedule; *d*, day; *IM*, intramuscular; *min*, minute; *mo*, month; *PB*, protein-binding; *PO*, by mouth; *subQ*, subcutaneous; *t½*, half-life; *UK*, unknown; *wk*, week.

20 years; however, in some families delayed growth causes significant emotional distress, despite reassurance from health professionals. The cause may be a deficiency of growth hormone, which can be associated with androgen deficiency, or it may be solely androgen deficiency. Treatment is not initiated before the age of 14 years. Therapy for 3 to 6 months or less before epiphyseal closure may result in linear growth without adverse permanent effects on hypothalamic, pituitary, or gonadal maturation. It is not known whether treatment has an effect on final adult height.

The selection of an androgen or anabolic steroid depends on the balance of growth and sexual maturation desired, as well as the preferred route of administration. Oxandrolone, an orally active testosterone analog, is effec-

tive for treating boys. Oxandrolone stimulates the onset of puberty. It is classified as an anabolic steroid and is regulated as such. The daily dosage is less than or equal to 0.1 mg/kg.

Studies have shown that men treated with human growth hormone (hGH) for nongrowth- hormone-dependent short stature showed reduced testicular volume and hypergonadotropic hypogonadism. They also have impaired spermatogenesis and altered testicular texture by ultrasound. Although no clinical or laboratory findings showed testicular dysfunction, an unfavorable gonadal outcome could occur in boys given growth hormone who did not have growth hormone deficiency.

Other Uses. Other uses of androgens include treatment of refractory anemias in men and women, the hereditary

Table 56–1

Androgens

Generic (Brand)	Route and Dosage	Uses and Considerations
Natural Androgens		
testosterone (Histerone, Tesamone, Testopel pellets, testosterone aqueous, testosterone powder)	IM: 10-25 mg 2-3 × wk subQ: 150-450 mg q3-6mo IM: 100 mg 3 × wk	Androgen replacement, delayed puberty, senile or postmenopausal osteoporosis. Started at full dose and adjusted according to tolerance and therapeutic response. Carcinoma of the breast. Therapy may be lifelong. *Pregnancy category:* X; PB: 98%; t½: 10-100 min
testosterone cypionate (Andro-Cyp, Andronate, Depandro, Depotest, Depo-Testosterone, Duratest, Testred cypionate, Virilon IM)	IM: 50-400 mg q2-6wk	Androgen replacement, delayed puberty. Therapy generally lasts 3-4 y. *Pregnancy category:* X; PB: 98%; t½: 10-100 min
testosterone enanthate (Andro, Andropository, Delatest, Delatestryl, Durathate, Everone, Testrin)	IM: 50-400 mg q2-6wk	Androgen replacement, delayed puberty. *Pregnancy category:* X; PB: 98%; t½: 10-100 min
testosterone propionate (Testex, testosterone propionate powder)	IM: 50 mg 3 × wk	Androgen replacement. *Pregnancy category:* X; PB: 98%; t½: 10-100 min
Transdermal testosterone (patch)	2.5 mg/24 h 5 mg/24 h	Apply to nonscrotal skin; avoid bony areas (Androderm)
Androderm	Apply to nonscrotal skin	
Synthetic Androgens		
Danazol	PO: 100-800 mg/d divided in 2 doses initially	Endometriosis, fibrocystic breast disease, angioedema. Initial doses are gradually reduced on an individual basis. Endometriosis therapy lasts 6-9 mo; fibrocystic breast disease therapy lasts 4-6 mo. *Pregnancy category:* X; PB: UK; t½: 4.5 h
fluoxymesterone (Halotestin)	PO: 10-30 mg/d divided in 1-4 doses	Androgen deficiency, carcinoma of the breast. *Pregnancy category:* X; PB: 98%; t½: 20-100 min
methyltestosterone (Android, Oreton Methyl, Testred, Virilon)	PO: 10-50 mg/d in divided doses initially, reduced for maintenance Buccal: 5-25 mg/d in divided doses PO: 50-200 mg/d Buccal: 2-25 mg/d in divided doses	Androgen deficiency Carcinoma of the breast. *Pregnancy category:* X; PB: UK; t½: UK
Anabolic Steroids		
nandrolone decanoate (Androlone-D, Deca-Durabolin, Hybolin Decanoate, Neo Durabolic)	IM: 50-200 mg q1-4wk C: IM: 25-50 mg q3-4wk	Anemia of renal disease. *Pregnancy category:* X; PB: UK; t½: UK
nandrolone phenpropionate (Durabolin, Hybolin improved, Nandrobolic LA)	IM: 50-100 mg/wk	Carcinoma of the breast. *Pregnancy category:* X; PB: UK; t½: 1-9 h
oxandrolone (Oxandrin)	PO: 5-20 mg/d, divided C: PO: 0.1 mg/kg/d	Delayed growth/puberty, osteoporotic pain, short stature, Turner's syndrome, alcoholic hepatitis. *Pregnancy category:* X; PB: UK; t½: 1-9 h
oxymetholone (Anadrol-50)	PO: 1-5 mg/kg/d	Anemias of deficient RBC production. *Pregnancy category:* X; PB: UK; t½: 9 h
stanozolol	PO: 2-6 mg/d	t½: UK

C, Child; *d,* day; *h,* hour; *IM,* intramuscular; *min,* minute; *mo,* month; *PB,* protein-binding; *PO,* by mouth; *RBC,* red blood cell; *subQ,* subcutaneous; *t½,* half-life; *UK,* unknown; *wk,* week; *y,* year.

autosomal clotting disorder angioneurotic edema, tissue wasting associated with severe or chronic illness, advanced carcinoma of the breast in women, and endometriosis. The effectiveness of androgens for treatment of **cryptorchidism** (undescended testis) and impotence has not been established. Androgens may be used in combination with estrogens for management of severe menopausal symptoms in women (see Chapter 55).

Side Effects

Side effects of androgen therapy include abdominal pain, nausea, insomnia, diarrhea or constipation, hives or redness at the injection site, increased salivation, mouth soreness, and increased or decreased sexual desire. If side effects persist, worsen, or disturb the individual, the health care provider should be notified.

Adverse Reactions

Virilizing effects (the development of secondary male sex characteristics) are inappropriate when the client is not a hypogonadal man. Women who use androgen therapy risk such manifestations, including acne and skin oiliness, the growth of facial hair, and vocal huskiness (**virilization**). Menstrual irregularities or amenorrhea, suppressed ovulation or lactation, baldness or increased hair growth (**hirsutism**), and hypertrophy of the clitoris may develop in women undergoing androgen therapy. Although most adverse effects slowly reverse themselves after short-term therapy is completed, vocal changes may be permanent. With long-term therapy, as in the treatment of breast cancer, adverse effects may be irreversible.

Children may experience profound virilization or feminization, as well as impaired bone growth. During pregnancy androgens can cross the placenta and cause masculinization of the fetus.

Hypogonadal men may experience frequent erections or **priapism**, **gynecomastia** (breast swelling or soreness), and urinary urgency. Continued use of androgens by normal men can halt **spermatogenesis** (formation of spermatozoa). The sperm count may be low (**oligospermia**) for 3 or more months after therapy is stopped. For this reason, androgens for contraceptive use by men are currently in development.

Less frequent adverse effects include dizziness, weakness, changes in skin color, frequent headaches, confusion, respiratory distress, depression, pruritus, allergic skin rash, edema of the lower extremities, jaundice, bleeding, paresthesias, chills, polycythemia, muscle cramps, and sodium and water retention. Hepatic carcinoma can occur in clients who have received 17-alpha-alkyl-substituted androgens over prolonged periods (i.e., 1 to 7 years).

Serum cholesterol may become elevated during androgen therapy. Other alterations in laboratory tests include altered thyroid and liver function tests, elevated urine 17-ketosteroids, and increased hematocrit.

Rare complications of long-term therapy include hepatic necrosis, hepatic peliosis, hepatic tumors, and leukopenia.

Contraindications

Androgen therapy is contraindicated during pregnancy and in individuals with nephrosis or the nephrotic phase of nephritis, hypercalcemia, pituitary insufficiency, hepatic dysfunction, benign prostatic hypertrophy, or prostate cancer. Men with breast cancer are not treated with androgens, nor are women whose breast cancer is not estrogen-dependent. A history of myocardial infarction is a contraindication.

Caution must be exercised when using androgen therapy in individuals with hypertension, hypercholesterolemia, coronary artery disease, gynecomastia, renal disease, or seizure disorder. It is used with caution in infants and prepubertal children because of the potential for growth disturbances and in older men because of their increased risk for benign prostatic hypertrophy and prostate cancer.

Drug Interactions

Androgens potentiate the effects of oral anticoagulants, necessitating a decrease in anticoagulant dosage. Androgens antagonize calcitonin and parathyroid hormones. Because androgens can decrease blood glucose in clients with diabetes, dosages of insulin or other antidiabetic agents may need to be reduced. Concurrent use of corticosteroids exacerbates the edema that can occur with androgen therapy. Barbiturates, phenytoin, and phenylbutazone decrease the effects of androgens.

Nursing Process

Androgens

ASSESSMENT

■ Assess the reason for androgen therapy and the client's perception of it. If delayed puberty is the indication, the nurse will assess client's and family's attitudes about the condition.

■ Monitor client's weight, blood pressure, liver and thyroid function, hemoglobin and hematocrit, creatinine, clotting factors, glucose tolerance, serum lipids and electrolytes, and blood count before and throughout treatment. The presence of liver or endocrine dysfunction should be noted.

■ Determine the pregnancy status of women of childbearing age. Concomitant anticoagulant therapy should be noted. When a prepubertal child is treated, radiographs are obtained before, every 6 months during, and after treatment to monitor growth.

■ Appraise client's expressive affect during therapy, particularly aggressiveness in clients taking large doses. Self-concept is an important consideration in client on androgen therapy, particularly in children with delayed puberty and in women.

NURSING DIAGNOSES

- Disturbed body image related to growth delay
- Delayed growth and development related to androgen deficiency
- Situational low self-esteem related to growth delay and/or virilizing effects of androgen therapy
- Sexual dysfunction related to androgen deficiency
- Ineffective sexuality pattern related to antiandrogen therapy and or delayed puberty
- Ineffective therapeutic regimen management related to a knowledge deficit regarding treatment protocol

PLANNING

- Clients will adhere to the prescribed regimen for taking the medication and for monitoring.
- Client will appropriately use the medication, avoid preventable adverse effects, and maintain a positive self-concept during long-term treatment.

NURSING INTERVENTIONS

Client Teaching

General

- Instruct client and family on proper administration of the medications, their reasons for use, and potential undesired effects. Inform them of which effects warrant prompt medical attention (e.g., urinary problems, priapism, respiratory distress).
- Teach client that an intermittent approach to treatment allows for monitoring of endocrine status between courses of androgen therapy. Explain the need to return to the health care facility for monitoring, and determine client's ability to do so. Make social service referrals if necessary.
- Instruct families pursuing treatment for a client with delayed puberty about the range of normal development.
- Urge individuals being treated for tissue wasting to reduce environmental stressors and promote rest and relaxation, because stress hormones are catabolic. Muscle strength will be monitored during treatment.

Self-Administration

- Oral androgens should be taken with food to decrease gastric distress.

Side Effects

- Women and prepubertal clients need instruction on good skin hygiene to decrease the severity of acne.
- Men undergoing androgen therapy are instructed to report priapism (painful, continuous erection) promptly. The drug dosage will be reduced to avoid subsequent erectile dysfunction. In addition, they are taught to report decreased urinary stream promptly, because androgens can stimulate prostatic hypertrophy.

Diet

- The nutritional intake of individuals with anemia, osteoporosis, or tissue wasting is assessed and revised as needed to ensure adequate intake of calories, protein, vitamins, iron, calcium and other minerals.
- Sodium may need to be restricted if edema develops. Client will be instructed to record body weight several times per week.
- Individuals with elevated serum calcium need 3 to 4L of fluid per day to prevent kidney stones. Individuals on bed rest need range-of-motion exercises, whereas ambulatory clients need to engage in active weight bearing. Indicators of hypercalcemia are shown in Box 56–1. Hypercalcemia needs prompt medical attention, because it can lead to cardiac arrest.

Cultural Considerations ❖

- Assess how the person's cultural group regards the expression of sexuality.
- Ascertain any culturally defined expectations about male-female or male-male relationships, including the health care relationship.
- Determine whether the person has any restrictions related to sexuality, exposure of body parts, or discussion of sexual functioning.
- If an interpreter is needed, meet these guidelines if possible:
  Use a trained medical interpreter from your agency if possible. A medical interpreter can help with advice about the cultural appropriateness of client's health care plan
  Use a family member only if absolutely necessary. Be aware that there may be limitations if the family member does not understand medical terms or is a different age or gender from the client. Family members may not be aware of medical procedures or medical ethics.
  Use simple language; try to use as few medical terms as possible.
  Speak in one or two sentences to allow easier translation.

EVALUATION

- Client's ability to adhere to the treatment regimen and response to prescribed drugs will be monitored.

Box 56–1

Signs of Hypercalcemia

- Nausea and vomiting
- Lethargy
- Decreased muscle tone
- Polyuria
- Increased urine and serum calcium

■ Client will be asked about therapeutic and adverse drug effects on follow-up visits. Monitoring of weight, blood pressure, and laboratory tests will continue throughout therapy, with alterations in the plan of care as needed.

■ Children and women who experience virilizing effects or acne will be periodically assessed for the ability to cope with these changes and maintain a positive self-concept.

■ Sexual function is assessed when appropriate.

■ Client's ability to adhere to the treatment plan and to discuss the treatment and its effects knowledgeably suggests that teaching has been effective and that client accepts the treatment.

Anabolic Steroids

Anabolic steroids are synthetic derivatives of testosterone developed to maximize the anabolic effects of androgens and to minimize their androgenic effects. Testosterone precursors available as nutritional supplements include androstenediol, androstenedione, and dehydroepiandrosterone (DHEA). Anabolic steroids increase strength and power, and artificially enhanced strength and power can lead to changes in performance. Older teens are the heaviest users, but more than half a million junior high school students use them. Marketed as "sport supplements" or "teen formulas," they can be purchased without a prescription in grocery stores, health food markets, and sports stores and on the Internet. Sudden dramatic increase in weight gain and body size, increased acne, and changes in mood and behavior can be signs of anabolic steroid use. Individuals using anabolic steroids may become more aggressive and physical. Side effects include water retention, which overloads the kidneys, and cardiovascular damage such as cardiomyopathy and stroke. There can also be hepatic problems, because anabolic steroids tend to lower HDL (good) cholesterol. The adverse effects may not be recognized until years later.

Two other steroids that have gained popularity, especially with athletes, are human chorionic gonadotropin (hCG, Pregnyl, Novarel, Ovidrel) and tetrahydrogestrinone (THG). Human chorionic gonadotropin is a hormone used to treat infertility; it also stimulates testosterone production. Tetrahydrogestrinone is a potent androgen developed to escape urine detection; THG is not approved by the Food and Drug Administration (FDA) and not legally marketed. All major athletic organizations prohibit the use of anabolic steroids, but their continued use despite bans has led to "anti-doping" investigations and punitive action.

Antiandrogens

Antiandrogens, or androgen antagonists, block the synthesis or action of androgens (Table 56–2). These drugs may be useful in the management of benign prostatic hypertrophy and carcinoma of the prostate. They have been used to treat male-pattern baldness, acne, hirsutism, viril-

Table 56–2

Antiandrogens

Mechanism	Drugs
Elevation of Gn-RH level	goserelin (Zoladex) nafarelin (Synarel) leuprolide acetate (Lupron, Lupron Depot)
Inhibition of testosterone synthesis	ketoconazole (Nizoral)
Blocks conversion of testosterone to dihydrotestosterone	finasteride (Proscar)
Receptor inhibitors	cyproterone, cyproterone acetate (orphan drug status in the United States) flutamide (Eulexin) spironolactone (generic, Aldactone)

Gn-RH, Gonadotropin-releasing hormone.

ization syndrome in women, and precocious puberty in boys, although their effectiveness is not well established. The effectiveness of these drugs to inhibit the sex drive of men who are sex offenders is controversial and not well documented.

Gonadotropin-releasing hormone (Gn-RH), or an analogue such as leuprolide, is the most effective inhibitor of testosterone synthesis. When such agents are given over time, LH and testosterone levels fall. Ketoconazole, an antimycotic, is used for treatment of prostatic carcinoma because of its inhibition of adrenal and gonadal steroid synthesis.

Two types of drugs have been developed to block testosterone action: androgen-receptor antagonists and agents that block conversion of testosterone to its active form, dihydrotestosterone. Cyproterone acetate, an orally active progesterone, is a potent androgen antagonist. It also suppresses LH and FSH secretion and has progestational qualities. Cyproterone acetate competes with dihydrotestosterone for binding to the androgen receptor. Cyproterone acetate can stunt growth in young people. Acne and baldness have been reported.

Flutamide (Eulexin) is a nonsteroidal drug that competes with androgens at androgen receptor sites. Men receiving flutamide show elevations in plasma LH and testosterone levels. Flutamide is used with Gn-RH blockade or estrogen to treat prostate cancer. Spironolactone also competes with dihydrotestosterone at the receptor site. It is used in doses of 50 to 100 mg/daily to treat hirsutism in women.

Finasteride, a steroid, inhibits conversion of testosterone to dihydrotestosterone. This orally active agent decreases the concentration of dihydrotestosterone in plasma and in the prostate without elevated plasma concentrations of LH or testosterone. Finasteride is used to treat benign prostatic hypertrophy (BPH). Other uses are under investigation. The recommended 5 mg daily dose for BPH needs to be reevaluated at 6 months and periodically thereafter. Women of childbearing potential should not be exposed to broken or crushed tablets. Adverse reactions include impotence, decreased libido, and decreased ejaculate.

Drugs Used in Other Male Reproductive Disorders

Developmental Disorders

Undescended testes are associated with subsequent infertility and testicular cancer. The primary treatment is orchidopexy (surgical placement of the testicle into the scrotum), which is usually performed by the time the child is 18 months old.

Delayed Puberty

In up to 5% of cases of **delayed puberty** (no signs of puberty by age 14 in a boy), there is insufficient secretion of Gn-RH, LH, or FSH. Once the cause is determined, Gn-RH, LH, or FSH replacement therapy is instituted.

Pituitary, Thyroid, and Adrenal Disorders

Inadequate pituitary function can result in hypogonadism. In a prepubertal boy, it results in lack of secondary sex characteristics and infertility; adult men may experience testicular atrophy and decreases in libido, potency, beard growth, and muscle tone. Menotropins, one ampule of which contains 75 international units each of LH and FSH, can stimulate testosterone production when injected intramuscularly (IM) three times a week over a period of years. Menotropins is indicated when both LH and FSH levels are low. It is given concomitantly with hCG 2000 international units IM twice a week for at least 3 months. Adverse effects include nausea, vomiting, diarrhea, gynecomastia, and fever. The drug is reconstituted with 1 to 2 ml sterile saline and must be used immediately.

Hypothyroidism, a deficiency in thyroid hormone, can be the result of insufficient thyroid hormone production or resistance to its effects at the target organs. The problem could be congenital. It can cause **inhibited sexual desire** (decreased or lack of interest in sexual activity) and erectile dysfunction. In **Addison's disease**, there is a deficit of both cortisol and the mineralocorticoid aldosterone. Men with Addison's disease may experience inhibited sexual desire, erectile dysfunction, or diminished fertility. Both these conditions are highly responsive to replacement therapy with the appropriate hormones (see Chapter 50).

The successful treatment of cancer with chemotherapy in boys and in young adults can be associated with impaired gonadal function as a result of damage to the Leydig cells, which can cause impaired spermatogenesis or sterility. Abnormalities of endocrine function and growth are common problems following bone marrow and peripheral stem cell transplantation in children. About 25% of children who receive total body irradiation experience hypothyroidism. Gonadal dysfunction is prevalent, and most males experience oligozoospermia. At this time the only clinical option for preserving male fertility is cryopreserv-ing sperm, also known as *sperm banking*, before the initiation of cancer therapy.

For young men with sickle cell disease, priapism is a complication that left untreated can result in irreversible fibrosis and impotency. The most common age for the first episode of priapism is 12, and most episodes are nocturnal. If an episode of priapism persists longer than 2 hours, the client should go to the emergency room for intravenous (IV) fluids and narcotics. After 4 hours, intracavernosal aspiration and instillation of an alpha-agonist should be performed.

Sexual Dysfunction

Sexual dysfunction is the inability to experience sexual desire, erection, ejaculation, and detumescence—the phases of the sexual response cycle. **Inhibited sexual desire** can result from androgen deficiency, an affective disorder, or discord in the sexual relationship. **Erectile dysfunction** (persistent inability to attain or maintain an erection satisfactory for sexual performance) may be caused by psychoemotional problems, diabetes, hypertension, lower urinary tract symptoms, and history of pelvic surgery, vascular insufficiency, neurologic disorders, androgen deficiency or resistance, or diseases of the penis. **Ejaculatory dysfunction** (impaired ejection of seminal fluid from the urethra of the male) can be psychogenic or a result of drug therapy, androgen deficiency, or sympathetic degeneration. Failure of detumescence (reduction of penile swelling) is most commonly caused by penile disease or systemic disease. Male sexual dysfunction may result from the use of various drugs, as listed in Table 56–3.

Individuals who experience premature ejaculation related to excessive anxiety about sexual intercourse may be helped by treatment with one of the monoamine oxidase (MAO) inhibitors in conjunction with psychotherapy (see Chapter 25). Erectile dysfunction caused by vascular insufficiency is occasionally treated on a short-term basis by local vasoactive drugs, including papaverine, phentolamine, prostaglandin E, nitroglycerin, or yohimbine, a systemic vasoactive drug.

A recently developed class of drugs, the phosphodiesterase (PDE) inhibitors, is now available. These agents facilitate erections by enhancing blood flow to the penis. The first drug of this group available is sildenafil citrate (Viagra). The PDE inhibitors potentiate the hypotensive effects of nitrates and are contraindicated for use by any client using organic nitrates in any form. Organic nitrates include nitroglycerin, isosorbide mononitrate, isosorbide nitrate, pentaerythritol tetranitrate, erythrityl tetranitrate, isosorbide dinitrate/phenobarbital, and illicit substances (amyl nitrate/nitrite, butyl nitrate). These PDE inhibitors are contraindicated in clients with significant cardiovascular disease or who have anatomic deformities or conditions predisposing them to priapism.

Other phosphodiesterase inhibitors are vardenafil (Levitra) and tadalafil (Cialis). Studies have shown that the newer agents are safe for clients with heart failure or a history of myocardial infarctions. Thus more men have the option of using a PDE inhibitor for the treatment of erec-

Table 56–3

Drugs Causing Sexual Dysfunction in Males

Drug Category	Drugs or Drug Families
Anticholinergics	atropine
	scopolamine
	benztropine
	trihexyphenidyl
Antidepressants	tricyclic antidepressants
	monoamine oxidase inhibitors
	serotonin reuptake inhibiting antidepressants (SSRIs)
Antihistamines	cimetidine
	diphenhydramine
	hydroxyzine
Antihypertensives	central sympathetic ganglion blockers
	postganglionic blockers
	alpha- and beta-receptor blockers
	diuretics
Antipsychotics	phenothiazines
	thioxanthenes
	butyrophenone
	lithium
Sedatives and social drugs	alcohol
	barbiturates
	diazepam
	chlordiazepoxide
	Cannabis
	cocaine
	opiates
	methadone
Others	aminocaproic acid
	baclofen
	steroids
	ethionamide
	perhexiline
	digoxin
	chemotherapeutic agents

tile dysfunction. Like sildenafil they are contraindicated if the client is taking nitrate-containing medications. Common side effect of the drugs are headache (most common), dyspepsia, nasal congestion, and nasopharyngitis. Other rare side effects can also occur, and the client should be taught about them; these effects include blurred vision; photosensitivity; changes in color perception (especially blue and green); and urinary tract symptoms such as frequency, painful urination, and cloudy or bloody urine. Clients are instructed to notify their health care provider of any side effects they experience.

The PDE inhibitors are taken before sexual activity. The differences are in the amount of time needed for the medication to start being effective and in the duration of the medication. Sildenafil has an onset of 30 to 60 minutes and a duration of 4 hours. Vardenafil's onset is 25 to 30 minutes and also has duration of 4 to 5 hours. Tadalafil has a quicker onset of 16 to 60 minutes but a duration of up to 36 hours.

For men who do not respond to oral medications or in whom these medications are contraindicated, drugs for both intracavernous and other routes of administration are available. Sublingual apomorphine (Uprima) and phentolamine (Vasomax) are examples of these medications. Some young hypogonadal men are able to resolve erectile dysfunction with testosterone replacement therapy by IM injection (testosterone cypionate, testosterone enanthate) or transdermal patches (Androderm). Since the 1980s, intracavernous injection using prostaglandin E (alprostadil), papaverine with phentolamine, or a combination of all three has been a successful treatment. Intraurethral prostaglandin E (Muse) has also been effective in some men. Given the success and high efficacy of the PDE inhibitors, the use of cavernous and intraurethral medications has decreased. Vasoactive drug injections may be associated with hypotension, dizziness, pain, and priapism. Papaverine can cause hepatotoxicity.

Certain drugs are often abused by individuals seeking a heightened sexual experience. Amyl nitrate is commonly believed to be an aphrodisiac. Sudden death, myocardial infarction, and methemoglobinemia have been reported with its use. Cantharides (Spanish fly) causes bladder and urethral irritation, accounting for its use as a sexual stimulant. Permanent penile damage has been reported with its use.

Natural Products. To self-treat sexual problems or to enhance their sexual performance, clients use a wide variety of herbs and plant-derived compounds (phytochemicals). Despite new scientific-based therapies, men are attracted to phytochemicals, because they are easy to obtain and may be cheaper than prescription medications, therapies, procedures, or surgeries not covered by insurance. The client may perceive natural products as providing health benefits beyond sexual performance because they can be purchased at nutrition centers or health food stores.

Some common herbs used for sexual health and performance are yohimbine, ginseng, damiana, ginkgo biloba, saw palmetto, muira puama, and *Tribulus terrestris*. With the exception of yohimbine, which has been scientifically studied, the other compounds do not have benefits proven by research. Rather their benefits appear to reflect popular or cultural beliefs. Reports in health magazines, booklets, and television/radio advertising are anecdotal and based on a small number of users or health care professionals.

Yohimbine, which is obtained from the bark of the African yohimbe tree, is an alpha-adrenergic antagonist that affects both the central and peripheral nervous system. Studies have shown that men experience a positive effect or improvement in erection. The side effects are headache, hypertension, sweating, anxiety, and sleeplessness. Men who have cardiovascular neurologic and psychologic problems should not take yohimbine.

Saw palmetto, a small palmlike plant found in the southeast United States, has been used to treat BPH. Studies show that it is helpful in reducing the symptoms of BPH (difficult or frequent urination) and can help shrink enlarged prostate glands. Although effective in the treatment of prostate enlargement, it has not shown to exert a positive effect on sexual response in men unless erections are inhibited by an enlarged prostate gland. In fact, saw palmetto may reduce androgen action and have a negative effect on sexual response.

Ginkgo biloba leaves have been shown to treat peripheral vascular disease and enhance cerebral blood flow. Recent research suggests that ginkgo biloba may reduce antidepressant (selective serotonin reuptake inhibitor [SSRI])-induced sexual dysfunction. It is not known how it achieves these effects, and further research is needed to substantiate its use.

Ginseng has been shown to improve sexual functioning in animals, but research in humans is contradictory. Like ginkgo biloba, further human research is warranted.

Nonsexually Transmitted Infections

Urinary tract infections are addressed in Chapter 33. If left untreated, acute or chronic prostatitis, orchitis, or epididymitis can develop.

Benign Prostate Hyperplasia

As a male ages, the glandular units in the prostate gland begin to undergo tissue hyperplasia (abnormal increase in the number of cells), resulting in prostatic hypertrophy (enlargement of the gland). The exact cause of BPH is unknown, but its development is almost universal in older men. The enlargement of the prostate gland causes pressure on the man's bladder, and he experiences lower urinary tract symptoms, such as a sensation of bladder fullness, frequency, nocturia, hesitation when trying to begin urinating, dribbling of urine, and erectile dysfunction. Because these are the same symptoms that prostate cancer may cause, the client will have a prostate-specific antigen (PSA) blood test and may undergo a prostate biopsy to make sure no cancer is present. Traditionally the only effective treatment was surgical, but now drug therapy has become the initial treatment of BPH.

Finasteride (Proscar) may be prescribed to shrink the prostate gland and relieve the client's symptoms. Finasteride lowers the client's level of dihydrotestosterone (DHT), a major cause of prostate growth, and decreasing DHT levels may shrink the size of the prostate gland. The client is taught that it may take as long as 6 months before he experiences relief of symptoms.

The prostate gland has alpha-adrenergic receptors in the prostatic smooth muscle. When alpha-blocking agents are given, the prostate gland constricts, thereby decreasing the size of the gland, reducing urethral and bladder pressure, and improving urine flow.

The client with an enlarged prostate should avoid medications that can cause urinary retention, such as anticholinergics, antihistamines, and decongestants.

Various medications used in the treatment of BPH are identified in Table 56–4.

Malignant Tumors

Prostatic cancer accounts for about 10% of all cancer deaths among American men. Most prostatic cancers are adenocarcinomas. Metastasis to lymph nodes, bone, lungs, liver, and adrenal glands is common. Prostatic cancer is often asymptomatic, but urinary obstruction is commonly the first sign. Treatment may include a combination of surgical resection, cryotherapy, antiandrogen administration, radiation therapy, chemotherapy, and pain management.

Testicular tumors peak in early adulthood. They include malignant germinal cell tumors and benign Leydig or Sertoli cell tumors. Treatment depends on the type and stage of tumor. Surgical excision, radiation therapy, and chemotherapy are used alone or in combination.

Of breast cancer cases, 1% occur in men—most commonly after the age of 60 years. Treatment, which is similar for men and women, entails surgery, radiation therapy, chemotherapy, and endocrine therapy. Carcinoma of the

---

Table 56–4

Medications Used for the Treatment of Benign Prostatic Hyperplasia

Generic (Brand)	Route and Dosage	Side Effects
5 Alpha-Reductase Inhibitors		
finasteride (Proscar)	A: PO: 5 mg daily	Decreased libido, erectile dysfunction
Duastride (Avodart, Duagen)	A: PO: 0.5 mg daily	
Alpha-Adrenergic Blocking Agents		
tamsulosin (Flomax)	A: PO: 0.4 mg daily 30 min after a meal	Hypotension, dizziness, fatigue
doxazosin (Cardura)	A: PO: Start 1 mg by mouth at bedtime; titrate up to 8 mg/d at bedtime	
terazosin (Hytrin)	A: PO: Start 1 mg by mouth at bedtime; titrate up to 10 mg/d with a maximum dose of 20 mg/d	
alfuzosin (Uroxatral)	A: PO: 10 mg daily after a meal	Postural hypotension, dizziness, fatigue
Safety in Administration		
Alpha-adrenergic blocking agents are also used to control blood pressure, so to prevent client from experiencing a hypotensive episode, ask for a list of all medications taken before adding another antihypertensive drug.		

d, Day; *min*, minute.

penis represents less than 1% of all malignancies among men. In situ, treatment entails local excision, radiation therapy, and local application of 5-fluorouracil cream or solution. Invasive carcinoma is treated by surgical resection of the penis and involved nodes. Radiation and chemotherapy follow as needed. Antineoplastic therapies are discussed in Unit IX, Immunologic Agents.

KEY WEBSITES

Nursing Center: www.nursingcenter.com
Office of Minority Health Resource Center: www.omhrc.gov
Sexuality Information and Education Council of the United States: www.siecus.org

Critical Thinking Case Study

MT, age 16, is a high school junior who is 59.30 inches and weighs 126 lb. He has increased feelings of discomfort about not fitting in with other students in his school, because he has not yet begun sexual maturation. He is a good student and an accomplished violinist in the school orchestra. His only brother is younger than he is. His father states that he also was a "late bloomer," but he and his wife are concerned about their son's increasing social withdrawal and seem determined to seek medical intervention for him. The nurse in the clinic assesses the needs and status of MT and his family.

1. What is the client's primary complaint? What concerns his family?
2. What information must be included in the history and physical examination?
3. What teaching should the nurse do before the parents decide whether to start their son on androgen therapy?

The decision is made to prescribe methyltestosterone 5 mg/d by buccal tablet (held inside the cheek until it dissolves). MT will be on this regimen for 4 months, during which time he is to come to the clinic at monthly intervals.

4. MT asks why he will be treated for 4 months. What will the nurse reply?
5. About what adverse effects do MT and his parents need to be taught?
6. What physical and psychosocial parameters will be monitored at his monthly visits?
7. What special hygiene needs does MT have while on this regimen?
8. When should he have radiographs taken? Why?
9. During a clinical visit, MT mentions that he has heard that the use of anabolic steroids might improve his chances of making the wrestling team. What should he be told about the safety and efficacy of anabolic steroid use?

AJ is a 70-year-old Hispanic man who came into the urgent care clinic complaining of being unable to empty his bladder. He has noticed over the past few months that he has had to get up two or three times during the night to urinate; sometimes he dribbles urine after he finishes urinat-

ing. He also mentions that his "plumbing isn't what it used to be" but does not seem to want to discuss it. He asks whether a male doctor is on duty today.

1. When interviewing this client, what should be the focus of the assessment?
2. How would you explain his symptoms to him?
3. What are some of the age and cultural issues affecting this client's ability to communicate?
4. What laboratory tests would be appropriate for this client?
5. What are some of the drug options available to AJ?

NCLEX Study Questions

1. Which of the following is the primary reason a male should take androgens?
   a. Hypogonadism
   b. Short stature
   c. Undescended testis
   d. Impotence

2. Common side effects associated with the use of medications used to treat benign prostatic hypertrophy (BPH) include:
   a. increased libido and hypertension
   b. hypertension and dizziness
   c. hypotension and dizziness
   d. decreased libido and urinary retention

3. What are some of the common symptoms of an enlarged prostate?
   a. Constipation
   b. Urinary frequency and nocturia
   c. Lower leg edema
   d. Abdominal pain

4. Which of the following is not a symptom of hypercalcemia?
   a. Nausea and vomiting
   b. Hypertension
   c. Polyuria
   d. Decreased mental status

5. Which of the following is a reason a woman would be prescribed androgens?
   a. To treat baldness
   b. To treat breast cancer
   c. To raise blood pressure
   d. To decrease cholesterol

6. Phosphodiesterase (PDE) inhibitors are drugs which facilitate erections by:
   a. increasing blood pressure
   b. shrinking the prostate gland
   c. increasing blood flow to the penis
   d. increasing libido

57

Drugs for Infertility and Sexually Transmitted Diseases

Sandra Elliott

ELECTRONIC RESOURCES

evolve

Evolve website (http://evolve.elsevier.com/KeeHayes/pharmacology/):
- Case Studies
- Content Updates
- Frequently Asked Questions
- Student Review Activities
- WebLinks
- Additional Reference Material

Companion CD-ROM:
- NCLEX Examination Review Questions
- Pharmacology Animations
- IV Therapy Checklists
- Medication Error Checklists
- Drug Calculation Problems
- Electronic Calculators
- Top 200 Drugs with Pronunciations
- References from the Textbook

Outline

Objectives

- Describe male, female, and couple causes of infertility.
- Instruct couples on the relationships among ovulatory stimulation therapy, fertility awareness, and timing of coitus.
- Describe the way in which ovulatory stimulants promote fertility.
- Describe clients at risk for acquiring sexually transmitted diseases (STDs).
- Describe the relationship between STDs and infertility.
- Instruct clients in regimens for common STDs.
- Plan management for STDs for which cures do not exist.
- Counsel health care workers about management of worksite exposure to blood-borne STDs.
- Describe the nursing process, including client teaching, related to drugs used for infertility and STDs.

Terms

This chapter discusses drug regimens for two broad categories of reproductive health alterations that are often interrelated: infertility and sexually transmitted diseases (STDs). Alterations in fertility reflect a wide range of developmental, endocrine, infectious, inflammatory, hypertrophic, and psychoemotional processes. Drug therapies used in the management of female and, briefly, male infertility are addressed, with emphasis on ovulation stimulants.

The broad category of diseases that are sexually transmitted constitutes a threat to reproductive tract integrity and functioning, as well as to neonatal health. Some STDs, such as the human immunodeficiency virus (HIV), are life-threatening in and of themselves. Drug therapies for these conditions are briefly reviewed.

Drugs Related to Infertility Treatment

Infertility is defined as the inability to conceive a child after 12 months of unprotected sexual intercourse. Women older than 35 years of age may be considered infertile after a shorter trial. Infertility is considered **primary infertility** if a couple has never conceived or has never carried a pregnancy to term. **Secondary infertility** affects couples who have conceived and carried a pregnancy to term, resulting in a live birth, but are unable to conceive after this. Approximately 10% to 15% of couples in the United States experience infertility. Most of infertility is age related.

Most pharmacologic approaches today are **ovulation-inducing agents**; that is, they stimulate the maturation and release of eggs.

Assessing Infertility

Causes of infertility (Table 57–1) are numerous. In about 15% of cases, no specific cause can be found. Up to 40% of cases are the result of STDs, which may result in neonatal death or altered reproductive tract integrity. Treatment of infertility depends on assessment of the cause.

General health is assessed; nutritional, reproductive, social drugs, and sexual histories are taken; and physical examinations with routine laboratory tests are conducted on both partners. Common tests to determine the specific causes of infertility are listed in Table 57–2.

Induction of Ovulation

Clomiphene citrate (Serophene, Clomid), an estrogen antagonist, blocks the negative hypothalamic-pituitary-gonadal feedback loop. The feedback mechanism is altered as clomiphene binds to estrogen receptors, resulting in increased gonadotropin-releasing hormone (Gn-RH) release and then increased luteinizing hormone (LH) and follicle-stimulating hormone (FSH) output. It is the most commonly used ovulation stimulant (Prototype Drug Chart 57–1). Some women may need concurrent treatment of hyperinsulinemia. Women with high circulatory androgens may be concurrently treated with dexamethasone.

Recombinant FSH, LH, and human chorionic gonadotropin (hCG) are now available to normalize hormone

Table 57–1
Causes of Infertility

Female Factors	
Genetic	Chromosomal abnormalities, enzyme defects
Tubal or peritoneal	Infection, occlusion, fimbrial damage, pelvic adhesions, endometriosis
Ovarian	Anovulation, oligoovulation, inadequate luteal phase, polycystic ovarian syndrome (PCOS)
Cervical	Cervicitis, poor-quality cervical mucus, diethylstilbestrol exposure
Uterine	Uterine fibromas, congenital malformations, adhesions, endometrial abnormalities
Endocrine	Panhypopituitarism, hypothyroidism, adrenal insufficiency, congenital adrenal hyperplasia, Cushing disease, cirrhosis, hyperprolactinemia, hormone receptor defects
Other	Age, drugs, malnutrition, excess alcohol intake, tobacco use
Male Factors	
Genetic	Chromosomal genetic abnormalities
Seminal	Failure of semen to liquefy, inadequate volume, low sperm count, decreased or erratic sperm motility, sperm dysmorphology, varicocele
Transport	Hypospadias, micropenis, retrograde ejaculation, epididymitis, impotence, ductal occlusion, ductal adhesions
Testicular	Oligospermia/azoospermia, cryptorchism, testicular agenesis, history of high fever, postpubertal orchitis, testicular injury/surgery, varicocele
Endocrine	Panhypopituitarism, hypothyroidism, adrenal insufficiency, congenital adrenal hyperplasia, Cushing disease, cirrhosis, hormone receptor abnormalities
Other	Age, drugs, excess alcohol intake, tobacco use, pollution, malnutrition, scrotal heat exposure, autoimmunity to sperm, infectious processes, allergies
Couple Factors	Sexual technique, frequency or timing of intercourse, immune response to sperm

Table 57–2

Common Tests for Infertility

Test	Purpose
Physical examination	Assess secondary sex characteristics, reproductive tract function, and patency by gross examination
Hematology, liver and renal function	Rule out disease processes
Hysterosalpingogram, tubal insufflation	Evaluate fallopian tube patency
Cervical mucus test	Assess viscosity of mucus and its effect on sperm motility
Plasma progesterone	Assess function of corpus luteum
Endometrial biopsy	Assess ovulatory status or adequacy of corpus luteum
Semen analysis	Check number, structure, movement of sperm
Basal body temperature	Determine whether ovulation occurs; document temperatures daily in chart
Sperm penetration assay	Determine ability of sperm to penetrate and fertilize ovum
Laparoscopy	Visualize female pelvic organs
Hysteroscopy	Visualize uterus
Echohysteroscopy	Assess structure of woman's internal reproductive organs
Hormone assays	Gn-RH, FSH, LH, progesterone, estrogen, prolactin, testosterone, thyroid hormone levels
Immunologic testing	Assess cervical immunity against sperm, seminal fluid immunity against sperm, serum antisperm antibodies in either partner
Imaging	Pituitary integrity

FSH, Follicle-stimulating hormone; *Gn-RH,* gonadotropin-releasing hormone; *LH,* luteinizing hormone.

Prototype DRUG CHART 57–1

CLOMIPHENE CITRATE

Drug Class	**Dosage**
Ovulation stimulant Trade names: Clomid, Serophene *Pregnancy Category:* X	**A: PO:** 50-100 mg/d for days 5-9 of cycle If ovulation does not occur with 50 mg/d, increase next course to 100 mg/d.
Contraindications	**Drug-Lab-Food Interactions**
Pregnancy, undiagnosed vaginal bleeding, depression, fibroids, hepatic dysfunction, thrombophlebitis, primary pituitary or ovarian failure	***Drug:*** None are significant; danazol may inhibit response; *decrease* effects of ethinyl estradiol ***Lab:*** *Increase* in serum thyroxine
Pharmacokinetics	**Pharmacodynamics**
Absorption: Readily absorbed from GI tract **Distribution:** PB: UK **Metabolism:** t½: 5-8 d **Excretion:** In feces	**PO:** Onset: 5-14 d Peak: UK Duration: UK

Therapeutic Effects/Uses

To stimulate ovarian follicle growth
Mode of Action: Stimulates release of follicle-stimulating hormone (FSH) and luteinizing hormone (LH)

Side Effects	**Adverse Reactions**
Breast discomfort, fatigue, dizziness, depression, anxiety, nausea, vomiting, constipation, increased appetite, headache, flatulence, multiple gestation, hot flashes, fluid retention	Visual disturbances, abdominal pain, weight gain, hair loss, ovarian hyperstimulation, anxiety, ovarian cysts, ectopic pregnancy

A, Adult; *d,* day; *GI,* gastrointestinal; *PB,* protein-binding; *PO,* by mouth; *t½,* half-life; *UK,* unknown.

levels with minimal adverse effects (Table 57–3). These drugs normalize FSH and LH levels to stimulate follicle maturation, ovulation, and development of the corpus luteum. The replacement of FSH or LH is enhanced in a few women by the use of leuprolide acetate before the administration of hCG and in other women by the use of a Gn-RH agonist such as progesterone after ovulation. In a small percentage of amenorrheic women, an elevated level of prolactin is the causative factor. A portion of these women can be treated with the ergot derivative bromocriptine (taken 2.5 mg twice daily). Bromocriptine binds to dopamine receptors in the pituitary and inhibits prolactin secretion; treatment continues until pregnancy is confirmed. Clomiphene can be introduced if needed after 2 months.

Pharmacokinetics

Data on the pharmacokinetics of clomiphene citrate are limited, but clomiphene is readily absorbed from the gastrointestinal (GI) tract. It is partially metabolized in the liver and excreted in the feces via biliary elimination. Clomiphene has a half-life of about 5 days.

Pharmacodynamics

The mechanism of action of clomiphene is unknown, but it is hypothesized that it competes with estrogen at receptor sites. The perception of decreased circulating estrogen by the hypothalamus and pituitary triggers the negative feedback response that increases the secretion of FSH and LH. The results are ovarian stimulation, maturation of the ovarian follicle, and development of the corpus luteum.

Side Effects

Side effects of clomiphene citrate include breast discomfort, fatigue, dizziness, depression, nausea, vomiting, increased appetite, weight gain, dermatitis, urticaria, anxiety, restlessness, weakness, heavier menses, vasomotor flushing, abdominal bloating or pain, and gas. Antiestrogenic effects include interference with endometrial maturation and cervical mucus production. Paradoxically this may interfere with fertilization or implantation.

Adverse Reactions

Adverse reactions include photophobia, mastalgia, diplopia, and decreased visual acuity. Ovarian hyperstimulation may result in ovarian enlargement, midcycle ovarian pain, and cysts. Reversible hair loss has been noted. Multiple gestation occurs in up to 12% of women who become pregnant. The effect of clomiphene citrate on fetal development is unclear. Neural tube defects have been reported but not confirmed by controlled studies. Adverse reactions of other ovulatory stimulants are listed in Table 57–4.

Contraindications

Contraindications for treatment with clomiphene citrate include undiagnosed vaginal bleeding, pregnancy, uterine fibroids, clinical depression, history of hepatic dysfunction or thromboembolic disease, and primary pituitary or ovarian failure. If the woman has ovarian cysts, clomiphene citrate may cause them to enlarge. Contraindications to the use of other ovulatory stimulants are listed in Table 57–4.

Drug Interactions

There are no known significant drug interactions with clomiphene citrate. Danazol may inhibit client response to clomiphene citrate, and clomiphene citrate may suppress response to ethinyl estradiol. There are no known drug interactions with human menopausal gonadotropin (hMG) or hCG.

Other Drug Treatments

Other pharmacologic approaches for the treatment of women with infertility include the use of pulsatile exogenous Gn-RH. In addition, hypothyroidism or hyperthyroidism and adrenal dysfunction must be treated. Endometriosis can be treated with a course of danazol to suppress gonadotropin output. Women with inadequate luteal-phase progesterone output are treated with progesterone 25 mg twice daily intravaginally or 12.5 mg intramuscularly (IM).

Table 57–3

Ovulatory Stimulants

Generic (Brand)	Route and Dosage	Use and Considerations
bromocriptine mesylate (Parlodel)	Up to 7.5 mg/d in divided doses	Normalizes prolactin levels. Possibly teratogenic. *Pregnancy category:* C; PB: 92%; t$^{1}/_{2}$: 50 h
clomiphene citrate (Clomid, Serophene)	(Prototype Drug Chart 57–1)	
Gn-RH	1-10 mcg/60-120 min via pump	Induces ovulation in women with hypothalamic amenorrhea. Ovarian hyperstimulation is a risk. Pregnancy loss is common. *Pregnancy category:* X; PB: UK; t$^{1}/_{2}$: 11-23 h
recombinant FSH (Puregon, Gonal-f, Follistim), recombinant LH (LHadi, Luveris), recombinant hCG (Ovidrel)	IM: 1-2 ampules/d × 5-12 d until follicle maturation; next day, CG (5000-10,000 international units IM) administered	Ovarian hyperstimulation remains a risk, though minimal, with recombinant products. Multiple gestation is a risk, which is reduced by careful monitoring. PB: UK; t$^{1}/_{2}$: 23-77 h IM, 13-35 h subQ

d, Day; *FSH*, follicle-stimulating hormone; *Gn-RH*, gonadotropin-releasing hormone; *h*, hour; *hCG*, human chorionic gonadotropin; *IM*, intramuscular; *LH*, luteinizing hormone; *min*, minute; *PB*, protein-binding; *subQ*, subcutaneous; *t$^{1}/_{2}$*, half-life; *UK*, unknown.

Table 57–4

Side Effects, Adverse Reactions, and Contraindications for Selected Infertility Drugs

Side Effects	Adverse Reactions	Contraindications
Human Chorionic Gonadotropin		
Headache, irritability, restlessness, fatigue, depression, fluid retention, pain at injection site	Ovarian hyperstimulation syndrome, rupture of ovarian cysts, multiple births, arterial thromboembolism	Androgen-dependent neoplasms. Caution in clients with asthma, cardiac or renal disease, epilepsy, migraine
Bromocriptine Mesylate		
Nausea, vomiting, headache, dizziness, drowsiness, fatigue, lightheadedness, nasal congestion, diarrhea, insomnia, depression	Confusion, visual disturbances, vertigo, shortness of breath, abdominal discomfort, involuntary movements, hypotension, anxiety, dysphagia, paresthesia, blepharospasm, mottling, urinary frequency, epileptiform seizures, ergotism	
Transient elevations in BUN, SGOT, SGPT, creatine phosphokinase, alkaline phosphatase, serum uric acid	Ischemic heart disease, peripheral vascular disease, pregnancy, lactation, ergot nervousness, sensitivity. Caution in hypotension, epilepsy, psychoses, cardiac arrhythmia, impaired hepatic or renal function	

BUN, Blood urea nitrogen; *SGOT,* serum glutamic-oxaloacetic transaminase; *SGPT,* serum glutamate pyruvate transaminase.

Drug Therapy for Male Infertility

For most infertile men, no specific causal factor can be identified. These clients are identified as having idiopathic oligospermia and asthenospermia. There is no documented cost-effective treatment for this large group of men. Most drug regimens used have shown little promise in controlled studies, with the exception of using testosterone (or other hormonal) therapy to attain physiologic levels. Assisted reproductive techniques currently appear to hold more promise than drug therapy. Some surgical techniques, such as removal of a varicocele, can sometimes improve male infertility. Intrauterine insemination and in-vitro fertilization (IVF) are beyond the scope of this chapter. Some herbal products contribute to male infertility problems (Herbal Alert 57–1).

Herbal ALERT 57–1

Herbs and Male Infertility
- *Saw palmetto* may cause metabolic changes in the sperm.
- *St. John's wort* may cause effects on sperm cells, decreased sperm motility, and decreased viability.

Nursing Process

Infertility

- Infertility management is a highly specialized field. Nurses are most likely to encounter clients when they are in the process of trying to identify the possible causes of their infertility. Nurses need to be sensitive to the grief, guilt, decreased self-esteem, and embarrassment that infertility may cause. Treatment of infertility requires that the health care team direct a couple's sexual life. Evaluation and intervention are often uncomfortable and expensive, and there is no guarantee that a viable pregnancy will result. The process drains the couple emotionally and economically.

ASSESSMENT

- A general health history, including documenting drug and herbal product use, and physical examination are required. Clients' reproductive and sexual histories are assessed, with attention to the timing and technique of coitus. A couple's mental health status should also be assessed, with a referral to a support group or counseling as needed. Infertility can be very isolating, because many couples may have several peers who are already pregnant or who already have children.
- The couple undergoes an exhaustive battery of diagnostic tests to evaluate the cause of infertility. Once this is determined, conditions that contraindicate the treatment of choice are ruled out.
- It is particularly important that the couple's interpretation of their infertility be explored, along with its impact on their relationship. The nurse should help the couple discuss their feelings in a safe, supportive environment.

NURSING DIAGNOSES

- Ineffective sexuality pattern related to infertility
- Disturbed body image related to infertility

- Situational low self-esteem related to infertility
- Deficient knowledge related to treatment regimen
- Anxiety related to infertility
- Powerlessness related to infertility
- Social isolation related to infertility
- Grieving related to the loss of the dream to have one's biological child.

PLANNING

- Short-term goals include clients' adherence to the medical regimen with minimal adverse effects.
- The long-term goal is the achievement of pregnancy or the consideration of alternatives to pregnancy with the partners' self-esteem and relationship intact.

NURSING INTERVENTIONS

General

- Interventions are aimed at helping clients understand the interrelationships among and timing of menses, ovulation, and coitus as they relate to conception. Couples need to know sexual techniques that enhance fertilization, such as the placement of a pillow under the woman's hips during coitus and the placement of the woman in a supine position with the hips elevated for about 30 minutes after her partner ejaculates. In addition, clients and their partners need to understand the treatment regimen.

Specific

- Female client is taught to report adverse effects such as abdominal pain or visual disturbances to her infertility specialist at once and to be cautious with tasks that require alertness. If she misses a dose of her medication, she should call her infertility specialist.
- Clients need to understand that treatment increases the chance of multiple births.

Client Teaching

- Couples need to be taught how to evaluate and record on a chart the basal body temperature and changes in the cervical mucus. The first day of menses is day 1 of the cycle. Ovulation is predicted by a 0.5° F drop in basal body temperature followed by a 1° F rise. In addition, over-the-counter diagnostic kits for assessing ovulatory status can be used to time coitus. The couple is advised to engage in coitus no more frequently than every other day from 4 days before to 3 days after ovulation to maximize the man's sperm count (Figure 57–1).
- The man is advised to wear boxer shorts during infertility treatment, because briefs hold the scrotum close to the body and the heat reduces sperm count. For the same reason, if he is seated all day in his work, he is counseled to take breaks every hour or so to walk about. Some women have conceived by taking guaifenesin (Robitussin), because it thins cervical mucus.
- The man is advised to avoid the use of certain herbs that impact sperm production (see Herbal Alert 57–1).
- The woman is advised to take her medication at the same time each day to maintain steady blood levels.

Cultural Considerations ❖

- The Catholic Church does not support the use of reproductive technologies. Many Catholic couples may opt instead for adoption or suffer additional anxiety if they go against the Church's teachings.
- Because of their modesty, many Chinese, Filipino and Muslim women will only be examined by a female health care provider. Individuals frequently combine traditional Chinese medicine with western medicine.
- Amish view pregnancy (and the anticipated baby) as a gift from God and want to have many gifts. They may be reluctant to seek help for infertility, especially to go to a health care provider "outside the community." They often use herbal remedies and folk practices.
- Use an interpreter as appropriate; one of the same gender and culture is preferred for sensitive topics.
- In male-dominated cultures, the male may be unwilling to undergo an infertility evaluation, because it is seen only as a female problem.

EVALUATION

- Successful outcomes of fertility treatment include avoidance of ovarian hyperstimulation as well as other untoward effects. The achievement of pregnancy that results in the birth of a live infant fulfills the objectives of treatment. If pregnancy is not achieved, intervention is aimed at helping the couple consider alternatives to childbearing without adverse impact on their self-esteem or harm to their relationship.

Drugs Used in the Treatment of Sexually Transmitted Diseases

Sexually transmitted diseases (STDs) are infections that are transmitted during sexual contact. Some pathogens are spread primarily through sexual contact. Others, such as *Shigella*, hepatitis A, or *Candida*, are transmitted primarily by other ways but can also be spread sexually. Pathogens implicated in STDs are listed in Table 57–5. Depending on the causative organism, STDs may be localized in lesions of the skin or mucosa. They may spread upward through the reproductive tract, resulting in **pelvic inflammatory disease (PID)** (infection of the uterus, fallopian tubes, and adjacent structures of the pelvic area usually caused by ascending infection) or **endometritis** (intrauterine infection) in women or in **prostatitis** (infection of the prostate), **epididymitis** (infection of the epididymis), or **orchitis** (infection of the testicles) in men. Finally, blood and

1. Purchase a special thermometer calibrated in tenths of degrees between 96° and 100° F.
2. Place the thermometer under the tongue for at least a full 3 minutes (preferably 5 minutes) after waking in the morning and before *any* activity (e.g., lifting your head off the pillow, shaking thermometer down, intercourse, or urinating) **or before you eat or drink anything.**
3. If you forget to take your temperature and have already gotten up, *do not take it.* Write *missed* on that day.
4. Take your temperature in the same manner about the same time each day.
5. Carefully record the reading on the graph by placing a dot at the proper location. Start this chart on the first day of your period.
6. Insert the month and day in the space provided.
7. The first day of menstrual flow is considered to be the start of a cycle (day 1). Each day of flow should be indicated with an M on the graph, starting at extreme left under number 1 day of cycle.
8. Record any obvious reason for temperature variation such as a cold, flu, or infection on the graph above the reading for that day.
9. If you are placed on medication, please indicate it in the space labeled medications on the days you take it.
10. If you feel you have menstrually related symptoms, such as breast tenderness or cramping, note these also.
11. If intercourse has taken place during the previous 24 hours, mark it with an (X).

Calendar for Thermal Method of Fertility Awareness

Day of Cycle: 1 2 3 4 5 6 7 8 9 10 11 12 13 14 15 16 17 18 19 20 21 22 23 24 25 26 27 28 29 30 31

Temperature
99.0
98.8
98.6
98.4
98.2
98.0
97.8
97.6
97.4
97.2
97.0

Menses (M):
Intercourse (X):

Mucus
   Color
   Consistency
   Amount

Other factors
   Medications
   Breast tenderness
   Cramps

FIGURE 57–1 Instructions for keeping a symptothermal record. (Adapted from Fogel CI, Lauver D: *Sexual health promotion,* Philadelphia, 1990, Saunders.)

Table 57–5

Pathogens Causing Sexually Transmitted Diseases

	Mode of Transmission		
Pathogen	**Predominantly Sexual**	**Can Be Sexual**	**Sexual Contact with Oral-Fecal Exposure**
Bacteria	*Calymmatobacterium granulomatis*	*Escherichia coli*	*Shigella*
	Chlamydia trachomatis	*Gardnerella vaginalis*	*Campylobacter*
	Haemophilus ducreyi	Other vaginal bacteria	
	Neisseria gonorrhoeae	Group B streptococcus	
	Treponema pallidum	*Mycoplasma hominis*	
	Ureaplasma urealyticum		
Viruses	Cytomegalovirus	Human T-lymphotrophic virus-1	HIV-1, HIV-2
	Hepatitis B	Herpes simplex virus type 1	Hepatitis C, D
	Herpes simplex virus type 2	Epstein-Barr virus	Hepatitis A
	Human papillomavirus		
	Molluscum contagiosum virus		
Protozoa, fungi, ectoparasites	*Trichomonas vaginalis*	*Candida albicans*	*Giardia lamblia*
	Phthirus pubis		*Entamoeba histolytica*
	Sarcoptes scabiei		

HIV, Human immunodeficiency virus.

secretions may spread STDs. If not treated, STDs can result in (1) damage to the male and female reproductive tracts, thus impairing fertility; (2) life-threatening illness and death; and (3) neonatal illness and death. The past 30 years have seen a dramatic increase in this problem. The emergence of STDs that are incurable or lethal in adults, such as genital herpes and HIV infection, has led to growing awareness of the seriousness of STDs, even in affluent, industrialized countries. Several infections, including those caused by HIV, human papillomavirus (HPV), human T-lymphotrophic virus, and Epstein-Barr virus, are associated with malignancies. *Chlamydia trachomatis* has been linked to increased risk for heart disease and cervical cancer. The human papillomavirus may also lead to cancer of the cervix, vulva, vagina, anus, or penis.

Transmission and Risk

Sexual transmission of pathogens can occur through breaks in the vaginal or cervical mucosa or the skin covering the shaft or glans of the penis. Each act of coitus results in tiny, friction-induced fissures on these surfaces. The problem is exacerbated by inadequate vaginal lubrication, which may occur after menopause, postpartum, just following menses, or when the woman is not sufficiently aroused before penetration.

Semen, sperm cells themselves, vaginal secretions, blood, and other body fluids can carry pathogens. Skin and mucosal lesions cannot only be penetrated by microorganisms but also shed them. Sexual contact can involve skin to skin, mouth to mouth, oral-genital, oral-anal, or hand-anal transmission of pathogens through breaks in the skin or mucosal surfaces or from inoculation by infectious body fluids. Anal penetration is particularly risky because of the likelihood of tissue trauma that results in the partner's exposure to enteric microorganisms.

One practice that places individuals at high risk for the transmission of STDs, particularly HIV, is engaging in sexual activity with multiple partners. Investigators at the National Institutes of Health suggest that the risk of acquiring STDs is markedly increased among individuals who have more than one sexual partner per year versus those who have fewer partners. Other high-risk practices are anal or vaginal intercourse without a condom, hand-anal contact, blood contact during sexual activity during menses, the use of an enema before anal intercourse, and urination on broken skin or inside the body. Risk-reducing behaviors are listed in Box 57–1.

STDs are often manifested as multiple infections. Individuals undergoing treatment for one STD should be assessed for others, including HIV. This is especially true if genital or perianal ulcerations are present.

Vertical transmission, or **perinatal infection**, occurs when a fetus or neonate is infected by the mother. Microbes can travel up the reproductive tract from the vagina or cervix and enter the intrauterine environment. Organisms that are of little consequence to healthy adults can be

---

Box 57–1

Risk-Reducing Behaviors for Avoidance of STDs

- Sexual abstinence or sexual contact with one faithful partner
- Consistently and correctly using a condom
- Washing and urinating before and after intercourse
- Avoiding sex with someone who has genital or anal lesions
- Reducing use of alcohol or drugs, both of which impair judgment about sexual risk and immune response
- Avoiding sexual contact with HIV-infected persons, users of intravenous drugs, immigrants from high-prevalence regions, or sexual partners of all such individuals
- Never sharing hypodermic needles or razors

---

devastating to a fetus. Transmission can occur through contact with the mother's blood at birth or through breast milk, as in the case of HIV and hepatitis B virus. Many STDs, such as syphilis, are transmitted transplacentally. Others, the herpes simplex virus type 2 (HSV-2) for example, require actual contact by the infant with microorganisms in the birth canal. Because of the risk of blindness caused by *Chlamydia trachomatis* and *Neisseria gonorrhoeae*, erythromycin is routinely used to treat the eyes of neonates.

Common STD syndromes and their causative pathogens are listed in Table 57–6. Current guidelines from the Centers for Disease Control and Prevention (CDC) for the primary treatment of various STDs are listed in Table 57–7. All sexual contacts of an infected individual should be informed of their exposure so they can be treated. Partners should refrain from sexual activity until each is clear of infection on follow-up evaluation or, at the very least, condoms should be used.

HIV Disease

Chapter 34 is devoted to the presentation of drugs used to treat HIV and acquired immunodeficiency syndrome (AIDS). These conditions involve the immune system and can be transmitted by means other than sexual contact.

Human Papillomavirus (HPV)

Gardasil is a vaccine indicated in girls and women ages 9 to 26 for the prevention of cervical cancer and genital warts caused by the human papillomavirus (HPV) Types 6, 11, 16, and 18. Gardasil should be administered in 3 separate intramuscular injections in the upper arm over a 6 month period with the first dose at an elected date, the second dose 2 months after the first dose, and the third dose 6 months after the first dose. Gardasil does not substitute for routine cancer screening, and women who receive Gardasil should continue to undergo screening per standard of care.

Table 57–6

Common Sexually Transmitted Disease Syndromes and Their Causative Pathogens

Syndrome	Pathogens
Acute arthritis	*Neisseria gonorrhoeae, Chlamydia trachomatis,* hepatitis B virus (HBV), human immunodeficiency virus (HIV)
Acquired immunodeficiency virus	HIV-1, HIV-2, and opportunistic pathogens
Cervicitis	*C. trachomatis, N. gonorrhoeae,* herpes simplex virus (HSV), *Candida albicans*
Cystitis, urethritis (female)	Gram-negative bacilli, gram-positive cocci, *C. trachomatis, N. gonorrhoeae*
Epididymitis	*C. trachomatis, N. gonorrhoeae*
Genital, anal warts	Human papillomavirus (HPV)
Lymphadenopathy	Cytomegalovirus (CMV), HIV, Epstein-Barr virus (EBV)
Neoplasias	HPV
Squamous cell cancers of cervix, anus, vulva, penis; Kaposi sarcoma; lymphoid neoplasia, hepatocellular carcinoma	HIV, EBV
HIV, human T-lymphotrophic virus (HTLV-1)	
Pelvic inflammatory disease	*Trichomonas vaginalis, N. gonorrhoeae, C. trachomatis, Bacteroides* spp, *Peptostreptococcus, Escherichia coli,* streptococci groups B and D, bacterial vaginitis-associated pathogens
Proctitis, proctocolitis or enterocolitis, enteritis	*N. gonorrhoeae,* HSV, *C. trachomatis, Treponema pallidum, Giardia lamblia, Campylobacter* spp, *Shigella* spp, *Entamoeba histolytica, Mycobacterium avium-intracellulare, Salmonella* spp, *Cryptosporidium, Isospora* (ingestion of intestinal flora)
Pubic lice	*Phthirus pubis*
Scabies	*Sarcoptes scabiei*
Ulcerative lesions of the genitalia	HSV-1, HSV-2, *T. pallidum, C. trachomatis, Calymmatobacterium granulomatis,* HPV, *Haemophilus ducreyi,* molluscum contagiosum virus
Urethritis, male	*N. gonorrhoeae, C. trachomatis, T. vaginalis,* HSV, *Ureaplasma urealyticum, Mycoplasma hominis, Bacteroides urealyticum*
Vulvovaginitis	Bacterial vaginosis: *Gardnerella vaginitis (Haemophilus vaginalis), M. hominis, U. urealyticum, Mobiluncus curtisii, Mobiluncus mulieris, Bacteroides* spp, *Peptostreptococcus, T. vaginalis, C. albicans, Torulopsis glabrata*

Table 57–7

Current Guidelines for Primary Therapies for Common Sexually Transmitted Diseases

Disease	Primary Therapy	Notes
Acute urethral syndrome	doxycycline 100 mg PO b.i.d. × 7 d *or* sulfamethoxazole 1.6 g *plus* trimethoprim 320 mg PO single dose	
Bacterial vaginosis	metronidazole 500 mg PO b.i.d. × 7 d *or* 2 g PO single dose *or* vaginal gel b.i.d. × 5 d	Avoid alcohol during therapy; contraindicated in pregnancy
Candidiasis	fluconazole 150 mg PO × 1 dose *or* miconazole nitrate 200 mg vaginal suppository qhs × 3 d *or* miconazole nitrate 2% vaginal cream, 5 g, qhs × 3 d *or* clotrimazole 200 mg, vaginal suppository, daily × 3 d	Recurrent candidiasis may be indicative of other disease, such as diabetes or HIV infection
Chancroid	azithromycin 1 g PO × 1 dose *or* ceftriaxone 250 mg IM × 1 *or* erythromycin base 500 mg PO q.i.d. × 7 d	Use compresses to remove necrotic material; clean ulcerative lesions t.i.d.
Chlamydia	A: doxycycline 100 mg PO b.i.d. × 7-10 d *or* azithromycin 1 g PO × 1	
	C: <45 kg: erythromycin 50 mg/kg/d PO divided in 4 doses × 10-14 d	
	C: >45 kg: erythromycin base 500 mg PO q.i.d. × 7 d *or* erythromycin succinate 800 mg PO b.i.d. × 7 d	
	Infants: erythromycin 50 mg/kg/d PO divided into 4 doses × 10-14 d	A second course of therapy may be required

A, Adult; *ACIP,* Advisory Committee on Immunization Practices; *b.i.d.,* twice a day; *C,* child; *CDC,* Centers for Disease Control and Prevention; *d,* day; *GI,* gastrointestinal; *h,* hour; *HAV,* hepatitis A virus; *HBV,* hepatitis B virus; *HCV,* hepatitis C virus; *HIV,* human immunodeficiency virus; *HPV,* human papillomavirus; *IM,* intramuscular; *IUD,* intrauterine device; *IV,* intravenous; *max,* maximum; *min,* minute; *mo,* month; *PO,* by mouth; *qhs,* daily at bedtime; *q.i.d.,* four times a day; *STD,* sexually transmitted disease; *t.i.d.,* three times a day; *wk,* week; *y,* year; >, greater than; <, less than. The most recent guidelines and alternative treatments are available from *www.cdc.gov/STD/treatment/*. *Continued*

Table 57–7

Current Guidelines for Primary Therapies for Common Sexually Transmitted Diseases—cont'd

Disease	Primary Therapy	Notes
Epididymitis	ceftriaxone 250 mg IM × 1 *and* doxycycline 100 mg PO b.i.d. × 10 d *or* ofloxacin 300 mg b.i.d. × 10 d	Treat for gonorrhea, then follow with treatment for nongonococcal urethritis
Genital warts	Cryotherapy *or* cryoprobe *or* podofilox 0.5% solution b.i.d. × 3 d, then 4 days off; repeat cycle × 4 *or* podophyllin 10%-25% in compound tincture of benzoin × 1/wk × 6 wk	Nothing eradicates HPV; podophyllin contraindicated during pregnancy
	Imiquimod 5% cream, applied once daily at bedtime, 3/wk for up to 16 wk. Treatment area should be washed with soap and water 6-10 h after application.	Safety during pregnancy has not been established
Gonorrhea	ceftriaxone 125 mg IM × 1 *or* ceftriaxone 50 mg/kg IM/IV (*max*: 1g) daily × 7d	*Plus* Azithromycin 1 g PO × 1 *or* doxycycline 100 mg PO b.i.d. × 7 *if chlamydia is not ruled out* *Pregnant women*: see complete CDC guidelines Treat for *Chlamydia* as well
	Ophthalmia neonatorum: ceftriaxone 25-50 mg/kg IM/IV × 1 (*max*: 125 mg) *Ophthalmia neonatorum prophylaxis*: silver nitrate (1%) aqueous × 1 *or* erythromycin (0.5%) ophthalmic ointment × 1 *or* tetracycline ophthalmic ointment (1%) × 1	Neonate may also have scalp abscess at site of fetal monitors, rhinitis, anorectal infection
Granuloma inguinale	doxycycline 100 mg PO b.i.d. × 7-28 d *or* erythromycin 500 mg q.i.d. PO × 14 d	
Hepatitis A	No specific therapy exists	Vaccine available. Should be offered to high-risk individuals (men who have sex with men, or injection drug users)
Hepatitis B	HAV and HBV are the two STDs for which a vaccine exists	The CDC recommends vaccination of all infants and adolescents. ACIP recommends vaccination of all persons with recent STD and those with more than one partner in the last 6 mo. A combined hepatitis A and B vaccine has been developed for adults
Hepatitis C	Alpha interferon and oral agent ribavirin may be used to treat HCV chronic liver disease	No vaccine available
Genital herpes simplex	*First episode:* acyclovir 400 mg PO t.i.d. × 7-10 d *or* famciclovir 250 mg PO t.i.d. × 7-10 d *or* valacyclovir 1 g PO b.i.d. × 7-10 d *Recurrent episode:* acyclovir 400 mg PO t.i.d. × 5 d *or* famciclovir 125 mg PO b.i.d. × 5 d *or* valacyclovir 500 mg PO b.i.d. × 3 d or valacyclovir 1 g orally once a day for 5 d *Suppressive therapy:* acyclovir 400 mg PO b.i.d. QD *or* famciclovir 250 mg b.i.d. QD *or* valacyclovir 500 mg PO QD or acyclovir 1 g PO QD *Severe:* acyclovir 5-10 mg/kg IV q8h × 5-7 d *Immunocompromised:* acyclovir 400 mg PO × 3-5/d until resolution *Neonatal:* acyclovir 30 mg/kg/d	Types 1 and 2 cannot be distinguished clinically. No cure is known. Systemic disease is life-threatening to neonates, and neurologic damage may result. Viral shedding is most prevalent when symptomatic; sexual relations should be avoided at that time
Lymphogranuloma venereum	doxycycline 100 mg PO b.i.d. × 21 d *or* erythromycin 0.5 gm PO q.i.d. × 21 d	
Molluscum contagiosum	Cryoanesthesia and curettage *or* caustic chemicals (podophyllin, trichloroacetic acid, silver nitrate) and cryotherapy	If all lesions not eradicated, may recur
Mucopurulent cervicitis	doxycycline 100 mg PO b.i.d. × 7-10 d	

Table 57–7

Current Guidelines for Primary Therapies for Common Sexually Transmitted Diseases—cont'd

Disease	Primary Therapy	Notes
Nongonococcal urethritis	doxycycline 100 mg PO b.i.d. × 7 d *or* erythromycin 500 mg PO q.i.d. × 7 d *or* azithromycin 1 g PO × 1 dose	
Pelvic inflammatory disease (PID)	*Inpatient:* doxycycline 100 mg IV b.i.d. *and* cefoxitin 2 g IV q.i.d. *or* cefotetan 2 g IV q.i.d. *48 h after clinical improvement:* doxycycline 100 mg PO b.i.d. for total of at least 14 d therapy *Ambulatory care:* metronidazole 500 mg b.i.d. × 14 d and ceftriaxone 250 mg IM × 1 *plus* doxycycline 100 mg PO b.i.d. × 14 d	Often polymicrobial. This regimen may not treat anaerobes, pelvic mass, or IUD-associated PID
Proctitis	ceftriaxone 125 mg IM × 1 *and* doxycycline 100 mg PO b.i.d. × 7 d	
Pubic lice	permethrin 1% cream rinse, apply for 10 min	Use lindane only if other therapy fails. Decontaminate clothes and bedding. Second treatment 7-10 d after first to kill newly hatched lice. Treat partner also
Scabies	permethrin cream 5% applied to all affected areas from neck down for 8-14 min *or* lindane 1% applied to all affected areas from neck down for 8 h	
Sexual assault	ceftriaxone 125 mg IM × 1 *and* metronidazole 2 g PO × 1 *and* doxycycline 100 mg PO b.i.d. × 7 d	Tetanus-booster and gamma globulin, as well as baseline HIV testing and follow-up are recommended
Syphilis	*Primary, secondary, or <1 y duration:* benzathine penicillin G, 2.4 million units IM *Unknown duration or >1 y:* benzathine penicillin G, 7.2 million units divided in 2.4 million IM weekly × 3 *Allergic to penicillin:* doxycycline 100 mg PO b.i.d. × 14-28 d *C:* benzathine penicillin G 50,000 units/kg IM × 1, up to 2.4 million units; repeat × 3 if unknown or >1 y duration	Pregnant women who are allergic to penicillin should be desensitized
Trichomoniasis	metronidazole 2 g PO × 1 *or* metronidazole 500 mg PO b.i.d. × 7 d Tindamax (tinidazole tablets); second-generation nitro-imidazole for the treatment of trichomoniasis, giardiasis, amebiasis, and amebic liver abscess; synthetic antiprotozoal agent with a longer half-life than metronidazole and has a lower incidence of GI side effects; should be taken with food, and clients should abstain from drinking alcohol for 72 h following therapy; because trichomoniasis is a sexually transmitted disease with potentially serious sequelae, partners of infected clients should be treated simultaneously to prevent reinfection.	Pregnant women can be treated after the first trimester Tindamax is contraindicated during the first trimester of pregnancy

 Nursing Process

Sexually Transmitted Diseases

■ Nurses need to be sensitive to clients' reasons for seeking or avoiding care for sexually transmitted diseases (STDs). Psychosocial reactions to a diagnosis of an STD may include feelings of anger, depression, shame, guilt, hurt, fear, and concern. Clients need privacy during the interview and examination, with attention to their comfort, such as warming the speculum before a pelvic examination. A second health professional should be present in the examination room during the physical examination of a female client.

ASSESSMENT

■ Before physical data are gathered, a history is elicited. Less sensitive issues are addressed first so that trust can be established. The term "partners" is used when discussing sexual activity rather than value-laden terms such as "wife" or "boyfriend." Include the following questions for all clients, regardless of gender or sexual orientation; "Do you have sex with women?" and "Do you have sex with men?"

■ The history includes the chief complaint, a description of the course of illness, a review of systems and general health history, a reproductive history, a sexual history, a review of lifestyle and social habits, and identification of allergies.

■ Physical examination includes inspection and palpation of the genitalia and other points of inoculation. Men may be allowed to swab themselves for cultures. Gonorrhea and chlamydia may now also be obtained from a urine specimen.

■ Laboratory tests include wet slides with microbe-specific setting agents, urinalysis, cultures, Papanicolaou smear, a complete blood count, syphilis serology, and herpes simplex virus types 1 and 2 antibodies.

NURSING DIAGNOSES

■ Deficient knowledge related to transmission and prevention as well as treatment

■ Noncompliance related to known prevention strategies

■ Pain related to inflammation and infection

■ Situational low self-esteem related to potential stigma of diagnosis

■ Ineffective sexuality patterns related to unsafe safe practices

■ Risk of infection related to unsafe sex practices

■ Medical diagnosis of HIV disease would bring with it these additional nursing diagnoses:

• Fatigue related to diagnosis

• Anxiety related to potential outcome of disease

• Anticipatory grieving related to fear of death

• Risk for loneliness related to possible stigma of diagnosis

• Ineffective therapeutic regimen management/health maintenance related to focus on daily concerns with diagnosis

PLANNING

■ Short-term goals include client's adherence to the treatment regimen and avoidance of adverse effects.

■ Long-term goals include client's return for follow-up evaluation and adoption of risk-reducing sexual behaviors.

NURSING INTERVENTIONS

■ Client needs to understand procedures performed during evaluation and how to administer prescribed medications and treatments. Side effects and adverse reactions that require immediate intervention are reviewed.

■ Specific interventions include providing needed support as client deals with the fact that the infection is sexually transmitted.

■ Client needs to notify sexual partners so they can be evaluated and treated.

■ Ideally, sexual contact is avoided during treatment. At the least, condoms should be used until both partners are shown to be clear of infection.

■ Individuals are scheduled for follow-up visits from 4 days to 4 weeks, depending on the type of infection and treatment.

■ Individuals with any STD are counseled about being tested for HIV infection.

Client Teaching

• The mode of transmission of STDs, the relationship of all STDs with HIV infection, and how HIV risk is avoided should all be reviewed.

• Teach how to use condoms

• Discuss condom negotiation

• Individuals are advised to plan periodic reproductive health check-ups.

Cultural Considerations ❖

• Because of their modesty, many Asian and Middle Eastern women will only be examined by a female health care provider.

• Use an interpreter as appropriate; one of same gender and culture is preferred for sensitive topics.

• In male-dominated cultures, the male may be unwilling to undergo testing or treatment.

EVALUATION

■ Intervention has been successful if the individual's infection is clear on reevaluation or, in the case of viral infections, the individual experiences quiescence of the virus.

■ One important outcome to evaluate is that the infection is not transmitted to other individuals. Another is that the individual is able to avoid sexual practices that carry risk for acquiring STDs, including promiscuity, intercourse without the use of a condom, and traumatic sexual practices.

Summary

Reproductive health and fertility require integrity of hormonal mechanisms and reproductive anatomy. Infertility can be caused by male, female, or couple factors. Often the use of drugs to stimulate ovulation is effective treatment. Clients need to understand the treatment regimen, and they need support in dealing with the psychologic impact of this condition.

Because STDs can threaten reproductive health, neonatal health, fertility, and even life, early diagnosis and treatment are crucial, but less effective than prevention. Numerous opportunistic infections and autoimmune processes complicate HIV and AIDS. For some, drug therapies may offer relief, although ultimately death is the result.

Critical Thinking Case Study

TD married DD, age 32, 3 years ago. DD is the only sexual partner TD has ever had. For the last year they have been trying to conceive without success. DD's nurse practitioner learns when taking DD's history that she had multiple sexual partners while in college and that she was once treated for gonorrhea. DD's menstrual history reveals an erratic pattern of unpredictable periods, about every 2 or 3 months. The nurse practitioner reviews the relationship between timing of coitus and conception, instructs DD to take her temperature each morning before she gets out of bed, and to maintain an ovulation record. She also suggests that a home test kit be used to identify when ovulation has occurred. DD and TD are referred to an infertility specialist.

1. What is the relevance of DD's past sexual history to the current complaint?
2. Why would the infertility specialist consider cultures for *Chlamydia trachomatis* and *Neisseria gonorrhoeae* years after exposure?
3. What other tests would reveal damage resulting from STDs?
4. What is positive about DD's menstrual history? What about her menstrual pattern makes conception difficult?
5. How can DD predict when she will ovulate?

After a complete evaluation of TD and DD, a course of clomiphene citrate is prescribed.

6. What side effects can DD expect?
7. When should DD take the medication?
8. When should TD and DD have sexual intercourse?
9. DD experiences midcycle abdominal pain. What should she do when this occurs? How will her infertility specialist interpret this?
10. DD becomes pregnant after four cycles on clomiphene citrate. What is one potential risk factor with this pregnancy?

DD becomes pregnant and gives birth to a boy following an uneventful pregnancy. The infant has numerous upper respiratory infections during his first 4 months of life—twice requiring hospitalization—and gains weight slowly. When the family is referred to a tertiary pediatric medical center, the medical staff asks DD if she would consider being tested for HIV.

11. What in her history puts DD at risk for HIV infection?

NCLEX Study Questions

1. The relationship between STDs and infertility include all but:
   a. damage to the male and female reproductive tracts
   b. increased risk of ovarian cancer
   c. life threatening illness and death
   d. neonatal illness and death

2. Adverse reactions of clomiphene citrate therapy include all but:
   a. ovarian hyperstimulation
   b. mastalgia
   c. hair growth
   d. weight gain

3. STDs that cannot be cured include all but:
   a. HIV
   b. Gonorrhea
   c. HPV
   d. Epstein Barr

4. STDs that are associated with life-threatening illness include all but:
   a. Syphilis
   b. HIV
   c. HPV
   d. Epstein Barr

5. What best describes why ulcerative STDs place an individual at risk for HIV infection?
   a. Transmission of pathogens are increased by a break in the skin
   b. They are commonly associated with other high-risk behaviors
   c. They are only found in individuals with multiple sexual partners
   d. They decrease the amount of lubrication

Answers: 1, b; 2, a; 3, b; 4, a; 5, a.

NINETEEN

Emergency Agents

This final unit focuses on adult and pediatric emergency drugs. Chapter 58 considers oxygen as an emergency drug and discusses pharmacologic treatment for four categories of emergency situations: (1) cardiac disorders, (2) neurosurgical disorders, (3) shock, and (4) hypertensive crises and pulmonary edema. Specific drug protocols and dosages for the pediatric client are included.

Photo courtesy Christiana Care Health System, Wilmington, Delaware.

58

Adult and Pediatric Emergency Drugs

Linda Laskowski-Jones

ELECTRONIC RESOURCES

Evolve website (http://evolve.elsevier.com/KeeHayes/pharmacology/):
- *Case Studies*
- *Content Updates*
- *Frequently Asked Questions*
- *Student Review Activities*
- *WebLinks*
- *Additional Reference Material*

Companion CD-ROM:
- *NCLEX Examination Review Questions*
- *Pharmacology Animations*
- *IV Therapy Checklists*
- *Medication Error Checklists*
- *Drug Calculation Problems*
- *Electronic Calculators*
- *Top 200 Drugs with Pronunciations*
- *References from the Textbook*

Outline

Objectives

- Describe indications for the emergency drugs listed in this chapter.
- Describe the basic mechanism of action for each emergency drug.
- Discuss pertinent nursing considerations and actions specific for each agent.
- Explain how to administer the drugs properly.
- Describe significant adverse effects of each drug.

Terms

The drugs described in this chapter are first-line agents commonly used to treat various medical emergencies. Nurses must have a ready knowledge of the indications and actions of these agents, because medical and surgical emergencies can occur in virtually any area of nursing practice. Learning key nursing implications *before* a crisis situation enables the nurse to function at the highest possible level when the client requires life-saving intervention.

At the end of each discussion of a group of emergency drugs is a summary prototype drug chart that contains dosages and indications. Common adult doses are listed in the drug charts; pediatric dosages may vary widely depending on the child's age and weight. The drug charts list only the most common indications and dosages for the emergency drugs discussed; they *do not* describe all possible uses and dosing regimens for the agents.

Oxygen as an Emergency Drug

Oxygen can be classified as a drug, because it can have both beneficial and adverse effects on the body based on the amount and manner in which it is administered. Oxygen is essential to life—without it brain death begins within 6 minutes. Inadequate oxygenation produces **hypoxemia** (inadequate oxygen in the blood) and significant physiologic sequelae to all body systems; therefore oxygen is a first-line drug for all emergency situations. Depending on the circumstances, adequate oxygenation may be all that is necessary to effectively treat physiologic disturbances such as chest pain, bradycardia, and cardiac dysrhythmias.

Before the other pharmacologic agents discussed in this chapter are administered, ensure that the client's airway and breathing are addressed to promote optimal oxygenation and ventilation. Giving a drug to treat a disorder brought on by hypoxemia without effectively correcting the cause of the hypoxemia is ineffective and ultimately does not produce the desired outcome. **Pulse oximetry**, which provides a digital display of oxygen saturation, is an essential monitoring tool that should be used in emergency situations to assess the adequacy of oxygenation and guide further interventions. Ideally oxygen saturation should be kept at or above 95%. It is important to recognize, however, that certain pathophysiologic states can make pulse oximetry readings inaccurate. These conditions include vasoconstriction, severe anemia, hypothermia, carbon monoxide poisoning, and shock.

The ambient room air contains approximately 21% oxygen. When clients breathe room air, the oxygen they inspire constitutes 21% of the total volume of gas they take in with each breath. This measure is termed the **fraction of inspired oxygen** (FiO$_2$). As a general rule, clients suffering from severe physiologic stress such as shock states, traumatic injury, acute myocardial infarction (AMI) with hemodynamic instability, and cardiac arrest initially require oxygen in high concentrations (i.e., an FiO$_2$ close to 100%). The oxygen devices of choice for these conditions include a nonrebreather mask with an oxygen reservoir (oxygen flow rate set at 10 to 15 L/min) for spontaneously breathing clients and a bag-valve-mask device attached to an oxygen source at a flow rate of 15 L/min for clients who require assisted ventilation. Although caution must be exercised for clients with chronic obstructive pulmonary disease (COPD), who may lose their hypoxic respiratory drive when given oxygen in high concentration, oxygen should never be denied to a client who needs it. In the case of COPD, the nurse should be prepared to ventilate the client manually with a bag-valve-mask if respiratory depression or arrest occurs. As the client's condition stabilizes, the oxygen concentration should be decreased. An FiO$_2$ above 50% for a prolonged period can lead to oxygen toxicity and other detrimental effects to the pulmonary system in adults and children.

For emergency situations that do not involve severe physiologic stress (e.g., angina, dysrhythmias, pulmonary disease), supplemental oxygen delivered by nasal cannula at 1 to 6 L/min or by simple face mask at 6 to 10 L/min may have significant physiologic benefit. Young children may better tolerate a face tent with a high oxygen flow of 10 to 15 L than a face mask.

Emergency Drugs for Cardiac Disorders

Drugs described in this section are indicated for cardiac emergencies such as angina, MI, disturbances of cardiac rate or rhythm, and cardiac arrest. In a resuscitation situation, the foundation of client therapy is based upon proper oxygenation and ventilation, performance of optimal CPR, and application of electrical therapy (cardioversion and defibrillation) according to established treatment algorithms and standards. Pharmacologic agents are used as adjuncts in synchrony with these efforts when indicated to enhance the likelihood of a successful outcome. These drugs often must be prepared and administered rapidly. A sound knowledge base as well as easy access to the drugs and necessary equipment is essential for the best client response in a cardiac emergency. Usually in an emergency, detailed personal, medical, drug, and herbal histories are unavailable (Herbal Alert 58–1). Treatment is based on client presentation. Drugs for cardiac emergencies are cross-referenced to the specialty chapter.

Nitroglycerin

Nitroglycerin dilates coronary arteries and improves blood flow to an ischemic myocardium. It is therefore the treatment of choice for **angina pectoris** (chest pain) and **myocardial infarction** (heart attack). A focused medication history is essential prior to administration, even in emergency situations, because nitroglycerin in combination with drugs for erectile dysfunction (i.e., sildenafil [Viagra], vardenafil [Levitra], tadalafil [Cialis]) causes profound hypotension when taken within a 24-48 hour period. This combination is contraindicated. Nitroglycerin is available in sublingual, translingual aerosol spray, oral, topical, and intravenous (IV) forms. Only the sublingual, translingual aerosol spray, and intravenous preparations are discussed.

Sublingual nitroglycerin (0.3-0.4 mg) and the translingual aerosol spray (0.4 mg-metered dose) preparations are indicated for clients experiencing an acute anginal attack. The client is taught to sit or lie down and place one sublingual nitroglycerin tablet under the tongue and allow it to dissolve slowly. Not all sublingual nitroglycerin preparations cause a burning sensation under the tongue, so a lack of burning sensation should not be relied on to indicate potency. If the chest pain is not relieved, sublingual nitroglycerin may be repeated at 5-minute intervals until a total of three tablets has been taken. Clients prescribed the translingual aerosol preparation should be reminded that the spray should not be inhaled. Instead, it should be sprayed onto or under the tongue. The client should be instructed not to swallow for approximately 10 seconds to allow absorption of the drug. As with sublingual nitroglycerin, up to three doses may be taken within 15 minutes. If pain persists despite three doses of the sublingual or aerosol forms, further interventions are necessary in an emergency or critical care setting. An ambulance should be called if the client is outside the hospital. Blood pressure and heart rate must be monitored closely. Hypotension is a common adverse effect, especially the first time a client takes nitroglycerin. **Tachycardia** (an abnormally high heart rate, in adults more than 100 beats per minute) or, uncommonly, bradycardia also may occur. Clients who take sublingual or translingual aerosol spray nitroglycerin while wearing a nitroglycerin patch may be at higher risk for hypotension. This situation warrants caution. Though tolerance to nitrates can develop in individuals who take nitroglycerin preparations daily and can offer some protection against hypotension, the nitroglycerin patch may need to be removed if blood pressure instability occurs. To prevent arcing and the potential for skin burns, the nitroglycerin patch must also be removed prior to cardioversion or defibrillation.

IV nitroglycerin is reserved for clients with unstable angina or an AMI. A continuous infusion is usually initiated at a rate of 10 to 20 mcg/min and increased by 5 to 10 mcg/min every 5 to 10 minutes, based on chest pain and blood pressure response. Continuous blood pressure and heart monitoring are required, because hypotension is a common adverse effect. Hypotension usually is treated by reducing or discontinuing the nitroglycerin infusion (see Chapter 41) and by placing the client in a supine position with legs elevated if tolerated.

Morphine Sulfate

Morphine sulfate, a narcotic analgesic, is used to treat the chest pain associated with an AMI. It also is indicated for acute cardiogenic pulmonary edema. Morphine relieves pain, dilates venous vessels, and reduces the workload on the heart. The standard dosage of morphine sulfate is 1 to 4 mg IV over 1 to 5 minutes, repeated every 5 to 30 minutes until chest pain is relieved. Because respiratory depression and hypotension are common adverse effects, the drug must be administered slowly and carefully titrated to achieve the desired therapeutic effects. Close client monitoring is essential. It is important to realize that although morphine can produce respiratory depression, this agent can relieve the dyspnea caused by pulmonary edema. In this situation, respiratory distress is not a contraindication to morphine administration. The narcotic antagonist naloxone (Narcan) may be ordered to reverse the action of morphine if adverse effects pose a significant risk to the client. The dose is 0.4 to 2 mg every 2 minutes as indicated (see Chapter 25).

Atropine Sulfate

Atropine sulfate is indicated in the treatment of hemodynamically significant **bradycardia** (slow heart rate) and some types of **heart block** (e.g., atrioventricular [AV] block at nodal level), as well as asystole and pulseless electrical activity. Atropine acts to increase heart rate by inhibiting the action of the vagus nerve (parasympatholytic effect).

Herbal ALERT 58–1

Herbs and Emergency Medications

In emergency situations a detailed personal health history is often not available; therefore treatment is based on client presentation. Herbal products with anticoagulation properties or those that interact with catecholamines (which may cause hypertensive crisis) could adversely influence the effectiveness of medications used to treat emergency conditions.

Atropine sulfate is also used as an emergency drug to reverse the toxic effects of organophosphate pesticide and nerve agent exposure, which include bradycardia and excessive secretions.

In symptomatic bradycardia, atropine is administered IV in 0.5- to 1-mg doses at 3- to 5-minute intervals until the desired heart rate is achieved or until 0.04 mg/kg (not more than 3 mg) is given. In **asystole** (cardiac arrest), atropine is given as a 1-mg bolus dose IV followed by a 20 ml IV fluid bolus and elevation of the extremity to speed drug delivery during CPR. Dosing in this manner may be repeated every 3 to 5 minutes up to a limit of 0.04 mg/kg (usually not more than 3 mg IV).

It is important to note that the adult IV atropine dose should never be less than 0.5 mg. Doses below 0.5 mg can produce a paradoxical bradycardia; at doses of 0.04 mg/kg or greater, vagal activity is considered completely blocked, and further atropine administration may have no benefit. However, in the case of organophosphate insecticide or nerve agent poisoning, *very high* doses of atropine may be necessary to counteract the pathophysiologic effects of these toxins. Therefore, the typical dosing range and limits do not apply under these circumstances.

If venous access is not available in an emergency situation, atropine sulfate should be administered through the intraosseous (IO) route. As a last resort, atropine may be given via the endotracheal tube (ETT) route if venous or intraosseous access can not be achieved. The dose for endotracheal administration is 2 to 2.5 times the venous dose, diluted with normal saline or sterile water. Accordingly, 2 to 3 mg of atropine would be diluted in 5-10 ml of normal saline or sterile water and instilled deep into the ETT via a feeding tube attached to a syringe. After endotracheal administration, the client should be ventilated vigorously with a bag-valve device to enhance absorption of the drug.

Continuous cardiac and blood pressure monitoring is essential for the client who receives atropine sulfate. Significant adverse effects include cardiac dysrhythmias, tachycardia, myocardial ischemia, restlessness, anxiety, mydriasis, thirst, and urinary retention. Chapter 18 has a full discussion of atropine and other anticholinergics.

Pediatric Implications

The definition of bradycardia is variable and age-specific for the pediatric population. Knowledge of normal ranges is essential. Because cardiac output is dependent on heart rate in infants younger than 6 months, bradycardia (heart rate <100 beats per minute [beats/min] for infants) must be treated. In fact a heart rate <60 beats/min in an infant requires performance of CPR. Before administration of drugs, efforts always should be targeted first toward restoring adequate ventilation and oxygenation. For the neonate in cardiac arrest or with a spontaneous heart rate of less than 80 beats/min, epinephrine 0.01 to 0.03 mg/kg IV or IO every 3 to 5 minutes as indicated should be given prior to atropine to elevate the heart rate, because stressed neo-

nates quickly deplete their own stores of catecholamines If these interventions do not produce the desired clinical response, then atropine is indicated in the presence of increased vagal tone or AV block.

The pediatric dose of atropine is 0.02 mg/kg IV or IO. It is important to be cognizant that the minimum single pediatric dose is 0.1 mg and the maximum single child dose is 0.5 mg IV. The maximum total pediatric dose is 1 mg in a child and 2 mg in an adolescent. Consult Chapter 10 for more information on pediatric medication dosing and monitoring.

Isoproterenol

Isoproterenol is a beta-adrenergic drug given to increase the heart rate. Because of the potential for significant deleterious effects, an infusion of isoproterenol is only initiated as a temporary measure while awaiting the availability of a transcutaneous pacemaker after the maximum dose of atropine (3 mg) has been given to clients with refractory hemodynamically significant bradycardia. It may also be administered to treat bradycardia in clients with beta-blocker poisoning or after a heart transplant. Because the transplanted heart is denervated, atropine will be ineffective in the treatment of bradycardia.

Isoproterenol is administered as an IV infusion, generally 1 mg diluted in 250 ml of 5% dextrose in water or normal saline, at 2 to 10 mcg/min titrated to heart rate (usually 60 beats/min). An electronic infusion device must be used to provide precise infusion control.

Myocardial oxygen consumption is greatly increased with isoproterenol administration; therefore the nurse must carefully monitor the client receiving isoproterenol. Significant adverse effects include myocardial ischemia, tachycardia, and life-threatening dysrhythmias such as ventricular tachycardia and ventricular fibrillation. The nurse should alert the physician promptly if any increase in premature ventricular contractions is noted on the cardiac monitor or if the heart rate exceeds 100 beats/min, because the dosage may need to be decreased or the infusion stopped. Isoproterenol should never be used to treat clients in cardiac arrest. For further review, Chapter 17 provides in-depth discussions of adrenergics and adrenergic blockers.

Pediatric Implications

Isoproterenol infusions are not indicated for treating bradycardia in children; epinephrine infusions are used instead.

Adenosine

Adenosine is the first-line drug of choice to treat **paroxysmal supraventricular tachycardia (PSVT)**, a sudden, uncontrolled, rapid rhythm (exceeding 150 beats/min in adults) that originates above the ventricles. The goal is to convert PSVT to sinus rhythm. A natural substance found in all body cells, adenosine slows impulse conduction through the heart's atrioventricular (AV) node, interrupts dysrhythmia-producing reentry pathways, and restores a normal rhythm in clients with PSVT. Because the half-life is less than 5 seconds, adenosine is administered rapidly as a 6-mg IV bolus over 1 to 3 seconds followed by a 20-ml saline flush. A 12-mg bolus may be given 1 to 2 minutes after the initial dose if PSVT persists. A third dose of 12 mg may be considered after 1 to 2 minutes if needed. Higher doses are not recommended.

Nursing considerations include continuous cardiac monitoring and frequent assessment of vital signs. Adenosine is inhibited by methylxanthines such as caffeine and theophylline, so higher doses may be needed. Though usually transient, ventricular ectopy, bradycardia, flushing, chest pain and dyspnea may occur. In addition, a short period of asystole may follow injection of adenosine (up to 15 seconds). Spontaneous cardiac activity typically resumes. Adenosine is contraindicated in clients with poison- or drug-related tachycardia, second- and third-degree heart block, and in clients with sick sinus syndrome, except those with functioning pacemakers. If the tachycardia originated in the ventricles, the client could deteriorate and become hypotensive after adenosine administration. Refer to Chapter 41 for a full discussion of antidysrhythmic drugs.

Verapamil

Verapamil, a calcium channel blocker, is indicated for the treatment of narrow complex paroxysmal supraventricular tachycardia (PSVT) as an alternative to adenosine in clients with normal blood pressure and adequate left ventricular function (i.e., no evidence of heart failure). Verapamil slows conduction (negative chronotropic) through the heart and has negative inotropic and vasodilating effects. In emergency situations, verapamil is administered as an IV bolus in variable age- and weight-dependent dosages, which should not exceed 2.5 to 5 mg given slowly over 2 minutes. Repeat doses of 5 to 10 mg may be ordered in 15 to 30 minutes. The maximum total dose with this regimen is 20 mg. Another approach is to give 5 mg of verapamil IV every 15 minutes until a total dose of 30 mg has been administered.

The nurse must carefully monitor heart rate and rhythm as well as blood pressure. Cardiac conduction disturbances and profound hypotension can occur, especially with concurrent use of beta-blockers. An IV injection of calcium may be ordered to prevent or treat calcium channel blocker-induced hypotension (see Chapters 41 and 42). Simultaneous use of calcium channel blockers and beta-blockers is contraindicated, because their negative inotropic and negative chronotropic effects are synergistic, causing myocardial depression and bradycardia. Other contraindications include preexisting heart block or sick sinus syndrome in the client without a pacemaker, Wolff-Parkinson-White syndrome, and heart failure.

Diltiazem

Diltiazem is a calcium channel blocker like verapamil and is administered as an IV bolus to treat PSVT and to slow the ventricular response rate in atrial fibrillation or flutter.

It is considered a second-line agent after adenosine. Diltiazem has less of a negative inotropic effect than verapamil, but it has strong negative chronotropic actions. Therefore IV diltiazem is less likely to cause cardiac depression, but is very effective in controlling heart rate.

The usual initial bolus dose of IV diltiazem is 0.25 mg/kg given over 2 minutes. If the supraventricular tachycardia does not convert to a normal sinus rhythm in 15 minutes, a second IV bolus of 0.35 mg/kg over 2 to 5 minutes may be necessary. For ongoing control of the ventricular rate in clients with atrial fibrillation or flutter, a continuous infusion of diltiazem is indicated at a dose range of 5 to 15 mg/hour, titrated according to the desired heart rate.

The nurse must carefully monitor blood pressure, heart rate, and rhythm after administering IV diltiazem. Arrhythmias, bradycardia, heart block and hypotension may develop. Diltiazem can elevate serum digoxin levels, predisposing the client to digitalis toxicity. Simultaneous use of calcium channel blockers and beta-blockers is contraindicated, because their negative inotropic and negative chronotropic effects are synergistic, causing myocardial depression and bradycardia. Other contraindications include preexisting heart block or sick sinus syndrome in the client without a pacemaker, Wolff-Parkinson-White syndrome, and heart failure.

Amiodarone

The IV form of amiodarone is considered a first-line agent in the advanced cardiac life support algorithms for the treatment of life-threatening ventricular dysrhythmias and cardiac arrest. It has alpha- and beta-adrenergic blocking effects and acts on sodium, potassium, and calcium channels. Indications for use include pulseless ventricular tachycardia and ventricular fibrillation (after defibrillation and epinephrine), hemodynamically stable ventricular tachycardia, PSVT refractory to adenosine, ventricular rate control in atrial fibrillation, and for pharmacologic treatment of atrial fibrillation.

Amiodarone is especially good for clients with impaired heart function who have atrial and ventricular dysrhythmias. It has been found to be more effective and to have fewer proarrhythmic properties than other agents with similar actions.

For clients who have a pulse (i.e., not in cardiac arrest), amiodarone 150 mg IV is given over 10 minutes, followed by a continuous infusion of 1 mg/min for 6 hours, then 0.5 mg/min over 18 hours as a maintenance infusion. For clients in cardiac arrest because of pulseless ventricular tachycardia or ventricular fibrillation, a dose of 300 mg diluted in 20 to 30 ml dextrose 5% in water (D_5W) is given as a rapid infusion followed by a continuous infusion as described earlier. Additional doses of 150 mg may be given by rapid infusion if ventricular fibrillation or ventricular tachycardia recurs. The maximum daily dose is 2.2 grams per 24-hour period.

Significant adverse effects include hypotension and bradycardia. The nurse should slow the infusion rate to prevent or treat these effects and be prepared to administer IV fluids, vasopressors, and agents to increase heart rate. A temporary pacemaker may be needed. Amiodarone has a very long half-life. It should not be given concurrently with pharmacologic agents that prolong the Q-T interval on the ECG (e.g., procainamide).

Pediatric Implications

Amiodarone is given for pulseless ventricular tachycardia and ventricular fibrillation as a 5 mg/kg rapid IV/IO bolus. For responsive children who have supraventricular (junctional and atrial) tachycardia and ventricular dysrhythmias with pulses present, amiodarone is given as a 5 mg/kg IV/IO loading dose over 20 to 60 minutes and repeated to a maximum daily IV dose of 15 mg/kg per 24-hour period.

Lidocaine

Lidocaine is commonly used to treat significant ventricular **dysrhythmias** (irregular heartbeats) such as frequent premature ventricular contractions (PVCs), ventricular tachycardia, and ventricular fibrillation, but is now considered an alternative agent to amiodarone. Lidocaine exerts a local anesthetic effect on the heart, thus decreasing myocardial irritability. Typically a client with ventricular dysrhythmias is given a 1- to 1.5-mg/kg bolus of lidocaine, followed by 0.5 mg/kg to 0.75 mg/kg every 5 to 10 minutes until the dysrhythmia is controlled or a total dose of 3 mg/kg has been administered via the IV or intraosseous (IO) route. A continuous lidocaine infusion is initiated at a rate of 1 to 4 mg/min to maintain a therapeutic serum level. Lidocaine may also be administered via the endotracheal route in doses of 2 to 4 mg/kg.

Important nursing considerations for the client receiving lidocaine include continuous cardiac monitoring and assessment for signs and symptoms of lidocaine toxicity (confusion, drowsiness, hearing impairment, cardiac conduction defects, myocardial depression, muscle twitching, and seizures). Because lidocaine is metabolized by the liver, clients with hepatic impairment, heart failure, shock, and advanced age (older than 70 years) are at higher risk for toxicity. In these clients, the lidocaine dose may need to be reduced by as much as 50% (see Chapter 41).

Pediatric Implications

Ventricular ectopy is uncommon in children. Metabolic causes should be suspected if ventricular dysrhythmias occur. The pediatric dose of lidocaine is 1 mg/kg IV or via the IO route. The endotracheal tube (ETT) dose is 2-3 mg/kg. A maintenance infusion of 20 to 50 mcg/kg/min is recommended following the bolus dose. Drug data for lidocaine are presented in Prototype Drug Chart 58–1.

Procainamide

Procainamide is an antidysrhythmic agent prescribed for ventricular tachycardia, PVCs, and rapid supraventricular dysrhythmias unresponsive to adenosine. The typical IV loading dose of procainamide is 20 mg/min until the dys-

rhythmia is successfully treated. Other endpoints to procainamide administration include a total administration of 17 mg/kg of the drug, the development of hypotension, and specific changes on the ECG (e.g., widening of the QRS complex by 50% or more). A continuous maintenance infusion of 1 to 4 mg/min may be ordered following the loading dose.

The nurse must monitor vital signs and the ECG with particular attention to heart rate and rhythm, as well as blood pressure and the width of the QRS complex. Procainamide administration can cause severe hypotension. Heart block, rhythm disturbances, and cardiac arrest can occur. Procainamide is contraindicated in clients with **torsades de pointes**, an unusual polymorphic ventricular tachycardia often associated with a prolonged Q-T interval. The drug is eliminated via the kidneys; therefore clients with renal failure are at higher risk of adverse effects and often require a lower dosage (see Chapter 41).

Pediatric Implications

Procainamide is given to children for ventricular tachycardia that is recurrent or refractory to other measures and for supraventricular tachycardia. The loading dose is 15 mg/kg/IV or IO given over 30 to 60 minutes. The same monitoring guidelines, adverse effects, and contraindications described for adults are relevant in the pediatric population.

Magnesium Sulfate

Magnesium is an essential element in multiple enzymatic reactions in the body, including function of the sodium-potassium adenosine triphosphatase (ATPase) pump. Its physiologic effects can be likened to a calcium channel blocker with neuromuscular blocking properties. Hypomagnesemia is associated with the development of atrial and ventricular dysrhythmias.

The primary indications for emergency administration of magnesium sulfate are refractory ventricular tachycardia, refractory ventricular fibrillation, cardiac arrest associated with **hypomagnesemia** (low serum magnesium level), and life-threatening ventricular dysrhythmias from digitalis toxicity. It is also the drug of choice for the treatment of torsades de pointes.

Magnesium is administered by diluting 1 to 2 g (2 to 4 ml of a 50% solution) in 10 ml of D_5W. For cardiac arrest caused by hypomagnesemia or torsades de pointes, magnesium is given by direct IV push or via the IO route over 5 to 20 minutes. For clients experiencing torsades de pointes who are not in cardiac arrest, a magnesium infusion of 1 to 2 g diluted in 50 to 100 ml of D_5W can be given IV/IO over 5 to 60 minutes followed by a continuous infusion of 0.5 to 1g/hour.

Although magnesium toxicity is rare, the nurse should monitor the client's response to magnesium administration. Hypotension is the most common adverse effect when magnesium is given by rapid IV push. Other effects include mild bradycardia, flush, and sweating. True hyper-

Prototype **DRUG CHART 58–1**

LIDOCAINE HCl

Drug Class

Antidysrhythmic, class IB
Trade name: Xylocaine
Pregnancy Category: C

Dosage

A: IV or IO: 1-1.5 mg/kg; may repeat 0.5 mg/kg
   q 5-10 min up to 3 mg/kg *(max)*
ETT*: 2-4 mg/kg
Drip: 1-4 mg/min
C: IV or IO: Initially: 1 mg/kg; maint: 20-50 mcg/kg/min is
   recommended after bolus
ETT*: 2-3 mg/kg
Therapeutic range: 1.5-5 mcg/ml

Contraindications

Hypersensitivity, advanced atrioventricular block
Caution: Liver disease, heart failure, elderly

Drug-Lab-Food Interactions

Drug: Increase effects with phenytoin, quinidine,
   procainamide, propranolol; *increase* risk of toxicity
   with cimetidine, beta-adrenergic blockers

Pharmacokinetics

Absorption: IV
Distribution: PB: 60%-80%; concentrates in
   adipose tissue
Metabolism: t½: Initial: 7-30 min; terminal: 9-120 min
Excretion: Through the liver

Pharmacodynamics

PO: Onset: 45-60 sec
   Peak: 45-60 sec
   Duration: 10-20 min

Therapeutic Effects/Uses

Antiarrhythmic drug to treat ventricular dysrhythmias such as premature ventricular contractions (PVCs), ventricular
   tachycardia, and ventricular fibrillation
Mode of Action: Decreases automaticity; increases electrical threshold of ventricle

Side Effects

Drowsiness, confusion, dyspnea, lethargy, hypotension,
   nausea, vomiting

Adverse Reactions

Life-threatening: Seizures, cardiac arrest

A, Adult; *C,* child; *ETT,* endotracheal tube; *IO,* intraosseous; *IV,* intravenous; *PB,* protein-binding; *maint,* maintenance; *max,* maximum; *min,* minute; *sec,* seconds; *t½,* half-life.
*Note: For endotracheal drug administration, dose should be 2 to 4 mg/kg in adults.

magnesemia can cause diarrhea, respiratory depression, deep tendon reflex impairment, flaccid paralysis, and circulatory collapse. Because magnesium is eliminated via the kidneys, it should be administered with caution in clients with renal impairment.

Pediatric Implications

Indications for magnesium sulfate in pediatric clients include torsades de pointes, hypomagnesemia, and status asthmaticus unresponsive to beta-adrenergic agents. The magnesium sulfate dose is 25 to 50 mg/kg IV/IO given slowly over 10 to 20 minutes with a maximum dose of 2 g. The drug may be pushed faster to treat torsades de pointes.

Epinephrine

Epinephrine is a catecholamine with alpha- and beta-adrenergic effects. It has multiple uses. Emergency cardiac indications for administration of IV/IO epinephrine include profound bradycardia and hypotension, asystole, pulseless ventricular tachycardia, and ventricular fibrillation. Epinephrine is thought to improve perfusion of the heart and brain in cardiac arrest states by constricting peripheral blood vessels. In addition, epinephrine increases the chances for successful electrical countershock (defibrillation) in ventricular fibrillation. It is important to be aware that epinephrine is available in two primary concentrations: 1:1000 and 1:10,000. The 1:10,000 concentration is used when administering a single IV/IO dose of epinephrine. The 1:1000 form is used when preparing a continuous epinephrine infusion or when giving epinephrine via the IM or subQ route.

For profound bradycardia or hypotension, an epinephrine infusion may be ordered at 2 to 10 mcg/min. For asystole, pulseless ventricular tachycardia, and ventricular fibrillation, epinephrine is administered in 1-mg doses (1:10,000 solution) IV/IO every 3 to 5 minutes until the desired clinical response is achieved (usually return of effective cardiac activity). Epinephrine also may be given via the ETT route in doses of 2 to 2.5 mg diluted in 10 ml of normal saline.

Nursing implications for clients receiving epinephrine include constant cardiac and hemodynamic monitoring. Epinephrine can cause myocardial ischemia and cardiac dysrhythmias. Epinephrine should never be administered in the same site as an alkaline solution such as sodium bicarbonate, because alkaline solutions inactivate epinephrine. In addition, the presence of metabolic or respiratory acidosis decreases the effectiveness of epinephrine. All efforts should be made to correct acid-base imbalances in the client. More drug information about epinephrine and other adrenergic drugs can be found in Chapter 17.

Pediatric Implications

The pediatric dose of epinephrine is 0.01 mg/kg (1:10,000 solution) given every 3 to 5 minutes IV or via the intraosseous (IO) route for cardiac arrest. The ETT dose of 0.1 mg/kg should be given using the 1:1000 solution.

Vasopressin

Vasopressin is indicated for the treatment of ventricular fibrillation that is refractory to defibrillation. It is found in the human body as endogenous antidiuretic hormone. The therapeutic dose is significantly higher than the amount normally present in humans. The effects of vasopressin as a cardiac emergency drug include nonadrenergic peripheral vasoconstriction. When used as an emergency agent, it appears to increase coronary artery perfusion during cardiopulmonary resuscitation (CPR) and to exhibit vasopressor effects. It is given to clients in cardiac arrest before or after epinephrine administration as a single 40 units IV or intraosseous dose. Although vasopressin can be given via the ETT route, a specific effective dose has not yet been established through research. Vasopressin is considered an adjunct to epinephrine and can replace either the first or second epinephrine dose in the cardiac arrest algorithm. Because vasopressin can induce myocardial ischemia and angina, it is contraindicated in responsive clients who have coronary artery disease (CAD), that is, clients with CAD who are not in cardiac arrest.

Pediatric Implications

Vasopressin administration is not recommended for the treatment of pediatric cardiac arrest at this time.

Sodium Bicarbonate

Sodium bicarbonate is prescribed to treat the metabolic acidosis that may accompany cardiac arrest and the hyperkalemia and acidotic states related to specific drug overdose situations. The current standard in resuscitation is to give sodium bicarbonate only *after* adequate ventilation, chest compressions, IV fluids, and drug therapy fail to correct the acidotic state. Sodium bicarbonate is not considered a first-line drug for the treatment of cardiac arrest; it is preferentially given based on results of arterial blood gas analysis when acidosis is severe. If a client has been in arrest for a prolonged period and blood gas analysis is not available, sodium bicarbonate may be ordered as part of the ongoing resuscitation attempt. The standard initial IV dose of sodium bicarbonate is 1 mEq/kg. The drug may be repeated at 0.5 mEq/kg every 10 minutes as needed.

Important nursing considerations relevant to sodium bicarbonate include careful monitoring of arterial blood gas analysis results. Sodium bicarbonate administration can lead to metabolic alkalosis, which may be very difficult to reverse and have deleterious physiologic effects. Catecholamines such as epinephrine, norepinephrine, and dopamine should not be infused in the same site as sodium bicarbonate, because they are inactivated by solutions containing sodium bicarbonate.

Table 58-1 lists emergency cardiac drugs and their dosages and indications.

Pediatric Implications

If severe metabolic acidosis persists after attention has been directed at maintaining optimal ventilation and oxygenation, sodium bicarbonate may be given to the pediatric client in a 1-mEq/kg dose via the IV or intraosseous route. Sodium bicarbonate is hyperosmolar and should be diluted from an 8.4% solution (1 mEq/ml) to a 4.2% solution (0.5 mEq/ml) for infants younger than 3 months of age.

Emergency Drugs for Neurosurgical Disorders

The neurosurgical drugs discussed in this section are commonly administered in emergency, trauma, and critical care settings. For maximum benefit, these agents must be given as early as possible when clinically indicated. Knowledge of proper administration techniques and guidelines enhances therapeutic effectiveness. These drugs are cross-referenced to their specialty chapters.

Mannitol

Mannitol is an osmotic diuretic used in the emergency and neurosurgical setting to treat cerebral edema and increased intracranial pressure, which may occur following head trauma, neurosurgery, and other types of intracranial pathology. Mannitol may be given as an IV bolus or via a continuous drip. The usual initial bolus dose of mannitol is 1g/kg IV of a 20% to 25% solution. Subsequent dosing is highly variable and is influenced by serum osmolality. In general, mannitol is held when serum osmolality exceeds 310 to 320. Mannitol is highly irritating to veins. The nurse must use a filter needle when administering mannitol, because crystals may form in the solution and syringe and be inadvertently injected. When a filter needle is used to draw up the mannitol, a *new* filter needle *must* be used to administer the mannitol IV. In addition, the nurse should carefully assess the client's neurologic status; monitor laboratory studies, including serum osmolality; and keep accurate intake and output records to assess fluid volume status, because diuresis may be substantial. Drug data for mannitol are presented in Prototype Drug Chart 58-2.

Table 58–1

Cardiac Emergency Drugs

Generic (Brand)	Route and Dosage	Uses and Considerations
adenosine	A: IV: Initially: 6 mg; then 12 mg in 1-2 min if needed; may repeat 12 mg × 1	Paroxysmal supraventricular tachycardia. *Pregnancy category:* C; PB: UK; $t^{1/2}$: <10 sec
amiodarone IV	A: IV: *with pulse:* 150 mg over 10 min; then continuous infusion 1 mg/min for 6 h; then 0.5 mg/min over 18 h *Cardiac arrest:* 300 mg diluted in 20-30 ml D_5W rapidly followed by continuous infusion as above; *max:* 2.2 g/d C: IV: *without pulse:* 5 mg/kg rapid IV/IO bolus. *With pulse:* 5 mg/kg IV/IO loading dose over 20-60 min; repeated to *max* daily dose of 15 mg/kg	Part of ACLS algorithm for treatment of both atrial and ventricular dysrhythmias. *Pregnancy category:* C; PB: UK; $t^{1/2}$: 26-107 d
atropine sulfate	IV or IO: 0.5-1 mg; can repeat up to 0.04 mg/kg or 3 mg *(max)* ETT: 2-3 mg diluted in 5-10 ml normal saline	Symptomatic bradycardia; asystole. *Pregnancy category:* C; PB: 60%-80%; $t^{1/2}$: 2-3 h
diltiazem	IV: 0.25 mg/kg; repeat in 15 min at 0.35 mg/kg IV: drip 5-15 mg/h	Supraventricular tachycardia, atrial fibrillation and flutter. *Pregnancy category:* C; PB: 80%; $t^{1/2}$: 2-5 h
epinephrine	IV or IO: 0.5-1 mg; may be repeated q3-5min ETT: 2.0-2.5 mg diluted in 10 ml normal saline (Prototype Drug Chart 58–1)	Cardiac arrest. *Pregnancy category:* C; PB: UK; $t^{1/2}$: UK
lidocaine		
magnesium sulfate	Dilute 1-2 g (2-4 ml of a 50% solution) in 10 ml of D_5W. Give IV/IO in cardiac arrest over 5-20 min. *Torsades de pointes:* 1-2 g diluted in 50-100 ml of D_5W given IV over 5-60 min, followed by a continuous infusion of 0.5-1 g	Used for hypomagnesemia, treatment of ventricular tachycardia and ventricular fibrillation. Drug of choice for torsades de pointes. Rapid infusion can cause hypotension. *Pregnancy category:* D; PB: 25%-35%; $t^{1/2}$: 30 min
morphine sulfate	IV: 1-4 mg q5-30min	Chest pain, unstable angina, pulmonary edema. *Pregnancy category:* C; PB: 35%; $t^{1/2}$: 2–2.5 h
nitroglycerin	SL: 0.3-0.4 mg; Translingual aerosol spray: 0.4 mg-metered dose, up to 3 sprays in 15 min onto or under the tongue IV: Drip: 10-20 mcg/min, increased 5-10 mcg/min q5-10min (titrated)	Chest pain, angina, unstable angina, MI. Hypotension can occur; contraindicated in clients taking drugs for erectile dysfunction (e.g., Viagra) *Pregnancy category:* C; PB: 60%; $t^{1/2}$: 1-4 min
procainamide HCl	IV: 20 mg/min; *max:* 17 mg/kg *Recognize endpoints:* • Hypotension • QRS widens >50% • Total dose of 17 mg/kg given Drip: 1-4 mg/min	PVCs, ventricular tachycardia, ventricular fibrillation, atrial dysrhythmias. *Pregnancy category:* C; PB: 20%; $t^{1/2}$: 3-4 h
sodium bicarbonate	IV: Initially: 1 mEq/kg; then 0.5 mEq/kg if needed q10min	Metabolic acidosis. *Pregnancy category:* C; PB: UK; $t^{1/2}$: UK
vasopressin	A: IV/IO/ETT: single 40-units dose after epinephrine administration	Ventricular fibrillation refractory to defibrillation. Contraindicated in responsive clients with CAD. *Pregnancy category:* C; PB: UK; $t^{1/2}$: 10-20 min
verapamil HCl	IV: Age- and weight-dependent dosages; should not exceed 5 mg; repeat doses may be needed to *max* of 20 mg-30 mg	Paroxysmal supraventricular tachycardia. *Pregnancy category:* C; PB: 90%; $t^{1/2}$: 3-8 h

A, Adult; *ACLS,* Advanced Cardiac Life Support; *C,* child; *CAD,* coronary artery disease; *d,* day; *ETT,* endotracheal tube; *h,* hour; *IO,* intraosseous; *IV,* intravenous; *max,* maximum; *MI,* myocardial infarction; *min,* minute; *PB,* protein-binding; *PVC,* premature ventricular contraction; *sec,* second; *SL,* sublingual; $t^{1/2}$, half-life; *UK,* unknown; >, greater than; <, less than.

Methylprednisolone

High-dose methylprednisolone may be administered as an option to clients with traumatic spinal cord injuries. However, its efficacy in regard to reducing sensory/motor deficits is controversial and not currently supported by evidence. When used, a strict pharmacologic protocol must be initiated within 8 hours of acute spinal cord injury: A bolus dose of 30 mg/kg of client's body weight is given IV over 15 minutes (mixed in 100 ml of normal saline solution); a maintenance infusion of 5.4 mg/kg/hour is then started within 45 minutes of the bolus and continued for 23 hours if the injury is less than 3 hours old. If the injury is between 3 and 8 hours old, the maintenance infusion must run for 48 hours.

Prototype DRUG CHART 58–2

MANNITOL

Drug Class

Osmotic diuretic
Trade name: Osmitrol
Pregnancy Category: C

Contraindications

Hypersensitivity, severe dehydration
Caution: Pregnancy, breastfeeding, current
intracranial bleeding

Dosage

A: IV: Initially 1g/kg of 20%-25% sol as a bolus
Highly individualized

Drug-Lab-Food Interactions

Drug: May *decrease* effectiveness with lithium

Pharmacokinetics

Absorption: IV
Distribution: PB: Confined to extracellular space
Metabolism: t½: 100 min
Excretion: In urine

Pharmacodynamics

Decrease in Intracranial Pressure:
IV: Onset: 30-60 min
  Peak: 1 h
  Duration: 6-8 h
Diuresis:
IV: Onset: 1-3 h
  Peak: 1 h
  Duration: 6-8 h

Therapeutic Effects/Uses

To treat increased intracranial pressure, cerebral edema
Mode of Action: Inhibition of reabsorption of electrolytes and water by affecting pressure of glomerular filtrate

Side Effects

Temporary volume expansion, hypo/hypernatremia,
hypo/hyperkalemia, dehydration, blurred vision,
dry mouth

Adverse Reactions

Pulmonary congestion, fluid/electrolyte imbalances
Life-threatening: Convulsions

A, Adult; *h,* hour; *IV,* intravenous; *min,* minute; *PB,* protein-binding; *sol,* solution; *t½,* half-life.

Contraindications include allergy to the drug, penetrating trauma to the spinal cord, human immunodeficiency virus (HIV) infection, severe infection, and a spinal cord injury more than 8 hours old. Relative contraindications include pregnancy and uncontrolled diabetes mellitus. Adverse effects include transient hypertension with administration of the loading dose and elevation of blood sugar during the infusion. The nurse must monitor vital signs and blood sugar and perform frequent and accurate neurologic assessments pertinent to spinal cord injury. Clients who have received methylprednisolone may be at a higher infection risk.

Table 58–2 lists neurosurgical emergency drugs and their dosages and indications (also see Chapters 26 and 49).

Emergency Drugs for Poisoning

Although there are numerous antidotes for specific types of poisoning, the drugs presented in this section are the most commonly prescribed agents in cases of drug overdose and ingestion of toxic substances, with pertinent exceptions noted. Particular attention must be given to administration guidelines to achieve the best possible clinical

Table 58–2

Neurosurgical Emergency Drugs

Generic (Brand)	Route and Dosage	Uses and Considerations
mannitol methylprednisolone (Solu-Medrol)	(Prototype Drug Chart 58–2) IV: bolus dose: 30 mg/kg in 100 ml NSS; then 5.4 mg/kg/h (23 h) or 48 h for SCI >3 h but <8 h old	For treatment of acute SCI (within 8 h of injury). Contraindicated in penetrating spinal cord trauma. *Pregnancy category:* C; PB: 80%-90%; t½: 2-4 h

h, Hour; *IV,* intravenous; *NSS,* normal saline solution; *PB,* protein-binding; *SCI,* spinal cord injury; *t½,* half-life; <, less than; >, greater than.

outcome for the client. These drugs are cross-referenced to their specialty chapters.

Naloxone

Naloxone is classified as an opiate antagonist. It reverses the effects of all opiate drugs (e.g., morphine, meperidine, codeine, propoxyphene, heroin) by competitively binding to opiate receptor sites in the body. Naloxone is indicated for individuals who have taken an overdose of opiate drugs, those experiencing respiratory or cardiovascular depression from therapeutic doses of opiates given in a health care setting, and those brought to the emergency department in a coma of unknown etiology (which may be drug induced).

The typical dose of naloxone for actual or suspected opiate overdose in adults is 0.4 to 2 mg IV administered every 2 minutes until the client's condition improves to an acceptable level. If there is no improvement within 10 minutes after 10 mg of the drug has been injected, nonopiate drugs or disease must be suspected. Although naloxone should be administered IV in emergency situations, it also may be given via the intramuscular (IM), intraosseous (IO) or subcutaneous (subQ) routes if IV access is not readily obtainable.

Because most opiate drugs have a longer duration of action than naloxone, the nurse must monitor the client closely for signs and symptoms of recurrent opiate effects such as respiratory depression and hypotension. In this situation, naloxone administration may need to be repeated several times or a continuous IV infusion ordered. Naloxone has no major adverse effects, but can precipitate withdrawal symptoms in clients addicted to opiate drugs and rarely cause anaphylaxis. In addition, pulmonary edema has been reported following naloxone administration in clients who have had an overdose of morphine (see Chapter 25). Drug data for naloxone are presented in Prototype Drug Chart 58–3.

Pediatric Implications

For narcotic reversal in children, give 0.01 mg/kg to 0.1 mg/kg, repeating the drug as necessary based upon desired therapeutic effects up to 2 mg. Naloxone can be administered IV, IO, IM or subQ in children.

Prototype **DRUG CHART 58–3**

NALOXONE HCl

Drug Class
Narcotic antagonist
Trade name: Narcan
Pregnancy Category: B

Contraindications
Hypersensitivity, respiratory depression
Caution: Opiate-dependent clients, cardiac disease, breastfeeding neonates of opiate-dependent mothers

Dosage
IV/IM/IO/subQ: 0.4-2 mg; repeat every 2-3 min as indicated

Drug-Lab-Food Interactions
Drug: Naloxone can precipitate withdrawal in a client dependent on narcotic analgesics
Lab: Urine vanillylmandelic acid (VMA), 5-hydroxyheptadecatrienoic acid (5-HIAA), urine glucose

Pharmacokinetics
Absorption: IM/subQ: Well absorbed
Distribution: PB: UK
Metabolism: t½: Adults: 1-4 h; neonates: 1-3 h
Excretion: In urine metabolites

Pharmacodynamics
subQ/IM: Onset: 2-5 min
　　　　Peak: UK
　　　　Duration: 1-4 h
IV/IO: Onset: 1-2 min
　　　　Peak: UK
　　　　Duration: 1-4 h

Therapeutic Effects/Uses
To treat respiratory depression caused by narcotics; to treat narcotic-induced depressant effects and narcotic overdose
Mode of Action: Blocks effects of narcotics by competing for the receptor sites

Side Effects
Negligible pharmacologic effect without narcotics in body

Adverse Reactions
Nausea, vomiting, tremulousness, sweating, tachycardia, elevated blood pressure
Life-threatening: Atrioventricular fibrillation, pulmonary edema (with overdose of morphine)

---

h, Hour; *IV,* intravenous; *IM,* intramuscular; *min,* minute; *PB,* protein-binding; *subQ,* subcutaneous; *t½,* half-life; *UK,* unknown.

Flumazenil

Flumazenil is the reversal agent for the respiratory depressant and sedative effects of benzodiazepine medications (e.g., diazepam [Valium], midazolam [Versed], chlordiazepoxide [Librium]). It is administered to counteract the effects of benzodiazepines given as sedative or anesthetic agents, as well as to treat accidental or intentional benzodiazepine overdose. Flumazenil does not reverse the central nervous system (CNS) depressant effects of nonbenzodiazepine agents such as alcohol, opiates, and barbiturates and may not reverse amnesia induced by benzodiazepines.

For suspected benzodiazepine overdose, flumazenil is given IV in an initial dose of 0.2 mg over 15 seconds. A second dose of 0.3 mg may be given over 30 seconds. A third dose and subsequent doses of 0.5 mg IV may be given every minute until the desired clinical response is achieved or until a total dose of 3 mg is given. If sedation occurs again, doses of flumazenil may be repeated at 20-minute intervals (not to exceed 1 mg at a time) to a total hourly dose of no more than 3 mg IV.

Nursing considerations include careful assessment of respiratory rate and effort, blood pressure, and mental status. If the benzodiazepine is reversed too rapidly, clients may have emergent reactions in which they become agitated and confused and experience perceptual distortions. Because seizures are precipitated by benzodiazepine withdrawal, seizure precautions must be implemented for clients at risk (those with long-standing benzodiazepine use or abuse) or for those who have a known seizure disorder.

Activated Charcoal

Activated charcoal may be prescribed for poisoning as a means to prevent absorption of toxins into the body if the ingested substance is known to be affected by charcoal in the gastrointestinal (GI) tract. A poison control center should be contacted as soon as possible to help guide medical therapy. In cases of known or suspected poisoning, activated charcoal is prepared as a slurry and given orally or via a gastric tube within 1 hour of ingestion, sometimes following gastric lavage. The dose is dependent on the amount of poison ingested; the typical adult and pediatric dose is 1 to 2 g/kg, up to 25 to 50 gm per dose.

Activated charcoal dosing may need to be repeated for certain types of poisoning, particularly from agents such as salicylates, slow-release drug preparations, and *Amanita phalloides* (death cap mushrooms), to name a few.

Vomiting is a common adverse reaction, and the nurse should use activated charcoal with extreme caution in the client with an impaired gag reflex or altered level of consciousness, because there is risk of aspiration. Activated charcoal should not be administered with milk products, because they decrease its adsorptive properties. Activated charcoal is ineffective and should not be given to clients who have ingested some forms of pesticides, hydrocarbons, alcohols, acids or alkalis, lithium, solvents and iron supplements. A **cathartic** (a purgative resulting in bowel movements) may be ordered following administration of activated charcoal to speed elimination of the charcoal-toxin complex from the body. The client should be told that charcoal produces black stools.

Table 58–3 lists the emergency drugs for poisoning and their dosages and indications.

Emergency Drugs for Shock

Drugs may be required to elevate blood pressure and to improve cardiac performance in various types of shock states. Therapeutic agents described in this section are indicated in conditions such as cardiogenic shock, neurogenic shock, septic shock, anaphylactic shock, and insulin shock. A noteworthy exception to the list of shock states is **hypovolemic shock** (shock resulting from loss of blood or fluid volume); drugs should not be used in an attempt to correct the hypotension associated with this condition. Administration of fluids or blood products or both is the only acceptable means to treat hypovolemic shock. The drugs that follow are cross-referenced to their specialty chapters.

Dopamine

Dopamine is a sympathomimetic agent often used to treat hypotension in shock states *not* caused by hypovolemia. Dopamine may also be used to increase heart rate (beta$_1$ effect) in bradycardic rhythms when atropine has not been effective. The dose range is 2 to 20 mcg/kg/min. Dopamine enhances

Table 58–3

Emergency Drugs for Poisoning

Generic (Brand)	Route and Dosage	Uses and Considerations
flumazenil	IV: Initial dose 0.2 mg over 15 sec. Additional doses of 0.3-0.5 mg over 30 sec every 1 min as indicated. For re-sedation, may be repeated at 20-min intervals to a total dose of no more than 3 mg.	Reversal agent for benzodiazepine overdose; may precipitate seizures in clients with long-term use or abuse of benzodiazepines and those with seizure disorders; may precipitate emergent reactions. *Pregnancy category:* C; PB: 50%; t$^{1/2}$: Variable (40-80 min)
naloxone (Narcan)	(Prototype Drug Chart 58–3)	
activated charcoal	A & C: 1-2 g/kg PO	To treat poisoning. Onset: <1 min. *Pregnancy category:* C; PB: NA; t$^{1/2}$: NA

A, Adult; *C*, child; *IV*, intravenous; *min*, minute; *NA*, not applicable; *PB*, protein-binding; *PO*, by mouth; *sec*, second; t$^{1/2}$, half-life; <, less than.

cardiac output by increasing myocardial contractility and increasing heart rate (beta₁ effect) and elevates blood pressure through vasoconstriction (alpha-adrenergic effect). Alpha effects predominate at higher doses—vasoconstriction of renal, mesenteric, and peripheral blood vessels occurs. Such vasoconstriction, although sometimes necessary to maintain adequate blood pressure in severe shock, can lead to poor organ and tissue perfusion, decreased cardiac performance, and reduction of urine output. The lowest effective dose of dopamine should be used. Clients must be weaned gradually from dopamine; abrupt discontinuation of the infusion can cause severe hypotension.

Dopamine is typically mixed as a concentration of 400 to 800 mg in 250 ml D₅W and administered IV by a volumetric infusion pump for precision, preferably in a central vein. Sodium bicarbonate will inactivate dopamine, so do not infuse dopamine in the same IV line. Continuous heart and blood pressure monitoring is essential. The nurse must carefully document vital signs and intake and output as ordered. Significant adverse effects include tachycardia, dysrhythmias, myocardial ischemia, nausea, and vomiting.

The IV site must be assessed hourly for signs of drug infiltration; **extravasation** (escape into tissues) of dopamine can produce tissue necrosis that may necessitate surgical debridement and skin grafting. If extravasation occurs, the site should be injected in multiple areas with phentolamine (Regitine), 5 to 10 mg diluted in 10 to 15 ml of normal saline, to reduce or prevent tissue damage. Drug data for dopamine are presented in Prototype Drug Chart 58–4.

Dobutamine

Dobutamine is a sympathomimetic drug with beta adrenergic activities. The beta₁ effects include enhancing the force of myocardial contraction (positive inotropic effect) and increasing heart rate (positive chronotropic effect). The beta₂ effects produce mild vasodilation. Dobutamine is indicated in shock states when improvement in cardiac output and overall cardiac performance is desired. Blood pressure is elevated only through the increase in cardiac output. The usual IV dose range of dobutamine is 2 to 20 mcg/kg/min administered via a volumetric infusion pump for precision. A typical concentration of dobutamine is 250 mg to

---

Prototype DRUG CHART 58–4

DOPAMINE HCl

Drug Class

Adrenergic
Trade name: Intropin
Pregnancy Category: C

Dosage

A: IV: Drip: 2-20 mcg/kg/min (>10 mcg/kg/min may be ordered if lower doses are ineffective)

Contraindications

Hypersensitivity, tachydysrhythmias, ventricular fibrillation, pheochromocytomas
Caution: Safety in children is not known.

Drug-Lab-Food Interactions

Drug: Used within 2 wk of MAOIs, may result in hypertensive crisis; concurrent IV administration of phenytoin may result in hypotension and bradycardia; sodium bicarbonate solutions inactive dopamine—do *not* administer through the save IV line

Pharmacokinetics

Absorption: IV
Distribution: PB: UK
Metabolism: t½: 2 min
Excretion: In urine

Pharmacodynamics

IV: Onset: 1-2 min
Peak: <5 min
Duration: <10 min

Therapeutic Effects/Uses

To treat hypotension in shock states not caused by hypovolemia; to increase heart rate in atropine-refractory bradycardia.
Mode of Action: Stimulates receptors to cause cardiac stimulation; increases systemic vascular resistance

Side Effects

Palpitations, tachycardia, hypertension, ectopic beats, angina, IV line site irritation, piloerection, nausea, vomiting

Adverse Reactions

Cardiac dysrhythmias, azotemia, tissue sloughing (from extravasation)
Life-threatening: MI, gangrene in extremities (from vasoconstriction)

A, Adult; *IV,* intravenous; *MAOIs,* monoamine oxidase inhibitors; *MI,* myocardial infarction; *min,* minute; *PB,* protein-binding; *t½,* half-life; *UK,* unknown; *wk,* week; *>,* greater than; *<,* less than.

1000 mg mixed in 250 ml of D$_5$W or normal saline. Like dopamine, dobutamine administration should be tapered gradually as the client's condition warrants.

Continuous cardiac and blood pressure monitoring are required for clients receiving dobutamine infusions. Adverse effects are dose-related and include myocardial ischemia, tachycardia, dysrhythmias, headache, nausea, and tremors. The nurse must carefully monitor intake and output and assess for any signs or symptoms of myocardial ischemia such as chest pain or development of dysrhythmias (see Chapter 17).

Norepinephrine

Norepinephrine is a catecholamine with extremely potent vasoconstrictor actions (alpha-adrenergic effect). It is used in shock states, often when drugs such as dopamine and dobutamine have failed to produce adequate blood pressure. Like high-dose dopamine, the peripheral vasoconstriction that results has the potential to impair cardiac performance and decrease organ and tissue perfusion. In general, 4 to 8 mg of norepinephrine are added to 250 ml D$_5$W or normal saline solution and infused at 0.5 to 30 mcg/min (titrated) for adults. Continuous cardiac monitoring and precise blood pressure monitoring are required. The drug must be tapered slowly; abrupt discontinuation can result in severe hypotension.

Nursing actions and considerations are the same as those for dopamine. Norepinephrine should not be used to treat hypotension in hypovolemic clients; fluid, blood, or both must be administered to restore adequate volume first. Adverse effects of norepinephrine include myocardial ischemia, dysrhythmias, and impaired organ perfusion. Extravasation of norepinephrine causes tissue necrosis, so attention to the IV site is essential. If extravasation occurs, the area should be infiltrated with phentolamine, as described for dopamine.

Epinephrine

Epinephrine is the drug of choice in the treatment of **anaphylactic shock**, an allergic response of the most serious type, brought about by an antibody-antigen reaction. Anaphylactic shock can be fatal if prompt treatment is not initiated. Severe bronchoconstriction and hypotension resulting from cardiovascular collapse are its hallmarks. Epinephrine is also indicated for an acute, severe asthmatic attack.

Administration of epinephrine causes bronchodilation, enhanced cardiac performance, and vasoconstriction to increase blood pressure. In severe asthma and anaphylactic shock, epinephrine is given in a dose range of 0.2 to 0.5 mg IM or subQ for adults via a tuberculin syringe for accuracy (1:1000 solution). IM administration is preferable to subQ administration, because the IM route has a more predictable pattern of absorption. As an alternative, epinephrine can be given in a dose of 0.1 to 0.25 mg IV over 5 to 10 minutes (1:10,000 solution). Epinephrine administration can be repeated every 5 to 15 minutes if necessary.

The client who receives epinephrine must be closely monitored for tachycardia, cardiac dysrhythmias, hypertension, and angina. Clients who are given IV epinephrine must be on a cardiac monitor, with resuscitation equipment immediately available. Other adverse effects include excitability, fear, anxiety, and restlessness. In addition, the nurse should be alert to the possibility that the anaphylactic response may recur and necessitate repeated treatment. For this reason steroids are commonly ordered and are slowly tapered over days to weeks to prevent recurrence. Examples of steroids are hydrocortisone sodium succinate, prednisone, and methylprednisolone. Client education should include strict avoidance of the agents responsible for the anaphylactic reaction and follow-up care with a physician. For some clients, such as those with severe allergic responses to bee stings, the physician may prescribe an epinephrine kit or pen to be carried with the client for self-medication in the event of contact with the antigen. Proper client education regarding the use of the kit or pen is essential. Refer to Chapters 17 and 40 for more information.

Albuterol

Albuterol is a beta-adrenergic bronchodilator used to reverse bronchoconstriction in anaphylactic shock, **asthma** (inflammation and narrowing of the airways caused by enhanced responsiveness of the tracheobronchial system to a variety of stimuli), and COPD. In emergency situations, it is typically administered via nebulizer (adults: 0.5 ml of 0.5% inhalation solution in 2.5 ml saline). Albuterol is also supplied as a metered-dose inhaler, which the client can carry to self-administer a "rescue" dose of the drug during an acute episode of bronchospasm. The nurse should assess breath sounds before and after administration; effectiveness is evidenced by relief of bronchospasm. In severe bronchospasm wheezing may not be audible. As the bronchospasm is relieved, wheezing may become more pronounced, indicating that the drug is producing the desired therapeutic effect. Assessment of the client's subjective feelings of respiratory distress before and after administration is especially important. Adverse effects of albuterol include tachycardia, tremor, nervousness, cardiac dysrhythmias, and hypertension.

Diphenhydramine Hydrochloride

Diphenhydramine, an antihistamine, is often administered with epinephrine to treat anaphylactic shock. This agent is effective for treating the histamine-induced tissue swelling and pruritus common to severe allergic reactions. The standard adult dose is 25 to 50 mg administered IV or deep IM. Oral pill and liquid forms of the drug exist, but the parenteral form is preferred in emergencies. However, the client may be instructed to keep an oral formulation on hand in the home setting for emergency self-administration during an allergic reaction prior to receiving medical assistance. An important tip for client teaching is that the liquid diphenhydramine is easier to swallow than a pill, especially in the presence of tissue edema in the mouth or throat. Adverse effects include drowsiness, sedation, confusion, vertigo, excitability, hypotension, tachycardia, GI disturbances, and dry mouth (see Chapter 39).

Dextrose 50%

Dextrose 50% is a concentrated, high-carbohydrate solution given to treat insulin-induced hypoglycemia or insulin shock. When insulin shock is known or suspected and the client's state of consciousness is impaired such that oral administration of sugar solutions is contraindicated, 50 ml of dextrose 50% is commonly ordered and given as an IV bolus. Dextrose 50% is highly irritating to veins and should be administered in a large peripheral or central vein whenever possible. Phlebitis can occur. Extravasation of the solution can cause tissue sloughing and necrosis. The nurse must monitor the client's blood sugar carefully; hyperglycemia is common, especially after rapid injection. Urine output should be accurately recorded, because osmotic diuresis can occur when blood sugar is elevated, and a hyperosmolar state can result. Client education must be centered on teaching about diabetes, nutrition, physical activity and insulin administration.

Pediatric Implications

Glycogen stores in infants and children may be quickly depleted in stress states produced by severe illness. Because adequate amounts of glucose are essential to strong myocardial function, hypoglycemia must be corrected to provide the greatest chance for successful resuscitation. After determining that hypoglycemia is present by the finger- or heel-stick method of rapid blood glucose testing, dextrose 25% or less may be administered per physician order. Because glucose is supplied in a 50% concentration, it must be diluted 1:1 in sterile water before administration to reduce its osmolarity and prevent sclerosis of peripheral veins. The standard dose is 0.5 to 1g/kg IV or IO (see Chapter 51).

Glucagon

Glucagon is a pancreas-produced hormone that elevates blood sugar by stimulating glycogen breakdown (**glycogenolysis**). Glucagon, like dextrose 50%, is indicated in the treatment of severe insulin-induced hypoglycemia or insulin shock. In an emergency when dextrose 50% is unavailable or cannot be administered IV, glucagon is an effective agent. Glucagon may be given subQ, IM, or IV. The standard dose for adults and children is 0.5 to 1 mg, which can be repeated in 15 minutes for persistent coma. If the coma has not resolved after two doses, dextrose 50% must be administered. Adverse effects from glucagon are uncommon, but can include nausea, vomiting, and a hypersensitivity reaction that may produce bronchospasm and respiratory distress. Glucagon can also be used as an agent to reverse the effects of calcium channel blocker and beta-blocker overdose; in this situation, 3 mg IV of glucagon is administered initially, followed by an IV infusion of 3 mg/hour.

Table 58–4 lists the emergency drugs for shock and their dosages and indications. Also consult Chapter 51 for expanded information on antidiabetic agents.

Emergency Drugs for Hypertensive Crises and Pulmonary Edema

A variety of pharmacologic agents may be prescribed to treat **hypertensive crisis**, generally defined as a diastolic blood pressure that exceeds 110 to 120 mm Hg, and pul-

Table 58–4		
Agents for Emergency Treatment of Shock		
Generic	**Route and Dosage**	**Uses and Considerations**
albuterol	A: nebulizer: 0.5 ml of 0.5% inhalation solution in 2.5 ml saline	Bronchoconstriction secondary to anaphylactic shock, asthma, and COPD. Tachycardia, tremor, nervousness, cardiac dysrhythmias, and hypertension. *Pregnancy category:* C; PB: UK; t½: 3.7-5 h
dextrose 50%	A: IV: 50 ml C: 0.5-1.0 g/kg IV of a dextrose 25% sol	Insulin shock; severe hypoglycemia. *Pregnancy category:* C; PB: UK; t½: UK
diphenhydramine	IM/IV: 25-50 mg	Anaphylactic shock; acute allergic reaction. *Pregnancy category:* C; PB: 98%-99%; t½: 3-8 h
dobutamine	IV: Drip: 2-20 mcg/kg/min	Low cardiac output. Effects antagonized by beta-blockers. *Pregnancy category:* C; PB: UK; t½: 2 min
dopamine HCl	(Prototype Drug Chart 58-4)	
epinephrine	IM/subQ: 0.2-0.5 mg (1:1000 sol) IV/IO: 0.1-0.25 mg (1:10,000 sol) ETT: 2.0-2.5 mg diluted in 10 ml normal saline	Anaphylactic shock; severe acute asthmatic attack. May cause hypertensive crisis with MAOIs, increased dysrhythmias with cardiac glycosides. *Pregnancy category:* C; PB: UK; t½: UK
glucagon	subQ/IM/IV: 0.5-1 mg; may repeat × 1	Insulin shock; severe hypoglycemia; beta-blocker overdose (reverses effects of beta-blockers). *Pregnancy category:* B; PB: UK; t½: 3-10 min
norepinephrine	IV: Drip: 0.5-30 mcg/min (titrated)	Hypotension not responsive to other therapies. *Pregnancy category:* D; PB: UK; t½: UK

A, Adult; *C*, child; *COPD*, chronic obstructive pulmonary disease; *ETT*, endotracheal tube; *h*, hour; *IM*, intramuscular; *IV*, intravenous; *MAOIs*, monoamine oxidase inhibitors; *min*, minute; *PB*, protein-binding; *sol*, solution; *subQ*, subcutaneous; *t½*, half-life; *UK*, unknown.

monary edema. Three of the most commonly prescribed drugs are discussed in this section. The drugs are cross-referenced to their specialty chapter.

Labetalol

Labetalol is an alpha- and beta-adrenergic blocker that acts by inhibiting the effects of the sympathetic nervous system. Its pharmacologic actions include lowering heart rate, blood pressure, myocardial contractility, myocardial oxygen consumption, and reducing the vasoconstriction that results from sympathetic nervous system stimulation. This agent is indicated for the acute management of clinically significant hypertension in the presence of ischemic and hemorrhagic stroke, as well as for hypertensive crisis.

Initially 10 to 20 mg of labetalol is administered IV push over 2 minutes. This starting dose can be repeated or doubled every 10 minutes until the desired clinical response is achieved, to a maximum dose of 300 mg. As an alternative approach, a continuous infusion of labetalol mixed with D_5W can be prepared to deliver 2 mg/min until the target therapeutic response is attained. The continuous infusion is then stopped, but may be repeated every 6 to 12 hours if needed.

Important nursing considerations during the administration of labetalol include the use of a volumetric infusion pump for accurate continuous infusion medication delivery, cardiac monitoring, and frequent blood pressure measurement. Documentation of blood pressure may need to be as often as every 5 minutes during IV push dosing or at the initiation of the continuous infusion. Serious adverse effects include hypotension, ventricular dysrhythmias, and bronchospasm. Dizziness is also a frequently reported adverse reaction. Labetalol is contraindicated in clients with bronchial asthma or COPD because of the risk of bronchospasm and in clients with severe bradycardia or apparent heart failure.

Nitroprusside Sodium

Nitroprusside sodium is an IV agent used to reduce arterial blood pressure in hypertensive emergencies. The mechanism of action is immediate direct arterial and venous vasodilation. Antihypertensive effects end when nitroprusside sodium is discontinued; blood pressure increases as soon as drug administration is stopped. Continuous and accurate blood pressure measurement is required. In general, 50 mg of nitroprusside sodium is mixed in 250 ml D_5W. The typical dose range for adults is 0.25 to 5 mcg/kg/min, titrated to the desired clinical response. The maximum dose is 10 mcg/kg/min.

There are several important nursing considerations:

- Nitroprusside sodium is rapidly inactivated by light; the IV bottle or bag must be wrapped with aluminum foil or another opaque material to protect the solution from degradation.
- Although a faint brown tint is typical, blue or brown discoloration of the solution indicates degradation and necessitates that the solution be discarded.
- When nitroprusside sodium therapy is prolonged, or infused at the maximum dose of 10 mcg/kg/min for more than 10 minutes, clients are at risk for toxicity resulting from elevated serum thiocyanate or cyanide levels (byproducts of drug metabolism). Signs and symptoms include metabolic acidosis, profound hypotension, dyspnea, dizziness, and vomiting. Serum thiocyanate levels should be monitored every 24 to 72 hours for clients receiving prolonged infusions of more than 3 mcg/kg/min. Clients with renal insufficiency or failure are at a higher risk, because the metabolites are excreted in the urine.
- Clients should be placed on an oral antihypertensive agent as soon as possible so that nitroprusside sodium can be tapered slowly. Drug data for nitroprusside sodium are presented in Prototype Drug Chart 58–5.

Furosemide

Furosemide is classified as a *loop diuretic* that acts by inhibiting sodium and chloride reabsorption from the ascending loop of Henle and the proximal and distal tubules. It promotes the renal excretion of water, sodium, chloride, magnesium, hydrogen, and calcium and depletes potassium. Furosemide also has peripheral and renal vasodilating effects that can lower blood pressure. The main indications for use of furosemide as an emergency drug are acute pulmonary edema from left ventricular dysfunction and hypertensive crisis.

Furosemide is given as an initial bolus of 0.5 to 1 mg/kg IV over 1 to 2 minutes. For clients who take furosemide on a regular basis, the effective dose may be much higher (up to 2 mg/kg). The vasodilatory effects occur *before* diuresis begins and act to lower blood pressure. Central venous pressure is reduced through a decrease in venous return to the heart once vasodilation is achieved. Diuresis should start within 10 minutes of drug administration and may continue for approximately 6 hours.

The most significant adverse effects are severe hypovolemia, dehydration, and electrolyte disturbances (hypokalemia, hypomagnesemia, hyponatremia, and hypochloremia). Clients on digitalis preparations are at an increased risk of digitalis toxicity from hypokalemia. The client's fluid and electrolyte status must be carefully assessed before and after furosemide administration, including auscultation of breath sounds for rales, strict surveillance of intake and output, and review of laboratory data when available. An indwelling urinary catheter might be necessary. Electrolyte and careful fluid replacement may be required during furosemide therapy to prevent physiologic consequences. The nurse must also exercise caution in administering the

---

Herbal ALERT 58–2

Furosemide

Ginseng can inhibit efficacy. *Licorice* can promote potassium loss, enhancing the potential for severe hypokalemia. These herbs should not be taken concurrently with furosemide.

Prototype DRUG CHART 58–5

NITROPRUSSIDE SODIUM

Drug Class	**Dosage**
Vasodilator Trade name: Nipride *Pregnancy Category:* C	**A: IV: Drip:** 0.25-5 mcg/kg/min; begin at 0.25 mcg/kg/min and titrate to desired effect

Contraindications	**Drug-Lab-Food Interactions**
Hypersensitivity, hypertension (compensatory), decreased cerebral perfusion, coarctation of aorta *Caution:* Increased intracranial pressure	*Drug:* Antihypertensives, general anesthetics Note: Do not mix with any other drug in syringe or solution. *Lab:* Decrease in PCO_2, pH

Pharmacokinetics	**Pharmacodynamics**

Absorption: IV only
Distribution: PB: UK
Metabolism: t½: <10 min
Excretion: In urine
	IV: Onset: 1-2 min
	  Peak: Rapid
	  Duration: 1-10 min

Therapeutic Effects/Uses

To treat hypertensive crisis and to decrease systemic vascular resistance to improve cardiac performance
Mode of Action: Stimulates smooth muscle of veins and arteries; produces peripheral vasodilation

Side Effects	**Adverse Reactions**
Dizziness, headache, nausea, abdominal pain, sweating, palpitations, weakness, vomiting	Thiocyanate toxicity: hypotension, tinnitus, dyspnea, blurred vision, metabolic acidosis *Life-threatening:* Severe hypotension, loss of consciousness, profound cardiovascular depression

A, Adult; *IV,* intravenous; *min,* minute; *PB,* protein-binding; *PCO₂,* partial pressure of carbon dioxide; *t½,* half-life; *UK,* unknown; <, less than.

---

drug to clients with sulfonamide sensitivity, because furosemide is a sulfonamide derivative and can produce an allergic reaction.

Morphine Sulfate

Like furosemide, morphine sulfate is also indicated for acute pulmonary edema, because it produces venous vasodilation that decreases cardiac **preload** (the amount of blood returning to the right ventricle). The net effect is a decrease in pulmonary venous congestion. Morphine has been discussed previously in this chapter.

Table 58–5 lists the emergency drugs for hypertensive crises and pulmonary edema and their dosages and considerations.

Table 58–5

Emergency Drugs for Hypertensive Crises and Pulmonary Edema

Generic (Brand)	Route and Dosage	Uses and Considerations
nitroprusside sodium (Nipride)	(Prototype Drug Chart 58–5)	
furosemide (Lasix)	IV: initial bolus of 0.5-1.0 mg/kg over 1-2 min, up to 2 mg/kg	Acute pulmonary edema from left ventricular dysfunction; hypertensive crisis *Adverse effects:* hypovolemia, dehydration, electrolyte disturbances
morphine	IV: 1-4 mg q5-30min	Pulmonary edema, chest pain, unstable angina, MI
labetalol hydrochloride	IV: Initial push 10-20 mg over 2 min, repeated or doubled q10min up to a *max* of 300 mg; continuous infusion 2 mg/min	Uses: Hypertension in CVA and hypertensive crisis. *Adverse effects:* ventricular dysrhythmias, hypotension, bronchospasm. *Contraindications:* bronchial asthma, COPD, severe bradycardia, heart failure

COPD, Chronic obstructive pulmonary disease; *CVA,* cerebrovascular accident; *IV,* intravenous; *max,* maximum; *min,* minute; *MI,* myocardial infarction.

FIGURE 58–1 Most severe injury-related emergencies are best managed at a Level I trauma center. (Courtesy Christiana Care Health System, Wilmington, Delaware.)

 ## Critical Thinking Case Study

JS, age 23, was assaulted during a gang fight 1 hour ago. He was stabbed in the back and suffered blows to the head with a baseball bat. He was transported immediately from the injury scene to the trauma center and has undergone initial resuscitation and a rapid diagnostic work-up. Imaging studies revealed that the knife penetrated the spinal cord at the T4 level. His admitting diagnoses include penetrating spinal cord injury with paraplegia at the T4 level and a closed head injury with cerebral edema diagnosed by computed tomography (CT) scan. At this time, JS opens his eyes spontaneously, is agitated, and does not follow commands. He moans and localizes to pain with his upper extremities only. His lower extremities exhibit no movement.

JS is HIV-positive and addicted to heroin. He also abuses oral diazepam (Valium) and other street drugs. His current vital signs are BP 88/56, HR 56, RR 24, temp 96.8° F (36° C). He has two functional IV catheters (one peripheral line in the right forearm and one central line in the left femoral vein), an oral gastric tube, and an indwelling urinary catheter.

1. On arrival to the trauma center, should JS have received supplemental oxygen based on his mechanism of injury? What type of oxygen device would be appropriate for JS upon initial presentation?

2. The physician orders 50 g of mannitol to be given now, IV push. On hand are several 50-ml vials of "mannitol, 25%" solution. How many milliliters of mannitol from this vial need to be drawn up into the syringe to administer 50 g?

3. Describe the type of needle that must be used when administering mannitol and why. What size syringe should be used? Which IV line should be used to administer the mannitol to JS?

4. Based on the case study, what are the indications for mannitol administration? List at least three nursing considerations when giving mannitol.

5. JS has a penetrating T4 spinal cord injury with paralysis. Should methylprednisolone be administered within 8 hours of injury in his case? Why or why not?

6. JS has a history of heroin and diazepam abuse. List the reversal agents that could be used if the trauma team believes recent illicit drug use may be a contributing factor to his altered mental state.

7. Because of JS's spinal cord injury, he is exhibiting signs of neurogenic shock: bradycardia, warm skin, hypotension. What is the drug of choice that the nurse should keep at the bedside in case JS requires emergency treatment for symptomatic bradycardia? Name the drug, its mechanism of action, and dosing considerations.

8. The physician orders a dopamine infusion, 800 mg/250 ml D₅W, to be titrated to maintain systolic BP >110 mmHg. Which IV site would be the best choice for a continuous dopamine infusion in JS? What is the consequence of dopamine extravasation? What is the treatment for dopamine extravasation?

9. What vital sign parameters must be monitored while JS receives dopamine? Name at least four adverse effects of dopamine.

Antibiotics are initiated to address the potential for infection in JS's stab wound, because the stab wound communicates with his spinal cord. Upon infusion of the antibiotic, a body-wide rash, swelling of the lips and tongue, wheezing, and hypotension develop.

10. After antibiotic administration, what condition has developed in JS?

11. What are the drugs of choice to treat JS's condition now?

12. How can the nurse evaluate the effectiveness of these drugs?

NCLEX Study Questions

1. The minimum intravenous dose of atropine that should be given to an adult with bradycardia is:
   a. 1 mg
   b. 0.5 mg
   c. .01 mg/kg
   d. 3 mg/kg

2. For what class of drug overdose is naloxone effective?
   a. benzodiazepine
   b. hallucinogenic
   c. narcotic
   d. anesthetic

3. For which of the following disorders is mannitol most clearly indicated in the neurosurgical setting?
   a. Spinal nerve root injury
   b. Concussion
   c. Elevated intracranial pressure
   d. Seizure activity

4. What is the antidote for extravasation of both norepinephrine and dopamine?
   a. phentolamine
   b. atropine
   c. sodium bicarbonate
   d. magnesium sulfate

5. Adenosine is indicated for the treatment of:
   a. sinus bradycardia
   b. ventricular tachycardia
   c. paroxysmal supraventricular tachycardia
   d. heart block

6. What drug is indicated to reverse significant respiratory depressant effects of morphine sulfate?
   a. naloxone
   b. flumazenil
   c. epinephrine
   d. activated charcoal

7. How should 50% dextrose solution best be prepared for safe administration to a child?
   a. Use a filter needle
   b. Draw the medication into a tuberculin syringe
   c. Dilute 1:1 with sterile water to produce dextrose 25%
   d. Shake the solution vigorously prior to injection

8. What is the reversal agent for benzodiazepine overdose?
   a. atropine
   b. naloxone
   c. activated charcoal
   d. flumazenil

9. The drug of choice for hypoxemia is:
   a. epinephrine
   b. sodium bicarbonate
   c. albuterol
   d. oxygen

10. The nurse practitioner orders epinephrine 0.3 mg IM for a severe allergic reaction to a bee sting in an adult. Which concentration of epinephrine should the nurse select to administer this particular dose?
    a. 1:10,000
    b. 1:1000
    c. 1:100
    d. 1:10

Answers: 1. b; 2. c; 3. c; 4. a; 5. c; 6. a; 7. c; 8. d; 9. d; 10. b.

A
Therapeutic Drug Monitoring (TDM)*

Selected drugs are monitored by serum and urine to achieve and maintain therapeutic drug effect and to prevent drug toxicity. Drugs with a wide therapeutic range (window), the difference between effective dose and toxic dose, are not usually monitored. Drug monitoring is important in maintaining a drug concentration–response relationship, especially when the serum drug range (window) is narrow, such as with digoxin and lithium. Therapeutic drug monitoring (TDM) is the process of following drug levels and adjusting them to maintain a therapeutic level. Not all drugs can be dosed and/or monitored by their blood levels alone.

Drug levels are obtained at peak time and trough time after a steady state of the drug has been achieved in the client. Steady state is reached after four to five half-lives of a drug and can be reached sooner if the drug has a short half-life. Once steady state is achieved, the serum drug level is checked at the peak level (maximum drug concentration) and/or at trough/residual level (minimum drug concentration). If the trough or residual level is at the high therapeutic point, toxicity might occur. Careful assessment is needed by both physical and laboratory means.

TDM is required for the following:
• Drugs with a narrow therapeutic index or range (window)
• When other methods for monitoring drugs are not effective, such as blood pressure (BP) monitoring
• To determine when adequate blood concentrations are reached
• To evaluate a client's compliance to drug therapy
• To determine whether other drugs have altered serum drug levels (increased or decreased) that could result in drug toxicity or lack of therapeutic effect
• To establish a new serum-drug level when the dosage is changed
• Drug groups for TDM include analgesics, antibiotics, anticonvulsants, antineoplastics, bronchodilators, cardiac drugs, hypoglycemics, sedatives, and tranquilizers. To effectively conduct TDM, the laboratory must be provided with the following information: the drug name and daily dosage, time and amount of last dose, time blood was drawn, route of administration, and client's age. Without complete information, serum drug reporting might be incorrect.

HIV drugs are primarily dosed based on the client's viral load or CD4 counts. Many of these drugs have dosage adjustments for renal and/or hepatic impairment.

From Kee JL: *Laboratory and diagnostic tests with nursing implications,* ed 6, Upper Saddle River, NJ, 2004, Prentice Hall Health.
*Revised by Ronald J. LeFever, RPh, Pharmacy Services, Medical College of Virginia, Richmond, Va.

Drug	Therapeutic Range	Peak Time	Toxic Level
acetaminophen (Tylenol)	10-20 mcg/ml	1-2.5 hours	>50 mcg/ml Hepatotoxicity: >200 mcg/ml
acetohexamide (Dymelor)	20-70 mcg/ml (should be dosed according to blood glucose levels)	2-4 hours	>75 mcg/ml
alcohol	Negative		Mild toxic: 150 mg/dl Marked toxic: >250 mg/dl
alprazolam (Xanax)	10-50 ng/ml	1-2 hours	>75 ng/ml
amikacin (Amikin)	Peak: 20-30 mcg/ml Trough: 10 mcg/ml	Intravenously: 0.5 hour Intramuscular: 0.5-1.5 hours	Peak: >35 mcg/ml Trough: >10 mcg/ml
aminocaproic acid (Amicar)	100-400 mcg/ml	1 hour	>400 mcg/ml
aminophylline (*see theophylline*)			
amiodarone (Cordarone)	0.5-2.5 mcg/ml	2-10 hours	>2.5 mcg/ml
amitriptyline (Elavil) + nortriptyline (parent and active metabolite)	110-225 ng/ml	2-4 hours (and up to 12 hours)	>500 ng/ml
amobarbital (Amytal)	1-5 mcg/ml	2 hours	>15 mcg/ml Severe toxicity: >30 mcg/ml
amphetamine: serum: urine	20-30 ng/ml	Detectable in urine after 3 hours; positive for 24-48 hours	0.2 mcg/ml >30 mcg/ml urine
aspirin (*see salicylates*)			
atenolol (Tenormin)	200-500 ng/ml	2-4 hours	>500 ng/ml
beta carotene	48-200 mcg/dl	Several weeks	>300 mcg/dl
bromide	20-80 mg/dl		>100 mg/dl
butabarbital (Butisol)	1-2 mcg/ml	3-4 hours	>10 mc g/ml
butalbital	10-20 mcg/ml		>40 mcg/ml
caffeine	Adult: 3-15 mcg/ml Infant: 8-20 mcg/ml	0.5-1 hour	>50 mcg/ml
carbamazepine (Tegretol)	4-12 mcg/ml	6 hours (range 2-24 hours)	>9-15 mcg/ml
chloral hydrate	2-12 mcg/ml	1-2 hours	>20 mcg/ml
chloramphenicol (Chloromycetin)	10-20 mg/L		>25 mg/L
chlordiazepoxide (Librium)	1-5 mcg/ml	2-3 hours	>5 mcg/ml
chlorpromazine (Thorazine)	50-300 ng/ml	2-4 hours	>750 ng/ml
chlorpropamide (Diabinese)	75-250 mcg/ml	3-6 hours	>250-750 mcg/ml
clonidine (Catapres)	0.2-2 ng/ml (hypotensive effect)	2-5 hours	>2 ng/ml
clorazepate (Tranxene)	0.12-1 mcg/ml	1-2 hours	>1 mcg/ml
cimetidine (Tagamet)	Trough: 0.5-1.2 mcg/ml	1-1.5 hours	Trough: >1.5 mcg/ml
clonazepam (Klonopin)	10-60 ng/ml	2 hours	>80 ng/ml
codeine	10-100 ng/ml	1-2 hours	>200 ng/ml
cyclosporine	100-300 ng/ml	3-4 hours	>400 ng/ml
dantrolene (Dantrium)	1-3 mcg/ml	5 hours	>5 mcg/ml
desipramine (Norpramin)	125-300 ng/ml	4-6 hours	>500 ng/ml
diazepam (Valium)	0.5-2 mg/L 400-600 ng/ml therapeutic	1-2 hours	>3 mg/L >3000 ng/ml
digitoxin (rarely administered)	10-25 ng/ml	Noticeable: 2-4 hours Peak: 12-24 hours	>30 ng/ml
digoxin	0.5-2 ng/ml	PO: 6-8 hours IV: 1.5-2 hours	2-3 ng/ml
Dilantin (*see phenytoin*)			
diltiazem (Cardizem)	50-200 ng/ml	2-3 hours	>200 ng/ml
disopyramide (Norpace)	2-4 mcg/ml	2 hours	>4 mcg/ml
doxepin (Sinequan)	150-300 ng/ml	2-4 hours	>500 ng/ml
ethosuximide (Zarontin)	40-100 mcg/ml	2-4 hours	>150 mcg/ml
flecainide (Tambocor)	0.2-1 mcg/ml	3 hours	>1 mcg/ml
5-Flucytosine	Peak: 100 mcg/ml Trough: 50 mcg/ml		125 mcg/ml 125 mcg/ml
fluoride			>15 μmol/L
fluoxetine	90-300 ng/ml	2-4 hours	>500 ng/ml
flurazepam (Dalmane)	20-110 ng/ml	0.5-1 hour	>1500 ng/ml
folate	>3.5 mcg/ml	1 hour	

>, Greater than; <, less than.

Drug	Therapeutic Range	Peak Time	Toxic Level
gentamicin (Garamycin)	Peak: 6-12 mcg/ml Trough: <2 mcg/ml	IV: 15-30 minutes	Peak: >12 mcg/ml Trough: >2 mcg/ml
gold	1-2 mcg/ml	2-6 hours	>5 mcg/ml
haloperidol (Haldol)	5-15 ng/ml	2-6 hours	>50 ng/ml
hydromorphone (Dilaudid)	1-30 ng/ml	0.5-1.5 hours	>100 ng/ml
ibuprofen (Motrin, etc.)	10-50 mcg/ml	1-2 hours	>100 mcg/ml
imipramine (Tofranil) + desipramine (parent and active metabolite)	200-350 ng/ml	PO: 1-2 hours IM: 30 minutes	>500 ng/ml
isoniazid (INH, Nydrazid)	1-7 mcg/ml (dose usually adjusted based on liver function tests)	1-2 hours	>20 mcg/ml
kanamycin (Kantrex)	Peak: 15-30 mcg/ml	PO: 1-2 hours IM: 30 minutes-1 hour	Peak: >35 mcg/ml Trough: >10 mcg/ml
lead	<20 mcg/dl Urine: <80 mcg/24 hours		>80 mcg/dl Urine: >125 mcg/24 hours
lidocaine (Xylocaine)	1.5-5 mcg/ml	IV: 10 minutes	>6 mcg/ml
lithium	0.8-1.2 mEq/L	0.5-4 hours	>1.5 mEq/L
lorazepam (Ativan)	50-240 ng/ml	1-3 hours	>300 ng/ml
meperidine (Demerol)	0.4-0.7 mcg/ml	2-4 hours	>1 mcg/ml
meprobamate (Equanil, Miltown)	15-25 mcg/ml	2 hours	>50 mcg/ml
methadone (Dolophine)	100-400 ng/ml	0.5-1 hour	>2000 ng/ml or >0.2 mcg/ml
methaqualone	1-5 mcg/ml		>10 mcg/ml
methotrexate	<0.1 μmol/L after 48 hours	1-2 hours	1×10^6 at 48 hours
methsuximide	<1 mcg/ml	1-4 hours	>40 mcg/ml
methyldopa (Aldomet)	1-5 mcg/ml	3-6 hours	>7 mcg/ml
methyprylon	8-10 mcg/ml	1-2 hours	>50 mcg/ml
metoprolol (Lopressor)	75-200 ng/ml	2-4 hours	>225 ng/ml
mexiletine (Mexitil)	<0.5-2 mcg/ml	2-3 hours	>2 mcg/ml
morphine	10-80 ng/ml	IV: Immediately IM: 0.5-1 hour subQ: 1-1.5 hours	>200 ng/ml
Netilmicin (Netromycin)	Peak: 0.5-10 mcg/ml Trough: <4 mcg/ml	IV: 30 minutes	Peak: >16 mcg/ml Trough: >4 mcg/ml
nifedipine (Procardia)	50-100 ng/ml	0.5-2 hours	>100 ng/ml
nortriptyline (Aventyl)	50-150 ng/ml	8 hours	>200 ng/ml
oxazepam (Serax)	0.2-1.4 mcg/ml	1-2 hours	
oxycodone (Percodan)	10-100 ng/ml	0.5-1 hour	>200 ng/ml
pentazocine (Talwin)	0.05-0.2 mcg/ml	1-2 hours	>1 mcg/ml Urine: >3 mcg/ml
pentobarbital (Nembutal)	1-5 mcg/ml	0.5-1 hour	>10 mcg/ml Severe toxicity: >30 mcg/ml
phenmetrazine (Preludin)	5-30 mcg/ml (urine)	2 hours	>50 mcg/ml (urine)
phenobarbital (Luminal)	15-40 mcg/ml	6-18 hours	>40 mcg/ml Severe toxicity: >80 mcg/ml
phenytoin (Dilantin)	10-20 mcg/ml	4-8 hours	>20-30 mcg/ml Severe toxicity: >40 mcg/ml
pindolol (Visken)	0.5-6 ng/ml	2-4 hours	>10 ng/ml
primidone (Mysoline)	5-12 mcg/ml	2-4 hours	>12-15 mcg/ml
procainamide (Pronestyl)	4-10 mcg/ml	1 hour	>10 mcg/ml
procaine (Novocain)	<11 mcg/ml	10-30 minutes	>20 mcg/ml
Prochlorperazine (Compazine)	50-300 ng/ml	2-4 hours	>1000 ng/ml
propoxyphene (Darvon)	0.1-0.4 mcg/ml	2-3 hours	>0.5 mcg/ml
propranolol (Inderal)	>100 ng/ml	1-2 hours	>150 ng/ml
protriptyline (Vivactil)	50-150 ng/ml	8-12 hours	>200 ng/ml
quinidine	2-5 mcg/ml	1-3 hours	>6 mcg/ml
ranitidine (Zantac)	100 ng/ml	2-3 hours	>100 ng/ml
Reserpine (Serpasil)	20 ng/ml	2-4 hours	>20 ng/ml

Drug	Therapeutic Range	Peak Time	Toxic Level
salicylates (aspirin)	10-30 mg/dl	1-2 hours	Tinnitus: 20-40 mg/ml Hyperventilation: >35 mg/dl Severe toxicity: >50 mg/dl
secobarbital (Seconal)	2-5 mcg/ml	1 hour	>15 mcg/ml Severe toxicity: >30 mcg/ml
streptomycin	Peak: 5-20 mcg/ml Trough: <5 mcg/ml		>40 mcg/ml >40 mcg/ml
sulfadiazine	100-120 mcg/ml		>300 mcg/ml
sulfamethoxazole	90-100 mcg/ml		>300 mcg/ml
sulfapyridine	75-90 mcg/ml		>300 mcg/ml
sulfisoxazole	90-100 mcg/ml		>300 mcg/ml
theophylline (Theo-Dur)	10-20 mcg/ml	PO: 2-3 hours IV: 15 minutes (depends on smoking or nonsmoking)	>20 mcg/ml
thiocyanate	4-20 mcg/ml		>60 mcg/ml
thioridazine (Mellaril)	100-600 ng/ml 1-1.5 mcg/ml	2-4 hours	>2000 ng/ml >10 mcg/ml
timolol (Blocadren)	3-55 ng/ml	1-2 hours	>60 ng/ml
tobramycin (Nebcin)	Peak: 5-10 mcg/ml Trough: 1-1.5 mcg/ml	IV: 15-30 minutes IM: 0.5-1.5 hours	Peak: >12 mcg/ml Trough: >2 mcg/ml
Tocainide (Tonocard)	4-10 mcg/ml	0.5-3 hours	>12 mcg/ml
tolbutamide (Orinase)	80-240 mcg/ml	3-5 hours	>640 mcg/ml
trazodone (Desyrel)	500-2500 ng/ml	1-2 weeks	>4000 ng/ml
trifluoperazine (Stelazine)	50-300 ng/ml	2-4 hours	>1000 ng/ml
trimethoprim/ sulfamethoxazole (TMP/SMX)	Peak: trimethoprim: >5 mcg/ml Peak: sulfamethoxazole: >100 mcg/ml		
valproic acid (Depakene)	50-100 mcg/ml	0.5-1.5 hours	>100 mcg/ml Severe toxicity: >150 mcg/ml
vancomycin (Vancocin)	Peak: 20-40 mcg/ml Trough: 5-10 mcg/ml	IV: Peak: 5 minutes IV: Trough: 12 hours	Peak: >80 mcg/ml
verapamil (Calan)	100-300 ng/ml	PO: 1-2 hours IV: 5 minutes	>500 ng/ml
warfarin (Coumadin)	1-10 mcg/ml (dose usually adjusted by patient: 1 to 2.5 × control) or INR: 2-3	1.5-3 days	>10 mcg/ml INR: >4

	Peak Time	Half-Life
Combination HIV Drugs for Monitoring Antiretroviral Protease Inhibitors		
lopinavir/ritonavir (Kaletra)	4 hours	5 to 6 hours
Nucleoside Analog Reverse Transcriptase Inhibitors (NARTIs)		
abacavir/lamivudine/zidovudine (Trizivir)		
lamivudine/zidovudine (Combivir)		
Single HIV Drugs for Monitoring Protease Inhibitors		
amprenavir (Agenerase)	1-2 hours	7 to 9.5 hours
indinavir (Crixivan)	0.8 hour	2 hours (hepatic impairment, 3 hours)
Antiretroviral		
stavudine (Zerit)	1 to 1.5 hours	1.5 hours (8 hours in renal impairment)
Antiretroviral Protease Inhibitors		
ritonavir (Norvir)	2 to 4 hours	3 to 5 hours
Guanosine Nucleoside Reverse Transcriptase Inhibitor		
abacavir (Ziagen)		1.5 hours
Nucleoside Reverse Transcriptase Inhibitors (NRTIs)		
didanosine (Videx)	0.25 to 1.5 hours	1.5 hours
lamivudine (Epivir)		5 to 7 hours (dose adjustment in renal impairment)
zidovudine (Retrovir)	0.5 to 1.5 hours	1 hour (1.4 to 2.9 hours in renal impairment)
Nonnucleoside Reverse Transcriptase Inhibitors (NNRTIs)		
efavirenz (Sustiva)	3 to 5 hours	40 to 55 hours
nevirapine (Viramune)	4 hours	25 to 30 hours

B

Potential Weapons of Bioterrorism

Note: Refer to online resources for the most current information.

Agent/Etiology	Transmission/Clinical Manifestations	Drug Treatment/Considerations
Bacteria and Viruses		
Anthrax, pulmonary/ *Bacillus anthracis*	Inhalation of spores; incubation up to 60 d. Initially ILS: fever, malaise, fatigue, non-productive cough, chest discomfort. Later, severe respiratory distress, stridor, cyanosis, septicemia, and hemorrhagic meningitis	Early treatment with antibiotics IMPORTANT, IV route preferred; ciprofloxacin and doxycycline drugs of choice; use of additional antibiotics to avoid drug resistance; duration for IV and PO 60 d. Low morbidity when treated early; with onset of respiratory distress, morbidity near 100%
Anthrax, cutaneous/ *Bacillus anthracis*	Spores enter through non-intact skin; incubation up to 60 d; papule becomes fluid-filled vesicle that dries and forms dark eschar	Ciprofloxacin or doxycycline PO for 7-10 d; with systemic symptoms or risk of inhalation, treat as above. Morbidity up to 24% if untreated; treated<1%
Smallpox/variola virus	Respiratory droplets and pustule drainage; incubation 7-17 d; prodrome 2-4 d of ILS; papular rash that becomes deep vesicles, then scabs; mostly face and extremities; does involve palms and soles	Supportive; research continues on new antivirals, e.g., cidofovir; proven treatment unknown. Treat corneal lesions with idoxuridine, vaccinate client, all contacts, and health care workers in facility. Morbidity: 30% likely; in rare hemorrhagic form: up to 90%
Plague, pneumonic/ *Yersinia pestis*	Inhaled droplets; incubation: 2-3 d; begins as ILS; rapid 24 h progression to severe pneumonia, hemoptysis, and then respiratory distress and failure	Antibiotics of choice streptomycin and gentamycin. In mass casualty environment PO administration is more usual with doxycycline or ciprofloxacin. No vaccine available. Morbidity 100% if untreated.
Tularemia/*Francisella tularensis*	Inhaled or through skin; incubation 2-5 d (up to 14 d); begins as ILS; progresses over days to pneumonia with dyspnea and hilar adenopathy	IV streptomycin, gentamycin, or ciprofloxacin. Morbidity <5%
Viral hemorrhagic fevers; Ebola	Blood or secretions; incubation 2-10 d; prodrome of ILS; bleeding day 3; desquamation day 5; progresses rapidly to multisystem organ failure and delirium	Supportive care; transfusions and fresh frozen plasma; dialysis

Adapted from Lehne R: *Pharmacology for nursing care*, ed 6, Philadelphia, 2007, Saunders.
ARDS, Adult respiratory distress syndrome; *d,* day; *FDA,* Food and Drug Administration; *GI,* gastrointestinal; *h,* hour; *ILS,* influenza-like syndrome; *IM,* intramuscular; *IV,* intravenous; *min,* minute; *mo,* month; *PEEP,* positive end-expiratory pressure; *PO,* by mouth; *PRN,* as needed; *y,* year; *>,* greater than; *<,* less than.
Note: All clients exposed to chemical agents should be decontaminated. Removal of clothing will remove up to 90% of contamination. Further decontamination should be performed with soap and water. All health care providers treating clients PRIOR to decontamination should wear protective equipment to prevent skin, mucous membrane, or respiratory exposure (i.e., impervious suit, gloves, boots, protective face shield with respirator).

Agent/Etiology	Transmission/Clinical Manifestations	Drug Treatment/Considerations
Biotoxins		
Botulinum	Inhaled; incubation of 24-72 h; symmetric descending flaccid paralysis; eyes, bulbar muscles, then respiratory and skeletal effects	Supportive; antitoxin (from Centers for Disease Control or Public Health) may decrease progress; no antibiotics. Morbidity uncertain; long recovery
Ricin/*Ricinus communis*	Inhalation: onset within hours; coughing, chest tightness, dyspnea, nausea, and muscle ache. Later, edematous airway; cyanosis and death may follow Ingested: GI hemorrhage, vomiting and diarrhea. Later, liver and kidney failure; may die within 10-12 d Injection: severe symptoms and death; route not available to terrorists	Supportive; no antidote for ricin. Vaccine in development
Chemical Weapons		
Nerve agents (e.g., Sarin, VX GA, GB)	Absorbed through skin and mucous membranes and inhaled; onset rapid when inhaled; skin or mucous membrane onset 30 min to 18 h. Early signs: eye pain, rhinorrhea, and local sweating if droplet. Classic toxidrome: diarrhea, urination, miosis, bronchospasm, bronchorrhea, bradycardia, emesis, lacrimation, and salivation	Mechanical ventilation support with oxygen. Atropine IV or IM in high doses: 2 mg q3-5min; pralidoxime chloride (2-PAM) 1-2 g IV over 30-60 min; may need drip of 500 mg over 24 h; valium or Versed PRN for seizures; homatropine for ciliary spasm. Morbidity potentially high depending on concentration and duration of exposure
Chlorine or phosgene	Inhaled, mucous membranes, and eyes; rapid irritant effects; pulmonary effects (distress and edema) may be seen in 6 to 24 h	Humidified oxygen; bronchodilators; ventilatory support with PEEP for ARDS; monitor for 24 h if suspected significant exposure. Morbidity depends on exposure level; phosgene higher than chlorine
Sulfur mustard (Mustard gas)	Mainly absorbed through skin; can affect airway, eyes, GI tract, & bone marrow. Delayed onset of >6 h with few warning symptoms of contact; blistering of affected areas. Later, seizures and dysrhythmias	Requires rapid decontamination. Intubation if severe airway damage. Wash with dilute sodium thiosulfate (2.5% solution); prednisone may have antidote effects; Neupogen for later leukopenia. Morbidity under 5%-10%.
Cyanide	Absorbed in GI tract via contaminated products; inhaled vapors or via skin; generally rapid onset of symptoms; delayed if low concentration; sudden loss of consciousness with high concentration; cyanosis and severe respiratory distress	Inhaled amyl nitrite, sodium nitrite IV, sodium thiosulfate. Morbidity varies by exposure level
Radiologic Agents		
Nuclear bombs	Immediate threat: blast; delayed threat: radioactive fallout	Potassium iodide blocks uptake by thyroid of radioactive iodine, thus reducing risk of cancer; tablets for this purpose are released by public health after determining presence of iodine-131. FDA recommended doses: Birth to 1 mo: 16 mg; >1 mo to 3 yr: 32 mg; >3 yr to 18 yr: 65 mg; >18 yr: 130 mg; Pregnant or lactating: 65 mg.

References

Abernathy E: Biological response modifiers, *Am J Nurs* 87(4):458, 1987.

Abrams AC, Lammon CB, Pennington SS: *Clinical drug therapy: rationales for nursing practice*, ed 8, Philadelphia, 2007, Lippincott Williams & Wilkins.

Adcock K: Prescribing principles for children: foundation of a rational approach, *Adv Nurse Pract* 14(3):30, 2006.

Adler CH, et al: Parkinson's disease: process along the continuum of care, *Patient Care Nurse Pract* 26:45, December 2000.

Agency for Healthcare Quality and Research: Eleven medications account for one-third of medication errors that harm hospitalized children, *Research Activities* 318:7, 2007.

Aggrenox: A combination of antiplatelet drugs for stroke prevention, *Med Lett Drugs Ther* 42(1071):11, 2000.

Aldosterone, *Mayo Clin Health Lett* 22(7):6, 2004.

Aliskiren (Tekturna) for hypertension, *Med Lett Drugs Ther* 49(1258):29, 2007.

American Academy of Pediatrics, American Heart Association: *PALS provider manual*, Dallas, 2002, American Heart Association.

American College of Obstetricians and Gynecologists: Nausea and vomiting of pregnancy, *ACOG practice bulletin* 52, Washington, DC, 2004, The College.

American Heart Association: *2005 American Heart Association guidelines for cardiopulmonary resuscitation and emergency cardiovascular care*, Circulation 112(Suppl 24), 2005.

American Heart Association: *Textbook of advanced cardiac life support*, Dallas, 1997, The Association.

American Society of Hospital Pharmacists: *AHFS drug information*, Bethesda, MD, 1995, The Society.

Anderson K: Targeted therapy of multiple myeloma based upon tumor-microenvironmental interactions, *Exp Hematol*, 35:155, 2007.

Anderson RJ: Hypopituitarism. In Rakel RE, editor: *Conn's current therapy 2000*, Philadelphia, 2000, Saunders.

Anticoagulants, *Mayo Clin Health Lett* 22(6):6, 2004.

Antihypertensive therapy choice impacts diabetes risk, *Nurs Spectr* 16(1):9, 2007.

Anttila T, et al: Serotypes of *Chlamydia trachomatis* and risk for development of cervical squamous cell carcinoma, *JAMA* 285(1):47, 2001.

Aschenbrenner DS: Drug watch: addiction treatment discontinued, *Am J Nurs* 103(12):65, 2003.

Aschenbrenner DS, Venable SJ: *Drug therapy in nursing*, ed 2, Philadelphia, 2006, Lippincott Williams & Wilkins.

Aspirin for primary prevention of cardiovascular disease, *Med Lett Drugs Ther* 42(1079):18, 2000.

AstraZeneca's Exanta fails to get OK: DE, *The News Journal*, A-1, A-5, Sept 11, 2004.

Atovaquone/Proquanil (Malarone) for malaria, *Med Lett Drugs Ther* 42(1093):109, 2000.

Avoid the risks of mixed medications, *The Cleveland Clinic Heart Advisor* 7(5):3, 2004.

AWHONN, Mattson S, Smith JE, editors: *Core curriculum for maternal newborn nursing*, ed 3, Philadelphia, 2004, Saunders.

Bangsi D, Zhou J, Sun Y, et al: Impact of a genetic variant in CYP3A4 on risk and clinical presentation of prostate cancer among white and African-American men, *Urol Oncol* 24:21, 2006.

Barbieri RL: Management of infertility caused by ovulatory dysfunction, ACOG practice bulletin 34, *Obstet Gynecol* 99(2):347, 2002.

Barsella RM: How to judge a failing heart, *Nurs Spectr* 16(8), April 9, 2007.

Bedell C: Pegfilgrastim for chemotherapy-induced neutropenia, *Clin J Oncol Nurs* 7(1):55, 2003.

Belew C: Herbs and the childbearing woman: guidelines for midwives, *J Nurse Midwifery* 44(3):231, 1999.

Bender S: Personal communication, letter from Professional Service Manager, Amgen, February 20, 1991.

Benenson AS: *Control of communicable disease in man*, ed 17, Washington, DC, 2000, American Public Health Association.

Blayney D, McGuire B, Cruickshank S, et al: Increasing chemotherapy dose density and intensity: phase I trials in non-small cell lung cancer and non-Hodgkin's lymphoma, *Oncologist* 10:138, 2005.

Blood pressure, *Mayo Clin Health Lett* 21(9):7, 2003.

Bongaerts B, de Goeij A, van den Brandt P, et al: Alcohol and the risk of colon and rectal cancer with mutations in the K-ras gene, *Alcohol* 38(3):147, 2006.

Brener T, Doyle R: *Nursing 2007 drug handbook*, ed 27, New York, 2007, Lippincott Williams & Wilkins.

Briggs G, Freeman RK, Yaffe SJ: *Drugs in pregnancy and lactation*, ed 7, Philadelphia, 2005, Lippincott Williams & Wilkins.

Brown M: Hypertension and ethnic group, *BMJ*, 2006 (online): www.bmj.com/cgi/content/full/332/7545/833.

Brunton LL, Lazo JS, Parker KL, editors: *Goodman and Gilman's the pharmacological basis of therapeutics*, ed 11, New York, 2006, McGraw-Hill.

Buck ML: Impact of new regulations for pediatric labeling by the Food and Drug Administration, *Pediatr Nurs* 26(1):95, 2000.

Buffum M, Buffum JC: Nonsteroidal anti-inflammatory drugs in the elderly, *Pain Manag Nurs* 1(2):40, 2000.

Buprenorphine, 2003, Washington, DC, Substance Abuse and Mental Health Services Administration (SAMHSA), Office of Applied Studies, US Department of Health and Human Services.

Burchard, E, et al: Latino populations: a unique opportunity for the study of race, genetics, and social environment in epidemiological research, *Am J Public Health*, 95(12):2161.

Burrow G, Duffy M, Copel J: *Medical complications during pregnancy*, ed 6, Philadelphia, 2004, Elsevier/Saunders.

Butler LD, Symons BK, Henderson SL, et al: Hypnosis reduces distress and duration of an invasive medical procedure for children, *Pediatrics* 115(1):e77, 2005.

Byrne M: Patients in poverty, *AORN Journal*, 84(5):837, 2006.

Campinha-Bacote J: African-Americans. In Purnell L, Paulanka B, editors: *Transcultural health care: a culturally competent approach*, ed 2, Philadelphia, 2003, FA Davis.

Camp-Sorrell D: Chemotherapy: toxicity management. In Groenwald SL, editor: *Cancer nursing: principles and practice*, Boston, 2000, Jones and Bartlett.

Carotid artery disease: a red flag for strike, *The Cleveland Clinic Men's Health Advisor* 6(1):1, 2004.

Carpenter C, Cantley L: Molecular targets in oncology: signal transduction systems. In DeVita V, Hellman S, Rosenberg S, editors: *Cancer: principles and practice of oncology*, ed 7, vol 2, Philadelphia, 2005, Lippincott Williams & Wilkins.

Carulli L, Rondinella S, Lombardini S, et al: Review article: Diabetes, genetics and ethnicity, *Aliment Pharmacol Ther* 22 (Suppl 2), 2005.

Centers for Disease Control and Prevention: Sexually transmitted diseases treatment guidelines, *MMWR Morbid Mortal Wkly Rep* 51, 2002 (website): www.cdc.gov/STD/treatment/.

Centers for Disease Control and Prevention: Guidelines for national human immunodeficiency virus case surveillance, including monitoring for human immunodeficiency virus infection and acquired immunodeficiency syndrome, *MMWR Recomm Rep* 487(RR-13):1-27, 29-31, December 10, 1999.

Chan PD, Johnson SM: Gynecology and obstetrics, Laguna Hills, CA, 2006, Current Clinical Strategies Publishing.

Chan PD, Johnson SM: *Gynecology and obstetrics*, Laguna Hills, CA, 2004, Current Clinical Strategies Publishing.

Chestnut D: *Obstetric anesthesia: principles and practice*, ed 3, Philadelphia, 2004, Elsevier Mosby.

Chlebowski RT: Reducing the risk of breast cancer, *N Engl J Med* 343(3):191, 2000.

Cholesterol: the good, the bad, and the balanced, *Nurs Spectr* 13(10):1, 2003.

Clayton BD, Stock YN, Harroun RD: *Basic pharmacology for nursing*, ed 14, St Louis, 2007, Mosby.

Committee on Trauma, American College of Surgeons: *Advanced trauma life support for doctors, student manual*, ed 7, Chicago, 2004, American College of Surgeons.

Compton P, McCaffery M: Treating acute pain in addicted patients, *Nursing* 31:17, 2001.

Connolly J, Goldsmith J, Wang J, et al: Principles of cancer pathology. In Kufe D, Bast JR, Hait W, et al, editors: *Cancer medicine*, ed 7, Hamilton, Ontario, 2006, BC Decker.

Conte JE: *Manual of antibiotics and infectious disease*, ed 9, Baltimore, 2002, Lippincott Williams & Wilkins.

Cooper M, Grywalski M, Lamp J, et al: Enhancing cultural competence: a model for nurses, *Nurs Womens Health* 11(2):148.

Cott J, Fugh-Berman AJ, Rakel D: Drug-herb interactions: how vigilant should you be?, *Patient Care Nurse Pract*, 17:46, Oct 2000.

Craig CR, Stitzel RE: *Modern pharmacology with clinical application*, ed 6, Boston, 2004, Lippincott Williams & Wilkins.

Cummins RO, editor: *ACLS: principles and practice*, Dallas, 2005, American Heart Association.

Cummins RO, editor: *ACLS: principles and practice*, Dallas, 2003, American Heart Association.

Cunningham FG, et al: *Williams obstetrics*, ed 22, New York, 2005, McGraw-Hill.

Darby S: Pre- and perinatal care of Hispanic families, *Nurs Womens Health* 11(2):161, 2007.

Davidson, JK: *Clinical diabetes mellitus: a problem-oriented approach*, Atlanta, 2000, Thieme Medical Publishers.

Davis R, Cook D, Cohen L: A community reliance approach to reducing ethnic and racial disparities in health, *Am J Public Health*, 95(12):2168.

Detrol LA and ditropan XL for overactive bladder, *Med Lett Drugs Ther* 43(1101):28, 2001.

DeVries C: Reflections:deception, *Am J Nurs* 104(2):39, 2004.

Diagnosis and management of preeclampsia and eclampsia, ACOG Practice Bulletin No. 33, American College of Obstetricians and Gynecologists, *Obstet Gynecol* 99:159, 2002.

DiPiro J, Talbert R, Yee G, et al: *Pharmacotherapy: a pathophysiologic approach*, ed 6, New York, 2005, McGraw-Hill.

Ditropano C: Arrival of ARBs: potential drugs in the treatment of hypertension and heart failure, *Adv for Nurses* 40, March 17, 2003.

Dlugocz CK, Chater RW, Engle JP: Appropriate use of nonprescription analgesics in pediatric patients, *J Pediatr Health Care* 20(5):316.

Doenges ME, Moorhouse MF, Murr AC: *Nurse's pocket guide: diagnoses, prioritized interventions and rationales*, ed 10, Philadelphia, 2004, FA Davis.

Dofetilide for atrial fibrillation, *Med Lett Drugs Ther* 42(1078):41, 2000.

Dombrowski KJ, Lantz PM, Freed GL: Risk factors for delay in age-appropriate vaccination, *Public Health Rep* 119(2):144.

Dominguez F, Jones J, Zabicki K, et al: Prevalence of hereditary breast/ovarian carcinoma risk in patients with a personal history of breast or ovarian carcinoma in a mammography population, *Cancer* 104:1849, 2005.

Donovan MD: Sex and racial differences in pharmacological response: effect of route of administration and drug delivery system on pharmacokinetics, *J Womens Health* 14(1):30, 2005.

Douglas MJ, Levinson G: Systemic medication for labor and delivery. In Hughes S, et al, editors: *Shnider and Levinson's anesthesia for obstetrics*, Philadelphia, 2002, Lippincott, Williams & Wilkins.

Dream of a do-it-all "polypill," *The Cleveland Clinic Men's Health Advisor* 10(6):1, 2003.

Drugs for asthma, *Med Lett Drugs Ther* 42(1073):19, 2000.

Drugs for hypertension, *Med Lett Drugs Ther* 43(1099):17, 2001.

Drugs for intermittent claudication, *Med Lett Drugs Ther* 46(1176):13, 2004.

Drugs for pain, *Med Lett Drugs Ther* 42(1085):73, 2000.

Drugs for rheumatoid arthritis, *Med Lett Drugs Ther* 42(1082):57, 2000.

Drugs of choice for cancer chemotherapy, *Med Lett Drugs Ther* 42(1087-1088):83, 2000.

Ebbert JO, et al: Treating tobacco dependence: review of the best and latest treatment options, *J Thorac Oncol* 2(3):249, 2007.

Entacapone for Parkinson's disease, *Med Lett Drugs Ther* 42(1070):7, 2000.

Epilepsy: two new drugs, *Med Lett Drugs Ther* 42(1076):33, 2000.

Epirubicin for adjuvant therapy in node-positive breast cancer, *Med Lett Drugs Ther* 42(1071):12, 2000.

Ettinger D: Amrubicin for the treatment of small cell lung cancer: does effectiveness cross the Pacific?, *J Thorac Oncol* 2(2):160, 2007.

Eyre H, Kahn R, Robertson RM: Preventing cancer, cardiovascular disease, and diabetes: a common agenda for the American Cancer Society, the American Diabetes Association, and the American Heart Association, *CA Cancer J Clin* 54(4):190, 2004.

Ezekial MR: *Handbook of anesthesiology, 2004-2005 edition*, Laguna Hills, CA, 2004, Current Clinical Strategies Publishing.

Fellows L, Miller E, Frederickson M, et al: Evidence-based practice for enteral feedings: aspiration prevention strategies, bedside detection, and practice change, *Medsurg Nurs*, 9(1):27, 2000.

Fernando R, Collis R: Mobile epidural techniques and new drugs in labour. In Reynolds R, editor: *Regional alegesia in obstetrics: a millennium update*, New York, 2001, Springer.

Fidler I, Langley R, Kerbel R, et al: Angiogenesis. In DeVita V, Hellman S, Rosenberg S, editors: *Cancer: principles and practice of oncology*, ed 7, vol 1, Philadelphia, 2005, Lippincott Williams & Wilkins.

Fitzpatrick A, Frank L: An integrative approach to female sexual dysfunction, *Intl J Integr Med* 3(2):8, 2001.

Fleming DR: Mightier than the syringe, *Am J Nurs* 100(11):44, 2000.

Fortner K, Szymanski L, Fox H, et al: *The Johns Hopkins manual of gynecology and obstetrics*, ed 3, Baltimore, 2007, Lippincott Williams & Wilkins.

Friedman DL, Constine LS: Late effects of treatment for Hodgkin lymphoma, *J Natl Compr Canc Netw* 4:249, 2006.

Gahart B: *Intravenous medications*, ed 23, St Louis, 2007, Mosby.

Gemmill R, Idell C, Biological advances for new treatment approaches, *Semin Oncol Nurs* 19(3): 162, 2003.

George TP, O'Malley SS: Current pharmacological treatments for nicotine dependence, *Trends Pharmacol Sci* 25(1):42, 2004.

Ghobrial I, Leleu X, Hatjiharissi E, et al: Emerging drugs in multiple myeloma, *Expert Opin on Emerg Drugs* 12:155, 2007.

Glyburide/metformin (Glucovance) for type 2 diabetes, *Med Lett* 42(1092):105, 2000.

Gonsalves MY: Coordinating care for patients with type 2 diabetes, *Patient Care Nurse Pract* 15-31, September 2000.

Goodman M: Chemotherapy: principles of administration. In Groenwald SL, editor: *Cancer nursing: principles and practice*, Boston, 2000, Jones and Bartlett.

Green MR: Targeting targeted therapy, *N Engl J Med* 350(21):2191, 2004.

Guyton AC, Hall JE: *Human physiology and mechanisms of disease*, ed 6, Philadelphia, 1997, Saunders.

Haber G: In some cases, two drugs better than one, *Delaware Sunday News Journal*, September 24, 2006.

Haifizi H, Lipson J: People of Iranian heritage. In Purnell L, Paulanka B, editors: *Transcultural health care: a culturally competent approach*, Philadelphia, 2003, FA Davis.

Halpern S, Douglas J: *Evidenced-based obstetric anesthesia*, Malden, MA, 2005, Blackwell Publishing.

Harper JP: New test and drugs boost success in managing heart failure, *Nurs Spectr* 15(1):19, 2006.

Hatcher RA, et al: *Contraceptive technology*, ed 18 rev, New York, 2005, Irvington.

Hatcher T: The proverbial herb, *Am J Nurs* 101(2):36, 2001.

Hayden FG, Gubareva LV, Monto AS, et al: Inhaled zanamivir for the prevention of influenza in families, *N Engl J Med* 343(18):1282, 2000.

Health consequences of involuntary exposure to tobacco smoke: a report of the Surgeon General, Washington, DC, 2006, U.S. Department of Health and Human Services.

Healthy heart checklist: are you doing all you can?, *Men's Health Advisor* 5(12):7, 2003.

Heart failure: a growing problem with age, *Mayo Clin Health Lett* 20(12):1, 2002.

Hemmings H, Hopkins P: *Foundations of anesthesia: basic sciences for clinical practice*, ed 2, Philadelphia, 2006, Elsevier Mosby.

High triglycerides: a red flag, *Mayo Clin Health Lett* 20(9):7, 2002.

Hill P, Lipson J, Meleis AI: *Caring for women cross-culturally*, Philadelphia, 2003, FA Davis.

Hill S, Blakely T, Kawachi I, et al: Mortality among lifelong nonsmokers exposed to secondhand smoke at home: cohort data and sensitivity analysis, *Am J Epidemiol* 165:530, 2007.

Hine S: Intelligent prescribing in diverse populations, *Patient Care* 9:133, 2000.

Hockenberry MJ, Wilson D: *Wong's nursing care of infants and children*, ed 8, St Louis, 2007, Mosby.

Hojilla C, Mohammed F, Khokha R: Matrix metalloproteinases and their tissue inhibitors direct cell fate during cancer development, *Br J Cancer* 89: 1817, 2003.

Homocysteine, *Mayo Clin Health Lett* (20)9:6, 2002.

How to read your blood test results, *The Cleveland Clinic Heart Advisor* 9(8):1, 2006.

Howe H, Wu X, Ries L, et al: Annual report to the nation on the status of cancer among U.S. Hispanic/Latino populations, *Cancer* 107:1711, 2006.

Hughes S, Levinson G, Rosen M: *Shnider and Levinson's anesthesia for obstetrics*, ed 4, Philadelphia, 2002, Lippincott Williams & Wilkins.

Human Nutrition Information Service: *USDA's food guide pyramid*, 2005.

Hypertension prevalence rising, *The Cleveland Clinic Heart Advisor* 6(11):6, 2003.

Inflammation and the heart, *The Cleveland Clinic Heart Advisor* 7(6):4, 2004.

InterNational Council on Infertility Information Dissemination: *The infertility Q&A: basic testing with a reproductive endocrinologist*, 2002, InterNational Council on Infertility Information Dissemination (online): www.inciid.org/bastest.html. Accessed May 4, 2004.

Jemal A, Siegel R, Ward E, et al: Cancer statistics: 2007, *CA Cancer J Clin* 57:43, 2007.

Jemal A, et al: Annual report for the nation on the status of cancer 1975-2001, with a special feature regarding survival, *Cancer* 101(1):3, 2004.

Jemal A, et al: Cancer statistics 2004, *CA Cancer J Clin* 54:8, 2004.

Johnson BA: The biologic basis of alcohol dependence, *Advanced Studies in Nursing* 2(2):48, 2004.

Joint Commission 2007 national patient safety goals, (online): www.jointcommission.org/NewsRoom/News Releases/nr_npsg_07.htm.

Jonat W, Hilpert F, Kaufmann M: Aromatase inhibitors: a safety comparison, *Expert Opin Drug Saf* 6:165, 2007.

Juliano LM, Griffiths RR: A critical review of caffeine withdrawal: empirical validation of symptoms and signs, incidence, severity, and associated features, *Psychopharmacology (Berl)* 176(1):1, 2004.

Karch AM: *Focus on nursing pharmacology*, ed 3, Philadelphia, 2006, Lippincott Williams & Wilkins.

Karig AW, Murray JL, Pray WS: Trends for self-care, *Patient Care Nurse Pract* 9-23, August 2000.

Katz R: Addressing the health care needs of American Indians and Alaskan natives, *Am J Public Health* 94(1):13, 2004.

Katzung BG, editor: *Basic and clinical pharmacology*, ed 10, Norwalk, 2007, McGraw-Hill.

Kay P: Targeted therapies: a nursing perspective, *Semin Oncol Nursing* 22(1):1, 2006.

Kee JL: *Handbook of laboratory and diagnostic tests*, ed 6, Upper Saddle River, NJ, 2008, Prentice Hall.

Kee JL: *Laboratory and diagnostic tests with nursing implications*, ed 7, Upper Saddle River, NJ, 2006, Prentice Hall Health.

Kee JL, Marshall SM: *Clinical calculations*, ed 6, Philadelphia, 2009, Elsevier.

Kee JL, Paulanka B, Purnell L: *Fluids and electrolytes with clinical applications*, ed 7, New York, 2004, Delmar.

Kelley WN, editor: *Textbook of internal medicine*, ed 2, vols 1 and 2, Philadelphia, 1992, JB Lippincott.

Kellick KA: Pharmacologic considerations in statin use, *Clinician Reviews (supplement), Therapeutic Spotlight*, April 2001.

Kelly AW, Saucier J: Is your patient suffering from alcohol withdrawal?, *RN* 67(2):27, 2004.

Kern KB, Halperin HR, Field J: New guidelines for cardiopulmonary resuscitation and emergency cardiac care: changes in the management of cardiac arrest, *JAMA* 285:1267, 2001.

Koda-Kimble MA, Young L, Kradjan W, et al: *Applied therapeutics: the clinical use of drugs*, ed 8, Philadelphia, 2005, Lippincott Williams & Wilkins.

Kosnik L: Retavase (reteplase): treatment option for myocardial infarction, *Adv Nurses* 37, January 29, 2001.

Kosten TR, Biegel D: Therapeutic vaccines for substance dependence, *Expert Rev Vaccines* 1(3):363, 2002.

Kowal-Vern A, Criswell B: Burn scar neoplasms: a literature review and statistical analysis, *Burns* 31:403, 2005.

Kreek MG, LaForge KS, Butelman E: Pharmacology of addictions, *Nat Rev Drug Discov* 1(9):710, 2002.

Krozely P: Epidermal growth factor receptor tyrosine kinase inhibitors: evolving role in the treatment of solid tumors, *Clin J Oncol Nurs* 8(2):163, 2004.

Kumar V, Abbas A, Fausto N: Neoplasia. In *Robbins and Cotran pathologic basis of disease*, ed 7, Philadelphia, 2005, Elsevier.

Kurjak A, Chervenak F: *Textbook of perinatal medicine*, ed 2, London, 2006, Informa Healthcare.

Lane C: Nausea and vomiting of pregnancy: a tailored approach to treatment. *Clin Obstet Gynecol* 50(1):100, 2007.

Languages spoken at home, 2002 (online): www.census.gov/population/cen2000/phc-t20/tab06.xls. Accessed February 28, 2004.

Lavanchy D: Worldwide epidemiology of HBV infection, disease burden, and vaccine prevention, *J Clin Virol* 34: S1-3, 2005.

Lawler S: Bacteria linked to colon cancer, *The Scientist* (online): www.biomedcentral.com/news/20031119/01. Accessed August 8, 2004

Lawler S: *Bacteria linked to colon cancer, The Scientist*, 2003.

Lawrence R, Lawrence R: *Breastfeeding: a guide for the medical profession*, ed 6, Philadelphia, 2005, Elsevier Mosby.

Lefever RJ: Therapeutic Drug Monitoring (TDM). In Kee JL: *Laboratory and diagnostic tests with nursing implications*, ed 7, Upper Saddle River, NJ, 2005, Prentice Hall Health.

Lehne RA: *Pharmacology for nursing care*, ed 6, Philadelphia, 2007, Elsevier.

Lehne RA: *Pharmacology for nursing care*, ed 5, Philadelphia, 2004, Saunders.

Leibowitz D, Hoffman J: *Control of communicable disease manual*, ed 18, Washington, DC, 2004, American Public Health Association.

Lembo D, Donalisio M, Cornaglia M, et al: Effect of high-risk human papillomavirus oncoproteins on p53R2 gene expression after DNA damage, *Virus Res*, 2006.

Lewin J, Lwaleed B, Cooper J, et al: The direct effect of nuclear pores on nuclear chemotherapeutic concentration in multidrug resistant bladder cancer: the nuclear sparing phenomenon, *J Urol* 177:1526, 2007.

Lewis SL, et al: *Medical-surgical nursing: assessment and management of clinical problems*, ed 7, St Louis, 2007, Mosby.

Lilley LL, Harrington S, Snyder JS: *Pharmacology and the nursing process*, ed 5, St Louis, 2007, Mosby.

Linezolid, *Med Lett Drugs Ther* 42(1079):45, 2000.

Lippincott Williams & Wilkins: *Nursing herbal medicine handbook*, ed 3, New York, 2006, Lippincott Williams & Wilkins.

Liu S, Dontu G, Wicha M: Mammary stem cells, self-renewal pathways, and carcinogenesis, *Breast Cancer Res* 7:86, 2005.

Lowdermilk DL, Perry SE: *Maternity nursing*, ed 7, St Louis, 2006, Mosby.

Ma B, Yeo W, Hui P, et al: Acute toxicity of adjuvant doxorubicin and cyclophosphamide for early breast cancer: a retrospective review of Chinese patients and comparison with an historic Western series, *Radiother Oncol* 62:185, 2002.

Mager D: Bacteria and cancer: cause, coincidence or cure? A review, *J Transl Med* 4, 2006.

March of Dimes: *Caffeine in pregnancy*, March of Dimes Fact Sheet (online): www.marchofdimes.com/printableArticles/681r1148.asp. Accessed August 17, 2004.

Marching to a different heartbeat:, *The Cleveland Clinic Men's Health Advisor* 8(9):1, 2006.

Marks F, Furstenberger G, Muller-Decker K: Tumor promotion as a target of cancer prevention, *Recent Results Cancer Res* 174:37, 2007.

Mathias R: Blood pressure medication can improve cocaine treatment results in patients with severe withdrawal symptoms, *NIDA Notes* 16(6), 2002.

Mattison D: *Herbal supplements: their safety: a concern for health care providers*, March of Dimes Fact Sheet (online): www/marchofdimes.com/professionals/681r1815.asp. Accessed August 17, 2004.

Mazanec P, Tyler MK: Cultural considerations in end-of-life care: how ethnicity, age, and spirituality affect decisions when death is imminent, *Am J Nurs* 103(3):50, 2003.

McCaul ME: Pharmacotherapy strategies for alcoholism treatment, *Advanced Studies in Nursing* 2(2):54-59, 2004.

McDonnell K, Wellstein A: Cancer metastasis. In Chang A, Ganz P, Hayes D, et al, editors: *Oncology: an evidence-based approach*, New York, 2006, Springer.

McDowell S, Coleman J, Ferner R: Systematic review and meta-analysis of ethnic differences in risks of adverse reactions to drugs used in cardiovascular medicine, 2006 (online): www.bmj.com/cgi/content/full/332/7551/1177. Accessed March 6, 2007.

McGuinness T: Methamphetamine abuse, *Am J Nurs* 106(12):54, 2006.

Moller A, Pedersen T, editors: *Evidence-based anaesthesia and intensive care*, New York, 2006, Cambridge University Press.

Monahan FD, et al: *Medical-surgical nursing: health and illness perspectives*, ed 8, St Louis, 2007, Mosby.

Morgan E, Mikhail M, Murray M: *Clinical anesthesiology*, ed 4, New York, 2006, Lange Medical Books/McGraw-Hill.

Morse L, Calarese P: EGRF-targeted therapy and related skin toxicity, Dana Farber Cancer Institute, Boston (online): www.dana-farber.org. Accessed August 5, 2006.

Mosby: *2007 Mosby's drug consult*, St Louis, 2007, Mosby.

Mosby: *2006 Mosby's Drug Consult*, St Louis, 2006, Elsevier Mosby.

Moss A: *HIV and AIDS: management by the primary team*, Oxford, 1992, Oxford University Press.

Munoz C, Hilenber C: Ethnopharmacology: understanding how ethnicity can affect drug response is essential to providing culturally competent care, *Holist Nurs Pract* 20(5):227, 2006.

Murphy P, Kronenburg F, Wade C: Complementary and alternative medicine in women's health: developing a research agenda, *J Nurse Midwifery* 44(3):192, 1999.

Musselwhite K, Faris P, Moore K, et al: Use of epidural anesthesia and the risk of acute postpartum urinary retention, *Am J Obstet Gynecol* 196(5): 472, 2007.

My Pyramid (online): www.mypyramid.gov/mypyramidmoms/index.html. Accessed November 1, 2007.

Nadeau C, et al: The challenges of oral anticoagulation, *Patient Care Nurse Pract*, 17-22, December 2000.

Nadler JL, Rude RK: Disorders of magnesium metabolism, *Endocrinol Metab Clin North Am* 24(3):623, 1995.

Nateglinide for type 2 diabetes, *Med Lett Drugs Ther* 43(1101):29, 2001.

National Academies Press: Folate in dietary reference intakes for thiamin, riboflavin, niacin, vitalin B$_6$, folate, vitamin B$_{12}$, pantothenic acid, biotin, and choline (online): www.nap.ecu/openbook/0309072794/html/196.html. Accessed 1998.

National Academies Press: Improving birth outcomes: meeting the challenge in the developing world (online): www.nap.ecu/openbook/0309086140/html/243.html. Accessed 2003.

National Academies Press: Iron in dietary reference intakes for vitamin A, vitamin K, arsenic, boron, chromium, copper, iodine, iron, manganese, molybdenum, nickel, silicon, vanadium, and zinc (online): www.nap.ecu/openbook/0309072794/html/290.html. Accessed 2000.

National Institute of Allergy and Infectious Diseases: *Understanding vaccines*, NIH Publication No 98-4219, Washington, DC, 1998, US Department of Health and Human Services.

National Institute on Drug Abuse: *Drugs, brains, and behavior—the science of addiction*, 2007 (online): www.drugabuse.gov/science of addiction/brain.html.

National Institute on Drug Abuse: Gender differences in drug abuse risks and treatment, *NIDA Notes* 15:4, 2000.

National Institute on Drug Abuse: *Bridging science and culture to improve drug abuse research in communities*, conference held Sept 24-26, 2001, Philadelphia (online): http://165.112.78.61/Meetings/Bridging/BridgeAbs1.html. Accessed June 1, 2004.

National survey on drug use and health, Washington DC, 2002, Substance Abuse and Mental Health Services Administration (SAMHSA), Office of Applied Studies, US Department of Health and Human Services.

Nebivolol (Bystolic) for hypertension, *The Medical Letter 50 (1281)*, 17-19, March 10, 2008.

New cholesterol-lowering drug makes its mark, *Mayo Clin Health Lett* 21(3):4, 2003.

New drug fights fluid build-up, *The Cleveland Clinic Heart Advisor* 7(4):3, 2003.

New hypertension guidelines, *The Cleveland Clinic Men's Health Advisor* 6(8):5, 2003.

Newberry L, editor: *Sheehy's emergency nursing principles and practice*, ed 5, St Louis, 2003, Mosby.

Ng R, Better N, Green M: Anticancer agents and cardiotoxicity, *Semin Oncol* 33:2, 2006.

Nichols R: Pain management in patients with addictive disease, *Am J Nurs* 103(3):87, 2003.

North American Nursing Diagnosis Association: *Nursing diagnoses: definitions and classifications 2003-2004*, Philadelphia, 2003, The Association.

Nurse practitioner prescribing reference—fall 2004, spring 2005, New York, 2004, Prescribing Reference.

O'Brien P: Addictive behaviors. In Lewis S, et al, editors: *Medical-surgical nursing: assessment and management of clinical problems*, ed 6, St Louis, 2004, Mosby.

Oncogenes and tumor suppressor genes, American Cancer Society, 2005 (online): www.cancer.org/docroot/ETO/content/ETO_1_4x_oncogenes_and_tumor_suppressor_genes.asp.

Oncology Education Services: *Molecular and targeted therapies in cancer care: from concept to chairside*, Pittsburgh, 2003, Oncology Education Services.

Oshima R, Lesperance J, Munoz V, et al: Angiogenic acceleration of Neu induced mammary tumor progression and metastasis, *Cancer Res* 64:169, 2004.

Oudin C, Bonnetain F, Boidot R, et al: Patterns of loss of heterozygosity in breast carcinoma during neoadjuvant chemotherapy, *Int J Oncology* 30:1145, 2007.

Overfield T: *Biologic variation in health and illness: race, age, and sex differences*, ed 2, Boca Raton, 1995, CRC Press.

Over-the-counter (OTC) cough remedies, *Med Lett Drugs Ther* 43(1100):23, 2001.

Pacquiao D: People of Filipino ancestry. In Purnell L, Paulanka B, editors: *Transcultural health care: a culturally competent approach*, Philadelphia, 2003, FA Davis.

Pain killers appear to weaken aspirin's primary protection, *The Cleveland Clinic Heart Advisor* 6(11):7, 2003.

Palacios S: The future of the new selective estrogen receptor modulators, *J Br Menopause Soc* 13:27, 2007.

Pallares J, Rojo F, Iriarte J, et al: Study of microvessel density and the expression of the angiogenic factors VEGF, bFGF and the receptors Flt-1 and FLK-1 in benign, premalignant and malignant prostate tissues, *Histol Histopathol* 21:857, 2006.

Pantoprazole (Protonix), *Med Lett Drugs Ther* 42(1083):65, 2000.

Papakosta V, Vairaktaris E, Vylliotis A, et al: The co-expression of c-myc and p53 increases and reaches a plateau early in oral oncogenesis, *Anticancer Res* 26:2957, 2006.

Papavassiliou A: Molecular medicine: transcription factors, *N Engl J Med* 332:45, 1995.

Paulino A: Late effects of radiotherapy for pediatric extremity sarcomas, *Int J Radiat Oncol Biol Phys* 60: 265, 2004.

Perey L, Paridaens R, Hawle H, et al: Clinical benefit of fulvestrant in postmenopausal women with advanced breast cancer and primary or acquired resistance to aromatase inhibitors: final results of phase II Swiss group for Clinical Cancer Research Trial (SAKK 21/00), *Ann Oncol* 18:64, 2007.

Plosker G, Keam S: Spotlight on trastuzumab in the management of HER2-positive metastatic and early-stage breast cancer, *BioDrugs* 20:259, 2006.

Pollack H: Screening for chronic hepatitis B among Asian/Pacific Islander populations, *MMWR Morb Mortal Wkly Rep* 55:505, 2005.

Polyak K, Meyerson M: Molecular biology, genomics, proteomics, and mouse models of human cancer. In Kufe D, Bast JR, Hait W, et al, editors: *Cancer Medicine*, ed 7, Hamilton, Ontario, 2006, BC Decker.

Porth CM: *Pathophysiology*, ed 7, Philadelphia, 2005, Lippincott Williams & Wilkins.

Prestor V, Rakovec P, Kozelj M, et al: Late cardiac damage of anthracycline therapy for acute lymphoblastic leukemia in childhood, *Pediatr Hematol Oncol* 17:527, 2000.

Prevention of malaria, *Med Lett Drugs Ther* 42(1070):8, 2000.

Prozac weekly, *Med Lett Drugs Ther* 43(1101):27, 2001.

Purnell L, Paulanka B, editors: *Transcultural health care: a culturally competent approach*, ed 3, Philadelphia, 2008, FA Davis.

Purnell L, Paulanka B, editors: *Transcultural health care: a culturally competent approach*, ed 4, Philadelphia, 2006, FA Davis.

Purohit SK, Hellstrom WJG: Erectile dysfunction. In Rakel RE, editor: *Conn's current therapy 2000*, Philadelphia, 2000, Saunders.

Raise your "good" cholesterol, *The Cleveland Clinic Heart Advisor* 7(5):3, 2003.

Rakel RE, editor: *Conn's current therapy 2000*, Philadelphia, 2000, Saunders.

Rapp CJ, Gordon DB: Understanding equianalgesic dosing, *Orthop Nurs* 19(3):65, 2000.

Recommended childhood immunization schedule, United States, *Clinician Reviews* 11(3):31, January-December 2001 (website): http://www.cdc.gov/nip.

Reed S: Cell cycle. In DeVita V, Hellman S, Rosenberg S, editors: *Cancer: principles and practice of oncology*, ed 7, vol 1, Philadelphia, 2005, Lippincott Williams & Wilkins.

Restifo N, Wunderlich J: Cancer immunology. In DeVita V, Hellman S, Rosenberg S, editors: *Cancer: principles and practice of oncology*, ed 7, vol 1, Philadelphia, 2005, Lippincott Williams & Wilkins.

Reviews (supplement), *Therapeutic Spotlight*, 10-13, April 2001.

Reya T, Clevers H: Wnt signaling in stem cells and cancer, *Nature* 434:843, 2005.

Roark D: Bar codes and drug administration, *Am J Nurs* 104(1):63, 2004

Robbins DC: Management of dyslipidemia, *Clinician Rev (suppl): Therapeutic Spotlight*, 4-9, April 2001.

Rock C: Primary dietary prevention: Is the fiber story over?, *Recent Results Cancer Res* 174: 171, 2007.

Rosen MA, Hughes SC, Levinson G: Regional anesthesia for labor and delivery. In Hughes S, et al, editors: *Shnider and Levinson's anesthesia for obstetrics*, Philadephia, 2002, Lippincott Williams & Wilkins.

Roshan F, Ostheimer G: What's new in obstetric anesthesia, Lecture, *Anesthesiology* 106(3): 615, 2007.

Rudin C, Thompson C: Apoptosis and cancer. In Vogelstein B, Kinzler K, editors: *The genetic basis of human cancer*, ed 2, New York, 2002, McGraw-Hill.

Ruhl JM: Myasthenia gravis: a baffling neuromuscular disorder, *Nurs Spectr* 9(12 PA):14, 2000.

Sagraves R: Increasing antibiotic resistance: its effect on the therapy for otitis media, *J Pediatr Health Care* 16(2):79, 2002.

Sanga S, Sinek J, Frieboes H, et al: Mathematical modeling of cancer progression and response to chemotherapy, *Expert Rev Anticancer Ther* 6:1361, 2006.

Saunders' nursing drug handbook 2007, Philadelphia, 2007, Saunders.

Schmiedeskamp M, Kockler D: Human papillomavirus vaccines, *Ann Pharmacother* 40:1344, 2006.

Science vs. a fabled heart threat, *The Cleveland Clinic Heart Advisor* 7(8):6, 2004.

Second opinion, *Mayo Clin Health Lett* 22(5):8, 2004.

Secondhand smoke: questions and answers, National Cancer Institute, 2007 (online): www.cancer.gov/cancertopics/factsheet/Tobacco/ETS.

Seeman M: Gender differences in the prescribing of antipsychotic drugs, *Am J Psychiatry* 161:1324, 2004.

Seymour FJ: A new program for the management of the chemically impaired nurse in Delaware, unpublished manuscript, executive position paper, 1991.

Shah J: Criteria influencing the clinical uptake of pharmacogenomic strategies, BMJ, 2004 (online): http://www.bmj.com/cgi/content/full/328/7454/1482.

Shields P: Understanding population and individual risk assessment: the case of polycholinated biphenyls, *Cancer Epidemiol Biomarkers Prev* 15:830, 2006.

Shute N: Over the limit: Americans young and old crave high-octane fuel and doctors are jittery, *U.S. News and World Report*, April 23, 2007.

Simbre V, Duffy S, Dadlani G, et al: Cardiotoxicity of cancer chemotherapy: implications for children, *Paediatr Drugs* 7:187, 2005.

Skaar J, DeCaprio J: Fundamental aspects of the cell cycle and signal transduction. In Chang A, Ganz P, Hayes D, et al, editors: *Oncology: an evidence-based approach*, New York, 2006, Springer.

Skidmore-Roth L: *Mosby's handbook of herbs and natural supplements*, St Louis, 2001, Mosby.

Smeltzer SC, Kelley L: Multiple sclerosis, *Adv for Nurses*, 10-12, July 31, 2001.

Smigal C, Ward E, Cokkinides V, et al: Trends in breast cancer by race and ethnicity: update 2006, *CA Cancer J Clin* 56:168, 2006.

Smith C, Marks A, Lieberman M: The molecular biology of cancer. In Smith C, Marks A, Lieberman, M, editors: *Marks' basic medical biochemistry: a clinical approach*, ed 2, Philadelphia, 2005, Lippincott Williams & Wilkins.

Smith R, Schlecht N, Childs G, et al: Pilot study of mucosal genetic differences in early smokers and nonsmokers, *Laryngoscope* 116:1375, 2006.

Sohn M, et al: Tobacco use and dependence, *Semin Oncol Nurs* 19(4):250, 2003.

Soo-Jin Lee S: Mountain J, Koenig A: The meanings of "race" in the new genomics: implications for health disparities research, *Yale J Health Policy Law Ethics*, vol 1, Spring 2001.

Speers A, Lwaleed B, Featherstone J, et al: Furosemide reverses multidrug resistance status in bladder cancer cells in vitro, *J Clin Pathol* 59:912, 2006.

Spratto GR, Woods AL: *Nurse's drug reference*, New York, 2004, Delmar.

Stamenkovic I: Extracellular matrix remodelling: the role of matrix metalloproteinases, *J Pathol* 200:448, 2003.

Starr C: The essentials of pediatric dosing, *Patient Care Nurse Pract*, 48-51, 62-66, 68, 72, 75, 2000.

Statin safety, *The Cleveland Clinic: Men's Health Advisor* 5(1):4, 2003.

Statins and your stroke risk, *The Cleveland Clinic: Men's Health Advisor* 8(3):4, 2006.

Steefel L: Epilepsy poses unique issues for women, *Nurs Spectr* 9(2 PA):6, January 24, 2000.

Stetler-Stevenson W: Invasion and metastases. In DeVita V, Hellman S, Rosenberg S, editors: *Cancer: principles and practice of oncology*, ed 7, vol 1, Philadelphia, 2005, Lippincott Williams & Wilkins.

Stockley IH: *Drug interactions*, ed 3, Oxford, 1994, Blackwell Scientific Publications.

Stoelting R, Miller R: *Basics of anesthesia*, ed 5, Philadelphia, 2007, Churchill Livingstone/Elsevier.

Stohr W, Paulides M, Bielack S, et al: Ifosfamide-induced nephrotoxicity in 593 sarcoma patients: a report from the Late Effects Surveillance System, *Pediatr Blood Cancer* 48(4):447, 2006.

Stohr W, Paulides M, Brecht I, et al: Comparison of epirubicin and doxorubicin cardiotoxicity in children and adolescents treated within the German Cooperative Soft Tissue Sarcoma Study (CWS), *J Cancer Res Clin Oncol* 132:35, 2005.

Stone JT, Wyman JF, Salisbury SA: *Clinical gerontological nursing*, ed 2, Philadelphia, 1999, Saunders.

Striking back at stroke, *The Cleveland Clinic: Men's Health Advisor* 8(11):3, 2006.

Stull D: Targeted therapies for the treatment of leukemia, *Semin Oncol Nurs* 19(2):90, 2003.

Suggs DM: Pharmacokinetics in children: history, considerations, and applications, *J Am Acad Nurse Pract* 12(6):236, 2000.

Swan N: The long road to medication development: cocaine treatment moves to clinical trials, *NIDA Notes* 18(6), 2004.

Systemic candidiasis. In *The Merck manual*, chapter 158, 1, 2000.

Tang G: Bridging languages and cultures, *Adv for Nurses*, 37-39, April 2, 2007.

Taniwaki M, Daigo Y, Ishikawa N, et al: Gene expression profiles of small-cell lung cancers: molecular signatures of lung cancer, *Int J Oncol* 29:567, 2006.

Tape S: Have targeted therapies lived up to their promise?, *Hematol Oncol* 395:15, 2004.

Targeted cancer therapies: questions and answers, National Cancer Institute, 2004 (online): http://cis.nci.nih.gov/fact/7r49.htm. Accessed August 5, 2004.

Thomas H: Overcoming mutidrug resistance in cancer: an update on the clinical strategy of inhibiting p-glycoprotein, CancerConsultants.com, 2004 (online): http://professional.cancerconsultants.com/print/aspx?id123711. Accessed August 3, 2004.

Thompson C, Bauer D, Lum J, et al: How do cancer cells acquire the fuel needed to support cell growth?, *Cold Spring Harb Symp Quant Biol* 70: 357, 2005.

Tokunaga E, Oki E, Nishida K, et al: Trastuzumab and breast cancer: developments and current status, *Int J Clin Oncol* 11:199, 2006.

Tortorice PV: Chemotherapy: principles of therapy. In Yarbro C, Frogge M, Goodman M, et al, editors: *Cancer nursing: principles and practice*, Boston, 2000, Johns and Bartlett.

"Trojan Horse" to fight clots, *The Cleveland Heart Advisor* 6(11):4, 2003.

Trossman S: Nurses' addictions, *Am J Nurs* 103(9):27, 2003.

Turkoski B, Lance B, Bonfiglio M: *Drug information handbook for advanced practice nursing*, ed 7, Hudson, OH, 2006, Lexi-Comp.

Twedell D: Genomics offer opportunities for nurses, *J Contin Educ Nurs* 34(5):195, 2003.

Two amlodipine? ARB combinations for hypertension. *The Medical Letter* 49 (1276), 101-103, December 17, 2007.

Umland EM: Applying pharmacokinetics: absorption, distribution, metabolism, and excretion of drugs, *Adv for Nurses* 29, 30, May 22, 2000.

U.S. Department of Health and Human Services: Naltrexone for extended-release injectable suspension for treatment of alcohol dependence, *Substance Abuse Treatment Advisory* 6(1), 2007 (online): www.kap.samhsa.gov/products/manuals/advisory/index.htm.

U.S. Department of Health and Human Services, Centers for Disease Control and Prevention, *Recommended immunization schedule for persons aged 0-6 years, United States 2007* (online): www.edc.gov/nip/acip. Accessed May 7, 2007.

U.S. Department of Health and Human Services, Centers for Disease Control and Prevention: *The guide to contraindications to vaccinations*, September 2003 (online): www.edc.gov/vaccines/recs/vac-admin/downloads/contraindications_guide.pdf. Accessed May 7, 2007.

U.S. Food and Drug Administration: FDA approves novel medication for smoking cessation, *FDA News*, Washington, DC, May 11, 2006.

United States Pharmacopeia drug information (USP-DI) for the health care professional, ed 27, vol 1, Rockville, MD, 2007, US Pharmacopeia Convention.

Varella L, Jones E, Meguid M: Drug-nutrient interactions in enteral feeding: a primary care focus, *Nurse Pract* 22(6):98.

Vaughn CJ, Gott AM: Update on statins, *Circulation* 110:886, 2003.

Volker D: Biology of cancer and carcinogenesis. In J. Itano J, Taoka, editors: *Core curriculum for oncology nursing*, ed 4, Philadelphia, 2005, Elsevier.

Vytorin: A combination of ezetimibe and simvastatin, *Med Lett Drugs Ther* 46(1191):73, 2004.

Waitman J, McCaffery M, Pasero C: Meperidine—a liability, *Am J Nurs* 101(1):57, 2001.

Wang Y: People of Chinese heritage. In Purnell L, Paulanka B, editors: *Transcultural health care: a culturally competent approach*, ed 2, Philadelphia, 2003, FA Davis.

Wang S, Peyrollier K, Bourguignon L: The influence of hyaluronan-CD44 interaction on topoisomerase II activity and etoposide cytotoxicity in head and neck cancer, *Arch Otolaryngol Head Neck Surg* 133:281, 2007.

Watson-Hurst K, Becker D: The role of N-cadherin, MCAM and beta3 integrin in melanoma progression, proliferation, migration and invasion, *Cancer Biology and Therapy*, 5:1375, 2006.

What readers say about statins, *The Cleveland Clinic Heart Advisor* 7(8):4, 2004.

Where most heart attacks begin, *The Cleveland Clinic Heart Advisor* 7(6):4, 2004.

Which beta-blocker?, *Med Lett Drugs Ther* 43(1097):9, 2001.

Which drug for hypertension?, *The Cleveland Clinic: Heart Advisor* 8(12):4, 2005.

Which medication is best for newly diagnosed hypertension?, *The Cleveland Clinic Men's Health Advisor* 5(5):4, 2003.

Whitten L: Disulfiram reduces cocaine abuse, *NIDA Notes* 20(2), 2005.

Whooley MA, Simon GE: Managing depression in medical outpatients, *N Engl J Med* 343(26):1942, 2000.

Wiese K, Nahata M: EMLA for painful procedures in infants, *J Pediatr Health Care* 19(1):42, 2005.

Wilkerson R, Northington LD, Fisher W: Ingestion of toxic substances by infants and children: what we don't know can hurt, *Crit Care Nurse* 25(4):35, 2005.

Williams JS: Cognitive deficits in marijuana smokers persist after use stops, *NIDA Notes* 18(5), 2003.

Wilson B, Shannon M, Stang C: *Nursing drug guide*, Upper Saddle River, NJ, Prentice Hall Health, 2007.

Wittert DD: Cholesterol: the good, the bad, and the balanced, *Nurs Spectr* 13(10):1, 2003.

Wong K, Depinho R: Telomerase. In DeVita V, Hellman S, Rosenberg S, editors: *Cancer: principles and practice of oncology*, ed 7, vol 1, Philadelphia, 2005, Lippincott Williams & Wilkins.

Xu J, Peng H, Zhang J: Human multidrug transporter ABCG2, a target for sensitizing drug resistance in cancer chemotherapy, *Current Medical Chemistry* 14: 689, 2007.

Yang H, Ma M, Vescio R, et al: Overcoming drug resistance in multiple myeloma: the emergence of therapeutic approaches to induce apoptosis, *J Clin Oncol* 21: 4239, 2003.

Zickler P: Nicotine medication also reduces craving in cocaine addicts, *NIDA Notes* 15(1), 2002.

Zickler P: In chronic drug abuse, acute dopamine surge may erode resolve to abstain, *NIDA Notes* 19(1), 2004.

Zickler P: Modafinil improves behavioral therapy results in cocaine addiction, *NIDA Notes* 20(3), 2005.

Zinkel S, Korsmeyer S: Apoptosis. In DeVita V, Hellman S, Rosenberg S, editors: *Cancer: principles and practice of oncology*, ed 7, vol 1, Philadelphia, 2005, Lippincott Williams & Wilkins.

Zonisamide for epilepsy, *Med Lett Drugs Ther* 42(1089):94, 2000.

Zoucha R, Purnell L: People of Mexican heritage. In Purnell L, Paulanka B, editors: *Transcultural health care: a culturally competent approach*, ed 2, Philadelphia, 2003, FA Davis.

Zurlinden J: FDA bans importing certain high-risk prescription drugs using the Internet, *Nurs Spectr* 12(3 PA):19, February 10, 2004.

Zurlinden J: New lab tests for CHF, kidney function, *Nurs Spectr* 12(16 PA):25, August 11, 2003.

Zurlinden J: Research deflates value of vitamin E for heart disease, *Nurs Spectr* 11(3 PA):26, February 11, 2002.

Zurlinden J: St John's wort popularity grows, but so do concerns, *Nurs Spectr* 9(7 PA):18, 19, 2000.

Index

Note: Entries followed by "b" indicate boxes; "f," figures; "t," tables.

957

List of Features—cont'd

Herbal Alerts

Preventing Medication Errors Boxes

List of Features

Prototype Drug Charts